ITEM	QUANTITIES FOR NUMBER OF PARTICIPANTS PER YEAR		
	UP TO 200	**200 TO 400**	**400 TO 600**
Germicides			
Alcohol (isopropyl)	5 pints	10 pints	15 pints
Boric acid (eyewash)	1 pint	2 pints	3 pints
Peroxide	1 pint	2 pints	3 pints
Heel cups (plastic)	5	10	15
Instant cold packs (dozen)	1	2	3
Massage lubricant	2 pints	4 pints	6 pints
Moleskin (12-inch [30 cm])	2 rolls	4 rolls	6 rolls
Neck and back board (emergency)	1	1	1
Neoprene knee sleeves			
Large	*	*	*
Medium	*	*	*
Small	*	*	*
Neoprene thigh caps			
Large	*	*	*
Medium	*	*	*
Small	*	*	*
Neoprene thigh guards			
Large	*	*	*
Medium	*	*	*
Small	*	*	*
Nonadhering sterile pads, 3 by 3 (100)	2	4	6
Orthotic plastic material	*	*	*
Powder	1	1	1
Prewrap, 3-inch (7.5 cm)	1 case	2 cases	3 cases
Shoulder harness	*	*	*
Skin lube (lubrication, 1-pound)	5	10	15
Slings (triangular bandages)	5	10	15
Splints, vacuum	1 set	1 set	1 set
Sponge rubber (vinyls), 36 by 44 inches (90 by 110 cm)			
⅛-inch (0.3 cm)	1 sheet	2 sheets	3 sheets
¼-inch (0.6 cm)	1 sheet	2 sheets	3 sheets
½-inch (1.25 cm)	1 sheet	2 sheets	3 sheets
Stockinette (3-inch [7.5 cm] roll)	1	3	6
Sun lotion, e.g., Paba (4-ounce)	4	8	12
Tape adherent (clear), spray cans (12 ounce)	1 can	2 cans	4 cans
Tape remover	½ gallon	¾ gallon	1 gallon
Thermo plastic (¼-inch [0.6 cm]) (Orthoplast)	2 sheets	3 sheets	4 sheets
Tongue depressors	500	1000	1500
Waterproof tape (1-inch [2.5 cm])	6 rolls	12 rolls	36 rolls

Principles of

ATHLETIC TRAINING

NINTH EDITION

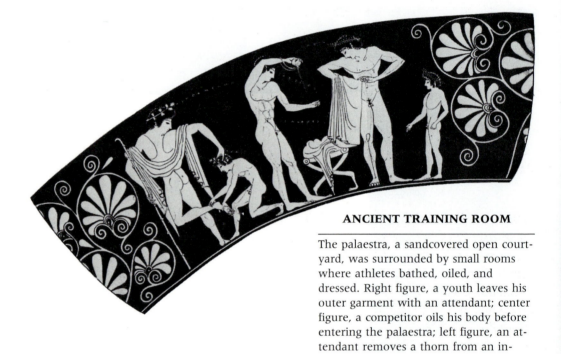

ANCIENT TRAINING ROOM

The palaestra, a sandcovered court-yard, was surrounded by small rooms where athletes bathed, oiled, and dressed. Right figure, a youth leaves his outer garment with an attendant; center figure, a competitor oils his body before entering the palaestra; left figure, an attendant removes a thorn from an injured athlete.

Principles of

ATHLETIC TRAINING

NINTH EDITION

Daniel D. Arnheim, D.P.E., A.T.C.
Fellow, American College of Sports Medicine
Professor Emeritus of Physical Education
California State University
Long Beach, California

William E. Prentice, Ph.D., P.T., A.T.C.
Professor, Coordinator of the Sports Medicine Specialization,
Department of Physical Education, Exercise, and Sport Science
Clinical Professor, Division of Physical Therapy,
Department of Medical Allied Health Professions,
Associate Professor, Department of Orthopaedics
School of Medicine
The University of North Carolina
Chapel Hill, North Carolina

Director, Sports Medicine Education and Fellowship Program
HEALTHSOUTH Corporation
Birmingham, Alabama

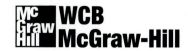

Boston, Massachusetts   Burr Ridge, Illinois   Dubuque, Iowa
Madison, Wisconsin   New York, New York   San Francisco, California   St. Louis, Missouri

WCB/McGraw-Hill

A Division of The McGraw-Hill Companies

Vice-President/Publisher James M. Smith
Senior Acquisitions Editor Vicki Malinee
Senior Developmental Editor Michelle Turenne
Project Manager Dana Peick
Project Specialist Catherine Albright
Designer Amy Buxton
Cover and Part Opener Photo Dennis O'Clair/
  Tony Stone Images
Photographer Missy Bello

Credits for all materials used by permission appear after Index.

This text was revised based on the most up-to-date research and suggestions made by individuals knowledgeable in the field of athletic training. The author and publisher disclaim any responsibility for any adverse effects or consequences from the misapplication or injudicious use of information contained within this text. It is also accepted as judicious that the athletic trainer performing his or her duties is, at all times, working under the guidance of a licensed physician.

NINTH EDITION

Copyright ©1997 by the McGraw-Hill Companies, Inc.
A Mosby imprint of Mosby-Year Book, Inc.

Previous editions copyrighted 1963, 1969, 1973, 1977, 1981, 1985, 1989, 1993

Printed in the United States of America
Composition by Clarinda
Printing/binding by Von Hoffmann

Mosby-Year Book, Inc.
11830 Westline Industrial Drive
St. Louis, Missouri 63146

International Standard Book Number 0-8151-0326-3

98 CL/VH 9 8 7 6 5 4 3

Believe it or not, this is the ninth edition of *Principles of Athletic Training*. Since the first edition of this text was published in 1963, the profession of athletic training has experienced amazing growth, not only in numbers but also in the associated body of knowledge. During those years the authors of this text have taken great care in providing the reader with the most current research-based information available in athletic training and sports medicine, and thus *Principles of Athletic Training* has always been considered the leading text in this field. Despite the new texts that have been recently introduced into the market, this edition remains the most comprehensive introductory text for the athletic trainer. Traditionally, this text has been the only one that covers all aspects of athletic training in an extremely clear, concise, and well-organized manner. The ninth edition of *Principles of Athletic Training* continues this tradition.

The essential philosophy of this edition of *Principles of Athletic Training* remains the same as in past editions. The text is designed to lead the student from general foundations to specific concepts relative to injury prevention, evaluation, management, and rehabilitation. As the student progresses from beginning to end, he or she will gradually begin to understand the complexities of the profession of athletic training and sports medicine. With this understanding, an increased grasp of medical and scientific terminology also results. As in past editions, a major premise is that the student should be able to apply the appropriate techniques and concepts in the day-to-day performance of his or her job.

A great deal of thought and planning always goes into the revision of *Principles of Athletic Training*. Developing the ninth edition included serious consideration and incorporation of suggestions made by students, as well as detailed feedback from reviewers and other respected authorities in the field. Consequently, the ninth edition reflects the major dynamic trends in the field of athletic training and sports medicine. Furthermore, it is our hope that this newest edition will help to prepare the student to become a competent professional who will continue to enhance the ongoing advancement of the athletic training profession.

Who Is It Written For?

Principles of Athletic Training is designed primarily as an introductory text to the field of athletic training. It may be used by both athletic trainers and coaches in courses concerned with the scientific and clinical foundations of athletic training and sports medicine. Practicing athletic trainers, physical therapists, and other health and safety specialists involved with physically active individuals will also find this text valuable.

What's New In This Edition?

Principles of Athletic Training has undergone significant changes in content with this newest edition. The changes and additions are reflective of the ever-increasing body of knowledge that is expanding the scope of practice for the athletic trainer. These include:

- A new Chapter 9, *Bloodborne Pathogens*, presents coverage of hepatitis B, HIV, and AIDS, and the universal precautions necessary in the athletic environment. This includes discussions of the symptoms and signs, prevention, and management for HBV and HIV, as well as personal precautions, testing, and precautions from exposure.
- Coverage of rehabilitation has been expanded in each of the body region chapters in Part V, *Specific Sports Conditions*, to include suggestions for general body conditioning, joint mobilization, flexibility exercises, muscular strength, neuromuscular control, functional progressions (when appropriate), and for return to activity. This offers the student the advantage of a consistent format to follow in studying rehabilitation for the different body regions.

- New *Critical Thinking Exercises* are included in every chapter and present brief case studies that help the student apply the content just studied. Solutions for each case are included at the end of each chapter.
- The majority of photographs are new to the ninth edition and will be useful in demonstrating correct techniques.
- Updated information on the certification process for athletic trainers and a detailed discussion of the competencies that are essential for the entry level athletic trainer are provided in Chapter 1, *The Athletic Trainer and the Sports Medicine Team.*
- *Organizational and Administrative Considerations,* has been moved to the front of the text in Chapter 2 and includes an expanded discussion of how the athletic trainer should handle important insurance and liability issues.
- Chapter 3, *Training and Conditioning Techniques,* has been revised to reflect the current philosophies regarding techniques for improving flexibility, muscular strength and endurance, and cardiorespiratory endurance.
- Nutrition is an increasingly important concern for successful athletic performance. Chapter 4, *Nutritional Considerations,* has been rewritten to include the most concise and current information available, including the Recommended Dietary Allowances (RDA).
- Chapter 5, *Protective Sports Equipment,* has been updated with many new photographs to show the latest equipment available for a variety of sports and includes expanded coverage of sports foot gear.
- New information covering sources of pain and soft-tissue healing in cartilage, ligaments, skeletal muscles, and nerve cells are included in Chapter 6, *Mechanisms and Characteristics of Sports Trauma,* and Chapter 7, *Tissue Response to Injury.* Additionally, Chapter 7 serves as a guide for sports management protocols for the regional sports injuries found in Part V.
- Guidelines for extracting an injured athlete from a pool have been added to Chapter 8, *Emergency Procedures.*
- Sports psychology is a rapidly expanding area of specialization in sports medicine. Chapter 11, *Psychology of Sport Injury and Illness,* has been revised beyond stresses to examine the athlete's psychological reactions to sudden serious injury requiring surgery and a prolonged period of rehabilitation. Personality factors leading to injury, staleness, "sudden exercise abstinence syndrome," and the psychological factors inherent in overtraining, as well as poor compliance during the rehabilitation process, are included. Psychological aspects as rehabilitation and intervention strategies used by the athletic trainer to facilitate return to activity have also been included.
- Chapter 12, *Environmental Considerations,* contains new information on the dangers of lightning during athletic practices and competitions and also on the importance of using sunscreens when competing outdoors.
- Chapter 13, *Bandaging and Taping,* has been reorganized to present bandaging before taping techniques. It has also been streamlined by eliminating little-used bandages and taping techniques and now includes taping for a turf toe.
- New information on ultrasound, diathermy, and electrical stimulating currents has been included in Chapter 14, *Therapeutic Modalities.*
- Chapter 15, *Rehabilitation Techniques,* now includes detailed discussion of the important components of a rehabilitation program including controlling pain, maintaining or improving flexibility, restoring or increasing strength, re-establishing neuromuscular control, and maintaining levels of cardiorespiratory fitness. Chapter 15 is also the basis for potential rehabilitation techniques that may be used in the three phases of the healing process in Part V, *Specific Sports Conditions.*
- The use of various medications by the athletic trainer is extremely controversial. Chapter 16, *Drugs and Sports,* has been completely revised to provide specific guidelines and detailed protocols for the athletic trainer to follow in administering over-the-counter medications to the athlete.

- Chapters 17 through 25 cover specific sports injuries to regional areas of the body. These chapters have been expanded to include new information and are now as comprehensive as possible within the scope of practice in athletic training.

  Each body region has been organized to include sections on anatomy, prevention, assessment, management of specific injuries, and rehabilitation (when appropriate).

  Each injury identified consistently discusses the associated etiology, symptoms and signs, and management.

  Coverage of rehabilitation techniques has been expanded to include suggestions for general body reconditioning, joint mobilization, flexibility exercises, muscular strength, neuromuscular control, functional progressions (when appropriate), and guidelines for return to activity.

- Chapter 17, *The Foot*, now includes coverage of sesamoiditis injuries to the great toe and includes a management plan for plantar fasciitis.
- Chapter 18, *The Ankle and Lower Leg*, now includes the syndesmotic ankle sprain and a management plan for medial tibial stress syndrome.
- Chapter 22, *The Elbow, Forearm, Wrist, and Hand*, now includes Little League elbow and wrist ganglion of the tendon sheath, as well as dislocations and fractures of the phalanges.
- Chapter 25, *The Head and Face*, includes new coverage of scalp injuries, skull fractures, postconcussion syndrome, cerebral contusion, "second injury syndrome," and provides helpful guidelines for returning the athlete to activity following a concussion. Additionally, coverage of acute conjunctivitis and the sty are now included in this chapter.
- Chapter 26, *Skin Disorders*, now includes coverage of dry (xerotic) skin.
- Chapter 27, *Additional Health Concerns*, includes expanded discussion of infectious mononucleosis, exercise-induced bronchial obstruction (asthma), and hypertension. Coverage of syphilis and "the female athlete triad" are now included.

PEDAGOGICAL AIDS

Numerous pedagogical devices are included in this edition:

- *Chapter objectives*   Goals begin each chapter to reinforce important key concepts to be learned.
- *Margin information*   Key concepts, selected definitions, helpful training tips, and illustrations are placed in the margins throughout the text for added emphasis and ease of reading and studying.
- *Anatomy*   Where applicable, extensive discussion of anatomy is presented and illustrated throughout the text.
- *Focus boxes*   Important information has been highlighted and boxed to make key information easier to find and to enhance the text's flexibility and appearance.
- *Critical Thinking Exercises*   New to this edition, 185 cases studies have been included that encourage the student to apply the content presented to the clinical setting.
- *Color throughout text*   Color is used throughout the text to accentuate and clarify illustrations and textual material.
- *New photographs and line drawings*   Many new photographs and color line drawings have been added.
- *Color illustrations*   Fourteen full-color photographs are included in Chapter 26 to depict common skin disorders.
- *Management plans*   In selected chapters, sample management plans are presented as examples of treatment procedures.
- *Chapter summaries*   Each chapter's salient points are summarized to reinforce key content.

- *Review questions and class activities*   Located at the end of each chapter, review questions and class activities are provided to enhance the learning process.
- *References*   References have been extensively updated to provide the most complete and current information available.
- *Annotated Bibliography*   For students and instructors who want to expand on the information presented in each chapter, an annotated bibliography has been provided.
- *A detailed Glossary*   An extensive list of key terms and their definitions is presented to reinforce information in one convenient location.
- *Appendix*   The Appendix contains Canada's *Food Guide for Healthy Living* and the Recommended Nutrient Intake (RNI).
- *Endpages*   Front and back endpages inside the covers of the text provide helpful lists of suggested supplies for the athletic training room and the athletic trainer's kit, along with charts for metric and celsius conversions.

ANCILLARIES

- **Instructor's Manual** and **Test Bank**
  Developed for the ninth edition, The *Instructor's Manual* was prepared by Meredith Busby, M.A., A.T.C. It includes:
  - Brief chapter overviews
  - Learning objectives
  - Key terminology
  - Discussion questions
  - Class activities
  - Worksheets
  - Worksheet answer keys
  - Test Bank
  - Appendixes of additional resources
  - Transparency masters
  - Perforated format, ready for immediate use

  In total, approximately 2000 examination questions are included. Reviewed by instructors of the course for accuracy and currency, each chapter contains true-false, multiple choice, and completion test questions. The worksheets in each chapter also include a separate *Test Bank* of matching, short answer, listing, essay, and personal or injury assessment questions that can be used as self-testing tools for students or as additional sources for examination questions.

- **Computerized Test Bank**
  A computerized version of the *Test Bank* from the *Instructor's Manual* is available for both IBM and Macintosh to qualified adopters. This software provides a unique combination of user-friendly aids and enables the instructor to select, edit, delete, or add questions and construct and print tests and answer keys.

- **Transparencies**
  Fifty-four acetate transparencies of important illustrations, tables, and charts are available to maximize the instructor's teaching and the student's learning process and are available to qualified adopters.

- **Photo CD**
  Photographs used in the text are available on CD-ROM, most in full-color, to qualified adopters.

Acknowledgements

The revision of this ninth edition of *Principles of Athletic Training* has been extremely interesting in light of the fact that Mosby, the company that has published eight previous editions since 1963, was purchased by McGraw-Hill as this newest edition was still in production. Those of us who have been Mosby authors for quite some time cannot begin to express the depth of our gratitude to the many Mosby editors and production personnel who have contributed to the metamorphosis of this text over the years. As with several past editions, we want to express our deepest gratitude to our developmental editor, Michelle Turenne, who has truly been the glue holding this whole project together. Her input and dedication to this project has been indispensable, and her loyalty to us as authors has never been questioned. Our editor, Vicki Malinee, has been a "rock" in keeping us focused and, as is the case with Michelle, we cannot thank her enough for her efforts on our behalf.

During the revision process for the ninth edition, we relied heavily on input solicited from our reviewers. Many personal thanks are extended to:

Andrew Paulin
Mt. San Antonio College

Steve Simpson
Tarleton State University

Gordon Stoddard
University of Wisconsin at Madison

Lorna R. Strong
University of Central Arkansas

We also wish to extend our sincere appreciation to our technical reviewers for their critique of selected chapters. Their input was most valuable to the completion of this edition.

Louis B. Almekinders, M.D.
The University of North Carolina at Chapel Hill

Daniel N. Hooker, Ph.D., P.T., A.T.C.
The University of North Carolina at Chapel Hill

Bryan W. Smith, M.D.
The University of North Carolina at Chapel Hill

O.E. Tillman, Jr., M.D.
The Hughston Orthopedic Clinic in Columbus, Georgia

Gordon M. Wardlaw, Ph.D.
The Ohio State University

Patsy Huff, Pharm.D.
The University of North Carolina at Chapel Hill

Sincere gratitude is also extended to Gary Nicholson, M.S., A.T.C., of Pacific Lutheran University, Tacoma, Washington, for his careful proofreading during the production process.

Finally, we wish to thank our families, and Dan's new bride, Lee, for their patience and support. Many thanks to Bill's wife, Tena, and our sons, Brian and Zach, for putting up with the old man during the writing of this edition.

Daniel D. Arnheim
William E. Prentice

BRIEF

Contents

DETAILED

Contents

PART V *Specific Sports Conditions*, 400

Introduction

The Athletic Trainer and the Sports Medicine Team

When you finish this chapter you should be able to

- Describe the historical foundations of athletic training.
- Identify the differences between professional organizations dedicated to athletic training and sports medicine.
- Differentiate among the role responsibilities of the athletic trainer, the team physician, and the coach.
- Explain the function of support personnel in sports medicine.
- Identify various employment settings for the athletic trainer.
- Discuss the certification and licensure of the athletic trainer.
- Discuss the role of the physical therapist in sports medicine.

An athletic trainer is concerned with the well-being of the athlete and generally assumes the responsibility for overseeing the total health care for the athlete. Participation in sports places the athlete in a situation in which injury is likely to occur. Fortunately, most of the injuries are not serious and lend themselves to rapid rehabilitation, but the athletic trainer must be capable of dealing with any type of trauma or catastrophic injury.

Although millions of individuals participate in organized and recreational sports, there is a relatively low incidence of fatalities and catastrophic injuries among them. A major problem, however, lies with the millions of sports participants who incur injuries or illnesses that could have been prevented and who later, as a consequence, develop more serious chronic conditions. Athletes in organized sports have every right to expect that their health and safety be kept as the highest of priorities. The field of athletic training, as a specialization, provides a major link between the sports program and the medical community for the implementation of injury prevention, emergency care, and rehabilitative procedures[13] (Figure 1-1).

HISTORICAL PERSPECTIVES
Early History

The drive to compete was important in many early societies. Sports developed over a period of time as a means of competing in a relatively peaceful and nonharmful way. Early civilizations show little evidence of highly organized sports. There is some evidence that in Greek and Roman civilizations there were coaches, trainers (people who helped the athlete reach top physical condition), and physicians to assist the athlete in reaching optimum performance.[32] Many of the roles that emerged during this early period are the same in modern sports.

For many centuries after the fall of the Roman Empire there was a complete lack of interest in sports activities. It was not until the beginning of the Renaissance that these activities slowly gained popularity. Athletic training as we know it came into existence during the late nineteenth century with the firm establishment of intercollegiate and interscholastic athletes in the United States. The first athletic trainers of this era were hangers-on who "rubbed down" the athlete. Because they possessed no technical knowledge, their athletic training techniques usually consisted of a rub, the application of some type of counterirritant, and occasionally the prescription of various home remedies and poultices. Many of those earlier athletic trainers were

The history of athletic training draws on the histories of exercise, medicine, physical therapy, physical education, and sports.

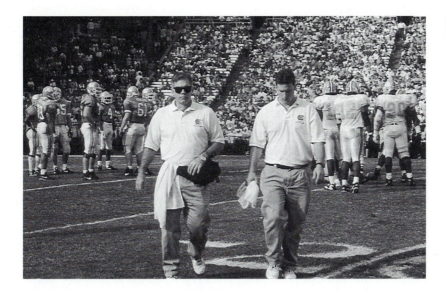

Figure 1-1

The field of athletic training is a major link between the sports program and the medical community.

persons of questionable background and experience. As a result, it has taken many years for the athletic trainer to attain the status of a well-qualified allied health care professional.[38]

Evolution of the Contemporary Athletic Trainer

The terms *training* and *athletic training, trainer* and *athletic trainer* are confused more often outside than inside the United States. Historically, training implies the act of coaching or teaching. In comparison, athletic training has traditionally been known as the field that is concerned with the athlete's health and safety. A trainer refers to someone who trains dogs or horses or functions in coaching or teaching areas. The athletic trainer is one who is a specialist in athletic training. Athletic training has evolved over the years to play a major role in the health care of the athlete. Growth of the athletic trainer's role from ancient times to the present has aptly been described thus: "The days of 'the rubber,' the know-it-all, the jack-of-all-trades and the master of all is over." This change occurred rapidly after World War I and the appearance of the athletic trainer in intercollegiate athletics. During this period the major influence in developing the athletic trainer as a specialist in preventing and managing athletic injuries resulted from the work of Dr. S.E. Bilik, a physician who wrote the first major text on athletic training and care of athletic injuries, called *The Trainer's Bible,* in 1917.[2]

In the early 1920s the Cramer family in Gardner, Kansas, started a chemical company and began producing a liniment to treat ankle sprains. Over the years, the Cramers realized that there was a market for products to treat injured athletes. In an effort to enhance communication and facilitate an exchange of ideas among coaches, trainers, and athletes, Cramer began publication of the *First Aider* in 1932. The members of this family were instrumental in early development of the athletic training profession and have always played a prominent role in the education of student athletic trainers.[32]

During the late 1930s an effort was made, primarily by several college and university trainers, to establish a national organization named the National Athletic Trainers Association (NATA). After struggling for existence from 1938 to 1944, the association essentially disappeared during the difficult years of World War II.

Between 1947 and 1950 university athletic trainers began once again to organize themselves into separate regional conferences, which would later become district organizations within NATA. In 1950 some 101 athletic trainers from the various conferences met in Kansas City, Missouri, and officially formed the National Athletic Trainers' Association. The primary purpose for its formation was to establish professional standards for the athletic trainer.[32] Since 1950 so many individuals have made contributions to the development of the profession that it is impossible to name them.

The growth of the profession of athletic training has been remarkable. Today NATA has more than 20,000 members, and the NATA-certified athletic trainer is widely recognized as a well-qualified allied health care provider.

SPORTS MEDICINE AND ATHLETIC TRAINING
The Field of Sports Medicine

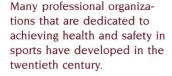

Sports medicine encompasses many different fields of study related to sport.

Sports medicine has become a term that has many connotations depending on which group is using it. It is a generic term that encompasses many different areas of sports related to both performance and injury. Among the areas of specialization within sports medicine are athletic training, biomechanics, exercise physiology, the practice of medicine relative to the athlete, physical therapy, sports nutrition, and sports psychology. The American College of Sports Medicine (ACSM) has defined sports medicine as multidisciplinary, including the physiological, biomechanical, psychological, and pathological phenomena associated with exercise and sports.[1] The clinical application of the work of these disciplines is performed to improve and maintain an individual's functional capacities for physical labor, exercise, and sports. It also includes the prevention and treatment of diseases and injuries related to exercise and sports.

Growth of Professional Sports Medicine Organizations

Many professional organizations that are dedicated to achieving health and safety in sports have developed in the twentieth century.

The twentieth century brought with it the development of a number of professional organizations dedicated to athletic training and sports medicine. Professional organizations have many goals: (1) to upgrade the field by devising and maintaining a set of professional standards, including a code of ethics; (2) to bring together professionally competent individuals to exchange ideas, stimulate research, and promote critical thinking; and (3) to give individuals an opportunity to work as a group with a singleness of purpose, thereby making it possible for them to achieve objectives that, separately, they could not accomplish. Addresses for these organizations are in the box below.

Federation of Sports Medicine

Among the first major organizations was the Federation of Sports Medicine, created in 1928 at the Olympic Winter Games in St. Moritz, Switzerland. This organization is multidisciplinary, including many disciplines that are concerned with the physically

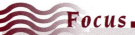

Focus

Addresses of professional organizations
American Academy of Pediatrics, Sports Committee, 1801 Hinman Ave., Evanston, IL 60204.
American Board of Physical Therapy Specialists, American Physical Therapy Association, 1111 North Fairfax St., Alexandria, VA 22314.
American College of Sports Medicine, 401 W. Michigan St. Indianapolis, IN 46202-3233.
American Orthopaedic Society for Sports Medicine, Suite 202, 70 West Hubbard, Chicago, IL 60610.
National Athletic Trainers Association, Inc., 2952 Stemmons Freeway Dallas, TX 75247.
National Collegiate Athletic Association, Competitive Safeguards and Medical Aspects of Sports Committee, P.O. Box 1906, Mission, KS 66201.
The National Federation of State High School Athletic Associations, 11724 Plaza Circle, P.O. Box 20626, Kansas City, MO 64195.

active individual. To some degree the ACSM has patterned itself after this organization.

American College of Sports Medicine

As discussed previously, the American College of Sports Medicine is interested in the study of all aspects of sports. Established in 1954, its membership is composed of medical doctors, doctors of philosophy, physical educators, athletic trainers, coaches, exercise physiologists, biomechanists, and others interested in sports. It holds national and regional conferences and meetings devoted to exploring the many aspects of sports medicine, and it publishes a quarterly magazine, *Medicine and Science in Sports and Exercise.* This journal includes articles in French, Italian, German, and English and provides complete translations in English of all articles. It reports recent developments in the field of sports medicine on a worldwide basis.

American Orthopaedic Society for Sports Medicine

The Orthopaedic Society for Sports Medicine was created in 1971 and is concerned with research and education. Its official bimonthly publication is the *American Journal of Sports Medicine.*

American Academy of Pediatrics, Sports Committee

The American Academy of Pediatrics, Sports Committee, was organized in 1979. Its primary goal is to educate all physicians, especially pediatricians, about the special needs of children who participate in sports. Between 1979 and 1983, this committee developed guidelines that were incorporated in a report, *Sports Medicine: Health Care for Young Athletes,* edited by Nathan J. Smith, M.D.

National Athletic Trainers Association

Before the formation of the National Athletic Trainers Association in 1950, athletic trainers occupied a somewhat insecure place in the athletic program. Since that time, as a result of the raising of professional standards and the establishment of a code of ethics, there has been considerable professional advancement. The association accepts as members only those who are properly qualified and who are prepared to subscribe to a code of ethics and to uphold the standards of the association. It publishes a quarterly journal, *The Journal of Athletic Training,* and holds an annual convention at which the members have an opportunity to keep abreast of new developments and to exchange ideas through clinical programs. The organization is constantly working to improve both the quality and the status of athletic training.

American Physical Therapy Association, Sports Physical Therapy Section

In 1981, the Sports Physical Therapy Section of the American Physical Therapy Association was officially established. Standards for clinical competence were proposed. Its official journal is the *Journal of Orthpaedic and Sports Physical Therapy.*[21]

Other Health-Related Organizations

Many other health-related professions have, over the years, become interested in the health and safety aspects of sports; thus dentists, podiatrists, and chiropractors also provide varied services to the athlete. Besides national organizations that are interested in athletic health and safety, there are state and local associations, which are extensions of the larger bodies. National, state, and local sports organizations have all provided extensive support to the reduction of illness and injury risk to the athlete.

Other journals that provide an excellent service to the field of athletic training and sports medicine are *The International Journal of Sports Medicine,* which is published in English by Thieme-Stratton, Inc., New York; *The Journal of Sports Medicine and Physical Fitness,* published by Edizioni Minerva Medica SPA, ADIS Press Ltd., Auckland 10,

New Zealand; the *Journal of Sport Rehabilitation,* published by Human Kinetics Publishers, Inc., Champaign, Illinois; the *Physician and Sportsmedicine,* published by McGraw-Hill, Inc.; *Physical Therapy* and *Clinical Management,* both published by the American Physical Therapy Association; the *Journal of Strength and Conditioning Research,* published by the National Strength Coaches Association; *Physical Medicine and Rehabilitation Clinics* and *Clinics in Sports Medicine,* both published by W.B. Saunders; and *Sports Medicine Update,* published by the Healthsouth Corporation.

THE SPORTS MEDICINE TEAM

The provision of health care to the athlete requires a group effort to be most effective.[20] The sports medicine team must involve a number of individuals, each of whom must perform specific functions relative to caring for the injured athlete. Those people having the closest relationship with the injured athlete are the athletic trainer, the team physician, and the coach.

The Athletic Trainer

Of all the professionals charged with injury prevention and health care provision for the athlete, perhaps none is more intimately involved than the athletic trainer.[9] The athletic trainer is the one individual who deals with the athlete throughout the period of rehabilitation, from the time of the initial injury until the athlete's complete, unrestricted return to practice or competition.[35] The athletic trainer is most directly responsible for all phases of health care in an athletic environment, including preventing injuries from occurring, providing initial first aid and injury management, evaluating injuries, and designing and supervising a timely and effective program of rehabilitation that can facilitate the safe and expeditious return of the athlete to activity.

The athletic trainer must be knowledgeable and competent in a variety of speciality areas encompassed under the umbrella of "sports medicine" if he or she is to be effective in preventing and treating injuries to the athlete.[7] The specific roles and responsibilities of the athletic trainer differ and to a certain extent are defined by the situation in which he or she works.[28]

Roles and Responsibilities of the Athletic Trainer

In December 1993 the NATA Board of Certification completed a role delineation study, which redefined the profession of athletic training.[29] This study was designed to examine the primary tasks performed by the entry level athletic trainer and the knowledge and skills required to perform each task. Recommendations made by a role delineation study panel were validated via a survey sent to 2000 certified athletic trainers. The panel determined that the roles of the present-day athletic trainer can be divided into five major areas or performance domains: (1) prevention of athletic injuries; (2) recognition, evaluation, and immediate care of injuries; (3) rehabilitation and reconditioning of athletic injuries; (4) health care administration; and (5) professional development and responsibility. The Focus box on the next page summarizes tasks that were identified as critical under each of the five domains.

The panel also identified certain elements of athletic training that "transcend" several domains. These elements were labeled as "universal competencies" and were included under several different domains. For example, a basic knowledge of anatomy is essential to the knowledge base in several different domains.[27] Table 1-1 is a matrix that represents how these universal competencies may be applied to the various domains.

Prevention of Athletic Injury

Participation in competitive sports places the athlete in a situation in which injuries are possible at any given time. One major responsibility of the athletic trainer is to make the competitive environment as safe as possible to reduce the likelihood of in-

---

Athletic training must be considered as a specialization under the broad field of sports medicine.

The primary athletic training team consists of the coach, the athletic trainer, and the team physician.

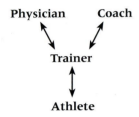

Physician   Coach

Trainer

Athlete

Five performance domains of the athletic trainer
- Prevention of athletic injuries
- Recognition, evaluation, and immediate care of injuries
- Rehabilitation and reconditioning of athletic injuries
- Health care administration
- Professional development and responsibility

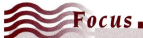

Focus

Domains and tasks

Domain 1. Prevention of athletic injuries

Task 1. Identify physical conditions predisposing the athlete or physically active individual to increased risk of injury and illness in athletic activity by following accepted preparticipation examination guidelines to ensure safe participation.

Task 2. Supervise conditioning programs and testing for athletes or physically active individuals using mechanical or other techniques to ensure readiness for safe participation in physical activity.

Task 3. Monitor environmental conditions (e.g., temperature, humidity, lightning) of playing or practice areas by following accepted guidelines to make recommendations regarding safe participation.

Task 4. Assess athletic apparatuses and athletic activity areas (e.g., playing surfaces, gyms, locker and athletic training room facilities) by periodic inspection and review of maintenance records to ensure a safe environment.

Task 5. Construct custom protective devices by fabricating and fitting with appropriate materials to protect specific parts of the body from injury during athletic activity.

Task 6. Apply specific and appropriate taping, wrapping, or prophylactic devices to the athlete or physically active individual by adhering to principles of biomechanics and injury mechanism to prevent injury or reinjury.

Task 7. Evaluate the use and maintenance of protective devices and athletic equipment (e.g., helmets, shoulder pads, shin guards) by inspecting and assessing the equipment to ensure optimal protection of the athlete or physically active individual.

Task 8. Educate parents, staff, coaches, athletes, and physically active individuals about the risks associated with participation and unsafe practices using direct communication to provide an opportunity for them to make an informed decision concerning physical activity.

Domain 2. Recognition, evaluation, and immediate care of athletic injuries

Task 1. Obtain a history from the athlete or physically active individual or witnesses through observation and interview to determine the pathology and extent of injury or illness.

Task 2. Inspect the involved area using bilateral comparison, if appropriate, to determine the extent of the injury or illness.

Task 3. Palpate the involved area using knowledge of human anatomy to determine the extent of the injury or illness.

Task 4. Perform specific tests on the involved area drawing on knowledge of anatomy, physiology, and biomechanics to determine the extent of the injury or illness.

Task 5. Determine the appropriate course of action by interpreting the signs and symptoms of the injury or illness to provide the necessary immediate care.

Task 6. Administer first aid using standard, approved techniques, and activate the emergency plan, if appropriate, to provide necessary medical care.

Task 7. Select and apply emergency equipment following standard, approved techniques to facilitate the athlete or physically active individual's safe, proper, and efficient transportation.

Task 8. Refer the athlete or physically active individual to the appropriate medical personnel or facility using standard procedures to continue proper medical care.

Domain 3. Rehabilitation and reconditioning of athletic injuries

Task 1. Identify injury or illness status by using standard techniques for evaluation and reassessment to determine appropriate rehabilitation programs.

Task 2. Construct rehabilitation or reconditioning programs for the injured or ill athlete or physically active individual using standard procedures for therapeutic exercise and modalities to restore functional status.

Task 3. Select appropriate rehabilitation equipment, manual techniques, and therapeutic modalities by evaluating the theory and use as defined by accepted standards of care to enhance recovery.

Task 4. Administer rehabilitation techniques and procedures to the injured or ill athlete or physically active individual by applying accepted standards of care and protocols to enhance recovery.

Task 5. Evaluate the readiness of the injured or ill athlete or physically active individual by assessing functional status to ensure a safe return to participation.

Task 6. Educate parents, staff, coaches, athletes, and physically active individuals about the rehabilitation process using direct communication to enhance rehabilitation.

Domain 4. Health care administration

Task 1. Maintain the health care records of the athlete or physically active individual using a recognized, comprehensive recording process to document procedures and services rendered by health care professionals.

Task 2. Comply with safety and sanitation standards by maintaining facilities and equipment to ensure a safe environment.

Continued

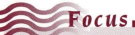

Focus

Domains and tasks—cont'd

Domain 4. Health care administration—cont'd

Task 3. Manage daily operations by implementing and maintaining standards for all personnel to ensure quality of service.

Task 4. Establish written guidelines for injury and illness management by standardizing operating procedures to provide a consistent quality of care.

Task 5. Obtain equipment and supplies by evaluating reliable product information to provide athletic training services for athletes and physically active individuals.

Task 6. Create a plan that includes emergency, management, and referral systems specific to the setting by involving appropriate health care professionals to facilitate proper care.

Task 7. Reduce the risk of exposure to infectious agents by following universal precautions to prevent the transmission of infectious diseases.

Domain 5. Professional development and responsibility

Task 1. Maintain knowledge of contemporary sports medicine issues by participating in continuing education activities to provide an appropriate standard of care.

Task 2. Develop interpersonal communication skills by interacting with others (e.g., parents, coaches, colleagues, athletes, physically active individuals) to enhance proficiency and professionalism.

Task 3. Adhere to ethical and legal parameters by following established guidelines that define the proper role of the certified athletic trainer to protect athletes, physically active individuals, and the public.

Task 4. Assimilate appropriate sports medicine research by using available resources to enhance professional growth.

Task 5. Educate the public by serving as a resource to enhance awareness of the roles and responsibilities of the certified athletic trainer.

Modified from National Athletic Trainers Association Board of Certification, Inc: *Study guide for the NATABOC entry level athletic trainer certification examination,* Philadelphia 1993, Davis.

1-1

Critical Thinking E x e r c i s e

A student of athletic training must develop a sound knowledge base in and demonstrate competent performance skills in five major domains: prevention of athletic injuries; recognition, evaluation, and immediate care of injuries; rehabilitation and reconditioning of athletic injuries; health care administration; and professional development and responsibility.

? How can student athletic trainers best prepare themselves to be competent professional athletic trainers?

jury. If injury can be prevented initially, there will be no need for first aid and subsequent rehabilitation.

Injury prevention includes (1) conducting physical examinations and preparticipation screenings to identify conditions that predispose an athlete to injury; (2) ensuring appropriate training and conditioning of the athlete; (3) monitoring environmental conditions to ensure safe participation; (4) selecting, properly fitting, and maintaining protective equipment; and (5) educating parents, coaches, and athletes about the risks inherent to sport participation.

Physical examinations   As previously mentioned, the athletic trainer, in cooperation with the team physician, should obtain a medical history and conduct physical examinations of the athletes before participation as a means of screening for existing or potential problems. (See Chapter 2.) The medical history should be reviewed closely and clarification given to any point of concern. The physical examination should include measurement of height, weight, blood pressure, and body composition. The physician examination should concentrate on cardiovascular, respiratory, abdominal, genital, dermatological, and ear, nose, and throat systems and may include blood work and urinalysis. A brief orthopedic evaluation would include range of motion, muscle strength, and functional tests to assess joint stability. If the athletic trainer knows at the beginning of a season that an athlete has a physical problem that may predispose the athlete to an injury during the course of the season, corrective measures that may significantly reduce the possibility of additional injury may be implemented immediately.

Developing training and conditioning programs   Perhaps the most important aspect of injury prevention is making certain that the athlete is fit and thus able to handle the physiological and psychological demands of athletic competition. The athletic trainer should work with the coaches to develop and implement an effective

TABLE 1-1 Role Delineation Matrix Identifying Competencies

Universal Competencies	Performance Domains				
	Prevention of Athletic Injuries	Recognition, Evaluation, and Immediate Care of Athletic Injuries	Rehabilitation and Reconditioning of Athletic Injuries	Health Care Administration	Professional Development and Responsibility
Domain-specific content	Knowledge and Skills Particular to Each Performance Domain				
Athletic training evaluation	Determination of an athlete's physical readiness to participate	Identification of underlying trauma	Ongoing evaluation of an athlete's progress through various stages of rehabilitation	Documentation of injury status and rehabilitation	Remains up-to-date with current evaluation skills, techniques, and knowledge
Human anatomy	Normal anatomical structure and function	Recognition of signs and symptoms of athletic injury and illness	Normal anatomical structure and function		Remains up-to-date in current human anatomical research and trends
Human physiology	Normal physiological function	Recognition of signs and symptoms of athletic injury and illness	Stages of injury response		Remains up-to-date in current human physiology research and trends
Exercise physiology	Physiological demand and response to exercise	Recognition of systemic and local metabolic failure	Musculoskeletal and cardiovascular demands placed on the injured athlete		Remains up-to-date with current exercise physiology research and trends
Biomechanics	Normal biomechanical demands of exercise	Identification of pathomechanics	Resolution of pathomechanical motion		Remains up-to-date with current biomechanical research and trends
Psychology/ counseling	Educational program for the healthy and injured athlete (i.e., alcohol and other drug abuse, performance anxiety)	Recognition of the psychological signs and symptoms of athletic injury and illness	Psychological implications of injury	Communication with and referral to the appropriate health care provider	Continues to develop interpersonal and communication skills
Nutrition	Nutritional demands of the athlete	Recognition of the effects of improper nutritional needs of the competing athlete (i.e., fluid replacement, diabetic shock)	Nutritional demands placed on the injured athlete	Referral to the appropriate health care provider	Remains up-to-date with current nutritional research and trends
Pharmacology	Contraindications and side effects of prescription and nonprescription medications	The role of prescription and nonprescription medication in the immediate/emergency care of athletic injury and illness	The role of prescription and nonprescription medications in the stages of injury response	Proper maintenance and documentation of records for the administration of prescription and nonprescription medication	Remains up-to-date with current pharmacological research and trends

Continued

TABLE 1-1   Role Delineation Matrix Identifying Competencies—cont'd

Universal Competencies	Performance Domains				
	Prevention of Athletic Injuries	Recognition, Evaluation, and Immediate Care of Athletic Injuries	Rehabilitation and Reconditioning of Athletic Injuries	Health Care Administration	Professional Development and Responsibility
Domain-specific content	Knowledge and Skills Particular to Each Performance Domain				
Physics	Absorption, dissipation, and transmission of energy of varying materials	The effect of stress loads on the human body (i.e., shear, tensile, compressive forces)	Physiological response to various energies imposed on the body		Remains up-to-date with current knowledge of physics as it relates to athletic training
Organization and administration	Legal requirements and rules of the sport	Planning, documentation, and communication of appropriate rehabilitation strategies to the necessary parties	Planning, documentation, and communication of appropriate rehabilitation strategies to the necessary parties	Development of operational policies and procedures	Remains up-to-date with current standards of professional practice

Modified from National Athletic Trainers Association Board of Certification, Inc. Role delineation matrix, *Certification Update* Fall (3):6,1994.

training and conditioning program for the athlete. (See Chapter 3.) It is essential that the athlete maintain a consistently high level of fitness during the preseason, the competitive season, and the off-season. This is critical not only for enhancing performance parameters but also for preventing injury and reinjury. An athletic trainer must be knowledgeable in the area of applied physiology of exercise, particularly with regard to strength training, flexibility, improvement of cardiorespiratory fitness, maintenance of body composition, weight control, and nutrition. Many colleges and most professional teams employ full-time strength coaches to oversee this aspect of the total program. The athletic trainer, however, must be acutely aware of any aspect of the program that may have a negative impact on an athlete or group of athletes and offer constructive suggestions for alternatives when appropriate. At the high school level, the athletic trainer may be totally responsible for designing, implementing, and overseeing the fitness and conditioning program for the athletes.

Ensuring a safe playing environment   To the best of his or her ability the athletic trainer must ensure a safe environment for competition. This may include duties not typically thought to belong to the athletic trainer, such as collecting trash, picking up rocks, or removing objects (e.g., hurdles, gymnastics equipment) from the perimeter of the practice area, all of which might pose potential danger to the athlete. The athletic trainer should call these potential safety hazards to the attention of an administrator. The interaction between the athletic trainer and a concerned and cooperative administrator can greatly enhance the effectiveness of the sports medicine team.

The athletic trainer should also be familiar with potential dangers associated with practicing or competing under inclement weather conditions, such as high heat and humidity, extreme cold, or electrical storms. Practice should be restricted, altered, or canceled if weather conditions threaten the health and safety of the athlete. If the team physician is not present, the athletic trainer must have the authority to curtail practice if the environmental conditions become severe. (See Chapter 12.)

Selecting, fitting, and maintaining protective equipment   The athletic trainer should work with coaches and equipment personnel to select protective equipment and be responsible for maintaining its condition and safety. (See Chapter 5.) In a time in which liability lawsuits have virtually become the rule rather than the exception,

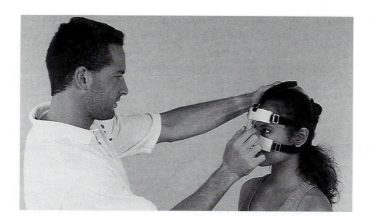

Figure 1-2

The trainer should be responsible for taping and also for fitting of protective devices.

the athletic trainer must make certain that high-quality equipment is being purchased initially and that it is constantly being worn, maintained, and reconditioned according to specific guidelines recommended by the manufacturers.

Protective equipment and devices can consume a significant portion of the athletic budget. The individual who is responsible for purchasing protective equipment is usually barraged with marketing literature on a variety of braces, supports, pads, and other types of protective equipment. Decisions on purchasing specific pieces or brands should be based on research data that clearly document effectiveness in reducing or preventing injury (Figure 1-2).

Equipment is generally relatively expensive, and schools are certainly subject to budgeting restrictions. However, decisions made on the equipment that is purchased should always be made in the best interest of the athlete. Most colleges and professional teams hire full-time equipment managers to oversee this area of responsibility, but it is imperative that the athletic trainer be knowledgeable about and aware of the equipment being worn by each athlete.

The design, building, and fitting of specific protective orthopedic devices are also responsibilities of the athletic trainer. Once the physician has indicated the problem and how it may be corrected, the athletic trainer should be able to construct an orthopedic device to correct it.

Counseling and guidance   The athletic trainer should take responsibility for educating parents and coaches about the nature of a specific injury and how it may affect the ability of the athlete to compete. But the athletic trainer should be concerned primarily with counseling and advising the athlete not only with regard to prevention, rehabilitation, and treatment of specific injuries but on any matter that might be of help to the athlete. Perhaps one of the most rewarding aspects of working as an athletic trainer can be found in the relationships that one develops with individual athletes. During the period of time that athletes are competing, the athletic trainer has the opportunity to get to know them very well on a personal basis because he or she spends a considerable amount of time with them. Athletes often develop a degree of respect and trust in the athletic trainer's judgment that carries over from their athletic life into their personal life. It is not uncommon for an athletic trainer to be asked questions about a number of personal matters, at which point he or she crosses a bridge from athletic trainer to friend and confidant. This is a considerable responsibility that is perhaps best handled by first listening to the problems, presenting several options, and then letting the athlete make his or her own decision. Certainly, the role of counselor and advisor cannot be taken lightly.[8]

Recognition, Evaluation, and Immediate Care of Injuries

Frequently, the athletic trainer is the first person to see an athlete who has sustained an injury. The athletic trainer must be skilled in recognizing the nature and extent of an injury through competency in injury evaluation. Once the injury has been evaluated, the athletic trainer must be able to provide the appropriate first aid and then refer the athlete to appropriate medical personnel.

Evaluation of athletic injuries   The athletic trainer must be able to efficiently and accurately evaluate an injury. Information obtained in this initial evaluation may be critical later on when swelling, pain, and guarding mask some of the functional signs of the injury.

It is essential that the athletic trainer be alert and observe, as much as possible, everything that goes on in practice. Invaluable information regarding the nature of an injury can be obtained by seeing the mechanism of the injury.

The subsequent on-field examination should include (1) obtaining a brief medical history of exactly what happened, according to the athlete, (2) observation, (3) palpation, (4) range of motion check, (5) muscle strength check, (6) functional joint stability tests, and (7) a brief neurological examination. Information obtained in this initial examination should be documented by the athletic trainer and given to the physician once the athlete is referred. The team physician is ultimately responsible for providing an accurate diagnosis of an injury. The initial evaluation often provides the basis for this diagnosis. (See Chapter 10.)

First aid and emergency care   The athletic trainer is responsible for administering appropriate first aid to the injured athlete and for making correct decisions in the management of acute injury. (See Chapter 8.) Although the team physician is frequently present at games or competitions, in most cases he or she cannot be at every practice session, where injuries are even more likely to occur. Thus the athletic trainer must possess sound skills not only in the initial recognition and evaluation of potentially serious or life-threatening injuries but also in emergency care.

The athletic trainer should be certified in cardiopulmonary resuscitation by the American Red Cross, the American Heart Association, or the National Safety Council. Athletic trainers should also be certified in first aid by the American Red Cross or the National Safety Council. Many athletic trainers have gone beyond these essential basic certifications and have completed requirements for emergency medical technician (EMT).

Emergency care procedures should be established by the athletic trainer in cooperation with local rescue squads and the community hospitals that can provide emergency treatment. Arrangements regarding transportation, logistics, billing procedures, and appropriate contacts made before having to deal with an injury help expedite emergency care and lessen the injured athlete's frustration and concern.

Referral to appropriate medical personnel   After the initial management of an injury, the athletic trainer should routinely refer the athlete to the team physician for further evaluation and accurate diagnosis. If an athlete requires treatment from medical personnel other than the team physician, such as a dentist or ophthalmologist, the athletic trainer should arrange appointments as necessary. Referrals should be made after consultation with the team physician.

Rehabilitation and Reconditioning

An athletic trainer must work closely with and under the supervision of the team physician with respect to designing rehabilitation and reconditioning protocols that make use of appropriate rehabilitative equipment, manual therapy techniques, or therapeutic modalities. The athletic trainer should then assume the responsibility of overseeing the rehabilitative process, ultimately returning the athlete to full activity. (See Chapter 15.)

Designing rehabilitation programs   Once the team physician has evaluated and diagnosed an injury, the rehabilitation process begins immediately. In most cases, the athletic trainer will design and supervise an injury rehabilitation program, modifying that program within the framework of the healing process. It is critical for an athletic trainer to have a sound background in anatomy. Without this background it is impossible to evaluate an injury. And if the athletic trainer cannot evaluate an injury,

---

1-2

Critical Thinking Exercise

A basketball player suffers a grade 2 ankle sprain during midseason of the competitive schedule. After a 3-week course of rehabilitation most of the pain and swelling has been eliminated. The athlete is anxious to get back into practice and competitive games as soon as possible, and subsequent injuries to other players have put pressure on the coach to force his return. Unfortunately the athlete is still unable to perform functional tasks (cutting and jumping) essential in basketball.

? Who is responsible for making the decision regarding when the athlete can fully return to practice and game situations?

there is no point in his or her knowing anything about rehabilitation because he or she will not know at what phase the injury is in the healing process. The athletic trainer must also understand how to incorporate therapeutic modalities and appropriate therapeutic exercise techniques if the rehabilitation program is to be successful.

Supervising rehabilitation programs   Too often in the past the athletic trainer has routinely referred the injured athlete to a physical therapist who will supervise the rehabilitation program. Although physical therapists are well qualified for this task, there is no reason for the well-trained athletic trainer to avoid this responsibility. In fact the athletic trainer should have a better understanding of how to design a series of activities related to the sport that allow the athlete to gradually progress to complete functional return.

Health Care Administration

The athletic trainer is responsible for the organization and administration of the training room facility, including the maintenance of health and injury records for each athlete, requisition and inventory of necessary supplies and equipment, the supervision of assistant or student trainers, and the establishment of policies and procedures for day-to-day operation of the athletic training program. (See Chapter 2.)

Record keeping   Accurate and detailed record keeping—including medical histories, preparticipation examinations, injury reports, treatment records, and rehabilitation programs—are critical for the athletic trainer, particularly in light of the number of lawsuits directed toward malpractice in health care. Although this may be difficult and time consuming for the athletic trainer who treats and deals with a large number of patients each day, it is an area that simply cannot be neglected.

Ordering equipment and supplies   Although tremendous variations in operating budgets exist, depending on the level and the institution, decisions regarding how available money may best be spent are always critical. The athletic trainer must keep on hand a wide range of supplies to enable him or her to handle whatever situation may arise. At institutions in which severe budgetary restrictions exist, prioritization based on experience and past needs must become the mode of operation. A creative athletic trainer can make do with very little equipment, which should at least include a taping and treatment table, an ice machine, and a few free weights. As in other professions the more tools available for use, the more effective the practitioner can be, as long as there is an understanding of how those tools are used most effectively.

Supervising assistants   In an athletic training environment the quality and efficiency of the assistant and student trainers in carrying out their specific responsibilities are absolutely essential. The person who supervises these assistants has a responsibility to design a reasonable work schedule that is consistent with other commitments and responsibilities they have outside of the training room. It is the responsibility of the head athletic trainer to provide an environment in which assistant and student trainers can continually learn and develop professionally.

Establishing policies for operation of an athletic training program   Although the athletic trainer must be able to easily adjust and adapt to a given situation, it is essential that specific policies, procedures, rules, and regulations be established to ensure smooth and consistent day-to-day operation of the athletic training program. A plan should be established for emergency management of injury. Appropriate channels for referral after injury and emergency treatment should be used consistently.

Policies and procedures must be established and implemented that reduce the likelihood of exposure to infectious agents by following universal precautions, which can prevent the transmission of infectious diseases.

Professional Development and Responsibility

The athletic trainer should assume personal responsibility for maintaining and expanding his or her own knowledge base and expertise within the chosen field. This

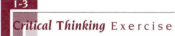

1-3

Critical Thinking Exercise

A young athletic trainer has taken his first job at All-American High School. The school administrators are extremely concerned about the number of athletes who get hurt playing various sports. They have charged the athletic trainer with the task of developing an athletic training program that can effectively help prevent the occurence of injury to athletes in all sports at that school.

? What things can the athletic trainer do in an attempt to reduce the number of injuries and to minimize the risk of injury in the competitive athletes at that high school?

may be accomplished by attending continuing education programs offered at state, district, and national meetings. Athletic trainers must also routinely review professional journals and consult current textbooks to stay abreast of the most up-to-date techniques.

The athletic trainer must take time to help educate student athletic trainers. There is little question that the continued success of any profession lies in its ability to educate its students. This should not simply be a responsibility but instead a priority. Students of athletic training must be given a sound academic background in a curriculum that stresses the competencies as outlined in this chapter. They must be able to translate the theoretical base presented in the classroom into practical application in a clinical setting if they are to be effective in treating patients.

The athletic trainer must also educate the general public, in addition to a large segment of the various allied medical health care professions, as to exactly what athletic trainers are and the scope of their roles and responsibilities. This is perhaps best accomplished by holding professional seminars, publishing research in scholarly journals, meeting with local and community organizations, and, most important, doing a good and professional job of providing health care to the injured athlete.

Personal Qualities of the Athletic Trainer

There is probably no field of endeavor that can provide more work excitement, variety of tasks, and personal satisfaction than athletic training. A person contemplating going into this field must love sports and enjoy the world of competition, in which there is a level of intensity seldom matched in any other area.

An athletic trainer's personal qualities, not the facilities and equipment, determine his or her success. Personal qualities are the many characteristics that identify individuals in regard to their actions and reactions as members of society. Personality is a complex of the many characteristics that together give an image of the individual to those with whom he or she associates. The personal qualities of athletic trainers are the most important because they in turn work with many complicated and diverse personalities. Although no attempt has been made to establish a rank order, the qualities discussed in the following paragraphs are essential if one desires to be a good athletic trainer.

Stamina and Ability to Adapt

Athletic training is not a field for a person who likes an 8-to-5 job. Long, arduous hours of often strenuous work will sap the reserve strength of anyone not in the best of physical and emotional health. Athletic training requires abundant energy, vitality, and physical and emotional stability. Every day brings new challenges and problems that must be solved. The athletic trainer must be able to adapt to new situations with ease. A problem that can happen in any "helping profession" and does on occasion occur among athletic trainers is burnout. This is a problem that can be avoided if addressed early.

A problem with burnout   The term *burnout* is commonly used to describe feelings of exhaustion and disinterest toward one's work.[10] Clinically, it is most often associated with the helping professions; however, it is seen in athletes and other types of individuals engaged in physically or emotionally demanding endeavors.[3] Most persons who have been associated with sports have known athletes, coaches, or athletic trainers who just "drop out."[4] They have become dissatisfied with and disinterested in the profession to which they have dedicated a major part of their lives. Signs of burnout include excessive anger, blaming others, guilt, being tired and exhausted all day, sleep problems, high absenteeism, family problems, and self-preoccupation.[11] Persons experiencing burnout may cope by consuming drugs or alcohol.

The very nature of athletic training is one of caring about and serving the athlete. When the emotional demands of work overcome the professional's resources to cope, burnout may occur. Too many athletes to care for, the expectations of coaches to

Athletic trainer's personal qualities
- Stamina and ability to adapt
- Empathy
- Sense of humor
- Ability to communicate
- Intellectual curiosity
- Ethics

As a member of a helping profession, the athletic trainer is subject to burnout.

return an injured athlete to action, difficulties in caring for chronic conditions, and personality conflicts involving athletes, coaches, physicians, or administrators can leave the athletic trainer physically and emotionally drained at the end of the day. Sources of emotional drain include little reward for one's efforts, role conflicts, lack of autonomy, and a feeling of powerlessness to deal with the problems at hand. Commonly, the professional athletic trainer is in a constant state of high emotional arousal and anxiety during the working day.

Individuals entering the field of athletic training must realize that it is extremely demanding. Even though the field is often difficult, they must learn that they cannot be "all things to all people." They must learn to say no when their health is at stake, and they must make leisure time for themselves beyond their work.[5]

Empathy   Empathy refers to the capacity to enter into the feeling or spirit of another person. Athletic training is a field that requires the ability to sense when an athlete is in distress, together with a desire to alleviate that stress.

Sense of humor   Many athletes rate having a sense of humor as the most important attribute that an athletic trainer can have. Humor and wit help release tension and provide a relaxed atmosphere. The athletic trainer who is too serious or too clinical will have problems in adapting to the often lighthearted setting of the sports world.

Communication   Athletic training requires a constant flow of both oral and written communication. As an educator, psychologist, counselor, therapist, and administrator, the athletic trainer must be a good communicator.

Intellectual curiosity   The athletic trainer must always be a student. The field of athletic training is so diverse and ever changing that it requires constant study. The athletic trainer must have an active intellectual curiosity. Through reading professional journals and books, communicating with the team physician, and attending professional meetings the athletic trainer stays abreast of the field.

Ethical practice   The athletic trainer must act at all times with the highest standards of conduct and integrity.[22] To ensure this behavior, NATA has developed a code of ethics, which was approved at the NATA annual symposium in 1993.[25] The five basic ethics principles are as follows:

1. Members shall respect the rights, welfare, and dignity of all individuals.
2. Members shall comply with the laws and regulations governing the practice of athletic training.
3. Members shall accept the responsibility for the exercise of sound judgment.
4. Members shall maintain and promote high standards in the provision of services.
5. Members shall not engage in conduct that constitutes a conflict of interest or that adversely reflects on the profession.

Members who act in a manner that is unethical or unbecoming to the profession can ultimately lose their certification.

Professional Memberships

It is essential that an athletic trainer become a member of and be active in professional organizations. Such organizations are continuously upgrading and refining the profession. They provide an ongoing source of information about changes occurring in the profession and include NATA, district associations within NATA, various state athletic training organizations, and ASCM. Some athletic trainers are also physical therapists. Over the years there has developed a closer relationship between NATA and the American Physical Therapy Association. Increasingly, physical therapists are becoming interested in working with physically active individuals.

As a professional, the athletic trainer must be a member of and be active in professional organizations.

The Athletic Trainer and the Athlete

The major concern of the athletic trainer should always be the athlete. If it were not for the athlete, the physician, the coach, and the athletic trainer would have nothing to do in sports. It is essential to realize that whatever decisions are made by the physician, coach, and athletic trainer, they ultimately affect the athlete. Athletes are frequently caught in the middle between coaches telling them to do one thing and medical staff telling them to do something else. Thus the injured athlete must always be informed and made aware of the why, how, and when that collectively dictate the course of an injury rehabilitation program.

The athletic trainer should educate the student athlete about injury prevention and management. Athletes should learn about techniques of training and conditioning that may reduce the likelihood of injury. They should be well informed about their injuries and taught how to listen to what their bodies are telling them to prevent reinjury.

In a high school setting the athletic trainer must also take the time to explain to and inform the parents about injury management and prevention. With an athlete of high school age, the parents' decisions regarding health care must be taken into consideration.

Each role and responsibility is critical if the athletic trainer is to be as effective as possible in treating people with injuries related to participation in sports.[31] Though a number of authorities can significantly affect the health care of the athlete, the athletic trainer is certainly an integral part of the sports medicine team.

The Team Physician

The athletic trainer works primarily under the supervision of the team physician, who is ultimately responsible for directing the total health care of the athlete (Figure 1-3). In cooperation with the team physician, the athletic trainer must make decisions that ultimately have a direct effect on the athlete who has sustained an injury.

From the viewpoint of the athletic trainer, there are a number of roles and responsibilities that the team physician should assume with regard to injury prevention and the health care of the athlete.[23,36] (See the Focus box on the next page.)

First, the physician should be a supervisor and an advisor to the athletic trainer and coach. However, the athletic trainer must be given flexibility to function independently in the decision-making process and must often act without the advice or direction of the physician. Therefore it is critical that the team physician and the athletic trainer share philosophical opinions regarding injury management and rehabilitation programs; this will help minimize any discrepancies or inconsistencies that may exist. Most athletic trainers would prefer to work with rather than for a team physician.

Figure 1-3

In treating the athlete, the athletic trainer carries out the directions of the physician.

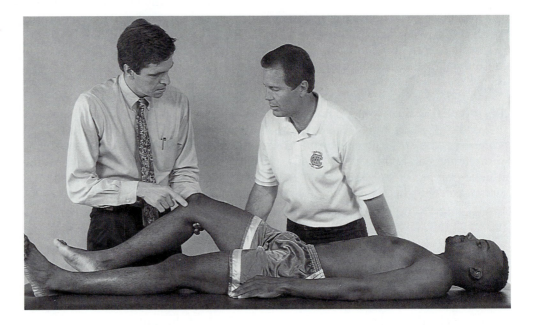

Compiling Medical Histories

The team physician should be responsible for compiling medical histories and conducting physical examinations for each athlete, both of which can provide critical information that may reduce the possibility of injury. Preparticipation screening done by both the athletic trainer and physician are important in establishing baseline information to be used for comparison should injury occur during the season.

Diagnosing Injury

The team physician should assume responsibility for diagnosing an injury and should be keenly aware of the program of rehabilitation as designed by the athletic trainer after the diagnosis. Athletic trainers should be capable of doing an accurate initial evaluation after acute injury. Input from that evaluation may be essential to the physician, who may not see the patient for several hours or perhaps days after the injury. However, the physician has been trained specifically to diagnose injuries and to make recommendations to the athletic trainer for treatment based on that diagnosis. The athletic trainer should have a sound background in injury rehabilitation and must be the one to design and supervise an effective rehabilitation scheme. These are two closely related yet distinct roles that require both cooperation and close communication if they are to be optimized.

Team physicians must have absolute authority in determining the health status of an athlete who wishes to participate in the sports program.

Deciding on Disqualification

The physician should determine when an athlete should be disqualified from competition on medical grounds and must have the final say in when an injured athlete may return to activity. Any decision to allow an athlete to resume activity should be based on recommendations from the athletic trainer. An athletic trainer most often has an advantage in that he or she knows the injured athlete well, including how the athlete responds to injury, how the athlete moves, and how hard to push to return the athlete safely to activity. The physician's judgment must be based not only on medical knowledge but also on knowledge of the psychophysiological demands of a particular sport.[19]

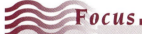

Focus

Duties of the team physician

- Seeing that a complete medical history of each athlete is compiled and is readily available
- Determining through a physical examination the athlete's health status
- Diagnosing and treating injuries and other illnesses
- Directing and advising the athletic trainer about health matters
- Acting, when necessary, as an instructor to the athletic trainer, assistant athletic trainer, and student athletic trainers about special therapeutic methods, therapeutic problems, and related procedures
- If possible, attending all games, athletic contests, scrimmages, and practices
- Deciding when, on medical grounds, athletes should be disqualified from participation and when they may be permitted to reenter competition
- Serving as an advisor to the athletic trainer and the coach and, when necessary, as a counselor to the athlete
- Working closely with the school administrator, school dentist, athletic trainer, coach, and health services personnel to promote and maintain consistently high standards for the care of the athlete

Attending Practices and Games

A team physician should make an effort to attend as many practices, scrimmages, and competitions as possible. This obviously becomes difficult at an institution where there may be 20 or more athletic teams. Thus the physician must be readily available should the athletic trainer (who generally is at most practices and games) require consultation or advice.

If it is not possible for the team physician to attend all practice sessions and competitive events or games, it is sometimes possible to establish a plan of rotation involving a number of physicians. In this plan any one physician need be present at only one or two activities a year. The rotation plan has proved practical in situations in which the school district is unable to afford a full-time physician or has so limited a budget that it must ask for volunteer medical coverage. In some instances the attending physician is paid a per-game stipend.

Commitment to Sports and the Athlete

Most important, the team physician must have a strong love of sports and must be generally interested in and concerned for the young people who compete. Colleges and universities typically employ someone to act as a full-time team physician. High schools most often rely on a local physician from within the community who volunteers his or her time. To serve as a team physician for the purpose of enhancing one's social standing in the community can be a frustrating and potentially dangerous situation for everyone involved in the athletic program.

When a physician is asked to serve as a team physician, arrangements must be made with the employing educational institution about specific required responsibilities. Policies must be established regarding emergency care, legal liability, facilities, personnel relationships, and duties.[37]

It is essential that the team physician promote and maintain consistently high-quality care for the athlete in all phases of the sports medicine program.

The Coach

The coach is directly responsible for preventing injuries by seeing that the athlete has undergone a preventive injury conditioning program. He or she must ensure that sports equipment, especially protective equipment, is of the highest quality and is properly fitted. The coach must also make sure that protective equipment is properly

Figure 1-4

The coach is directly responsible for preventing injuries in his or her sport.

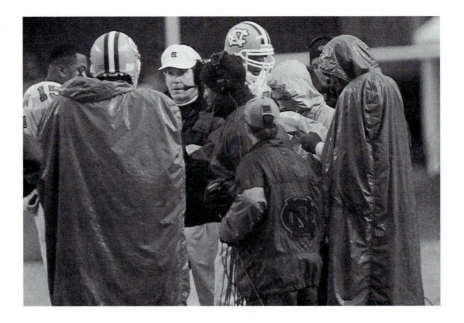

maintained.[18] A coach must be keenly aware of what produces injuries in his or her particular sport and what measures must be taken to avoid them (Figure 1-4). A coach should be able to apply proper first aid when called on to do so. This is especially true in cases of serious head and spinal injuries.

It is essential that a coach have a thorough understanding of the skill techniques and environmental factors that may adversely affect the athlete. Poor biomechanics in skill areas such as throwing and running can lead to overuse injuries of the arms and legs, and overexposure to heat and humidity may cause death. Just because a coach is experienced in coaching does not mean that he or she knows proper skill techniques. It is essential that coaches engage in a continual process of education to further their knowledge in their particular sport. When a sports program or specific sport is without an athletic trainer, the coach often takes over this role.

Coaches work closely with athletic trainers; therefore both must develop an awareness and an insight into each other's problems so that they can function as effectively as possible. The athletic trainer must develop patience and must earn the respect of the coaches so that his or her judgment in all training matters is fully accepted. In turn, the athletic trainer must avoid questioning the abilities of the coaches in their particular fields and must restrict opinions to athletic training matters. To avoid frustration and hard feelings, the coach must coach, and the athletic trainer must conduct athletic training matters. In terms of the health and well-being of the athlete, the physician and the athletic trainer have the last word. This position must be backed at all times by the athletic director.

Other Sports Medicine Support Personnel

A number of support health services may be used by a sports program. They may include a nurse, school health services, team orthopedist, team dentist, team podiatrist, team nutritionist, equipment personnel, and referees.

The Nurse

As a rule, the nurse is not usually responsible for the recognition of sports injuries. Education and background, however, render the nurse capable in the recognition of skin disease, infections, and minor irritations. The nurse works under the direction of the physician and in liaison with the athletic trainer and the school health services.

School Health Services

Colleges and universities maintain school health services that range from a department operating with one or two nurses and a physician available on a part-time basis to an elaborate setup comprised of a full complement of nursing services with a staff of full-time medical specialists and complete laboratory and hospital facilities. At the high school level health services are usually organized so that one or two nurses conduct the program under the direction of the school physician, who may serve a number of schools in a given area or district. This organization poses a problem, because it is often difficult to have qualified medical help at hand when it is needed. Local policy determines the procedure for referral for medical care. If such policies are lacking, the athletic trainer should see to it that an effective method is established for handling all athletes requiring medical care or opinion. The ultimate source of health care is the physician. The effectiveness of athletic health care service can be evaluated only to the extent to which it meets the following criteria:

1. Availability at every scheduled practice or contest of a person qualified and delegated to render emergency care to an injured or ill participant
2. Planned access to a physician by phone or nearby presence for prompt medical evaluation of the health care problems that warrant this attention
3. Planned access to a medical facility, including plans for communication and transportation

Support personnel concerned with the athlete's health and safety
- Nurse
- School health services
- Team orthopedist
- Team dentist
- Team podiatrist
- Physician's assistant
- Biomechanist
- Strength and conditioning coach
- Sport psychologist
- Physical therapist
- Exercise physiologist
- Team nutritionist
- Equipment personnel
- Referees

Team Orthopedist

Often the team physician has a speciality in family medicine or is an internist. In such cases serious musculoskeletal injuries are referred to an orthopedic surgeon who specializes in these disorders. Many colleges and universities have a team orthopedist on their staff.

Team Dentist

The role of team dentist is somewhat analogous to that of team physician. He or she serves as a dental consultant for the team and should be available for first aid and emergency care. Good communication between the dentist and the coach or athletic trainer should ensure a good dental program. There are three areas of responsibility for the team dentist:

1. Organizing and performing the preseason dental examination
2. Being available to provide emergency care when needed
3. Conducting the fitting of mouth protectors

Team Podiatrist

Podiatry, the specialized field dealing with the study and care of the foot, has become an integral part of sports health care. Many podiatrists are trained in surgical procedures, foot biomechanics, and the fitting and construction of orthotic devices for the shoe. Like the team dentist, a podiatrist should be available on a consulting basis.

Physician's Assistants

Physician's assistants (PAs) are trained to assume some of the responsibilities for patient care traditionally done by a physician. They assist the physician by conducting preliminary patient evaluations, arranging for various hospital-based diagnostic tests, and dispensing appropriate medications. A number of athletic trainers have also become PAs in recent years.

Biomechanist

An individual who possesses some expertise in the analysis of human motion can also be a great aid to the athletic trainer. The biomechanist uses sophisticated video and computer-enhanced digital analysis equipment to study movement. By advising the athlete, coach, and athletic trainer on matters such as faulty gait patterns or improper throwing mechanics, the biomechanist can reduce the likelihood of injury to the athlete.

Strength and Conditioning Coach

Many colleges and universities and some high schools employ full-time strength coaches to advise athletes on training and conditioning programs. Athletic trainers should routinely consult with these individuals to advise them about injuries to a particular athlete and exercises that should be avoided or modified relative to a specific injury. Strength coaches can now be certified by the National Strength Coaches Association.

Sports Psychologists

The sports psychologist can advise the athletic trainer on matters related to the psychological aspects of the rehabilitation process. The way the athlete feels about his or her injury and how it affects his or her social, emotional, intellectual, and physical dimensions can have a substantial effect on the course of a treatment program and how quickly the athlete may return to competition. The sports psychologist uses different intervention strategies to help the athlete cope with injury. Sport psychologists can seek certification through the Association for the Advancement of Sport Psychology.

Physical Therapists

Some athletic trainers use physical therapists to supervise the rehabilitation programs for injured athletes while the athletic trainer concentrates primarily on getting a player ready to practice or compete. A number of athletic trainers are also physical therapists.

Exercise Physiologists

The exercise physiologist can significantly influence the athletic training program by giving input to the trainer regarding training and conditioning techniques, body composition analysis, and nutritional considerations.

Team Nutritionist

Increasingly, individuals in the field of nutrition are becoming interested in athletics. Some large athletic training programs engage a nutritionist as a consultant who plans eating programs that are geared to the needs of a particular sport. He or she also assists individual athletes who need special nutritional counseling.

Equipment Personnel

Sports equipment personnel are becoming specialists in the purchase and proper fitting of protective equipment. They work closely with the coach and the athletic trainer.

Referees

Referees must be highly knowledgeable regarding rules and regulations, especially those that relate to the health and welfare of the athlete. They work cooperatively with the coach and the athletic trainer. They must be capable of checking the playing facility for dangerous situations and equipment that may predispose the athlete to injury. They must routinely check athletes to ensure that they are wearing adequate protective pads.

EMPLOYMENT SETTINGS FOR THE ATHLETIC TRAINER

Opportunities for employment as an athletic trainer have changed dramatically during recent years. Since the 1950s the traditional employment setting for the athletic trainer has been in a training room at the college, university, or professional levels. During the 1980s—primarily because of intensive public relations efforts by NATA— the majority of jobs available were at the high school level. Today the largest percentage of certified athletic trainers are employed in sports medicine clinics or in industry, areas that until recently had been considered nontraditional settings.

Secondary Schools

It would be ideal to have certified athletic trainers serve every secondary school in the United States.[14] Many of the physical problems that occur later from improperly managed sports injuries could be avoided initially if proper care from an athletic trainer had been provided. Many times a coach does all of his or her own athletic training, although in some cases, a coach is assigned additional athletic training responsibilities and is assisted by a student athletic trainer. If a secondary school hires an athletic trainer, it is commonly in a faculty-trainer capacity. This individual is usually employed as a teacher in one of the school's classroom disciplines and performs athletic training duties on a part-time or extracurricular basis.[34] In this instance compensation usually is on the basis of released time from teaching, a stipend as a coach, or both.[17]

Another means of obtaining high school or community college athletic training coverage is using a certified graduate student from a nearby college or university. The graduate student receives a graduate assistantship with a stipend paid by the secondary school or community college. In this situation both the graduate student and

Athletic trainers work in a number of different settings
- Secondary schools
- School districts
- Colleges and universities
- Professional sports
- Sports medicine clinics
- Industrial settings

the school benefit.[12] However, this practice may prevent a school from employing an athletic trainer on a full-time basis.

School Districts

Some school districts have found it effective to employ a centrally placed certified athletic trainer. In this case the athletic trainer, who may be full- or part-time, is a nonteacher who serves a number of schools. The advantage is savings; the disadvantage is that one individual cannot provide the level of service usually required by a typical school.

Colleges or Universities

At the college or university level the athletic training position varies considerably from institution to institution. In smaller institutions, the athletic trainer may be a half-time teacher in physical education and half-time athletic trainer. In some cases, if the athletic trainer is a physical therapist rather than a teacher, he or she may spend part of the time in the school health center and part of the time in athletic training. Increasingly at the college level, athletic training services are being offered to members of the general student body who participate in intramural and club sports. In most colleges and universities the athletic trainer is full-time, does not teach, works in the department of athletics, and is paid by the state or from student union or alumni funds.

Professional Teams

The athletic trainer for professional sports teams usually performs specific team training duties for 6 months out of the year; the other 6 months are spent in off-season conditioning and individual rehabilitation. The athletic trainer working with a professional team is involved with only one sport and is paid according to contract, much like a player. Playoff and championship money may add substantially to the yearly income.

Sports Medicine Clinics

For years, sports medicine clinics have been considered a nontraditional setting for employment as an athletic trainer. Today, more athletic trainers are employed in sports medicine clinics than in any other employment setting. The role of the athletic trainer is extremely variable from one clinic to the next. Most clinical athletic trainers see patients with sports-related injuries during the morning hours in the clinic. In the afternoons, trainers' services are contracted out to local high schools or small colleges for game or practice coverage. For the most part, private clinics have well-equipped facilities in which to work, and salaries for their trainers are generally somewhat higher than in the more traditional settings.

Industrial Settings

It is becoming relatively common for corporations or industries to employ athletic trainers to oversee fitness and injury rehabilitation programs for their employees. In addition to these responsibilities trainers may be assigned to conduct wellness programs and provide education and individual counseling. It is likely that many job opportunities will exist for the athletic trainer in industry in the next few years.

RECOGNITION OF THE ATHLETIC TRAINER AS AN ALLIED HEALTH PROFESSIONAL

In June 1991 the American Medical Association (AMA) officially recognized athletic training as an allied health profession. The primary purpose of this recognition was for accrediting educational programs. The AMA's Committee on Allied Health Education and Accreditation (CAHEA) was charged with the responsibility of developing essentials and guidelines for academic programs to use in preparation of individuals

---

1-4

Critical Thinking Exercise

An athletic trainer has taken a job working in a sports medicine clinic. There are four physical therapists and two physical therapy assistants. There has never been an athletic trainer in this clinic before, and there is some uncertainty among the physical therapists as to exactly what role the athletic trainer will play in the function of the clinic.

? How does the role of the athletic trainer working in the clinic differ from the responsibilities of the athletic trainer working in a university setting?

for entry into the profession through the Joint Review Committee on Athletic Training (JRC-AT). As of 1993, all entry-level athletic training education programs became subject to the CAHEA accreditation process.[6]

In June 1994 CAHEA was dissolved and was replaced immediately by the Commission on Accreditation of Allied Health Education Programs (CAAHEP). Currently there are 17 professional review committees sponsored by the 49 separate organizations, including NATA, which make up CAAHEP. The CAAHEP is recognized as an accreditation agency for allied health education programs by the U.S. Department of Education. Entry level college and university athletic training education programs at both the undergraduate and graduate levels that were at one time approved by NATA and subsequently by CAHEA must now be accreditated by CAAHEP. The JRC-AT is currently made up of representatives from NATA, the American Academy of Pediatrics, the American Association of Sports Medicine, and the American Academy of Family Practice.

The effects of CAAHEP accreditation are not limited to the educational aspects. In the future, this recognition may potentially affect regulatory legislation, the practice of athletic training in nontraditional settings, and insurance considerations. This recognition will continue to be a positive step in the development of the athletic training profession.

Requirements for Certification as an Athletic Trainer

An athletic trainer who is certified by NATA is a highly qualified paramedical professional educated and experienced in dealing with the injuries that occur with participation in sports. Candidates for certification are required to have an extensive background of both formal academic preparation and supervised practical experience in a clinical setting, according to CAAHEP guidelines. The guidelines listed in the Focus box on the next page have been established by the National Athletic Trainers Association Board of Certification.[30]

The Certification Examination

Once the requirements have been fulfilled, applicants are eligible to sit for the certification examination. The certification examination has been developed by the National Athletic Trainers Association Board of Certification (NATABOC) in conjunction with Columbia Assessment Services, Inc., and is administered four times each year at various locations throughout the United States.[30] The examination consists of three sections: a written portion, an oral-practical portion, and a written-simulation portion. The examination tests for knowledge and skill in five major domains: (1) prevention of athletic injuries; (2) recognition, evaluation, and immediate care of injuries; (3) rehabilitation and reconditioning of athletic injuries; (4) health care administration; and (5) professional development and responsibility. Successful performance on the certification examination leads to certification as an athletic trainer.

Continuing Education Requirements

To ensure ongoing professional growth and involvement by the certified athletic trainer, NATABOC has established requirements for continuing education.[26] To maintain certification, all certified trainers must document a minimum of eight Continuing Education Units (CEUs) attained during each 3-year recertification term. CEUs may be awarded for attending symposiums, seminars, workshops, or conferences; serving as a speaker, panelist, or certification exam model; participating in the USOC program; authoring a research article in a professional journal; completing a NATA journal quiz; completing postgraduate course work; and obtaining CPR, first aid, or EMT certification. All certified athletic trainers must also demonstrate proof of CPR certification at least once during the 3-year term.

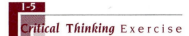

1-5

Critical Thinking Exercise

A second-semester college sophomore has decided that she is interested in becoming a certified athletic trainer. She happens to be in an institution that offers an advanced master's degree in athletic training yet does not offer an entry level CAAHEP-approved curriculum. However, the institution does sponsor an internship program that currently has about 15 students.

? How can this student most effectively achieve her goal of becoming a certified athletic trainer?

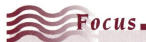

NATA certification

Purpose of certification

The National Athletic Trainers Association Board of Certification (NATABOC) was established in 1970 to implement a program of certification for entry level athletic trainers. The purpose of the certification program is to establish standards for entry into the profession of athletic training.

To attain certification as an athletic trainer, an applicant must fulfill the following core requirements and must either complete a CAAHEP-accredited entry level program or an internship program.

Core requirements

Note: If one or more of the core requirements are not fulfilled at the time of application, the application will be returned.

1. The athletic training student must have a high school diploma to begin accumulating directly supervised clinical hours that are to be used to meet requirements for NATABOC certification.
2. Proof of graduation (an official transcript) at the baccalaureate level from an accredited college or university located in the United States of America. Foreign-degreed applicants who wish to credit this degree toward a bachelor's degree requirement will be evaluated, at the candidate's expense, by an independent consultant selected by the NATABOC. Students who have begun their last semester or quarter of college are eligible to take the certification examination before graduation, provided the other core and section requirements have been fulfilled at the time of application. Verification of intent to graduate must be provided to the Board of Certification by the dean or department chairperson of the college or university the applicant is attending. Certification will not be issued until an official transcript indicating date of degree is received by the Board of Certification.
3. Proof of current American National Red Cross Standard First Aid Certification and current Basic CPR (American Red Cross or American Heart Association); EMT equivalent instead of First Aid and CPR will be accepted. Both cards must be current at the time of application.
4. At the time of application, all candidates for certification (curriculum and internship) must verify that at least 25% of their athletic training experience hours credited in fulfilling the certification requirements were attained in actual (on location) practice or game coverage with one or more of the following sports: football, soccer, hockey, wrestling, basketball, gymnastics, lacrosse, volleyball, and rugby.
5. Endorsement of certification application by a NATA-certified athletic trainer.
6. Subsequent passing of the certification examination (written, oral-practical, and written-simulation sections).

Section requirements

CAAHEP accredited program

The candidate must graduate from an undergraduate or graduate program accredited by the Commission on Accreditation of Allied Health Education Programs (CAAHEP). Students applying to take the certification exam must complete formal instruction in the following core curriculum subject areas:

Human anatomy
Human physiology
Psychology
Kinesiology/biomechanics
Exercise physiology
Prevention of athletic injuries/illness
Evaluation of athletic injuries/illness
First aid and emergency care
Therapeutic modalities
Therapeutic exercise
Personal community health
Nutrition
Administration of athletic training programs

It is recommended that students complete coursework in physics, chemistry, pharmacology, research design, and statistics. In addition, students are required to complete a minimum of 800 clinical hours under the direct supervision of a NATA-certified athletic trainer at that college or an affiliated site. Applicants who are applying for NATA certification from a CAAHEP-accredited undergraduate or graduate program must receive their degree from that college or university.

Continued

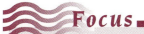*Focus*

State Regulation of the Athletic Trainer

During the mid-1970s the membership of NATA realized the necessity of obtaining some type of official recognition by other medical allied health organizations of the athletic trainer as a health care professional. Laws and statutes specifically governing the practice of athletic training were nonexistent in virtually every state.

State regulation: certification, registration, licensing, exemption.

Based on this perceived need, the athletic trainers in many individual states organized their efforts to secure recognition by seeking some type of regulation of the athletic trainer by state licensing agencies. To date, this ongoing effort has resulted in 36 of the 50 states enacting some type of regulatory statutes governing the practice of athletic training.[24]

Rules and regulations governing the practice of athletic training vary tremendously from state to state. Regulation may be in the form of certification, registration, licensure, or exemption. (See the following Focus box.) Certification indicates that a person possesses basic knowledge and skills that are required in the profession. Both individual states and national organizations can certify individuals. Registration means that before an individual can practice athletic training he or she must register in that state. There may or may not be any mechanism for assessing competency. Licensing limits the practice of athletic training to those who have met minimal requirements of a licensing board and is the most restrictive of all the forms of regulation. Certain states have exempted athletic trainers from complying with the practice acts of other professions, although they still may be required to meet certification standards.

For the most part, legislation regulating the practice of athletic training has been positive and to some extent protects the athletic trainer from litigation. However, in some instances, legislation has restricted the limits of practice for the athletic trainer. The leadership of NATA has strongly encouraged athletic trainers in all states to seek some form of state regulation.

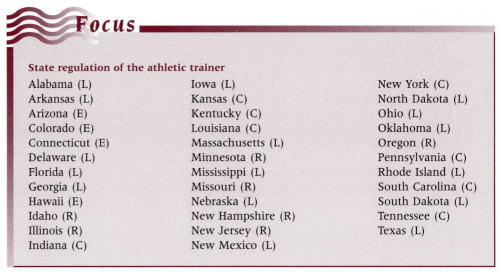

State regulation of the athletic trainer

Alabama (L)	Iowa (L)	New York (C)
Arkansas (L)	Kansas (C)	North Dakota (L)
Arizona (E)	Kentucky (C)	Ohio (L)
Colorado (E)	Louisiana (C)	Oklahoma (L)
Connecticut (E)	Massachusetts (L)	Oregon (R)
Delaware (L)	Minnesota (R)	Pennsylvania (C)
Florida (L)	Mississippi (L)	Rhode Island (L)
Georgia (L)	Missouri (R)	South Carolina (C)
Hawaii (E)	Nebraska (L)	South Dakota (L)
Idaho (R)	New Hampshire (R)	Tennessee (C)
Illinois (R)	New Jersey (R)	Texas (L)
Indiana (C)	New Mexico (L)	

E, Exempt from existing licensure standards; C, certification; R, registration; L, licensure.

The Physical Therapist and Athletic Trainer

As the certified athletic trainer continues to gain recognition among the health care professions, interest on the part of many individuals with backgrounds in other health-related professions likewise continues to increase. In particular, it is not unusual to find a physical therapist interested in sports and athletics who is working toward certification as an athletic trainer.[16] Conversely, the certified trainer who is interested in working with patients outside of the athletic population is often looking toward licensure as a physical therapist.

Historically, the relationship between athletic trainers and physical therapists has been less than cooperative. Many reasons underlie this lack of cooperation, and they all too often result from misunderstanding. Recently, efforts of a joint task force composed of members from NATA and the American Physical Therapy Association (APTA) failed in their attempt to formulate a proposal to clarify the roles of each group in injury rehabilitation.

Athletic trainers have been trained to deal specifically with those injuries that occur in sports, whereas physical therapists have a much broader expertise in injury rehabilitation across many different patient populations. The physical therapist who has not been exposed to the athletic training environment is as inefficient in that setting as the athletic trainer who might want to work with stroke patients in a rehabilitation setting.

The academic curricula required for the athletic trainer and for the physical therapist are similar, particularly in the basic sciences and in the clinical methods courses. Without question the physical therapy curriculum provides a significantly broader background in treating patients of all ages who have a wide variety of physical problems. However, it is essential that the physical therapist receive additional clinical instruction in an athletic training environment above and beyond that which is typically offered in a physical therapy curriculum. Otherwise the period of adjustment and orientation to a nontraditional physical therapy setting is often difficult.

The individual who achieves both certification as an athletic trainer and licensure as a physical therapist is extremely well qualified to function in various sports medicine settings, including both the private clinic and the colleges and universities. Today, the person who holds a dual credential is in high demand in the job market.

Certification as a sports physical therapist   In the late 1970s the sports physical therapy section of the American Physical Therapy Association began identifying competencies specific to the practice of physical therapy in a sports medicine setting. In

1985 the Professional Examination Service was contracted by APTA to develop a specialty examination based on specifically identified competencies.[21]

Candidates for the examination must fulfill the minimal criteria as outlined in the document *Minimal Criteria for Therapist to Sit for the Initial Certification Examination*. This includes the completion of a required number of hours of clinical practice in patient care, education, and administration. In addition, written evidence of competency in these areas and research must be submitted.

FUTURE DIRECTIONS FOR THE ATHLETIC TRAINER

The athletic training profession has made remarkable gains during the past two decades. Today, certified athletic trainers possess a strong, highly structured academic background in addition to a substantial amount of closely supervised clinical experience in their chosen area of expertise. The athletic trainer continues to gain credibility and recognition as a health care professional trained to deal with injuries that occur in sports.

As with any profession, the future directions for athletic training will be determined by the efforts of NATA and its membership. Athletic trainers must continue to enhance their visibility through research efforts and scholarly publication[13,15,33] and by making themselves available for local and community meetings to discuss the health care of the athlete. They must continue to provide and refine quality educational programs for student athletic trainers. Most important, the athletic trainer must continue efforts in injury prevention and provide appropriate, high-quality health care to athletes who are injured while participating in a sport.

SUMMARY

- Athletic training is a specialization within sports medicine, with its major concern being the health and safety of athletes. The primary athletic training team consists of the coach, the athletic trainer, and the team physician. The coach must ensure that the environment and the equipment that is worn are the safest possible, that all injuries and illnesses are properly cared for, that skills are properly taught, and that conditioning is at the highest level.
- The athletic trainer must be a highly educated, well-trained professional. The athletic trainer must be certified and, if possible, have a state license to practice. The successful athletic trainer loves sports and the competitive environment. He or she must have an abundance of vitality and emotional stability and empathy for people who are in physical or emotional pain, as well as a sense of humor, the ability to communicate, and a desire to learn. All of the athletic trainer's actions must follow the highest standards of conduct.
- The team physician can be in varied specializations. Team physicians, depending on the time they are committed to a specific sports program, can perform a variety of responsibilities. Some key responsibilities are performing the preparticipation health examination, diagnosing and treating illnesses and injuries, advising and teaching the athletic training staff, attending games, scrimmages, and practices, and counseling the athlete about health matters.

....

█ *Solutions to Critical Thinking* Exercises

1-1 Students of athletic training must be "sponges" who are willing to soak up whatever knowledge they can attain to make themselves more efficient in performing their chosen profession. That knowledge may come from the classroom, reading books or

journals, attending lectures and conferences, and actively learning the "tricks of the trade" during the hours spent in the training room and on the field. Students must be able to apply theoretical knowledge to a practical setting if they are to be competent clinicians.

1-2 Ultimately the team physician is responsible for making that decision. However, that decision must be made based on collective input from the athletic trainer, the coach, and the athlete. Remember that everyone in the sports medicine team has the same ultimate goal, that being to return the athlete to full competitive levels as quickly and safely as possible.

1-3 To help prevent injury the athletic trainer should (1) arrange for physical examinations and preparticipation screenings to identify conditions that predispose an athlete to injury, (2) ensure appropriate training and conditioning of the athlete, (3) monitor environmental conditions to ensure safe participation, (4) select and maintain properly fitting protective equipment, and (5) educate parents, coaches, and athletes about the risks inherent to sport participation.

1-4 To some extent, the role of the clinical athletic trainer is dictated by the type of regulation of the practice of athletic training in a particular state. Certainly the clinical and academic preparation of athletic trainers should enable them to effectively evaluate an injured patient and guide that patient through a rehabilitative program. The athletic trainer should treat only those individuals who have sustained injury related to physical activity and not patients with neurological or orthopedic conditions. The athletic trainer may work part time in the clinic and then cover one or several high schools around the area. The athletic trainer and physical therapist should work as a team to maximize the effectiveness of patient care.

1-5 To be eligible for certification through the internship route, the student must complete 1500 hours of directly supervised clinical experience and course work in each of seven areas. It is possible to complete this in 2 years, although realistically it will be difficult. It is likely that at this point, an additional year may be necessary to complete the requirements. An alternative would be to transfer to an institution that offers an entry level CAAHEP-approved program in which the student must complete course work covering 14 subject matter areas and 800 hours of directly supervised clinical experience.

REVIEW QUESTIONS AND CLASS ACTIVITIES

1. How do modern athletic training and sports medicine compare with early Greek and Roman approaches for the care of the athlete?
2. What professional organizations are important to the field of athletic training?
3. Why is athletic training considered a team endeavor? Contrast the coach's, athletic trainer's, and team physician's roles in athletic training.
4. What qualifications should the athletic trainer have in terms of education, certification, and personality?
5. What are the various employment opportunities available to the athletic trainer?
6. Explain the criteria for becoming certified as an athletic trainer.

REFERENCES

1. American College of Sports Medicine: 1987 annual meeting, Las Vegas, Nev, May 27-30, 1987.
2. Bilik SE: *The trainer's bible,* New York, 1956, Reed (originally published 1917).
3. Campbell D, Miller M, Robinson W: The prevalance of burnout among athletic trainers, *Ath Train* 20(2):110, 1985.
4. Capel S: Attrition of athletic trainers, *Ath Train* 25(1):34, 1990.
5. Capel S: Psychological and organizational factors related to burnout in athletic trainers, *Ath Train* 21(4):322, 1986.
6. Committee on Allied Health Education and Accreditation: *Essentials and guidelines for an accreditated educational program for athletic trainers,* Chicago, 1992, American Medical Association.
7. Cramer C: A preferred sequence of competencies for athletic training education programs, *Ath Train* 25(2):123, 1990.
8. Furney SR, Patton B: An examination of health counseling practices of athletic trainers, *Ath Train* 21(4):294, 1985.
9. Gaunya ST: The role of the trainer. In Vinger PF, Hoerner EF, editors: *Sports injuries: the unthwarted epidemic,* Boston, 1982, John Wright, PSG.
10. Geick J: The burnout syndrome among athletic trainers, *Ath Train* 17(1):36, 1982.
11. Geick J: Athletic training burnout: a case study, *Ath Train* 21(1):43, 1986.
12. Hossler P: How to acquire athletic trainers on the high school level, *Ath Train* 20(3):199, 1985.
13. Kegerreis S: Professional advancement of athletic training via documentation and publication, *Ath Train* 15(1):47, 1980.
14. Knight K: Athletic trainers for secondary schools, *Ath Train* 23(4):313, 1988.
15. Knight K: Research in athletic training: a frill or a necessity, *Ath Train* 23(3):212, 1988.
16. Knight K: Roles and relationships between sports PTs and ATCs, *Ath Train* 23(2):153, 1988.
17. Lephart S, Metz K: Financial and appointment trends of the athletic trainer clinician/educator, *Ath Train* 25(2):118, 1990.
18. Lester RA: The coach as codefendant: football in the 1980s. In Appenzeller H, editor: *Sports and law: contemporary issues,* Charlottesville, Va, 1985, Michie.
19. Loeffler RD: On being a team physician, *Sports Med Dig* 9(2):1, 1987.
20. Lombardo JA: Sports medicine: a team effort, *Phys Sportsmed* 13(2):72, 1985.
21. Malone T: Sports physical therapy specialization, *J Orthop Sports Phys Ther* 7(5):273, 1986.
22. Mangus BC, Ingersoll CD: Approaches to ethical decision making in athletic training, *Ath Train* 25(4):340, 1990.
23. Mellion, MB, Walsh WM: The team physician. In Mellion MB, Walsh WM, editors: *The team physician's handbook,* Philadelphia, 1990, Hanley & Belfus.
24. National Athletic Trainers Association Governmental Affairs Committee: Personal communication, July 1995.
25. National Athletic Trainers Association: New NATA code of ethics approved, *NATA News* 4(7):15, 1992.
26. National Athletic Trainers Association Board of Certification, Inc., Continuing Education Office: *Continuing education file 1994-96,* Dallas, 1994, NATABOC.
27. National Athletic Trainers Association Board of Certification, Inc.: Role delineation matrix, *Certification Update* Fall (3):6, 1994.
28. National Athletic Trainers Association Board of Certification, Inc.: *Role delineation study of the entry level athletic trainer certification examination,* Philadelphia, 1994, Davis.
29. National Athletic Trainers Association Board of Certification, Inc.: *Role delineation study,* Raleigh, NC, 1995, Columbia Assessment Services.
30. National Athletic Trainers Association Board of Certification, Inc.: *Study guide for the NATABOC entry level athletic trainer certification examination,* Philadelphia, 1993, Davis.
31. National Athletic Trainers Association Professional Education Committee: *Competencies in athletic training,* Dallas, 1992, National Athletic Trainers Association.
32. O'Shea M: *A history of the National Athletic Trainers Association,* Greenville, NC, 1980, National Athletic Trainers Association.
33. Osternig L: Research in athletic training: the missing ingredient, *Ath Train* 23(3):323, 1988.

34. Prentice W, Mischler B: A national survey of employment opportunities for athletic trainers in the public schools, *Ath Train* 21(3):215, 1986.

35. Prentice W: The athletic trainer. In Mueller F, Ryan A, editors: *Prevention of athletic injuries: the role of the sports medicine team*, Philadelphia, 1991, Davis.

36. Rich BS: All physicians are not created equal: understanding the educational background of the sports medicine physician, *J Ath Train* 28(2):177, 1993.

37. Schneiderer L: A survey of appointing and utilizing intercollegiate athletic team physicians, *Ath Train* 22(3):211, 1987.

38. Snook GA: The history of sports medicine, part 1, *Am J Sports Med* 12(3):252, 1984.

ANNOTATED BIBLIOGRAPHY

Bilik SE: *The trainer's bible*, ed 9, New York, 1956, Reed.

A classic book, first published in 1917, by a major pioneer in athletic training and sports medicine.

National Athletic Trainers Association Board of Certification, Inc.: *Role delineation study of the entry level athletic trainer certification examination*, Philadelphia, 1994, Davis.

Contains a complete discussion of the 1993 role delineation study that redefined the responsibilities of the athletic trainer.

National Athletic Trainers Association, Inc.: *Code of ethics 1993* National Athletics Trainers Association.

Contains a revision of the previous code of ethics of 1983. Includes ethical principles, membership standards, and certification standards.

O'Shea ME: *A history of the National Athletic Trainers Association*, Greenville, NC, 1980, National Athletic Trainers Association.

An interesting text about the history of NATA that any student interested in athletic training as a career should read.

Organizational and Administrative Considerations

When you finish this chapter, you should be able to

- Describe a functional, well-designed athletic training facility.
- Identify policies and procedures that should be enforced in the athletic training room.
- Explain budgetary concerns for ordering supplies and equipment.
- Explain the importance of the preparticipation physical examination.
- Identify the necessary records that must be maintained by the athletic trainer.
- Describe current systems for gathering data on injuries.
- Identify the essential insurance requirements for protection of the athlete.
- Explain legal considerations for the athletic trainer.

Operating an effective athletic training program requires careful organization and administration regardless of whether the setting is in a high school, college, or university, at the professional level, or in a clinical or industrial setting. Besides being a clinical practitioner, the athletic trainer must be an administrator who performs both managerial and supervisory duties. This chapter looks at the administrative tasks required of the athletic trainer for successful operation of the program, including facility design, policies and procedures, budget considerations, administration of physical examinations, record keeping, insurance requirements, and legal considerations.

FACILITIES

The maximum use of facilities and the most effective use of equipment and supplies are essential to any sports program. The athletic training facility must be specially designed to meet the many requirements of the sports athletic training program (Figure 2-1). The size and the layout of the athletic training facility depends on the scope of the athletic training program, including the size and number of teams and athletes and what sports are offered. In the clinical setting there is a much broader patient population and thus the requirements for equipment and supplies will be somewhat different. To accommodate the various functions of an athletic training program, it must serve as a health care center for athletes.[11]

Size and Construction

An athletic training area of less than 1000 square feet is impractical. An athletic training facility 1000 to 1200 square feet in size is satisfactory for most schools. The 1200 square foot area (40 by 30 feet) permits the handling of a sizable number of athletes at one time and allows ample room for the bulky equipment needed. A facility of this size is well suited for pregame preparation. Careful planning will determine whether a larger area is needed or desirable.

Windows are to some extent desirable in a training room facility. However, most contemporary training rooms must rely on artificial lighting and air-conditioned ventilation systems. The walls and ceiling should be of drywall, plaster, or concrete block construction and should be painted in a light color with a washable paint.

The floor should be of smooth-finished concrete or terrazzo with a nonslip texture. Cleats are sometimes worn in the facility, and a wooden floor may in time splin-

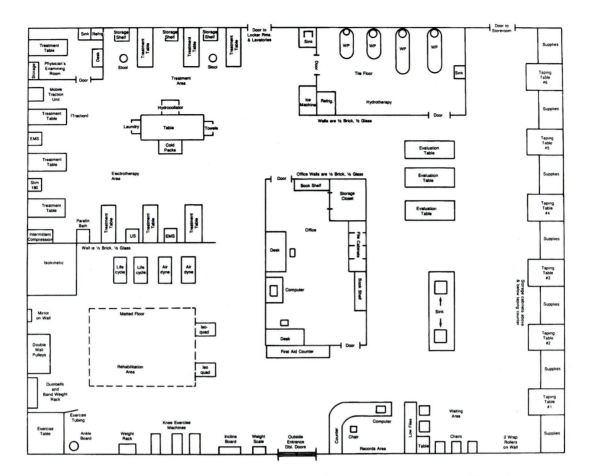

Figure 2-1

The ideal training room facility should be well designed to maximize its use.

ter and warp. Vinyl tile, although somewhat expensive, has been used as a floor covering with considerable success. The floors should be graded to slope toward strategically placed drain outlets.

Location

The athletic training facility should be located immediately adjacent to the dressing quarters of the athletes and should have three entrances: an outside entrance from the sports field and two inside entrances leading from the men's and women's locker rooms. This arrangement makes it unnecessary to bring injured athletes in through the building and possibly through several doors; it also permits access when the rest of the building is not in use. Entrance doorways should be at least 44 inches wide; a double door at each entrance is preferable to allow easy passage of a wheelchair or a stretcher. A ramp at the outside entrance is safer and far more functional than are stairs. If an outside entrance is present, provisions should be made to protect against drafts, particularly during cold or inclement weather.

Toilet facilities should be located adjacent to the athletic training room and should be readily accessible through a door in the training room. The athletic training room should be located close to the shower rooms so that showers are readily available to dirt- or mud-covered athletes coming in for treatment.

Because the athletic training facility is the place where emergency treatment is given, its light, heat, and water sources should be independent from those for the rest of the building.

Illumination

The athletic training facility should be well lighted throughout. Artificial lighting should be planned with the advice of a technical lighting engineer. The standard level

2-1

Critical Thinking Exercise

The members of the school board at All-American High School voted to allocate $25,000 dollars to renovate a 25' × 40' storage space and to purchase new equipment for an athletic training room. The athletic trainer has been asked to provide the school principle with a "wish list" of what should be included in this facility. It has been estimated that the physical renovation will cost approximately $17,000.

? How may this space be best used and what type of equipment should be purchased to maximize the effectiveness of this new facility?

The training facility is a multi-purpose area used for first aid, therapy and exercise rehabilitation, injury prevention, medical procedures such as the physical examination, and athletic training administration.

of illumination recommended for athletic training facilities is 30 foot-candles at the height of 4 feet above the floor. Ceilings and walls acting as reflective surfaces aid in achieving an equable distribution and balance of light.

Light fixtures may be of several types. Because an even, nonglaring light is desired, a fixture that illuminates indirectly by casting direct light on the ceiling, from which it is reflected down and outward, is excellent. Fluorescent lights, when used with a diffuser, also provide a good source of light. Diffusers eliminate the flickering that is often an objectionable feature.

Special Service Sections

Apart from the storage and office space, a portion of the athletic training room should be divided into special sections, preferably by low walls or partial glass walls. It should be noted, however, that space may not permit a separate area for each service section, and an overlapping of functions may be required.

Treatment Area

The treatment area should include four to six treatment tables, preferably of adjustable height, which can be used during the application of ice packs or hydrocollator packs or for manual therapy techniques such as massage, mobilization, or proprioceptive neuromuscular facilitation (PNF). Three or four adjustable stools on rollers should also be readily available. The hydrocollator unit and ice bags should be easily accessible to this area.

Electrotherapy Area

The electrotherapy area should constitute approximately 20% of the total special service area and is used for treatment by ultrasound, diathermy, or electrical stimulating units. Equipment should include at least two treatment tables, several wooden chairs, one or two dispensing tables for holding supplies, shelves, and a storage cabinet for supplies and equipment. The area should contain a sufficient number of grounded outlets, preferably in the walls and several feet above the floor. It is advisable to place rubber mats or runners on each side of the treatment tables as a precautionary measure. This area must be under supervision at all times, and the storage cabinet should be kept locked when not in use.

Hydrotherapy Area

The hydrotherapy area should constitute approximately 15% of the total special service area. The floor should slope toward a centrally located drain to prevent water from standing. Equipment should include two or three whirlpool baths (one permitting complete immersion of the body), several lavatories, and storage shelves. Because some of this equipment is electrically operated, considerable precaution must be observed. All electrical outlets should be placed 4 to 5 feet above the floor and should have spring-locked covers and water spray deflectors. All cords and wires must be kept clear of the floor to eliminate any possibility of electrical shock. To prevent water from entering the other areas, a slightly raised, rounded curb should be built at the entrance to the area. When an athletic training room is planned, ample outlets must be provided—under no circumstances should two or more devices be operated from the same outlet. All outlets must be properly grounded using ground fault interruptors (GFI).

Exercise Rehabilitation Area

Ideally, an athletic training facility should accommodate injury reconditioning under the strict supervision of the athletic trainer. Selected pieces of resistance equipment should be made available. Depending on the existing space, dumbbells and free weights, exercise machines for knee, ankle, shoulder, hip, and so forth, isokinetic equipment, devices for balance and proprioception, and space for using surgical tubing may all be available for use.

Taping, Bandaging, and Orthotics Area

Each athletic training room should provide a place where taping, bandaging, and applying orthotic devices can be executed. This area should have three or four taping tables adjacent to a sink and a storage cabinet.

Physician's Examination Room

In colleges and universities the team physician has a special room. In this facility examinations and treatments may be given. This room contains an examining table, sink, locking storage cabinets, refrigerator, and small desk with a telephone. At all times, this facility must be kept locked to outsiders.

Records Area

There should be some space either in the office or at the entrance to the training room that is devoted to record keeping. This may range from a filing system to a more sophisticated computer-based system. Records should be accessible to sports medicine personnel only.

Storage Facilities

Many athletic training facilities lack ample storage space. Often storage facilities are located a considerable distance away, which is extremely inconvenient. In addition to the storage cabinets and shelves provided in each of the three special service areas, a small storage closet should be placed in the athletic trainer's office. All of these cabinets should be used for the storage of general supplies, as well as for the small specialized equipment used in the respective areas. A large walk-in closet, 80 to 100 square feet in area, is a necessity for the storage of bulky equipment, medical supplies, adhesive tape, bandages, and protective devices (Figure 2-2). A refrigerator for the storage of frozen water in styrofoam cups for ice massage and other necessities is also an important piece of equipment. Many athletic trainers prefer to place the refrigerator in their office, where it is readily accessible but still under close supervision. In small sports programs, a large refrigerator will probably be sufficient for all ice needs. If at all possible, an ice-making machine should be installed in an auxiliary area to provide an ample and continuous supply of ice for treatment purposes.

> It is essential to have adequate storage space available for supplies and equipment.

Athletic Trainer's Office

A space at least 10 feet by 12 feet is ample for the athletic trainer's office. It should be located so that all areas of the training room can be well supervised without the athletic trainer's having to leave the office. Glass partitions on two sides permit the athletic trainer, even while seated at the desk, to observe all activities. A desk, chair, tack board for clippings and other information, telephones, and a record file are the basic equipment. In some cases a computer is also housed in this office.

Figure 2-2

An effective athletic training program must have appropriate storage facilities that are highly organized.

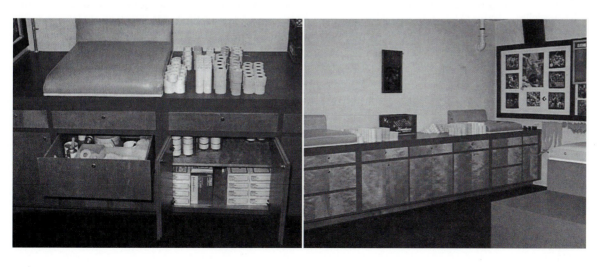

Because of the nature and character of the athletic training room and of the equipment and supplies within, this room should have an independent lock-and-key system so that it is accessible only to authorized personnel.

Additional Areas

If space is available there are several other areas that could potentially be included as part of a training room facility.

Pharmacy Area

A separate room that can be secured for storing and dispensing medications is helpful. All medications, including over-the-counter drugs, should be kept under lock and key. If prescription medications are kept in the training room, only the team physician or pharmacist from a campus health center should have access to the storage cabinet. Records for administering medications to athletes should be kept in this area.

Rehabilitation Pool

It is rare that a pool is located in the training room; however, if the facility has the space and can afford one, it can be an extremely useful rehabilitation tool. The pool should be accessible to individuals with various types of injuries. It should have a graduated depth to at least 7 feet, the deck should have a nonslip surface, and the filter system should be in a separate room.[24]

X-Ray Room

A separate room for x-ray equipment must have lead shielding in the walls. The x-ray room must be large enough to house all the necessary equipment (x-ray unit, processing unit, etc.).

PROGRAM OPERATIONS

It is imperative that every athletic training program develop policies and procedures that carefully delineate the daily routine of the program. This is especially true for handling health problems and injuries.

Who Should Be Served?

A major factor in any athletic training program is the establishment of limits as to who is to be served by the athletic training staff. The individual athlete, the institution, and the community are considered.

The Athlete

The athletic trainer must decide the extent to which the athlete will be served. For example, will prevention and care activities be extended to athletes for the entire year, including summer and other vacations, or only during the competitive season? Also, the athletic trainer must decide what care will be rendered. Will it extend to all systemic illnesses or to just musculoskeletal problems?

The Institution

A policy must be established as to who will be served by the athletic training program. Often legal concerns and the school liability insurance dictate who, other than the athlete, is to be served. A policy should make it clear whether students other than athletes, athletes from other schools, faculty, and staff are to receive care. If so, how are they to be referred and medically directed? Also, it must be decided whether the athletic training program will act as a clinical setting for student athletic trainers.

The Community

A decision must be made as to which, if any, outside group or person in the community will be served by the athletic training staff. Again, legality and the institution's

> Every athletic training program must develop policies and procedures that carefully delineate the daily routine of the program.

insurance program must be taken into consideration. If a policy is not delineated in this matter, outside persons may abuse the services of the athletic training facilities and staff.

Clinical and Industrial Setting Considerations

The athletic trainer working in the clinical or industrial setting will likely be working with patients other than high school or college athletes. The scope of practice within an individual clinic may include pediatric, work hardening, orthopedic, or even occasionally neurological patients. Athletic trainers in the clinical setting should be assigned to work only with patient populations that may generally be classified as "physically active." Clinical administrators should not require athletic trainers to treat other patient populations because there has been no formal education or training geared toward those patient problems.

Athletic trainers in the industrial setting, in addition to overseeing preventative and rehabilitation programs, are frequently asked to take on responsibility for employee fitness programs. Therefore a more advanced understanding of the principles of training and conditioning will be necessary. (See Chapter 3.)

Providing Coverage

Facility Personnel Coverage

A major concern of any athletic department is that there is proper personnel coverage provided for the athletic training facility and specific sports. Depending on whether a school has a full-time athletic training staff, an athletic training facility may operate from 7 AM to 10 PM. Mornings are commonly reserved for treatments and exercise rehabilitation; early afternoons are for treatment, exercise rehabilitation, and preparation for practice or a contest; and late afternoons and early evenings are spent in injury management. High schools with limited available supervision may be able to provide athletic training facility coverage only in the afternoons and during vacation periods.

Sports Coverage

Ideally, all sports should have a certified or at least a student athletic trainer in attendance at all practices and contests, both at home and away. Ideally, high-risk sports should have a certified athletic trainer and physician present at all practices and contests.

Hygiene and Sanitation

The practice of good hygiene and sanitation is of the utmost importance in an athletic training program. The prevention of infectious diseases is a direct responsibility of the athletic trainer, whose duty it is to see that all athletes are surrounded by as hygienic an environment as is possible and that each individual is practicing sound health habits. Chapter 9 discusses the management of bloodborne pathogens. The athletic trainer must be aware of and adhere to guidelines for the operation of an athletic care facility as dictated by the Occupational Safety and Health Administration (OSHA).

Good hygiene and sanitation are essential for an athletic training program.

The Athletic Training Facility

The athletic training room should be used only for the prevention and care of sports injuries. Too often the athletic training facility becomes a meeting or club room for the coaches and athletes. Unless definite rules are established and practiced, room cleanliness and sanitation become an impossible chore. Unsanitary practices or conditions must not be tolerated. The following are some important athletic training room policies:

1. No cleated shoes are allowed. Dirt and debris tend to cling to cleated shoes; therefore cleated shoes should be removed before athletes enter the athletic training facility.

2. Game equipment is kept outside. Because game equipment such as balls and bats adds to the sanitation problem, it should be kept out of the athletic training room. Coaches and athletes must be continually reminded that the athletic training room is not a storage room for sports equipment.

3. Shoes must be kept off treatment tables. Because of the tendency of shoes to contaminate treatment tables, they must be removed before any care is given to the athlete.

4. Athletes should shower before receiving treatment. The athlete should make it a habit to shower before being treated if the treatment is not an emergency. This procedure helps keep tables and therapeutic modalities sanitary.

5. Roughhousing and profanity should not be allowed. Athletes must be continually reminded that the athletic training facility is for injury care and prevention. Horseplay and foul language lower the basic purpose of the athletic training room.

6. No food or smokeless tobacco should be allowed.

General cleanliness of the athletic training room cannot be stressed enough. Through the athletic trainer's example, the athlete may develop an appreciation for cleanliness and in turn develop wholesome personal health habits. Cleaning responsibilities in most schools are divided between the athletic training staff and the maintenance crew. Care of permanent building structures and trash disposal are usually the responsibilities of maintenance, whereas upkeep of specialized equipment falls within the province of the training staff.

Division of routine cleaning responsibilities may be organized as follows:

1. Maintenance crew
   a. Sweep floors daily.
   b. Clean and disinfect sinks and built-in tubs daily.
   c. Mop and disinfect hydrotherapy area twice a week.
   d. Refill paper towel and drinking cup dispensers as needed.
   e. Empty wastebaskets and dispose of trash daily.
2. Athletic training staff
   a. Clean and disinfect treatment table daily.
   b. Clean and disinfect hydrotherapy modalities daily.
   c. Clean and polish other therapeutic modalities weekly.

The Gymnasium

Maintaining sanitation in sports is a continual battle in the athletic training environment. Practices such as passing a common towel to wipe off perspiration, using common water dispensers, or failing to change dirty clothing for clean are prevalent violations of sanitation in sports. The following is a suggested health practice checklist that may be used by the coach and the athletic trainer:

1. Facilities sanitation
   a. Are the gymnasium floors swept daily?
   b. Are drinking fountains, showers, sinks, urinals, and toilets cleaned and disinfected daily?
   c. Are lockers aired and sanitized frequently?
   d. Are mats cleaned routinely (wrestling mats and wall mats cleaned daily)?
2. Equipment and clothing issuance
   a. Are equipment and clothing fitted to the athlete to avoid skin irritations?
   b. Is swapping of equipment and clothes prevented?
   c. Is clothing laundered and changed frequently?
   d. Is wet clothing allowed to dry thoroughly before the athlete wears it again?
   e. Is individual attention given to proper shoe fit and upkeep?
   f. Is protective clothing provided during inclement weather or when the athlete is waiting on the sidelines?
   g. Are clean, dry towels provided each day for each individual athlete?

Emergency Phone

The installation of an emergency phone adjacent to all major activity areas is also desirable. It should be possible to use this phone to call outside for emergency aid and to contact the athletic training facilities when additional assistance is required. Two-way radios or preferably cellular telephones provide flexibility in the communication system and should be bought if the budget permits.

The Athlete

To promote good health among the athletes, the coach or the athletic trainer should encourage sound health habits. The following checklist may be a useful guide for coaches, athletic trainers, and athletes:

1. Are the athletes medically cleared to participate?
2. Is each athlete insured?
3. Does the athlete promptly report injuries, illnesses, and skin disorders to the coach or the athletic trainer?
4. Are good daily living habits of resting, sleeping, and proper nutrition practiced?
5. Do the athletes shower after practice?
6. Do they dry thoroughly and cool off before departing from the gymnasium?
7. Do they avoid drinking from a common water dispenser?
8. Do they avoid using a common towel?
9. Do they avoid exchanging gym clothes with teammates?
10. Do they practice good foot hygiene?
11. Do they avoid contact with teammates who have a contagious disease or infection?

Budgetary Concerns

One of the major problems faced by athletic trainers is to obtain a budget of sufficient size to permit them to perform a creditable job of athletic training. Most high schools fail to make any budgetary provisions for athletic training except for the purchase of tape, ankle wraps, and a training bag that contains a minimum amount of equipment. Many fail to provide a room and any of the special facilities that are needed to establish an effective athletic training program. Some school boards and administrators fail to recognize that the functions performed in the athletic training facility are an essential component of the athletic program and that even if no specialist is used, the facilities are nonetheless necessary. Colleges and universities are not usually faced with this problem to the extent of high schools. By and large, athletic training is recognized as an important aspect of the athletic program.

A major problem often facing athletic trainers is a budget of sufficient size.

Budgetary needs vary considerably within programs; some require only a few thousand dollars, whereas others spend hundreds of thousands of dollars. The amount spent on building and equipping a training facility, of course, is entirely a matter of local option. In purchasing equipment, immediate needs and availability of personnel to operate specialized equipment should be kept in mind.

Budget records should be kept on file so that they are available for use in projecting the following year's budgetary needs. They present a picture of the distribution of current funds and serve to substantiate future budgetary requests.

Expenditures for individual items vary in accordance with different training philosophies. Some athletic trainers may spend much of their budget on expendable supplies such as adhesive tape. An annual inventory must be conducted at the end of the year or before the ordering of supplies and equipment takes place. Accurate records must be kept to justify future requests.

Supplies

Supplies are expendable and usually are for injury prevention, first aid, and management. Examples of supplies are athletic training tape, germicides, and massage lubricants.

Equipment

The term *equipment* refers to items that are not expendable. Equipment may be further divided into fixed and nonfixed. Fixed equipment does not necessarily mean that it cannot be moved but that it is not usually removed from the athletic training facility. Examples of fixed equipment are icemakers, isokinetic exercise devices, and electrical therapeutic modalities. Nonfixed equipment refers to nonexpendable items that are less fixed, that may be part of an athletic trainer's kit, or that may be at the site where a sport is being held. Examples are blankets, scissors, and training kits.

Purchasing Systems

Purchasing of supplies and equipment must be done through either direct buy or competitive bid. For expensive purchases an institutional purchasing agent is sent out to competing vendors who quote a price on specified supplies or equipment. Orders are generally placed with the lowest bidder. Smaller purchases or emergency purchases may be made directly from one single vendor.[23]

An alternative to purchasing expensive equipment is to arrange for a lease. Many manufacturers and distributors are now willing to lease equipment on a monthly or yearly basis. Over the long run, purchasing equipment will be less costly. However, in the short term, if a large capital expenditure is not possible a leasing agreement should be considered.[24]

Additional Budget Considerations

In addition to supplies and equipment, the athletic trainer must also consider other costs that may be included in the operation of an athletic training program; these include telephone and postage, contracts with physicians or clinics for services, professional liability insurance, memberships in professional organizations, the purchase of professional journals or textbooks, travel and expenses for attending professional meetings, and clothing to be worn in the training room.[24,25]

RECORD KEEPING

Record keeping is a major responsibility of the athletic training program. Some athletic trainers object to keeping records and filling out forms, stating that they have neither the time nor the inclination to be bookkeepers. Nevertheless in a time when lawsuits are the rule rather than the exception, accurate and up-to-date records are an absolute necessity. Medical records, injury reports, treatment logs, personal information cards, injury evaluations and progress notes, supply and equipment inventories, and annual reports are essential records that should be maintained by the athletic trainer.

Administering Preparticipation Health Examinations

The primary purpose of the preseason health examination is to identify if an athlete is at risk before he or she participates in a specific sport.[15] The preparticipation examination should consist of a medical history, a physical examination, and a brief orthopedic screening. Information obtained during this examination will establish a baseline to which comparisons may be made after injury. It may also reveal conditions that could warrant disqualification from certain sports. The examination will also satisfy insurance and liability issues.

The preparticipation physical may be administered on an individual basis by a personal physician, or it may be done using a station examination system with a team of examiners.[4]

Medical History

A medical history form should be completed before the physical examination and orthopedic screening; its purpose is to identify any past or existing medical problems.[1] This form should be updated for each athlete every year. Medical histories should be closely reviewed by both the physician and the athletic trainer so that they may be prepared should some medical emergency arise. Necessary participation release forms and insurance information should be collected along with the medical history[16] (Figure 2-3).

Physical Examination

The physical examination should include assessment of height, weight, body composition, blood pressure, pulse, vision, skin, dental, ear, nose, throat, heart and lung function, abdomen, lymphatics, genitalia, maturation index, urinalysis, and blood work[17] (Figure 2-4).

Maturity Assessment

Maturity assessment should be part of the physical examination as a means of protecting the young athlete.[5] The most commonly used methods are the circumpubertal (sexual maturity), skeletal, and dental assessments. Of the three, Tanner's five stages of assessment, indicating maturity of secondary sexual characteristics, is the most expedient for use in the station method of examination. The Tanner approach evaluates pubic hair and genitalia development in boys and pubic hair and breast development in girls. Other indicators that may be noted are facial and axillary hair. Stage one indicates that puberty is not evident, and stage five indicates full development. The crucial stage in terms of collision and high-intensity noncontact sports is stage three, in which there is the fastest bone growth. In this stage, the growth plates are two to five times weaker than the joint capsule and tendon attachments.[5] Young athletes in grades 7 to 12 must be matched by maturity, not age.[19]

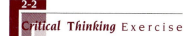

2-2

Critical Thinking Exercise

All-American High School offers 18 sports, which may basically be divided in 6 fall, 6 winter, and 6 spring sports. There are a total of approximately 500 athletes, and approximately 200 of them are involved in the fall sports. The athletic trainer is charged with the responsibility of arranging and administering preparticipation examinations so that each athlete can be cleared for competition.

? How can the athletic trainer most efficiently set up the preparticipation exams to clear 200 athletes for competition in the fall sports?

Figure 2-3

Sample medical history examination form.

MEDICAL HISTORY FORM

HEAD
1. Do you experience headaches? _____
   If yes, how frequently do they appear? _____
   Where are they located? _____
   Do you take any medicine to relieve them? _____
   If yes, what do you use? _____
2. Do you have any episodes of dizziness, seizures, or convulsions? _____
3. Have you ever fainted? _____
4. Have you ever had a head or neck injury? _____
   If yes, did you lose consciousness? _____
   If yes, how long? _____
   Were you under the care of a doctor? _____
   Were you hospitalized? _____
   Paralysis? _____ Numbness, tingling, or weakness of any extremity? _____
   How long before you resumed normal activity? _____

EYES
1. Have you ever had a problem with your eyes? Trauma? _____
   Loss of vision? _____ Pink eye? _____ Pain? _____

EARS
1. Have you ever had a problem with your ears? _____
   Infection? _____ Swimmer's ear? _____ Pain? _____
   Drainage? _____ Loss of hearing? _____

NOSE
1. Have you ever had a problem with your nose? _____
   Broken? _____ Sneezing? _____ Nosebleeds? _____

THROAT
1. How often do you have colds or sore throats? _____

SKIN
1. Do you ever have a skin rash? _____
   If yes, explain. _____

CHEST
1. Do you ever have chest pain? _____
   If yes, explain. _____
2. Do you have chronic cough? _____ Asthma? _____
   Hay fever? _____ Have you ever coughed up blood? _____

HEART
1. Have you ever been told you had a heart murmur? _____
   If yes, explain. _____
2. Have you ever been told you had elevated blood pressure? _____
   If yes, explain. _____
3. Is heart disease present in your family? _____
   If yes, explain. _____
4. Have you ever been told that a member of your family died suddenly or had a heart attack at a young age? _____

GI
1. Do you have trouble with heartburn? _____ Indigestion _____
   Nausea? _____ Vomiting? _____ Constipation? _____
   Diarrhea? _____ Have you ever vomited blood? _____
   If yes, explain. _____
2. Have you ever passed blood in your stools? _____
   If yes, explain. _____

GU
1. Have you ever noted burning on urination? _____
   Urgency? _____ Frequency? _____ Wake up at night to pass urine? _____ Penile discharge? _____ Passed blood on urination? _____ Kidney stone? _____

SKELETAL
1. Have you ever had arthritis? _____
   Sprained ankle? _____ If yes, explain. _____
   Knee injury? _____ If yes, explain. _____
   Shoulder injury? _____ If yes, explain. _____
   Broken Bone? _____ If yes, explain. _____
   Neck injury? _____ If yes, explain. _____
   Back trouble? _____ If yes, explain. _____
   Have you ever had surgery? _____ If yes, explain. _____
   Have you ever had a dislocation? If yes, explain. _____
2. Does any joint feel as if it is slipping? _____
3. Do you have a pin, plate, screw, or anything metal in your body? _____ If yes, explain. _____

GENERAL
1. Do you have drug allergy? _____
2. Are you allergic to insect bites? _____
3. Are you allergic to anything? _____
4. Have you ever had hepatitis? _____ Mononucleosis? _____
   Diabetes? _____ Does any family member have diabetes? _____
5. Have you ever had any serious disease? _____ If yes, explain. _____
6. Have you ever had heat exhaustion or heat stroke? _____
   If yes, explain. _____
7. Has any member of your family ever had heat exhaustion or heat stroke? _____
8. Has any member of our family been told they were allergic to medication used as anesthesia? _____
9. Have you ever been allergic to local anesthetics used by doctors or dentists? _____
10. Has your weight changed in the last three months? _____
    If yes, explain. _____

Figure 2-4

Sample physical examination form.

Name _____ SS# _____ Date _____
Height _____ Weight _____ Percent body fat _____

Check if Negative

1. Blood pressure _____ /_____
2. Pulse _____
3. Vision
   Without glasses R 20/_____ L 20/_____
   With glasses R 20/_____ L 20/_____
4. Skin _____
5. Dental/mouth _____
6. Ears _____
7. Nose _____
8. Throat _____
9. Chest
   Heart rhythm _____
   Lungs _____
   Breasts _____
10. Abdomen
    Liver _____
    Spleen _____
    Kidneys _____
    Stomach _____
    Bowel _____
11. Lymphatics
    Cervical _____
    Axillary _____
    Femoral _____
12. Genitalia _____
13. Maturation Index _____
14. Urinalysis
    Protein _____
    Sugar _____
15. Blood
    Hematocrit _____
16. Other _____
Disposition
        No participation
        Limited participation
        Clearance withheld
        Cleared for participation
Comments _____
_____
_____

_____
Physician's Signature
_____
Date

Orthopedic Screening

Orthopedic screening may be done as part of the physical examination or separately by the athletic trainer. An example of a quick orthopedic screening examination appears in Figure 2-5 and usually will take about 90 seconds.[2] A more detailed orthopedic examination may be conducted to assess strength, range of motion, and stability at various joints (Figure 2-6).

Orthopedic Screening Examination

Activity and Instruction	To Determine
Stand facing examiner	Acromioclavicular joints; general habitus
Look at ceiling, floor, over both shoulders; touch ears to shoulders	Cervical spine motion
Shrug shoulders (examiner resists)	Trapezius strength
Abduct shoulders 90° (examiner resists at 90°)	Deltoid strength
Full external rotation of arms	Shoulder motion
Flex and extend elbows	Elbow motion
Arms at sides, elbows 90° flexed; pronate and supinate wrists	Elbow and wrist motion
Spread fingers; make fist	Hand or finger motion and deformities
Tighten (contract) quadriceps; relax quadriceps	Symmetry and knee effusion; ankle effusion
"Duck walk" four steps (away from examiner with buttocks on heels)	Hip, knee, and ankle motion
Stand with back to examiner	Shoulder symmetry; scoliosis
Knees straight, touch toes	Scoliosis, hip motion, hamstring tightness
Raise up on toes, raise heels	Calf symmetry, leg strength

Figure 2-5

The orthopedic screening examination. Equipment that may be needed includes reflex hammer, tape measure, pin, and examining table.

Personal Physician

Examination by a personal physician has the advantage of yielding an in-depth history and an ideal physician-patient relationship. A disadvantage of this type of examination is that it may not be directed to detection of factors that predispose the athlete to a sports injury.[27]

Station Examination

The most thorough and sport-specific type of preparticipation examination is the station examination.[21] This method can provide the athlete with a detailed examination in a short period of time. A team of nine people is needed to examine 30 or more athletes. The team should include two physicians, two medically trained non-physicians (nurse, athletic trainer, physical therapist, or physician assistant), and five managers, student athletic trainers, or assistant coaches[27] (Table 2-1).

Sport Disqualification

As discussed previously, sports participation involves risks. Most disqualification conditions that are ascertained by a preparticipation health evaluation are noted in the medical history[21] (Table 2-2).

In general, the athlete who has lost one of two paired organs such as eyes or kidneys is cautioned against playing a collision or contact sport.[10] Such an athlete should be counseled into participating in a noncontact sport. The athlete with one testicle or one or two undescended testicles must be informed that there is a small risk, which is substantially minimized with the use of an athletic supporter and a protective device.[21]

Injury Reports and Injury Disposition

An injury report serves as a record for future reference (Figure 2-7). If the emergency procedures followed are questioned at a later date, one's memory of the details may be somewhat hazy, but a report completed on the spot provides specific

Figure 2-6

Sample of a detailed orthopedic screening examination form.

Orthopedic Screening Form

Name: _____ SS#: _____

FLEXIBILITY		Check if Normal
Shoulder:		Abduction
		Adduction
		Flexion
		Extension
		Internal rot.
		External rot.
Hip:		Ext. (flex knee)
		Flex. (flex knee)
		Ext. (str. leg)
		Flex. (str. leg)
		Abduction
		Adduction
Knee:		Flexion
		Extension
Ankle:		Dorsiflexion
		Plantar flexion
Trunk:		Flexion
		Extension
		Rotation
		Lat. Flexion

Joint Stability

Knee:		Lachman
		Pivot shift
		Anterior drawer
		Posterior drawer
		Valgus
		Varus
		McMurray
		Apley's grind
Ankle:		Anterior drawer
		Talor tilt

Leg Length

Posture:		Pelvis height
		Shoulder height
		Spine

Previous Injury: _____

Comments: _____

information. It should be noted that in a litigation situation questions may be asked of an athletic trainer about an injury that occurred 3 years in the past. All injury reports of this nature should be filed in the athletic trainer's office. It is well advised to make them out in triplicate so that one copy may be sent to the school health office, one to the physician, and one retained.

TABLE 2-1 Suggested Station Preparticipation Examination

Station	Points Noted	Personnel
1. Individual history; height, weight, body composition	"Yes" answers are probed in depth; height and weight relationships	Physician, nurse, or athletic trainer
2. Blood pressure, pulse	Upper limits: age 6 to 11—130/80; 12 and older—140/90; right arm is measured while athlete is seated	Student athletic trainer or manager
3. Snellen test, vision	Upper limits of visual acuity—20/40	Student athletic trainer or manager
4. Skin, mouth, ears, nose, throat	Suspicious-looking skin infections or rashes, dental prosthesis or caries, abnormalities of the ears, nose, throat	Physician, nurse, or athletic trainer
5. Chest, heart, lungs, breasts	Heart abnormalities (e.g., murmurs, latent bronchospasm), clarity of lungs	Physician
6. Lymphatics, abdomen, male genitalia	Adenopathy (cervical and axillary), abnormalities of genitalia, hernia	Physician or physician's assistant
7. Orthopedics	Postural asymmetry, decreased range of motion or strength, abnormal joint laxity	Physician, athletic trainer, physical therapist, or nurse practitioner
8. Urinalysis	After its collection in a paper cup, urine is tested in a lab for sugar and protein	Student athletic trainer or manager
9. Blood work	Lab test to determine hematocrit	Nurse or physician
10. Review	History and physical examination reports are evaluated and the following decisions are made: (a) No sports participation (b) Limited participation (no participation in specific sports such as football or ice hockey) (c) Clearance withheld until certain conditions are met (e.g., additional tests are taken, rehabilitation is completed) (d) Full, unlimited participation is allowed	Physician and athletic trainer

TABLE 2-2 Disqualifying Conditions for Sports Participation

Conditions	Collision*	Contact†	Noncontact‡	Others§
General health				
Acute infections	X	X	X	X
Respiratory, genitourinary, infectious mononucleosis, hepatitis, active rheumatic fever, active tuberculosis				
Obvious physical immaturity in comparison with other competitors	X	X		
Hemorrhagic disease	X	X	X	
Hemophilia, purpura, and other serious bleeding tendencies				
Diabetes, inadequately controlled	X	X	X	X
Diabetes, controlled	‖	‖	‖	‖
Jaundice	X	X	X	X
Eyes				
Absence or loss of function of one eye	X	X		
Respiratory				
Tuberculosis (active or symptomatic)	X	X	X	X
Severe pulmonary insufficiency	X	X	X	X
Cardiovascular				
Mitral stenosis, aortic stenosis, aortic insufficiency, coarctation of aorta, cyanotic heart disease, recent carditis of any etiology	X	X	X	X
Hypertension on organic basis	X	X	X	X
Previous heart surgery for congenital or acquired heart disease	¶	¶	¶	¶
Liver, enlarged	X	X		
Skin				
Boils, impetigo, and herpes simplex gladiatorum	X	X		
Spleen, enlarged	X	X		
Hernia				
Inguinal or femoral hernia	X	X	X	
Musculoskeletal				
Symptomatic abnormalities of inflammations	X	X	X	X
Functional inadequacy of the musculoskeletal system, congenital or acquired, incompatible with the contact or skill demands of the sport	X	X	X	

Continued

*Football, rugby, hockey, lacrosse, and so forth.
†Baseball, soccer, basketball, wrestling, and so forth.
‡Cross country, track, tennis, crew, swimming, and so forth.
§Bowling, golf, archery, field events, and so forth.
‖No exclusions.
¶Each individual should be judged on an individual basis in conjunction with his or her cardiologist and surgeon.
**Each patient should be judged on an individual basis. All things being equal, it is probably better to encourage a young boy or girl to participate in a noncontact sport rather than a contact sport. However, if a patient has a desire to play a contact sport and this is deemed a major ameliorating factor in his or her adjustment to school, associates, and the seizure disorder, serious consideration should be given to letting him or her participate if the seizures are moderately well controlled or the patient is under good medical management.
††The Committee approves the concept of contact sports participation for youths with only one testicle or with an undescended testicle(s), except in specific instances such as an inguinal canal undescended testicle(s), after appropriate medical evaluation to rule out unusual injury risk. However, the athlete, parents, and school authorities should be fully informed that participation in contact sports for youths with only one testicle carries a slight injury risk to the remaining healthy testicle. Fertility may be adversely affected after an injury. But the chances of an injury to a descended testicle are rare, and the injury risk can be further substantially minimized with an athletic supporter and protective device.

TABLE 2-2 Disqualifying Conditions for Sports Participation—cont'd

Conditions	Collision*	Contact†	Noncontact‡	Others§
Neurological				
History of symptoms of previous serious head trauma or repeated concussions	X			
Controlled convulsive disorder	**	**	**	**
Convulsive disorder not moderately well controlled by medication	X			
Previous surgery on head	X	X		
Renal				
Absence of one kidney	X	X		
Renal disease	X	X	X	X
Genitalia				
Absence of one testicle	††	††	††	††
Undescended testicle	††	††	††	††

The Treatment Log

Each athletic facility should have a sign-in log available for the athlete who receives any service. Emphasis is placed on recording the treatments for the athlete who is receiving daily therapy for an injury. As with accident records and injury disposition, these records often have the status of legal documents and are used to establish certain facts in a civil litigation, an insurance action, or a criminal action after injury.

Personal Information Card

Always on file in athletic trainer's office is the athlete's personal information card. This card is completed by the athlete at the time of the health examination and serves as a means of contacting the family, personal physician, and insurance company in case of emergency.

Injury Evaluation and Progress Notes

Injuries should be evaluated by the athletic trainer who must record information obtained in some consistent format. The subjective, objective, assessment, plan for treatment (SOAP) format is a concise method of recording the evaluation and the treatment plan for the injured athlete. (See Chapter 10.) The subjective portion of the SOAP note refers to what the athlete tells the athletic trainer about the injury relative to the history or what he or she felt. The objective portion documents information that the athletic trainer gathers during the evaluation such as range of motion, strength levels, patterns of pain, and so forth. The assessment records the athletic trainer's professional opinion about the injury based on information obtained during the subjective and objective portions. The plan for treatment indicates how the injury will be managed and includes short- and long-term goals for rehabilitation.

Supply and Equipment Inventory

A major responsibility of the athletic trainer is to manage a budget, most of which is spent on equipment and supplies. Every year an inventory must be conducted and recorded on such items as new equipment needed, equipment that needs to be replaced or repaired, and the expendable supplies that need replenishing.

Annual Reports

Most athletic departments require an annual report on the functions of the athletic training program. This report serves as a means for making program changes and improvements. It commonly includes the number of athletes served, a survey of the

Figure 2-7

Athletic injury record form.

Name _____ Sport _____ Date: ___ /___ /___ Time: _____ Injury number: _____

Player I.D. _____ Age: _____ Location: _____ Intercollegiate-nonintercollegiate

Initial injury   Recheck   Reinjury   Preseason—Practice—Game   Incurred while participating in sport: yes ___ no ___

Description: How did it happen? _____

_____

Initial impression: _____

_____

_____

Site of injury	Body part	Structure	Treatment _____
1 Right	1 Head 25 MP joint	1 Skin	_____
2 Left	2 Face 26 PIP joint	2 Muscle	_____
3 Proximal	3 Eye 27 Abdomen	3 Fascia	_____
4 Distal	4 Nose 28 Hip	4 Bone	_____
5 Anterior	5 Ear 29 Thigh	5 Nerve	_____
6 Posterior	6 Mouth 30 Knee	6 Fat pad	_____
7 Medial	7 Neck 31 Patella	7 Tendon	_____
8 Lateral	8 Thorax 32 Lower leg	8 Ligament	_____
9 Other	9 Ribs 33 Ankle	9 Cartilage	_____
_____	10 Sternum 34 Achilles tendon	10 Capsule	_____
_____	11 Upper back 35 Foot	11 Compartment	_____
Site of evaluation	12 Lower back 36 Toes	12 Dental	_____
1 SHS	13 Shoulder 37 Other	13 _____	_____
2 Athletic Trn Rm.	14 Rotator cuff		**Medication** _____
3 Site-Competition	15 AC joint		_____
4 _____	16 Glenohumeral	**Nature of injury**	_____
_____	17 Sternoclavicular	1 Contusion	_____
Procedures	18 Upper arm **Nontraumatic**	2 Strain	_____
1 Physical exam	19 Elbow 1 Dermatological	3 Sprain	_____
2 X-ray	20 Forearm 2 Allergy	4 Fracture	_____
3 Splint	21 Wrist 3 Influenza	5 Rupture	_____
4 Wrap	22 Hand 4 URI	6 Tendonitis	_____
5 Cast	23 Thumb 5 GU	7 Bursitis	_____
6 Aspiration	24 Finger 6 Systemic infect.	8 Myositis	**Prescription dispensed**
7 Other	7 Local infect.	9 Laceration	1 Antibiotics 5 Muscle relaxant
_____	8 Other	10 Concussion	2 Antiinflammatory 6 Enzyme
_____	_____	11 Avulsion	3 Decongestant 7 _____
Disposition	**Referral**	12 Abrasion	4 Analgesic
1 SHS	1 Arthrogram **Disposition of injury**	13 _____	**Injections**
2 Trainer	2 Neurological 1 No part.		1 Steroids
3 Hospital	3 Int. Med. 2 Part part.	**Degree**	2 Antibiotics
4 H.D.	4 Orthopedic 3 Full part.	1° 2° 3°	3 Steroids-xylo
5 Other	5 EENT		4 _____
_____	6 Dentist		
	7 Other		

_____   Previous injury _____

_____

number and types of injuries, an analysis of the program, and recommendations for future improvements.

Release of Medical Records

The athletic trainer may not release an athlete's medical records to anyone without written consent. If the athlete wishes to have medical records released to professional sports organizations, insurance companies, the news media, or any other group or individual, the athlete must sign a waiver that specifies which information is to be released.

Computer Use

Increasingly, computers are becoming an indispensible tool for the athletic trainer (Figure 2-8). Athletic trainers who have access to a computer find that a great deal of information can be efficiently stored for immediate and future use because of large storage and retrieval capacities. Hardware and software are available for most of the functions that need storing.

Record keeping is a time-consuming but essential chore for all athletic trainers regardless of whether they work at a college or university, at a high school, in the clinical setting, or in industry. Several software programs are available specifically for managing injury records in the athletic training setting. Among these are the Integrated Injury Tracking System (Micro Integration Services); Athletic Injury Management (Cramer, Inc.); Sports Injury Monitoring System (Med Sport Systems, Inc.); and SportsWare Injury Tracking System (Computer Sports Medicine Inc.).[24,25]

Besides record keeping, computer software can be used for planning a budget, managing a personal schedule or calender, or creating a database from which injury data can be organized, retrieved, or related to specific injury situations or other injury records for analysis. Other software can provide analysis and information relative to nutrition, body composition, injury risk profiles based on other anthropometric measures, and the recording of isokinetic evaluation and exercise.[26]

The use of educational software to assist in teaching and the academic preparation of student athletic trainers will be an important component of the education program. As new software becomes available the use of CD-ROM, with its interactive capabilities, will make learning more interesting and memorable for the student.

The use of electronic mail (E-mail) to share information and communicate with colleagues or other computers has opened up a new world of possibilities for education. By using a modem, a telephone line, and appropriate communications software one can gather and disseminate information and communicate with other individu-

Computers facilitate the record-keeping process.

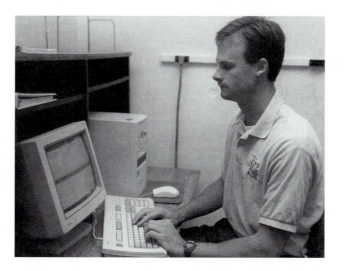

Figure 2-8

Computers are becoming an essential tool in athletic training.

2-3

Critical Thinking Exercise

During a high school gymnastics meet, a gymnast fell off the uneven parallel bars and landed on her forearm. The athletic trainer suspected a fracture and decided an x-ray was needed. The gymnast's parents had general health insurance through a PPO, but because she was in severe pain she was sent to the nearest emergency room to be treated. Unfortunately, the emergency facility was not on the list of preferred providers, and the insurance company denied the claim. The athletic trainer assured the parents that the school would take care of whatever medical costs were not covered by their insurance policy.

? Because the PPO denied the claim, what type of insurance policy should the school carry to cover the medical costs?

Every athlete should have a general health insurance policy that covers illness, hospitalization, and emergency care.

Figure 2-9

Sample insurance information form.

als interested in sports medicine all over the world. There are over 100 informational networks that connect educational and research institutions.[25]

INSURANCE REQUIREMENTS

Since 1971 there has been a significant increase in the number of lawsuits filed, caused in part by the steady increase in individuals who have become active in sports. The costs of insurance have also significantly increased during this period. With more lawsuits and much higher medical costs there is a crisis in the insurance industry.[6] Medical insurance is a contract between an insurance company and a policy holder that agrees to reimburse a portion of the total medical bill after some deductible has been paid by the policy holder. The major types of insurance about which individuals concerned with athletic training and sports medicine should have some understanding are general health insurance, catastrophic insurance, accident insurance, and liability insurance, as well as insurance for errors and omissions. There is a need to protect adequately all who are concerned with sports health and safety.

General Health Insurance

Every athlete should have a general health insurance policy that covers illness, hospitalization, and emergency care. Some institutions offer primary insurance coverage in which all medical expenses are paid for by the athletic department. The institutions pay an extremely high premium for this type of coverage. Most institutions offer secondary insurance coverage, which pays the athlete's remaining medical bills once the athlete's personal insurance company has made its payment. Secondary insurance always includes a deductible that will not be covered by the plan.

Many athletes are covered under some type of family health insurance policy. However, the school or university must make certain that personal health insurance is arranged for or purchased by athletes not covered under family policies.[24] A form letter directed to the parents of all athletes should be completed and returned to the institution to make certain that appropriate coverage is provided (Figure 2-9). Some so-called comprehensive plans do not cover every health need. For example, they may cover physicians' care but not hospital charges. Many of these plans require large prepayments before the insurance takes effect. Supplemental policies such as accident insurance and catastrophic insurance are designed to take over where general health insurance stops.

Insurance Information on Student Athletes
Student's Name _____ Date of Birth _____
Address _____
Social Security Number _____ Sex: M _____ F _____
Names of Insurance Companies _____
Address of Insurance Company _____
Certificate Number _____ Group _____ Type _____
Policy Holder _____ Relationship to Student _____
Employer or Policyholder _____
Should my son/daughter require services beyond those covered by the Sports Medicine Program, I give permission to the Division of Sports Medicine to file a claim for such services with the above health care insurer.
According to NCAA regulations, I understand that any insurance payments I receive must be returned to be placed on my child's account.
Date _____   _____
                                    Parent's Signature

Third-party reimbursement   Third-party reimbursement is the primary mechanism of payment for medical services in the United States.[25] Health care professionals are reimbursed for services performed by the policy holder's insurance company. Medical insurance companies may provide group and individual coverage for employees and dependents. Managed care involves a prearranged system for delivering health care that is designed to control cost while continuing to provide quality care. To cut pay-out costs, many insurance companies have begun to pay for preventive care (to reduce the need for hospitalization) and to limit where the individual can go for care. A number of different health care systems have been developed to contain costs.

Health maintenance organizations   Health maintenance organizations (HMOs) provide preventive measures and limit where the individual can receive care. With the exception of an emergency, permission must be obtained before the individual can go to another provider. Health maintenance organizations generally pay 100% of the medical costs as long as care is rendered at an HMO facility. Many supplemental policies do not cover the medical costs that would normally be paid by the general policy. Therefore an athlete treated outside the HMO may be ineligible for any insurance benefits. Many HMOs determine fees using a capitation system, which limits the amount that will be reimbursed for a specific service. It is essential for the athletic trainer to understand the limits of and restrictions on coverage at his or her institution.

Preferred provider organizations   Preferred provider organizations (PPOs) provide discount health care but also limit where a person can go for treatment of an illness. The coach or athletic trainer must be apprised in advance where the ill athlete should be sent. Athletes sent to a facility not on the approved list may be required to pay for care, whereas if they are sent to a preferred facility, all costs are paid.[6] Added services such as physical therapy may be more easily attained, and at no cost or at much lower cost, than with another insurance policy. Preferred provider organizations pay on a fee-for-service basis.

Point of service plan   The point of service plan is a combination of the HMO and PPO plans. It is based on an HMO structure, yet it allows members to go outside of the HMO to obtain services. This flexibility is allowed only with certain conditions and under special circumstances.

Fee-for-service   Fee-for-service is the most traditional form of billing for health care, in which the provider charges the patient or a third-party payer for services provided. Charges are based on a set fee schedule.

Capitation   Capitation is a form of reimbursement used by managed care providers in which members make a standard payment each month regardless of how much service is rendered to the member by the provider.

Third-party reimbursement for athletic trainers   Currently, unless the athletic trainer is also a licensed physical therapist, it is difficult if not impossible to obtain third-party reimbursement for health care services provided. Because the majority of athletic trainers are now employed in a clinical or industrial setting, this has become a major concern for the future of athletic trainers working in a for-profit private clinic. State licensing or credentialing of the athletic trainer has, to date, not helped with obtaining reimbursement. Insurance companies have not been willing to cover services provided by the athletic trainer. Athletic trainers working in the clinical setting perform many of the same functions as physical therapists in the clinic and are also responsible for obtaining referrals to the clinic through contacts in local high schools. Certainly, securing third-party reimbursement for athletic training services should be a priority, especially for the clinical athletic trainer.[25]

Accident Insurance

Besides general health insurance, low-cost accident insurance is available to the student. It often covers accidents on school grounds while the student is in attendance.

Third-party reimbursement involves reimbursement for services performed by the policy holder's insurance company.

Third-party payers: private insurance carriers, HMOs, and PPOs.

The purpose of this insurance is to protect against financial loss from medical and hospital bills, encourage an injured student to receive prompt medical care, encourage prompt reporting of injuries, and relieve a school of financial responsibility.

The school's general insurance may be limited; thus accident insurance for a specific activity such as sports may be needed to provide additional protection.[6] This type of coverage is limited and does not require knowledge of fault, and the amount it pays is limited. For serious sport injuries requiring surgery and lengthy rehabilitation, accident insurance is usually not adequate. This inadequacy can put families with limited budgets into a real financial bind. Of particular concern is insurance that does not adequately cover catastrophic injuries.

Personal Liability Insurance

Most individual schools and school districts have general liability insurance to protect against damages that may arise from injuries occurring on school property. Liability insurance covers claims of negligence on the part of individuals. Its major concern is whether supervision was reasonable and if unreasonable risk of harm was perceived by the sports participant.[24]

Because of the amount of litigation based on alleged negligence, premiums have become almost prohibitive for some schools. Typically, when a victim sues, the lawsuit has been a "shotgun approach," with the coach, athletic trainer, physician, school administrator, and school district all involved. If a protective piece of equipment is involved, the product manufacturer is also sued.

All athletic trainers should carry professional liability insurance and must clearly understand the limits of coverage. Liability insurance typically covers negligence in a civil case. If there is also a criminal complaint, liability insurance will not cover the athletic trainer.

Catastrophic Insurance

Although catastrophic injuries in sports participation are relatively uncommon, when they do occur the consequences to the athlete, family, and institution, as well as society, can be staggering. In the past when available funds have been completely diminished, the family was forced to seek funding elsewhere, usually through a lawsuit. Organizations such as the National Collegiate Athletic Association (NCAA) and National Association of Intercollegiate Athletics (NAIA) provide plans that deal with the problem of a lifetime that requires extensive medical and rehabilitative care because of a permanent disability.[6] Benefits begin when expenses have reached $25,000 and are then extended for a lifetime. At the secondary school level a program is offered to districts by the National Federation of State High School Associations (NFSHSA). This plan provides medical, rehabilitation, and transportation costs in excess of $10,000 not covered by other insurance benefits.[24] Costs for catastrophic insurance are based on the number of sports and the number of hazardous sports offered by the institution.

To offset this shotgun mentality and to cover what is not covered by a general liability policy, errors and omissions liability insurance has evolved. It is designed to cover school employees, officers, and the district against suits claiming malpractice, wrongful actions, errors and omissions, and acts of negligence.[24] Even when working in a program that has good liability coverage, each person within that program who works directly with students must have his or her own personal liability insurance.

As indicated, insurance that covers the athlete's health and safety can be complex. It must be the concern of the coach and the athletic trainer that every athlete is adequately covered by a reliable insurance company. In some athletic programs the filing of claims becomes the responsibility of the athletic trainer. This task can be highly time consuming, taking the athletic trainer away from his or her major role of working directly with the athlete. Because of the intricacies and time involved with

Because of the amount of litigation for alleged negligence, all professionals involved with the sports program must be fully protected by personal liability insurance.

claim filing and follow-up communications with parents, doctors, and vendors, a staff person other than the athletic trainer should be assigned this responsibility.

Insurance Billing

It is essential that the athletic trainer file insurance claims immediately and correctly.[25] The athletic trainer working in an educational setting can facilitate this process by collecting insurance information on every athlete at the beginning of the year. A letter should also be drafted to the parents of the athlete explaining the limits of the school insurance policy and what the parents must do to process a claim if injury does occur. If the school has a secondary policy it should be stressed that the parents must submit all bills to their insurance company before submitting the remainder to the school. In educational institutions, most claims will be filed with a single insurance company, which will pay for medical services provided by individual health care providers.

Athletic trainers working in the clinical setting should understand that the clinic must be able to collect reimbursement from third-party payers for services provided. The athletic trainer should request approval from insurance companies before treating patients. The athletic trainer must bill the patient's insurance company according to the Current Procedural Terminology (CPT) codes published by the American Medical Association, which lists appropriate number codes for specific procedures or services delivered to the patient. In 1994 the American Physical Therapy Association proposed a new coding scheme that specifically addressed the inequities of the physical therapy and sports medicine reimbursement system.[25]

> The athletic trainer must bill an insurance company according to CPT codes.

LEGAL CONCERNS OF THE COACH AND ATHLETIC TRAINER

In recent years negligence suits against teachers, coaches, athletic trainers, school officials, and physicians because of sports injuries have increased both in frequency and in the amount of damages awarded. An increasing awareness of the many risk factors present in physical activities has had a major effect on the coach and the athletic trainer in particular. A great deal of care must be taken in following coaching and athletic training procedures that conform to the legal guidelines governing liability.[18]

Liability

Liability is the state of being legally responsible for the harm one causes another person.[13] It assumes that the coach or athletic trainer would act according to the standards of care of any individual with similar educational background or training. In most cases in which someone has been charged with negligence, the actions of a hypothetical, reasonably prudent person have been compared with the actions of the defendant to ascertain whether the course of action followed by the defendant was in conformity with the judgment exercised by such a reasonably prudent person.[13] The key phrase has been "reasonable care." Individuals who have many years of experience, who are well-educated in their field, and who are certified or licensed must act in accordance with this background.

> Liability is the state of being legally responsible for the harm one causes another person.

Negligence is the failure to use ordinary or reasonable care—care that persons would normally exercise to avoid injury to themselves or to others under similar circumstances. This standard assumes that the individual is neither an exceptionally skillful individual nor an extraordinarily cautious one but is a person of reasonable and ordinary prudence. Put another way, it is expected that the individual will bring a commonsense approach to the situation at hand and will exercise due care in its handling. An example of negligence is when an athletic trainer, through improper or careless handling of a therapeutic agent, seriously burns an athlete. Another illustration, occurring all too often in sports, is one in which a coach or an athletic trainer moves a possibly seriously injured athlete from the field of play to permit competition or practice to continue and does so either in an improper manner or before con-

> Negligence is the failure to use ordinary or reasonable care.

2-4

Critical Thinking E x e r c i s e

A baseball batter was struck with a pitched ball directly in the orbit of the right eye and fell immediately to the ground. The athletic trainer ran to the player to examine the eye. There was some immediate swelling and discoloration around the orbit, but the eye appeared to be normal. The player insisted that he was fine and told the trainer he could continue to bat. After the game the athletic trainer told the athlete to go back to his room, put ice on his eye, and check in tomorrow. That night the baseball player began to hemorrhage into the anterior chamber of the eye and suffered irreparable damage to his eye.

? An opthalmologist stated that if the athlete's eye had been examined immediately after the injury the bleeding could have been controlled and there would not have been any damage to his vision. If the athlete brings a lawsuit against the athletic trainer, what must he prove if he is to win a judgment?

Torts are legal wrongs committed against a person.

sulting those qualified to know the proper course of action. Should a serious or disabling injury result, the coach or the athletic trainer is liable.

Assumption of Risk

The courts generally acknowledge that hazards are present in sports through the concept of assumption of risk. In other words, the individual, either by expressed or implied agreement, assumes the danger and hence relieves the other individual of legal responsibility to protect him or her; by so doing he or she agrees to take his or her own chances.[14] This concept, however, is subject to many and varied interpretations in the courts, especially when a minor is involved, because he or she is not considered able to render a mature judgment about the risks inherent in the situation. Although athletes participating in a sports program are considered to assume a normal risk, this in no way exempts those in charge from exercising reasonable care and prudence in the conduct of such activities or from foreseeing and taking precautionary measures against accident-provoking circumstances. In general, the courts have been fairly consistent in upholding waivers and releases of liability for adults unless there is evidence of fraud, misrepresentation, or duress.[13]

Torts

Torts are legal wrongs committed against the person or property of another.[13] Such wrongs may emanate from an act of omission, wherein the individual fails to perform a legal duty, or from an act of commission, wherein he or she commits an act that is not legally his or hers to perform. In either instance, if injury results, the person can be held liable. In the case of omission a coach or athletic trainer may fail to refer a seriously injured athlete for the proper medical attention. In the case of commission, the coach or athletic trainer may perform a medical treatment not within his or her legal province and from which serious medical complications develop.

Negligence

The tort concept of negligence is held by the courts when it is shown that an individual (1) does something that a reasonably prudent person would not do or (2) fails to do something that a reasonably prudent person would do under circumstances similar to those shown by the evidence.[3]

Athletic trainers employed by an institution have a duty to provide athletic training care to athletes at that institution. Clinical athletic trainers have a greater choice of who they may choose to treat as a patient. Once the athletic trainer assumes the duty of caring for an athlete there is an obligation to make sure that appropriate care is given.

It is expected that a person possessing more training in a given field or area will possess a correspondingly higher level of competence than, for example, a student. An individual will therefore be judged in terms of his or her performance in any situation in which legal liability may be assessed. It must be recognized that liability per se in all of its various aspects is not assessed at the same level nationally but varies in interpretation from state to state and from area to area. It is therefore good to know and to acquire the level of competence expected in one's particular area. In essence, negligence is conduct that results in the creation of an "unreasonable risk of harm to others."[29]

If the athletic trainer fails to provide an acceptable standard of care, there is a breach of duty on the part of the athletic trainer, and the athlete must then prove that this breach caused the injury or made the injury worse. If the athletic trainer breaches a duty yet no harm was done, there is no negligence.

Statutes of Limitation

Statutes of limitation set a specific length of time that individuals may sue for damages from negligence. These statutes vary from state to state, but in general in states where athletic trainers are covered by malpractice laws, the statute of limitation is between 1 and 3 years. In states where there is no regulation, there may be no statute of limitation for athletic trainers.

Avoiding Litigation

The athletic trainer or coach can significantly decrease risk of litigation by paying attention to several key points.[12] The coach must follow these guidelines:

1. Warn the athlete of the potential dangers inherent in the sport.
2. Supervise constantly and attentively.
3. Properly prepare and condition the athlete.
4. Properly instruct the athlete in the skills of the sport.
5. Ensure that proper and safe equipment and facilities are used by the athlete at all times.

The athletic trainer should do as follows:

1. Work to establish good personal relationships with athletes, parents, and co-workers.
2. Establish specific policies and guidelines for operation of an athletic training facility, and maintain qualified and adequate supervision of the training room, its environs, facilities, and equipment at all times.
3. Develop and carefully follow an emergency plan.
4. Make it a point to become familiar with the health status and medical history of the athletes under his or her care so as to be aware of the particular problems that they may have that could present a need for additional care or caution.
5. Keep good records that document all injuries and rehabilitation steps.
6. Document efforts to create a safe playing environment.
7. Have a detailed job description in writing.
8. Obtain written consent for providing health care, particularly when minors are involved.
9. Maintain confidentiality of medical records.
10. If allowed by law, exercise extreme caution in the administration of nonprescription medications; athletic trainers may not dispense prescription drugs.
11. Use only those therapeutic methods that he or she is qualified to use and that the law states may be used.
12. Not use or permit the presence of faulty or hazardous equipment.
13. Work cooperatively with the coach and the team physician in the selection and use of sports protective equipment, and insist that the best be obtained, properly fitted, and properly maintained.
14. Not permit injured players to participate unless cleared by the team physician. Players suffering a head injury should not be permitted to reenter the game. In some states a player who has suffered a concussion may not continue in the sport for the balance of the season.
15. Develop an understanding with the coaches that an injured athlete will not be allowed to reenter competition until, in the opinion of the team physician or the athletic trainer, he or she is psychologically and physically able. Athletic trainers should not allow themselves to be pressured to clear an athlete until he or she is fully cleared by the physician.
16. Follow the expressed orders of the team physician at all times.
17. Purchase liability insurance to protect against litigation and be aware of the limitations of the policy.
18. Know the limitations of his or her expertise as well as the applicable state regulations and restrictions that limit the athletic trainer's scope of practice.
19. Use common sense in making decisions about the athlete's health and safety.

In the case of an injury the coach or athletic trainer must use reasonable care to prevent further injury until medical care is obtained.[15] (See Chapter 8 for additional comments.)

Product Liability

Manufacturers of athletic equipment have a duty to design and produce equipment that will not cause injury as long as it is used as intended. An expressed warranty is the manufacturer's written guarantee that a product is safe. Warning labels on football helmets inform the player of possible dangers inherent in using the product. Athletes must read and sign a form indicating that they have read and understand the warning. The National Operating Committee on Standards for Athletic Equipment (NOCSAE) establishes minimum standards for equipment that must be met to ensure its safety.

INJURY DATA COLLECTION AND SURVEILLANCE

By their very nature sports activities invite injury. The "all-out" exertion required, the numerous situations requiring body contact, and play that involves the striking and throwing of missiles establish hazards that are either directly or indirectly responsible for the many different injuries suffered by athletes.

Because of the vast number of people involved with organized and recreational sports and the number of injuries sustained from these activities, accurate data acquisition is essential. Although methods are much improved over the past, many weaknesses exist in systematic data collection and analysis of sports injuries.[20]

The state of the art of sports injury surveillance is at this time unsatisfactory.[7] Currently most local, state, and federal systems are concerned with the accident or injury only after it has happened, and they focus on injuries requiring medical assistance or those that cause time loss or restricted activity.

The ideal system takes an epidemiological approach that studies the relationship of various factors that influence the frequency and distribution of sports injuries.[22] When considering the risks inherent in a particular sport, both extrinsic and intrinsic factors must be studied.[24] Thus information is gleaned from epidemiological data and the individual measurements of the athlete. The term *extrinsic factor* refers to the type of activity that is performed, the amount of exposure to injury, factors in the environment, and the equipment. The term *intrinsic factor* refers directly to the athlete and includes his or her age, gender, neuromuscular aspects, structural aspects, performance aspects, and mental and psychological aspects.

Using Injury Data

Valid, reliable sports injury data can materially help decrease injuries. If properly interpreted, the data can be used to modify rules, assist coaches and players in understanding risks, and help manufacturers evaluate their product against the overall market.[22] The public, especially parents, should understand the risks inherent in a particular sport, and insurance companies that insure athletes must know risks to set reasonable costs.

Current National Injury Data-Gathering Systems

A number of data collection systems tabulate the incidence of sports injuries. The most often mentioned systems are the National Safety Council, the Annual Survey of Football Injury Research, the National Electronic Injury Surveillance System (NEISS), the NCAA Injury Surveillance System, the National Center for Catastrophic Sports Injury Research, and the National High School Sports Injuries Registry.

National Safety Council

The National Safety Council* is a nongovernmental, nonprofit public service organization. It draws sports injuries data from a variety of sources, including educational institutions.

*National Safety Council, 444 North Michigan Avenue, Chicago, IL 60611.

2-5

Critical Thinking Exercise

A basketball coach at All-American High School is concerned about what seems to be an abnormally high frequency of ankle sprains on her varsity team. Her philosophy is to require all of her players to wear high-top shoes, yet the budget will not permit all players' ankles to be taped by the athletic trainer for practices and games. Together the coach and athletic trainer decide to purchase a number of lace-up ankle braces to see if they will help limit the number of ankle sprains.

? How can the athletic trainer determine if the braces are helping to decrease the frequency of ankle sprains in these basketball players?

Annual Survey of Football Injury Research

In 1931 the American Football Coaches Association (AFCA) conducted its first Annual Survey of Football Fatalities. Since 1965 this research has been conducted at the University of North Carolina. In 1980 the survey's title was changed to Annual Survey of Football Injury Research. Every year, with the exception of 1942, data have been collected about public school, college, professional, and sandlot football. Information is gathered through personal contact interviews and question-naires.[27] The sponsoring organizations of this survey are the AFCA, NCAA, and NFSHSA.

This survey classifies football fatalities as being direct or indirect. Direct fatalities are those resulting directly from participation in football. Indirect fatalities are produced by systemic failure caused by the exertion of playing football or by a complication that arose from a nonfatal football injury.

National Center for Catastrophic Sports Injury Research

In 1977 the NCAA initiated the National Survey of Catastrophic Football Injuries. As a result of the injury data collected from this organization, several significant rules changes have been incorporated into collegiate football. Because of the success of this football project, the research was expanded to all sports for both men and women, and a National Center for Catastrophic Sports Injury Research was established at the University of North Carolina under the direction of Dr. Fred Mueller. With support from the NCAA, the NFSHSA, the AFCA, and the Section on Sports Medicine of the American Association of Neurological Sciences, this center compiles data on catastrophic injuries at all levels of sport.[20]

National Collegiate Athletic Association Injury Surveillance System

The National Collegiate Athletic Association Injury Surveillance System was established in 1982 primarily for the purpose of studying the incidence of football injuries so that rule change recommendations could be made to reduce injury rate. Since that time this system has been greatly expanded and now collects data on most major sports. For the most part athletic trainers are primarily involved in the collection and transmission of injury data.

National Electronic Injury Surveillance System

In 1972 the federal government established the Consumer Product Safety Act (CPSA), which created and granted broad authority to the Consumer Product Safety Commission to enforce the safety standards of more than 10,000 products that may be risky to the consumer.[6] To perform this mission, the National Electronic Injury Surveillance System (NEISS)** was established. Data on injuries related to consumer products are monitored 24 hours a day from a selected sample of 5000 hospital emergency rooms nationwide. Sports injuries represent 25% of all injuries reported by NEISS. It should be noted that a product may be related to an injury but not be the direct cause of that injury.

Once a product is considered hazardous, the commission can seize the product or create standards to decrease the risk.[7] Also, manufacturers and distributors of sports recreational equipment must report to the commission any product that is potentially hazardous or defective.[7] The commission can also research the reasons that a sports or recreational product is hazardous.

National High School Sports Injuries Registry

In fall 1995 the National High School Sports Injuries Registry began tracking injuries in 10 different sports at 150 to 200 high schools in each sport. The registry is under

---

**National Electronic Injury Surveillance System, U.S. Consumer Products Safety Commission, Directorate for Epidemiology, National Injury Information Clearinghouse, Washington, DC.

the direction of Dr. John Powell and is being administered by Med Sport Systems Inc. and funded by the NATA. Data collection will continue through spring 1998.

The Incidence of Injuries

accident
An act that occurs by chance or without intention.

injury
An act that damages or hurts.

Risk of injury is determined by the type of sport—collision, contact, or noncontact.

The epidemiological approach toward injury data collection provides the most information.

An **accident** is defined as an unplanned event capable of resulting in loss of time, property damage, injury, disablement, or even death.[22] An **injury** may be defined as damage to the body that restricts activity or causes disability to such an extent that the athlete is confined to his or her bed.[9] In general, the incidence of sports injuries can be studied epidemiologically from many points of view—in terms of age of occurrence, gender, body regions that sustain injuries, or the occurrence in different sports. When examined, sports are usually classified according to the risk, or chances, of their occurring under similar circumstances. Sports classified as the collision type have a higher risk potential for fatalities, catastrophic neck injuries, and severe musculoskeletal injuries when compared with sports that are categorized as contact or noncontact.

In collision sports, athletes use their bodies to deter or punish opponents. Collision sports include football, ice hockey, and rugby. Contact sports include basketball, baseball, field hockey, judo, lacrosse, soccer, softball, and touch or flag football. A great number of sports are classified as noncontact activities, including archery, badminton, bowling, crew or rowing, cross-country running, curling, fencing, golf, gymnastics, riflery, skiing, squash, swimming and diving, tennis, track and field, and volleyball.

When considering athletes in all sports, recreational and organized, who participate in sports in 1 year's time, there is a 50% chance of their sustaining some injury. Of the 50 million estimated sports injuries per year, 50% require only minor care and no restriction of activity.[9] Approximately 90% of injuries are muscle contusions, minor joint sprains, and muscle strains; however, 10% of these injuries lead to microtrauma complications and eventually to a severe, chronic condition in later life.

Of the sports injuries that must be medically treated, sprains or strains, fractures, dislocations, and contusions are the most common.[9] In terms of the body regions most often injured, the knee has the highest incidence, with the ankle second and the upper limb third. For both males and females the most commonly injured body part is the knee, followed by the ankle; however, males have a much higher incidence of shoulder and upper-arm injuries than females.[9]

Catastrophic Injuries

As previously indicated, although millions of individuals participate in organized and recreational sports, there is a relatively low incidence of fatalities or catastrophic injuries. Ninety-eight percent of individuals with injuries requiring hospital emergency room medical attention are treated and released.[20] Deaths have been attributed to chest or trunk impact with thrown objects, other players, or nonyielding objects (e.g., goalposts). Deaths have occurred when players were struck in the head by sports implements (bats, golf clubs, hockey sticks) or by missiles (baseballs, soccer balls, golf balls, hockey pucks). Deaths have also resulted when an individual received a direct blow to the head from another player or the ground. On record are a number of sports deaths in which a playing structure, such as a goalpost or backstop, fell on a participant.

The highest incidence of indirect sports death stems from heatstroke. Less common indirect causes include cardiovascular and respiratory problems or congenital conditions not previously known.

Catastrophic injuries leading to cervical injury and quadriplegia are seen mainly in American football. Although the incidence is low for the number of players involved, it could be lowered even further if more precautions were taken.

In most popular organized and recreational sports activities, the legs and arms have the highest risk factor, with the head and face next. Muscle strains, joint sprains, contusions, and abrasions are the most frequent injuries sustained by the active sports participant.[9]

It is the major goal of this text to provide the reader with the fundamental principles necessary for preventing and managing illnesses and injuries common to the athlete.

SUMMARY

- Organization and administration of the athletic training program demands a significant portion of the athletic trainer's time and effort. The efficiency and success of the athletic training program depend in large part on the administrative abilities of the athletic trainer in addition to the clinical skills required to treat the injured athlete.
- The athletic training program can certainly be enhanced by designing or renovating a facility to maximize the potential use of the space available. Space designed for injury treatment, rehabilitation, modality use, office space, physician examination, record keeping, and storage of supplies should be designated within each facility.
- The athletic training program may best serve the athlete, the institution, and the community by establishing specific policies and regulations governing the use of available services.
- Budgets should allow for the purchase of equipment and supplies essential for providing appropriate preventive and rehabilitative care for the athlete.
- Preparticipation exams must be given to athletes and should include a medical history, a general physical examination, and orthopedic screenings. The athletic trainer must maintain accurate and up-to-date medical records in addition to the other paperwork that is necessary for the operation of the athletic training program. Computers are extremely useful tools that enable athletic trainers to retrieve and store a variety of records.
- Because of the high cost of medical care, every athlete should be covered by appropriate insurance policies that maximize the benefits should injury occur. The athletic trainer should be keenly aware of the legal issues involved in providing care for the athlete.
- In recent years negligence suits against teachers, coaches, athletic trainers, school officials, and physicians because of sports injuries have increased both in frequency and in the amount of damages awarded. A great deal of care must be taken in following coaching and athletic training procedures that conform to the legal guidelines governing liability.
- A number of data collection systems tabulate the incidence of sports injuries. The most often mentioned systems are the National Safety Council, the Annual Survey of Football Injury Research, the National Electronic Injury Surveillance System, the NCAA Injury Surveillance System, the National Center for Catastrophic Sports Injury Research, and the National High School Sports Injuries Registry.

....

Solutions to Critical Thinking Exercises

2-1 The training room should have specific areas designated for taping and preparation, treatment and rehabilitation, and hydrotherapy. There should be an office for the athletic trainer and adequate storage facilities positioned within the space to allow for an efficient traffic flow. Equipment purchases might include four or five treatment tables and two or three taping tables (these could be made in house if possible), a large capacity ice machine, a combination ultrasound/electrical stimulating unit, a whirlpool, and various free weights and exercise tubing.

2-2 The preparticipation examination should consist of a medical history, a physical examination, and a brief orthopedic screening. The preparticipation physical may be effectively administered using a station examination system with a team of examiners. A station examination can provide the athlete with a detailed examination in a short period of time. A "team" of people is needed to examine this many athletes. The team should include several physicians, medically trained nonphysicians (nurses, athletic trainers, physical therapists, or physician assistants), and managers, student athletic trainers, or assistant coaches.

2-3 Besides general health insurance, low-cost accident insurance often covers accidents on school grounds while the athlete is competing. The purpose of this insurance is to protect against financial loss from medical and hospital bills, encourage an injured athlete to receive prompt medical care, encourage prompt reporting of injuries, and relieve a school of financial responsibility.

2-4 When the athletic trainer assumes the duty of caring for an athlete there is an obligation to make sure that appropriate care is given. If the athletic trainer fails to provide an acceptable standard of care, there is a breach of duty on the part of the athletic trainer, and the athlete must then prove that this breach caused the injury or made the injury worse.

2-5 The athletic trainer should do a simple study in which one half of the team is randomly placed in the ankle braces while the other half continues to play in their high-top shoes. By comparing the number of ankle injuries in the group wearing the braces with those in the group without the braces, the athletic trainer can make some decision as to the effectiveness of the braces in preventing ankle injuries. Collecting and analyzing injury data are helpful in determining the efficacy of many of the techniques used by the athletic trainer.

REVIEW QUESTIONS AND CLASS ACTIVITIES

1. What are the major administrative functions that an athletic trainer must perform?
2. Design two athletic training facilities—one for a medium-sized university and one for a large university.
3. Observe the activities in the athletic training facility. Pick both a slow time and a busy time to observe.
4. Why do hygiene and sanitation play an important role in athletic training? How should the athletic training facility be maintained?
5. Fully equip a new medium-size high school, college athletic training facility, or clinical facility. Pick equipment from current catalogs.
6. Establish a reasonable budget for a small high school, a large high school, and a large college or university.
7. Identify the groups of individuals to be served in the athletic training facility.
8. Organize a preparticipation health examination for 90 football players.
9. Record keeping is a major function in athletic training. What records is it necessary to keep? How can a computer help?
10. Debate what conditions constitute good grounds for medical disqualification from a sport.
11. Define the types of insurance necessary in sports.
12. What are the major legal concerns of the coach and the athletic trainer in terms of liability, assumption of risk, torts, and negligence?
13. Discuss the epidemiological approach to recording sports injury data.

REFERENCES

1. Abdenour TE, Weir NJ: Medical assessment of the prospective student athlete, *Ath Train* 21:122-123, 186, 1986.
2. American Academy of Pediatrics Policy Statement: Recommendations for participation in competitive sports, *Phys Sportsmed* 16(5):51-59, 1988.
3. Appenzeller H: *Sports and the law: contemporary issues*, Charlottesville, Va, 1985, Michie.
4. Bonci CM, Ryan R: Pre-participation screening in intercollegiate athletics, *Postgrad Adv Sports Med* 3:3-6, 1988.
5. Caine DJ, Broekhoff J: Maturity assessment: a viable preventive measure against physical and psychological insult to the young athlete? *Phys Sportsmed* 15(3):67, 1987.
6. Chambers RL: Insurance types and coverages: knowledge to plan for the future (with a focus on motor skill activities and athletics), *Phys Educator* 44:233, 1986.
7. Damron CF: Injury surveillance systems for sports. In Vinger PF, Hoerner EF, editors: *Sports injuries*, Boston, 1986, Year Book Medical Publishers.
8. Dean CH, Hoerner EF: Injury rates in team sports and individual recreation. In Vinger PF, Hoerner EF, editors: *Sports injuries*, Boston, 1986, Year Book Medical Publishers.
9. DeHaven JE, Lintner DM: Athletic injuries: comparison by age, sport, and gender, *Am J Sports Med* 14(3):218, 1986.
10. Dorsen PJ: Should athletes with one eye, kidney, or testicle play contact sports? *Phys Sportsmed* 14(7):130, 1986.
11. Forseth EA: Consideration in planning small college athletic training facilities, *Ath Train* 21(1):22, 1986.
12. Graham L: Ten ways to dodge the malpractice bullet, *Ath Train* 20(2):117-119, 1985.
13. Hawkins J, Appenzeller H: Legal aspects of sports medicine. In Mueller F, Ryan A: *Prevention of athletic injuries: the role of the sports medicine team*, Philadelphia, 1991, Davis.
14. Herbert D: Legal aspects of sports medicine, Canton, Ohio, 1990, Professional Reports Corporation.
15. Herbert D: Professional considerations related to conduct of preparticipation exams, *Sports Med Standards Malpractice Reporter* 6(4):49-52, 1994.
16. Jones R: The prepaticipation, sport-specific athletic profile examination, *Semin Adolesc Med* 3:169-175, 1987.
17. Kibler W: *The sports participation fitness examination,* Champaign, Ill, 1990, Human Kinetics.
18. Leverenz L, Helms L: Suing athletic trainers, parts I and II, *Ath Train* 25(3):212-226, 1990.
19. McKeag DB: Preseason physical examination for the prevention of sports injuries, *Sports Med* 2:413, 1985.
20. Mueller F: Catastrophic sports injuries. In Mueller F, Ryan A: *Prevention of athletic injuries: the role of the sports medicine team*, Philadelphia, 1991, Davis.
21. Myers GC, Garrick JG: The preseason examination of school and college athletes. In Strauss RH, editor: *Sports medicine*, Philadelphia, 1984, Saunders.
22. Powell J: Epidemiologic research for injury prevention programs in sports. In Mueller F, Ryan A: *Prevention of athletic injuries: the role of the sports medicine team*, Philadelphia, 1991, Davis.
23. Rankin J: Financial resources for conducting athletic training programs in the collegiate and high school settings, *J Ath Train* 27(4):344-349, 1992.
24. Rankin J, Ingersoll C: *Athletic training management: concepts and applications,* St Louis, 1995, Mosby.
25. Ray R: *Management strategies in athletic training,* Champaign, Ill, 1994, Human Kinetics.
26. Ray R, Shire TL: An athletic training program in the computer age, *Ath Train* 21:212, 1986.
27. Swander H: *Preparticipation physical examination,* Kansas City, 1992, American Academy of Family Physicians, American Academy of Pediatrics, American Orthopedic Society for Sports Medicine, American Osteopathic Academy for Sports Medicine.

28. Torg J: *Athletic injuries to the head, neck, and face,* St Louis, 1991, Mosby.
29. Yasser R: Calculating risk, *Sports Med Dig* 9(2):5, 1987.

ANNOTATED BIBLIOGRAPHY

Appenzeller H: *Sports and the law: contemporary issues,* Charlottesville, Va, 1985, Michie.

Exposes sports litigation from the perspectives of the athletic director, athlete, athletic trainer, coach, officials, and products liability expert. A chapter on the athletic trainer emphasizes the use of modalities and how this use relates to the practice of physical therapy in different states.

Rankin J, Ingersoll C: *Athletic training management: concepts and applications,* St Louis, 1995, Mosby.

This text is designed for upper-division undergraduate or graduate students interested in all aspects of organization and administration of an athletic training program.

Ray R: *Management strategies in athletic training,* Champaign, Ill, 1994, Human Kinetics.

This was the first text available to cover the principles of organization and administration as they apply to many different employment settings in athletic training. It contains many examples and case studies based on principles of administration presented in the text.

Smith NJ, editor: *Sports medicine: health care for young athletes,* Evanston, Ill, 1983, American Academy of Pediatrics.

Based on the concerns and needs of children who engage in sports. Covers the major health and safety aspects at this level.

Injury Prevention

Training and Conditioning Techniques

When you finish this chapter, you should be able to

- Identify the major conditioning seasons and the types of exercise that are performed in each season.
- Identify the principles of conditioning.
- Discuss the importance of the warm-up and cool-down periods.
- Describe the importance of flexibility, strength, and cardiorespiratory endurance for both athletic performance and injury prevention.
- Identify specific techniques and principles for improving flexibility, muscular strength, and cardiorespiratory endurance.

P reventing injury to the athlete is one of the primary functions of the athletic trainer. To compete successfully at a high level, the athlete must be fit. An athlete who is not fit is more likely to sustain an injury. Coaches and athletic trainers recognize that improper conditioning is one of the major causes of sports injuries (Figure 3-1). Thus coaches and athletic trainers should work cooperatively to supervise training and conditioning programs that minimize the possibility of injury and maximize performance.[34]

It takes time and careful preparation to bring an athlete into competition at a level of fitness that will preclude early-season injury. The athletic trainer must possess sound understanding of the principles of training and conditioning relative to flexibility, strength, and cardiorespiratory endurance.

Lack of physical fitness is one of the primary causes of sports injury.

CONDITIONING SEASONS AND PERIODIZATION

No longer do serious athletes engage only in preseason conditioning and in-season competition. Sports conditioning is a year-round endeavor. The concept of periodization is an approach to conditioning that attempts to bring about peak performance while reducing injuries and overtraining in the athlete by developing a training and conditioning program to be followed throughout the various seasons. The idea of periodization takes into account that athletes have different needs relative to training and conditioning during different seasons and modifies the program according to individual needs. For the athlete, the conditioning program often encompasses four training seasons: postseason, off-season, preseason, and in-season. This plan is especially appropriate for collision-type sports such as football. This approach is referred to as the quadratic training cycle.[14] For American tackle football, the postseason generally is from February to May; off-season, May to July; preseason, July to September; and in-season, September to January.

Sports conditioning often falls into four seasons: postseason, off-season, preseason, and in-season.

Postseason Conditioning

Conditioning during the postseason is commonly dedicated to physical restoration. This period is particularly appropriate when the athlete has been injured during the in-season. This is a time when postsurgical rehabilitation takes place and detailed medical evaluations can be obtained.[14]

Off-Season Conditioning

It is essential that athletes continue with a conditioning program during the off-season. It is usually a good idea for the athletic trainer and coach to encourage

Figure 3-1

Modern sports programs often require elaborate conditioning facilities and equipment to apply sound injury prevention methods.

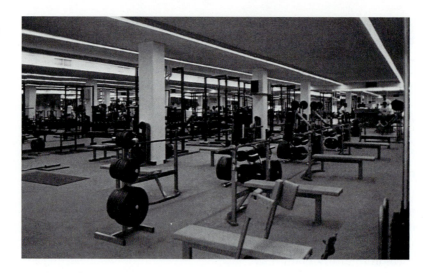

athletes to participate in another sport during this period. Such an activity should make certain physical demands embodying strength, endurance, and flexibility by means of running and general all-around physical performance. This activity will assist athletes in maintaining their level of fitness. In other words, the sport must be sufficiently demanding to require a good level of fitness to participate effectively. An excellent off-season sport for the football player would be wrestling or gymnastics. Track, especially cross-country, is a conditioner.

A weekly workout of moderate-to-strong intensity is usually all that is required because physical fitness is retained for a considerable length of time after an active program of competition ends. The physically vigorous athlete tends to be active in the off-season too and, as a rule, will stay in reasonably good condition throughout the year.[14]

Establishing regular training routines for the off-season enables the athletic trainer to keep a close check on athletes even if they are seen only at 2- or 3-week intervals.

Preseason

Athletic trainers should impress on their athletes the need for maintaining a reasonably high level of physical fitness during the off-season. If such advice is followed, the athlete will find preseason work relatively rewarding and any proneness to potential injury considerably diminished. No difficulty in reaching a state of athletic fitness suitable for competition within 6 to 8 weeks should then be experienced. During this preliminary period flexibility, endurance, and strength should be emphasized in a carefully graded developmental program. In such a program there must be wise and constant use of established physiological bases for improving physical condition and performance.

Many athletes, particularly in one-season sports, tend to reach their highest level of performance halfway through the season. As a result, they are truly efficient only half of the time. Conference and federation restrictions often hamper or prohibit effective preseason training, especially in football, and therefore compel the athlete to come into early-season competition before being physically fit for it. At the high school level 6 to 8 weeks of preseason conditioning afford the best insurance against susceptibility to injury and permit the athlete to enter competition in a good state of physical fitness, provided a carefully graded program is established and adhered to conscientiously. Recently, physicians have been adding their voices to the demands for a realistic approach to proper conditioning, and school administrators and the general public may see the need and effectiveness of permitting adequate and properly controlled preseason training.

In-Season

Intensive preseason conditioning programs, which bring the athlete to the competitive season, may not be maintained by the sport itself. Unless there is strenuous conditioning throughout the season, a problem of deconditioning may occur. Athletes who do not undergo maintenance conditioning may lose their entry level of physiological fitness.[14]

Cross-training

The concept of cross-training is an approach to training and conditioning for a specific sport that involves substitution of alternative activities that have some carryover value to that sport. For example, a swimmer could engage in jogging, running, or aerobic exercise to maintain levels of cardiorespiratory conditioning. Cross-training is particularly useful in both the postseason and the off-season for maintaining fitness levels and avoiding boredom that would typically occur by following the same training regimen and using the same techniques for conditioning as in the preseason and competitive season.

PRINCIPLES OF CONDITIONING

The following principles should be applied in all programs of training and conditioning to minimize the likelihood of injury:

1. *Warm-up/cool-down.* Take time to do an appropriate warm-up before engaging in any activity. Do not neglect the cool-down period after a training bout.
2. *Motivation.* Athletes are generally highly motivated to work hard because they want to be successful in their sport. By varying the training program and incorporating different aspects of conditioning, the program can remain enjoyable rather than becoming routine and boring.
3. *Overload.* To see improvement in any physiological component, the system must work harder than it is accustomed to working. Gradually, that system will adapt to the imposed demands.
4. *Consistency.* The athlete must engage in a training and conditioning program on a consistent, regularly scheduled basis if it is to be effective.
5. *Progression.* Increase the intensity of the conditioning program gradually and within the individual athlete's ability to adapt to increasing workloads.
6. *Intensity.* Stress the intensity of the work rather than the quantity. Coaches and athletic trainers too often confuse working hard with working for long periods of time. They make the mistake of prolonging the workout rather than increasing tempo or workload. The tired athlete is prone to injury.
7. *Specificity.* Specific goals for the training program must be identified. The program must be designed to address specific components of fitness (i.e., strength, flexibility, cardiorespiratory endurance) relative to the sport in which the athlete is competing.
8. *Individuality.* The needs of individual athletes vary considerably. The successful coach is one who recognizes these individual differences and adjusts or alters the training and conditioning program accordingly to best accommodate the athlete.
9. *Minimize stress.* Expect that athletes will train as close to their physiological limits as possible. Push the athletes as far as possible but consider other stressful aspects of their lives, allowing time for them to be away from the conditioning demands of their sport.
10. *Safety.* Make the training environment as safe as possible. Take time to educate athletes regarding proper techniques, how they should feel during the workout, and when they should push harder or back off.

3-1

Critical Thinking Exercise

A professional football player sustained a grade 2 hamstring strain during week 6 of the season. Just before the playoffs he reinjured the muscle while doing some slow-speed cutting drills. Unfortunately, he was forced to remain on the injured reserve list for the duration of the season despite his best efforts to return. Because he has been unable to run he has lost a great deal of cardiorespiratory fitness, and he exhibits weakness in lower extremity muscular strength because lifting has been difficult.

? Given that he will be required to attend two minicamps during the spring and early summer with preseason practice officially beginning in July, what should be his conditioning plan during the postseason and the off-season?

FOUNDATIONS OF CONDITIONING

The SAID principle indicates that the body will gradually adapt to the specific demands imposed on it.

Logan and Wallis[21] identified the SAID principle, which expressly relates to the process of training and conditioning. SAID is an acronym for *specific adaptation to imposed demands.* The SAID principle states that when the body is subjected to stresses and overloads of varying intensities it will gradually adapt over time to overcome whatever demands are placed on it.

Although overload is a critical factor in training and conditioning, the stress must not be great enough to produce damage or injury before the body has had a chance to adjust specifically to the increased demands. Therefore it is essential that the athletic trainer be aware of the principles of training and conditioning to reduce the likelihood of injury.

WARM-UP AND COOL-DOWN

A period of warm-up exercises should take place before a training session begins. The warm-up increases body temperature, stretches ligaments and muscles, and increases flexibility. Related warm-ups, those similar to the activity engaged in, are preferable to unrelated ones because of the rehearsal or practice effect that results.

3-2

Critical Thinking Exercise

A track athlete constantly complains of feelings of tightness in her lower extremity during workouts. She states that she has a difficult time during her warm-up and cannot seem to "get loose" until her workout is almost complete. She feels that she is always on the verge of "pulling a muscle."

? What should the athletic trainer recommend as a specific warm-up routine that should consistently be done before this athlete begins her workout?

Warm-ups have been found to be important in preventing injury and muscle soreness.[32] It appears that muscle injury can result when vigorous exercises are not preceded by a related warm-up. An effective, quick warm-up can also be an effective motivator. An athlete who gets satisfaction from a warm-up probably will have a stronger desire to participate in the activity. By contrast, a poor warm-up can lead to fatigue and boredom, limiting attention and ultimately resulting in a poor program. There is some evidence that a good warm-up may also improve certain aspects of performance.[8]

The function of the warm-up is to prepare the body physiologically for some upcoming physical work. Most athletic trainers view the warm-up period as a precaution against unnecessary musculoskeletal injury and possible muscle soreness. The purpose is to gradually stimulate the cardiorespiratory system to a moderate degree, thus producing an increased blood flow to working skeletal muscles and resulting in an increase in muscle temperature.

Moderate activity speeds up the metabolic processes that produce an increase in core body temperature. An increase in the temperature of skeletal muscle causes an increased speed of contraction and relaxation, probably because nerve impulse conduction velocity is increased. The elastic properties (the length of stretch) of the muscle are increased, whereas the viscous properties (the rate at which the muscle can change shape) are decreased.

Before any workout activities there should be a warm-up. This warm-up should include a general warm-up followed by a specific warm-up. The general warm-up involves elevating the core temperature and static stretching exercises. The specific warm-up involves activities related to the activity to be performed. These activities are sport specific and should gradually increase in intensity.

Warming up involves general body warming and warming specific body areas for the demands of the sport.

The type of warm-up should be related to the activity. For example, a soccer player uses the upper extremity considerably less than the lower extremity, so his or her warm-up should be directed more toward the lower extremity, perhaps by adding some stretching exercises for the lower extremity. The warm-up should also be sport specific; for example, a basketball player should warm up by shooting layups and jump shots and dribbling; a tennis player should hit forehand and backhand shots and serves.

The warm-up should last approximately 10 to 15 minutes. The athlete should not wait longer than 15 minutes to get started in the activity after the warm-up, although the effects will generally last up to about 45 minutes. Thus the third-string football player who warms up before the game and then does nothing more than stand around until he gets into the game during the fourth quarter is running a much higher risk of injury. This player should be encouraged to stay warmed up and ready to play throughout the course of a game. In general, sweating is a good indication that the body has been sufficiently warmed up and is ready for more strenuous activity.

The warm-up should begin with 2 or 3 minutes of light jogging to increase metabolic rate and core temperature. This should be followed by a period of flexibility exercises in which the muscles are stretched to take advantage of the increase in muscle elasticity. Finally, the intensity of the warm-up should be increased gradually by performing body movements and skills associated with the specific activity in which the athlete is going to participate.

Cool-down

After a vigorous workout, a cool-down period is essential. This part of the training program helps in returning the blood to the heart for reoxygenation, thus preventing a pooling of the blood in the muscles of the arms and legs. Pooling of the blood in the extremities places additional unnecessary stress and strain on the heart. After vigorous activity, enough blood may not circulate back to the brain, heart, and intestines, and symptoms such as dizziness or faintness may occur without a cool-down period. The cool-down period enables the body to cool and return to a resting state. Such a period should last about 5 to 10 minutes.

Proper cooling down decreases blood and muscle lactic acid levels more rapidly.

Although the value of warm-up and workout periods is well accepted, the importance of a cool-down period afterward is often ignored. Again, experience and observation seem to indicate that persons who stretch during the cool-down period tend to have fewer problems with muscle soreness after strenuous activity.

Conditioning should be performed gradually, with work added in small increments.

IMPROVING AND MAINTAINING FLEXIBILITY

Flexibility is the ability to move a joint or series of joints smoothly and easily throughout a full range of motion.[1] An athlete who has a restricted range of motion will probably realize a decrease in performance capabilities. For example, a sprinter with tight, inelastic hamstring muscles probably loses some speed because the hamstring muscles restrict the ability to flex the hip joint, thus shortening stride length.

The "tight" or inflexible athlete performs with a considerable handicap in terms of movement.

Lack of flexibility may result in uncoordinated or awkward movements and probably predisposes the athlete to muscle strain. Low back pain is frequently associated with tightness of the musculature in the lower spine and also of the hamstring muscles.

Most activities require relatively "normal" amounts of flexibility.[15] However, some activities, such as gymnastics, ballet, diving, karate, and yoga, require increased flexibility for superior performance (Figure 3-2). Increased flexibility may increase one's performance through balance and reaction time.

Good flexibility is essential to successful physical performance.[35] Most athletic trainers feel that maintaining good flexibility is important in prevention of injury to the musculotendinous unit, and they will generally insist that stretching exercises be

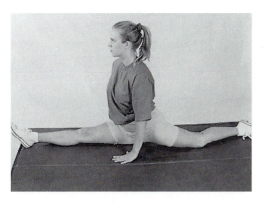

Figure 3-2

Flexibility can be an important factor in decreasing sports injuries.

included as part of the warm-up before engaging in strenuous activity, although little or no research evidence is available to support this.

Flexibility may best be defined as the range of motion possible about a given joint or series of joints. Flexibility can be discussed in relation to movement involving only one joint, such as in the knees, or movement involving a whole series of joints, such as the spinal vertebral joints, which must all move together to allow smooth bending or rotation of the trunk.

Factors that Limit Flexibility

A number of factors may limit the ability of a joint to move through a full, unrestricted range of motion. The *bony structure* may restrict the endpoint in the range. An elbow that has been fractured through the joint may deposit excess calcium in the joint space, causing the joint to lose its ability to fully extend. However, in many instances bony prominences stop movements at normal endpoints in the range.

Excessive *fat* may also limit the ability to move through a full range of motion. An athlete who has a large amount of fat on the abdomen may have severely restricted trunk flexion when asked to bend forward and touch the toes. The fat may act as a wedge between two lever arms, restricting movement wherever it is found. *Skin* might also be responsible for limiting movement. For example, an athlete who has had some type of injury or surgery involving a tearing incision or laceration of the skin, particularly over a joint, will have inelastic scar tissue formed at that site. This scar tissue is incapable of stretching with joint movement. *Muscles and their tendons,* along with their surrounding fascial sheaths, are most often responsible for limiting range of motion. When performing stretching exercises for the purpose of improving flexibility about a particular joint, one is attempting to take advantage of the highly elastic properties of a muscle. Over time it is possible to increase the elasticity, or the length that a given muscle can be stretched. Athletes who have a good deal of movement at a particular joint tend to have highly elastic and flexible muscles. *Connective tissue* surrounding the joint, such as ligaments on the joint capsule, may be subject to contractures. Ligaments and joint capsules do have some elasticity; however, if a joint is immobilized for a period of time, these structures tend to lose some elasticity and shorten. This condition is most commonly seen after surgical repair of an unstable joint, but it can also result from long periods of inactivity.

It is also possible for an athlete to have relatively slack ligaments and joint capsules. These individuals are generally referred to as being loose-jointed. Examples of this would be an elbow or knee that hyperextends beyond 180 degrees (Figure 3-3). Frequently there is instability associated with loose-jointedness that may present as great a problem in movement as ligamentous or capsular contractures.

Skin contractures caused by scarring, ligaments, joint capsules, and musculotendinous units are each capable of improving elasticity to varying degrees through

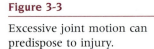

Figure 3-3

Excessive joint motion can predispose to injury.

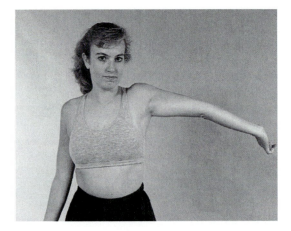

stretching over time. With the exception of bony structure, age, and gender, all the other factors that limit flexibility may be altered to increase range of joint motion.

Active and Passive Range of Motion

Active range of motion, also called dynamic flexibility, refers to the degree to which a joint can be moved by a muscle contraction, usually through the midrange of movement. Dynamic flexibility is not necessarily a good indicator of the stiffness or looseness of a joint because it applies to the ability to move a joint efficiently, with little resistance to motion.[27]

Passive range of motion, sometimes called static flexibility, refers to the degree to which a joint may be passively moved to the endpoints in the range of motion. No muscle contraction is involved to move a joint through a passive range.

When a muscle actively contracts, it produces a joint movement through a specific range of motion. However, if passive pressure is applied to an extremity, it is capable of moving farther in the range of motion. It is essential in sport activities that an extremity be capable of moving through a nonrestricted range of motion. For example, a hurdler who cannot fully extend the knee joint in a normal stride is at considerable disadvantage because stride length and thus speed will be reduced significantly (Figure 3-4).

Passive range of motion is important for injury prevention. There are many situations in sport in which a muscle is forced to stretch beyond its normal active limits. If the muscle does not have enough elasticity to compensate for this additional stretch, it is likely that the musculotendinous unit will be injured.

Stretching Techniques

The maintenance of a full, nonrestricted range of motion has long been recognized as critical to injury prevention and as an essential component of a conditioning program[4] (see the Focus box on the next page).

The goal of any effective flexibility program should be to improve the range of motion at a given articulation by altering the extensibility of the musculotendinous units that produce movement at that joint. It is well documented that exercises that stretch these musculotendinous units over a period of time increase the range of movement possible about a given joint.[26]

Stretching techniques for improving flexibility have evolved over the years. The oldest technique for stretching is called ballistic stretching, which makes use of repetitive bouncing motions. A second technique, known as static stretching, involves stretching a muscle to the point of discomfort and then holding it at the point for an extended time. This technique has been used for many years. Recently another group of stretching techniques known collectively as proprioceptive neuromuscular facilitation (PNF), involving alternating contractions and stretches, has been recommended.[25]

Researchers have had considerable discussion about which of these techniques is most effective for improving range of motion.

Agonist Versus Antagonist Muscles

Before discussing the three different stretching techniques it is essential to define the terms *agonist* and *antagonist*. Most joints in the body are capable of more than one movement. The knee joint, for example, is capable of flexion and extension. Contraction of the quadriceps group of muscles on the front of the thigh causes knee extension, whereas contraction of the hamstring muscles on the back of the thigh produces knee flexion.

To achieve knee extension, the quadriceps group contracts while the hamstring muscles relax and stretch. The muscle that contracts to produce a movement, in this case the quadriceps, is referred to as the agonist muscle. The muscle being stretched in response to contraction of the agonist muscle is called the antagonist muscle. In

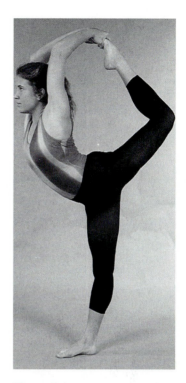

Figure 3-4

Good flexibility is essential to successful performance in many sport activities.

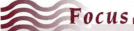

Focus

Guidelines and precautions for stretching

The following guidelines and precautions should be incorporated into a sound stretching program:

Warm up using a slow jog or fast walk before stretching vigorously.

To increase flexibility, the muscle must be overloaded or stretched beyond its normal range but not to the point of pain.

Stretch only to the point where you feel tightness or resistance to stretch or perhaps some discomfort. Stretching should not be painful.

Increases in range of motion will be specific to whatever joint is being stretched.

Exercise caution when stretching muscles that surround painful joints. Pain is an indication that something is wrong and should not be ignored.

Avoid overstretching the ligaments and capsules that surround joints.

Exercise caution when stretching the low back and neck. Exercises that compress the vertebrae and their disks may cause damage.

Stretching from a seated position rather than a standing position takes stress off the low back and decreases the chances of back injury.

Stretch those muscles that are tight and inflexible.

Strengthen those muscles that are weak and loose.

Always stretch slowly and with control.

Be sure to continue normal breathing during a stretch. Do not hold your breath.

Static and PNF techniques are most often recommended for individuals who want to improve their range of motion.

Ballistic stretching should be done only by those who are already flexible or are accustomed to stretching and done only after static stretching.

Stretching should be done at least three times per week to see minimal improvement. It is recommended that you stretch five or six times per week to see maximum results.

knee extension, the antagonist muscle would be the hamstring group. Some degree of balance in strength between agonist and antagonist muscle groups is necessary for normal smooth coordinated movement and for reducing the likelihood of muscle strain caused by muscular imbalance.

Ballistic Stretching

ballistic stretching
Older stretching technique that uses repetitive bouncing motions.

Ballistic stretching involves a bouncing movement in which repetitive contractions of the agonist muscle are used to produce quick stretches of the antagonist muscle. The ballistic stretching technique, although apparently effective in improving range of motion, has been criticized because increased range of motion is achieved through a series of jerks or pulls on the resistant muscle tissue. If the forces generated by the jerks are greater than the tissues' extensibility, muscle injury may result.

Successive forceful contractions of the agonist that results in stretching of the antagonist may cause muscle soreness. For example, forcefully kicking a soccer ball 50 times may result in muscular soreness of the hamstrings (antagonist muscle) as a result of eccentric contraction of the hamstrings to control the dynamic movement of the quadriceps (agonist muscle). Ballistic stretching that is controlled usually does not cause muscle soreness.

Static Stretching

static stretching
Passively stretching an antagonist muscle by placing it in a maximal stretch and holding it there.

The **static stretching** technique is a widely used and effective technique of stretching. This technique involves passively stretching a given antagonist muscle by placing it in a maximal position of stretch and holding it there for an extended time.

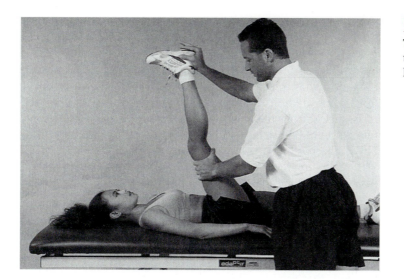

Figure 3-5

The slow-reversal-hold-relax technique for stretching the hamstring muscles.

Recommendations for the optimal time for holding this stretched position vary, ranging from as short as 3 seconds to as long as 60 seconds.[20] Data are inconclusive at present; however, it appears that 30 seconds may be a good time. The static stretch of each muscle should be repeated three or four times.

Much research has been done comparing ballistic and static stretching techniques for the improvement of flexibility. It has been shown that both static and ballistic stretching are effective in increasing flexibility and that there is no significant difference between the two. However, with static stretching there is less danger of exceeding the extensibility limits of the involved joints because the stretch is more controlled. Ballistic stretching is apt to cause muscular soreness, whereas static stretching generally does not and is commonly used in injury rehabilitation of sore or strained muscles.[8]

Static stretching is certainly a much safer stretching technique, especially for sedentary or untrained individuals. However, many physical activities involve dynamic movement. Thus stretching as a warm-up for these types of activity should begin with static stretching followed by ballistic stretching, which more closely resembles the dynamic activity.

PNF Stretching Techniques

The **PNF techniques** were first used by physical therapists for treating patients who had various types of neuromuscular paralysis.[20] Only recently have PNF stretching exercises been used as a stretching technique for increasing flexibility.

There are a number of different PNF techniques currently being used for stretching, including slow-reversal-hold-relax, contract-relax, and hold-relax techniques.[20] All involve some combination of alternating contraction and relaxation of both agonist and antagonist muscles (a 10-second pushing phase followed by a 10-second relaxing phase). Using a hamstring stretching technique as an example (Figure 3-5), the slow-reversal-hold-relax technique would be done as follows. With the athlete lying supine with the knee extended and the ankle flexed to 90 degrees, the athletic trainer passively flexes the hip joint to the point at which there is slight discomfort in the muscle. At this point the athlete begins pushing against the athletic trainer's resistance by contracting the hamstring muscle. After pushing for 10 seconds, the hamstring muscles are relaxed and the agonist quadriceps muscle is contracted while the athletic trainer applies passive pressure to further stretch the antagonist hamstrings. This should move the leg so that there is increased hip joint flexion. The relaxing phase lasts for 10 seconds, at which time the athlete pushes against the ath-

proprioceptive neuromuscular facilitation (PNF)
Stretching techniques that involve combinations of alternating contractions and stretches.

letic trainer's resistance, beginning at this new joint angle. The push-relax sequence is repeated at least three times.[28]

The contract-relax and hold-relax techniques are variations on the slow-reversal-hold-relax method. In the contract-relax method, the hamstrings are isotonically contracted so that the leg actually moves toward the floor during the push phase. The hold-relax method involves an isometric hamstring contraction against immovable resistance during the push phase. During the relax phase, both techniques involve relaxation of hamstrings and quadriceps while the hamstrings are passively stretched. This same basic PNF technique can be used to stretch any muscle in the body. The PNF stretching techniques are perhaps best performed with a partner, although they may also be done using a wall as resistance. (See Chapter 15.)

Neurophysiologic Basis of Stretching

All three stretching techniques are based on a neurophysiologic phenomenon involving the *stretch reflex* (Figure 3-6).[28] Every muscle in the body contains mechanoreceptors that when stimulated inform the central nervous system of what is happening with that muscle. Two of these receptors are important in the stretch reflex: the *muscle spindles* and the *Golgi tendon organs.* Both types of receptors are sensitive to changes in muscle length. The Golgi tendon organs are also affected by changes in muscle tension.

When a muscle is stretched, the muscle spindles are also stretched, sending a volley of sensory impulses to the spinal cord that informs the central nervous system that the muscle is being stretched. Impulses return to the muscle from the spinal cord, which causes the muscle to reflexively contract, thus resisting the stretch.[28] If the stretch of the muscle continues for an extended period of time (at least 6 seconds), the Golgi tendon organs respond to the change in length and the increase in tension

Figure 3-6

Stretch reflex. The muscle spindle produces a reflex resistance to stretch, and the Golgi tendon organ causes a reflex relaxation of the muscle in response to stretch.

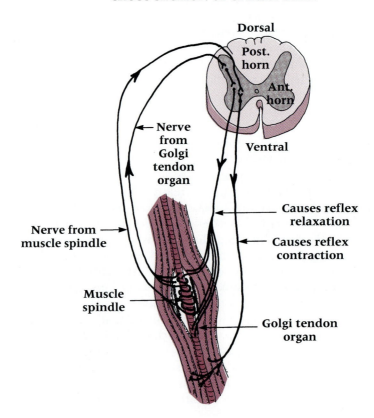

CROSS SECTION OF SPINAL CORD

Dorsal

Post. horn

Ant. horn

Ventral

Nerve from Golgi tendon organ

Nerve from muscle spindle

Causes reflex relaxation

Causes reflex contraction

Muscle spindle

Golgi tendon organ

by firing off sensory impulses of their own to the spinal cord. The impulses from the Golgi tendon organs, unlike the signals from the muscle spindle, cause a reflex relaxation of the antagonist muscle. This reflex relaxation serves as a protective mechanism that will allow the muscle to stretch through relaxation before the extensibility limits are exceeded, causing damage to the muscle fibers.

With the jerking, bouncing motion of ballistic stretching the muscle spindles are being repetitively stretched; thus there is continuous resistance by the muscle to further stretch. The ballistic stretch is not continued long enough to allow the Golgi tendon organs to have any relaxing effect.

The static stretch involves a continuous sustained stretch lasting anywhere from 6 to 60 seconds, which is sufficient time for the Golgi tendon organs to begin responding to the increase in tension. The impulses from the Golgi tendon organs have the ability to override the impulses coming from the muscle spindles, allowing the muscle to reflexively relax after the initial reflex resistance to the change in length. Thus lengthening the muscle and allowing it to remain in a stretched position for an extended period of time is unlikely to produce any injury to the muscle.

The effectiveness of the PNF techniques may be attributed in part to these same neurophysiologic principles. The slow-reversal-hold technique discussed previously takes advantage of two additional neurophysiologic phenomena.[28] The maximal isometric contraction of the muscle that will be stretched during the 10-second push phase again causes an increase in tension, which stimulates the Golgi tendon organs to effect a reflex relaxation of the antagonist even before the muscle is placed in a position of stretch. This relaxation of the antagonist muscle during contractions is referred to as **autogenic inhibition.**

During the relaxing phase the antagonist is relaxed and passively stretched while there is a maximal isotonic contraction of the agonist muscle pulling the extremity further into the agonist pattern. In any synergistic muscle group, a contraction of the agonist causes a reflex relaxation in the antagonist muscle, allowing it to stretch and protecting it from injury. This phenomenon is referred to as *reciprocal inhibition* (Figure 3-7). Thus with the PNF techniques the additive effects of autogenic inhibition and reciprocal inhibition should theoretically allow the muscle to be stretched to a greater degree than is possible with static stretching or the ballistic technique.[28]

autogenic inhibition
The relaxation of the antagonist muscle during contractions.

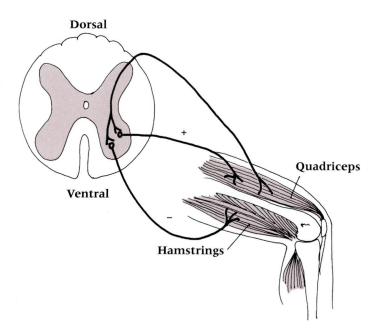

Figure 3-7

A contraction of the agonist will produce relaxation in the antagonist.

Practical Application

Although all three stretching techniques have been demonstrated to effectively improve flexibility, there is still considerable debate as to which technique produces the greatest increases in range of movement. The ballistic technique is seldom recommended because of the potential for causing muscle soreness. However, it must be added that most sport activities are ballistic in nature (e.g., kicking, running), and those activities use the stretch reflex to enhance performance. In highly trained individuals, it is unlikely that ballistic stretching will result in muscle soreness. Static stretching is perhaps the most widely used technique. It is a simple technique and does not require a partner. A fully nonrestricted range of motion can be attained through static stretching over time.[3]

The PNF stretching techniques are capable of producing dramatic increases in range of motion during one stretching session. Studies comparing static and PNF stretching suggest that PNF stretching is capable of producing greater improvement in flexibility over an extended training period.[28] The major disadvantage of PNF stretching is that a partner is required for stretching, although stretching with a partner may have some motivational advantages. An increasing number of athletic teams are adopting the PNF technique as the method of choice for improving flexibility.

The Relationship between Strength and Flexibility

It is often said that strength training has a negative effect on flexibility. For example, someone who develops large bulk through strength training is often referred to as "muscle-bound." The term *muscle-bound* has negative connotations in terms of the ability of that athlete to move. We tend to think of athletes who have highly developed muscles as having lost much of their ability to move freely through a full range of motion. Occasionally an athlete develops so much bulk that the physical size of the muscle prevents a normal range of motion. It is certainly true that strength training that is not properly done can impair movement; however, there is no reason to believe that weight training, if done properly through a full range of motion, will impair flexibility. Proper strength training probably improves dynamic flexibility and, if combined with a rigorous stretching program, can greatly enhance powerful and coordinated movements that are essential for success in many athletic activities. In all cases a heavy weight-training program should be accompanied by a strong flexibility program.

Assessment of Flexibility

Accurate measurement of the range of joint motion is difficult. Various devices have been designed to accommodate variations in the size of the joints and the complexity of movements in articulations that involve more than one joint. Of these devices, the simplest and most widely used is the goniometer (Figure 3-8). A goniometer is a large protractor with measurements in degrees. By aligning the two arms parallel to the longitudinal axis of the two segments involved in motion about a specific joint, it is possible to obtain relatively accurate measures of range of movement. The goniometer has its place in a rehabilitation setting, where it is essential to assess improvement in joint flexibility for the purpose of modifying injury rehabilitation programs.

THE IMPORTANCE OF MUSCULAR STRENGTH

The development of **muscular strength** is an essential component of a training program for every athlete. By definition, strength is the ability of a muscle to generate force against some resistance. Most movements in sports are explosive and must include elements of both strength and speed if they are to be effective. If a large amount of force is generated quickly, the movement can be referred to as a power movement. Without the ability to generate power, an athlete will be limited in his or her performance capabilities.[18,27,29]

3-3

Critical Thinking Exercise

A college swimmer has been engaged in an offseason weight-training program to increase her muscular strength and endurance. Although she has seen some improvement in her strength she is concerned that she also seems to be losing flexibility in her shoulders, which she feels is critical to her performance as a swimmer. She has also noticed that her muscles are hypertrophying to some degree and is worried that that may be causing her to lose flexibility. She has just about decided to abandon her weight-training program altogether.

? What can the athletic trainer recommend to her that will allow her to continue to improve her muscular strength and endurance while simultaneously maintaining or perhaps even improving her flexibility?

muscular strength
The maximum force that can be applied by a muscle during a single maximum contraction.

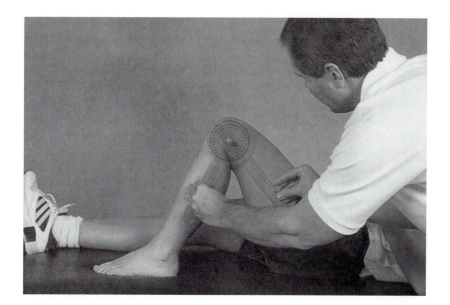

Figure 3-8
A goniometer can be used to measure joint angles.

Muscular strength is closely associated with muscular endurance. **Muscular endurance** is the ability to perform repetitive muscular contractions against some resistance for an extended period of time. As muscular strength increases, there tends to be a corresponding increase in endurance. For example, an athlete can lift a weight 25 times. If muscular strength is increased by 10% through weight training, it is likely that the maximum number of repetitions would be increased because it is easier for the athlete to lift the weight.

muscular endurance
The ability to perform repetitive muscular contractions against some resistance.

Skeletal Muscle Contractions

Skeletal muscle is capable of three different types of contraction: *isometric contraction,* *concentric contraction,* and *eccentric contraction.*[31] An isometric contraction occurs when the muscle contracts to produce tension but there is no change in length of the muscle. Considerable force can be generated against some immovable resistance even though no movement occurs. In concentric contraction the muscle shortens in length as tension is developed to overcome or move some resistance. In eccentric contraction the resistance is greater than the muscular force being produced and the muscle lengthens while producing tension. Concentric and eccentric contractions are both considered to be dynamic movements.[31]

Skeletal muscle is capable of three types of contractions:
  Isometric
  Concentric
  Eccentric

Fast-Twitch versus Slow-Twitch Fibers

All fibers in a particular motor unit are either *slow-twitch* or *fast-twitch* fibers, each of which has distinctive metabolic and contractile capabilities. Slow-twitch fibers are also referred to as type I fibers. They are more resistant to fatigue than are fast-twitch fibers; however, the time required to generate force is much greater in slow-twitch fibers.[23] Because they are relatively fatigue resistant, slow-twitch fibers are associated primarily with long-duration, aerobic-type activities.

There are three basic types of muscle fibers:
  Slow-twitch type I
  Fast-twitch type IIa
  Fast-twitch type IIb

Fast-twitch fibers (also referred to as type II fibers) are capable of producing quick, forceful contractions but have a tendency to fatigue more rapidly than do slow-twitch fibers. Fast-twitch fibers are useful in short-term, high-intensity activities, which mainly involve the anaerobic system. Fast-twitch fibers are capable of producing powerful contractions, whereas slow-twitch fibers produce a long-endurance type of force. There are two subdivisions of fast-twitch fibers. Although both types of fast-twitch fibers are capable of rapid contraction, type IIa fibers are moderately resistant to fatigue whereas type IIb fibers fatigue rapidly and are considered the "true" fast-twitch fibers.

Within a particular muscle are both types of fibers, and the ratio in an individual muscle varies with each person.[23] Those muscles whose primary function is to maintain posture against gravity require more endurance and have a higher percentage of slow-twitch fibers. Muscles that produce powerful, rapid, explosive strength movements tend to have a much greater percentage of fast-twitch fibers. Because this ratio is genetically determined, it may play a large role in determining ability for a given sport activity. Sprinters and weight lifters, for example, have a large percentage of fast-twitch fibers in relation to slow-twitch fibers.[6] Conversely, marathon runners generally have a higher percentage of slow-twitch fibers.

The metabolic capabilities of both fast-twitch and slow-twitch fibers may be improved through specific strength and endurance training. It now appears that there can be an almost complete change from slow-twitch to fast-twitch and from fast-twitch to slow-twitch fiber types in response to training.[23]

Factors that Determine Levels of Muscular Strength

Muscular strength is proportional to the cross-sectional diameter of the muscle fibers. The greater the cross-sectional diameter or the bigger a particular muscle, the stronger it is, and thus the more force it is capable of generating. The size of a muscle tends to increase in cross-sectional diameter with weight training. This increase in muscle size is referred to as **hypertrophy.**[16] Conversely, a decrease in the size of a muscle is referred to as **atrophy.**

hypertrophy
Enlargement of a muscle caused by an increase in the size of its cells in response to training.

atrophy
Decrease of a muscle caused by the decrease in the size of its cells because of inactivity.

Strength is a function of the number and diameter of muscle fibers composing a given muscle. The number of fibers is an inherited characteristic; thus an athlete with a large number of muscle fibers to begin with has the potential to hypertrophy to a much greater degree than does someone with relatively fewer fibers.[14]

Strength is also directly related to the efficiency of the neuromuscular system and the function of the motor unit in producing muscular force. Initial increases in strength during a weight-training program can be attributed primarily to increased neuromuscular efficiency.

Strength in a given muscle is determined not only by the physical properties of the muscle itself but also by biomechanical factors that dictate how much force can be generated through a system of levers to an external object. If we think of the elbow joint as one of these lever systems, we would have the biceps and muscle producing flexion of this joint (Figure 3-9). The position of attachment of the biceps muscle on the lever arm, in this case the forearm, will largely determine how much force this muscle is capable of generating. If there are two persons, **A** and **B,** and **A** has a biceps attachment that is closer to the fulcrum (the elbow joint) than **B,** **A** must produce a greater effort with the biceps muscle to hold the weight at a right angle because the length of the lever arm will be greater than with **B.**

The length of a muscle determines the tension that can be generated. By varying the length of a muscle different tensions may be produced. This length-tension relationship is illustrated in Figure 3-10. At position **B** in the curve, the interaction of the crossbridges between the actin and myosin myofilaments within the sarcomere is at a maximum. Setting a muscle at this particular length will produce the greatest amount of tension. At position **A** the muscle is shortened, and at position **C** the muscle is lengthened. In either case the interaction between the actin and myosin myofilaments through the crossbridges is greatly reduced and the muscle is not capable of generating significant tension.

Overtraining can have a negative effect on the development of muscular strength. The statement "if you abuse it you will lose it" is applicable. Overtraining can result in psychological breakdown (staleness) or physiological breakdown, which may involve musculoskeletal injury, fatigue, or sickness. Engaging in proper and efficient resistance training, eating a proper diet, and getting appropriate rest can minimize the potential negative effects of overtraining.

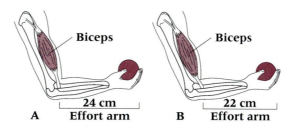

Figure 3-9

The position of attachment of the muscle tendon on the arm can affect the ability of that muscle to generate force. **B** should be able to generate greater force than **A** because the tendon attachment is closer to the resistance.

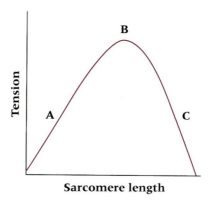

Figure 3-10

Because of the length-tension relation in muscle, the greatest tension is developed at point **B** with less tension developed at points **A** and **C.**

Gains in muscular strength resulting from resistance training are reversible. Athletes who interrupt or stop resistance training altogether will see rapid decreases in strength gains. "If you don't use it you'll lose it."

Physiology of Strength Development

A number of theories have been proposed to explain why a muscle hypertrophies in response to strength training.[10] Some evidence exists that there is an increase in the number of muscle fibers because fibers split in response to training.[14] However, this research has been conducted in animals and should not be generalized to humans. It is generally accepted that the number of fibers is genetically determined and does not seem to increase with training.

It has been hypothesized that because the muscle is working harder in weight training, more blood is required to supply that muscle with oxygen and other nutrients. Thus it is thought that the number of capillaries is increased. This hypothesis is only partially correct; few new capillaries are formed during strength training, but a number of dormant capillaries may become filled with blood to meet this increased demand for blood supply.

A third theory to explain this increase in muscle size seems the most credible. Muscle fibers are composed primarily of small protein filaments, called myofilaments, which are the contractile elements in muscle. These myofilaments increase in both size and number as a result of strength training, causing the individual muscle fibers themselves to increase in cross-sectional diameter.[23] This is particularly true in men, although women also see some increase in muscle size.[5] More research is needed to further clarify and determine the specific causes of muscle hypertrophy.

Other Physiological Adaptations to Resistance Exercise

In addition to muscle hypertrophy there are a number of other physiological adaptations to resistance training. The strength of noncontractile structures, including tendons and ligaments, is increased. The mineral content of bone is increased, making the bone stronger and more resistant to fracture. Maximal oxygen uptake is improved when resistance training is of sufficient intensity to elicit heart rates at or above training levels. There is also an increase in several enzymes important in aerobic and anaerobic metabolism.[12]

Techniques of Resistance Training

There are a number of different techniques of resistance training for strength improvement, including isometric exercise, progressive resistive exercise, isokinetic training, circuit training, and plyometric exercise. Regardless of which of these techniques is used, one basic principle of training is extremely important. For a muscle to improve in strength, it must be forced to work at a higher level than that to which it is accustomed. In other words, the muscle must be *overloaded*. Without overload the muscle will be able to maintain strength as long as training is continued against a resistance the muscle is accustomed to. To most effectively build muscular strength, weight training requires a consistent, increasing effort against progressively increasing resistance. Progressive resistive exercise is based primarily on the principles of overload and progression. If this principle of overload is applied, all three training techniques will produce improvement of muscular strength over a period of time.

Isometric Exercise

isometric exercise
Contracts the muscle statically without changing its length.

An **isometric exercise** involves a muscle contraction in which the length of the muscle remains constant while tension develops toward a maximal force against an immovable resistance.[12,30] The muscle should generate a maximal force for 10 seconds at a time, and this contraction should be repeated 5 to 10 times per day. Isometric exercises are capable of increasing muscular strength; unfortunately, strength gains are specific to the joint angle at which training is performed. At other angles, the strength curve drops off dramatically because of a lack of motor activity at that angle.

Another major disadvantage of isometric exercises is that they tend to produce a spike in blood pressure that can result in potentially life-threatening cardiovascular accidents.[12] This sharp increase in blood pressure results from holding one's breath and increasing intrathoracic pressure. Consequently, the blood pressure experienced by the heart is increased significantly. This has been referred to as the Valsalva effect. To avoid or minimize this effect, it is recommended that breathing be done during the maximal contraction to prevent this increase in pressure.

Isometric exercises are useful in the rehabilitation of certain injuries as will be discussed in later chapters.

Progressive Resistive Exercise

A second technique of resistance training is perhaps the most commonly used and most popular technique for improving muscular strength. Progressive resistive exercise training uses exercises that strengthen muscles through a contraction that overcomes some fixed resistance such as with dumbells, barbells, or various weight machines (Figure 3-11). Progressive resistive exercise uses isotonic contractions in which force is generated while the muscle is changing in length.[7]

concentric (positive) contraction
The muscle shortens while contracting against resistance.

Isotonic contractions may be either concentric or eccentric. If an athlete is performing a biceps curl, to lift the weight from the starting position the biceps muscle must contract and shorten in length. This shortening contraction is referred to as a **concentric** or **positive contraction.** If the biceps muscle does not remain contracted when the weight is being lowered, gravity will cause the weight to simply fall back to the starting position. Thus to control the weight as it is being lowered, the biceps muscle must continue to contract while at the same time gradually lengthening. A contraction in which the muscle is lengthening while still applying force is called an **eccentric** or **negative contraction.**

eccentric (negative) contraction
The muscle lengthens while contracting against resistance.

It is possible to generate greater amounts of force against resistance with an eccentric contraction than with a concentric contraction. This may be explained by the fact that eccentric contractions require a much lower level of motor unit activity to achieve a certain force than do concentric contractions. Because fewer motor units

CHAPTER 3 Training and Conditioning Techniques

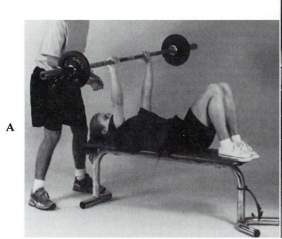

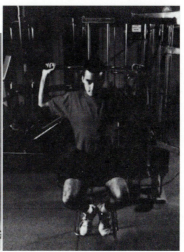

A   **B**

Figure 3-11

A, Barbells and dumbells are free weights that assist the athlete in developing isotonic strength. **B,** Many machine exercise systems provide a variety of exercise possibilities for the athlete.

are firing to produce a specific force, additional motor units may be recruited to generate increased force. In addition, oxygen utilization is much lower during eccentric exercise than in comparable concentric exercise. Thus eccentric contractions are less resistant to fatigue than are concentric contractions. The mechanical efficiency of eccentric exercise may be several times higher than that of concentric exercise.[31]

Various types of exercise equipment can be used with progressive resistive exercise, including free weights (barbells and dumbells) or exercise machines such as Universal, Nautilus, Cybex, Eagle, and Body Master. Dumbells and barbells require the use of iron plates of varying weights that can be easily changed by adding or subtracting equal amounts of weight to both sides of the bar. The exercise machines have a stack of weights that are lifted through a series of levers or pulleys. The stack of weights slides up and down on a pair of bars that restrict the movement to only one plane. Weight can be increased or decreased simply by changing the position of a weight key.

There are advantages and disadvantages to both free weights and machines. The exercise machines are relatively safe to use in comparison with free weights. It is also a simple process to increase or decrease the weight by moving a single weight key with the exercise machines, although changes can generally be made only in increments of 10 or 15 pounds. With free weights, iron plates must be added or removed from each side of the barbell.

Regardless of which type of equipment is used, the same principles of **isotonic training** may be applied. In progressive resistive exercise it is essential to incorporate both concentric and eccentric contractions. Research has clearly demonstrated that the muscle should be overloaded and fatigued both concentrically and eccentrically for the greatest strength improvement to occur.[11,23]

When training specifically for the development of muscular strength, the concentric or positive portion of the exercise should require 1 to 2 seconds and the eccentric or negative portion of the lift should require 2 to 4 seconds. The ratio of negative to positive should be approximately 1 to 2. Physiologically, the muscle will fatigue much more rapidly concentrically than eccentrically.

Athletes who have strength trained using both free weights and machines realize the difference in the amount of weight that can be lifted. Unlike the machines, free weights have no restricted motion and can thus move in many different directions, depending on the forces applied. With free weights, an element of muscular control on the part of the lifter to prevent the weight from moving in any direction other than vertical will usually decrease the amount of weight that can be lifted.[33]

One problem often mentioned in relation to isotonic training is that the amount of force necessary to move a weight through a range of motion changes according to

isotonic exercise
Shortens and lengthens the muscle through a complete range of motion.

the angle of pull of the contracting muscle. It is greatest when the angle of pull is approximately 90 degrees. In addition, once the inertia of the weight has been overcome and momentum has been established, the force required to move the resistance varies according to the force that the muscle can produce through the range of motion. Thus it has been argued that a disadvantage of any type of isotonic exercise is that force required to move the resistance is constantly changing throughout the range of movement.

The design of certain exercise machines tries to minimize this change in resistance by using a cam system (Figure 3-12). The cam has been individually designed for each piece of equipment so that the resistance is variable throughout the movement. It attempts to alter resistance so that the muscle can handle a greater load, but at the points where the joint angle or muscle length is mechanically disadvantageous, it reduces the resistance to muscle movement. Whether this design does what it claims is debatable. This change in resistance at different points in the range has been labeled accommodating resistance, or variable resistance.

Progressive Resistive Exercise Techniques

Perhaps the single most confusing aspect of progressive resistive exercise is the terminology used to describe specific programs. The following list of terms with their operational definitions may help clarify the confusion:

- Repetitions—number of times a specific movement is repeated.
- Repetitions maximum (RM)—maximum number of repetitions at a given weight.
- Set—a particular number of repetitions.
- Intensity—the amount of weight or resistance lifted.
- Recovery period—the rest interval between sets.
- Frequency—the number of times an exercise is done in 1 week.

A considerable amount of research has been done in the area of resistance training to determine optimal techniques in terms of the intensity or the amount of weight to be used, the number of repetitions, the number of sets, the recovery period, and the frequency of training. It is important to realize that there are many different effective techniques and training regimens. Regardless of specific techniques used, it is certain that to improve strength the muscle must be overloaded in a progressive manner. This is the basis of progressive resistive exercise. The amount of weight used and the number of repetitions must be enough to make the muscle work at a higher intensity than it is used to. This is the single most critical factor in any strength-training program. It is also essential to design the strength-training program to meet the specific needs of the athlete.

There is no such thing as an optimal strength training program. Achieving total agreement on a program of resistance training that includes specific recommendations relative to repetitions, sets, intensity, recovery time, and frequency among re-

Figure 3-12

The cam system on the Nautilus equipment is designed to equalize the resistance throughout the full range of motion.

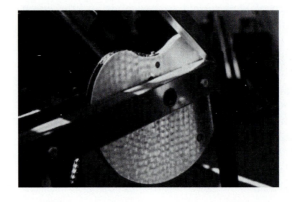

searchers or other experts in resistance training is impossible. However, the following general recommendations will provide an effective resistance training program.

For any given exercise, the amount of weight selected should be sufficient to allow six to eight repetitions maximum (RM) in each of the three sets with a recovery period of 60 to 90 seconds between sets. Initial selection of a starting weight may require some trial and error to achieve this 6 to 8 RM range. If at least three sets of six repetitions cannot be completed, the weight is too heavy and should be reduced. If it is possible to do more than three sets of eight repetitions, the weight is too light and should be increased.[5] Progression to heavier weights is determined by the ability to perform at least 8 RM in each of three sets. An increase of about 10% of the current weight being lifted should still allow at least 6 RM in each of three sets.

A particular muscle or muscle group should be exercised consistently every other day. Thus the frequency of weight training should be at least three times per week but no more than four times per week. It is common for serious weight trainers to lift every day; however, they exercise different muscle groups on successive days. For example, Monday, Wednesday, and Friday may be used for upper body muscles, whereas Tuesday, Thursday, and Saturday are used for lower body muscles.

Training for muscular strength versus endurance   Muscular endurance is the ability to perform repeated muscle contractions against resistance for an extended period of time. Most weight-training experts believe that muscular strength and muscular endurance are closely related.[27] As one improves, there is a tendency for the other to improve also.

It is generally accepted that when weight training for strength, heavier weights with a lower number of repetitions should be used. Conversely, endurance training uses relatively lighter weights with a greater number of repetitions.

It has been suggested that endurance training should consist of three sets of 10 to 15 repetitions using the same criteria for weight selection, progression, and frequency as recommended for progressive resistive exercise.[5] Thus suggested training regimens for muscular strength and endurance are similar in terms of sets and numbers of repetitions. Persons who possess great levels of strength tend to also exhibit greater muscular endurance when asked to perform repeated contractions against resistance.

Isokinetic Exercise

An **isokinetic exercise** involves a muscle contraction in which the length of the muscle is changing while the contraction is performed at a constant velocity.[25] In theory, maximal resistance is provided throughout the range of motion by the machine. The resistance provided by the machine will move only at some preset speed regardless of the force applied to it by the individual. Thus the key to isokinetic exercise is not the resistance but the speed at which resistance can be moved.

Several isokinetic devices are available commercially; Cybex, Biodex, Kin-Com, and Lido are among the more common isokinetic machines (Figure 3-13). In gen-

isokinetic exercise
Resistance is given at a fixed velocity of movement with accommodating resistance.

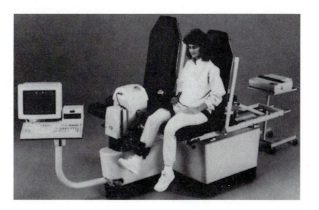

Figure 3-13
During isokinetic exercising the amount of resistance depends on the extent of force applied by the athlete.

eral, they rely on hydraulic, pneumatic, and mechanical pressure systems to produce constant velocity of motion. The majority of the isokinetic devices are capable of resisting both concentric and eccentric contractions at a fixed speed to exercise a muscle.

A major disadvantage of these units is their cost. Many of them come with a computer and printing device and are used primarily as diagnostic and rehabilitative tools in the treatment of various injuries.

Isokinetic devices are designed so that regardless of the amount of force applied against a resistance, it can be moved only at a certain speed. That speed will be the same whether maximal force or only half the maximal force is applied. Consequently, when training isokinetically, it is absolutely necessary to exert as much force against the resistance as possible (maximal effort) for maximal strength gains to occur. This is one of the major problems with an isokinetic strength-training program.

Anyone who has been involved in a weight-training program knows that on some days it is difficult to find the motivation to work out. Because isokinetic training requires a maximal effort, it is easy to "cheat" and not go through the workout at a high level of intensity. In a progressive resistive exercise program, one knows how much weight has to be lifted with how many repetitions. Thus isokinetic training is often more effective if a partner system is used primarily as a means of motivation toward a maximal effort.

When isokinetic training is done properly with a maximal effort, it is theoretically possible that maximal strength gains are best achieved through the isokinetic training method in which the velocity and force of the resistance are equal throughout the range of motion. However, there is no conclusive research to support this theory. Whether changing force capability is in fact a deterrent to improving the ability to generate force against some resistance is debatable.

In the athletic training setting, isokinetics are perhaps best used as a rehabilitative and diagnostic tool rather than as a training device.[19]

Circuit Training

circuit training

Exercise stations that consist of various combinations of weight training, flexibility, calisthenics, and aerobic exercises.

Circuit training employs a series of exercise stations that consist of various combinations of weight training, flexibility, calisthenics, and brief aerobic exercises. Circuits may be designed to accomplish many different training goals. With circuit training one moves rapidly from one station to the next and performs whatever exercise is to be done at that station within a specified time period. A typical circuit would consist of 8 to 12 stations, and the entire circuit would be repeated three times.

Circuit training is most definitely an effective technique for improving strength and flexibility. Certainly, if the pace or the time interval between stations is rapid and if workload is maintained at a high level of intensity with heart rate at or above target training levels, the cardiorespiratory system may benefit from this circuit. However, there is little research evidence that shows that circuit training is effective in improving cardiorespiratory endurance. It should be and is most often used as a technique for developing and improving muscular strength and endurance.

Calisthenic Strengthening Exercises

Calisthenics, or free exercise, is one of the more easily available means of developing strength. Isotonic movement exercises can be graded according to intensity by using gravity as an aid, ruling gravity out, moving against gravity, or using the body or body part as a resistance against gravity. Most calisthenics require the athlete to support the body or move the total body against the force of gravity. Push-ups are a good example of a vigorous antigravity free exercise. To be considered maximally effective, the isotonic calisthenic exercise, as in all types of exercise, must be performed in an exacting manner and in full range of motion. In most cases, 10 or more repetitions are performed for each exercise and are repeated in sets of two or three.

Some free exercises have an isometric or holding phase instead of using a full range of motion. Examples of these are back extensions and sit-ups. When the exercise produces maximum muscle tension, it is held between 6 and 10 seconds and then repeated one to three times.

Plyometric Exercise

Plyometric exercise is a technique that includes specific exercises which encompass a rapid stretch of a muscle eccentrically, followed immediately by a rapid concentric contraction of that muscle for the purpose of facilitating and developing a forceful explosive movement over a short period of time.[9] The greater the stretch put on the muscle from its resting length immediately before the concentric contraction, the greater the resistance the muscle can overcome. Plyometric exercises emphasize the speed of the eccentric phase. The rate of stretch is more critical than the magnitude of the stretch. An advantage to using plyometric exercises is that they can help develop eccentric control in dynamic movements.

Plyometric exercises involve hops, bounds, and depth jumping for the lower extremity and the use of medicine balls and other types of weighted equipment for the upper extremity. Depth jumping is an example of a plyometric exercise in which an individual jumps to the ground from a specified height and then quickly jumps again as soon as ground contact is made.[9]

Plyometrics place a great deal of stress on the musculoskeletal system. The learning and perfection of specific jumping skills and other plyometric exercises must be technically correct and specific to one's age, activity, and physical and skill development.

STRENGTH TRAINING FOR THE FEMALE ATHLETE

Strength training is critical for the female athlete.[24] The average female is incapable of building significant muscle bulk through weight training. Significant muscle hypertrophy is dependent on the presence of the anabolic steroidal hormone testosterone. Testosterone is considered a male hormone, although all women possess some testosterone in their systems. Women with higher testosterone levels tend to have more masculine characteristics such as increased facial and body hair, a deeper voice, and the potential to develop a little more muscle bulk.[23]

With weight training, the female sees some remarkable gains in strength initially, even though muscle bulk does not increase. For a muscle to contract, an impulse must be transmitted from the nervous system to the muscle. Each muscle fiber is innervated by a specific motor unit. By overloading a particular muscle, as in weight training, the muscle is forced to work efficiently. Efficiency is achieved by getting more motor units to fire, causing a stronger contraction of the muscle. Consequently, it is not uncommon for a female to see extremely rapid gains in strength when a weight-training program is first begun. These tremendous initial strength gains, which can be attributed to improved neuromuscular system efficiency, tend to plateau, and minimal improvement in muscular strength will be realized during a continuing strength-training program. These initial neuromuscular strength gains will also be seen in men, although their strength will continue to increase with appropriate training.

Perhaps the most critical difference between males and females regarding physical performance is the ratio of strength to body weight. The reduced **strength–body weight ratio** in women is the result of their higher percentage of body fat. The strength–body weight ratio may be significantly improved through weight training by decreasing the body fat percentage while increasing lean weight.

CARDIORESPIRATORY ENDURANCE

By definition, **cardiorespiratory endurance** is the ability to perform whole-body large muscle activities for extended periods of time. The cardiorespiratory system provides a means by which oxygen is supplied to the various tissues of the body. For the athlete it is critical for both performance and preventing undue fatigue that may predispose to injury.

plyometric exercise
This type of exercise maximizes the myotatic or stretch reflex.

3-4
Critical Thinking Exercise

A high school shot-putter has been working intensely on weight training to improve his muscular power. In particular he has been concentrating on lifting extremely heavy free weights using a low number of repetitions (three sets of six to eight repetitions). Although his strength has improved significantly over the last several months he is not seeing the same degree of improvement in his throws even though his coach says that his technique is very good.

? The athlete is frustrated with his performance and wants to know if there is anything else he can do in his training program that might enhance his performance.

cardiorespiratory endurance
Ability to perform activities for extended periods of time.

Transport and Utilization of Oxygen

Basically, transport of oxygen throughout the body involves the coordinated function of four components: the heart, the lungs, the blood vessels, and the blood. The improvement of cardiorespiratory endurance through training occurs because of the increased capability of each of these four elements in providing necessary oxygen to the working tissues. The greatest rate at which oxygen can be taken in and used during exercise is referred to as maximal oxygen consumption ($\dot{V}O_2$max).[2] The performance of any activity requires a certain rate of oxygen consumption that is about the same for all persons, depending on the level of fitness. Generally, the greater the rate or intensity of the performance of an activity, the greater the oxygen consumption. Each person has his or her own maximal rate of oxygen consumption. That person's ability to perform an activity (or to fatigue) is closely related to the amount of oxygen required by that activity and is limited by the maximal rate of oxygen consumption of which the person is capable. Apparently, the greater the percentage of maximum oxygen consumption required during an activity, the less time the activity may be performed (Figure 3-14).

The maximal rate at which oxygen can be used is a genetically determined characteristic; one inherits a certain range of $\dot{V}O_2$max, and the more active one is, the higher the existing $\dot{V}O_2$max will be in that range. A training program is capable of increasing $\dot{V}O_2$max to its highest limit within that range. Maximal oxygen consumption is most often presented in terms of the volume of oxygen used relative to body weight per unit of time (ml/kg/min). A normal $\dot{V}O_2$max for most college-age athletes would fall somewhere in the range of 45 to 60 ml/kg/min.[2] A world-class male marathon runner may have a $\dot{V}O_2$max in the 70 to 80 ml/kg/min range.

Three factors determine the maximal rate at which oxygen can be used: external respiration, involving the ventilatory process, or pulmonary function; gas transport, which is accomplished by the cardiovascular system (i.e., the heart, blood vessels, and blood); and internal respiration, which involves the use of oxygen by the cells to produce energy. Of these three factors the most limiting is generally the ability to transport oxygen through the system; thus the cardiovascular system limits the overall rate of oxygen consumption. A high $\dot{V}O_2$max within an athlete's inherited range indicates that all three systems are working well.

Effects on the Heart

The heart is the main pumping mechanism and circulates oxygenated blood throughout the body to the working tissues. As the body begins to exercise, the muscles use oxygen at a much higher rate, and the heart must pump more oxygenated blood to meet this increased demand. The heart is capable of adapting to this increased demand through several mechanisms. Heart rate shows a gradual adaptation to an increased workload by increasing proportionally to the intensity of the exercise and will plateau at a given level after about 2 to 3 minutes (Figure 3-15).

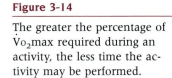

Figure 3-14

The greater the percentage of $\dot{V}O_2$max required during an activity, the less time the activity may be performed.

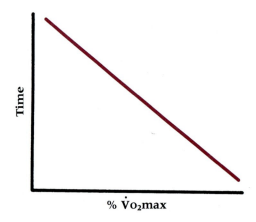

Monitoring heart rate is an indirect method of estimating oxygen consumption. In general, heart rate and oxygen consumption have a linear relationship, although at very low intensities and at high intensities this linear relationship breaks down (Figure 3-16). During higher-intensity activities maximal heart rate may be achieved before maximal oxygen consumption, which will continue to rise.[23] The greater the intensity of the exercise, the higher the heart rate. Because of these existing relationships it should become apparent that the rate of oxygen consumption can be estimated by taking heart rate.[8]

A second mechanism by which the heart is able to adapt to increased demands during exercise is to increase the stroke volume, the volume of blood being pumped out with each beat. The heart pumps out approximately 70 ml of blood per beat. Stroke volume can continue to increase only to the point at which there is simply not enough time between beats for the heart to fill up. This occurs at about 40% of maximal heart rate, and above this level increases in the volume of blood being pumped out per unit of time must be caused entirely by increases in heart rate[23] (Figure 3-17).

Stroke volume and heart rate together determine the volume of blood being pumped through the heart in a given unit of time. Approximately 5 L of blood are

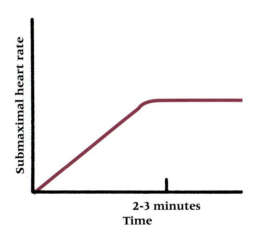

Figure 3-15

Two to three minutes are required for heart rate to plateau at a given workload.

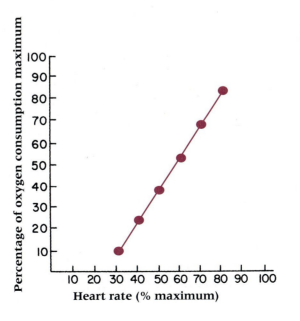

Figure 3-16

Maximal heart rate is achieved at about the same time as $\dot{V}o_2max$.

Figure 3-17

Stroke volume plateaus at
40% of maximal heart rate.

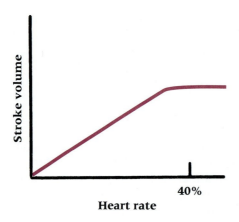

Figure 3-18

Cardiac output limits $\dot{V}_{O_2}$max.

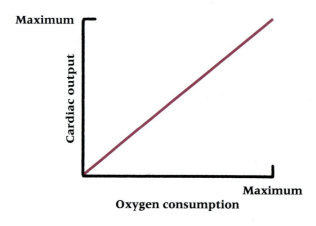

pumped through the heart during each minute at rest. This is referred to as the cardiac output, which indicates how much blood the heart is capable of pumping in exactly 1 minute. Thus cardiac output is the primary determinant of the maximal rate of oxygen consumption possible (Figure 3-18). During exercise, cardiac output increases to approximately four times that experienced during rest in the normal individual and may increase as much as six times in the elite endurance athlete.

A **training effect** that occurs with regard to cardiac output of the heart is that the stroke volume increases while exercise heart rate is reduced at a given standard exercise load. The heart becomes more efficient because it is capable of pumping more blood with each stroke. Because the heart is a muscle, it will hypertrophy to some extent, but this is in no way a negative effect of training.

training effect
Stroke volume increases while heart rate is reduced at a given exercise load.

Training Effect

$$\frac{\text{Cardiac}}{\text{output}} = \frac{\text{Increased}}{\text{stroke volume}} \times \frac{\text{Decreased}}{\text{heart rate}}$$

Effects on Work Ability

Cardiorespiratory endurance plays a critical role in our ability to resist fatigue. Fatigue is closely related to the percentage of $\dot{V}_{O_2}$max that a particular workload demands.[27] For example, Figure 3-19 presents two athletes, **A** and **B**. Athlete **A** has a $\dot{V}_{O_2}$max of 50 ml/kg/min, whereas athlete **B** has a $\dot{V}_{O_2}$max of only 40 ml/kg/min. If both **A** and **B** are exercising at the same intensity, **A** will be working at a much lower percentage of $\dot{V}_{O_2}$max than **B** is. Consequently, **A** should be able to sustain his or her activity over a much longer period of time. Athletic performance may be impaired if the ability to use oxygen efficiently is impaired. Thus improvement of cardiorespiratory endurance should be an essential component of any training program.

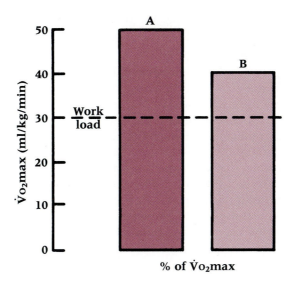

Figure 3-19

Athlete **A** should be able to work longer than Athlete **B** as a result of lower utilization of $\dot{V}o_2max$.

The Energy Systems

Various sports activities involve specific demands for energy. For example, sprinting and jumping are high-energy activities, requiring a relatively large production of energy for a short time. Long-distance running and swimming, on the other hand, are mostly low-energy activities per unit of time, requiring energy production for a prolonged time. Other physical activities demand a blend of both high- and low-energy output. These various energy demands can be met by the different processes in which energy can be supplied to the skeletal muscles.

ATP: The Immediate Energy Source

Energy is produced from the breakdown of nutrient foodstuffs.[23] This energy is used to produce adenosine triphosphate (ATP), which is the ultimate usable form of energy for muscular activity. Adenosine triphosphate is produced in the muscle tissue from blood glucose or glycogen. Glucose is derived from the breakdown of dietary carbohydrates. Glucose not needed immediately is stored as glycogen in the resting muscle and liver. Stored glycogen in the liver can later be converted back to glucose and transferred to the blood to meet the body's energy needs. Fats and proteins can also be metabolized to generate ATP.

Once much of the muscle and liver glycogen is depleted, the body relies more heavily on fats stored in adipose tissue to meet its energy needs. The longer the duration of an activity, the greater the amount of fat that is used, especially during the later stages of endurance events. During rest and submaximal exertion, both fat and carbohydrates are used as energy substrate in approximately a 60% to 40% ratio.[23]

Regardless of the nutrient source that produces ATP, it is always available in the cell as an immediate energy source. When all available sources of ATP are depleted, more must be regenerated for muscular contraction to continue.

Aerobic versus Anaerobic Metabolism

Two major energy systems function in muscle tissue: anaerobic and aerobic metabolism. Each of these systems generates ATP. During sudden outbursts of activity in intensive, short-term exercise, ATP can be rapidly metabolized to meet energy needs. After a few seconds of intensive exercise, however, the small stores of ATP are used up. The body then turns to glycogen as an energy source. Glycogen can be metabolized within the muscle cells to generate ATP for muscle contractions.

Both ATP and muscle glycogen can be metabolized without the need for oxygen. Thus this energy system involves anaerobic metabolism (occurring in the absence of oxygen). As exercise continues, the body has to rely on the metabolism of carbohydrates (more specifically, glucose) and fats to generate ATP. This second energy system requires oxygen and is therefore referred to as aerobic metabolism (occurring in the presence of oxygen).

In most activities both aerobic and anaerobic systems function simultaneously. The degree to which the two major energy systems are involved is determined by the intensity and duration of the activity. If the intensity of the activity is such that sufficient oxygen can be supplied to meet the demands of working tissues, the activity is considered to be aerobic. Conversely, if the activity is of high enough intensity or the duration is such that there is insufficient oxygen available to meet energy demands, the activity becomes anaerobic. Consequently, an oxygen debt is incurred that must be paid back during the recovery period. For example, short bursts of muscle contraction, as in running or swimming sprints, use predominantly the anaerobic system. However, endurance events depend a great deal on the aerobic system. Most sports use a combination of both anaerobic and aerobic metabolism (Table 3-1).

Training Techniques for Improving Cardiorespiratory Endurance

Cardiorespiratory endurance may be improved through a number of different methods. Largely, the amount of improvement possible will be determined by initial levels of cardiorespiratory endurance.

Continuous Training

Continuous training involves four considerations:
- *Mode* or type of activity
- *Frequency* of the activity
- *Duration* of the activity
- *Intensity* of the activity

Mode The type of activity used in continuous training must be aerobic. Aerobic activities are those that elevate the heart rate and maintain it at that level for an extended time. Aerobic activities generally involve repetitive, whole-body, large-muscle movements performed over an extended time. Examples of aerobic activities are running, jogging, walking, cycling, swimming, rope skipping, stair climbing, and cross-country skiing. The advantage of these aerobic activities as opposed to more intermittent activities, such as racquetball, squash, basketball, or tennis, is that aerobic activities are easy to regulate by either speeding up or slowing down the pace. Because we already know that the given intensity of the workload elicits a given heart rate, these aerobic activities allow us to maintain heart rate at a specified or target level. Intermittent activities involve variable speeds and intensities that cause the heart rate to fluctuate considerably. Although these intermittent activities improve cardiorespiratory endurance, they are much more difficult to monitor in terms of intensity.

Frequency To see at least minimal improvement in cardiorespiratory endurance, it is necessary for the average person to engage in no less than three sessions per week. If possible, one should aim for four or five sessions per week. A competitive

3-5

Critical Thinking Exercise

A female soccer player has a grade I ankle sprain that is likely to keep her out of practice for about a week. She has worked extremely hard on her fitness levels and is concerned that not being able to run for an entire week will hurt her cardiorespiratory fitness.

? What types of activity should the athletic trainer recommend during her rehabilitation period that can help her maintain her existing level of cardiorespiratory endurance?

TABLE 3-1 Comparison of Aerobic versus Anaerobic Activities

	Mode	Relative Intensity	Performance	Frequency	Duration	Miscellaneous
Aerobic activities	Continuous, long duration, sustained activities	Less intense	60% to 80% of maximum range	At least three but not more than six times per week	20 to 60 min	Less risk to sedentary or older individuals
Anaerobic activities	Explosive, short duration, burst-type activities	More intense	85% to 100% range	Three to four days per week	10 sec to 2 min	Used in sport and team activities

athlete should be prepared to train as often as six times per week. Everyone should take off at least 1 day per week to allow for both psychological and physiological rest.

Duration   For minimal improvement to occur, an individual must participate in at least 20 minutes of continuous activity with the heart rate elevated to its working level. Recent evidence suggests that even shorter exercise bouts of as little as 12 minutes may be sufficient to show improvement. Generally, the greater the duration of the workout, the greater the improvement in cardiorespiratory endurance. The competitive athlete should train for at least 45 minutes with the heart rate elevated to training levels.

Intensity   Of the four factors being considered, the most critical factor is the intensity of training, even though recommendations regarding training intensities vary. This is particularly true in the early stages of training, when the body is forced to make a lot of adjustments to increase workload demands.

Because heart rate is linearly related to the intensity of the exercise and to the rate of oxygen consumption, it becomes a relatively simple process to identify a specific workload (pace) that will make the heart rate plateau at the desired level. By monitoring heart rate, we know whether the pace is too fast or too slow to get heart rate into a target range.

Several formulas identify a target training heart rate. Exact determination of maximal heart rate involves exercising an individual at a maximal level and monitoring the heart rate using an electrocardiogram. This is a difficult process outside a laboratory. However, an approximate estimate of maximal heart rate for both males and females is that maximal heart rate is thought to be about 220 beats per minute. Maximal heart rate is related to age. As age increases, maximal heart rate decreases. Thus a relatively simple estimation of maximal heart rate (HR) would be Maximal HR = 220 − Age. If an athlete is working at 70% of maximal rate, the target heart rate can be calculated by multiplying 0.7 × (220 − Age).

Another commonly used formula that takes into account current level of fitness is the Karvonen equation.[17]

$$\text{Target training HR} = \text{Resting HR} + (0.6\,[\text{Maximal HR} - \text{Resting HR}])$$

Regardless of the formula used, it should be clear that to see minimal improvement in cardiorespiratory endurance, the heart rate should be elevated to at least 70% of its maximal rate.[2] In a trained individual it is not difficult to sustain a heart rate at the 85% level.

Interval Training

Unlike continuous training, interval training involves more intermittent activities. **Interval training** consists of alternating periods of relatively intense work and active recovery. It allows for performance of much more work at a more intense workload over a longer period of time than if working continuously.[22]

It is most desirable in continuous training to work at an intensity of about 60% to 80% of maximal heart rate. Obviously, sustaining activity at a relatively high intensity over a 20-minute period would be extremely difficult. The advantage of interval training is that it allows work at this 80% or higher level for a short period of time followed by an active period of recovery during which an individual may be working at only 30% to 45% of maximum heart rate.[13] Thus the intensity of the workout and its duration can be greater than with continuous training.

Most sports are anaerobic, involving short bursts of intense activity followed by a sort of active recovery period (for example, football, basketball, soccer, or tennis). Training with the interval technique allows the athlete to be more sport specific during the workout. With interval training the overload principle is applied by making the training period much more intense.

There are several important considerations in interval training. The training period is the amount of time that continuous activity is actually being performed, and

interval training
Alternating periods of work with active recovery.

the recovery period is the time between training periods. A set is a group of combined training and recovery periods, and a repetition is the number of training and recovery periods per set. Training time or distance refers to the rate or distance of the training period. The training-recovery ratio indicates a time ratio for training versus recovery.

An example of interval training would be a soccer player running sprints. An interval workout would involve running two sets of four 440-yard dashes in under 70 seconds, with a 2-minute 20-second walking recovery period between each dash. During this training session the soccer player's heart rate would probably increase to 85% to 90% of maximal level during the dash and should probably fall to the 30% to 45% level during the recovery period.

Fartlek Training

Fartlek is a training technique that is a type of cross-country running originated in Sweden. Fartlek literally means "speed play." It is similar to interval training in that one must run for a specified period of time; however, specific pace and speed are not identified. It is recommended that the course for a fartlek workout be some type of varied terrain with some level running, some uphill and downhill running, and some running through obstacles such as trees or rocks. The object is to put surges into a running workout, varying the length of the surges according to individual purposes.

One advantage of fartlek training is that because the terrain is always changing, the course may prevent boredom and may actually turn out to be relaxing.

Again, if fartlek training is going to improve cardiorespiratory endurance, it must elevate the heart rate to at least minimal training levels. Fartlek may best be utilized as an off-season conditioning activity or as a change of pace activity to counteract the boredom of training using the same activity day after day.

SUMMARY

- Proper physical conditioning for sports participation should prepare the athlete for a high-level performance while helping to prevent injuries inherent to that sport.
- Year-round conditioning is essential in most sports to assist in preventing injuries. Postseason conditioning is concerned with injury rehabilitation, off-season conditioning with a degree of physical maintenance, and preseason with conditioning that meets the demands of a particular sport.
- Physical conditioning must follow the SAID principle—an acronym for specific adaptation to imposed demands. It must work toward making the body as lean as possible, commensurate with the athlete's sport.
- A proper warm-up should precede conditioning, and a proper cool-down should follow. It takes at least 15 to 30 minutes of gradual warm-up to bring the body to a state of readiness for vigorous sports training and participation. Warming up consists of general unrelated activity followed by a specific related activity.
- Optimum flexibility is necessary for success in most sports. However, too much flexibility can allow joint trauma to occur, whereas too little flexibility can result in muscle tears or strains. Ballistic stretching exercises should be avoided. The safest means of increasing flexibility are static stretching and the proprioceptive neuromuscular facilitation (PNF) technique, consisting of slow-reversal-hold-relax, contract-relax, and hold-relax methods.
- Strength is the capacity to exert a force or the ability to perform work against a resistance. There are numerous means to develop strength, including isometric, isotonic, and isokinetic muscle contraction. Isometric exercise generates heat energy by forcefully contracting the muscle in a stable position that produces no change in the length of the muscle. Isotonic exercise involves shortening and lengthening a muscle through a complete range of motion. Isokinetic exercise allows resisted movement through a full range at a specific velocity. Circuit training uses a series

of exercise stations to improve strength and flexibility. Plyometric training uses a quick eccentric contraction to facilitate a more explosive concentric contraction.

■ Cardiorespiratory endurance is the ability to perform whole-body, large-muscle activities repeatedly for long periods of time. Maximal oxygen consumption is the greatest determinant of the level of cardiorespiratory endurance. Most sport activities involve some combination of both aerobic and anaerobic metabolism. Improvement of cardiorespiratory endurance may be accomplished through continuous, interval, or fartlek training.

. . . .

Solutions to Critical Thinking Exercises

3-1 Despite the fact that every effort was made to maintain existing levels of fitness during the rehabilitation period, it is important to understand that an athlete in any sport must practice or engage in that specific activity to improve his fitness to competitive levels. The athlete must begin a heavy strength-training program for the upper body immediately in the postseason and continue to progressively return to heavy lifting with the lower extremity as soon as the healing process will allow. It is essential for him to progressively increase the intensity and variety of conditioning drills that specifically relate to performance at his particular position.

3-2 The warm-up should begin with a 5 to 7 minute slow jog during which the athlete should break into a light sweat. At that point, she should engage in stretching (using either static or PNF techniques) concentrating on quadriceps, hamstrings, groin, and hip abductor muscles. Each specific stretch should be repeated four times holding the stretch for 15 to 20 seconds. Once the workout begins, gradually and moderately increase the intensity of the activity. Remember that it may be equally as important if not more effective to stretch during the cool-down period after the workout.

3-3 There is no reason to think that weight training will have a negative effect on flexibility as long as the lifting technique is done properly. Lifting the weight through a full range of motion will serve to improve strength and simultaneously maintain range of motion. Chances are that a female swimmer is not likely to "bulk up" to the point where range of motion will be affected by muscle size. It is also important to recommend that she continue to incorporate active stretching into her training regimen.

3-4 The shot put, like many other dynamic movements in sport, requires not only great strength, but also the ability to generate that strength rapidly. To develop muscular power the athlete must engage in dynamic, "explosive" training techniques, which will help him develop his ability. Power lifting techniques such as squats and power cleans should be helpful. Plyometric exercises using weights for added resistance will help him learn to improve his speed of muscular contraction against some resistive force.

3-5 In the case of a lower extremity injury where weight bearing is limited, alternative activities such as swimming or riding a stationary exercise bike should be incorporated into the rehabilitation program immediately. If the pressure on the ankle when riding an exercise bike is too painful, using a bike that incorporates upper extremity exercise may be initially helpful. The athletic trainer should recommend that the soccer play engage in a minimum of 30 minutes of continuous training, as well as some higher-intensity interval training, to maintain both aerobic and anaerobic fitness.

REVIEW QUESTIONS AND CLASS ACTIVITIES

1. Why is year-round conditioning so important for injury prevention?
2. In terms of injury prevention, list as many advantages as you can for conditioning.
3. How does the SAID principle relate to sports conditioning and injury prevention?
4. What is the value of proper warm-up and cool-down to sports injury prevention?
5. Critically observe how a variety of sports use warm-up and cool-down procedures.
6. Compare ways to increase flexibility and how they may decrease or increase the athlete's susceptibility to injury.
7. How may increasing strength decrease susceptibility to injury?
8. Compare different techniques of increasing strength. How may each technique be an advantage or a disadvantage to the athlete in terms of injury prevention?
9. Discuss the relationships among maximal oxygen consumption, heart rate, stroke volume, and cardiac output.
10. Differentiate between aerobic and anaerobic training methods.
11. How is continuous training different from interval training?

REFERENCES

1. Anderson B: *Stretching,* Bolinas, Calif, 1986, Shelter.
2. Astrand PO, Rodahl K: *Textbook of work physiology,* New York, 1986, McGraw-Hill.
3. Bealieu JE: Developing a stretching program, *Phys Sportsmed* 9(11):59, 1981.
4. Bealieu JE: *Stretching for all sports,* Pasadena, Calif, 1980, Athletic Press.
5. Berger R: *Conditioning for men,* Boston, 1973, Allyn & Bacon.
6. Costill D et al: Skeletal muscle enzymes and fiber compositions in male and female track athletes, *J Appl Physiol* 40:149, 1976.
7. De Lorme TL, Watkins AL: *Progressive resistance exercise,* New York, 1951, Appleton-Century-Crofts.
8. deVries H: *Physiology of exercise for physical education and athletics,* Dubuque, Iowa, 1986, William C Brown.
9. Duda M: Plyometrics: a legitimate form of power training, *Phys Sportsmed* 16:213, 1988.
10. Dudley GA, Fleck SJ: Strength and endurance training: are they mutually exclusive? *Sports Med* 4(2):79, 1987 (review).
11. Etheridge G, Thomas T: Physiological and biomedical changes of human skeletal muscle induced by different strength training programs, *Med Sci Sports Exerc* 14:141, 1982.

12. Fleck SJ, Kramer WJ: Resistance training: physiological responses and adaptations, *Phys Sportsmed* 16:108, 1988.
13. Fox E, Bowers R, Foss M: *The physiological basis of physical education and athletics*, Philadelphia, 1988, Saunders College.
14. Gollnick P, Sembrowich W: Adaptations in human skeletal muscle as a result of training. In Amsterdam EA, editor: *Exercise in cardiovascular health and disease*, New York, 1977, York Medical Books.
15. Hunter ST et al: Standards and norms of fitness and flexibility in high school athletes, *Ath Train* 20(3):210, 1985.
16. Jensen C, Fisher G: *Scientific basis of athletic conditioning*, Philadelphia, 1979, Lea & Febiger.
17. Karvonen MJ, Kentala E, Mustala O: The effects of training on heart rate: a longitudinal study, *Ann Med Exp Biol* 35:305, 1957.
18. Kirkendall DT: Mobility: conditioning programs. In Gould JA, Davies GJ, editors: *Orthopaedic and sports physical therapy*, vol 2, St Louis, 1990, Mosby.
19. Knight KL: Guidelines for rehabilitation of sports injuries. In Harvey JS, editor: *Clinics in sports medicine*, vol 4, no 3, Philadelphia, 1985, Saunders.
20. Knott M, Voss P: *Proprioceptive neuromuscular facilitation*, ed 3, New York, 1985, Harper & Row.
21. Logan GA, Wallis EL: Recent findings in learning and performance. Paper presented at the Southern Section Meeting, California Association for Health, Physical Education and Recreation, Pasadena, Calif, 1960.
22. MacDougall D, Sale D: Continuous vs. interval training: a review for the athlete and coach, *Can J Appl Sport Sci* 6:93, 1981.
23. McArdle W, Katch F, Katch V: *Exercise physiology, energy, nutrition, and human performance*, Philadelphia, 1994, Lea & Febiger.
24. O'Shea JP: Power weight training and the female athlete, *Phys Sportsmed* 9(6):109, 1981.
25. Perrin DH: *Isokinetic exercise and assessment*, Champaign, Ill, 1993, Human Kinetics.
26. Prentice W: A comparison of static and PNF stretching for improvement of hip joint flexibility, *Ath Train* 18(1):56, 1983.
27. Prentice W: *Fitness for college and life*, ed 5, St Louis, 1997, Mosby.
28. Prentice WE: A review of PNF techniques—implications for athletic rehabilitation and performance, *Forum Medicum* 51:1-13, 1989.
29. President's Council on Physical Fitness and Sports: *Weight training for strength and power*, Washington, DC, 1980, US Government Printing Office.
30. Rehfeldt H et al: Force, endurance time, and cardiovascular responses in voluntary isometric contractions of different muscle groups, *Biomed Biochim Acta* 48(5-6):S509, 1989.
31. Sanders B: *Sports physical therapy*, Norwalk, Conn, 1990, Appleton & Lange.
32. Shellock F, Prentice WE: Warm-up and stretching for improved physical performance and prevention of sport related injury, *Sports Med* 2:267, 1985.
33. Weltman A, Stamford B: Strength training: free weights vs. machines, *Phys Sportsmed* 10:197, 1982.
34. Wilmore JH: *Training for sport and activity*, Boston, 1985, Allyn & Bacon.
35. Zezoney F: Stretching and flexibility in athletics, *Sports Med Guide* 4(3):8, 1985.

ANNOTATED BIBLIOGRAPHY

Alter J: *The science of stretching*, Boston, 1988, Houghton Mifflin.

This text explains the principles and techniques of stretching and details the anatomy and physiology of muscle and connective tissue. It includes guidelines for developing a flexibility program and illustrated stretching exercises and warm-up drills.

Anderson B: *Stretching*, Bolinas, Calif, 1986, Shelter.

An extremely comprehensive best-selling text on stretching exercises for the entire body.

Chu D: *Jumping into plyometrics*, Champaign, Ill, 1992, Human Kinetics.

This text helps you develop a safe plyometric training program with exercises designed to improve your quickness, speed, upper body strength, jumping ability, balance, and coordination. It is well illustrated.

Cooper K: *The aerobics program for total well-being*, New York, 1982, Bantam Books.

Perhaps the bible for aerobics. Well written and documented, this book is an expansion of several earlier efforts dealing with aerobic exercise by Dr. Cooper.

Garhamner J: Sports Illustrated *strength training*, New York, 1987, Harper & Row.

A comprehensive look at weight training, including recommendations on a high-quality strength and conditioning program, various types of equipment, places to train, nutrition, and individualized training programs.

Prentice W: *Fitness for college and life*, St Louis, 1997, Mosby.

A comprehensive fitness text that covers all aspects of a training and conditioning program.

Sharkey BJ: *Physiology of fitness*, Champaign, Ill, 1984, Human Kinetics.

Written as a "how and why" of physical conditioning.

Tobias M, Sullivan JP: *Complete stretching*, New York, 1992, Knopf.

A colorful and well-illustrated guide to maximum mental and physical energy, increased flexibility, improved body shape, and enhanced relaxation.

Wolf M: *The Nautilus home fitness workout*, rev ed, Chicago, 1986, Contemporary Books.

Examines strength training using Nautilus exercise equipment. Good illustrations and step-by-step instructions.

Nutritional Considerations

When you finish this chapter, you should be able to

- Identify the six classes of nutrients and describe their major functions.
- Explain the importance of good nutrition in enhancing performance and preventing injuries.
- Describe the advantages or disadvantages of supplementing nutrients in the athlete's diet.
- Explain the advantages and disadvantages of a preevent meal.
- Explain the distinction between body weight and body composition.
- Explain the principle of caloric balance and how to assess it.
- Assess body composition using skinfold calipers.
- Describe methods for losing and gaining weight.
- List the signs of bulimia and anorexia nervosa.

The relation of nutrition, diet, and weight control to overall health and fitness is an important aspect of any training and conditioning program for an athlete. Athletes who practice sound nutritional habits reduce the likelihood of injury by maintaining a higher standard of healthful living. We know that eating a well-balanced diet can positively contribute to the development of strength, flexibility, and cardiorespiratory endurance. Unfortunately, misconceptions, fads, and in many cases superstitions regarding nutrition affect dietary habits, particularly in the athletic population.

Many athletes associate successful performance with the consumption of special foods or supplements. If the athlete is performing well, there may be a reluctance to change dietary habits regardless of whether the diet is physiologically beneficial to overall health. There is no question that the psychologic aspect of allowing the athlete to eat whatever he or she is most comfortable with can greatly affect performance. The problem is that these eating habits tend to become accepted as beneficial and may become traditional when in fact they may be physiologically detrimental to athletic performance. Thus there is a tendency for many nutrition "experts" to disseminate nutritional information based on traditional rather than experimental information. The athletic trainer must possess a strong knowledge base in nutrition so that he or she may serve as an informational resource for the athlete.

NUTRITION BASICS

Nutrition is the science of the substances that are found in food that are essential to life. A substance is essential if it must be supplied by the diet.[9] There are six classes of nutrients: carbohydrates (CHO), fats, proteins, vitamins, minerals, and water. Nutrients are necessary for three major roles: growth, repair, and maintenance of all tissues; regulation of body processes; and providing energy.[29]

Nutrient density describes foods that supply adequate amounts of vitamins and minerals in relation to their caloric value. The so-called junk foods provide excessive amounts of calories from fat and sugar in relation to vitamins and minerals and therefore are not nutrient dense. However, many people live on junk foods that displace more nutrient-dense foods from their diet. This is not a healthful behavior in the long run.[13]

The six classes of nutrients are carbohydrates, fat, protein, vitamins, minerals, and water.

Nutrient-dense foods supply adequate amounts of vitamins and minerals in relation to caloric value.

ENERGY SOURCES
Carbohydrates

Athletes have increased energy needs. Carbohydrates are the body's most efficient source of energy and should be relied on to fill that need.[7] For the athlete, carbohydrates should account for 55% to 60% or more of total caloric intake. The following describes different forms of carbohydrates and their role in the production of energy and maintenance of health.[29]

Sugars

Carbohydrates are sugar, starches, or fiber.

Carbohydrates are classified as simple (sugars) or complex (starch and most forms of fiber). Sugars are further divided into monosaccharides and disaccharides. Monosaccharides, single sugars, are found mostly in fruits, syrups, and honey. Glucose (blood sugar) is a monosaccharide. Milk sugar (lactose) and table sugar (sucrose) are combinations of two monosaccharides and are called disaccharides. Because it contributes little in the way of other nutrients, the amount of sugar eaten should account for less than 15% of the total caloric intake.

Starches

Starches are complex carbohydrates. A starch is made up of long chains of glucose units. During the digestion process, the starch chain is broken down and the glucose units are free to be absorbed. Food sources of starch, such as rice, potatoes, and breads, often provide vitamins and minerals in addition to serving as the body's principal source of glucose. Many people believe that starchy foods contribute to obesity. However, most of these foods are eaten with fats from butter, margarine, sauces, and gravies that make the food more enjoyable but contribute an excess of calories.

Glycolysis is the process that breaks down glucose to produce energy.

The body cannot use starches and many sugars directly from food for energy. It must obtain the simple sugar glucose (blood sugar). During digestion and metabolism, starches and disaccharide sugars are broken down and converted to glucose. The glucose that is not needed for immediate energy is stored as glycogen in the liver and muscle cells. Glucose can be released from glycogen later if needed. The body, however, can store only a limited amount of glucose as glycogen. Any extra amount of glucose is converted to body fat. When there is an inadequate intake of dietary carbohydrate, the body can use protein to make glucose. Thus protein is diverted from its own important functions. Therefore a supply of glucose must be kept available to prevent the use of protein for energy. This is called the protein-sparing action of glucose.

Fiber

In recent years, researchers have given considerable attention to the importance of fiber in the diet. Fiber forms the structural parts of plants and is not digested by humans. Fiber is not found in animal sources of food. There are two kinds of dietary fiber: soluble and insoluble. Soluble fiber includes gums and pectins; cellulose is the primary insoluble form. Sources of soluble fiber are oatmeal, legumes, and some fruits. Food sources of insoluble fiber include whole grain breads and bran cereals.

Because it is not digested, fiber passes through the intestinal tract and adds bulk. Fiber aids normal elimination by reducing the amount of time required for wastes to move through the digestive tract. This is believed to reduce the risk of colon cancer. Also, increased fiber intake is thought to reduce the risk of coronary artery disease. Soluble forms of fiber bind to cholesterol passing through the digestive tract and prevent its absorption. This can reduce blood cholesterol levels. In addition, foods rich in saturated fats (meats, in particular) often take the place of fiber-rich foods in the diet, thus increasing cholesterol absorption and formation. Also, consumption of adequate amounts of fiber has been associated with lowered incidences of obesity, constipation, colitis, appendicitis, and diabetes.

The recommended amount of fiber in the diet is approximately 25 grams per day. Unfortunately, the average person consumes only 10 to 15 grams per day. It is recommended that fiber intake be increased by increasing the amount of whole grain cereal products and fruits and vegetables in the diet rather than using fiber supplements. Excessive consumption of fiber may cause intestinal discomfort, as well as increased losses of calcium and iron.

Fats

Fats are another essential component of the diet. They are the most concentrated source of energy, providing more than twice the calories per gram when compared with carbohydrates or proteins. Fat is used as a primary source of energy. Some dietary fat is needed to make food more flavorful and for sources of the fat-soluble vitamins. Also, a minimal amount of fat is essential for normal growth and development.

Saturated versus Unsaturated Fat

Both plant and animal foods provide sources of dietary fat. About 95% of the fat consumed is in the form of triglycerides. Depending on their chemical nature, fatty acids may be saturated or unsaturated. The unsaturated fatty acids can be subdivided into monounsaturates or polyunsaturates. Therefore the terms *saturated, monounsaturated,* and *polyunsaturated* are used to describe the chemical nature of the fat in foods. The triglycerides that make up food fats are usually mixtures of saturated and unsaturated fatty acids but are classified according to the type that predominates. In general, fats containing more unsaturated fatty acids are from plants and are liquid at room temperature. Saturated fatty acids are derived mainly from animal sources.

Other Fats

Phospholipids and sterols represent the remaining 5% of fats. Phospholipids include lecithin; cholesterol is the best known sterol. Cholesterol is consumed in the diet from animal foods, and it is not supplied by plant sources of food. Generally, it is wise to avoid eating foods high in cholesterol. Although it is essential to many body functions, it is also true that the body can manufacture cholesterol from CHO, proteins, and especially saturated fat. Thus there is little if any need to consume additional amounts of cholesterol in the diet. The American Heart Association recommends consuming less than 300 mg per day.

A type of unsaturated fatty acid that seems to serve as a protective mechanism against certain disease processes are the omega-3 fatty acids, which apparently have the capability of reducing the likelihood of diseases such as heart disease, stroke, and hypertension. These fatty acids are found in cold-water fish. However, experts do not recommend the use of fish oil supplements as a source of omega-3 fatty acids.

Dietary fat represents approximately 40% to 50% of the total caloric intake. A substantial amount of the fat is from saturated fatty acids. This intake is believed to be too high and may contribute to the prevalence of obesity, certain cancers, and coronary artery disease. The recommended intake should be limited to less than 30% of total calories with saturated fat reduced to less than 10% of total calories.

Proteins

Proteins make up the major structural components of the body. They are needed for growth, maintenance, and repair of all body tissues. In addition, proteins are needed to make enzymes, many hormones, and antibodies that help fight infection. In general, the body prefers not to use much protein for energy; instead it relies on fats and carbohydrates. Protein intake should be around 12% to 15% of total calories.

Amino Acids

The basic units that make up proteins are smaller compounds called amino acids. Most of the body's proteins are made up of about 20 amino acids. Amino acids can

---

4-1

Critical Thinking Exercise

A female softball player has been told by her coach that she is slightly overweight and needs to lose a few pounds. The athlete has been watching TV and reading about how important it is to limit the dietary intake of fat for losing weight. She has decided to go on a diet that is essentially fat free and is totally convinced that this will help her lose weight.

? What should the athletic trainer tell her about avoiding the excessive intake of fat as a means of losing weight?

Fats may be saturated or unsaturated

Dietary recommendations: CHO 55%, fats 30%, proteins 15%.

Proteins are made up of amino acids.

Critical Thinking Exercise

A volleyball player complains that she constantly feels tired and lethargic even though she feels that she is eating well and getting a sufficient amount of sleep. A teammate has suggested that she begin taking vitamin supplements, which she claims gives her more energy and makes her more resistant to fatigue. The athlete comes to the athletic trainer to ask advice about what kind of vitamins she needs to take.

? What facts should the athletic trainer explain to the athlete about vitamin supplementation, and what recommendations should be made?

be linked together in a wide variety of combinations, which is why there are so many different forms and uses of proteins. Most of the amino acids can be produced as needed in the body. The others cannot be made to any significant degree and therefore must be supplied by the diet. These are referred to as the essential amino acids. The amount of protein, as well as the levels of the individual essential amino acids, is important for determining the quality of one's diet. A diet that contains large amounts of protein will not support growth, repair, and maintenance of tissues if the essential amino acids are not available in the proper proportions.[11]

Most of the proteins from animal foods contain all of the essential amino acids that humans require and are called complete or high-quality proteins. Incomplete proteins, that is, those sources of protein that do not contain all of the essential amino acids, usually are from plant sources of food.

Protein Sources and Need

Most athletes do not have difficulty meeting protein needs because the typical diet is rich in protein and many athletes consume more than twice the recommended levels of protein. There is no advantage to consuming more protein, particularly in the form of protein supplements. If more protein is supplied than needed, the body must convert the excess to fat for storage. This can create a situation in which excess water is removed from cells, leading to dehydration and possible damage to the kidneys or liver. Protein supplements may also create imbalances of the chemicals that make up proteins, the amino acids, which is not desirable. A condition of the bones, osteoporosis, has been linked to a diet that contains too much protein.[16]

Increased physical activity increases one's need for energy, not protein. The increases in muscle mass that result from conditioning and training are associated with only a small increase in protein requirements that can easily be met with the usual diet. Therefore no supplements are needed by an athlete.

REGULATOR NUTRIENTS
Vitamins

Although they are required in extremely small amounts when compared with water, proteins, carbohydrates, and fats, vitamins perform essential roles primarily as regulators of body processes. There are 13 with specific roles in the body. Many of these roles are still being explored. In the past, letters were assigned as names for vitamins. Today, most are known by their scientific names. Vitamins are classified into two groups: fat-soluble vitamins, which are dissolved in fats and stored in the body, and water-soluble vitamins, which are dissolved in watery solutions and are not stored. Table 4-1 lists the vitamins and indicates their primary functions.

Fat-Soluble Vitamins

Fat-soluble vitamins: A, D, E, and K.

Vitamins A, D, E, and K are fat soluble. They are found in the fatty portions of foods and in oils. Because they are stored in the body's fat, it is possible to consume excess amounts and show the effects of vitamin poisoning.

Water-Soluble Vitamins

Water-soluble vitamins: C, thiamin, riboflavin, niacin, folate, biotin, and panothenic acid.

The water-soluble vitamins consist of vitamin C, known as ascorbic acid, and the B-complex vitamins, most now referred to by their scientific names. B-complex vitamins include thiamin, riboflavin, niacin, B_6, folate, B_{12}, biotin, and pantothenic acid. Although vitamins are not metabolized for energy, thiamin, riboflavin, niacin, biotin, and pantothenic acid are used to regulate the metabolism of CHO, proteins, and fats to obtain energy. Vitamin B_6 regulates the body's use of amino acids. Folate and vitamin B_{12} are important in normal blood formation. Vitamin C is used for building bones and teeth, maintaining connective tissues, and strengthening the immune system. Unlike fat-soluble vitamins, water-soluble vitamins cannot be stored to any significant extent in the body and should be supplied in the diet each day.

TABLE 4-1 Vitamins

Vitamin	Major Function	Most Reliable Sources	Deficiency	Excess (Toxicity)
A	Maintains skin and other cells that line the inside of the body; bone and tooth development; growth; vision in dim light	Liver, milk, egg yolk, deep green and yellow fruits and vegetables	Night blindness; dry skin; growth failure	Headaches, nausea, loss of hair, dry skin, diarrhea
D	Normal bone growth and development	Exposure to sunlight; fortified dairy products; eggs and fish liver oils	"Rickets" in children—defective bone formation leading to deformed bones	Appetite loss, weight loss, failure to grow
E	Prevents destruction of polyunsaturated fats caused by exposure to oxidizing agents; protects cell membranes from destruction	Vegetable oils, some in fruits and vegetables, whole grains	Breakage of red blood cells leading to anemia	Nausea and diarrhea; interferes with vitamin K if vitamin D is also deficient; not as toxic as other fat-soluble vitamins
K	Production of blood-clotting substances	Green leafy vegetables; normal bacteria that live in intestines produce K that is absorbed	Increased bleeding time	
Thiamin	Needed for release of energy from carbohydrates, fats, and proteins	Cereal products, pork, peas, and dried beans	Lack of energy, nerve problems	
Riboflavin	Energy from carbohydrates, fats, and proteins	Milk, liver, fruits and vegetables, enriched breads and cereals	Dry skin, cracked lips	
Niacin	Energy from carbohydrates, fats, and proteins	Liver, meat, poultry, peanut butter, legumes, enriched breads and cereals	Skin problems, diarrhea, mental depression, and eventually death (rarely occurs in U.S.)	Skin flushing, intestinal upset, nervousness, intestinal ulcers
B$_6$	Metabolism of protein; production of hemoglobin	White meats, whole grains, liver, egg yolk, bananas	Poor growth, anemia	Severe loss of coordination from nerve damage
B$_{12}$	Production of genetic material; maintains central nervous system	Foods of animal origin	Neurological problems, anemia	
Folate (Folic acid)	Production of genetic material	Wheat germ, liver, yeast, mushrooms, green leafy vegetables, fruits	Anemia	
C (Ascorbic acid)	Formation and maintenance of connective tissue; tooth and bone formation; immune function	Fruits and vegetables	"Scurvy" (rare); swollen joints, bleeding gums, fatigue, bruising	Kidney stones, diarrhea
Pantothenic acid	Energy from carbohydrates, fats, proteins	Widely found in foods	Not observed in humans under normal conditions	
Biotin	Use of fats	Widely found in foods	Rare under normal conditions	

Antioxidants

Certain nutrients, called antioxidants, may prevent premature aging, certain cancers, heart disease, and other health problems.[28] An antioxidant protects vital cell components from the destructive effects of certain agents, including oxygen. Vitamin C, vitamin E, and beta-carotene are antioxidants. Beta-carotene is a plant pigment that is found in dark green, deep yellow, or orange fruits and vegetables. The body can convert beta-carotene to vitamin A. In the early 1980s researchers reported that smokers who ate large quantities of fruits and vegetables rich in beta-carotene were less likely to develop lung cancer than other smokers. Since that time, more evidence is accumulating about the benefits of a diet rich in the antioxidant nutrients.

Some experts believe athletes should increase their intake of antioxidants, even if it means taking supplements. Others are more cautious. Excess beta-carotene pigments circulate throughout the body and may turn the skin yellow. However, the pigment is not believed to be toxic as is its nutrient cousin, vitamin A. On the other hand, increasing intake of vitamins C and E is not without some risk. Excess vitamin C is not well absorbed; the excess is irritating to the intestines and creates diarrhea. Although less toxic than vitamins A or D, too much vitamin E causes health problems.

Vitamin Deficiencies

The illness that results from a lack of any nutrient, especially those needed in such small amounts as the vitamins, is referred to as a deficiency disease.[25] Vitamin deficiency diseases are rare. As with the other nutrients, adequate amounts of the differ-

TABLE 4-2 Minerals

Mineral	Major Role	Most Reliable Sources	Deficiency	Excess
Calcium	Bone and tooth formation; blood clotting; muscle contraction; nerve function	Dairy products	May lead to osteoporosis	Calcium deposits in soft tissues
Phosphorus	Skeletal development; tooth formation	Meats, dairy products, and other protein-rich foods	Rarely seen	
Sodium	Maintenance of fluid balance	Salt (sodium chloride) added to foods and sodium-containing preservatives		May contribute to the development of hypertension
Iron	Formation of hemoglobin; energy from carbohydrates, fats, and proteins	Liver and red meats, enriched breads and cereals	Iron-deficiency anemia	Can cause death in children from supplement overdose
Copper	Formation of hemoglobin	Liver, nuts, shellfish, cherries, mushrooms, whole grain breads and cereals	Anemia	Nausea and vomiting
Zinc	Normal growth and development	Seafood and meats	Skin problems, delayed development, growth problems	Interferes with copper use; may decrease high-density lipoprotein levels
Iodine	Production of the hormone thyroxin	Iodized salt, seafood	Mental and growth retardation; lack of energy	
Fluorine	Strengthens bones and teeth	Fluoridated water	Teeth are less resistant to decay	Damage to tooth enamel

ent vitamins can be obtained if a wide variety of foods is eaten. For most people, vitamin supplements are a waste of money and can cause toxic effects if too many are taken. Many individuals think that vitamins are "foods" and are safe. However, in large doses, vitamins have druglike effects on the body. Table 4-1 describes some of the vitamins, including toxicity problems.

Minerals

More than 20 mineral elements have an essential role in the body and therefore must be supplied in the diet. These include the minerals listed in Table 4-2. Most minerals are stored in the body, especially in the liver and bones. Magnesium is needed in energy-supplying reactions; sodium and potassium are important for the transmission of nerve impulses. Iron plays a role in energy metabolism but is also combined with a protein to form hemoglobin, the compound that transports oxygen in red blood cells. Calcium has many important functions. It is necessary for proper bone and teeth formation, blood clotting, and muscle contraction. In general, minerals have roles that are too numerous to detail within the scope of this book. As with the vitamins, eating a wide variety of foods is the best way to obtain the minerals needed in the proper concentrations.

Water

Water is the most essential of all the nutrients and should be the nutrient of greatest concern to the athlete.[15] It is the most abundant nutrient of the body, accounting for approximately 60% of the body weight. Water is essential for all the chemical processes that occur in the body, and an adequate supply of water is necessary for energy production and normal digestion of other nutrients. It is also necessary for temperature control and for elimination of waste products of nutrient and body metabolism. Too little water leads to dehydration, and severe dehydration frequently leads to death. The average adult requires a minimum of 2.5 liters of water per day.

The body has a number of mechanisms designed specifically to maintain body water at near-normal level. Too little water leads to accumulation of solutes in the blood. These signal the brain that the body is thirsty while signaling the kidney to conserve water. Excessive water dilutes these solutes. This signals the brain to stop drinking and the kidneys to get rid of the excess water.

Water is the only nutrient of greater importance to the athlete than to those who are more sedentary, especially during prolonged exercise carried out in a hot, humid environment. Such a situation may cause excessive sweating and subsequent losses of large amounts of water. Restriction of water during this time will result in dehydration. Symptoms of dehydration include fatigue, vomiting, nausea, exhaustion, fainting, and possibly death.

Replacing fluid after heavy sweating is far more important than replacing electrolytes.

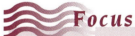

Focus

Directions for fluid ingestion

When conditioning, training, or competing, the athlete should:
- Drink a pint (500 to 600 ml) of cold (40° to 50° F) water 15 to 30 minutes before exercise.
- Avoid highly sugared drinks ingested within an hour of exercise (this drink elevates blood glucose and insulin and may lead to hyperglycemia).
- Ingest fluid that contains less than or equal to 2.5 g glucose per 100 ml water.
- Ingest fluid that contains a low concentration of ions (e.g., less than 0.2 g of sodium chloride and less than 0.2 g of potassium per quart [1000 ml] of fluid).

TABLE 4-3 Recommended Dietary Allowances[a] *Revised* **1989**

Category	Age (Years) or Condition	Weight[b] (kg)	Weight[b] (lb)	Height[b] (cm)	Height[b] (in)	Protein (g)	Fat-Soluble Vitamins Vitamin A (µg RE)[c]	Vitamin D (µg)[d]	Vitamin E (mg α-TE)[e]	Vitamin K (µg)	Water-Soluble Vitamins Vitamin C (mg)	Thiamin (mg)
Males	15-18	66	145	176	69	59	1000	10	10	65	60	1.5
	19-24	72	160	177	70	58	1000	10	10	70	60	1.5
	25-50	79	174	176	70	63	1000	5	10	80	60	1.5
	51+	77	170	173	68	63	1000	5	10	80	60	1.2
Females	15-18	55	120	163	64	44	800	10	8	55	60	1.1
	19-24	58	128	164	65	46	800	10	8	60	60	1.1
	25-50	63	138	163	64	50	800	5	8	65	60	1.1
	51+	65	143	160	63	50	800	5	8	65	60	1.0
Pregnant						60	800	10	10	65	70	1.5
Lactating												
First 6 months						65	1300	10	12	65	95	1.6
Second 6 months						62	1200	10	11	65	90	1.6

[a]The allowances, expressed as average daily intakes over time, are intended to provide for individual variations among most normal persons who live in the United States under usual environmental stresses. Diets should be based on a variety of common foods to provide other nutrients for which human requirements have been less well defined.

[b]Weights and heights of reference adults are actual median for the U.S. population of the designated age, as reported by NHANES II. The use of these figures does not imply that the height-to-weight ratios are ideal.

[c]Retinol equivalents. 1 retinol equivalent = 1 µg retinol or 6 µg beta-carotene.

[d]As cholecalciferol. 10 µg cholecalciferol = 400 IU of vitamin D.

[e]α-Tocopherol equivalents. 1 mg d-α tocopherol = 1 α-TE.

[f]1 NE (niacin equivalent) is equal to 1 mg of niacin or 60 mg of dietary tryptophan.

Electrolyte Requirements

Electrolytes: sodium, chloride, potassium, magnesium, and calcium.

Electrolytes, including sodium, chloride, potassium, magnesium, and calcium, are electrically charged ions. They maintain the balance of water outside the cell. There may be a need for electrolyte replenishment when a person is not fit, suffers from extreme water loss, participates in a marathon, or has just completed an exercise period and is expected to perform at near-maximum effort within the next few hours. In most cases, electrolytes can be sufficiently replaced with a balanced diet, which can if necessary be salted slightly more than usual. Free access to water (ad libitum) before, during, and after activity should be the rule. Electrolyte losses are primarily responsible for muscle cramping and intolerance to heat. Sweating results not only in body water loss but in some electrolyte loss as well.[8]

In most cases, plain water is an effective and inexpensive means of fluid replacement for most types of exercise. Commercial drinks, rather than adequately hydrating the athlete, may in fact hinder water absorption because of their high sugar content. Drinks containing too much glucose, fructose, or sucrose are hypertonic and may draw water from blood plasma into the intestinal tract, dehydrating the athlete even more. For most sports, electrolytes provided by commercial sports drinks are not needed unless the athlete is engaging in events such as ultramarathons.[10]

polymers
Natural or synthetic substances formed by the combination of two or more molecules of the same substance.

A new group of sports drinks that uses glucose **polymers** has been introduced. These drinks have the advantage of not causing the hypertonic problems of other commercial solutions. These drinks are most appropriate for highly intense and prolonged events that severely deplete glycogen stores.[10]

During cold weather water is not as critical as in hot weather. Therefore a stronger electrolyte solution that allows a slower, more steady release of fluid from the stomach should be used. As in hot weather, thirst is not an indicator of hydration.

Water-Soluble Vitamins					Minerals						
Riboflavin (mg)	Niacin (mg NE)[f]	Vitamin B$_6$ (mg)	Folate (μg)	Vitamin B$_{12}$ (μg)	Calcium (mg)	Phosphorus (mg)	Magnesium (mg)	Iron (mg)	Zinc (mg)	Iodine (μg)	Selenium (μg)
1.8	20	2.0	200	2.0	1200	1200	400	12	15	150	50
1.7	19	2.0	200	2.0	1200	1200	350	10	15	150	70
1.7	19	2.0	200	2.0	800	800	350	10	15	150	70
1.4	15	2.0	200	2.0	800	800	350	10	15	150	70
1.3	15	1.5	180	2.0	1200	1200	300	15	12	150	50
1.3	15	1.6	180	2.0	1200	1200	280	15	12	150	55
1.3	15	1.6	180	2.0	800	800	280	15	12	150	55
1.2	13	1.6	180	2.0	800	800	280	10	12	150	55
1.6	17	2.2	400	2.2	1200	1200	320	30	15	175	65
1.8	20	2.1	280	2.6	1200	1200	355	15	19	200	75
1.7	20	2.1	260	2.6	1200	1200	340	15	16	200	75

NUTRIENT REQUIREMENTS AND RECOMMENDATIONS

A nutrient requirement is that amount of the nutrient that is needed to prevent the nutrient's deficiency disease. Nutrient needs vary among individuals within a population. A recommendation for a nutrient is different than the requirement. Scientists establish recommendations for nutrients and calories based on extensive scientific research and assessment of present dietary intakes.[28]

The U.S. Recommended Daily Allowances (US RDA) were designed to help consumers compare the nutritional value of many food products (Table 4-3). For over a decade, the US RDA appeared on nutrient labels. However, this information is presently being replaced by a new nutrient label format that uses new standards, Reference Daily Intakes (RDI).

The new label will help consumers make more informed food selections (Figure 4-1). Concern over the amount of fat, cholesterol, sodium, and fiber in the typical American diet led the drive for a more health-conscious label. Instead of amounts of certain nutrients, the new format presents the information in the form of percentages that are based on a standard 2000 calories and the "percent daily values" that are shown on the new label.

The US RDA helps consumers compare nutritional values of foods.

THE FOOD PYRAMID

Most people are familiar with the basic four food groups plan, which was introduced in the mid-1950s. More recently, the basic four has been redesigned into a food pyramid concept that is believed to do a better job in educating Americans about the relationship of food choices to health. Figure 4-2 shows the food pyramid. For most of the food groupings, the minimum number of servings that should be eaten daily is specified, as well as examples of members of foods from this group. Carbohydrate-rich foods (the breads and cereals group) form the foundation of the diet. The other food groups are shown according to their relative importance in a healthy diet. One major change from the basic four plan is that the fruits and vegetables are separated into two distinct groups, each with a specified number of servings. Note that fats and sugars form the small apex of the pyramid. This indicates that foods rich in fat and sugar should provide the smallest proportion of total calories; no minimum number of servings is suggested because many people consume far too much fat and sugars.

NUTRITION AND PHYSICAL ACTIVITY

Vitamin requirements do not increase during exercise.

Athletes often believe that exercise increases requirements for nutrients such as proteins, vitamins, and minerals and that it is possible and desirable to saturate the body with these nutrients. There is no scientific basis for ingesting levels of these nutrients above RDA levels.[31] Exercise increases the need for energy, not for proteins, vitamins, and minerals.[24] Thus it is necessary to explore some of the more common myths that surround the subject of nutrition's role in physical performance.

Vitamin Supplementation

Many athletes believe that taking large amounts of vitamin supplements can lead to superior health and performance. A megadose of a nutrient supplement is essentially an overdose; the amount ingested far exceeds the RDA levels. The rationale used for such excessive intakes is that if a pill that contains the RDA for each vitamin and mineral makes you healthy, taking a pill that has 10 times the RDA should make you 10 times healthier.

An example of a popular practice among athletes is to take megadoses of vitamin C. Such doses do not prevent the common cold or slow aging. They do cause diarrhea and possibly the development of painful kidney stones. As with the other nutrients, an athlete has no increased need for vitamin C. Fruits, juices, and vegetables are reliable sources of vitamin C and also supply other vitamins and minerals.

Taking megadoses of vitamin E has become popular among people of all ages. The vitamin functions to protect certain fatty acids in cell membranes from being damaged. There is not much evidence to support the notion that this vitamin can extend life expectancy or enhance physical performance. Vitamin E does not enhance sexual ability, prevent graying hair, or cure muscular dystrophy. A person can obtain adequate amounts of vitamin E by consuming whole grain products, vegetable oils, and nuts.

The B-complex vitamins that are involved in obtaining energy from CHO, fats, and proteins are often abused by athletes who believe that vitamins provide energy. Any increased need for these nutrients is easily fulfilled when the athlete eats more nutritious foods while training. If athletes do not increase their food consumption, they will lose weight because of their high level of caloric expenditure.

Mineral Supplementation

Obtaining adequate levels of certain minerals can be a problem for some athletes. Calcium and iron intakes may be low for those who do not include dairy products, red meats, or enriched breads and cereals in their diet. However, one must be careful to first determine whether one needs extra minerals to prevent wasting money and overdosing. The following explores some of the minerals that can be low in the diet and some suggestions for improving the quality of the diet so that supplements may not be necessary.[15]

Calcium

Calcium is the most abundant mineral in the body. It is essential for bones and teeth, as well as for muscle contraction and conduction of nerve impulses. However, the importance of obtaining adequate calcium supplies throughout life has become more recognized. If calcium intake is too low to meet needs, the body can remove calcium from the bones. Over periods of time, the bones become weakened and appear porous on x-ray films. These bones are brittle and often break spontaneously. This condition is called **osteoporosis** and is estimated to be eight times more common among women than men. It becomes a serious problem for women after menopause.

osteoporosis
A decrease in bone density.

The RDA for young adults is 1200 mg (an 8-ounce glass of milk contains about 300 mg of calcium). Unfortunately about 25% of all females in the United States consume less than 300 mg of calcium per day, well below the RDA. High-protein diets and alcohol consumption also increase calcium excretion from the body. Exer-

Figure 4-1

A food label provides nutritional information.

Nutrition Facts
Serving Size ½ cup (114g)
Servings Per Container 4

Amount Per Serving

Calories 260	Calories from Fat 120

	% Daily Value*
Total Fat 13g	20%
Saturated Fat 5g	25%
Cholesterol 30mg	10%
Sodium 660mg	28%
Total Carbohydrate 31g	11%
Dietary Fiber 0g	0%
Sugars 5g	
Protein 5g	

Vitamin A 4%	Vitamin C 2%
Calcium 15%	Iron 4%

*Percent Daily Values are based on a 2000 Calorie diet. Your daily values may be higher or lower depending on your calorie needs.

	Calories: 2000	2500
Total Fat	Less than 65g	80g
Sat. Fat	Less than 20g	25g
Cholesterol	Less than 300mg	300mg
Sodium	Less than 2,400mg	2,400mg
Total Carbohydrate	300g	375g
Dietary Fiber	25g	30g

Calories per gram
Fat 9 · Carbohydrate 4 · Protein 4

cise causes calcium to be retained in bones, so physical activity is beneficial. However, younger females who exercise to extremes so that their normal hormonal balance is upset are prone to develop premature osteoporosis. For females who have a family history of osteoporosis, calcium supplementation, preferably as calcium carbonate or citrate rather than phosphate, may be advisable.

Milk products are the most reliable sources of calcium. Many athletes dislike milk. They may complain that it "upsets their stomach." They may lack an enzyme called lactase that is needed to digest milk sugar, lactose. This is referred to as lactose intolerance or **lactase deficiency.** The undigested lactose enters the large intestine, where the bacteria that normally reside there use it for energy. The bacteria produce large quantities of intestinal gas, which causes discomfort and cramps. Many lactose-intolerant people also suffer from diarrhea. Fortunately, scientists have produced the missing enzyme, lactase. Lactase is available without prescription in forms that can be added to foods before eating or taken along with meals.

lactase deficiency
Difficulty digesting dairy products.

Figure 4-2

The food pyramid offers examples of appropriate food selections important to an athlete's diet.

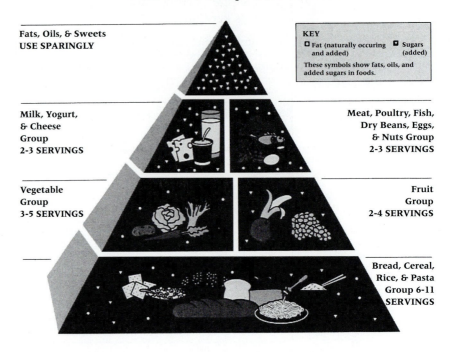

Food Guide Pyramid
A Guide to Daily Food Choices

Fats, Oils, & Sweets
USE SPARINGLY

KEY
☐ Fat (naturally occuring   ☐ Sugars
and added)   (added)
These symbols show fats, oils, and
added sugars in foods.

Milk, Yogurt,
& Cheese
Group
2-3 SERVINGS

Meat, Poultry, Fish,
Dry Beans, Eggs,
& Nuts Group
2-3 SERVINGS

Vegetable
Group
3-5 SERVINGS

Fruit
Group
2-4 SERVINGS

Bread, Cereal,
Rice, & Pasta
Group 6-11
SERVINGS

anemia

Lack of iron.

Iron Deficiency

Iron deficiency is also a common problem, especially for young females. Lack of iron can result in iron-deficiency **anemia.** (See Chapter 27.) Iron is needed to properly form hemoglobin. In this condition, the oxygen-carrying ability of the red blood cells is reduced so that muscles cannot obtain enough oxygen to generate energy. One feels tired and weak. Obviously, a person cannot compete at peak level while suffering from an iron deficiency.

Sugar and Performance

It has been suggested that ingesting large quantities of glucose in the form of honey, candy bars, or pure sugar immediately before physical activity has a significant impact on performance. As carbohydrates are digested, large quantities of glucose enter the blood. This increase in blood sugar (glucose) levels stimulates the release of the hormone insulin. Insulin allows the cells to use the circulating glucose so that blood glucose levels soon return to normal. It was hypothesized that this decline in blood sugar levels was detrimental to performance and endurance. However, recent evidence indicates that the effect of eating large quantities of carbohydrates is beneficial rather than negative.[23]

Nevertheless, some athletes are sensitive to high-carbohydrate feedings and experience problems with increased levels of insulin. Also, some athletes cannot tolerate large amounts of the simple sugar fructose. For these individuals, too much fructose leads to intestinal upset and diarrhea. Therefore it is suggested that athletes test themselves with various high-carbohydrate foods to see if they are affected (but not before a competitive event).[23]

Caffeine

Caffeine is a central nervous system stimulant. Most people who consume caffeine in coffee, tea, or carbonated beverages are aware of its effect of increasing alertness and decreasing fatigue. Chocolate contains compounds that are related to caffeine and have the same stimulating effects. However, large amounts of caffeine cause nervousness, irritability, increased heart rate, and headaches. Also, headaches are a withdrawal symptom experienced when one tries to stop consuming caffeinated products.

Although small amounts of caffeine do not appear to harm physical performance, cases of nausea and light-headedness have been reported. There is evidence that caffeine enhances the use of fat during endurance exercise, thus delaying the depletion of glycogen stores. This would help endurance performance. There is also some evidence that caffeine helps make calcium more available to the muscle during contraction. The muscle would be able to work more efficiently. However, Olympic officials rightfully consider caffeine to be a drug. It should not be present in an Olympic competitor's blood in levels greater than that resulting from drinking 5 or 6 cups of coffee.

Alcohol

Alcohol provides energy for the body; each gram of pure alcohol (ethanol) supplies 7 calories. However, sources of alcohol provide little other nutritional value with regard to vitamins, minerals, and proteins. The depressant effects of alcohol on the central nervous system include decreased physical coordination, slowed reaction times, and decreased mental alertness. Also, this drug increases the production of urine, resulting in body water losses (diuretic effect). Therefore use of alcoholic beverages by the athlete cannot be recommended before, during, or after physical activity.

Organic, Natural, or Health Foods

Many athletes are concerned about the quality of the foods they eat, not just the nutritional value of the food but also its safety. Organic foods are grown without the use of synthetic fertilizers and pesticides. Those who advocate the use of organic farming methods claim that these foods are nutritionally superior and safer than the same products grown using chemicals, such as pesticides and synthetic fertilizers.

Technically, the description of organic food is meaningless. All foods (except water) are organic, that is, contain the element carbon. Organically produced foods are often more expensive than the same foods that have been produced by conventional means. There is no advantage to consuming organic food products. They are not more nutritious than foods produced by conventional methods. Nevertheless, for some, the psychological benefit of believing that they are doing something "good" for their bodies justifies the extra cost.

Natural foods have been subjected to little processing and contain no additives, such as preservatives or artificial flavors. Processing can protect nutritional value. Preservatives save food that would otherwise spoil and have to be destroyed. Furthermore, many foods in their natural form are poisonous. The green layer often found under the skin of potatoes is poisonous if eaten in large amounts. There are poisonous mushrooms and molds in peanuts that cause liver cancer.

Both organic and natural foods could be described as health foods. However, there is no benefit derived from eating a diet consisting of health foods, even for the athlete.

Vegetarianism

Many athletes are health conscious and try to do things that are good for their bodies. Vegetarianism has emerged as an alternative to the usual American diet. All vegetarians use plant foods to form the foundation of their diet; animal foods are either totally excluded or included in a variety of eating patterns. Athletes who choose to become vegetarians do so for economic, philosophical, religious, cultural, or health reasons. Vegetarianism is no longer considered to be a fad if it is practiced intelligently. However, the vegetarian diet may create deficiencies if nutrient needs are not carefully considered. Athletes who follow this eating pattern must plan their diet care-

Vegetarians: total vegetarians, lactovegitarians, ovolactovegetarians, and semivegetarians.

fully so that their calorie needs are met. Types of vegetarian dietary patterns are categorized as follows:

- *Total vegetarians, or vegans:* People who consume plant but no animal foods; meat, fish, poultry, eggs, and dairy products are excluded. This diet has been found to be adequate for most adults if they give careful consideration to obtaining enough calories, vitamin B_{12}, and the minerals calcium, zinc, and iron.
- *Lactovegetarians:* Individuals who consume milk products along with plant foods. Meat, fish, poultry, and eggs are excluded. Iron and zinc levels can be low in this form of vegetarianism.
- *Ovolactovegetarians:* People who consume dairy products and eggs in their diet along with plant foods. Meat, fish, and poultry are excluded. Again, iron could be a problem.
- *Semivegetarians:* People who consume animal products but exclude red meats. Plant products still form an important part of the diet. This diet is usually adequate.

Preevent Nutrition

The importance and content of the preevent meal has been heatedly debated among coaches, athletic trainers, and athletes. The trend has been to ignore logical thinking about what should be eaten before competition in favor of upholding the tradition of "rewarding" the athlete for hard work by serving foods that may hamper performance. For example, the traditional steak-and-eggs meal before football games is great for coaches and trainers; however, the athlete gains nothing from this meal. The important point is that too often people are concerned primarily with the preevent meal and fail to realize that those nutrients consumed over several days before competition are much more important than what is eaten 3 hours before an event. The purpose of the preevent meal should be to provide the competitor with sufficient nutrient energy and fluids for competition while taking into consideration the digestibility of the food and, most important, the eating preferences of the individual athlete (see the Focus box on the next page). Figure 4-3 gives an example of a preevent meal.

The athlete should be encouraged to be conscious of his or her diet. However, there is no experimental evidence to indicate that performance may be enhanced by altering a diet that is basically sound. There are a number of ways that a nutritious diet may be achieved, and the diet that is optimal for one athlete may not be the best for another. In many instances, the individual will be the best judge of what he or she should or should not eat in the preevent meal or before exercising. It seems that a person's best guide is to eat whatever he or she is most comfortable with.

Liquid Food Supplements

Recently, liquid meals have been recommended as extremely effective preevent meals and are being used by high school, college, university, and professional teams with some indications of success. These supplements supply from 225 to 400 calories per average serving. Athletes who have used these supplements report elimination of the usual pregame symptoms of "dry mouth," abdominal cramps, leg cramps, nervous defecation, and nausea.

Under ordinary conditions it usually takes approximately 4 hours for a full meal to pass through the stomach and the small intestine. Pregame emotional tension often delays the emptying of the stomach; therefore the undigested food mass remains in the stomach and upper bowel for a prolonged time, even up to or through the actual period of competition, and frequently results in nausea, vomiting, and cramps. This unabsorbed food mass is of no value to the athlete. According to team physicians who have experimented with the liquid food supplements, one of their major advantages is that they clear both the stomach and the upper bowel before game time, thus making available the caloric energy that would otherwise still be in an unassimilated state. There is merit in the use of such food supplements for pregame meals.

4-3

Critical Thinking Exercise

A recreational runner has been training to run his first marathon. He feels good about his level of conditioning but wants to make certain that he does everything that he can do to maximize his performance. He is concerned about eating the right type of foods both before and during the marathon to help ensure that he does not become excessively fatigued.

? What recommendations should the athletic trainer make regarding glycogen supercompensation, the preevent meal, and food consumption during the event?

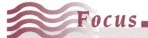 *Focus*

The pregame meal

- Try to achieve the largest possible storage of carbohydrates (glycogen) in both resting muscle and the liver. This is particularly important for endurance activities but may be beneficial for intense, short-duration exercise.
- A stomach that is full of food during contact sports is subject to injury. Therefore the type of food eaten should allow the stomach to empty quickly. Carbohydrates are easier to digest than fats or proteins. A meal that contains plenty of carbohydrates will leave the stomach and be digested faster than a fatty meal. It would be wise to replace the traditional steak-and-eggs preevent meal with a low-fat one containing a small amount of pasta, tomato sauce, and bread.
- Foods should not cause irritation or upset to the gastrointestinal tract. Foods high in cellulose and other forms of fiber, such as whole grain products, fruits, and vegetables, increase the need for defecation. Highly spiced foods or gas-forming foods (such as onions, baked beans, or peppers) must also be avoided because any type of disturbance in the gastrointestinal tract may be detrimental to performance. Carbonated beverages and chewing gum also contribute to the formation of gas.
- Liquids consumed should be easily absorbed and low in fat content and should not act as a laxative. Whole milk, coffee, and tea should be avoided. Water intake should be increased, particularly if the temperature is high.
- A meal should be eaten approximately 3 to 4 hours before the event or before exercising. This allows for adequate stomach emptying, but the individual will not feel hungry during activity.
- Any food that is disliked should not be eaten. Most important, the individual must feel psychologically satisfied by any preevent meal. If not, performance may be impaired more by psychological factors than by physiological factors.
- Prolonged fasting and diet programs that severely restrict caloric intake are scientifically undesirable and can be medically dangerous.
- Fasting and diet programs that severely restrict caloric intake result in the loss of large amounts of water, electrolytes, minerals, glycogen stores, and other fat-free tissue (including proteins within fat-free tissues), with minimal amounts of fat loss.
- Mild calorie restriction (500 to 1000 calories less than the usual daily intake) results in a smaller loss of water, electrolytes, minerals, and other fat-free tissue and is less likely to cause malnutrition.
- Dynamic exercise of large muscles helps maintain fat-free tissue, including muscle mass and bone density, and results in losses of body weight. Weight loss resulting from an increase in energy expenditure is primarily in the form of fat weight.
- A nutritionally sound diet resulting in mild calorie restriction coupled with an endurance exercise program, along with behavioral modification of existing eating habits, is recommended for weight reduction. The rate of sustained weight loss should not exceed 1 kg (2 lb) per week.
- To maintain proper weight control and optimal body fat levels, a lifetime commitment to proper eating habits and regular physical activity is required.

Glycogen Supercompensation

For endurance events, maximizing the amount of glycogen that can be stored, especially in muscles, may make the difference between finishing first or at the "end of the pack." Glycogen supplies in muscle and liver can be increased by reducing the training program a few days before competing and by significantly increasing carbohydrate intake during the week before the event.[3] By reducing training for at least 48 hours before the competition, the body is able to eliminate any metabolic waste products that may hinder performance. The high-carbohydrate diet restores glycogen levels in muscle and the liver. This practice is called **glycogen supercompensa-**

Glycogen supercompensation
High-carbohydrate diet.

Figure 4-3

Sample preevent meals.

Meal 1

¾ c Orange juice	¾ c Orange juice
½ c Cereal with 1 tsp sugar	1-2 Pancakes with:
1 Slice whole wheat toast with:	1 tsp Margarine
1 tsp Margarine	2 tbsp Syrup
1 tsp Honey or jelly	8 oz Skim or lowfat milk
8 oz Skim or lowfat milk	Water
Water	(Approximately 450-500 kcal)
(Approximately 450-500 kcal)	

Meal 2

1 c Vegetable soup	1 c Spaghetti with tomato sauce and cheese
1 Turkey sandwich with:	½ c Sliced pears (canned) on ¼ c cottage cheese
2 Slices bread	1-2 Slices (Italian) bread with 1-2 tsp margarine
2 oz Turkey (white or dark)	(avoid garlic)
1 oz Cheese slice	½ c Sherbet
2 tsp Mayonnaise	1-2 Sugar cookies
8 oz Skim or lowfat milk	4 oz Skim or lowfat milk
Water	Water
(Approximately 550-600 kcal)	(Approximately 700 kcal)

tion. The basis for the practice is that the quantity of glycogen stored in muscle directly affects the endurance of that muscle.[19]

Glycogen supercompensation is accomplished over a 6-day period divided into three phases. In phase 1 (days 1 and 2), training should be hard and dietary intake of carbohydrates restricted. During phase 2 (days 3 through 5), training is cut back and the individual eats plenty of carbohydrates. Studies have indicated that glycogen stores may be increased from 50% to 100%, theoretically enhancing endurance during a long-term event. Phase 3 (day 6) is the day of the event, during which a normal diet must be consumed.

The effect of glycogen supercompensation in improving performance during endurance activities has not as yet been clearly demonstrated. It has been recommended that glycogen supercompensation not be done more than two to three times during the course of a year. It must be added that glycogen supercompensation is only of value in long-duration events that produce glycogen depletion, such as a marathon.[21]

Fat Loading

Recently some endurance athletes have tried fat loading in place of carbohydrate loading. Their intent was to have a better source of energy at their disposal. The deleterious effects of this procedure outweigh any benefits that may be derived. Associated with fat loading is cardiac protein and potassium depletion, causing arrhythmias and increased levels of serum cholesterol as a result of the ingestion of butter, cheese, cream, and marbled beef.

WEIGHT CONTROL AND BODY COMPOSITION

Gain or loss of weight in an athlete often poses a problem because the individual's ingrained eating habits are difficult to change. The athletic trainer's inability to adequately supervise the athlete's meal program in terms of balance and quantity further complicates the problem. An intelligent and conscientious approach to weight control requires, on the part of both athletic trainer and athlete, some knowledge of what is involved. Such understanding allows athletes to better discipline themselves as to the quantity and kinds of foods they should eat.

BODY COMPOSITION

Ideal body weight is most often determined by consulting age-related height and weight charts such as those published by life insurance companies. Unfortunately, these charts are inaccurate because they involve broad ranges and often fail to take individual body types into account. Because they are based solely on gross body weight, their accuracy is questionable. Thus health and performance may best be related to body composition rather than body weight.[30]

Body composition refers to both the fat and nonfat components of the body. That portion of total body weight that is composed of fat tissue is referred to as the percent body fat. That portion of the total body weight that is composed of nonfat or lean tissue, which includes muscles, tendons, bones, and connective tissue, is referred to as lean body weight. Body composition measurements are more accurate in attempting to determine precisely how much weight an athlete may gain or lose.[6]

The average college-age female has between 20% and 25% of her total body weight made up of fat. The average college-age male has between 12% and 15% body fat. Male endurance athletes may get their fat percentage as low as 8% to 12%, and female endurance athletes may reach 10% to 18%. It is recommended that body fat percentage not go below 3% in males and 12% in females, because below these percentages the internal organs tend to lose their protective padding of essential fat, potentially subjecting them to injury.[5]

Being overweight and being obese are different conditions. Being overweight implies having excess body weight relative to physical size and stature. This may not be a problem unless one is also overfat, which means that the percentage of total body weight that is made up of fat is excessive. **Obesity** implies an extreme amount of excessive fat, much greater than what would be considered normal. A female with percent body fat over 30% and males with percent body fat over 20% are considered to be obese.

obesity
Excessive amount of body fat.

Two factors determine the amount of fat in the body: the number of fat, or adipose, cells and the size of the adipose cell. Proliferation, or hyperplagia, of adipose cells begins at birth and continues to puberty. It is thought that after early adulthood the number of fat cells remains fixed, although there is some recent evidence to suggest that the number of cells is not necessarily fixed.[17] Adipose cell size also increases gradually, or hypertrophies, to early adulthood and can increase or decrease as a function of caloric balance. In adults, weight loss or gain is primarily a function of the change in cell size, not cell number. Obese adults tend to exhibit a great deal of adipose cell hypertrophy.

The **adipose cell** stores triglyceride (a form of liquid fat). This liquid fat moves in and out of the cell according to the energy needs of the body, which are determined to some extent by the type of activity. The greatest amount of fat is used in activities of moderate intensity and long duration. The greater the amount of triglyceride contained in the adipose cell, the greater the amount of total body weight composed of fat. One pound of body fat is made up of approximately 3500 calories stored as triglyceride within the adipose cell.

adipose cell
Stores triglyceride.

Assessing Body Composition

Among the several methods of assessing **body composition** are hydrostatic, or underwater, weighing; measurement of electrical impedance; and measurement of skinfold thickness.[1]

body composition
Percent body fat plus lean body weight.

Measuring the thickness of skinfolds is based on the fact that about 50% of the fat in the body is contained in the subcutaneous fat layers and is closely related to total fat. The remainder of the fat in the body is found around organs and vessels and serves a shock-absorptive function. The skinfold technique involves measurement of the thickness of the subcutaneous fat layer with a skinfold caliper (Figure 4-4). Its accuracy is relatively low; however, expertise in measurement is easily developed and the time required for this technique is considerably less than for the others. It has been estimated that error in skinfold measurement is ±3% to 5%.[17]

A number of different methods have been described for measuring body composition using the skinfold technique. A technique proposed by McArdle and

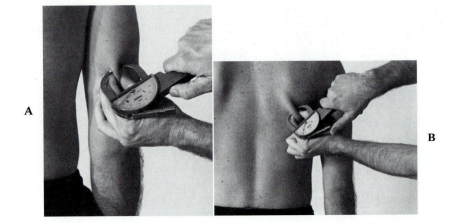

co-workers,[19] which measures the triceps skinfold and the subscapular skinfold, is widely used.

Assessing Caloric Balance

Changes in body weight are almost entirely the result of changes in caloric balance.

$$\text{Caloric balance} = \text{Number of calories consumed} - \text{Number of calories expended}$$

Positive caloric balance leads to weight gain; negative caloric balance leads to weight loss.

Calories may be expended by three different processes: basal metabolism; work (work may be defined as any activity that requires more energy than sleeping); and excretion. If more calories are consumed than expended, there is a positive caloric balance resulting in weight gain. Conversely, weight loss results from a negative caloric balance in which more calories are expended than are consumed.

Caloric balance is determined by the number of calories consumed regardless of whether the calories are contained in fat, carbohydrate, or protein. There are differences in the caloric content of these foodstuffs:

- Carbohydrate = 4 calories per gram
- Protein = 4 calories per gram
- Fat = 9 calories per gram
- Alcohol = 7 calories per gram

Estimations of caloric intake for college athletes range between 2000 and 5000 calories per day. Estimations of caloric expenditure range between 2200 and 4400 calories on the average. Energy demands will be considerably higher in endurance-type athletes, who may require as many as 7000 calories.[18]

METHODS OF WEIGHT LOSS

There are several ways that one can go about losing weight: dieting, increasing the amount of physical exercise, or a combination of diet and exercise.

Weight loss through dieting alone is difficult, and in most cases dieting alone is an ineffective means of weight control. Long-term weight control through dieting alone is successful only 2% of the time.[29] Through dieting, 35% to 45% of the weight decrease results from a loss of lean tissue. It is recommended that the minimum caloric intake for a female not go below 1000 to 1200 calories per day and for a male not below 1200 to 1400 calories per day.[17]

Weight loss through exercise involves an 80% to 90% loss of fat tissue with almost no loss of lean tissue. Weight loss through exercise alone is almost as difficult as losing weight through dieting. However, exercise will not only result in weight reduction but may also enhance cardiorespiratory endurance, improve strength, and increase flexibility.[12] For this reason, exercise has some distinct advantages over dieting in any weight-loss program.

The most efficient method of decreasing the percentage of body weight that is fat is through some combination of diet and exercise. A moderate caloric restriction combined with a moderate increase in caloric expenditure will result in a negative caloric balance. This method is relatively fast and easy compared with either of the others because habits are being moderately changed.

In any weight-loss program, the goal should be to lose 1½ to 2 pounds per week. Weight loss of more than 4 to 5 pounds per week may be attributed to dehydration as opposed to a loss of body fat.

In any weight-loss program the "long-haul" approach must be emphasized. It generally takes a long time to put on extra weight, and there is no reason to expect that true loss of excess body fat can be accomplished in a relatively short time. The American College of Sports Medicine has made specific recommendations for weight loss.[2]

METHODS FOR GAINING WEIGHT

The aim of a weight-gaining program should be to increase lean body mass, that is, muscle, as opposed to body fat. Muscle mass should be increased only by muscle work combined with an appropriate increase in dietary intake. It cannot be increased by the intake of any special food or vitamin.

The recommended rate of weight gain is approximately one to two pounds per week. Each pound of lean body mass gained represents a positive caloric balance. This is an intake in excess of an expenditure of approximately 2500 calories. One pound of fat represents the equivalent of 3500 calories; lean body tissue contains less fat, more protein, and more water and represents approximately 2500 calories. To gain one pound of muscle, an excess of approximately 2500 calories is needed; to lose one pound of fat, approximately 3500 calories must be expended in activities in excess of intake. Adding 500 to 1000 calories daily to the usual diet will provide the energy needs of gaining one to two pounds per week and fuel the increased energy expenditure of the weight-training program. Weight training must be part of the program. Otherwise, the excess intake of energy will be converted to fat.

EATING DISORDERS

There is an epidemic in our society, especially in sports. This problem is the inordinate concern with being overweight. Out of this obsession has emerged the eating disorders bulimia and anorexia nervosa. Both of these disorders are increasingly seen in athletes.[4,27]

Bulimia

The bulimic person is commonly female, ranging in age from adolescence to middle age. It is estimated that 1 out of every 200 American girls, ages 12 to 18 years (1% to 2% of the population), will develop patterns of bulimia, anorexia nervosa, or both.[22] The bulimic individual typically gorges herself with thousands of calories after a period of starvation and then "purges" herself through induced vomiting and further fasting or through the use of laxatives or diuretics. This secretive binge-eating-purging cycle may go on for years.

Typically the bulimic athlete is white and belongs to a middle-class or upper-middle-class family. She is perfectionistic, obedient, overcompliant, highly motivated, successful academically, well liked by her peers, and a good athlete.[14] She most commonly participates in gymnastics, track, and dance. Male wrestlers and gymnasts may also develop bulimia. (See the Focus box on the next page.) The formal definition of bulimia is as follows: recurrent episodes of rapid, uncontrollable ingestion of large amounts of food in a short period of time, usually followed by purging, either by forced vomiting or abuse of laxatives or diuretics.

Binge-purge patterns of eating can cause stomach rupture, disruption of heart rhythm, and liver damage. Stomach acids brought up by vomiting cause tooth decay and chronically inflame the mucous lining of the mouth and throat.

4-4
Critical Thinking Exercise

An ice hockey attackman has an excellent level of fitness and has superb skating ability and stick work. He is convinced that the only thing keeping him from moving to the next level is his body weight. In recent years he has engaged more in weight training activities to improve his endurance and to a lesser extent to increase strength.

? What recommendations should the athletic trainer make for him to be successful in his weight-gaining efforts?

4-5

Critical Thinking Exercise

A tennis coach observes that one of her tennis players has lost a significant amount of weight. It seems that along with this loss of weight her level of play has begun to decrease. The coach becomes seriously concerned when another player comes to the coach and tells her that she thinks that her roommate was purposely throwing up after a team meal on a recent road trip.

? After briefly questioning the athlete about her eating habits the coach decided to ask the athletic trainer to become involved in dealing with this situation. How should the athletic trainer respond to this request?

Anorexia Nervosa

It has been estimated that 30% to 50% of all individuals diagnosed as having anorexia nervosa also develop some symptoms of bulimia. Anorexia nervosa is characterized by a distorted body image and a major concern about weight gain. As with bulimia, anorexia nervosa affects mostly females. It usually begins in adolescence and can be mild without major consequences or can become life threatening. As many as 15% to 21% of individuals diagnosed as anorexic ultimately die from this disorder. Despite being extremely thin, the athlete sees herself as too fat. These individuals deny hunger and are hyperactive, engaging in abnormal amounts of exercise such as aerobics or distance running.[14] In general, the anorexic individual is highly secretive, and the coach and athletic trainer must be sensitive to eating problems. Early intervention is essential. Any athlete with signs of bulimia or anorexia nervosa must be confronted in a kind, empathetic manner by the coach or athletic trainer. When detected, individuals with eating disorders must be referred for psychological or psychiatric treatment. Unfortunately, simply referring an anorexic person to a health education clinic is not usually effective. The key to treatment of anorexia seems to be getting the patient to realize that a problem exists and that he or she could benefit from professional help. The individual must voluntarily accept such help if treatment is to be successful.[26]

Female Athlete Triad Syndrome

Female athlete triad syndrome is a potentially fatal problem that involves a combination of an eating disorder (either bulimia or anorexia), amenorrhea, and osteoporosis (diminished bone density) and that occurs primarily in female athletes. The incidence of this syndrome is uncertain; however, some studies have suggested that eating disorders in female athletes may be as high as 62% in certain sports, with amenorrhea being common in at least 60%. However, the major risk of this syndrome is that the bone lost in osteoporosis may not be regained.

SUMMARY

- The classes of nutrients are carbohydrates, fats, proteins, vitamins, minerals, and water. Carbohydrates, fats, and proteins provide the energy required for muscular work during activity and also play a role in the function and maintenance of body tissues. Vitamins are substances found in food that have no caloric value but are necessary to regulate body processes. Vitamins may be either fat soluble (vitamins A, D, E, and K) or water soluble (B-complex vitamins and vitamin C). The essential minerals are nec essary in most physiological functions of the body. Water is the most essential of all the nutrients and should be of great concern to anyone involved in physical activity.

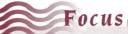

Focus

Identifying the athlete with an eating disorder

Signs to look for are athletes who display

- Social isolation and withdrawal from friends and family.
- A lack of confidence in athletic abilities.
- Ritualistic eating behavior (e.g., organizing food on plate).
- An obsession with counting calories.
- An obsession with constantly exercising, especially just before a meal.
- An obsession with weighing self.
- A constant overestimation of body size.
- Patterns of leaving the table directly after eating to go into the restroom.
- Problems related to eating disorders (e.g., malnutrition, menstrual irregularities, or chronic fatigue).
- Family history of eating disorders.

- A nutritious diet consists of eating a variety of foods in amounts recommended in the food pyramid. If your diet meets those recommended amounts, nutrient supplementation is not necessary.
- Protein supplementation during weight training is not necessary if a nutritious diet is maintained. Many males and especially females may require calcium supplementation to prevent osteoporosis. It may be necessary to supplement the diet with extra iron to prevent iron-deficiency anemia.
- Organic or natural foods have no beneficial effect on performance. Vegetarian diets can provide all of the essential nutrients if care is taken and the diet is well thought out and properly prepared.
- The preevent meal should be higher in carbohydrates, easily digested, eaten 3 to 4 hours before an event, and psychologically pleasing.
- Glycogen supercompensation involves maximizing resting stores of glucose in the muscle, blood, and liver before a competitive event.
- Body composition indicates the percentage of total body weight composed of fat tissue versus the percentage composed of lean tissue. The size and number of adipose cells determine percent body fat. Measurement of percent body fat can be done by measuring the thickness of the subcutaneous fat with a skinfold caliper at specific areas.
- Changes in body weight are caused almost entirely by a change in caloric balance, which is a function of the number of calories taken in and the number of calories expended. Weight can be lost either by increasing caloric expenditure through exercise or by decreasing caloric intake through dieting. Diets generally do not work. The recommended technique for losing weight involves a combination of moderate calorie restriction and a moderate increase in physical exercise during the course of each day. Weight gain should be accomplished by increasing caloric intake and engaging in a weight-training program. It is possible to gain weight and lose fat, thus changing body composition. Equal volumes of muscle weigh more than fat.
- Anorexia is a disease in which a person suffers a pathological weight loss because of a psychological aversion to food and eating. Bulimia is an eating disorder that involves binging and subsequent purging.

Solutions to Critical Thinking Exercises

4-1 In terms of weight control the important consideration is the total number of calories that one consumes relative to the total number of calories expended. It makes no difference whether the calories consumed are CHO, fat, or protein. Fat contains more than twice the number of calories as either CHO or protein, so one can eat significantly more food and still have about the same caloric intake if the diet is high in CHO. It is also essential to consume at least some fat, which is necessary for the production of several enzymes and hormones.

4-2 For an athlete who is truly consuming anything close to a well-balanced diet, vitamin supplementation is generally not necessary. However, if taking a one-a-day type of vitamin supplement makes the athlete feel better, there will be no harm. The fact that she feels tired could be related to a number of medical conditions (e.g., mononucleosis). An iron-deficiency anemia may be detected through a laboratory blood test. The athletic trainer should refer the athlete to a physician for blood work.

4-3 The amount of glycogen that can be stored in muscle and liver can be increased by reducing the training program a few days before competing and by significantly increasing carbohydrate intake during the week before the event. Nutrients consumed over several days before competition are much more important than what is eaten 3 hours before an event. The purpose of the preevent meal should be to provide the competitor with sufficient nutrient energy and fluids for competition while taking into consideration the digestibility of the food. Glucose-rich drinks taken at regular intervals are beneficial for highly intense and prolonged events that severely deplete glycogen stores.

4-4 The athlete must understand the importance of adding lean tissue muscle mass rather than increasing his percent body fat. It is true that caloric intake must be increased so that he is in a positive caloric balance of about 500 calories per day. Additional calorie intake should consist primarily of CHO. Additional supplementation with protein is not necessary. It is absolutely essential to incorporate a weight-training program using heavy weights that will overload the muscle, forcing it to hypertrophy over a period of time.

4-5 Treating eating disorders is difficult even for health care professionals specifically trained to counsel these individuals. The athletic trainer should approach the athlete as a support person and not with accusation, showing concern about her weight loss and expressing a desire to help her secure appropriate counseling. Remember that the athlete must first be willing to admit that she has an eating disorder before treatment and counseling will be effective. Eliciting the support of close friends and family can help with treatment.

REVIEW QUESTIONS AND CLASS ACTIVITIES

1. What is the value of good nutrition in terms of an athlete's performance and injury prevention?
2. Ask coaches of different sports about the type of diet they recommend for their athletes and their rationale for doing so.
3. Have a nutritionist talk to the class about food myths and fallacies.
4. Have each member of the class prepare a week's food diary; then compare it with other class members' diaries.
5. What are the daily dietary requirements according to the food pyramid? Should the requirements of the typical athlete's diet differ from them? If so, in what ways?
6. Have the class debate the value of vitamin and mineral supplements.
7. Describe the advantages and disadvantages of supplementing iron and calcium.
8. Is there some advantage to preevent nutrition?
9. Are there advantages or disadvantages in the vegetarian diet for the athlete?
10. Discuss the importance of the athlete monitoring body composition.
11. Explain the most effective technique for losing weight.
12. Contrast the signs and symptoms of bulimia and anorexia nervosa. If a coach or athletic trainer is aware of an athlete who may have an eating disorder, what should he or she do?

REFERENCES

1. Amato H, Wenos D: Bioelectrical impedance of hydration effects on muscular strength and endurance in college wrestlers, *J Ath Train* 28(2):170, 1993.
2. American College of Sports Medicine: Proper and improper weight loss programs, *Med Sci Sports Exerc* 15:ix, 1983.
3. Astrand PO, Rodahl K: *Textbook of work physiology*, New York, 1986, McGraw-Hill.
4. Black DR, Burckes-Miller ME: Male and female college athletes: use of anorexia and bulemia nervosa weight loss methods, *Res Q Exerc Sport* 59:252, 1988.
5. Brownell KD, Steen SN, Wilmore JH: Weight regulation practices in athletes: analysis of metabolic and health effects, *Med Sci Sports Exerc* 19(6):546, 1987 (review).
6. Champaign BN: Body fat distribution: metabolic consequences and implications for weight loss, *Med Sci Sport Exerc* 22:291, 1990.
7. Coyle EF, Coyle E: CHOs that speed recovery from training, *Phys Sportsmed* 21:111, 1993.
8. deVries H: *Physiology of exercise for physical education and athletics*, Dubuque, Iowa, 1986, William C Brown.
9. First International Conference on Nutrition and Fitness: Proceedings of a conference, Ancient Olympia, Greece, May 21-26, 1988, *Am J Clin Nutr* 49(5 suppl):909, 1989.
10. Harrelson G: Factors affecting the gastric emptying of athletic drinks, *Ath Train* 20:21, 1986.
11. Hegarty V: *Decisions in nutrition*, St Louis, 1988, Mosby.
12. Hoerr SL: Exercise: an alternative to fad diets for adolescent girls, *Phys Sportsmed* 12(2):76, 1984.
13. James WP: The role of nutrition and fitness in chronic diseases, *Am J Clin Nutr* 49(5 suppl):933, 1989.
14. Jones J: Bulemia: determining prevalence and examining intervention, *J Am College Health* 37(5):23, 1989.
15. Koszuta LE: Experts speak out on fitness and nutrition, *Phys Sports Med* 16(6):42, 1988.
16. Leaf A, Frisa KB: Eating for health or for athletic performance? *Am J Clin Nutr* 49(5 suppl):1066, 1989.
17. Liang MTC, McKeigue ME, Walker C: Nutrition for athletes and physically active adults, *J Osteopath Sports Med* 2(2):15, 1988.
18. Lohman T: *Advances in body composition assessment*, Champaign, Ill, 1992, Human Kinetics.
19. McArdle W, Katch F, Katch V: *Exercise physiology, energy, nutrition and human performance*, Philadelphia, 1994, Lea & Febiger.
20. Moore M: Carbohydrate loading: eating through the wall, *Phys Sports Med* 9(10):97, 1981.
21. Payne W, Hahn D: *Focus on health*, St Louis, 1997, Mosby.
22. Schlabach G: Carbohydrate strategies for injury prevention, *J Ath Train* 29(3):244, 1994.
23. Sherman WM, Lamb DR: Nutrition and prolonged exercise. In Lamb DR, Murray R, editors: *Perspectives in exercise science and sports medicine*, vol 1, Indianapolis, 1988, Benchmark.
24. Sherman WM, Peden MC, Wright DA: Carbohydrate feedings 1 hour before exercise improves exercise performance, *Am J Clin Nutr* 54:866, 1991.
25. Simopoulos AP: Nutrition and fitness, *JAMA* 261(19):2862, 1989.
26. Thames K: Teaching nutrition: serve up a nutritional stew to fill students' appetite for health information, *Idea Today* 6(8):15, 1988.
27. Thornton JS: Feast or famine: eating disorders in athletes, *Phys Sportsmed* 18:116, 1990.
28. US Department of Health and Human Services, Public Health Service: *Surgeon General's report on nutrition and health*, Washington, DC, 1988, US Government Printing Office.
29. Wardlaw GM, Insel PM: *Perspectives in nutrition*, St Louis, 1996, Mosby.
30. Wheeler KB: Sports nutrition for the primary care physician: the importance of carbohydrate, *Phys Sports Med* 17(1):106, 1989.
31. Williams M: *Nutrition for fitness and sports*, Dubuque, Iowa, 1992, William C Brown.

ANNOTATED BIBLIOGRAPHY

Becker G, Hammock D: *Eat well, be well cookbook*, New York, 1986, Simon & Schuster.

Provides sound nutritional information, fitness and weight control guidance, recipes, and food tips that help to establish a nutritional program and a life-long pattern of eating to promote good health.

Byrne K: *A parent's guide to anorexia and bulimia*, New York, 1987, Henry Holt.

Provides a list of resources and services available, as well as a guide to helping and understanding individuals with eating disorders.

Clark N: *The athlete's kitchen*, New York, 1987, Bantam Books.

A well-written, easy-to-read guide to nutrition for the physically active person. Includes a long list of over 200 recipes.

Haas R: *Eat to win*, New York, 1985, Signet.

The best seller that provides nutritional recommendations for athletes based on a healthier style of living.

Lohman T: *Advances in body composition assessment*, Champaign, Ill, 1992, Human Kinetics.

Explores the latest issues, concepts, and controversies in body composition assessment.

McArdle W, Katch F, Katch V: *Exercise physiology, energy, nutrition and human performance*, Philadelphia, 1994, Lea & Febiger.

An excellent text on the subject of exercise, nutrition, and weight control.

Wardlaw GM, Insel PM: *Perspectives in nutrition*, St Louis, 1996, Mosby.

A comprehensive text dealing with all aspects of nutrition.

Williams M: *Nutrition for fitness and sport*, Dubuque, Iowa, 1992, William C Brown.

An excellent and comprehensive guide to the concepts of sound nutrition for individuals engaging in sport or fitness activities.

Protective Sports Equipment

When you finish this chapter, you should be able to

- Identify the major legal ramifications related to manufacturing, buying, and issuing commercial protective equipment.
- Fit selected protective equipment properly (e.g., football helmets, shoulder pads, and running shoes).
- Differentiate between good and bad features of selected protective devices.
- Compare the advantages and disadvantages of customized versus commercial foot and ankle protective devices.
- Describe the controversies surrounding the use of certain protective devices—are they in fact weapons against opposing players, or do they really work?
- Rate the protective value of various materials used in sports to make pads and orthotic devices.
- List the order of steps in making a customized foam pad with a thermomoldable shell.

M odifications and improvements in sports equipment are continually being made, especially for sports in which injury is common. In this chapter, both commercial and preventive, or **prophylactic,** techniques are discussed. Protective sports equipment should be used for preventing initial injury and reinjury.

prophylactic
Refers to prevention, preservation, or protection.

COMMERCIAL EQUIPMENT

Proper selection and fit of sports equipment are essential in the prevention of many sports injuries. This is particularly true in direct contact and collision sports such as football, hockey, and lacrosse, but it can also be true in indirect contact sports such as basketball and soccer. Whenever protective sports equipment is selected and purchased, a major decision in the safeguarding of the athletes' health and welfare is being made.

Currently there is serious concern about the standards for protective sports equipment, particularly material durability standards—concerns that include who should set these standards, mass production of equipment, equipment testing methods, and requirements for wearing protective equipment. Some people are concerned that a piece of equipment that is protective to one athlete might in turn be used as a weapon against another athlete.

Standards are also needed for protective equipment maintenance, both to keep it in good repair and to determine when to throw it away. Too often old, worn-out, and ill-fitting equipment is passed down from the varsity players to the younger and often less-experienced players, compounding their risk of injury. Coaches must learn to be less concerned with the color, look, and style of a piece of equipment and more concerned with its ability to prevent injury. Many national organizations are addressing these issues (see the Focus box on the next page). Engineering, chemistry, biomechanics, anatomy, physiology, physics, computer science, and other related disciplines are applied to solve problems inherent in safety standardization of sports equipment and facilities.

Old, worn-out, ill-fitting equipment should never be passed down to younger, less-experienced players; it compounds their chances for injury.

Legal Concerns

As with other aspects of sports participation, there is increasing litigation related to equipment. Manufacturers and purchasers of sports equipment must foresee all pos-

5-1

Critical Thinking Exercise

A student athletic trainer must acquire a basic understanding of protective sports equipment.

? What competencies in protective sports equipment must student athletic trainers have?

Focus

Protective sports equipment regulatory organizations

Athletic Equipment Manager Association (AEMA)
723 Keil Court
Bowling Green, OH 43402
(419) 352-1207

National Association of Intercollegiate Athletics (NAIA)
1221 Baltimore
Kansas City, MO 64105
(816) 842-5050

National Collegiate Athletic Association (NCAA)
P.O. Box 1906
Nall at 63rd Street
Mission, KS 66201
(913) 384-3220

National Federation of State High School Associations (NFSHSA)
P.O. Box 20626
11724 Plaza Circle
Kansas City, MO 64195
(816) 464-5400

American National Standards Institute (ANSI)
1430 Broadway
New York, NY 10018
(212) 354-3300

National Operating Committee on Standards for Athletic Equipment (NOCSAE)
11724 Plaza Circle
P.O. Box 11724
Kansas City, MO 64195
(816) 464-5470

United States Olympic Committee (USOC)
1750 E. Boulder Street
Colorado Springs, CO 80909
(719) 632-5551

5-2

Critical Thinking Exercise

C- and B-level high school football players are issued their equipment. These athletes and their parents know very little about the equipment's potential for preventing injury.

? The athletic trainer is given the responsibility to educate the team and their parents about the equipment safety limits. The purpose is to reduce legal liability.

---

sible uses and misuses of the equipment and must warn the user of any potential risks inherent in the use or misuse of that equipment.[2]

To decrease the possibilities of sports injuries and litigation stemming from equipment, the practitioner should do the following:
1. Buy sports equipment from reputable manufacturers.
2. Buy the safest equipment that resources will permit.
3. Make sure that all equipment is assembled correctly. The person who assembles equipment must be competent to do so and must follow the manufacturer's instructions "to the letter."
4. Maintain all equipment properly, according to the manufacturer's guidelines.
5. Use equipment only for the purpose for which it was designed.
6. Warn athletes who use the equipment about all possible risks that using the equipment could entail.
7. Use great caution in the construction or customizing of any piece of equipment.
8. Use no defective equipment. All equipment must routinely be inspected for defects, and all defective equipment must be rendered unusable.

Commercial stock and custom protective devices differ considerably. Stock devices are premade and packaged and are for immediate use. Customized devices are constructed according to the individual characteristics of an athlete. Stock items may have problems with their sizing. In contrast, a custom device can be specifically sized and made to fit the protection and support needs of the individual. Both commercial and customizing devices are discussed in this chapter.

HEAD PROTECTION

Direct collision sports such as football and hockey require special protective equipment, especially for the head. Football provides more frequent opportunities for body contact than does hockey, but hockey players generally move faster and therefore create greater impact forces. Besides direct head contact, hockey has the added injury elements of swinging sticks and fast-moving pucks. Other sports using fast-moving projectiles are baseball, with its pitched ball and swinging bat, and track and field, with the javelin, discus, and shot, which can also produce serious head injuries. In recent years most helmet research has been conducted for football and ice hockey; however, some research has been performed on baseball headgear.[1]

Football Helmets

The National Operating Committee on Standards for Athletic Equipment (NOCSAE) has developed standards for football helmet certification. An approved helmet must protect against concussive forces that may injure the brain. Collision that causes concussion is usually from another player or striking the turf.[7]

Schools must provide the athlete with quality equipment. This especially is true of the football helmet. All helmets must have a NOCSAE certification. Even though a helmet is certified does not mean that it is completely "fail-safe." Athletes, as well as their parents, must be apprised of the dangers that are inherent in any sport, particularly football.[7] To make this especially clear, the NOCSAE has adopted the following recommended warning to be placed on all football helmets:

> WARNING: Do not strike an opponent with any part of this helmet or face mask. This is a violation of football rules and may cause you to suffer severe brain or neck injury, including paralysis or death. Severe brain or neck injury may also occur accidentally while playing football. NO HELMET CAN PREVENT ALL SUCH INJURIES. USE THIS HELMET AT YOUR OWN RISK.

Each player's helmet must have a visible exterior warning label ensuring that players have been made aware of the risks involved in the game of American football. The label must be attached to each helmet by both the manufacturer and the reconditioner.[6]

It is important to have each player read this warning, after which it is read aloud by the equipment manager. The athlete then signs a statement, agreeing that he understands this warning. A popular type of helmet is the air and fluid helmet (Figure 5-1). When fitting helmets, always wet the player's hair to simulate playing conditions; this makes the initial fitting easier. Closely follow the manufacturer's directions for a proper fit. (See the Focus box on the next page.)

The football helmet must be routinely checked for proper fit, especially in the first few days that it is worn. A check for snugness should be made by inserting a tongue depressor between the head and the liner. Fit is proper when the tongue depressor is resisted firmly when moved back and forth. If air bladder helmets are used by a team that travels to a different altitude and air pressure, the helmet fit must be routinely rechecked.

Chin straps are also important in maintaining the proper head and helmet relationship. Two basic types of chin straps are in use today—a two-snap and a four-snap strap. Many coaches prefer the four-snap chin strap because it keeps the helmet

Football helmets must withstand repeated blows that are of high mass and low velocity.

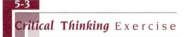

5-3

Critical Thinking Exercise

The athletic trainer explains the helmet's limitations to a football team.

? Why does the football helmet have a warning label?

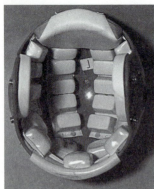

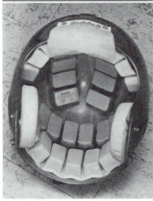

Figure 5-1

The air- and fluid-filled padded football helmet.

Even high-quality helmets are of no use if not properly fitted or maintained.

Ice hockey helmets must withstand the high-velocity impact of a stick or puck and the low-velocity forces from falling or hitting a sideboard.

from tilting forward and backward. The chin strap should always be locked so that it cannot be released by a hard external force to the helmet (Figure 5-2).

Jaw pads are also essential to keep the helmet from rocking laterally. They should fit snugly against the player's cheekbones. Even if a helmet's ability to withstand the forces of the game is certified, it is of no avail if the helmet is not properly fitted or maintained.

Ice Hockey Helmets

As with football helmets, there has been a concerted effort to upgrade and standardize ice hockey helmets.[2] In contrast to football, blows to the head in ice hockey are usually singular rather than multiple. An ice hockey helmet must withstand both high-velocity impacts (e.g., being hit with a stick or a puck, which produces low mass and high velocity), as well as the high-mass–low-velocity forces produced by running into the sideboard or falling on the ice. In each instance, the hockey helmet, like the football helmet, must be able to spread the impact over a large surface area through a firm exterior shell and, at the same time, be able to decelerate forces that act on the head through a proper energy-absorbing liner. It is essential for all hockey players to wear protective helmets that carry the stamp of approval from the Canadian Standards Association (CSA).

Baseball Batting Helmets

Like ice hockey helmets, the baseball batting helmet must withstand high-velocity impacts. Unlike football and ice hockey, baseball has not produced a great deal of data on batting helmets.[2] It has been suggested, however, that baseball helmets do little to adequately dissipate the energy of the ball during impact (Figure 5-3). A possible answer is to add external padding or to improve the helmet's suspension.[2] The use of a helmet with an ear flap can afford some additional protection to the batter. Each runner and on-deck batter is required to wear a baseball or softball helmet that carries the NOCSAE stamp, similar to that on football helmets.

FACE PROTECTION

Devices that provide face protection fall into four categories: full face guards, mouth guards, ear guards, and eye protection devices.

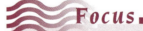
Focus

Properly fitting the helmet

In general, the helmet should adhere to the following fit standards:
- The helmet should fit snugly around all parts of the player's head (front, sides, and crown), and there should be no gaps between the pads and the head or face.
- It should cover the base of the skull. The pads placed at the back of the neck should be snug but not to the extent of discomfort.
- It should not come down over the eyes. It should set (front edge) ¾ inch (1.91 cm) above the player's eyebrows (approximately two finger widths).
- The ear holes should match.
- It should not shift when manual pressure is applied.
- It should not recoil on impact.
- The chin strap should be an equal distance from the center of the helmet. Straps must keep the helmet from moving up and down or side to side.
- The cheek pads should fit snugly against the sides of the face.
- The face mask should be attached securely to the helmet, allowing a complete field of vision, and positioned three finger widths from the nose.

A   B   C

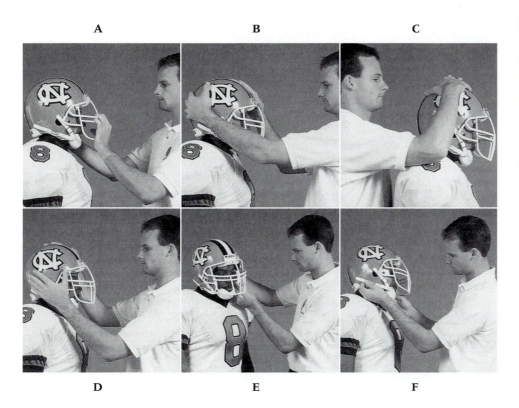

D   E   F

Figure 5-2

Fitting a football helmet. **A,** Pull down on face mask; helmet must not move. **B,** Turn helmet to position on the athlete's head. **C,** Push down on helmet; there must be no movement. **D,** Try to rock helmet back and forth; there must be no movement. **E,** Check for a snug jaw pad fit. **F,** Proper adjustment of the chin strap is necessary to ensure proper helmet fit.

Face Guards

Face guards are used in a variety of sports to protect against flying or carried objects during a collision with another player (Figure 5-4). Since the adoption of face guards and mouth guards for use in football, mouth injuries have been reduced more than 50% (Figure 5-5), but the incidence of neck injuries has increased significantly. The catcher in baseball, the goalie in hockey, and the lacrosse player should all be adequately protected against facial injuries, particularly lacerations and fractures (Figure 5-6).

A great variety of face masks and bars is available to the player, depending on the position played and the protection needed. In football no face protection should have less than two bars. Proper mounting of the face mask and bars is imperative for maximum safety. All mountings should be made in such a way that the bar attachments are flush with the helmet. A 3-inch (7.62 cm) space should exist between the top of the face guard and the lower edge of the helmet. No helmet should be drilled more than one time on each side, and this must be done by a factory-authorized reconditioner. Attachment of a bar or face mask not specifically designed for the helmet can invalidate the manufacturer's warranty.

Ice hockey face masks have been shown to reduce the incidence of facial injuries. In high school they are required not only for the goalie but also for all players. The rule stipulates that helmets be equipped with commercial plastic-coated wire mask guards, which must meet standards set by the Hockey Equipment Certification Council (HECC) and the American Society for Testing Materials (ASTM).[6] The openings in the guard must be small enough to prevent a hockey stick from entering. Plastic guards such as polycarbonate face shields have been approved by the HECC and ASTM and the CSA Committee on Hockey Protective Equipment. The rule also requires that, in addition to face protectors, goalkeepers wear commercial throat protectors. The National Federation of High School Associations (NFHSA) rule is similar to the National Collegiate Athletic Association (NCAA) rule requiring players to wear face guards. There should be a space of 1 to 1½ inches (3.81 cm) between the play-

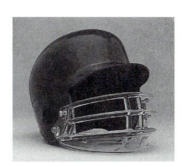

Figure 5-3

There is some question about how well baseball batting helmets protect against high-velocity impacts.

In sports, the face may be protected by
    Face guards
    Mouth guards
    Ear guards
    Eye-protection devices

Figure 5-4

Sports such as fencing require complete face protection.

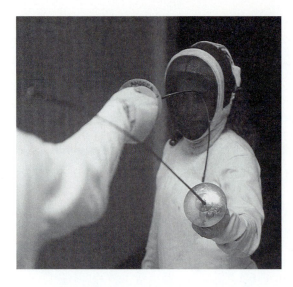

Figure 5-5

Face guards used for football.

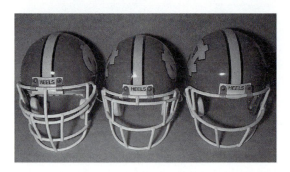

er's nose and the face guard. As with the helmet shell, pads, and chin strap, the face guard must be checked daily for defects.

Laryngotracheal Protection

A laryngotracheal injury, though relatively uncommon, can be fatal.[7] Baseball catchers, lacrosse goalies, and ice hockey goalies are most at risk. Throat protection should be mandatory for these sports.

Mouth Protection

A properly fitted mouth guard protects the teeth, absorbs blows to the chin, and can prevent concussion.

The majority of dental traumas can be prevented if the athlete wears a correctly fitted customized intraoral mouth guard (Figure 5-7). In addition to protecting the teeth, the intraoral mouth guard absorbs the shock of chin blows and helps prevent a possible cerebral concussion. Mouth guards serve also to prevent lacerations to lips and cheeks and fractures to the mandible. The mouth protector should give the athlete proper and tight fit, comfort, unrestricted breathing, and unimpeded speech during competition. A loose mouthpiece will soon be ejected onto the ground or left unused in the locker room. The athlete's air passages should not be obstructed in any way by the mouthpiece. It is best when the mouthpiece is retained on the upper jaw and projects backward only as far as the last molar, thus permitting speech. Maximum protection is afforded when the mouth guard is composed of a flexible, resilient material and is form fitted to the teeth and upper jaw.

Cutting down mouth guards to cover only the front four teeth should never be permitted. It invalidates the manufacturer's warranty against dental injuries, and a cut-down mouth guard can easily become dislodged and lead to an obstructed airway, which poses a serious life-threatening situation for the athlete.

Three types of mouth guards generally used in sports include the stock variety, a commercial mouth guard formed after submersion in boiling water, and the custom-fabricated type, which is formed over a model made from an impression of the athlete's maxillary arch.[2]

Many high schools and colleges now require that mouth guards be worn at all times during participation. For example, the NCAA football rules mandate that all players wear a properly manufactured mouth guard. A time-out is charged a team if a player fails to wear the mouth guard. To assist enforcement, official mouth guards are increasingly made in the most visible color possible—yellow.[2] It is important that coaches and athletic trainers measure the arch length of the mouth guards to ensure adequate protection for the athlete and to be in compliance with the NCAA rule.[2]

Ear Guards

With the exception of wrestling, water polo, and boxing, most contact sports do not make a special practice of protecting the ears. All these sports can cause irritation of the ears to the point that permanent deformity can ensue. To avoid this problem special ear guards should be routinely worn (Figure 5-8).

Eye Protection Devices

The National Society to Prevent Blindness estimates that the highest percentage of eye injuries are sports or play related. Most injuries are from blunt trauma. Protective devices must be sport specific.

Spectacles

For the athlete who must wear corrective lenses, glasses can be both a blessing and a nuisance. They may slip on sweat, get bent when hit, fog from perspiration, detract from peripheral vision, or be difficult to wear with protective headgear. Even with all these disadvantages, properly fitted and designed glasses can provide adequate protection and withstand the rigors of the sport. If the athlete has glass lenses, they must be case-hardened to prevent them from splintering on impact. When a case-hardened

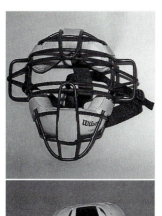
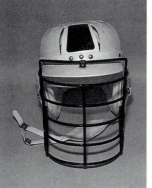

Figure 5-6

A, Baseball catcher's mask. **B,** Lacrosse helmet and faceguard.

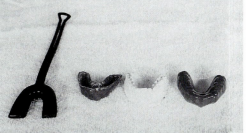
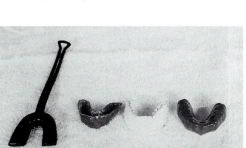

Figure 5-7

Moldable and customized mouth protectors.

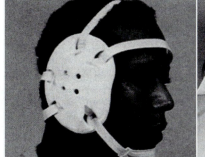
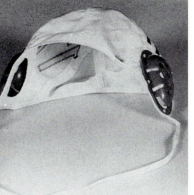

Figure 5-8

Ear protection. **A,** The wrestler's ear guard. **B,** Water polo player's ear protection.

Eye protection must be worn by all athletes who play sports that use fast-moving projectiles.

lens breaks, it crumbles, eliminating the sharp edges that may penetrate the eye. The cost of this process is relatively low. The only disadvantages involved are that the weight of the glasses is heavier than average, and they may be scratched more easily than regular glasses.

Another possible sports advantage of glass lenses is a process through which the lenses can become color tinted when exposed to ultraviolet rays from the sun and then return to a clear state when removed from the sun's rays. They are known as *photochromic lenses.*

Plastic lenses for glasses are becoming increasingly popular with athletes. They are much lighter in weight than glass lenses; however, they are much more prone to scratching.

Contact Lenses

In many ways the athlete who is able to wear contact lenses without discomfort can avoid many of the inconveniences of glasses. Their greatest advantage is probably the fact that they "become a part of the eye" and move with it.

Contact lenses come mainly in two types: the corneal type, which covers just the iris of the eye, and the scleral type, which covers the entire front of the eye, including the white. Peripheral vision, as well as astigmatism and corneal waviness, is improved through the use of contact lenses. Unlike regular glasses, contact lenses do not normally cloud during temperature changes. They also can be tinted to reduce glare. For example, yellow lenses can be used against ice glare and blue ones against glare from snow. One of the main difficulties with contact lenses is their high cost compared with regular glasses. Some other serious disadvantages of wearing contact lenses are the possibility of corneal irritation caused by dust getting under the lens and the possibility of a lens becoming dislodged during body contact. In addition, only certain individuals are able to wear contacts with comfort, and some individuals are unable to ever wear them because of certain eye idiosyncrasies. There is currently a trend toward athletes' preferring the soft, hydrophilic lenses to the hard type. Adjustment time for the soft lenses is shorter than for the hard, they can be more easily replaced, and they are more adaptable to the sports environment. There are also disposable lenses and lenses that can be worn for an extended period. In the last few years, the cost of contact lenses has dropped significantly.

Eye and Glass Guards

It is essential that athletes take special precautions to protect their eyes, especially in sports that use fast-moving projectiles and implements, such as handball or racquetball (Figure 5-9). Besides the more obvious sports of ice hockey, lacrosse, and base-

Figure 5-9

Athletes playing sports that involve small, fast projectiles should wear the closed type of eye guards.

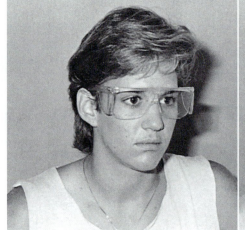 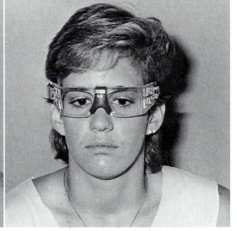

A   B

ball, the racquet sports also cause serious eye injury. Athletes not wearing glasses should wear closed eye guards to protect the orbital cavity. Athletes who normally wear glasses with plastic or case-hardened lenses are to some degree already protected against eye injury from an implement or projectile; however, greater safety is afforded by the metal-rimmed frame that surrounds and fits over the athlete's glasses. The protection the guard affords is excellent, but it hinders vision in some planes. Polycarbonate eye shields that have recently been developed can be attached to football face masks, hockey helmets, and baseball and softball helmets.

Neck Protection

Restrictive neck straps are being used by some football teams. A semielastic strap 1½-inches (3.75 cm) wide is fixed to the back of the helmet and shoulder pad to restrict excessive flexion. Experts in cervical injuries consider the major value of commercial and customized cervical collars to be mostly a reminder to the athlete to be cautious rather than to provide a definitive restriction.[2]

TRUNK AND THORAX PROTECTION

Trunk and thorax protection is essential in many contact and collision sports. Sports such as football, ice hockey, and lacrosse use extensive body protection. Areas that are most exposed to impact forces must be properly covered with some material that offers protection against soft-tissue compression. Of particular concern are the exposed bony protuberances of the body that have insufficient soft tissue for protection, such as shoulders, ribs, and spine, as well as external genitalia (Figures 5-10 and 5-11).

As discussed earlier, the problem that arises in the wearing of protective equipment is that, although it is armor against injury to the athlete wearing it, it can also serve as a weapon against all opponents. Standards must become more stringent in determining what equipment is absolutely necessary for body protection and at the same time is not itself a source of trauma. Proper fit and maintenance of equipment are essential.

Football Shoulder Pads

Manufacturers of shoulder pads have made great strides toward protecting the football player against direct force to the shoulder muscle complex (Figure 5-12). There

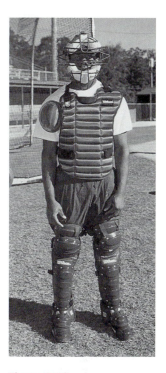

Figure 5-10

Full-body protection. Baseball chest protector for catchers.

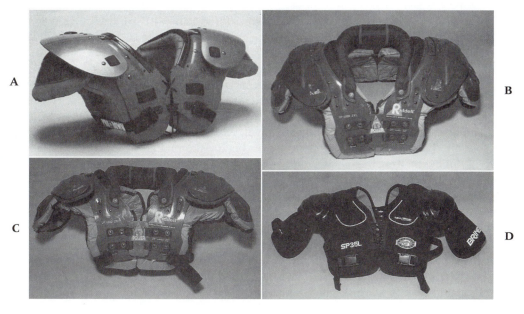

Figure 5-11

Shoulder pads protect both the shoulder and thorax. **A, B, C,** Football shoulder pads. **D,** Lacrosse shoulder pad.

Figure 5-12

Football shoulder pads should be made to protect the player against direct force to the entire shoulder complex.

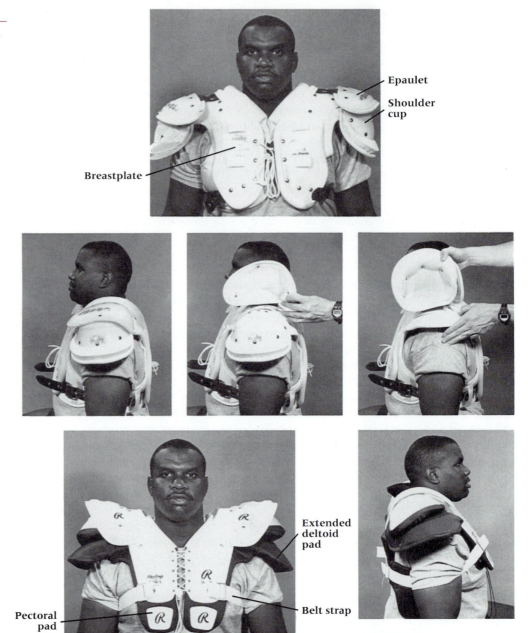

are two general types of pads: flat and cantilevered. The player who uses the shoulder a great deal in blocking and tackling requires the bulkier cantilevered type as compared with the quarterback or ball receiver, who use the flat type. Over the years the shoulder pad's front and rear panels have been extended along with the cantilever. The following are rules for fitting the football shoulder pad:

- The width of the shoulder is measured to determine the proper size of pad.
- The inside shoulder pad should cover the tip of the shoulder in a direct line with the lateral aspect of the shoulder.
- The epaulets and cups should cover the deltoid muscle and allow movements required by the athlete's specific position.
- The neck opening must allow the athlete to raise the arm overhead but not allow the pad to slide back and forth.
- If a split-clavicle shoulder pad is used, the channel for the top of the shoulder must be in the proper position.

■ Straps underneath the arm must hold the pads firmly in place, but not so they constrict soft tissue. A collar and drop-down pads may be added to provide additional protection.

Some athletic trainers use a combination of football and ice hockey shoulder pads to prevent injuries high on the upper arm and shoulder. A pair of supplemental shoulder pads are placed under the football pads (Figure 5-13). The deltoid cap of the hockey pad is connected to the main body of the hockey pad by an adjustable lace. The distal end of the deltoid cap is held in place by a Velcro strap. The chest pad is adjustable to ensure proper fit for any size athlete. The football shoulder pads are placed over the hockey pads. The athletic trainer should observe for a proper fit. Larger football pads may be needed.

Breast Support

Until recently the primary concern for female breast protection had been against external forces that could cause bruising. With the vast increase in the number of physically active women, concern has been redirected to protecting the breasts against movement that stems from running and jumping. This is a particular problem for women with large breasts. Many girls and women in the past may have avoided vigorous physical activity because of the discomfort felt from the uncontrolled movement of their breasts. Manufacturers are making a concerted effort to develop specialized bras for women who participate in all types of physical activity. The athletic clothing industry has produced an array of stylish, comfortable, and supportive sports bras.

A bra should hold the breasts to the chest and prevent stretching of the Cooper's ligament, which causes premature sagging (Figure 5-14).

Most regular bras do not provide sufficient support to prevent excessive breast motion, and many are poorly designed. Sports bras fall into three categories:

1. Bras with good upward support with elastic material have wide bands under the breasts with wide shoulder straps that are attached close to the hooks in the back (Figure 5-15, *A*).
2. Compressive bras function like wide elastic bandages, binding the breasts to the chest wall (Figure 5-15, *B*).
3. To be effective a bra should hold the breasts to the chest and prevent stretching of the Cooper's ligament, which causes premature sagging (Figure 5-14). Metal parts (snaps, fasteners, underwire support) rub and abrade the skin. They lack suffi-

To be effective, a bra should hold the breasts tightly to the chest.

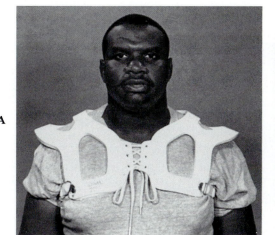
A

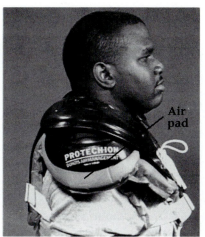
B

Figure 5-13

Customized foam is placed on the underside of the shoulder pad to provide additional protection.

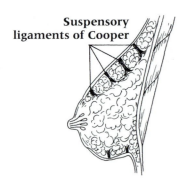

Figure 5-14

Stretching of Cooper's ligament causes premature sagging.

cient padding. Seams over nipples compound the rubbing of the bra on the nipple, leading to irritation.

For women with small breasts no special type of bra is required except to protect the nipple area. Women with medium-sized breasts generally prefer the compressive bras, but women with a size C cup or larger should wear a firm supportive bra. Fabric, fabric weight, and firmness of construction depend on the intensity of activity, support needed, sensitivity to the fabric, and climate. In contact sports additional padding may be placed inside the cup if needed. Women competing in ice hockey, for example, wear protective plastic chest pieces that attach to their shoulder pads to protect the breast tissue from contusions. Women should look for a bra with these features:

- No irritating seams or fasteners next to the skin
- Nonslip straps
- Good support or compression that holds the breasts close to the body
- Firm, durable construction

Thorax

Manufacturers such as Bike Company and Casco provide similar equipment for thorax protection. Many of the thorax protectors and rib belts can be modified, replacing stock pads with customized thermomoldable plastic protective devices.[2] Recently many lightweight pads have been developed to protect the athlete against external forces. A jacket developed by Byron Donzis for the protection of a rib injury incorporates a pad composed of air-inflated, interconnected cylinders that protect against severe external forces (Figure 5-16). This same principle has been used in the development of other protective pads.

Hips and Buttocks

Pads in the region of the hips and buttocks are often needed in collision and high-velocity sports such as hockey and football. Other athletes needing protection in this region are amateur boxers, snow skiers, equestrians, jockeys, and water skiers.[2] Two popular commercial pads are the girdle and belt types (Figure 5-17).

Groin and Genitalia

Sports involving high-velocity projectiles (e.g., hockey, lacrosse, and baseball) require cup protection for male participants. It comes as a stock item that fits into place in a jockstrap, or athletic supporter[2] (Figure 5-18).

Figure 5-15

Female athletes should wear sports bras made of elastic material. **A,** Support bra. **B,** Compressive bra.

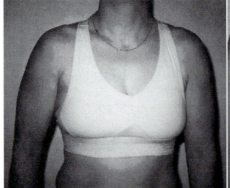
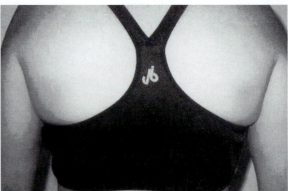

A

B

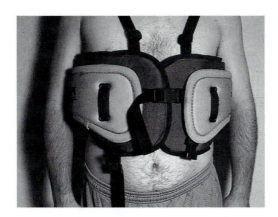

Figure 5-16

Protective rib belt.

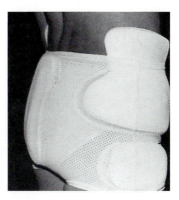

Figure 5-17

Girdle-style hip and coccygeal pad.

LIMB PROTECTION

Limbs, as with other areas of the body, can be exposed a great deal to sports injuries and can require protection or, where there is weakness, support. Compression and mild soft-tissue support can be provided by neoprene sleeves, and hard bony areas of the body can be protected by commercial pads (Figure 5-19). In contrast, the athlete with a history of injury that needs special protection and support may require a commercial brace.

Footwear

Footwear can mean the difference between success, failure, or injury in competition. It is essential that the coach, athletic trainer, and equipment personnel make every effort to fit their athletes with proper shoes and socks.

Socks

Poorly fitted socks can cause abnormal stresses on the foot. For example, socks that are too short crowd the toes, especially the fourth and fifth ones. Socks that are too long can wrinkle and cause skin irritation. All athletic socks should be clean, dry, and without holes to avoid irritations. Manufacturers are now providing different types of socks for various sports. The composition of the sock's material also should be noted. Cotton socks can be too bulky, whereas a combination of materials such as cotton and polyester is less bulky and dries faster.

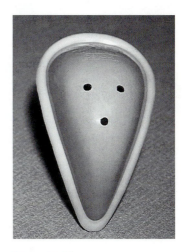

Figure 5-18

A cup, held in place by an athletic supporter, used for protecting the genitals against high-velocity projectiles.

All athletic socks should be clean and dry and without holes. Socks of the wrong size can irritate the skin.

Shoes

Even more damaging than improperly fitted socks are improperly fitted shoes. Chronic abnormal pressures to the foot can often cause permanent structural deformities, as well as potentially dangerous calluses and blisters. Besides these local problems, improperly fitted shoes result in mechanical disturbances that affect the body's total postural balance and may eventually lead to pathological conditions of the muscles and joints. It also should be noted that worn or broken-down shoes predispose the athlete to injuries of the foot and leg. Badly worn shoes have also been known to create hip and low back problems.

Shoe composition   The bare human foot is designed to function on uneven surfaces. Shoes were created to protect against harmful surfaces, but they should never interfere with natural functioning. Sports shoes, like all shoes, are constructed of different parts, each of which is designed to provide function, protection, and durability. Each sport places unique stresses and performance demands on the foot. In general, all sport shoes, like street shoes, are made of similar parts—a sole, uppers, heel counter, and toe box.

Sole   The sole, or bottom, of a shoe is divided into a center, middle, and inner section, each of which must be sturdy and flexible and provide a degree of cushion-

A properly fitted shoe will bend where the foot bends.

Figure 5-19

Types of neoprene sleeves.

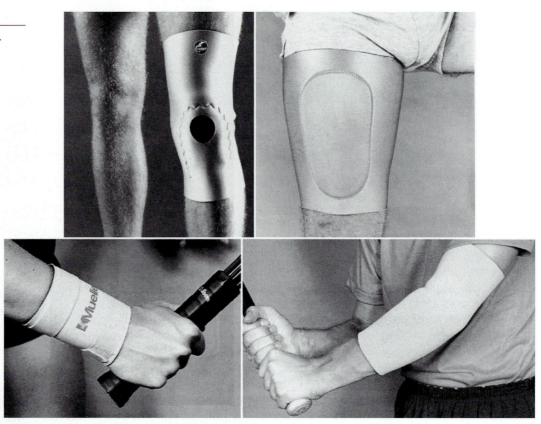

ing.[10] Most shoes have three layers on the sole: a thick spongy layer, which absorbs the force of the foot strike under the heel; a midsole, which cushions the midfoot and toes; and a hard rubber layer, which comes in contact with the ground. The average runner's feet strike the ground between 1500 and 1700 times per mile. Thus it is essential that the force of the heel strike be absorbed by the spongy layer to prevent overuse injuries from occurring in the ankles and knees. Heel wedges are sometimes inserted either on the inside or outside surface of the sole underneath the heel counter to accommodate and correct for various structural deformities of the foot that may alter normal biomechanics of the running gait.

Shoe uppers The upper part of the shoe is made of some combination of nylon and leather. The uppers should be lightweight, capable of quick drying, and well-ventilated. The uppers should have some type of extra support in the saddle area, and there should also be some extra padding in the area of the Achilles tendon just above the heel counter.

Heel counters The heel counter is the portion of the shoe that prevents the foot from rolling from side to side at heel strike. The heel counter should be firm but well fitted to minimize movement of the heel up and down or side to side. A good heel counter may prevent ankle sprains and painful blisters.[10]

Toe box There should be plenty of room for your toes in the fitness shoe. Most experts recommend a ½- to ¾-inch distance between toes and the front of the shoe made in varying widths or narrow widths. Most shoe salespersons can recommend a specific shoe for the athlete's foot. The best way to make sure there is adequate room in the toe box is to have one's foot measured and then try on the shoe (Figure 5-20).[10]

Shoe fitting Fitting sports footgear is always difficult, mainly because the individual's left foot varies in size and shape from the right foot. Therefore measuring

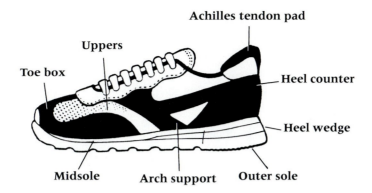

Figure 5-20

Parts of a well-designed sport shoe.

both feet is imperative. To fit the sports shoe properly, the athlete should approximate the conditions under which he or she will perform, such as wearing athletic socks, jumping up and down, or running. It is also desirable to fit the athlete's shoes at the end of the day to accommodate the gradual increase in size that occurs from the time of awakening. The athlete must carefully consider this shoe choice because he or she will be spending countless hours in those shoes (see the Focus box on the next page for suggestions concerning shoe fitting).[4]

During performance conditions the new shoe should feel snug but not too tight.[2] The sports shoe should be long enough that all toes can be fully extended without being cramped. Its width should permit full movement of the toes, including flexion, extension, and some spreading. A good point to remember is that the wide part of the shoe should match the wide part of the foot to allow the shoe to crease evenly when the athlete is on the balls of the feet. The shoe should bend (or "break") at its widest part; when the break of the shoe and the ball joint coincide, the fit is correct. However, if the break of the shoe is in back or in front of the normal bend of the foot (metatarsophalangeal joint), the shoe and the foot will oppose one another, causing abnormal skin and structural stresses to occur. Two measurements must be considered when fitting shoes: the distance from the heel to the metatarsophalangeal joint and the distance from the heel to the end of the longest toe. An individual's feet may be equal in length from the heels to the balls of the feet but different between heels and toes. It should be noted that one type of shoe is not appropriate for all athletes in a particular sport. Shoes therefore should be selected for the longer of the two measurements. Other factors to consider when buying the sports shoe are the stiffness of the sole and the width of the shank, or narrowest part of the sole. A shoe with a too rigid, nonyielding sole places a great deal of extra strain on the foot tendons. A shoe with too narrow a shank also places extra strain because it fails to adequately support the athlete's inner, longitudinal arches.[2]

The specially soled shoe The cleated or specially soled sports shoe presents some additional problems in fitting. For example, American football uses the multi–short-cleated polyurethane sole with the soccer-type sole with cleats no longer than 0.5 inches (1.27 cm) (Figure 5-21). Specially soled shoes are also worn when playing on a synthetic surface. Whenever cleated shoes are used, the cleats must be properly positioned under the two major weight-bearing joints and must not be felt through the soles of the shoes. (See Table 1-1 for shoe comparisons.[10])

Commercial Foot Pads

Commercial foot pads are intended for use by the general public and are not usually designed to withstand the rigors of sports activities. Commercial pads that are suited

5-4

Critical Thinking Exercise

A high school basketball player is given advice on purchasing a pair of basketball shoes.

? What fitting factors must be taken into consideration when purchasing basketball shoes?

Indiscriminate use of commercial foot orthotics may give the athlete a false sense of security.

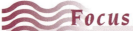

Focus

Proper running shoe design and construction

To avoid injury, the running shoe should[7]

- Have a strong heel counter that fits well around the foot and locks the shoe around the foot.
- Always have good flexibility in the forefoot where toes bend.
- Preferably have a fairly high heel for the athlete with a tight Achilles tendon.
- Have a midsole that is moderately soft but does not flatten easily.
- Have a heel counter that is high enough to surround the foot but still allows room for an orthotic insert, if needed.
- Have a counter that is attached to the sole to avoid the possibility of its coming loose from attachment.
- Always be of quality construction.

for sports are generally not durable enough for hard, extended use. If money is no object, the ready-made commercial pad has the advantage of saving time. Commercial pads are manufactured for almost every type of common structural foot condition, ranging from corns and bunions to fallen arches and pronated feet.[2] In general, excessive foot pronation often eventually leads to overuse injuries. Available to the athlete commercially are preorthotic and arch supports (Figure 5-22). Scholl 610.2, Spenco arch supports, Shea devices, and Foothotics "Ready to Dispense" orthotics are commonly used before more formal customized orthotic devices are made. They offer a compromise to the custom-made foot orthotics, providing some biomechanical control.[4] Indiscriminate use of these aids, however, may intensify the pathological condition or cause the athlete to delay seeing the team physician or team podiatrist for evaluation.

For the most part, foot devices are fabricated and customized from a variety of materials such as foam, felt, plaster, aluminum, and spring steel (see under Construction of Protective and Supportive Devices, later in this chapter). The heel cup, designed to reduce tissue shearing and shock (Figure 5-23), is one item that began as a prefabricated device but now is commercial.

Commercial Ankle Supports

Currently, semirigid orthoses such as the Air Stirrup are being used successfully to restrain ankle motion. Compared with ankle taping, these devices do not loosen significantly during exercise[3] (Figure 5-24). Commercial ankle stabilizers, either alone or in combination with ankle taping, are becoming increasingly popular in sports.[3]

Figure 5-21

Variations in cleated shoes: the longer the cleat, the higher the incidence of injury.

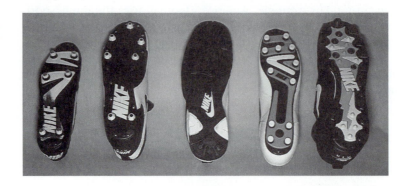

TABLE 5-1 **Shoe Comparisons**

	Tennis	Aerobic	Running
Flexibility	Firm sole, more rigid than running shoe	Sole between running and tennis shoe	Flexible ball of foot
Uppers	Leather or leather with nylon	Leather or leather with nylon	Nylon or nylon mesh
Heel flare	None	Very little	Flared for stability
Cushioning	Less than a running shoe	Between running and tennis shoe	Heel and sole well padded
Soles	Polyurethane	Rubber or polyurethane	Carbon-based material for greater durability
Tread	Flattened	Flat or pivot dot	Deep grooves for grip

Shin and Lower Leg

The shin is an area of the body that is commonly neglected in contact and collision-type sports. Commercially marketed hard-shelled, molded shin guards are used in field hockey and soccer (Figure 5-25).

Thigh and Upper Leg

Thigh and upper leg protection is necessary in collision-type sports such as hockey and football. Generally, pads slip into ready-made pockets in the sports suit or uniform (Figure 5-26). To prevent abnormal slipping within the pocket and to protect from injury, customized pads are constructed.

Knee Supports and Protective Devices

Knees follow ankles and feet in terms of incidence of sports injury. As a result of the variety and high frequency of knee afflictions, many protective and supportive devices have been devised. The devices most frequently used in sports today are sleeves, pads, and braces.

Elastic knee pads or guards are extremely valuable in sports in which the athlete falls or receives a direct blow to the anterior aspect of the knee. An elastic sleeve

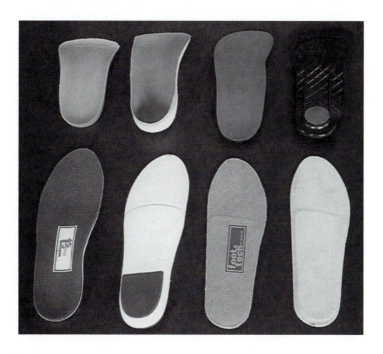

Figure 5-22

Commercially manufactured orthotic devices.

Figure 5-23

Heel cups and pads including lifts of orthopedic felt.

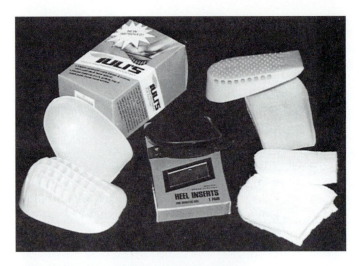

Figure 5-24

Commercial ankle supports for an injured ankle.

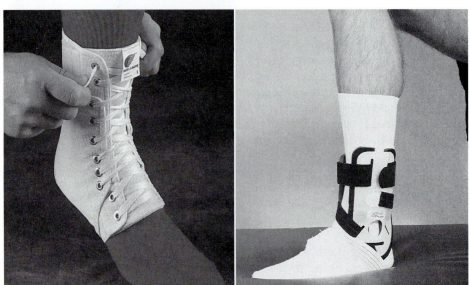

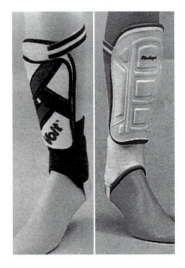

Figure 5-25

Soccer shin guards.

containing a resilient pad may help dissipate an anterior striking force but fails to protect the knee against lateral, medial, or twisting forces.

Knee Braces

There are a number of different knee braces on the market. Some consist of vertical rigid strips held in an elastic sleeve or an elastic sleeve containing rigid hinges to be placed on either side of the knee joint. The ability of these braces to act as a protection against initial or recurrent injury is extremely questionable. Braces of the wraparound type with rigid strips contained in less elastic material hold the knee more firmly in place.

Prophylactic knee brace The American Academy of Orthopaedic Surgeons (AAOS) and the American Orthopaedic Society for Sports Medicine have voiced reservations about knee braces.[1] As discussed in Chapter 19, knee braces are classified into three types: prophylactic, functional, and rehabilitative. The prophylactic knee brace will be addressed here. The AAOS Committee on Sports Medicine indicates that the ideal prophylactic knee brace should have all of the following criteria[9]:

■ It should adapt to various anatomic shapes and sizes.
■ It should supplement the stiffness of the knee, reducing loads from contact and noncontact stresses.

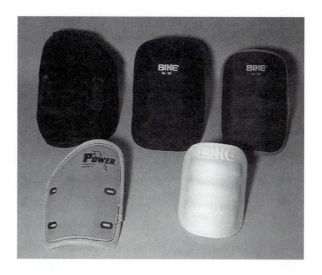

Figure 5-26
Protective thigh pads.

- It should be cost effective and durable.
- It should not interfere with normal knee function.
- It should not harm other players.
- It should not increase injuries to the lower extremity.
- It should have documented efficacy in preventing injuries.

Currently no brace on the market fulfills all of these criteria. Therefore use of the prophylactic knee brace is controversial and should be employed on an individual basis.[9]

Other popular knee devices are sleeves composed of elastic or neoprene material. Sleeves of this type provide mild soft-tissue support and to some extent retain body heat and help reduce edema caused by tissue compression (Figure 5-27).

Hand, Wrist, and Elbow Protection

As with the lower limbs, the upper limbs require initial protection from injury, as well as prevention of further injury after a trauma. One of the finest physical instruments, the human hand, is perhaps one of the most neglected in terms of injury, especially in sports. Special attention must be paid to protecting the integrity of all aspects of the hand when encountering high-speed projectiles or receiving external forces that contuse or shear (Figure 5-28). Constant stress to the hand, as characterized by the force received by the hand of the baseball catcher, can lead to irreversible

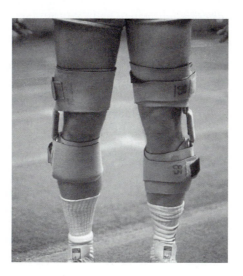

Figure 5-27
A prophylactic knee brace designed to protect against a lateral force and to distribute load away from joint.

Figure 5-28

The hand is an often neglected area of the body in sports.

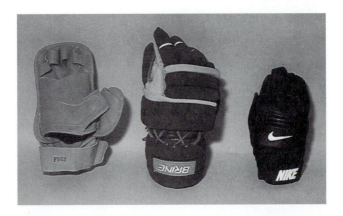

Figure 5-29

Commercial wrist and elbow pads and braces.

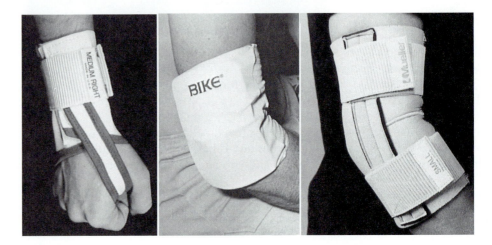

pathological damage in later life). The wrist and the elbow are also vulnerable to sports trauma and often need compression or support for protection (Figure 5-29).

CONSTRUCTION OF PROTECTIVE AND SUPPORTIVE DEVICES

Being able to construct protective and supportive devices is of considerable value in sports. The primary materials used are sponge rubber, felt, adhesive sponge rubber, adhesive felt, gauze pads, cotton, lamb's wool, and plastic.

Custom Pad and Orthotic Materials

There are many different materials available to the athletic trainer desiring to protect or support an injured area. In general, they can be divided into soft and hard materials (Figure 5-30).

Soft Materials

The major soft-material mediums found in training rooms are lamb's wool, cotton, gauze pads, adhesive felt or adhesive foam rubber felt, and an assortment of foam rubber in bulk.

Lamb's wool is a material commonly used on and around the athlete's toes when circular protection is required. In contrast to cotton, lamb's wool does not pack but keeps its resiliency over a long period of time.

Gauze padding is less versatile than other pad materials. It is assembled in varying thicknesses and can be used as an absorbent or protective pad.

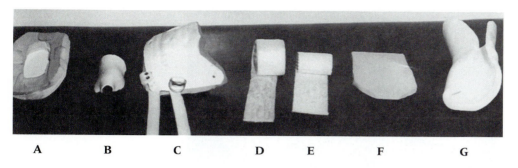

A   B   C   D   E   F   G

Figure 5-30

Types of sports orthoses. **A,** Orthoplast with a foam rubber doughnut. **B,** Orthoplast splint. **C,** Orthoplast rib protector with a foam rubber pad. **D,** Fiberglass material for splint construction. **E,** Plaster of paris material for cast construction. **F,** Foam rubber pad. **G,** Aloplast foam moldable material for protective pad construction.

Cotton is probably the cheapest and most widely used material in sports. It has the ability to absorb, to hold emollients, and to offer a mild padding effect.

Adhesive felt (moleskin) or *sponge rubber* material contains an adhesive mass on one side, thus combining a cushioning effect with the ability to be held in a specific spot by the adhesive mass. It is a versatile material that is useful on all body parts.

Felt is a material composed of matted wool fibers pressed into varying thicknesses that range from ¼ to 1 inch (0.6 to 2.5 cm). Its benefit lies in its comfortable, semiresilient surface, which gives a firmer pressure than most sponge rubbers. Because felt absorbs perspiration, it clings to the skin, and it has less tendency to move than sponge rubber (Figure 5-31). Because of its absorbent qualities, it must be replaced daily. Currently, it is used as support and protection for some foot conditions.

Foams are currently the major materials used for providing injury protection in sports. They come in many different thicknesses and densities (Figure 5-32). They are usually resilient, nonabsorbent, and able to protect the body against compressive forces. Some foams are open celled, whereas others are closed. The closed-cell type is preferable in sports because it rebounds and returns to its original shape quickly. Foams can be easily worked, through cutting, shaping, and faceting.[2] Some foams are *thermomoldable* and, when heated, become highly pliant and easy to shape. When cooled, they retain the shape in which they were formed. A new class of foams are composed of viscoelastic polymers, of which Sorbothane is an example.[2] This foam has a high energy-absorbing quality, but it also has a high density, making it heavy (Figure 5-33). Used in innersoles in sports shoes, it helps prevent blisters and also effectively absorbs vertical, front-to-back, and rotary shock caused by the foot. Foams generally range from ⅛ to ½ inch (0.3 to 1.25 cm) in thickness.

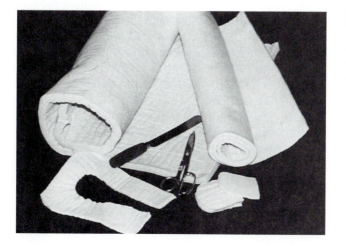

Figure 5-31

Orthopedic felt, both ½- and ¼-inch wide, with broad-blade knife and large scissors for contouring.

Figure 5-32

Foam assortment: *left*, thermo-moldable, *center*, closed celled, *right*, open celled.

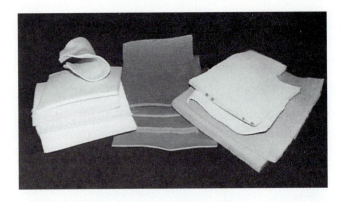

Figure 5-33

Sorbothane products: *left*, sheet stock and insoles; *right*, knee pads.

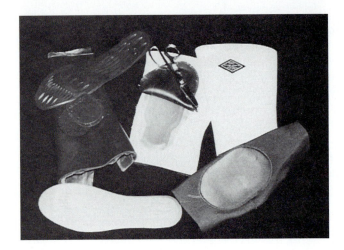

Nonyielding Materials

A number of hard, nonyielding materials are used in athletic training for making protective shells and splints.

Thermomoldable plastics A number of plastic materials are becoming widely used in sports medicine for customized orthotics. They can brace, splint, and shield a body area. They can provide casting for a fracture, support for a foot defect, or a firm, nonyielding surface to protect a severe contusion.

Plastics used for these purposes differ in their chemical composition and reaction to heat. The three major categories are heatforming plastics, heatsetting plastics, and heatplastic foams.

Heatforming plastics are of the low-temperature variety and are the most popular in athletic training. When heated to 140° to 180° F (60° to 82.2° C), depending on the material, the plastic can be accurately molded to a body part. Aquaplast (polyester sheets) and Orthoplast (synthetic rubber thermoplast) are popular types.

Heatsetting plastics require relatively higher temperatures for shaping. They are rigid and difficult to form, usually requiring a mold rather than being formed directly to the body part. High-impact vinyl (polyvinyl chloride), Kydex (polyvinyl chloride acrylic), and Nyloplex (heatplastic acrylic) are examples of the more commonly used thermoforming plastics.

Heatplastic foams are plastics that have differences in density as a result of the addition of liquids, gas, or crystals. They are commonly used as shoe inserts and other body padding. Aloplast (polyethylene foam) and Plastazote (polyethylene foam) are two commonly used products.

Usually the plastic is heated until soft and malleable. It is then molded into the desired shape and allowed to cool, thereby retaining its shape. Various pads and other

Heatforming plastics of the low-temperature variety are the most popular in athletic training.

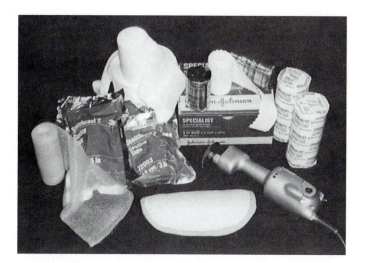

Figure 5-34

Casting material: *left*, fiberglass; *right*, plaster including cast saw used to trim pictured skin guard.

materials can also be fastened in place. There may be limitations in the use of rigid thermomoldable plastics based on rules and regulations of various sport activities.

Casting materials   Applying casts to injured body areas has long been a practice in sports medicine. The material of choice is fiberglass, using resin and a catalytic converter, plus water, to produce hardening. Besides casts, this material makes effective shells for splints and protective pads. Once hardened, the fiberglass is trimmed to shape with a cast saw (Figure 5-34).

Tools Used for Customizing

Working with the various materials used to customize protective equipment requires the use of many different tools.[2] They include adhesives, adhesive tapes, heat sources, and shaping tools.

Adhesives   A number of adhesives are used in constructing custom protective equipment. Many cements and glues join plastic to plastic or join other combinations of materials (Figure 5-35).

Adhesive tape   Adhesive tape is a major tool in holding various materials in place. Linen and elastic tape can hold pads to a rigid backing or to adhesive felt (moleskin) and can be used to protect against sharp edges.

Heat sources   To form thermomoldable plastics, a heat source must be available. Three sources are commonly found in training rooms: the commercial moist heat unit, a hot air gun or hair dryer, and an electric skillet or portable oven with a temperature control. The usual desired temperature is 160° F (71° C) or higher.

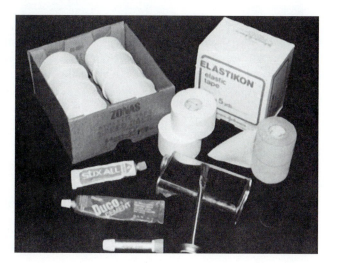

Figure 5-35

Glues and adhesive tapes.

Figure 5-36

Fastening materials, including Velcro, Wet Wrap, leather, laces, rubber wraps, and hardware.

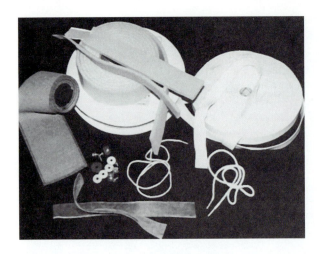

Figure 5-37

Constructing a hard-shell pad. **A,** Marking the area to be protected. **B,** Temporary foam insert to provide "bubble" relief. **C,** Heating plastic and wrapping it over temporary relief pad. **D,** Removing foam used to create bubble. **E,** Trimmed shell. *(continued)*

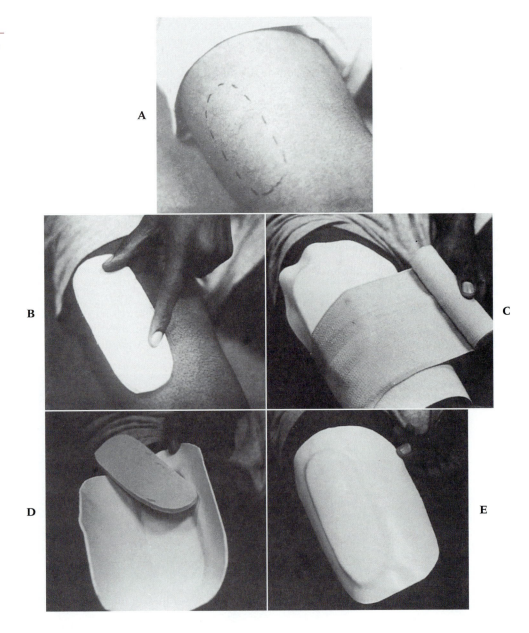

Shaping tools   Commonly, the tools required to shape custom devices are heavy-duty scissors, sharp-blade knives, and cast saws.

Holding materials in place   Once formed, customized protective equipment often must be secured in place. Fastening materials requires the availability of a great variety of different materials. For example, if something is to be held securely, cotton herringbone–weave straps that are cut and riveted to the device may be desired. On the other hand, a Velcro fastener can be used when a device must be continually put on and removed. Leather can be cut and riveted in place to form hinge straps with buckles attached. Various types of laces can be laced through eyelets to hold something in place (Figure 5-36). Tools that allow for this type of construction include a portable drill, a hole punch, and an ice pick.

Customized Hard-Shell Pads

Commonly, an athlete who needs a hard-shell pad has acquired an injury, such as a painful contusion (bruise), that must be completely protected from further injury. To customize such a pad, follow the procedures presented in the Focus box on the next page and in Figure 5-37.

Custom Foot Orthotics

The athlete with serious biomechanical foot problems often requires a customized foot orthotic device. Measurement for this device is usually performed by an orthopedic surgeon or podiatrist. Foot orthotic devices prescribed by a professional are semisoft, semirigid, and rigid.

Semisoft orthotic device   This orthotic device is similar in its construction to the preorthotic device. The major advantage of this device is that it is easily made in the doctor's office, is inexpensive, and is almost immediately comfortable, having a relatively short "break-in" period. It can easily be modified with cork shims.

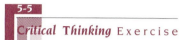

5-5

Critical Thinking E x e r c i s e

A soccer player has incurred a number of contusions to the right quadriceps muscle.

? The athletic trainer must customize a hard-shell protective thigh pad for the soccer player. How is this done?

Figure 5-37—cont'd

F, Doughnut-shaped foam lining. **G,** Doughnut combined with softer foam. **H,** Using an elastic wrap to secure pad.

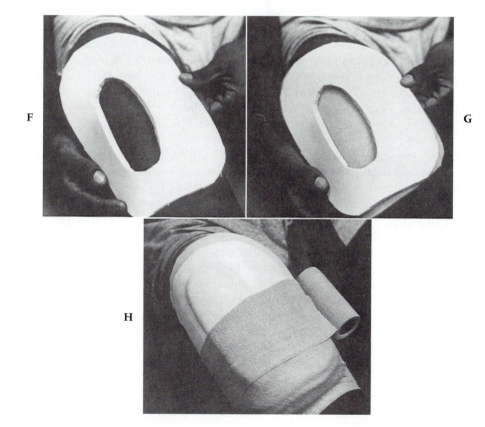

F

G

H

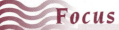

How to construct a hard-shell pad

1. Select proper material and tools, which might include
   a. Thermomoldable plastic sheet.
   b. Scissors.
   c. Felt material.
2. Palpate and mark the margins of the tender area that needs protection.
3. Cut a felt piece to fit in the area of tenderness.
4. Heat plastic until malleable.
5. Place heated plastic over felt and wrap in place with an elastic wrap.
6. When cooled, remove elastic wrap and felt pad.
7. Trim shell to desired shape; a protective shell has now been made to provide a "bubble" relief.
8. If needed, add a softer inner layer of foam to distribute and lessen force further.
   a. Cut a doughnut-type hole in softer foam material the same size as the injury site.
   b. Cut foam the same shape as the hard shell.
   c. Use tape or an adhesive to affix the foam to the shell.

Construction of a semisoft orthotic device requires picking the correct size blank with the appropriate thickness and density. The foot is measured on the blank, followed by shaping and smoothing by a drum grinding wheel.[2]

Semirigid orthotic device   The semirigid orthotic device is constructed from malleable plastics such as polyethylene, polypropylene, and polyvinyl chloride. As the name implies, semirigid orthotic devices will "give" under great force.

Construction of this device requires casting the foot in a neutral position, then sending the cast to an outside laboratory for construction. The break-in period for this orthotic device is much longer than for the semisoft one.

Rigid orthotic device   The rigid orthotic device is the most expensive and most difficult one to construct. Providing the most rigid control, it is made from a cast of the foot in a neutral position. Rigid acrylic plastic is used by heating and pressing it over the mold. Of all three orthotic devices, the rigid one is the most difficult to fit, and its use has the highest degree of complications.[2]

SUMMARY

- The proper selection and fitting of sports equipment are essential in the prevention of many sports injuries. Because of the number of current litigations, sports equipment standards are of serious concern regarding the durability of the material and the fit and wear requirements of the equipment. Manufacturers must foresee all of the possible uses and misuses of their equipment and warn the user of any potential risks.
- Head protection in many collision and contact sports is of concern to sports professionals. A major concern is that the football helmet be used for its intended purpose and not as a weapon. To avoid unwarranted litigation, a warning label must be placed on the outside of the helmet indicating that it is not fail-safe and must be used as intended. Proper fit is also a major requirement.
- Face protection is of major importance in sports that have fast-moving projectiles, use implements that are in close proximity to other athletes, and facilitate body collisions. Protecting teeth and eyes is of particular significance. The customized mouth guard, fitted to individual requirements, provides the best protection for the teeth and also protects against concussions. Eyes must be protected against projectiles and sports implements. The safest eye guard for the athlete not wearing

contact lenses or spectacles is the closed type that completely protects the orbital cavity.

■ Many sports require protection of various parts of the athlete's body. American football players, ice hockey players, and baseball catchers are examples of players who require body protection. Commonly, the protection is for the shoulders, chest, thighs, ribs, hips, buttocks, groin, genitalia (male athletes), and breasts (female athletes).

■ Quality sportswear, properly fitted, is essential to prevent injuries. Socks must be clean, without holes, and made of appropriate materials. Shoes must be suited to the sport and must be fitted to the largest foot. The wide part of the foot must match the wide part of the shoe. If the shoe has cleats, they must be positioned at the metatarsophalangeal joints.

■ Currently, there are many stock pieces of specialized, protective equipment on the market. They may be designed to support ankles, knees, or other body parts. In addition to stock equipment, athletic trainers often construct customized equipment out of a variety of materials to pad injuries or support feet. Professionals such as orthopedists and podiatrists may devise orthopedic footwear and orthotic devices to improve the biomechanics of the athlete's foot.

....

Solutions to Critical Thinking Exercises

5-1 The student athletic trainer must acquire the following protective equipment competencies:
- Identify good-quality and poor-quality commercial protective equipment.
- Properly fit commercial protective equipment.
- Construct protective and supportive devices.

5-2 The athletic trainer initiates the following steps:
1. A team meeting is called in which the risks entailed in the use and fitting of the equipment is fully explained.
2. A defective piece of equipment must be immediately reported and repaired.
3. A letter is sent out to each parent or guardian explaining equipment limitations. This letter is signed and returned to the athletic trainer.
4. A meeting of parents, team members, and coaches is called to further explain equipment limitations.

5-3 The athletic trainer explains that the helmet cannot prevent serious neck injuries. Striking an opponent with any part of the helmet or face mask can place abnormal stress on cervical structures. Most severe neck injuries occur from striking an opponent with the top of the helmet; this is known as axial loading.

5-4 The athletic trainer advises the following:
- Purchase shoes to fit the large foot.
- Fit shoes wearing athletic socks.
- Purchase shoes at the end of the day.
- Shoes feel snug but comfortable when jumping up and down and performing cutting motions.
- Shoe length and width allow full toe function.
- Wide part of foot matches the wide part of the shoe.
- Shoe bends at widest part of shoe.
- Each foot is measured from the heel to the end of the largest toe.

5-5 To construct a hard-shell pad the athletic trainer
1. Marks the area on the athlete to be protected.
2. Cuts a foam piece to temporarily cover the injury.
3. Heats thermomoldable plastic and forms over the foam piece to form a bubble.
4. Cuts a plastic sheet to form to the athlete's thigh.
5. Creates a doughnut-shaped foam lining to surround the injury.
6. Secures the foam doughnut to the plastic piece.
7. Secures the pad in place with elastic wrap.

REVIEW QUESTIONS AND CLASS ACTIVITIES

1. What are the legal responsibilities of the equipment manager, coach, and athletic trainer in terms of protective equipment?
2. Have the equipment manager of your sports program talk to your class about the purchase and fitting of equipment (e.g., football helmets and shoulder pads).
3. What are the differences between the helmet that protects against a fast-moving projectile and the one that protects against hard blows from an opponent?
4. What are the advantages of a custom-made mouth guard over the stock type?
5. What sports require ear guards?
6. Why are proper eye protection devices necessary in different sports? Identify the different types and their corresponding sports.
7. Which sports require trunk protection? Why? Which types of equipment are necessary?
8. Why is proper breast support so important to the woman with large breasts?
9. On what basis should different sports shoes be evaluated?
10. How should sports shoes be fitted?
11. When would you suggest a commercial foot pad to be used by an athlete?
12. Have a class debate about one of the following: the benefits of prophylactic taping versus the uselessness of prophylactic taping; commercial ankle supports versus no supports;

and the current trend of using prophylactic knee braces versus not using braces.

13. What are the advantages and disadvantages of the *fitted* knee brace?

14. What is the relative value of commercial braces for the hand, wrist, and elbow?

15. You are given the responsibility to purchase materials that can be used for general padding or can be customized into special pads or other protective devices. What materials would you buy and why?

16. What steps would you take in making a hard-shell plastic pad?

REFERENCES

1. American Academy of Orthopaedic Surgeons: *Athletic training and sports medicine,* ed 2, Park Ridge, Ill, 1991, American Academy of Orthopaedic Surgeons.

2. American Society for Testing and Materials, Committee F-8 on Sports Equipment and Facilities: *Member information packet,* Philadelphia, 1978.

3. Davis PF, Trevino SG: Ankle injuries. In Baxter DE, editor: *The foot and ankle in sport,* St Louis, 1995, Mosby.

4. Frey C: The shoe in sports. In Baxter DE, editor: *The foot and ankle in sport,* St Louis, 1995, Mosby.

5. Hermann TJ: Taping and padding of the foot and ankle. In Sammarco GI, editor: *Rehabilitation of the foot and ankle,* St Louis, 1995, Mosby.

6. Hodgson VR, Thomas LM: Biomechanical study of football head impacts using a head model—condensed version. Final report prepared for National Operating Committee on Standards for Athletic Equipment (NOCSAE), 1975.

7. Lord JL: Protective equipment in high-risk sports. In Berrer RB, editor: *Sports medicine for primary care physician,* ed 2, Boca Raton, Fla, 1994, CRC Press.

8. *National Federation of State High School Football Rules, National Federation Publication,* Kansas City, Mo, 1989, Brice B. Durlan.

9. Montgomery DL: Prophylactic knee braces. In Torg JS, Shephard RJ, editors: *Current therapy in sports medicine,* St Louis, 1995, Mosby.

10. Prentice W: *Fitness for college and life,* ed 5, St Louis, 1997, Mosby.

ANNOTATED BIBLIOGRAPHY

Baxter DE, editor: *The foot and ankle in sport,* St Louis, 1995, Mosby.

An in-depth medical text covering all aspects of foot and ankle conditions in sport.

Ellison AE, editor: *Athletic training and sports medicine,* Chicago, 1984, American Academy of Orthopaedic Surgeons.

Discusses all aspects of buying, fitting, and constructing protective equipment in Part 4, Protective Equipment.

Nicholas JA, Hershman EB, editors: *The upper extremity in sports medicine,* St Louis, 1990, Mosby.

Includes a special chapter on protective equipment for the shoulder, elbow, wrist, and hand.

Wu K: *Foot orthoses: principles and clinical applications,* Baltimore, 1990, Williams & Wilkins.

A complete text on examination, fabrication, and application of foot orthoses.

PART III

Basic Foundations of Sports Trauma

Mechanisms and Characteristics of Sports Trauma

When you finish this chapter, you should be able to

- Explain the biomechanical factors in sports injuries.
- Describe the major biomechanical forces occurring in sports injuries.
- Identify the most common exposed skin injuries.
- Explain the normal structures of soft tissue and the specific mechanical forces that cause skin, internal soft-tissue, synovial joint, and bone injuries.
- Define the terms that describe the major injuries incurred during sports participation.
- Describe how epiphyseal injuries occur.
- Explain how microtraumas and overuse injuries occur.

To effectively present and manage sports injuries the athletic trainer must understand tissue susceptibility to sports trauma.

? What should the athletic trainer know about tissue properties?

A physical injury or wound sustained in sport produced by an external or internal force is defined as trauma.

This chapter is concerned with the many factors that produce mechanical injuries or trauma in sports. Trauma is defined as *a physical injury or wound sustained in sport and produced by an external or internal force or violence* (Figure 6-1). The primary purpose of this chapter is to provide a foundation for the identification, understanding, and management of sports injuries. It examines mechanical forces and tissue characteristics of sports injuries and the classification of these injuries.

MECHANICAL INJURY

"Force or mechanical energy is that which changes the state of rest or uniform motion of matter. When a force applied to any part of the body results in a harmful disturbance in function and or structure, a mechanical injury is said to have been sustained."[12] Injuries related to sports participation can be caused by external forces directed on the body or can occur internally within the body. To understand sports injuries there must be a knowledge of tissue susceptibility to trauma and the mechanical forces involved.

Figure 6-1

A sport injury can be sustained from an external or internal force.

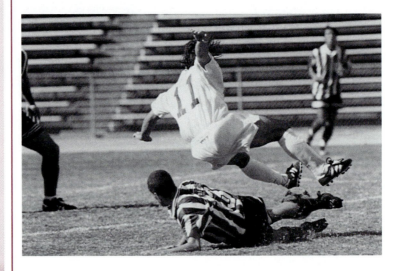

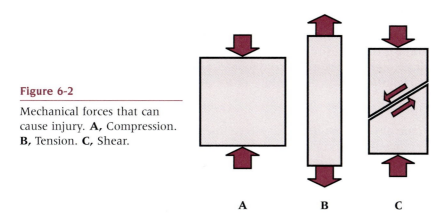

Figure 6-2

Mechanical forces that can cause injury. **A,** Compression. **B,** Tension. **C,** Shear.

A   B   C

load
Outside force or forces acting on tissue.

stress
The internal reaction or resistance to an external load.

strain
Extent of deformation of tissue under loading.

viscoelastic
Any material whose mechanical properties vary depending on rate of a load.

Human tissue is viscoelastic—it has both viscous and elastic properties.

yield point
Elastic limit of tissue.

mechanical failure
Elastic limit of tissue is exceeded, causing tissue to break.

The three tissue mechanical stresses that can lead to sports injuries are tension, compression, and shearing.

Tissue Properties

Tissues have relative abilities to resist a particular load. The stronger the tissue, the greater magnitude of load it can withstand. Strength pressure, or power, is often used to imply a *force*. A force can be described as a push or pull.[13] Tissue properties are described according to engineering terminology. A **load** can be a singular or group of outside or internal forces acting on the body. The resistance to a load is called a mechanical **stress,** and the internal response is a *deformation,* or change in dimensions. Deformation is also defined as a mechanical **strain.** All human tissue is **viscoelastic;** it has both viscous and elastic properties, allowing for deformation. Tissue such as bone is brittle and has much fewer viscoelastic properties when compared to softer tissue. Tissue also is *anisotropic,* responding with greater or lesser strength depending on the direction of the load that is being applied. When tissue is deformed to the extent that its elasticity is almost fully exceeded a **yield point** has been reached. When the yield point has been exceeded **mechanical failure** occurs, resulting in tissue damage.[2]

There are three primary tissue stresses leading to sports injuries: tension, compression, and shear.

Tension is that force that pulls or stretches tissue.

Stretching beyond the yield point leads to rupturing of soft tissue or fracturing of a bone. Examples of stretching injuries are sprains, strains, and avulsion fractures.

Compression is a force that, with enough energy, crushes tissue. When the force can no longer be absorbed, injury occurs. Where there is constant submaximum compression over a period of time, the contacted tissue can develop abnormal "wear." Compression occurs when a muscle or bone is stretched directly or when cartilage bone is directly loaded. Arthritic changes, fractures, and contusions are commonly caused by compression force.

Shearing is a force that moves across the parallel organization of the tissue. Injury occurs once shearing has exceeded the inherent strength of a tissue. Shearing stress can result in skin injuries such as blisters, rips of the hands, abrasions, or vertebral disks injuries (Figure 6-2).

BENDING STRAIN

A force placed on a horizontal beam or bone places stresses within the structure, causing it to bend or strain.[13] This is known as three-point bending (Figure 6-3). Compression occurs parallel to the beam's length if on the concave side and tension if on its convex side. Shear stress is also caused in two directions within the bending beam.[13] Bending strain can also occur perpendicular to or along the length of a beam, with compression, tension, and shearing occurring. The hip and femur are examples of this type of bending strain. A torsion, or twisting, load causes compression and tension in a spiral pattern, with shearing stresses occurring parallel to the long axes. An example of a torsion injury is the spiral fracture that occurs in skiing[9] (Figure 6-4).

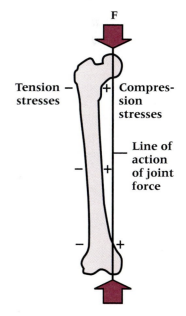

F

Tension — stresses

Compression stresses

Line of action of joint force

Figure 6-3

Bending strain. Compression and tension stress caused by a bending of the femur.

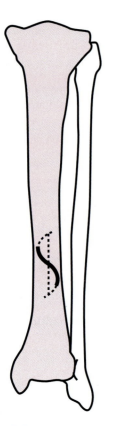

Figure 6-4

A torsion force could lead to a spiral fracture.

6-2

Critical Thinking Exercise

A baseball player slides into home base, severely scraping the skin on the left side.

? What is the force and type of injury produced?

SOFT-TISSUE TRAUMA

Soft tissue, or nonbony tissue, falls generally under the category of noncontractile and contractile. Noncontractile tissues are skin, joint capsules, ligaments, fascia, cartilage, dura mater, and nerve roots. Contractile tissues are those structures that are a part of the muscle, its tendon, or its bony insertion.[3]

SKIN INJURIES

Generally, trauma that happens to the skin is visually exposed and is categorized as a skin wound. It is defined as a break in the continuity of the soft parts of body structures caused by a trauma to these tissues.

Anatomical Characteristics

The skin, or integument, is the external covering of the body. It represents the body's largest organ system and essentially consists of two layers—the epidermis and the dermis (corium). Because of the soft, pliable nature of skin, it can be easily traumatized. (See Chapter 26 for a more in-depth discussion of anatomy.)

Injurious Mechanical Forces

Numerous mechanical forces can adversely affect the skin's integrity. These forces are friction or rubbing, scraping, compression or pressure, tearing, cutting, and penetrating.

Wound Classification

Wounds are classified according to the mechanical force that causes them (Table 6-1).

Friction Blisters

Continuous rubbing over the surface of the skin causes a collection of fluid below or within the epidermal layer called a blister.

Abrasions

Abrasions are common conditions in which the skin is scraped against a rough surface. The epidermis and dermis are worn away, exposing numerous blood capillaries.

Skin Bruise

When a blow compresses or crushes the skin surface and produces bleeding under the skin, the condition is identified as a bruise, or contusion.

TABLE 6-1 Soft-Tissue Trauma

Primary Tissue	Type	Mechanical Forces	Condition
Skin	Acute	Rubbing/friction	Blister
		Compression/contusion	Bruise
		Tearing	Laceration
		Tearing/ripping	Avulsion
		Penetrating	Puncture
Muscle/tendon	Acute	Compressional	Contusion
		Tension	Strain
	Chronic	Tension/shearing	Myositis/fasciitis
		Tension	Tendinitis/tenosynovitis
		Compression/tension	Bursitis
		Compression/tension	Ectopic calcification—myositis ossificans, calcific tendinitis

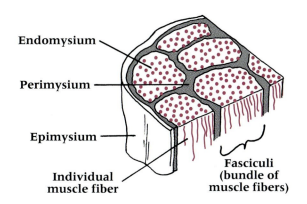

Figure 6-5

Connective tissue related to a skeletal muscle.

Laceration

A laceration is a wound in which the flesh has been irregularly torn.

Skin Avulsion

Skin that is torn by the same mechanism as a laceration to the extent that tissue is completely ripped from its source is considered an avulsion injury.

Incision

An incision wound is one in which the skin has been sharply cut.

Puncture Wound

Puncture wounds, as the name implies, are penetrations of the skin by a sharp object.

NOTE: The care of skin wounds is discussed in Chapter 26.

SKELETAL MUSCLE INJURIES

Skeletal muscles have an extremely high percentage of sports injuries.

Anatomical Characteristics

Muscles are composed of contractile cells, or fibers, that produce movement. Muscle fibers have the ability to contract, plus the properties of irritability, conductivity, and elasticity. Three types of muscles are within the body—smooth, cardiac, and striated. Of major concern in sports medicine are conditions that affect striated, or skeletal, muscles. Within the fiber cell is a semifluid substance called sarcoplasm (cytoplasm). Myofibrils are surrounded by the endomysium, fiber bundles are surrounded by the perimysium, and the entire muscle is covered by the epimysium (Figure 6-5). The epimysium, perimysium, and endomysium may be combined with the fibrous tendon. The fibrous wrapping of a muscle may become a flat sheet of connective tissue (aponeurosis) that attaches to other muscles. Tendons and aponeuroses are extremely resilient to injuries. They will pull away from a bone, a bone will break, or a muscle will tear before tendons and aponeuroses are injured.[18] Skeletal muscles are generally well supplied with blood vessels that permeate throughout their structure. Arteries, veins, lymph vessels, and bundles of nerve fibers spread into the perimysium. A complex capillary network goes throughout the endomysium, coming into direct contact with the muscle fibers.

Muscle Injury Classification

Acute Muscle Injuries

The two categories of acute muscle injuries are contusions and strains.

Contusions   A bruise or contusion is received because of a sudden traumatic blow to the body. The intensity of a contusion can range from superficial to deep tissue compression and hemorrhage (Figure 6-6).

6-3

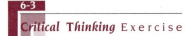

Critical Thinking Exercise

A shortstop is hit in the shin by a batted ball that took a bad hop.

? What is the force and type of injury sustained by this athlete?

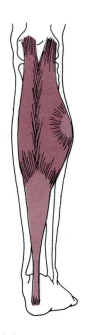

Figure 6-6

A contusion is caused by a severe compression force.

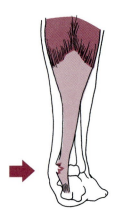

Figure 6-7

A strain is produced by severe tension force.

Interrupting the continuity of the circulatory system results in a flow of blood and lymph into the surrounding tissues. A hematoma (blood tumor) is formed by the localization of the extravasated blood into a clot, which becomes encapsulated by a connective tissue membrane. The speed of healing, as with all soft-tissue injuries, depends on the extent of tissue damage and internal bleeding.

A contusion can penetrate to the skeletal structures, causing a bone bruise. The extent to which an athlete may be hampered by this condition depends on the location of the bruise and the force of the blow. Typical in cases of severe contusion are the following:

1. The athlete reports being struck a hard blow.
2. The blow causes pain and a transitory paralysis caused by pressure on and shock to the motor and sensory nerves.
3. Palpation often reveals a hard area, indurated because of internal hemorrhage.
4. Ecchymosis, or tissue discoloration, may take place.

Muscle contusions are usually rated by the extent the muscle is able to produce range of motion in a part. (See Chapter 7.) It is noteworthy that a blow to a muscle can be so great that the related fascia is ruptured, allowing muscle tissue to protrude through it.

Strains   A strain is a stretch, tear, or rip in the muscle or adjacent tissue such as the fascia or muscle tendons (Figure 6-7). The cause of muscle strain is often obscure. Most often a strain is produced by an abnormal muscular contraction. The cause of this abnormality has been attributed to many factors. One popular theory suggests that a fault in the reciprocal coordination of the agonist and antagonist muscles takes place. The cause of this fault or incoordination is more or less a mystery. However, among the possible explanations advanced are that it may be related to a mineral imbalance caused by profuse sweating, fatigue metabolites collected in the muscle itself, or a strength imbalance between agonist and antagonist muscles.

A strain may range from a minute separation of connective tissue and muscle fibers to a complete tendinous avulsion or muscle rupture (grade 1, 2, or 3). The resulting pathology is similar to that of the contusion or sprain, with capillary or blood vessel hemorrhage. A grade 1 strain is accompanied by local pain, which is increased by tension of the muscle, and a minor loss of strength. There is mild swelling, ecchymosis and local tenderness.[18] A grade 2 strain is similar to the mild strain but has moderate signs and symptoms and impaired muscle function.[16] A grade 3 strain has signs and symptoms that are severe, with a loss of muscle function and commonly a palpable defect in the muscle.[16] The muscles that have the highest incidence of strains in sports are the hamstring group, gastrocnemius, quadriceps group, hip flexors, hip adductor group, spinalis group of the back, deltoid, and rotator cuff group of the shoulder.

Tendon Injuries

The tendon contains wavy parallel collagenous fibers that are organized in bundles surrounded by a gelatinous material that decreases friction. A tendon attaches a muscle to a bone and concentrates a pulling force in a limited area. Tendons can produce and maintain a pull from 8700 to 18,000 pounds per square inch. When a tendon is loaded by tension, the wavy collagenous fibers straighten in the direction of the load; when the tension is released, the collagen returns to its original shape. In tendons, collagen fibers will break if their physiological limits have been reached. A breaking point occurs after a 6% to 8% increase in length. Because a tendon is usually double the strength of the muscle it serves, tears commonly occur at the muscle belly, musculotendinous junction, or bony attachment. Clinically, however, a constant abnormal tension on tendons increases elongation by the infiltration of fibroblasts, which will cause more collagenous tissue to be produced. Repeated microtraumas can evolve into chronic muscle strain that resorbs collagen fibers and eventually weakens the tendon. Collagen resorption occurs in the early period of sports conditioning and during the immobilization of a part. During resorption collagenous tissues are weakened and susceptible to injury; therefore a gradually paced conditioning program and early mobilization in the rehabilitation process are necessary.

Muscle Cramps and Spasms

Muscle cramps and spasms lead to muscle and tendon injuries. A cramp is usually a painful involuntary contraction of a skeletal muscle or muscle group. Cramps have been attributed to a lack of water or other electrolytes in relation to muscle fatigue. A reflex reaction caused by trauma of the musculoskeletal system is commonly called a spasm. The two types of cramps or spasms are the *clonic* type, with alternating involuntary muscular contraction and relaxation in quick succession, and the *tonic* type, with rigid muscle contraction that lasts over a period of time.

Overexertion Muscle Problems

One constant problem in physical conditioning and training is overexertion. Even though the gradual pattern of overloading the body is the best way for ultimate success, many athletes and even coaches believe that if there is no pain, there is no gain.

Exercise "overdosage" is reflected in muscle soreness, decreased joint flexibility, and general fatigue 24 hours after activity. Four specific indicators of possible overexertion are acute muscle soreness, muscle stiffness, delayed muscle soreness, and muscle cramping.

Muscle soreness has long been a problem for the person engaging in physical conditioning. Two major types of muscle soreness are associated with severe exercise. The first, occurring immediately after exercise, is acute soreness, which is resolved when exercise has ceased. The second and more serious problem is delayed soreness, which is related mainly to early-season or unaccustomed work. Severe muscular discomfort occurs 24 to 48 hours after exercise.

Acute-onset muscle soreness   Acute-onset muscle soreness is related to an impedance of circulation, causing muscular ischemia. Lactic acid and potassium collect in the muscle and stimulate pain receptors.[6]

Delayed-onset muscle soreness   Delayed-onset muscle soreness (DOMS) increases in intensity for 2 to 3 days and then decreases in intensity until it has completely disappeared within 7 days.[5]

The cause of DOMS apparently is sublethal and lethal damage to a small group of recruited muscle fibers.[5] The perception of soreness is caused by the activation of free nerve endings around selected muscle fibers.[6] The type of activity that causes the most soreness is eccentric exercise. Muscle fibers may take as long as 12 weeks to repair; therefore athletes need abundant recovery time.[6]

There are many ways to reduce the possibility of delayed-onset muscle soreness. One is a gradual and complete warm-up before engaging in vigorous activity, followed by a careful cool-down. In the early part of training, careful attention should be paid to static stretching before and after activity. If there is extreme soreness, the application of ice packs or ice massage to the point of numbness (approximately 5 to 8 minutes) followed by a static stretch often provides relief.

Muscle stiffness   Muscle stiffness does not produce pain. It occurs when a group of muscles have been worked hard for a long period of time. The fluids that collect in the muscles during and after exercise are absorbed into the bloodstream at a slow rate. As a result the muscle becomes swollen, shorter, and thicker and therefore resists stretching. Light exercise, massage, and passive mobilization assist in reducing stiffness.

Muscle cramps   Like muscle soreness and stiffness, muscle cramps can be a problem related to hard conditioning. The most common cramp is **tonic,** in which there

The two major types of muscle soreness associated with severe exercise are acute and delayed.

tonic
Muscle contraction characterized by constant contraction that lasts for a period of time.

clonic
Involuntary muscle contraction characterized by alternate contraction and relaxation in rapid succession.

tendinitis
Inflammation of tendon-muscle attachments, tendons, or both.

6-5

Critical Thinking Exercise

A tennis player with a pronounced topspin style of hitting a backhand stroke sustains a painful elbow.

? What are the forces and type of elbow injury sustained by the tennis player, and what are ways to prevent this problem?

---

bursitis
Inflammation of bursa at sites of bony prominences between muscle and tendon.

ectopic
Located in a place different from normal.

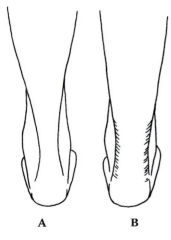

A   **B**

Figure 6-8

Tenosynovitis is an inflammation of the sheath covering a tendon. **A,** Normal. **B,** Strained.

---

is continuous muscle contraction. It is caused by the body's depletion of essential electrolytes or an interruption of synergism between opposing muscles. **Clonic,** or intermittent, contraction stemming from nerve irritation may rarely occur.

Chronic Muscle Injuries

As discussed previously, chronic injuries usually come with a slow progression over a long period of time. Often, repeated acute injuries can lead to a chronic condition. A constant irritation caused by poor performance techniques or a constant stress beyond physiological limits can eventually result in a chronic condition. These injuries are often attributed to overuse microtraumas.[15]

Chronic muscle injuries are representative of a low-grade inflammatory process with a proliferation of fibroblasts and scarring. The acute injury that is improperly managed or that allows an athlete to return to activity before healing has completely occurred can cause chronic injury. The student should be especially knowledgeable about six chronic muscle conditions: myositis, tendinitis, tenosynovitis, bursitis, ectopic calcification, and muscle atrophy and contracture.

Myositis/fascitis   In general, the term *myositis* means inflammation of muscle tissue. More specifically, it can be considered as a fibrositis or connective tissue inflammation. Fascia that supports and separates muscle can also become chronically inflamed after injury. A typical example of this condition is plantar fascitis.

Tendinitis   Tendinitis has a gradual onset, diffuse tenderness because of repeated microtraumas, and degenerative changes. Obvious signs of tendinitis are swelling and pain that move with the tendon.

Tenosynovitis   Tenosynovitis is inflammation of the synovial sheath surrounding a tendon. In its acute state there is rapid onset, articular crepitus, and diffuse swelling. In chronic tenosynovitis the tendons become locally thickened, with pain and articular crepitus present during movement (Figure 6-8).

Bursitis   The bursa is the fluid-filled sac found in places where friction might occur within body tissues. Bursae are predominantly located between bony prominences and muscles or tendons. Sudden irritation can cause acute **bursitis,** and overuse of muscles or tendons, as well as constant external compression or trauma, can result in chronic bursitis. The signs and symptoms of bursitis include swelling, pain, and some loss of function. Repeated trauma may lead to calcific deposits and degeneration of the internal lining of the bursa.

Ectopic calcification   Voluntary muscles can become chronically inflamed, resulting in myositis. An **ectopic** calcification known as *myositis ossificans* can occur in a muscle that directly overlies a bone. Two common sites for this condition are the quadriceps region of the thigh and the brachial muscle of the arm. In myositis ossificans osteoid material that resembles bone rapidly accumulates. If there is no repeated injury, the growth may subside completely in 9 to 12 months, or it may mature into a calcified area, at which time surgical removal can be accomplished with little fear of recurrence. Occasionally, tendinitis leads to deposits of minerals, primarily lime, and is known as *calcific tendinitis*.

Atrophy and contracture   Two complications of muscle and tendon conditions are atrophy and contracture. Muscle atrophy is the wasting away of muscle tissue. Its main cause in athletes is immobilization of a body part, inactivity, or loss of nerve stimulation. A second complication in sport injuries is *muscle contracture*, an abnormal shortening of muscle tissue in which there is a great deal of resistance to passive stretch. Commonly associated with muscle injury, a contracture is associated with a joint that has developed unyielding and resisting scar tissue.

SYNOVIAL JOINTS

A joint in the human body is defined as the point where two bones join together. A joint must also transmit forces between participating bones.[12]

Anatomical Characteristics

The joint consists of cartilage and fibrous connective tissue. Joints are classified as immovable (synarthrotic), slightly movable (amphiarthrotic), and freely movable (diarthrotic). Diarthrotic joints are also called synovial articulations. Because of their ability to move freely and thus become more susceptible to trauma, joints are of major concern to the coach, the athletic trainer, and the physician. Anatomical characteristics of the synovial articulations consist of four features: they have a capsule or ligaments; the capsule is lined with a synovial membrane; the opposing bone surfaces contain hyaline cartilage; and there is a joint space (joint cavity) containing a small amount of fluid (synovial fluid) (Figure 6-9). In addition, there are nerves and blood supplied to the synovial articulation, and there are muscles that cross the joint or are intrinsic to it.[18]

Joint Capsule

Bones of the diarthrotic joint are held together by a cuff of fibrous tissue known as the capsule, or capsular ligament. It consists of bundles of collagen and functions primarily to hold the bones together. It is extremely strong and can withstand cross-sectional forces of 500 kg/cm². Parts of the capsule become slack or taut depending on the joint movements.

Ligaments

Ligaments are sheets or bundles of collagen fibers that form a connection between two bones. Ligaments fall into two categories: ones that are considered intrinsic and ones that are extrinsic to the joint. Intrinsic ligaments occur where the articular capsule has become thickened in some places. Extrinsic ligaments are separate from the capsular thickening.

Ligaments and capsules, found in synovial joints, are similar in composition to tendons; however, in contrast they contain elastic fibers and collagen fibers that have a wavy, irregular, and spiral configuration. Attaching bone to bone, ligaments are strongest in their middle and weakest at their ends. When an intact ligament is traumatically stretched, the injury often produces an avulsion-type fracture or tear at the ends, rather than in the middle. Avulsion fractures are more common when bone tissue is comparatively weaker than ligamentous tissue, as is evidenced in older individuals or postmenopausal women in whom significant osteoporosis has occurred or in children in whom the epiphyseal plates are relatively wide and soft.

A major factor in ligamentous injury is the viscoelastic tissue properties of ligaments and capsules. Viscoelasticity refers to extensibility when loaded that is time dependent. Constant compression or tension causes ligaments to deteriorate, whereas intermittent compression and tension increases strength, especially at the bony attachment. Chronic inflammation of ligamentous, capsular,

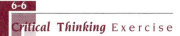

6-6

Critical Thinking Exercise

A football player who plays wide end sustains repeated blows to his left quadriceps muscle.

? What type of injury could be sustained from repeated compressive forces to the quadriceps muscle?

Constant compression or tension will cause ligaments to deteriorate; intermittent compression and tension will increase strength and growth.

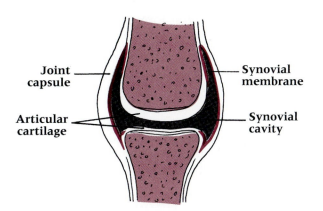

Figure 6-9

General anatomy of a diarthrodial joint.

Joint capsule

Synovial membrane

Articular cartilage

Synovial cavity

and fascial tissue causes a shrinkage of collagen fibers; therefore repeated microtraumas over time make capsules and ligaments highly susceptible to major acute injuries.

Ligaments act as protective backups for the joint. Primary protection occurs from the dynamic aspect of muscles and their tendons.[1] In a fast-loading situation, ligament failure ultimately will occur; however, the capsule and ligament provide maximum protection during rapid movements. Nevertheless, capsular and ligamentous tissues are highly sensitive to movement deprivation stress through joint immobilization.[1] Capsular and ligamentous tissue respond to *Roux's law* of functional adaptation: an organ will adapt itself structurally to an alteration, quantitative or qualitative, of function.[16]

Synovial Membrane and Synovial Fluid

Lining the synovial articular capsule is a synovial membrane made of connective tissue with flattened cells and villi (small projections) on its inner aspect. Fluid is secreted and absorbed by the synovial membrane. Synovial fluid has the consistency of egg white and acts as a joint lubricant. It has the ability to vary its viscosity. During slow movement, the fluid thickens; during fast movement it thins to a greater or lesser extent, both produced by the presence of hyaluronic acid.

Articular Cartilage

In general cartilage, as a connective tissue, provides firm and flexible support. It occurs throughout the body and consists of hyaline, fibrous, and elastic types. Cartilage is a semifirm type of connective tissue with a predominance of ground substance in the extracellular matrix. Within the ground substance are inset varying amounts of collagenous and elastic fibers. Cartilage has a bluish white or gray color and is semiopaque. It has no direct blood or nerve supply. Hyaline cartilage composes part of the nasal septum, the larynx, the trachea, the bronchi, and the articular ends of bones of the synovial joints. Fibrocartilage makes up the vertebral disks, symphysis pubis, and menisci of the knee joint. Elastic cartilage is found in the external ear and the eustachian tube.

As mentioned previously, the ends of the bones in a diarthrotic joint are covered by hyaline cartilage, which acts as a cushion for the bone ends. Its general appearance is smooth and pearly. Hyaline cartilage acts like a sponge in relation to synovial fluid. As movement occurs, it absorbs and squeezes out the fluid as pressures vary between the joint surfaces. Because of its great strength, the cartilage can be deformed without damage and can still return to its original shape. However, cartilaginous degeneration, producing microtrauma, may occur during the abnormal compressional forces that occur over a period of time. Hyaline cartilage has no direct blood supply, receiving its nourishment from the synovial fluid—more specifically, from the synovial membrane located at its edges. Deeper aspects of the cartilage are fed by spaces (lacunae) in the adjacent bone.

Additional Synovial Joint Structures

Fat

In some joints, such as the knee and elbow, there are pads of fat that lie between the synovial membrane and the capsule. They tend to fill in the spaces between the bones that form joints. As movement occurs, they move in and out of these spaces.

Articular Disks

Some diarthrotic joints have an additional fibrocartilaginous disk. These disks vary in shape and are connected to the capsule. They are found in joints where two planes of movement exist and may act as "spreaders" of the synovial fluid between the joint surfaces.

Nerve Supply

The articular capsule, ligaments, outer aspects of the synovial membrane, and fat pads of the synovial joint are well supplied with nerves. The inner aspect of the synovial membrane, cartilage, and articular disks, if present, have nerves as well. Mechano-receptors (encapsulated nerve endings) provide information about the relative position of the joint and are found in the fibrous capsule and ligaments. They are myelinated, whereas nonmyelinated fibers are pain receptors or blood vessel suppliers.

Types of Synovial Joints

Synovial joints are subdivided into six types—ball-and-socket, hinge, pivot, ellipsoidal, saddle, and gliding. *Ball-and-socket* joints allow all possible movement (e.g., shoulder and hip joints). *Hinge* joints allow only flexion and extension (e.g., elbow joint). *Pivot* joints permit rotation around an axis (e.g., cervical atlas and axis, proximal ends of radius and ulna). *Ellipsoidal* joints have an elliptical convex head in an elliptical concave socket (e.g., wrist joint). *Saddle-shaped* joints are reciprocally concavoconvex (e.g., carpometacarpal joint of the thumb). *Gliding* joints allow a small amount of gliding back and forth or sideways (e.g., joints between the carpal and tarsal bones and all of the joints between the articular processes of the vertebrae).

Functional Synovial Joint Characteristics

Synovial joints differ in their ability to withstand trauma, depending on their skeletal, ligamentous, and muscular organization. Table 6-2 provides a general guide to the relative strength of selected articulations in terms of sports participation.

Synovial Joint Stabilization

Muscle tension is important in limiting synovial joint movement. Limitation may be the result of contacting another body. When the joint capsule is overstretched, a reflex contraction of muscles in the area occurs to prevent overstretching. This reaction demonstrates Hilton's law, which states that the joint capsule, the muscles moving that joint, and the skin overlying the insertion of the muscles have the same nerve supply. Ligaments, for the most part, are not extensible but can be extended as a result of the collagen fibers being arranged in bundles at right angles to one another. As the angles of the bundles are changed, ligaments can be extended without lengthening the collagen fiber.

TABLE 6-2 **General Relative Strength Grades in Selected Articulations**

Articulation	Skeleton	Ligaments	Muscles
Ankle	Strong	Moderate	Weak
Knee	Weak	Moderate	Strong
Hip	Strong	Strong	Strong
Lumbosacral	Weak	Strong	Moderate
Lumbar vertebrae	Strong	Strong	Moderate
Thoracic vertebrae	Strong	Strong	Moderate
Cervical vertebrae	Weak	Moderate	Strong
Sternoclavicular	Weak	Weak	Weak
Acromioclavicular	Weak	Moderate	Weak
Glenohumeral	Weak	Moderate	Moderate
Elbow	Moderate	Strong	Strong
Wrist	Weak	Moderate	Moderate
Phalanges (toes and fingers)	Weak	Moderate	Moderate

In terms of stability, ligaments and capsular structures are highly important to joints. Characteristically, joints that are shallow and relatively poor fitting must depend on their capsular structures or muscles for major support. The knee is an example of an articulation that lacks bony congruence and depends mainly on muscles and ligaments for its support.

Besides moving limbs, muscles also provide joint stabilization to a greater or lesser extent and absorb the forces of load transmission. Muscles help stabilize joints in the following ways: muscles that cross joints assist in maintaining proper articular alignment; and some muscles attach directly to the articular capsule (shunt muscles) and, when stretched, also tighten the capsule. By becoming taut the shunt muscles prevent the articulations from separating and also assist in maintaining proper alignment.

Articular Capsule and Ligaments

Capsular and ligamentous tissue maintain anatomical integrity and structural alignment of synovial joints. Both of these structures are similar in composition to tendons. However, they contain elastic fibers, and their collagenous fibers, although having many configurations, are irregular and have a spiral arrangement. Attaching bone to bone, ligaments are generally strongest in the middle and weakest at the ends. In comparison with the fast, protective response of ligaments and capsular tissues, muscles respond much more slowly. For example, a muscle begins to develop protective tension within just a few hundredths of a second when overly stretched but will not fully respond until approximately one tenth of a second has elapsed.[7] The articular cartilage, which is classified as soft tissue, has three major mechanical functions: control of joint motion, joint stability, and force or load transmission.

Motion control   The shape of the articular cartilage determines what motion will occur. An enarthrodial joint or a ball-and-socket joint such as the hip is considered a universal joint, allowing movement in all planes. In contrast, a hinge joint such as the interphalangeal joint allows movement in only one plane.

Stability   In general, bones that form a joint normally closely match with one another and produce varying degrees of stability, depending on their particular shape.

Load transmission   The articular cartilage assists in transmitting a joint load smoothly and uniformly. The atmospheric pressure within the joint space must be kept constant at all times.

Synovial Joint Trauma

A major factor in joint injuries is the viscoelastic tissue properties of ligaments and capsules (Table 6-3). As mentioned previously, *viscoelastic* refers to the extensibility of collagen fibers that is time dependent. This extensibility is dependent on the rapidity of the movement. Constant compression or tension can cause ligaments or capsular tissue to deteriorate. In contrast, intermittent compression and tension will, over time, increase the overall strength, including that of the bony attachments of the connec-

TABLE 6-3 Synovial Joint Trauma

Primary Tissue	Type	Mechanical Forces	Condition
Capsule	Acute	Tension/compression	Sprains Dislocation/subluxation Synovial swelling
	Chronic	Tension/compression/shearing	Capsulitis Synovitis Bursitis
Articular cartilage (hyaline)	Chronic	Compression/shearing	Osteochondrosis Traumatic arthritis

tive tissue. Much like tension forces, torsional or twisting forces, when exceeding the relative strength of collagen fibers, can produce injury. Although occurring less often, a shearing action that cuts across the collagen fiber can traumatize capsular and ligamentous tissue. When articular cartilage fails to properly transmit the applied loads, tissue damage may occur. In other words, the bones and hyaline cartilage that form a joint become out of accordance with each other's compressional forces over a period of time and predispose the joint to degenerative changes.

Synovial Joint Injury Classification

Acute Joint Injuries

The major injuries that happen to synovial joints are sprains, subluxations, and dislocations.

Sprains   The sprain, one of the most common and disabling injuries seen in sports, is a traumatic joint twist that results in stretching or total tearing of the stabilizing connective tissues (Figure 6-10). When a joint is forced beyond its normal anatomical limits, microscopic and gross pathologies occur. Specifically, there is injury to ligaments and to the articular capsule and synovial membrane. According to the extent of injury, sprains are graded in three degrees. A grade 1 sprain is characterized by some pain, minimum loss of function, mild point tenderness, little or no swelling, and no abnormal motion when tested. With a grade 2 sprain there is pain, moderate loss of function, swelling, and in some cases slight to moderate instability.[16] A grade 3 (or severe) sprain is extremely painful, with major loss of function, severe instability, tenderness, and swelling. A grade 3 sprain may also represent a subluxation that has been reduced spontaneously.

Effusion of blood and synovial fluid into the joint cavity during a sprain produces joint swelling, local temperature increase, pain or point tenderness, and skin discoloration (ecchymosis). As with tendons, ligaments and capsules can experience forces that completely rupture or produce an avulsion fracture. Ligaments and capsules heal slowly because of a relatively poor blood supply; however, their nerves are plentiful, often producing a great deal of pain when injured.

The joints that are most vulnerable to sprains in sports are the ankles, knees, and shoulders. Sprains occur least often to the wrists and elbows. Because it is often difficult to distinguish between joint sprains and tendon strains, the examiner should expect the worst possible condition and manage it accordingly. Repeated joint twisting can eventually result in chronic inflammation, degeneration, and arthritis.

Acute synovitis   The synovial membrane of a joint can be acutely injured by a contusion or a sprain. Irritation of the membrane causes an increase in fluid production, and swelling occurs. The result is joint pain during motion, along with skin sensitivity from pressure at certain points. In a few days, with proper care, effusion and extravasated blood are absorbed, and swelling and pain diminish.

Subluxations, dislocations, and diastasis   Dislocations are second to fractures in terms of disabling the athlete. The highest incidence of dislocations involves the fingers and, next, the shoulder joint (Figure 6-11). Dislocations, which result primarily from forces causing the joint to go beyond its normal anatomical limits, are divided

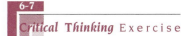

6-7

Critical Thinking E x e r c i s e

A basketball player steps on another player's foot, causing a lateral ankle injury.

? What forces are applied, and what type of injury has been incurred?

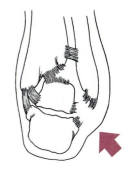

Figure 6-10

A sprain mainly involves injury to ligamentous and capsular tissue; however, muscle tendons can be secondarily strained.

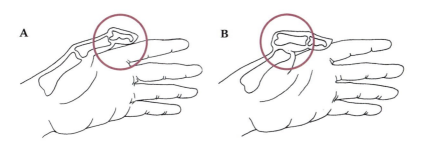

A   B

Figure 6-11

A point that is forced beyond its anatomical limits can become **A,** partially dislocated (subluxated); or **B,** completely dislocated (luxated).

into two classes: *subluxations* and *luxations.* Subluxations are partial dislocations in which an incomplete separation between two articulating bones occurs. Luxations are complete dislocations, presenting a total disunion of bone apposition between the articulating surfaces. A diastasis, in contrast to subluxations and luxations, is of two types: a disjointing of two bones parallel to one another, such as the radius and ulna; and the rupture of a "solid" joint, such as the symphysis pubis.[1] A diastasis occurs commonly with a fracture.

Several factors are important in recognizing and evaluating dislocations:

1. There is a loss of limb function. The athlete usually complains of having fallen or of having received a severe blow to a particular joint and then suddenly being unable to move that part.
2. Deformity is almost always apparent. Because the deformity can often be obscured by heavy musculature, it is important for the examiner to palpate the injured site to determine the loss of normal body contour. Comparison of the injured side with its normal counterpart often reveals distortions.
3. Swelling and point tenderness are immediately present.

At times, as with a fracture, x-ray examination is the only absolute diagnostic measure. First-time dislocations or joint separations may result in a rupture of the stabilizing ligamentous and tendinous tissues surrounding the joint and avulsion or pulling away from the bone. Trauma is often so violent that small chips of bone are torn away with the supporting structures, or the force may separate growth epiphyses or cause a complete fracture of the neck in long bones. These possibilities indicate the importance of administering complete and thorough medical attention to first-time dislocations. It has often been said, "Once a dislocation, always a dislocation." In most cases this statement is true because once a joint has been either subluxated or completely luxated, the connective tissues that bind and hold it in its correct alignment are stretched to such an extent that the joint will be extremely vulnerable to subsequent dislocations. Chronic, recurring dislocations may take place without severe pain because of the somewhat slack condition of the stabilizing tissues.

A first-time dislocation should always be considered and treated as a possible fracture. Once it has been ascertained that the injury is a dislocation, a physician should be consulted for further evaluation. However, before the patient is taken to the physician, the injury should be properly splinted and supported to prevent any further damage.

Chronic Joint Injuries

As with other chronic physical injuries or problems occurring from sports participation, chronic synovial joint injuries stem from microtraumas and overuse. The two major categories in which they fall are osteochondrosis and traumatic arthritis (osteoarthritis or inflammation of surrounding soft tissues such as the bursal capsule and the synovium).[8] Another general expression for the chronic synovial conditions of the child or adolescent is articular epiphyseal injury. It should be noted that a major cause of chronic joint injury such as osteoarthritis is failure of the muscle control of limit deceleration. Athletes can avoid such injuries by avoiding chronic fatigue and training when tired and by wearing protective gear to enhance active absorption of impact forces.[14]

Osteochondrosis   Osteochondrosis is a category of conditions of which the causes are not well understood. A synonym for this condition, if it is located in a point such as the knee, is *osteochondritis dissecans* and, if located at a tubercle or tuberosity, *apophysitis.* Apophysial conditions are discussed in the section on skeletal trauma.

One suggested cause of osteochondrosis is *aseptic necrosis* in which circulation to the epiphysis has been disrupted. Another suggestion is that trauma causes particles of the articular cartilage to fracture, eventually resulting in fissures that penetrate to the subchondral bone. If trauma to a joint occurs, pieces of cartilage may be dislodged, which can cause joint locking, swelling, and pain. If the condition occurs in an ap-

---

A first-time dislocation should always be considered a possible fracture.

6-8

Critical Thinking Exercise

A young female gymnast has a pronounced knee malalignment.

? The athlete complains of a left knee locking, pain, and swelling. What is the gymnast's possible condition?

ophysis, there may be an avulsion-type fracture and fragmentation of the epiphysis, along with pain, swelling, and disability.

Traumatic arthritis   Traumatic arthritis is usually the result of microtraumas. With repeated trauma to the articular joint surfaces, the bone and synovium thicken and pain, muscle spasm, and articular crepitus, or grating on movement, occur. Joint insult leading to arthritis can come from repeated sprains that leave a joint with weakened ligaments. There can be malalignment of the skeleton, which stresses joints, or it can arise from an irregular joint surface that stems from repeated articular chondral injuries. Loose bodies that have been dislodged from the articular surface can also irritate and produce arthritis. Athletes with joint injuries that are improperly immobilized or who are allowed to return to activity before proper healing has occurred may eventually be afflicted with arthritis.

Bursitis, capsulitis, and synovitis   The soft tissues that are an integral part of the synovial joint can develop chronic problems.

Bursitis   As discussed previously, bursae provide protection between tendons and bones, between tendons and ligaments, and between other structures where there is friction. Bursae located in and around synovial joints can become acutely or, over a period of time, chronically inflamed. Bursitis in the knee, elbow, and shoulder is common among athletes.

Capsulitis and synovitis   After repeated joint sprains or microtraumas, a chronic inflammatory condition called capsulitis may occur. Usually associated with capsulitis is synovitis. Synovitis also occurs acutely, but with repeated joint injury or with joint injury that is improperly managed, a chronic condition can arise. Chronic synovitis involves active joint congestion with edema. As with the synovial lining of the bursa, the synovium of a joint can undergo degenerative tissue changes. The synovium becomes irregularly thickened, exudation is present, and a fibrous underlying tissue is present. Several movements may be restricted, and there may be joint noises such as grinding or creaking.

SKELETAL TRAUMA

Bone provides shape and support for the body. As with soft tissue, it can be traumatized during sports participation.

Anatomical Characteristics

As discussed previously, bone is a specialized type of dense connective tissue, consisting of bone cells (osteocytes) that are fixed in a matrix, which consists of an intercellular material. The outer surface of a bone is composed of compact tissue, and the inner aspect is composed of a more porous tissue known as cancellous bone (Figure 6-12). Compact tissue is tunneled by a marrow cavity. Throughout the bone run countless branching canals, which contain blood vessels and lymphatic vessels. These canals form the Haversian system. On the outside of a bone is a tissue covering, the periosteum, which contains the blood supply to the bone.

Bone Functions

Bones perform five basic functions: body support, organ protection, movement (through joints and levers), a reservoir for calcium, and the formation of blood cells (hemopoiesis).

Types of Bone

Bones are classified according to their shapes. They include bones that are flat, irregular, short, and long. Flat bones are in the skull, the ribs, and the scapulae; irregular bones are in the vertebral column and the skull. Short bones are primarily in the wrist and the ankle. Long bones are the most commonly injured bones in sports. They consist of the humerus, ulna, femur, tibia, fibula, and phalanges.

Flat, irregular, and short bones have the same inner cancellous bone over which

Athletes with improperly immobilized joint injuries or who are allowed to return to activity before proper healing has occurred may eventually be afflicted with arthritis.

Figure 6-12

Anatomical characteristics of bone. **A,** Longitudinal section. **B,** Cutaway section.

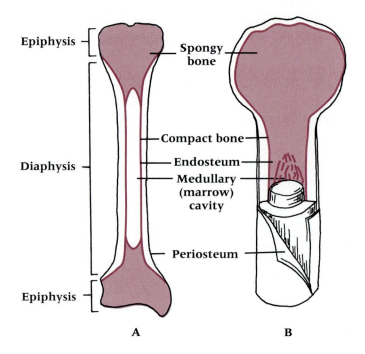

Epiphysis

Spongy bone

Diaphysis

Compact bone

Endosteum

Medullary (marrow) cavity

Periosteum

Epiphysis

A   B

there is a layer of compact bone. A few irregular and flat bones (e.g., the vertebrae and the sternum) have some space in the cancellous bone that is filled with red marrow and sesamoid bones.

Gross Structures

The gross structures of bone that are visible to the naked eye include the diaphysis, epiphysis, articular cartilage, periosteum, medullary (marrow) cavity, and endosteum. The *diaphysis* is the main shaft of the long bone. It is hollow, cylindrical, and covered by compact bone. The *epiphysis* is located at the ends of long bones. It is bulbous in shape, providing space for the muscle attachments. The epiphysis is composed primarily of cancellous bone, giving it a spongelike appearance. As discussed previously, the ends of long bones are covered with a layer of *hyaline cartilage* that covers the joint surfaces of the epiphysis. This cartilage provides protection during movement and cushions jars and blows to the joint. A dense, white fibrous membrane, the *periosteum*, covers long bones except at joint surfaces. Many fibers, called Sharpey's fibers, from the periosteum penetrate the underlying bone. Interlacing with the periosteum are fibers from the muscle tendons. Throughout the periosteum on its inner layer exist countless blood vessels and osteoblasts (bone-forming cells). The blood vessels provide nutrition to the bone, and the osteoblasts provide bone growth and repair. The *medullar cavity,* a hollow tube in the long bone diaphysis, contains a yellow, fatty marrow in adults. Lining the medullar cavity is the *endosteum.*

Microscopic Structures

Calcium salts impregnate the intercellular substance of bone, making it hard. Osteocytes are found in small, hollow spaces called *lacunae.* Running throughout the bone is the Haversian system, consisting of a central tube (Haversian canal) with alternate layers of intercellular matrix surrounding it in concentric cylinders. Haversian systems are the structural units of compact bone. Compact and cancellous bones differ in their structures. In bone that is compact, interspersed lamellae fill the spaces between adjacent Haversian systems. In cancellous bone, there are numerous open spaces located between thin processes called *trabeculae.* Trabeculae act like a scaffold, joining cancellous bone. They arrange themselves along the line of greatest stress, providing additional structural strength to the bone. The blood circulation connects the periosteum with the Haversian canal through the Volkmann's canal. The medullary cavity and the bone marrow are supplied directly by one or more arteries.

Bone Growth

In general, bone ossification occurs from the synthesis of bone's organic matrix by osteoblasts, followed immediately by the calcification of this matrix.

The epiphyseal growth plate is a cartilaginous disk located near the end of each long bone. Growth of the long bones depends on these plates. Ossification in long bones begins in the diaphysis and in both epiphyses. It proceeds from the diaphysis toward each epiphysis and from each epiphysis toward the diaphysis. The growth plate has layers of cartilage cells in different stages of maturity with the more immature cells at one end and mature ones at the other end. As the cartilage cells mature, immature osteoblasts replace them later to produce solid bone. Epiphyseal growth plates are often less resistant to deforming forces than are ligaments of nearby joints or the outer shaft of the long bones; therefore severe twisting or a blow to an arm or leg can result in disruption in growth. Injury can prematurely close the growth plate, causing a loss of length in the bone. Growth plate dislocation can also cause deformity of the long bone.[11]

Bone diameter increases as a result of the combined action of osteoblasts and osteoclasts. *Osteoblasts* build new bone on the outside of the bone; at the same time *osteoclasts* increase the medullary cavity by breaking down bony tissue. Once a bone has reached its full size, there occurs a balance of bone formation and bone destruction, or osteogenesis and resorption, respectively. This process may be disrupted by factors in sports conditioning or participation. These factors may cause greater osteogenesis than resorption. Conversely, resorption may exceed osteogenesis in situations in which the athlete is out of shape but overtrains. On the other hand, women whose estrogen is decreased as a result of training may experience bone loss.[3] (See Chapter 27.) In general, bone loss begins to exceed bone gain by ages 35 to 40. Gradually, bone is lost in the endosteal surfaces and then is gained on the outer surfaces. As the thickness of long bones decreases, they are less able to resist the forces of compression. This process also leads to increased bone porosity, known as osteoporosis.

As with other structures in the human body, bones are morphologically, biochemically, and biomechanically highly sensitive to both stress and stress deprivation. With this in mind, bone's functional adaptation follows Wolff's law.[19] Every change in the form and function of a bone, or of its function alone, is followed by certain definite changes in its internal architecture and equally definite secondary alterations in its mathematical laws.

Bone Injuries

Because of its viscoelastic properties, bone will bend slightly. However, bone is generally brittle and is a poor shock absorber because of its mineral content. This brittleness increases under tension forces as opposed to compression forces.

Many factors of bone structure affect its strength. Anatomical strength or weakness can be affected by a bone's shape and its changes in shape or direction. A hollow cylinder is one of the strongest structures for resisting both bending and twisting, as compared with a solid rod, which has much less resistance to such forces.[10] This may be why bones such as the tibia are primarily cylinders. Most spiral fractures of the tibia occur at its middle and distal third, where the bone is most solid (Figure 6-13).

Anatomical Weak Points

Stress forces become concentrated where a long bone suddenly changes shape and direction. Long bones that change shape gradually are less prone to injury than those that change suddenly. The clavicle, for example, is prone to fracture because it changes from round to flat at the same time it changes direction.

Figure 6-13

Anatomical strengths or weaknesses of a long bone can be affected by its shape, changes of direction, and hollowness.

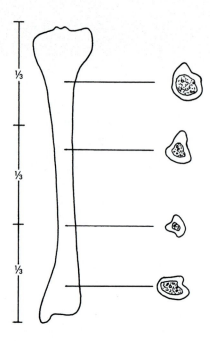

Load Characteristics

Long bones can be stressed by tension, compression, bending, torsion, and shearing.

Long bones can be stressed or loaded to fail by *tension, compression, bending, twisting* (torsion), and *shearing*. These forces, either singularly or in combination, can cause a variety of fractures. For example, spiral fractures are caused by twisting, whereas oblique fractures are caused by the combined forces of axial compression, bending, and torsion. Transverse fractures occur by bending (Figure 6-14).

Along with the type of stress, the amount of the load must be considered. The more complex the fracture, the more energy is required. Energy is used in deforming the bone and breaking the bony tissue, and some energy becomes dissipated in adjacent soft tissue.[9]

The rate of energy at which a force is applied to a long bone can cause tissue failure. Depending on the type of bony tissue, more energy is generally required to cause fracture in a shorter period of time than over a longer period of time.[5]

A bone's magnitude of stress and strain is most prevalent at its outer surface, gradually decreasing to zero at its center.[14]

Bone Trauma Classification

Bone trauma can generally be classified as periostitis, acute fractures, stress fractures, and epiphyseal conditions.

Periostitis   An inflammation of the periosteum can result from various sports traumas, mainly contusion. It often appears as skin rigidity of the overlying muscles. It can occur as an acute episode or can become chronic.

Acute bone fractures   A bone fracture can be a partial or complete interruption in a bone's continuity and can occur without external exposure or can extend through the skin, creating an external wound (open fracture). Fractures can result from direct trauma; in other words, the bone breaks directly at the site where a force is applied. When the fracture occurs some distance from where force is applied, it is called an indirect fracture. A sudden, violent muscle contraction or repetitive abnormal stress to a bone can also cause a fracture. Fractures must be considered one of the most serious hazards of sports and should be routinely suspected in musculoskeletal injuries. The following are more detailed descriptions of acute fractures.

Depressed fracture   Depressed fractures occur most often in flat bones such as those found in the skull. They are caused by falling and striking the head on a hard, im-

6-9

Critical Thinking Exercise

An alpine skier catches his right ski tip and severely twists the lower leg.

? What type of serious injury could be created by this mechanism?

MECHANISM	PATTERN	APPEARANCE	Figure 6-14

Mechanisms, patterns, and appearances of acute bone fractures.

MECHANISM	PATTERN
Bending	Transverse
Torsion	Spiral
Compression plus bending	Oblique-transverse or butterfly
Compression plus bending plus torsion	Oblique
Variable	Comminuted
Compression	Metaphyseal compression

movable surface or by being hit with a hard object. Such injuries also result in gross pathology of soft areas.

Greenstick fracture Greenstick fractures are incomplete breaks in bones that have not completely ossified, as is the case in adolescence. They occur most frequently in the convex bone surface, with the concave surface remaining intact. The name is derived from the similarity of the fracture to the break in a green twig taken from a tree.

Impacted fracture Impacted fractures can result from a fall from a height, which causes a long bone to receive, directly on its long axis, a force of such magnitude that the osseous tissue is compressed. This telescopes one part of the bone on the other. Impacted fractures require immediate splinting by the athletic trainer and traction by the physician to ensure a normal length of the injured limb.

Longitudinal fracture Longitudinal fractures are those in which the bone splits along its length, often the result of jumping from a height and landing in such a way as to impact force or stress to the long axis.

Oblique fracture Oblique fractures are similar to spiral fractures and occur when one end receives sudden torsion or twisting and the other end is fixed or stabilized.

Serrated fracture Serrated fractures in which the two bony fragments have a sawtooth, sharp-edged fracture line are usually caused by a direct blow. Because of the sharp and jagged edges, extensive internal damage, such as the severance of vital blood vessels and nerves, often occurs.

Spiral fracture Spiral fractures have an S-shaped separation. They are common in football and skiing, in which the foot is firmly planted and then the body is suddenly rotated in an opposing direction.

Transverse fracture Transverse fractures occur in a straight line, more or less at right angles to the bone shaft. A direct outside blow usually causes this injury.

Comminuted fracture Comminuted fractures consist of three or more fragments at the fracture site. They could be caused by a hard blow or a fall in an awkward position. From the physician's point of view, these fractures impose a difficult healing situation because of the displacement of the bone fragments. Soft tissues are often interposed between the fragments, causing incomplete healing. Such cases may need surgical intervention.

Contrecoup fracture Contrecoup fractures occur on the side opposite to the part where trauma was initiated. Fracture of the skull is at times an example of the contrecoup. An athlete may be hit on one side of the head with such force that the brain and internal structures compress against the opposite side of the skull, causing a fracture.

Blowout fracture Blowout fractures occur to the wall of the eye orbit as the result of a blow to the eye.

Avulsion fracture An avulsion fracture is the separation of a bone fragment from its cortex at an attachment of a ligament or tendon. This fracture usually occurs as a result of a sudden, powerful twist or stretch of a body part. An example of a ligamentous episode is a sudden eversion of the foot that causes the deltoid ligament to avulse bone away from the medial malleolus. An example of a tendinous avulsion is one that causes a patellar fracture, which occurs when an athlete falls forward while suddenly bending a knee. The stretch of the patellar tendon pulls a portion of the inferior patellar pole apart (Figure 6-15).

Stress fractures Stress fractures have been variously called march, fatigue, and spontaneous fractures, although stress fracture is the most commonly used term. The exact cause of this fracture is not known, but there are a number of likely possibilities such as an overload caused by muscle contraction, an altered stress distribution in the bone accompanying muscle fatigue, a change in the ground reaction force such as going from a wood surface to a grass surface, and performing a rhythmically repetitive stress leading up to a vibratory summation point. The last possibility is favored by many authorities.[17] Rhythmic muscle action performed over a period of time at a subthreshold level causes the stress-bearing capacity of the bone to be exceeded, hence a stress fracture. A bone may become vulnerable to fracture during the first few weeks of intense physical activity or training. Weight-bearing bones undergo bone resorption and become weaker before they become stronger. The sequence of events is suggested by Stanitski and co-workers[17] as resulting from increased muscular forces plus an increased rate of remodeling that leads to bone resorption and rarefaction, which progresses to produce increasingly more severe fractures. The four progressively severe fractures are focal microfractures, periosteal or endosteal response (stress fractures), linear fractures (stress fractures), and displaced fractures.

Typical responses for stress fractures in sports are as follows:
1. Coming back into competition too soon after an injury or illness.
2. Going from one event to another without proper training in the second event.
3. Starting initial training too quickly.
4. Changing habits or the environment (e.g., running surfaces, the bank of a track, or shoes).

In addition to these stresses, susceptibility to fracture can be increased by a variety of postural and foot conditions. Flatfeet, a short first metatarsal bone, or a hypermobile metatarsal region can predispose an athlete to stress fractures. (See Chapter 17.)

Early detection of the stress fracture may be difficult. Because of their frequency in a wide range of sports, stress fractures always must be suspected in susceptible body areas that fail to respond to usual management. Until there is an obvious reaction in the bone, which may take several weeks, x-ray examination may fail to reveal any change. Although nonspecific, a bone scan can provide early indications in a given area.

The major signs of a stress fracture are swelling, focal tenderness, and pain. In the early stages of the fracture the athlete complains of pain when active but not at rest. Later, the pain is constant and becomes more intense at night. Percussion, by light tapping on the bone at a site other than the suspected fracture, will produce pain at the fracture site.

The most common sites of stress fracture are the tibia, fibula, metatarsal shaft, calcaneus, femur, pars interarticularis of the lumbar vertebrae, ribs, and humerus (Figure 6-16).

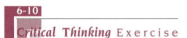

6-10

Critical Thinking Exercise

A long jumper experiences a sudden sharp pain in the region of the left ischial tuberosity during a jump.

? What injuries are possible through this mechanism?

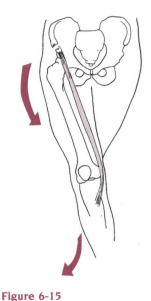

Figure 6-15

Tendinous avulsion fracture of the sartorius muscle.

Figure 6-16

The most common stress fracture sites.

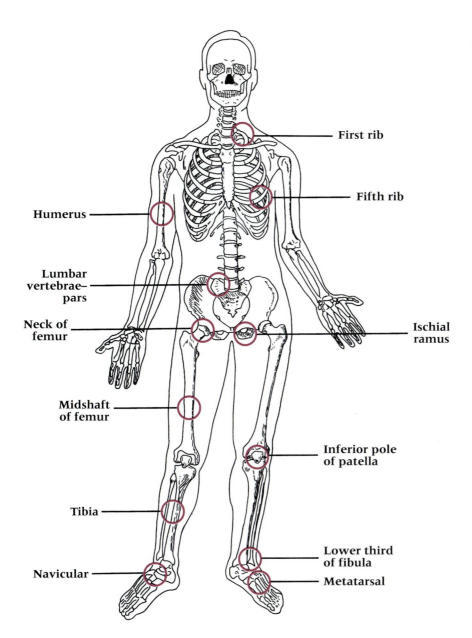

The management of stress fractures varies with the individual athlete, injury site, and extent of injury. Stress fractures that occur on the compression side of bone heal more rapidly and are managed more easily compared with those on the tension side. Stress fractures on the tension side can rapidly produce a complete fracture.

Epiphyseal conditions   Three types of epiphyseal growth site injuries can be sustained by children and adolescents performing sports activities. They consist of injury to the epiphyseal growth plate, articular epiphyseal injuries, and apophyseal injuries. The most prevalent age range for these injuries is from 10 to 16 years.

Epiphyseal growth plate injuries (Figure 6-17) have been classified by Salter-Harris[4] into five types as follows:

- Type I—complete separation of the epiphysis in relation to the metaphysis without fracture to the bone.
- Type II—separation of the growth plate and a small portion of the metaphysis.
- Type III—fracture of the epiphysis.
- Type IV—fracture of a portion of the epiphysis and metaphysis.

Figure 6-17

Salter-Harris classification of long bone epiphyseal injuries in children.

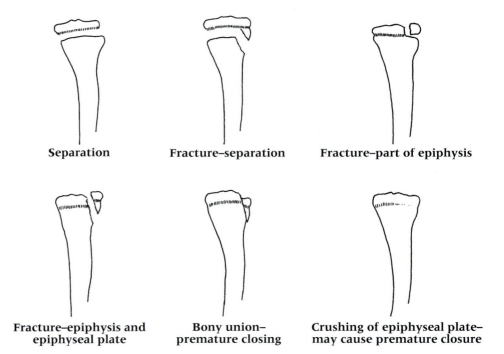

| Separation | Fracture–separation | Fracture–part of epiphysis |

| Fracture–epiphysis and epiphyseal plate | Bony union–premature closing | Crushing of epiphyseal plate–may cause premature closure |

A musculoskeletal injury to a child or adolescent should always be considered a possible epiphyseal condition.

- Type V—no displacement of the epiphysis, but the crushing force can cause a growth deformity.

Apophyseal injuries The young, physically immature athlete is particularly prone to apophyseal injuries. The apophyses are traction epiphyses in contrast to the pressure epiphyses of the long bones. These apophyses serve as origins or insertions for muscles on growing bone that provide bone shape but not length. Common apophyseal avulsion conditions found in sports are Sever's disease and Osgood-Schlatter disease. (See Chapter 18.)

NERVE TRAUMA

A number of abnormal nerve responses can be attributed to athletic participation or injury. The most frequent type of nerve injury is neuropraxia produced by a direct flow. A laceration can cut nerves, causing complications in healing of the injury. Fractures and dislocation can avulse or abnormally compress nerves.

Anatomical Characteristics

The tissue that makes up the nervous system occurs throughout the body. It is composed of neurons; interstitial tissues, including neuroglia (supporting elements); neurilemma cells (the membranous sheath enveloping a nerve fiber); and satellite cells (flat epithelium-like cells forming the inner aspect of a double-layered capsule covering the neuron). Nerve tissue provides the body with its reception and response to stimuli.

Nerve Injuries

The two main forces that cause major nerve injury responses are compression and tension. As with other tissues in the body, the injurious forces may be acute or chronic.

Physical trauma, to nerves in general, produces pain as part of the inflammatory process. (See Chapter 7.) Any number of traumas directly affecting nerves can also produce a variety of sensory responses, including pain. For example, a sudden nerve stretch or pinch can produce a sharp burning pain that radiates down a limb along with muscle weakness. *Neuritis,* a chronic nerve problem, can be caused by a variety of forces that usually have been repeated or continued for a long period of time. Symptoms of neuritis can range from minor nerve problems to paralysis.

Pain that is felt at a point of the body other than at its actual origin is commonly known as *referred pain.* Another potential cause of referred pain is a trigger point, which occurs in the muscular system but refers pain to some other distant body part.

BODY MECHANICS AND INJURY SUSCEPTIBILITY

If we carefully study the mechanical structure of the human body, it is amazing that humans can move so effectively in the upright posture. Not only must constant gravitational force be overcome, but the body also must be manipulated through space by a complex system of somewhat inefficient levers, fueled by a machinery that operates at an efficiency level of approximately 30%. The bony levers that move the body must overcome considerable resistance in the form of inertia and muscle viscosity and must work in most instances at an extremely unfavorable angle of pull. All these factors mitigate the effectiveness of lever action to the extent that most movement is achieved at an efficiency level of less than 25%.

When determining the mechanical reasons for sports injuries to the musculoskeletal system, many factors stand out. Hereditary, congenital, or acquired defects may predispose an athlete to a specific type of injury. Anomalies in anatomical structure or in body build (somatotype) may make an athlete prone to injuries. The habitually incorrect application of skill is a common cause of overuse injuries.

Microtrauma and Overuse Syndrome

Injuries as a result of abnormal and repetitive stress and microtraumas fall into a class with certain identifiable syndromes. Such stress injuries frequently result in either limitation or curtailment of sports performance. Most of these injuries in athletes are directly related to the dynamics of running, throwing, or jumping. The injuries may result from constant and repetitive stresses placed on bones, joints, or soft tissues; from forcing a joint into an extreme range of motion; or from prolonged strenuous activity. Some of the injuries falling into this category may be relatively minor; still, they can be disabling.[19] Among injuries classified as repetitive stress and microtrauma are Achilles tendinitis; splints; stress fractures, particularly of the fibula and second and fifth metatarsal bones; Osgood-Schlatter disease; runner's and jumper's knee; patellar chondromalacia; apophyseal avulsion, especially in the lower extremities of growing athletes; and intertarsal neuroma.

Postural Deviations

Postural deviations are often a major underlying cause of sports injuries. Postural malalignment may be the result of unilateral muscle and soft-tissue asymmetries or bony asymmetries. As a result, the athlete engages in poor mechanics of movement (pathomechanics). Many sports activities are unilateral, thus leading to asymmetries in body development. The resulting imbalance is manifested by a postural deviation as the body seeks to reestablish itself in relation to its center of gravity. Often such deviations are a primary cause of injury. For example, a consistent pattern of knee injury may be related to asymmetries within the pelvis and the legs (short-leg syndrome). Unfortunately, not much in the form of remedial work is usually performed. As a result, an injury often becomes chronic—sometimes to the point that participation in a sport must be halted. When possible, the athletic trainer should seek to ameliorate or eliminate faulty postural conditions through therapy, working under the direction of an orthopedist or other qualified medical personnel. A number of postural conditions offer genuine hazards to athletes by making them exceedingly prone to specific injuries. Some of the more important are discussed in the chapters on foot and leg anomalies, spinal anomalies, and various stress syndromes.

SUMMARY

- "When a force applied to any part of the body results in a harmful disturbance in function or structure, a mechanical injury is said to have been sustained."[12] Engineering terminology is used to describe tissue properties and sport injuries.

Examples are load, stress, deformation, viscoelastic, anisotropic, yield point, and tissue failure.

- The three primary stresses leading to tissue trauma are stretching, compression, and shearing. Bending strain can produce a torque on a bone followed by injury. A torsion, or twisting, load can produce a spiral fracture along the long axis of a bone.

- Soft tissue (nonbony tissue) is categorized as being noncontractile and contractile (muscle) tissues.

- Skin trauma can occur from a variety of forces (e.g., friction, scraping, compression, tearing, cutting, and puncturing) that produce blisters, skin bruises, lacerations, skin avulsions, incisions, and puncture wounds.

- Skeletal muscle trauma from sports participation can involve any aspect of the muscle-tension unit. Forces that injure muscles are compression, tension, and shearing. Acute muscle injuries include contusions and strains. Avulsion fractures and muscle ruptures can occur from an acute episode. Chronic muscle conditions are myositis, fascitis, tendinitis, tenosynovitis, and bursitis. Chronic muscle irritation can cause ectopic calcification; muscle disuse can cause atrophy; and immobilization can cause joint contracture.

- Sports injuries to the synovial joints are common. Anatomically, synovial joints have relative strengths or weaknesses based on their ligamentous or capsular type and their muscle arrangements. Forces that can injure synovial joints are tension, compression, torsion, and shear. Sprains involve acute injury to ligaments or the joint capsule. A grade 3 sprain may cause ligament rupture or an avulsion fracture. Acute synovial joint injuries that go beyond the third degree may result in a dislocation. Two major chronic synovial joint conditions are osteochondrosis and traumatic arthritis. Other chronic conditions are bursitis, capsulitis, and synovitis.

- Long bones can be anatomically susceptible to fractures because of their shape and as a result of changes in direction of the force applied to them. Mechanical forces that cause injury are compression, tension, bending, torsion, and shear. Bending and torsional forces are forms of tension. Acute fractures include avulsion, blowout, comminuted, depressed, greenstick, impacted, longitudinal, oblique, serrated, spiral, transverse, and contrecoup types. Stress fractures are commonly the result of overload to a given bone area. Stress fractures are apparently caused by an altered stress distribution or by the performance of a rhythmically repetitive action that leads to a vibratory summation and thus a fracture. Three major epiphyseal injuries in sports occur to the growth plate, the articular cartilage, and the apophysis.

- Nerve trauma can be produced by overstretching or compression. As with other injuries, they can be acute or chronic. The sudden stretch of a nerve can cause a burning sensation. A variety of traumas to nerves can produce acute pain or a chronic pain such as neuritis.

- An athlete who has faulty body mechanics has an increased potential for injury.

Solutions to Critical Thinking EXERCISES

6-1 All human tissue has viscous and elastic properties. The resistance of tissue is dependent on its viscoelastic characteristic and the types of forces that are applied.

6-2 The friction force produced by sliding into home base causes a serious abrasion skin injury.

6-3 The ball created a compressive force that crushed tissue causing a secondary contusion.

6-4 The football player could have sustained a tension force to the long head of the biceps tendon that caused a rupture or severe strain.

6-5 The mechanism of this elbow injury is repeated tension to the extensor tendons attached to the lateral epicondyle, causing microtraumas. Stress to this area can be reduced by increasing the grip circumference and flattening the backhand stroke.

6-6 Repeated contusions to the quadriceps could produce an ectopic calcification known as myositis ossificous.

6-7 In stepping on another player's foot the basketball player produces an abnormal ankle torsion and lateral ankle tension, stretching and tearing ligaments.

6-8 Knee malalignment produces abnormal compression and shearing forces on the lateral menisci, leading to osteochondritis dissecans and osteochondritis.

6-9 Catching the ski tip produces a torsional force that causes a boot-top spiral fracture.

6-10 During the jump a powerful stretch of the biceps femoris causes a serious strain or an avulsion fracture in the region of the ischial tuberosity.

REVIEW QUESTIONS AND CLASS ACTIVITIES

1. Describe the mechanics that produce noncontractile and contractile sports injuries.
2. Describe the injurious mechanical forces that injure skin.
3. What forces injure muscle tissue?
4. Describe all types of acute muscle injuries.
5. Describe all types of chronic muscle injuries.
6. Describe the major acute injuries occurring to joints.
7. What mechanical forces traumatize the musculotendinous unit and the synovial joint? How are the forces similar to one another, and how are they different?
8. What forces gradually weaken tendons and ligaments?
9. Contrast two chronic synovial joint injuries.
10. List the structural characteristics that make a long bone susceptible to fracture.
11. What mechanical forces cause acute fracture of a bone?
12. How do stress fractures probably occur?
13. Describe the most common epiphyseal conditions that result from sports participation.
14. What are the relationships of postural deviations to sports injuries?
15. Discuss the concept of pathomechanics as it relates to microtraumas and overuse syndromes.

REFERENCES

1. Akeson WH et al: The biology of ligaments. In Hunter LY, Funk FJ Jr, editors: *Rehabilitation of the injured knee,* St Louis, 1984, Mosby.
2. American Academy of Orthopaedic Surgeons: *Athletic training and sports medicine,* Park Ridge, Ill, 1991, American Academy of Orthopaedic Surgeons.
3. Barak T et al: *Basics concepts of orthopaedic manual therapy,* ed 2, In Gould JA III, editor: St Louis, 1990, Mosby.
4. Blavelt CT, Nelson FRT: *A manual of orthopaedic terminology,* ed 4, St Louis, 1990, Mosby.
5. Byrnes WB, Clarkson PM: Delayed onset muscle soreness and training. In Katch FL, Freedson PS, editors: *Clinics in sports medicine,* vol 5, Philadelphia, 1986, Saunders.
6. Evans WJ: Exercise-induced skeletal muscle damage, *Phys Sportsmed* 15(1):89, 1987.
7. Fine PG: The biology of pain. In Heil J, editor: *Psychology of sport injury,* Champaign, Ill, 1993, Human Kinetics.
8. Geesink RGT et al: Stress response of articular cartilage, *Int J Sports Med* 5:100, 1984.
9. Gould JA III, Davies GJ, editors: *Orthopaedic and sports physical therapy,* ed 2, St Louis, 1990, Mosby.
10. Gonza ER: Biomechanics of long bone injuries. In Gonza ER, Harrington IJ, editors: *Biomechanics of musculoskeletal injury,* Baltimore, 1982, Williams & Wilkins.
11. Hirsch CS, Lumwalt RE: Injuries caused by physical agents. In Kissane JM, editor: *Anderson's pathology,* ed 9, vol 1, St Louis, 1990, Mosby.
12. Huson A: Mechanics of joints, *Int J Sports Med* 5:83, 1984.
13. Leaveau BF: Basic biomechanics in sports and orthopaedic therapy. In Gould JA III, Davies GJ, editors: *Orthopaedic and sports physical therapy,* St Louis, 1990, Mosby.
14. Markey KL: Stress fractures. In Hunter-Griffin LY, editor: *Overuse injuries, clinics in sports medicine,* vol 6, Philadelphia, 1987, Saunders.
15. Porth CM: *Pathophysiology,* ed 4, Philadelphia, 1994, Lippincott.
16. Roux W: *Die entwichlungsmechanic,* Leipzig, Germany, 1905, Englemann.
17. Stanitski CL, McMaster JH, Scranton PE: On the nature of stress fractures, *Am J Sports Med* 6:391, 1978.
18. Thibodeau GA, Patton KT: *Anatomy and physiology,* ed 3, St Louis, 1996, Mosby.
19. Wolff J: *Das geset der transformation der knockan,* Berlin, 1892, Hirschwald.

ANNOTATED BIBLIOGRAPHY

Blavelt CT, Nelson RRT: *A manual of orthopaedic terminology,* ed 4, St Louis, 1990, Mosby.

A resource book for all individuals who need to identify medical words or their acronyms.

Booher JM, Thibodeau GA: *Athletic injury assessment,* St Louis, 1994, Times Mirror/Mosby College.

An excellent guide to the recognition, assessment, classification, and evaluation of athletic injuries.

Brown LO, Yavorsky P: Locomotor biomechanics and pathomechanics: a review, *J Orthop Sports Phys Ther* 9:3, 1987.

A review of current knowledge regarding clinical anatomy and arthrokinematics of the foot and ankle.

Gunta KE: Alterations in skeletal functions: trauma and infection. In Porth CM, editor: *Pathophysiology,* Philadelphia, 1994, Lippincott.

Chapter 56 is dedicated to major soft and bony tissue trauma and infection.

Haubrich WS: Medical meanings: a glossary of word origins, San Diego, 1984, Harcourt Brace Jovanovich.

Medical meaning provides the reader with derivation and definition of medical terms beyond the medical dictionary.

Peacinn M, Bojanic I: *Overuse injuries of musculoskeletal system,* Boca Raton, Fla, 1993, CRC Press.

A comprehensive text describing overuse injuries of tendons, tendon sheath, bursae, muscles, muscle-tendon function, cartilage, and nerve.

Williams JGP: *Color atlas of injury in sport,* Chicago, 1990, Mosby.

An excellent visual guide to the area of sports injuries. It covers the nature and incidence of sport injury, types of tissue damage, and regional injuries caused by a variety of sports activities.

Tissue Response to Injury

When you finish this chapter, you should be able to

■ Describe the major events of acute and chronic inflammation.
■ Identify the process of repair and regeneration.
■ List the differences between soft tissue and bone healing.
■ Identify the management concepts designed for healing and pain modulation.
■ List the major characteristics of a stress fracture.
■ Explain pain perception.
■ Describe pain transmission and management.

This chapter presents the reaction of vascularized living tissue to sports trauma, including the inflammatory response and the healing process. It provides a foundation for therapeutically managing the sports injury (Figure 7-1).

THE INFLAMMATORY RESPONSE

Inflammatory response can be acute or chronic (Figure 7-2). Acute inflammation has a short onset and a short duration. It consists of hemodynamic changes, production of an exudate, and the presence of granular leukocytes.[12] Chronic inflammation has a long onset and a long duration. It displays a presence of nongranular leukocytes and a more extensive formation of scar tissue.

The Roman physician Celsus in the first century AD described the local reactions to an injury, which are now known as the cardinal signs of inflammation. They are *rubor* (redness), *tumor* (swelling), *color* (heat), and *dolor* (pain). Galen, a Greek physician in the second century AD, added a fifth cardinal sign, *functio laesa* (loss of function).

Acute inflammation in general is divided into two categories: vascular events and cellular events.

SOFT-TISSUE INJURIES

Soft tissue refers to all tissues other than bone.

Acute Inflammation

Acute musculoskeletal injuries sustained in sports generally fall into three phases: the acute, reactive, or substrate inflammatory phase; the repair and regeneration phase; and the remodeling phase.

Phase I: Acute Phase

Acute phase:
Redness
Heat
Swelling
Pain
Loss of function

The acute phase of inflammation is the initial reaction of body tissue to an irritant or injury and is characteristic of the first 3 or 4 days after injury. Acute inflammation is the fundamental reaction designed to protect, localize, and rid the body of some injurious agent in preparation for healing and repair. The main causes of inflammation are trauma, chemical agents, thermal extremes, and pathogenic organisms.[13] The tissue irritants leading to the inflammatory process impose a number of vascular, cellular, and chemical responses.[11]

An external or internal injury is associated with tissue death. In an acute phase, tissue death occurs from the actual trauma. After trauma, cellular death may continue as a result of a lack of oxygen in the area. Continued death also occurs when

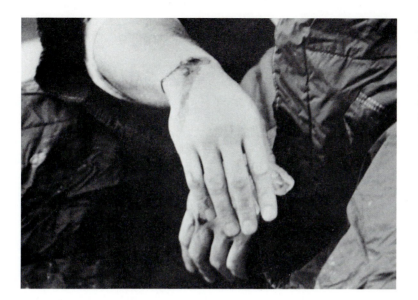

Figure 7-1

Tissue healing and the causation of pain are not clearly understood. However, what is not known must be studied as a foundation for proper injury management.

the digestive enzymes of engulfing phagocytes spill over and kill normal cells. This fact points to the major importance of proper immediate care using rest, ice, compression, and elevation (RICE).

Vascular response

First hour   At the time of trauma, before the usual signs of inflammation appear, a transitory **vasoconstriction** occurs, causing decreased blood flow. At the moment of vasoconstriction, coagulation begins to seal broken blood vessels, followed by the activation of chemical influences. Vasoconstriction is replaced by the dilation of venules, arterioles, and capillaries in the immediate area of the injury.

Second hour   **Vasodilation** brings with it a slowing of blood flow, increased blood viscosity, and stasis, which leads to swelling (edema). With dilation also comes exudation of plasma and concentration of red blood cells (hemoconcentration). Much of the plasma **exudate** results from fluid seepage through the intact vessel lining, which becomes more **permeable,** and from higher pressure within the vessel. Permeability is relatively transient in mild injuries, lasting only a few minutes, with restoration to a preinjury state in 15 to 30 minutes. In slightly more severe situations there may be a delayed response with a late onset of permeability. In such cases, permeability may not appear for many hours and then appears with some additional irritation and a display of rapid swelling lasting for an extended period.

A redistribution of leukocytes occurs within the intact vessels, caused in part by a slowing of circulation. These leukocytes move from the center of the blood flow to become concentrated and then line up and adhere to the endothelial walls. This process is known as *margination,* or *pavementing,* and occurs mainly in venules. The leukocytes pass through the wall of the blood vessel by ameboid action, known as *diapedesis,* and are directed to the injury site by chemotaxis (a chemical attraction to the injury). It should be noted that ameboid motion is a slow process, taking about 6 hours.[17] With an injury there is also an increase in lymph flow because of a high interstitial tissue pressure.

Cellular response

In phase I of acute inflammation, **mast cells** and **leukocytes** are in abundance. Mast cells are connective tissue cells that contain heparin (a blood anticoagulant) and histamine. Basophils, monocytes, and neutrophils are the major leukocytes. Basophil leukocytes are believed to bring anticoagulant substances to tissues that are inflamed and are present during both acute and chronic inflammatory healing phases. The neutrophils representing about 60% to 70% of the leukocytes arrive at the injury site before the larger monocytes. They immigrate from the blood-

Cellular death continues after initial injury because of the following:
   Lack of oxygen caused by disruption of circulation
   Digestive enzymes of the engulfing phagocytes spill over to kill normal cells

vasoconstriction
Decrease in the diameter of a blood vessel.

vasodilation
Increase in the diameter of a blood vessel.

exudate
fluid with a high protein content and containing cellular debris that comes from blood vessels and accumulates in the area of the injury.

permeable
Permitting the passage of a substance through a vessel wall.

mast cells
Connective tissue cells that contain heparin and histamine.

Figure 7-2

Severe pain can be the outcome of serious sports injuries.

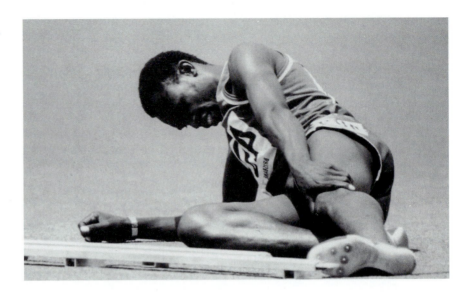

leukocytes

Consist of two types—granulocytes (e.g., basophils and neutrophils) and agranulocytes (e.g., monocytes and lymphocytes).

phagocytosis

Process of ingesting microorganisms, other cells, or foreign particles, commonly performed by monocytes (white blood cells).

Chemical mediators:
   Histamine
   Serotonin
   Bradykinin
   Prostaglandins
   Leukotrienes

7-1

Critical Thinking Exercise

A wrestler receives a sudden twist to his right shoulder causing a grade 2 strain to the teres minor muscle.

? What hemodynamic changes occur in the first hour of this acute injury?

Complement system:
   Leukocyte chemotaxis
   Phagocytosis

stream. Neutrophils emigrate from the bloodstream through diapedesis and **phagocytosis** to ingest smaller debris than do monocytes. Phagocytosis is the process of ingesting material such as bacteria, dead cells, and other debris associated with disease, infection, or injury. Opsonin is a protein substance in the blood serum that coats microorganisms and other cells, making them more amenable to phagocytosis. The phagocyte commonly accomplishes this process by projecting cytoplasmic pseudopods, which engulf the object and ingest the particle through enzymes. When the neutrophil disintegrates, it gives off enzymes called lysozomes, which digest engulfed material. These enzymes act as irritants and continue the inflammatory process. Neutrophils also have *chemotactic* properties, attracting other leukocytes to the injured area (Figure 7-3). The monocyte, which is a nongranular leukocyte, arrives on the scene after the neutrophils, about 5 hours after injury. Monocytes transform themselves into large macrophages that have the ability to ingest large particles of bacteria or cellular debris.

Chemical mediators   Chemical mediators for the inflammatory process are stored and given off by various cells. *Histamine,* the first chemical to appear in inflammation, is given off by blood platelets, basophil leukocytes, and mast cells. It is a major producer of arterial dilation, venule, and capillary permeability. *Serotonin* is a powerful vasoconstrictor found in platelets and mast cells. With an increase in blood there is an increase in local metabolism. Permeability is produced by the contraction of the endothelial cells of the capillary wall, producing a gap between cells. Gaps allow plasma to leak plasma proteins, platelets, and leukocytes. Plasma proteases, with their ability to produce polypeptides, act as chemical mediators. A major plasma protease in inflammation is *bradykinin,* which increases permeability and causes pain.[19]

Heparin is also given off by mast cells and basophils and temporarily prevents blood coagulation. In addition, in the early stages of acute injury, *prostaglandins* and *leukotrienes* are produced. Both of these substances stem from arachidonic acid; however, prostaglandins are produced in almost all body tissues. They are stored in the cell membranes' phospholipids. Leukotrienes alter capillary permeability and, it is believed, play a significant role, along with prostaglandins, in all aspects of the inflammatory process. Prostaglandins apparently encourage, as well as inhibit, inflammation, depending on the conditions that are prevalent at the time.[11] Table 7-1 summarizes the chemical responses to the various kinds of inflammation.

Complement system   The complement system is a series of enzymatic proteins in normal serum that, in the presence of a specific sensitizer, destroys bacteria and other cells. Fourteen components combine with the antigen-antibody complex to effect cell lysis. Once activated, the components are involved in a great number of immune

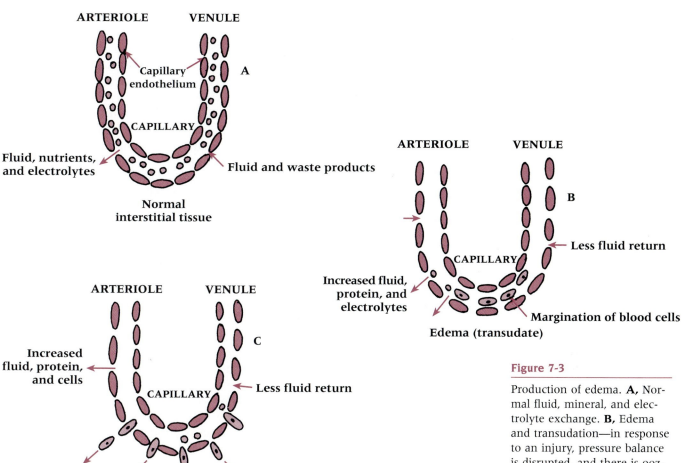

Figure 7-3

Production of edema. **A,** Normal fluid, mineral, and electrolyte exchange. **B,** Edema and transudation—in response to an injury, pressure balance is disrupted, and there is oozing of fluids, proteins, and electrolytes through the blood vessel walls. **C,** Edema and exudate—as inflammation continues, neutrophils and other blood cells emigrate into the surrounding tissue to form an exudate.

Blood coagulation: Thromboplastin + Calcium = Prothrombin = Thrombin = Fibrinogen = Insoluble fibrin clot

defense mechanisms, including anaphylaxis, leukocyte chemotaxis, and phagocytosis.

Bleeding and exudate   The extent of fluid in the injured area is highly dependent on the extent of damaged vessels and the permeability of the intact vessel. Blood coagulates in three stages. In the initial stage *thromboplastin* is formed. In the second stage *prothrombin* is converted into *thrombin* under the influence of thromboplastin with calcium. In the third stage thrombin changes from soluble *fibrinogen* into insoluble *fibrin*. The plasma exudate then coagulates into a network of fibrin and localizes the injured area.

TABLE 7-1   Inflammation and Chemical Response

Inflammation Response	Mediators
Vasoconstriction	Serotonin from platelets and most cells
Vasodilation	Histamine from platelets, basophils, and most cells
	Protoglandin from arachidonic acid
	Leukotrienes from arachidonic acid
	Bradykinin from body fluids
Margination and pavementing	Loss of microcirculation and increase in blood viscosity
Emigration of leukocytes	Leukocytes pass through capillary walls (diapedesis)
Chemotaxis	Leukocytes attract other leukocytes
Phagocytosis	Leukocytes, debris, complement, opsonization

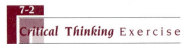

7-2

Critical Thinking Exercise

An athlete sustained a grade 2 lateral ankle sprain 3 weeks ago. It was given proper immediate and follow-up care.

? What repair has taken place during this time?

Phase II: Repair Phase

The term *repair* is synonymous with healing, whereas *regeneration* refers to the restoration of destroyed or lost tissue. Healing, which extends from the inflammatory phase (48 to 72 hours to approximately 6 weeks), occurs when the area has become clean through the removal of cellular debris, erythrocytes, and the fibrin clot. Tissue repair is accomplished through three processes: by resolution, in which there is little tissue damage and normal restoration; by the formation of granulation tissue, occurring if resolution is delayed; and by regeneration, the replacement of tissue by the same tissue.[9] The formation of scar tissue after trauma is a common occurrence; however, because scar tissue is less viable than normal tissue, the less scarring the better. When mature, scar tissue represents tissue that is firm, fibrous, inelastic, and devoid of capillary circulation. The type of scar tissue known as adhesion can complicate the recovery of joint or organ disabilities. Healing by scar tissue begins with an exudate, a fluid with a large content of protein and cellular debris that collects in the area of the injury site. From the exudate, a highly vascular mass develops known as granulation tissue. Infiltrating this mass is a proliferation of immature connective tissue (fibroblasts) and endothelial cells. Gradually the collagen protein substance, stemming from fibroblasts, forms a dense, fibrous scar. Collagenous fibers have the capacity to contract approximately 3 to 14 weeks after an injury and even as long as 6 months afterward in more severe cases.[4]

During this stage, two types of healing occur. *Primary healing,* healing by first intention, takes place in an injury that has even and closely opposed edges, such as a cut or incision. With this type of injury, if the edges are held in very close approximation, a minimum of granulation tissue is produced. *Secondary healing,* healing by secondary intention, results when there is a gaping lesion and large tissue loss leading to replacement by scar tissue. External wounds such as lacerations and internal musculoskeletal injuries commonly heal by secondary intention.[16]

Regeneration   The ability to regenerate is associated with nutrition, general health of the individual, and, most important, the type of tissue that has been injured. Repair and regeneration depend on three major factors: elimination of debris, the regeneration of endothelial cells, and the production of fibroblasts, which compose connective tissue throughout the body and form the basis of scar tissue.

Typically in a traumatic event injured blood vessels become deprived of oxygen and die. Before repair and regeneration can occur, debris must be removed by phagocytosis. Stimulated by a lack of oxygen (hypoxia) and the action of macrophages, capillary buds begin to form in the walls of the intact vessels (Figure 7-4). From these buds grow immature vessels that form connections with other vessels. As these vessels become mature, more oxygenated blood is brought to the injured area. From the perivascular cells come the fibroblasts (immature fibrocytes) that migrate to the injury and form collagen substances, often within a few days of the injury. The development of collagen is stimulated by lactic acid and vitamin C as well as the proper amount of oxygen.

Phase III: Remodeling Phase

Remodeling of the traumatized area overlaps that of repair and regeneration. Normally in acute injuries the first 3 to 6 weeks are characterized by increased production of scar tissue and increased strength of its fibers. Strength of scar tissue continues to increase from 3 months to 2 years after injury. Ligamentous tissue takes as long as 1 year to become completely remodeled. To avoid a rigid, nonyielding scar, there must be a physiological balance between **synthesis** and **lysis.** There is simultaneous synthesis of collagen by fibrablasts and lysis by collagenase enzymes.[17] The tensile strength of collagen apparently is specific to the mechanical forces imposed during the remodeling phase. Forces applied to the ligament during rehabilitative exercise will develop strength specifically in the direction that force is applied. If too early or excessive strain is placed on the injury, the healing process is extended. For

synthesis
The process of forming or building up.

lysis
A process of breaking down.

Remodeling depends on the amount and type of scar tissue present.

Macrophage   Polymorphonuclear   Mast   Fibrocyte
              leukocytes   cell   (fibroblast)

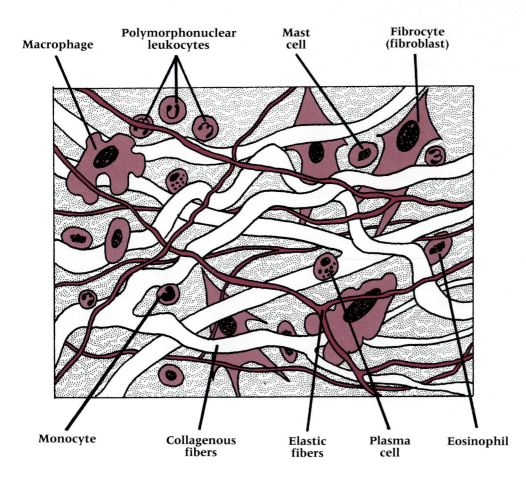

Monocyte   Collagenous   Elastic   Plasma   Eosinophil
            fibers   fibers   cell

Figure 7-4

Stimulated by hypoxia and the action of macrophages, capillary buds begin to form in the walls of the intact vessels.

proper healing of muscles and tendons, there must be careful consideration of when to mobilize the site. Early mobilization can assist in producing a more viable injury site; on the other hand, too long a period of immobilization can delay healing. The ideal of collagen remodeling is to have the healed area contain a preponderance of mature collagenous fibers that have a number of cross-linkages. As stated, collagen content and quality may be deficient for months after injury.[15]

Chronic Inflammation

The chronic muscle and joint problem is an ever-present, self-perpetuating concern in sports. If an acute inflammation reaction fails to be resolved in 1 month, it is termed a subacute inflammation. If it lasts for months or even years, the condition is termed chronic. Chronic inflammation results from repeated acute microtraumas and overuse. Prominent features that are distinct from acute inflammation are proliferation of connective tissue and tissue degeneration. The primary cells during chronic inflammation are lymphocytes, plasma cells, and macrophages (monocytes), in contrast to neutrophil leukocytes in acute inflammation. It has been suggested that lymphocytes, although not normally phagocytic, may be used to stimulate fibroblasts to heal and to form scar tissue. The role of plasma cells is not clearly understood, however. Macrophages, present in both acute and chronic inflammation, are definitely phagocytic and actively engaged in repair and healing.

Major chemicals found during chronic inflammation are the kinins (especially bradykinin), which also cause vasodilation, increased permeability, and pain. Prostaglandin, also seen in chronic conditions, causes vasodilation. Prostaglandin can be inhibited by aspirin.

Chronic inflammation can stem from repeated acute microtraumas and overuse.

7-3

Critical Thinking Exercise

A lacrosse player complains of a swollen ankle that never became completely resolved since a sprain was sustained 9 months ago.

? What is the reason for this chronic swelling?

Healing of Soft-Tissue Types

Cartilage Healing

Articular cartilage has limited capacity to heal. Cartilage in general has little if any direct blood supply. When chondrocytes are destroyed and the matrix is disrupted, healing is variable. Failing to clot and with no perichondrum, articular cartilage heals and repairs slowly. On the other hand, if the subchondral bone having a greater blood supply is affected, granulation tissue is formed and the healing process proceeds normally.

Ligament Healing

Ligament healing follows the same course of healing as other vascular tissue. If proper immediate and follow-up management is done, a sprained ligament will undergo the acute, repair, and remodeling phases in approximately the same time period as other vascular tissues.

During the repair phase collagen or connective tissue fibers are arranged in a random woven pattern with little organization. Gradually a scar is formed. In the next months the scar matures along with a realignment of collagen fibers in reaction to joint stress and strains. Full ligament healing with scar maturation may take as long as 12 months.

Skeletal Muscle Healing

Skeletal muscles are unable to undergo the mitotic activity required to replace cells that have been injured. In other words, regeneration of new myofibers is minimal. Skeletal muscle healing and repair follow the same process as other soft tissue. Collagen fibers mature and become oriented along lines of tensile strength according to Wolff's law.[15]

Nerve Healing

Because of the special nature of nerve cells, once they die regeneration cannot take place. If a nerve fiber is involved rather than the cell, regeneration can take place. The closer the injury is to the cell, the more difficult regeneration becomes.

For nerve regeneration to occur an optimal environment must be present. If peripheral nerve regeneration occurs it is at a rate of only 3 to 4 mm per day. Injured nerves within the central nervous system regenerate poorly when compared with peripheral nerves.

Modifying Soft-Tissue Healing

The healing process is unique in each athlete. In addition, different tissues vary in their ability to regenerate. For example, cartilage regenerates to some degree from the perichondrium, striated muscle is limited in its regeneration, and peripheral nerve fibers can regenerate only if their damaged ends are opposed. Usually connective tissue will readily regenerate, but, as with all tissue, this possibility is dependent on the availability of nutrients.

Age and general nutrition can play a role in healing. The older athlete may be delayed in healing when compared with younger athletes. The injuries of an athlete with a poor nutritional status may heal more slowly than normal. Athletes with certain organic disorders may heal slowly. For example, blood conditions such as anemia and diabetes often inhibit the healing process.

Management Concepts

Methods to modify soft-tissue healing include
   Drugs to treat inflammation
   Superficial thermal agents
   Physical modalities
   Exercise and rehabilitation

Many of the current treatment approaches are designed to enhance the healing process. They generally come under the headings of drugs to combat inflammation, thermal agents, physical modalities, mobilization, and exercise rehabilitation.

Drugs to treat inflammation   There is a current trend toward the use of antiprostaglandin medications, or nonsteroidal antiinflammatory drugs (NSAIDs). The intent of this practice is to decrease vasodilation and capillary permeability.

Physical modalities   Both cold and heat are used for different conditions. In general, heat stimulates acute inflammation and cold acts as a depressant. Conversely, in chronic conditions, heat may serve as a depressant.

A number of electrical procedures are increasing in popularity for the treatment of inflammation stemming from sports injuries. They come under the headings of penetrating heat devices such as microwave and ultrasound therapy and electrical stimulation, including transcutaneous electrical nerve stimulation (TENS) and electrical muscle stimulation (EMS).

Exercise rehabilitation   A major aim of soft-tissue rehabilitation through exercise is pain-free movement, full-strength power, and full extensibility of associated muscles. The ligamentous tissue, if related to the injury, should become pain free, have full tensile strength, and full range of motion. The dynamic joint stabilizers should regain full strength and power.

Immobilization of a part after injury or surgery is not always good for all injuries. When a part is immobilized over an extended period of time, adverse biochemical changes occur in collagenous tissue. Early mobilization used in exercise rehabilitation that is highly controlled may enhance the healing process. (See Chapter 15.)

FRACTURE HEALING

Those concerned with sports must fully realize the potential seriousness of a bone fracture. Coaches often become impatient for the athlete with a fracture to return to competition and sometimes become unjust in their criticism of the physician for being conservative. Time is required for proper bone union to take place.

The osteoblast is the cellular component of bone and forms its matrix; the osteocyte both forms and destroys bone, and osteoclasts destroy and resorb bone. The constant ongoing remodeling of bone is caused by osteocytes; osteoclasts are related mainly to pathological responses (Figure 7-5). Osteoclasts come from the cambium layer of the periosteum, which is the fibrous covering of the bone, and are involved in bone healing. The inner cambium layer, in contrast to the highly vascular and dense external layer, is more cellular and less vascular. It serves as a foundation for blood vessels and provides a place for attaching muscles, tendons, and ligaments.

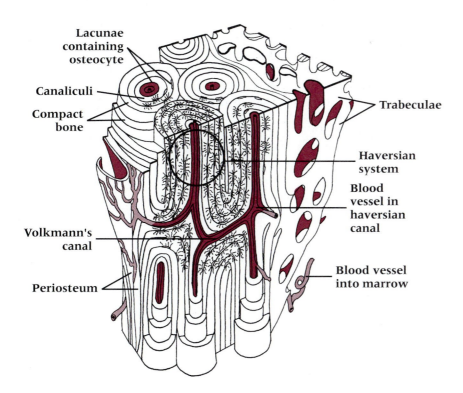

Figure 7-5

Bone is a complex organ in both growth and healing.

Skeletal fractures are discussed under the general headings of acute fractures and stress fractures of the bone.[8]

Acute Fractures of the Bone

Acute fracture healing follows similar phases as soft tissue but is more complex. In general there are five stages; hematoma formation, cellular proliferation, callus formation, ossification, and remodeling.[8]

Hematoma Formation

Acute inflammation usually lasts approximately 4 days. When a bone fractures, there is trauma to the periosteum and surrounding soft tissue. With hemorrhaging, a hematoma accumulates in the medullary canal and surrounding soft tissue in the first 48 to 72 hours. The exposed ends of vascular channels become occluded with clotted blood accompanied by dying of the osteocytes, disrupting the intact blood supply. The dead bone and related soft tissue begin to elicit a typical inflammatory reaction, including vasodilation, plasma exudate, and inflammatory cells.

Cellular Formation

As with a soft-tissue injury, the hematoma begins its organization in granulation tissue and gradually builds a fibrous junction between the fractured ends. At this time the environment is acid, but it will slowly change to neutral or slightly alkaline. A major influx of capillary buds that carry endosteal cells from the bone's cambium layer occurs. These cells first produce a fibrous callus, then cartilage, and finally a woven bone. When there is an environment of high oxygen tension, fibrous tissue predominates, whereas when oxygen tension is low, cartilage develops. Bone will develop at the fracture site when oxygen tension and compression are in the proper amounts.

Callus Formation

The soft callus, in general, is an unorganized network of woven bone formed at the ends of the broken bone that is later absorbed and replaced by bone. At the soft-callus stage, both internal and external calluses are produced that bring an influx of osteoblasts that begin to immobilize the fracture site. The internal and external calluses are formed by bone fragments that grow to bridge the fracture gap. The internal callus grows rapidly to create a rigid immobilization. Beginning in 3 to 4 weeks, and lasting 3 or 4 months, the hard callus forms. Hard callus is depicted by a gradual connecting of bone filament to the woven bone at the fractured ends. If there is less than satisfactory immobilization, a cartilagenous rather than bony union is produced.

Ossification

With adequate immobilization and compression, the bone ends become crossed with a new Haversian system that will eventually lead to the laying down of primary bone. The ossification stage is the completion of laying down bone. The fracture has been bridged and firmly united. Excess callus has been resorbed by osteoclasts.

Remodeling

Remodeling occurs after the callus has been resorbed and trabecular bone is laid down along the lines of stress. Complete remodeling may take many years. The influence of bioelectrical stimulation (piezoelectric effect) is the basis for development of new trabecular bone to be laid down at the point of greatest stress. This influence is predicated on the fact that bone is electropositive on its convex side and electronegative on its concave side. The convex is considered the tension side, whereas the concave is the compression side. Significantly, osteoclasts are drawn to a positive electrical charge and osteoblasts to a negative electrical charge. Remodeling is considered com-

---

acute fracture healing

Phase I: acute phase
  Trauma
  Hemorrhage
  Bone death
Phase II: repair and regeneration phase
  Granulation
  Woven bone
  Soft callus
  Hard callus
Phase III: remodeling phase
  Callus resorbed
  Trabecular bone
  Bone

7-4

Critical Thinking Exercise

A field hockey player falls and sustains an acute fracture of the left humerus.

? What are the healing events typical of this acute bone fracture?

plete when a fractured bone has been restored to its former shape or has developed a shape that can withstand imposed stresses.

Management of Acute Fractures

In the treatment of acute fractures the bones commonly must be immobilized completely until x-ray studies reveal that the hard callus has been formed. It is up to the physician to know the various types of fractures and the best form of immobilization for each specific fracture. During healing, fractures can keep an athlete out of participation in his or her particular sport for several weeks or months, depending on the nature, extent, and site of the fracture. During this period, certain conditions can seriously interfere with the healing process:

- If there is a *poor blood supply to the fractured area* and one of the parts of the broken bone is not properly supplied by the blood, that part will die and union or healing of the fracture will not take place. This condition is known as aseptic necrosis and often occurs in the head of the femur, the navicular bone in the wrist, the talus in the ankle, and isolated bone fragments. The condition is relatively rare among vital, healthy, young athletes except in the navicular bone of the wrist.

- *Poor immobilization of the fracture site,* resulting from poor casting by the physician and permitting motion between the bone parts, may not only prevent proper union but may also, in the event that union does transpire, cause deformity to develop.

- *Infection* can materially interfere with the normal healing process, particularly in the case of a compound fracture, which offers an ideal situation for development of a severe streptococcal or staphylococcal infection. The increased use of modern antibiotics has considerably reduced the prevalence of these infections coincidental with or immediately after a fracture. The closed fracture is not immune to contamination because infections within the body or poor blood supply can render it susceptible. If the fracture site should become and remain infected, the infection could interfere with the proper union of the bone. The interposition of soft parts between the severed ends of the bone—such as muscle, connective tissue, or other soft tissue immediately adjacent to the fracture—can prevent proper bone union, often necessitating surgical cleansing of the area of such tissues by a surgeon.

Conditions that interfere with fracture healing:
Poor blood supply
Poor immobilization
Infection

Healing of Stress Fractures

As discussed in Chapter 6, stress fractures may be created by cyclic forces that adversely load a bone at a susceptible site. Fractures may be the result of axial compression or tension created by the pull of muscles. As indicated, stress on ligamentous and bony tissue can be positive and can increase relative strength or can be negative and lead to tissue weakness. As discussed previously, bone produces an electrical potential in response to the stress of tension and compression. As a bone bends, tension is created on its convex side along with a positive electrical charge; conversely, on the concave or compressional side, a negative electrical charge is created. Torsional forces produce tension circumferentially. Constant tension caused by axial compression or stress by muscular activity can result in an increase in bone resorption and subsequently a microfracture. In other words, if the osteoclastic activity is greater than the osteoblastic activity the bone becomes increasingly susceptible to stress fractures.[10]

As with the healing of acute fractures, healing of stress fractures involves restoring a balance of osteoclastic and osteoblastic activity. Achieving this balance requires recognition of the situation as early as possible. Stress fractures that go unhealed will eventually develop into complete cortical fractures that may, over a period of time, become displaced. A decrease in activity and elimination of other factors in training that cause stress will allow bone remodeling and the ability to withstand stress.[10]

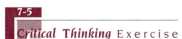

7-5

Critical Thinking Exercise

A female cross-country runner sustains a stress fracture of her left tibia. Her left leg is ¾ inch shorter than the right leg.

? What is a possible cause of this injury?

PAIN

Pain is one of the major indicators of the presence of injury. Many complex factors are inherent in pain, including anatomical structures; physiological reactions; and psychological, social, cultural, and cognitive factors.[2] The experience of pain is an individual experience and is subjective.[6]

Nociception

Pain receptors, known as *nociceptors,* or free nerve endings, are sensitive to extreme mechanical, thermal, and chemical energy.[5] They are commonly found in meninges, periosteum, skin, teeth, and some organs.

A nociceptive neuron transmits pain information to the spinal cord via the unmyelinated C fibers and the myelinated A-delta fibers. The smaller C fibers carry impulses at a rate of 0.5 to 2.0 m per second and the larger A-delta fibers at a rate of 5 to 30 m per second. When a nociceptor is stimulated there is release of a neuropeptide (substance P) that initiates an electrical impulse along the afferent fiber toward the spinal cord.[5] The faster A-delta afferent fiber impulse moves up the spinal cord at a moderately rapid speed to the thalamus, which gives a precise location of the acute pain, which is perceived as being bright, sharp, or stabbing.[2] In contrast the slower-conducting smaller unmyelinated C fibers are concerned with pain that is diffused, dull, aching, and unpleasant.[2,6] It also terminates in the thalamus, with projections to the limbic cortex that provide an emotional aspect to this pain. Nociceptive stimuli are at or close to an intensity that produces tissue damage.[2]

Endogenous Analgesics

The nervous system is powered electrochemically. Chemicals released by a presynaptic cell cross a synapse, stimulating or inhibiting a postsynaptic cell. This is called a neurotransmitter. Two types of chemical neurotransmitters that mediate pain are the endorphins and serotonin. They are generated by noxious stimuli, which activate inhibition of pain transmission.[6]

Stimulation of the periaqueductal gray area (PGA) of the midbrain and the raphe nucleus in the pons and medulla causes analgesia. Analgesia is produced by the stimulation of opioids, morphine-like substances manufactured in the PGA and many other areas of the central nervous system. These endogenous opioid peptides are known as endorphins and enkephalins.

Noradrenergic neurons stimulating norepinephrine can also inhibit pain transmission. Serotonin has also been identified as a neuromodulator.[2]

Pain Categories

Pain can be described according to a number of different categories, such as pain sources, fast versus slow pain, acute versus chronic, and projected (referred) pain.[2]

Pain Sources

Pain sources are cutaneous, deep somatic, visceral, and psychogenic. Cutaneous pain is usually sharp, bright, and "burning" and can have a fast or slow onset. Deep somatic pain stems from structures such as tendons, muscles, joints, periosteum, and blood vessels. Visceral pain originates from internal organs. Visceral pain is diffused at first and later may be localized, as in appendicitis. In psychogenic pain the individual feels pain, but the cause is emotional rather than physical.

Fast versus Slow Pain

As discussed earlier, fast pain is localized and carried through A-delta axons located in the skin. Slow pain, in contrast, is perceived as aching, throbbing, or burning. It is conducted through the C fibers.

7-6

Critical Thinking Exercise

A butterfly swimmer has been experiencing low back pain for over 6 months. The pain is described as aching and throbbing.

? What type of pain is this athlete experiencing?

Acute versus Chronic Pain

Acute pain is pain that is less than 6 months in duration. Tissue damage occurs and serves as a warning to the athlete. Chronic pain, on the other hand, has a duration longer than 6 months. The International Association for the Study of Pain describes chronic pain as that which continues beyond the usual normal healing time.[2,7]

Projected (Referred) Pain

One major category of pain that professionals in the field of sports medicine and athletic training commonly encounter is projected, or referred, pain. Such pain occurs away from the actual site of irritation. This pain has been called an error in perception. Each projected pain site must also be considered unique to each individual. Symptoms and signs vary according to the nerve fibers affected. Response may be motor, sensory, or both. The larger myelinated fibers (A-alpha) are the most sensitive to pressure (e.g., in a nerve root) and can produce paresthesia. Three types of referred pain that may be common to athletes are myofascial, sclerotomic, and dermatomic pain.

Myofascial pain   Acute and chronic musculoskeletal pain can be caused by myofascial trigger points. A **trigger point** is a specific sensitive area that has been referred to soft tissue. Such pain sites have variously been described as fibrositis, myositis, myalgia, myofascitis, and muscular strain. Trigger points are small hyperirritable areas within a muscle in which nerve impulses bombard the central nervous system and are expressed as a referred pain.

trigger points
Small hyperirritable areas within a muscle.

There are two types of trigger points—active and latent. The active trigger point is hyperirritable and causes an obvious complaint. The latent trigger point, on the other hand, is dormant, producing no complaint except perhaps a loss of range of motion. The trigger point does not follow a usual area of distribution such as sclerotomes, dermatomes, or peripheral nerves. The trigger point pain area is called the *reference zone,* which could be close to the point or a considerable distance from the point.

Sclerotomic and dermatomic pain   Deep pain, which can be either slow or fast, may originate from sclerotomic, myotomic, or dermatomic nerve irritation or injury. A sclerotome is an area of bone or fascia that is supplied by a single nerve root. Myotomes are muscles supplied by a single nerve root. Dermatomes also are in an area of skin supplied by a single nerve root.

Sclerotomic pain is often transmitted by the unmyelinated (C) fibers. Irritation of these fibers can cause deep, aching, and poorly localized pain. Sclerotomic pain impulses can be projected to regions in the brain such as the hypothalamus, limbic system, and reticular formation and cause depression, anxiety, fear, or anger. Autonomic changes may also occur, producing changes in vasomotor tone, blood pressure, and sweating.

Irritation of the A-delta fiber can produce dermatomic pain. This pain, in contrast to sclerotomic pain, is sharp and well localized. Unlike sclerotomic pain, dermatomic pain projects mainly to the thalamus and is relayed directly to the cortex, skipping autonomic and affective responses.

Variations in Pain Sensitivity

There are numerous variations in sensitivity to the pain stimuli. Hyperexcitability of sensory nerve fibers can cause *hyperesthesia.* Unpleasant sensations from severe nerve irritation produces *paresthesia. Analgesia* is the absence of pain.

Pain modulation   Because pain is a mixture of both physiological and psychological factors, management can be a major challenge for the athletic trainer. In most cases pain in the athletic training setting is acute.[18]

Pain assessment   Assessing pain can be a difficult task for the athletic trainer. The Agency for Health Care Policy and Research (AHCPR) indicates that the patient's self-report is the best reflection of pain and discomfort.[1]

Methods for pain assessment include the numerical value scale, the visual analog scale, and verbal descriptor scales. The numeric value scale is most commonly used in sports medicine. The athlete is asked to rate his or her pain on a scale of 1 to 10 with 1 representing the least pain and 10 representing the worst possible pain. The visual analog scale uses a line 10 cm in length. One end is labeled no pain and the other end is labeled severe pain. The athlete then marks along the line to indicate the pain's severity.[5] This same approach can be used to determine the effectiveness of treatment. In other words, one end of the line indicates no pain relief and the other complete pain relief.

Verbal descriptor scales use words such as none, slight, mild, moderate, and severe.

Pain treatment   The athletic trainer is primarily concerned with acute pain. A number of approaches are used separately or in combination. Common to musculoskeletal injuries is the cyclic condition of *pain-spasm-hypoxia-pain*. Disrupting this cycle can occur through a variety of means such as heat or cold, electrical stimulation–induced analgesia, or selected pharmacological approaches.

Heat and cold   Heat and cold are commonly used to address pain in sports medicine. Heat increases blood circulation through blood vessel dilation, reduces nociception and ischemia caused by muscle spasm, and may release endogenous opioids.[2]

In acute injury cold is applied to cause vasoconstriction and prevent extravasation of blood into the tissues. Pain is relieved by reducing swelling and muscle spasm.

Induced analgesia   In sports therapy there are a number of electrical devices that are designed to reduce pain. They are discussed in some detail in Chapter 14. Two that will be discussed here are TENS using the gate theory and acupuncture.

The gate theory and TENS   The gate theory, as developed by Melzack and Wall,[14] sets forth the idea that the spinal cord is organized in such a way that pain or other sensations may be experienced. An area located in the dorsal horn causes inhibition of the pain impulses ascending to the cortex for perception. The area, or gate, within the dorsal horn is composed of T cells and the *substantia gelatinosa.* T cells apparently are neurons that organize stimulus input and transmit the stimulus to the brain. The substantia gelatinosa functions as a gate-control system. It determines the stimulus input sent to the T cells from peripheral nerves. If the stimulus from a noxious material exceeds a certain threshold, pain is experienced (Figure 7-6). Apparently the smaller and slower nerve fibers carry pain impulses, and larger and faster nerve fibers carry other sensations. Impulses from the faster fibers arriving at the gate first inhibit pain impulses. In other words, stimulation of large, rapidly conducting fibers can selectively close the gate against the smaller pain fiber input. This concept explains why acupuncture, acupressure, cold, heat, and chemical skin irritation can provide some relief against pain. It also provides a rationale for the current success of TENS.

Acupuncture   Acupuncture dates back thousands of years to ancient China. Acupuncture has been found to cause analgesia when needles are applied to specific points on the body.

Acupuncture points lie along a series of meridians that run throughout the body. These points are named according to the meridian on which they lie. Whenever there is pain or illness, certain points on the surface of the body become tender. When pain is eliminated or the disease is cured, these tender points apparently disappear. According to acupuncture theory, stimulation of specific points through needling can dramatically reduce pain in areas of the body known to be associated with a particular point. Thousands of acupuncture points have been identified by the Chinese.

Acupressure is the application of digital pressure over acupuncture points. Using acupuncture charts, specific points are selected, which are described in the literature as having some relationship to the area of pain. The charts provide the athletic trainer with a general idea of where these points are located. Two techniques may be used to specifically locate acupressure points. Because it is known that electrical imped-

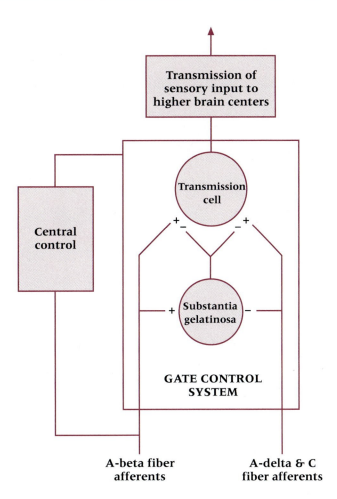

Figure 7-6

Scheme of the pain-modulating system in the dorsal horn of the spinal cord.

ance is reduced at acupuncture points, an ohmmeter may be used to locate the points. Perhaps the easiest technique is simply to palpate the area until either a small fibrous nodule or a strip of tense muscle tissue that is tender to the touch is felt.

Once the point is located, massage is begun using the index or middle fingers, the thumb, or the elbow. Small, circular motions are used on the point. The amount of pressure applied to the acupressure points should be determined by patient tolerance; however, it must be intense and will likely be painful to the patient. Generally, the more pressure the patient can tolerate, the more effective the treatment.

Effective treatment times range from 1 to 5 minutes at a single point per treatment. It may be necessary to massage several points during the treatment to obtain the greatest effect. If this is the case, it is best to work distal points first and to move proximally. During the massage, the patient will report a dulling or numbing effect and will frequently indicate that the pain has diminished or has subsided totally during the massage. The lingering effects of acupressure massage vary tremendously from patient to patient. The effects may last for only a few minutes in some but may persist in others for several hours.

Pharmacological agents The athlete may be prescribed oral or injectable medications for pain. The most common of these medications are analgesics and antiinflammatory agents.[3]

Psychological Aspect of Pain

Pain, especially chronic pain, is a subjective, psychological phenomenon. When painful injuries are treated, the total athlete must be considered, not just the pain or condition. Even in the most well-adjusted person, pain will create emotional changes.

Figure 7-7

Coping with pain in sports is as much psychological as it is physical.

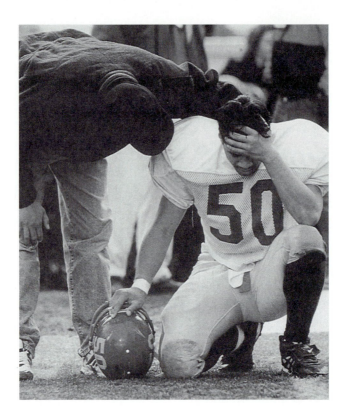

Constant pain will often cause self-centeredness and an increased sense of dependency.

Athletes, like nonathletes, vary in their pain thresholds (Figure 7-7). Some can tolerate enormous pain, whereas others find mild pain almost unbearable. Pain apparently is worse at night because persons are alone, more aware of themselves, and devoid of external diversions. Personality differences can also cause differences in pain toleration. For example, athletes who are anxious, dependent, and immature have less tolerance for pain than those who are relaxed and emotionally in control.

A number of theories about how pain is produced and perceived by the brain have been advanced. Only in the last few decades has science demonstrated that pain is both a psychological and physiological phenomenon and is therefore unique to each individual. Sports activities demonstrate this fact clearly. Through conditioning, an athlete learns to endure the pain of rigorous activity and to block the sensations of a minor injury.

SUMMARY

- Inflammation can be acute or chronic based on vascular and cellular events and biochemical mediators.
- Acute soft-tissue healing consists of the acute, repair and regeneration, and remodeling phases. The acute phase lasts 3 to 4 days. During initial trauma transitory vasoconstriction occurs, followed by vasodilation and increased permeability. Through the process of chemotaxis, leukocytes, by means of diapedesis, are attracted to the injured area. Throughout the acute phase major cellular and chemical events are occurring. A complement system that consists of enzymatic proteins is also involved. An integral part of the acute phase is blood coagulation, which occurs in three stages.
- The second phase of soft-tissue healing, repair and regeneration, extends from the inflammatory phase of 48 to 72 hours to approximately 6 weeks. It consists of resolution, development of granulation tissue, and finally regeneration of lost tissue, depending on the extent of the injury. The two types of healing are gen-

erally known as primary, or first intention, and secondary, or second intention. Secondary healing develops more granulation tissue and subsequently has a greater possibility of producing more scar tissue. Remodeling is the final phase of the healing process of soft tissue. Remodeling refers to a balance of tissue synthesis and lysis. To maximize this phase concern must be given to determining the extent of immobilization and mobilization of the injured part.

■ Inflammation that lasts for a long period of time is chronic, lasting for months or even years. It may occur as a result of acute microtrauma and overuse. The typical cells that are involved are lymphocytes, plasma cells, and monocytes. Scar tissue and degeneration are associated with chronic inflammation. A number of factors such as nutrition and blood supply can modify the healing process. Antiinflammatory drugs, thermal agents, physical modalities, and proper exercise procedures can positively alter the healing process.

■ Fractures can be acute or stress related. Healing of an acute fracture follows many of the phases of acute soft-tissue healing, with the exception of replacing osteocytes. Proper management, including immobilization when called for, is essential for bone healing and remodeling.

■ Pain is both a psychological and physiological phenomenon. Pain perception is subjective and may be described as fast or slow. Acute pain is designed to protect the body, whereas chronic pain serves no useful purpose. Chronic pain is believed to be caused by a noxious stimulus that affects the high-threshold nociceptors in various tissue. Pain is managed by interrupting some aspect of the pain-spasm-ischemia-hypoxia-pain cycle. Interruption can be accomplished by certain drugs and therapeutic approaches such as TENS.

Solutions to Critical Thinking EXERCISES

7-1 Initially, a transitory vasoconstriction with the start of blood coagulation of the broken blood vessels occurs. Dilation of the vessels in the region of injury follow, along with activation of chemical mediators via key cells.

7-2 A grade II lateral ankle sprain implies that the joint capsule and ligaments are partially torn. At 3 weeks the injury has been cleaned of debris and is undergoing the process of secondary healing. Granulation tissue fills the torn areas, and fibroblasts are beginning to form scar tissue.

7-3 The athlete's injury in its acute phase was not allowed to heal properly. As a result, the injury became chronic with a proliferation of scar tissue, lymphocytes, plasma cells, and macrophages.

7-4 Uncomplicated acute bone healing goes through five stages: hematoma formation, cellular proliferation, callus formation, ossification, and remodeling.

7-5 Because it is shorter, the left leg has the greater stress during running. This creates an increase of tension on the tibia's concave side, causing an increase in osteoclastic activity.

7-6 The pain is considered to be chronic, deep somatic pain stemming from the low back muscles. It is conducted primarily by the C-type nerve fibers.

REVIEW QUESTIONS AND CLASS ACTIVITIES

1. Identify the outward signs of inflammation.
2. Describe the vascular, cellular, chemical, and complement system events that occur during acute soft-tissue healing.
3. How does soft tissue repair and regenerate itself after an acute injury?
4. What are the major implications of soft-tissue remodeling after injury?
5. Differentiate between acute and chronic inflammatory processes.
6. What are the reasons for using drugs, thermal agents, physical modalities, and exercise rehabilitation during the healing process?
7. Differentiate between acute soft-tissue healing and acute bone-fracture healing.
8. How does a stress fracture heal?
9. How does pain occur? Why is it generally described as pain perception?
10. What is projected, or referred, pain?
11. What are the major management concepts used in treating pain?

REFERENCES

1. Acute Pain Management Guideline Panel: *Acute pain management: operative or medical procedures and trauma,* AHCPR Pub. No. 92-0032, Rockville, Md, 1992, Agency for Health Care Policy and Research, Public Health Service, US Department of Health and Human Services.
2. Curtis SM, Curtis RL: Somatosensory function and pain. In Porth CM, editor: *Pathophysiology,* ed 4, Philadelphia, 1994, Lippincott.
3. Clark WG: *Goth's medical pharmacology,* ed 13, St Louis, 1992, Mosby.
4. Daly TJ: The repair phase of wound healing—reepithelialization and contraction. In Kloth LC, McCulloch JM, Feedar JH, editors: *Wound healing: alternatives in management,* Philadelphia, 1990, Davis.

5. Donley PB, Denegar CR: Managing pain with therapeutic modalities. In Prentice WE, editor: *Therapeutic modalities in sports medicine*, ed 3, St Louis, 1994, Mosby.

6. Fine PG: The biology of pain. In Heil J, editor: *Psychology of sport injury*, Champaign, Ill, 1993, Human Kinetics.

7. Grichnick K, Ferrante FM: The difference between acute and chronic pain, *Mt Sinai J Med* 58:217-220, 1991.

8. Gunta KE: Alterations in skeletal function: trauma and infection. In Porth CM, editor: *Pathophysiology*, ed 4, Philadelphia, 1994, Lippincott.

9. Hettinga DL: Inflammatory response of synovial joint structures. In Gould JA III, editor *Orthopaedic and sports physical therapy*, St Louis, 1990, Mosby.

10. Hershman EB, Mailly T: Stress fractures. In Watson JT, Bergfeld JA, editors: *Fractures, clinics in sports medicine*, vol 9, no 1, Philadelphia, 1990, Saunders.

11. Kloth CL, Miller KH: The inflammatory response. In Kloth LE, McCulloch JM, Feedar JA, editors: *Wound healing: alternatives in management*, Philadelphia, 1990, Davis.

12. Larocco M: Inflammation and immunity. In Porth CM, editor: *Pathophysiology*, ed 4, Philadelphia, 1994, Lippincott.

13. Madri JA: Inflammation and healing. In Kissane JM, editor: *Anderson's pathology*, vol 1, ed 9, St Louis, 1990, Mosby.

14. Melzack R, Wall PD: Pain mechanisms: a new theory, *Science* 150:971, 1965.

15. Prentice NE: The healing process and the pathophysiology of musculoskeletal injuries. In Prentice WE, editor: *Rehabilitation technique in sports medicine*, ed 2, St Louis, 1994, Mosby.

16. Price H: Connective tissue in wound healing. In Kloth LE, McCulloch, JM, Feedar JA, editors: *Wound healing: alternatives in management*, Philadelphia, 1990, Davis.

17. Porth CM: Cellular adaptation/injury and wound healing/repair. In Porth CM, editor: *Pathophysiology*, ed 4, Philadelphia, 1994, Lippincott.

18. Santiesleban AJ: Physical agents and musculoskeletal pain. In Gould JA III, editor: *Orthopaedic and sports physical therapy*, ed 2, St Louis, 1990, Mosby.

19. Thibodeau GA, Patton KT: *Anatomy and physiology*, ed 2, St Louis, 1993, Mosby.

ANNOTATED BIBLIOGRAPHY

Kissane JM, editor: *Anderson's pathology*, vol 1, ed 9, St Louis, 1990, Mosby.

A major text in pathology discussing inflammation and healing in depth.

Kloth LE, McCulloch JM, Feedar JA: *Wound healing: alternative in management*, Philadelphia, 1990, Davis.

An excellent discussion of factors influencing wound healing, evaluation, and methods of treatment.

Porth CM: *Pathophysiology*, ed 4, Philadelphia, 1994, Lippincott.

An in-depth text on the physiology of altered health with an excellent discussion on inflammation, healing, and pain.

Management Skills

Emergency Procedures

When you finish this chapter, you should be able to

- Establish a plan for handling an emergency situation at your institution.
- Explain the importance of knowing cardiopulmonary resuscitation and how to manage an obstructed airway.
- Describe the types of hemorrhage and their management.
- Assess the types of shock and their management.
- Describe the emergency management of musculoskeletal injuries.
- Describe techniques for moving and transporting the injured athlete.

Most sports injuries do not result in life-or-death emergency situations, but when such situations do arise, prompt care is essential. An emergency is defined as "an unforeseen combination of circumstances and the resulting state that calls for immediate action."[12] Time becomes the critical factor, and assistance to the injured individual must be based on knowledge of what to do and how to do it—how to perform effective aid immediately. There is no room for uncertainty, indecision, or error. A mistake in the initial management of injury can prolong the length of time required for rehabilitation and can potentially create a life-threatening situation for the athlete.

THE EMERGENCY PLAN

The prime concern of emergency aid is to maintain cardiovascular function, and indirectly central nervous system function, because failure of either of these systems may lead to death. The key to emergency aid in the sports setting is the initial evaluation of the injured athlete. Time is of the essence, so this evaluation must be done rapidly and accurately so that proper aid can be rendered without delay. In some instances these first steps not only will be lifesaving but also may determine the degree and extent of permanent disability. Injury assessment is discussed in detail in Chapter 10.

As discussed in Chapter 1, the athletic training team—the coach, the athletic trainer, and the team physician—must at all times act reasonably and prudently. This behavior is especially important during emergencies.

All sports programs must have a prearranged emergency plan that can be implemented immediately when necessary. The following issues must be addressed when developing the emergency system:

1. Phones should be readily accessible. Cellular phones are best because the athletic trainer can carry them at all times. If cellular phones are not available, the location of the telephone should be well known by student athletic trainers, coaches, and athletes and clearly marked. (Use 911 if available.)
2. Someone should be specifically assigned to make an emergency phone call. The emergency medical system can be accessed by dialing 911. This number gets you a dispatcher who has access to rescue squad, police, and fire. The person making the emergency phone call must provide the following information:
   a. Type of emergency situation
   b. Type of suspected injury
   c. Present condition of the athlete
   d. Current assistance being given (e.g., cardiopulmonary resuscitation)
   e. Location of telephone being used
   f. Exact location of emergency (give names of streets and cross streets) and how to enter facility

Time becomes critical in an emergency situation.

All sports programs must have an emergency plan.

3. Keys to gates or padlocks must be easily accessible. Both the coach and the athletic trainer should have the appropriate key.
4. There should be separate emergency plans for each sport's fields, courts, or gymnasiums.
5. All coaches, athletic trainers, athletic directors, school nurses, and maintenance personnel should be apprised of the emergency plan at a meeting held annually before the beginning of the school year. Each individual must know his or her responsibilities should an emergency occur.
6. Someone should be assigned to accompany the injured athlete to the hospital.

It is essential that individuals providing emergency care to the injured athlete cooperate and act professionally. Too often, the rescue squad personnel, the physician, and the athletic trainer disagree over exactly how the injured athlete should be handled and transported. The athletic trainer is usually the first individual to deal with the emergency situation. The athletic trainer has generally had more training and experience in moving and transporting an injured athlete than the physician. If the rescue squad is called and responds, the emergency medical technicians (EMTs) should have the final say on how that athlete is to be transported while the athletic trainers assume an assistive role.

To alleviate potential conflicts, the athletic trainer should establish procedures and guidelines and arrange practice sessions at least once a year with all parties concerned for handling the injured athlete. The rescue squad may not be experienced in dealing with someone who is wearing a helmet or other protective equipment. The athletic trainer should make sure before an incident occurs that the EMTs understand how athletes wearing various types of athletic equipment should be managed. When dealing with the injured athlete, all egos should be put aside. The most important consideration is what is the best for the athlete.

Parent Notification

If the injured athlete is a minor, the athletic trainer should try to obtain consent from the parent to treat the athlete during an emergency. Consent may be given in writing either before or during an emergency. This is notification that the parent has been informed about what the athletic trainer thinks is wrong and what the athletic trainer intends to do, and parental permission is granted to give treatment for a specific incident. If the athlete's parents cannot be contacted, the predetermined wishes of the parent given at the beginning of a season or school year can be enacted. If there is no informed consent, implied consent on the part of the athlete to save the athlete's life takes precedence.

PRINCIPLES OF ASSESSMENT

The athletic trainer cannot deliver appropriate medical care to the injured athlete until some systematic assessment of the situation has been made. This assessment (Figure 8-1) helps determine the nature of the injury and provides direction in the decision-making process concerning the emergency care that must be rendered. The primary survey refers to assessment of potentially life-threatening problems, including airway, breathing, and circulation (ABCs), severe bleeding, and shock. It takes precedence over all other aspects of victim assessment and should be used to correct life-threatening situations.[7] Once the condition of the victim is stabilized, the secondary survey takes a closer look at the injury sustained by the athlete. The secondary survey gathers specific information about the injury from the athlete, systematically assesses vital signs and symptoms, and allows for a more detailed evaluation of the injury. The secondary survey is done to uncover problems that do not pose an immediate threat to life but that may do so if they remain uncorrected.[7]

An injured athlete who is conscious and stable will not require a primary survey. However, the unconscious athlete must be monitored for life-threatening problems throughout the assessment process.

Figure 8-1

Flowchart showing the appropriate emergency procedures for the injured athlete.

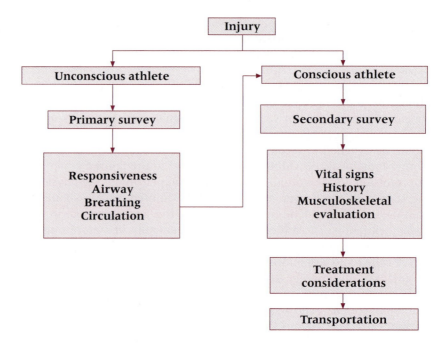

The Unconscious Athlete

The state of unconsciousness provides one of the greatest dilemmas in sports. Whether it is advisable to move the athlete and allow the game to resume or to await the arrival of a physician is a question that too often is resolved hastily and without much forethought. Unconsciousness may be defined as a state of insensibility in which there is a lack of conscious awareness. This condition can be brought about by a blow to either the head or the solar plexus, or it may result from general shock. It is often difficult to determine the exact cause of unconsciousness (Table 8-1).

The unconscious athlete must always be considered to have a life-threatening injury, which requires an immediate primary survey. The following guidelines should be used when working with the unconscious athlete:

1. The athletic trainer should immediately note the body position, and determine the level of consciousness and unresponsiveness.
2. Airway, breathing, and circulation should be established immediately.
3. Injury to the neck and spine is always a possibility in the unconscious athlete.
4. If the athlete is wearing a helmet, it should never be removed until neck and spine injury have been unequivocally ruled out. However, the face mask must be cut away and removed to allow for cardiopulmonary resuscitation (CPR).
5. If the athlete is supine and not breathing, establish ABC immediately.
6. If the athlete is supine and breathing, do nothing until consciousness returns.
7. If the athlete is prone and not breathing, logroll him or her carefully to the supine position and establish ABC immediately.
8. If the athlete is prone and breathing, do nothing until consciousness returns, then carefully logroll him or her onto a spine board because CPR could be necessary at any time.
9. Monitor and maintain life support for the unconscious athlete until emergency medical personnel arrive.
10. Once the athlete is stabilized the athletic trainer should begin a secondary survey.

TABLE 8-1　Evaluating the Unconscious Athlete

Functional Signs	Fainting	Concussion	Grand Mal Epilepsy	Brain Compression and Injury	Heat stroke	Diabetic Coma	Shock
Onset	Usually sudden	Usually sudden	Sudden	Usually gradual	Gradual or sudden	Gradual	Gradual
Mental	Complete unconsciousness	Confusion or unconsciousness	Unconsciousness	Unconsciousness gradually deepening	Delirium or unconsciousness	Drowsiness, later unconsciousness	Listlessness, later unconsciousness
Pulse	Feeble and fast	Feeble and irregular	Fast	Gradually slower	Fast and feeble	Fast and feeble	Fast and feeble
Respiration	Quick and shallow	Shallow and irregular	Noisy, later deep and slow	Slow and noisy	Difficult	Deep and sighing	Rapid and shallow, with occasional deep sigh
Skin	Pale, cold, and clammy	Pale and cold	Livid, later pale	Hot and flushed	Hot and relatively dry	Livid, later pale	Pale, cold, and clammy
Pupils	Equal and dilated	Equal	Equal and dilated	Unequal	Equal	Equal	Equal and dilated
Paralysis	None	None	None	May be present in leg, arm, or both	None	None	None
Convulsions	None	None	None	Present in some cases	Present in some cases	None	None
Breath	N/A	N/A	N/A	N/A	N/A	Acetone smell	N/A
Special features	Giddiness and sway before collapse	Signs of head injury, vomiting during recovery	Bites tongue, voids urine and feces, may injure self while falling	Signs of head injury, delayed onset of symptoms	Vomiting in some cases	In early stages, headache, restlessness, and nausea	May vomit; early stages shivering, thirst, defective vision, and ear noises

PRIMARY SURVEY
Treatment of Life-Threatening Injuries

Life-threatening injuries take precedence over all other injuries sustained by the athlete. Situations that are considered life-threatening include those that require cardiopulmonary resuscitation (i.e., obstruction of the airway, no breathing, no circulation), profuse bleeding, and shock.

Overview of Emergency Cardiopulmonary Resuscitation

It is essential that a careful evaluation of the injured person be made to determine whether CPR should be conducted. The following is an overview of adult CPR and is not intended to be used by persons who are not certified in CPR. It should also be noted that, because of the serious nature of CPR, updates should routinely be studied through the American Red Cross, the American Heart Association, or the National Safety Council.

First, establish unresponsiveness of the athlete by tapping or gently shaking his or her shoulder and shouting, "Are you okay?" Note that shaking should be avoided if there is a possible neck injury. If the athlete is unresponsive, the Emergency Medical System (EMS) should be activated immediately by dialing 911. Carefully position the athlete in the supine position. If the athlete is in a position other than supine, he or she must be carefully rolled over as a unit, avoiding any twisting of the body, because CPR can be administered only with the athlete lying flat on the back with knees straight or slightly flexed (see Figure 8-6). In cases of suspected cervical spine injury care must be taken to minimize cervical movement during logrolling. Then proceed with CPR.[12]

Equipment Considerations

Protective equipment worn by an athlete may complicate lifesaving CPR procedures. There is a great deal of controversy among athletic trainers as to whether equipment should be removed or left in place. The presence of a football, ice hockey, or lacrosse helmet, with a face mask and various types of shoulder pads associated with each sport, will obviously make CPR more difficult if not impossible.

It has been proposed that removing the face mask should be the first step.[10] The face mask does not hinder the evaluation of the airway, but it may hinder treatment.[3] A number of techniques using various instruments have been recommended to remove the face mask, including electric screwdrivers, which work well as long as the screws are not rusted, and wire cutters, bolt cutters, trainer's scissors, and scalpels, none of which work very well. Recently, two devices, the Anvil Pruner and the Trainer's Angel, have been recommended as being effective in quickly cutting the plastic clips[8] (Figure 8-2). It has also been suggested that the athletic trainer must be proficient in removing the face mask within 30 seconds.[8]

In 1992 the Occupational Safety and Health Administration (OSHA) mandated the use of barrier devices to protect the athletic trainer from transmission of bloodborne pathogens during CPR. It is possible to slip the barrier mask under the face mask, attach the one-way mouthpiece or valve through the bars of the face mask, and begin CPR within 5 to 10 seconds without removing the face mask.[11]

Decisions to remove the helmet and shoulder pads before initiating CPR should be based on the potential of injury to the cervical spine. If it is reasonably certain that no injury has occurred to the cervical spine, both the helmet and shoulder pads can be quickly removed before initiating CPR. If injury to the cervical spine is a possibility, care must be taken to minimize movement of the head and neck while permitting CPR to be performed. Again, controversy exists as to whether the helmet and shoulder pads should be left in place or removed. The athletic trainer must either remove both the helmet and shoulder pads or leave them both in place. Removing one or the other independently will force the cervical spine into either flexion or extension. If they are left in place, the face mask should be dealt with as

8-1
Critical Thinking Exercise

A football defensive back is making a tackle and on contact drops his head to tackle the ball carrier. He hits the ground and does not move. When the athletic trainer gets to him, the athlete is lying prone, is unconscious, but is breathing.

? How should the athletic trainer manage this situation?

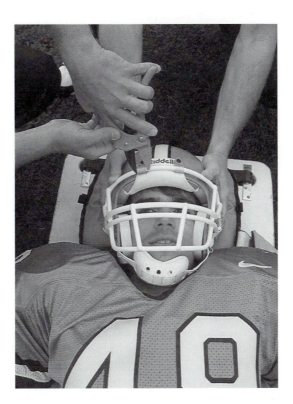

Figure 8-2

Various clipping devices such as the Anvil Pruner and the Athletic Trainer's Angel have been recommended as being effective in quickly cutting plastic clips.

recommended previously, and the jersey and shoulder pad strings or straps should be cut, spreading the shoulder pads apart so that the chest may be compressed according to CPR guidelines. Although removal of the helmet and shoulder pads has been recommended,[3] it seems that no matter how much care is taken, removal would create unnecessary movement of the cervical spine and would delay initiation of CPR, neither of which is best for the injured athlete.

It should also be added that if cervical neck injury is suspected, yet the athlete is conscious and breathing and does not require CPR, the athlete should be transported with the helmet, chin strap, and shoulder pads in place. The face mask should be removed in case CPR becomes necessary.

The ABCs of CPR

The ABCs of CPR are easily remembered and indicate the sequential steps used for basic life support:[1]

1. A—airway opened.
2. B—breathing restored.
3. C—circulation restored.

Frequently, when A is restored, B and C will resume spontaneously, and it is then unnecessary to perform them. In some instances, the restoration of A and B obviates the necessity for step C. When performing CPR on an adult victim, the following sequence should be followed.

Opening the Airway

Open the airway by using the head tilt–chin lift method. Lift chin with one hand while pushing down on victim's forehead with the other, avoiding the use of excessive force. The tongue is the most common cause of respiratory obstruction; the forward lift of the jaw raises the tongue away from the back of the throat, thus clearing the airway.

NOTE: On victims with suspected head or neck injuries, perform a modified jaw thrust maneuver by grasping each side of the lower jaw at the angles, thus displacing the lower mandible forward as the head is tilted backward. In executing this maneuver both elbows should rest on the same surface as that on which the victim is lying. Should the lips close, they can be opened by retracting the lower lip with a thumb. If there is no breathing, additional forward displacement of the jaw may help.

Establishing Breathing

1. To determine if the victim is breathing, maintain the open airway, place your ear over the victim's mouth, observe the chest, and look, listen, and feel for breath sounds.
2. With the hand that is on the athlete's forehead, pinch the nose shut, keeping the heel of the hand in place to hold the head back (if there is no neck injury) (Figure 8-3). Taking a deep breath, place your mouth over the athlete's mouth to provide an airtight seal and give two slow full breaths at a rate of 1½ to 2 seconds per inflation. Observe the chest rise and fall. Remove your mouth, and listen for the air to escape through passive exhalation. If the airway is obstructed, reposition the victim's head and try again to ventilate. If still obstructed, give up to five abdominal thrusts followed by a finger sweep with the index finger to clear objects from the mouth. Be careful not to push the object further into the throat. Continue to repeat this sequence until ventilation occurs. NOTE: OSHA has mandated the use of barrier shields by athletic trainers to minimize the risk of transmitting bloodborne pathogens (Figure 8-4). These shields have a plastic or silicone sheet that spreads over the face and separates the athletic trainer from the athlete. Some models have a tubelike mouthpiece, which may help in situations in which the athlete is wearing a face mask.

Establishing Circulation

1. To determine pulselessness, locate the Adam's apple with the index and middle fingers of the hand closest to the head. Then slide them down into the groove on the side of the body on which you are kneeling to locate the carotid artery. Palpate the carotid pulse with one hand (allow 5 to 10 seconds) while maintaining head tilt with the other.
2. Maintain open airway. Position yourself close to the side of the athlete's chest. With the middle and index fingers of the hand closest to the waist, locate the lower margin of the athlete's rib cage on the side next to you (Figure 8-5).

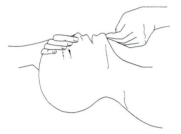

Figure 8-3

Head tilt–chin lift technique for establishing an airway.

Figure 8-4

A barrier mask protects the athletic trainer from potential exposure to bloodborne pathogens.

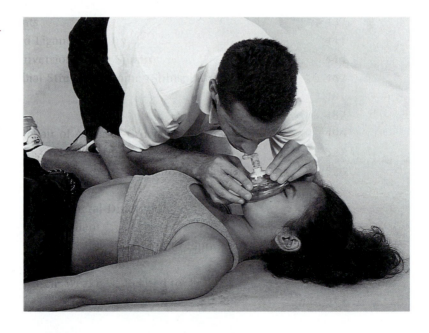

3. Run the fingers up along the rib cage to the xiphoid notch where the ribs meet the sternum.

4. Place the middle finger on the notch and the index finger next to it on the lower end of the sternum.

5. Next, the hand closest to the athlete's head is positioned on the lower half of the sternum next to the index finger of the first hand that located the notch; then the heel of that hand is placed on the long axis of the sternum.

6. The first hand is then removed from the notch and placed on top of the hand on the sternum so that the heels of both hands are parallel and the fingers are directed straight away from the coach or athletic trainer (Figure 8-6).

7. Fingers can be extended or interlaced, but they must be kept off of the chest wall.

8. Elbows are kept in a locked position with arms straight and shoulders positioned over the hands, enabling the thrust to be straight down.

9. In a normal-sized adult, enough force must be applied to depress the sternum 1½ to 2 inches (4 to 5 cm). After depression, there must be complete release of the sternum to allow the heart to refill. The time of release should equal the time of compression. For one rescuer compression must be given at the rate of 80 to 100 times per minute, maintaining a rate of 15 chest compressions to 2 full breaths.

10. After 4 cycles of 15 compressions and 2 breaths (15:2) or about 1 minute, recheck the pulse at the carotid artery (allow 5 seconds) while maintaining head tilt. If there is no pulse continue the 15:2 cycle beginning with chest compressions.

Every coach and athletic trainer should be certified in CPR and should take a refresher examination at least once a year. It is wise to have all training assistants certified as well.

Obstructed Airway Management

Choking on foreign objects claims close to 3000 lives every year. Choking is a possibility in many sports activities; for example, an athlete may choke on a mouth guard, a broken bit of dental work, chewing gum, or even a "chaw" of tobacco. When such emergencies arise, early recognition and prompt, knowledgeable action are necessary to avert a tragedy. An unconscious athlete can have an obstructed airway when the tongue falls back in the throat, thus blocking the upper airway. Blood clots resulting from head, facial, or dental injuries may impede normal breathing, as may vomiting. When complete airway obstruction occurs, the individual is unable to speak, cough, or breathe. If the athlete is conscious, there is a tremendous effort made to breathe, the head is forced back, and the face initially is flushed and then becomes cyanotic as oxygen deprivation occurs. If partial airway obstruction is causing the choking, some air passage can be detected, but during a complete obstruction no air movement is discernible.

To relieve airway obstruction caused by foreign bodies, two maneuvers are recommended: the Heimlich maneuver and finger sweeps of the mouth and throat.

Heimlich maneuver   As with CPR, the Heimlich maneuver (subdiaphragmatic abdominal thrusts) requires practice before proficiency is acquired. There are two methods of obstructed airway management, depending on whether the victim is in an erect position or has collapsed and is either unconscious or too heavy to lift. For the conscious victim the standing Heimlich maneuver is performed until he or she is relieved. In cases of unconsciousness, five abdominal thrusts are applied, followed by a finger sweep with an attempt at ventilation.

Method A   Stand behind and to one side of the athlete. Place both arms around the waist just above the belt line, and permit the athlete's head, arms, and upper trunk to hang forward (Figure 8-7, *A*). Grasp one of your fists with the other, placing the thumb side of the grasped fist immediately below the xiphoid process of the

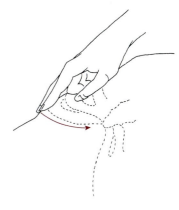

Figure 8-5

With the middle and index fingers of the hand closest to the waist, the lower margin of the victim's rib cage is located. The fingers are then run along the rib cage to the notch where the ribs meet the sternum. The middle finger is placed on the notch with the index finger next to it on the lower end of the sternum.

All coaches and athletic trainers must have current CPR certification.

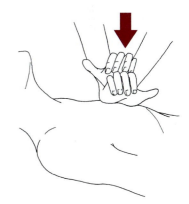

Figure 8-6

The heel of the headward hand is placed on the long axis of the lower half of the sternum next to the index finger of the first hand. The first hand is removed from the notch and placed on top of the hand on the sternum with fingers interlaced.

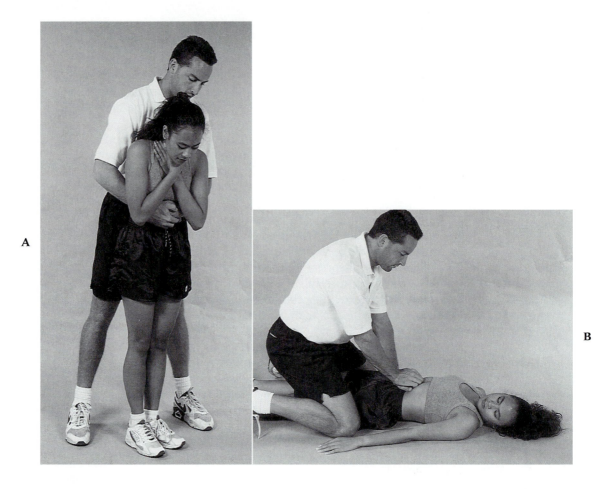

Figure 8-7

The Heimlich maneuver for an obstructed airway. **A,** Manual thrust maneuver for the conscious athlete. **B,** Manual thrust maneuver for the unconscious athlete.

sternum, clear of the rib cage. Now sharply and forcefully thrust the fists into the abdomen, inward and upward, several times. This "hug" pushes up on the diaphragm, compressing the air in the lungs, creating forceful pressure against the blockage, and thus usually causing the obstruction to be promptly expelled. Repeat the maneuver until the athlete is relieved or becomes unconscious. If the athlete loses consciousness, activate the EMS system, perform a finger sweep, open the airway, and try to ventilate. If the airway is still obstructed reposition the head and try again. Then give up to five abdominal thrusts. Repeat this sequence as long as necessary.

Method B   If the athlete is on the ground or on the floor, place him or her on the back and straddle the victim's hips, keeping your weight centered over your knees. Place the heel of your left hand against the back of your right hand and push sharply into the abdomen just above the umbilicus (note the position, Figure 8-7, *B*). Repeat this maneuver up to five times, and then repeat the finger sweep. Care must be taken in either of these methods to avoid extreme force or applying force over the rib cage because fractures of the ribs and damage to the organs can result.

Finger sweeping   If a foreign object such as a mouth guard is lodged in the mouth or the throat and is visible, it may be possible to remove or release it with the fingers. Care must be taken that the probing does not drive the object deeper into the throat. It is usually impossible to open the mouth of a conscious victim who is in distress, so the Heimlich maneuver technique should be used immediately. In the unconscious athlete, turn the head either to the side or face up, open the mouth by grasping the tongue and the lower jaw, hold them firmly between the thumb and fingers, and lift—an action that pulls the tongue away from the back of the throat and from the impediment. If this is difficult to do, the crossed finger method can usually be used effectively. The index finger of the free hand (or if both hands are

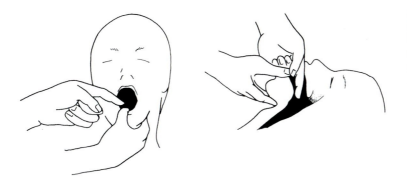

Figure 8-8

Finger sweeping of the mouth is essential in attempting to remove a foreign object from a choking victim.

used, an assistant can probe) should be inserted into one side of the mouth along the cheek deeply into the throat; using a hooking maneuver, attempt to free the impediment, moving it into a position from which it can be removed (Figure 8-8). Attempt to ventilate after each sweep until the airway is open. Once the object is removed, if the athlete is not already breathing, an attempt is made to ventilate him or her.

Control of Hemorrhage

An abnormal discharge of blood is called a hemorrhage. The hemorrhage may be venous, capillary, or arterial and may be external or internal. Venous blood is characteristically dark red with a continuous flow, capillary bleeding exudes from tissue and is a reddish color, and arterial bleeding flows in spurts and is bright red. NOTE: The athletic trainer must be concerned with exposure to bloodborne pathogens and other diseases when coming into contact with blood or other body fluids. It is essential to take universal precautions to minimize this risk. Disposable latex gloves should be used routinely whenever the athletic trainer comes into contact with blood or other body fluids. This topic is discussed in detail in Chapter 9.

External Bleeding

External bleeding stems from open skin wounds such as abrasions, incisions, lacerations, punctures, or avulsions. (See Chapter 26 for further discussion.) The control of external bleeding includes the use of direct pressure, elevation, and pressure points.

Direct pressure   Pressure is directly applied with the hand over a sterile gauze pad. The pressure is applied firmly against the resistance of a bone (Figure 8-9).

Elevation   Elevation, in combination with direct pressure, provides an additional means for the reduction of external hemorrhage. Elevating a hemorrhaging part against gravity reduces hydrostatic blood pressure and facilitates venous and lymphatic drainage, which slows bleeding.[15]

Pressure points   When direct pressure combined with elevation fails to slow hemorrhage, the use of pressure points may be the method of choice. Eleven points on each side of the body have been identified for controlling external bleeding; the two most commonly used are the brachial artery in the upper limb and the femoral artery in the lower limb. The brachial artery is compressed against the medial aspect of the humerus, and the femoral artery is compressed as it is detected within the femoral triangle (Figure 8-10).

Internal Hemorrhage

Internal hemorrhage is invisible to the eye unless manifested through some body opening or identified through x-ray studies or other diagnostic techniques. Its danger lies in the difficulty of diagnosis. When internal hemorrhaging occurs, either subcutaneously such as in a bruise or contusion, intramuscularly, or in joints, the athlete may be moved without danger in most instances. However, the detection of bleeding within a body cavity such as the skull, thorax, or abdomen is of the utmost

8-2

Critical Thinking Exercise

A soccer player jumps to win a head ball and an opponent's head smashes his right eyebrow, creating a significant laceration. The athlete is conscious but is bleeding profusely from the wound.

? What techniques may be most effectively used to control the bleeding, and what should be done to close the wound?

External bleeding can usually be managed by using direct pressure, elevation, or pressure points.

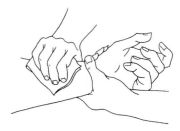

Figure 8-9

Direct pressure for the control of bleeding is applied with the hand over a sterile gauze pad.

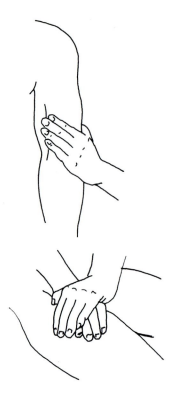

Figure 8-10

The two most common sites for direct pressure are the brachial artery and the femoral artery.

8-3

Critical Thinking E x e r c i s e

A wrestler is thrown to the mat and suffers an open fracture of both the radius and ulna in the forearm. There is significant bleeding from the wound. The athlete begins to complain of light-headedness, his skin is pale and feels cool and clammy, and his pulse becomes rapid and weak.

? What potential problem may be developing, and how should the athletic trainer manage this situation?

importance because it could mean the difference between life and death. Because the symptoms are obscure, internal hemorrhage is difficult to diagnose properly. It has been said that, as a result of this difficulty, athletes with internal injuries require hospitalization under complete and constant observation by a medical staff to determine the nature and extent of the injuries. All severe hemorrhaging will eventually result in shock and should therefore be treated on this premise. Even if there is no outward indication of shock, the athlete should be kept quiet and body heat should be maintained at a constant and suitable temperature. (See the following section on shock for the preferred body position.)

Shock

With any injury shock is a possibility. But when severe bleeding, fractures, or internal injuries are present, the development of shock is more likely. Shock occurs when there is a diminished amount of blood available to the circulatory system. As a result there are not enough oxygen-carrying blood cells available to the tissues, particularly those of the nervous system. This situation occurs when the vascular system loses its capacity to hold the fluid portion of the blood within its system because of dilation of the blood vessels within the body and disruption of the osmotic fluid balance. When this occurs, a quantity of plasma is lost from the blood vessels to the tissue spaces of the body, leaving the blood cells within the vessels, causing stagnation, and slowing the blood flow. With this general collapse of the vascular system there is widespread tissue death, which will eventually cause the death of the individual unless treatment is given.

Certain conditions, such as extreme fatigue, extreme exposure to heat or cold, extreme dehydration of fluids and mineral loss, or illness, predispose an athlete to shock. In a situation in which there is a potential shock condition, there are other signs by which the athletic trainer or coach should assess the possibility of the athlete's lapsing into a state of shock as an aftermath of the injury. The most important clue to potential shock is the recognition of a severe injury. It may happen that none of the usual signs of shock is present.

The main types of shock are hypovolemic, respiratory, neurogenic, psychogenic, cardiogenic, septic, anaphylactic, and metabolic.[15]

Hypovolemic shock stems from trauma in which there is blood loss. With decreased blood volume there will be a decrease in blood pressure. Without enough blood in the circulatory system organs are not properly supplied with oxygen.

Respiratory shock occurs when the lungs are unable to supply enough oxygen to the circulating blood. Trauma that produces a pneumothorax or injury to the breathing control mechanism can produce respiratory shock.

Neurogenic shock is caused by the general dilation of blood vessels within the cardiovascular system. When it occurs, the typical 6 L of blood can no longer fill the system. As a result the cardiovascular system can no longer supply oxygen to the body.

Psychogenic shock refers to what is commonly known as fainting (syncope). It is caused when there is temporary dilation of blood vessels, reducing the normal amount of blood in the brain.

Cardiogenic shock refers to the inability of the heart to pump enough blood to the body.

Septic shock occurs from a severe, usually bacterial, infection. Toxins liberated from the bacteria cause small blood vessels in the body to dilate.

Anaphylactic shock is the result of a severe allergic reaction caused by foods, insect stings, drugs, or inhaling dusts, pollens, or other substances.

Metabolic shock happens when a severe illness such as diabetes goes untreated. Another cause is an extreme loss of bodily fluid (e.g., through urination, vomiting, or diarrhea).

Symptoms and Signs

The major signs of shock are moist, pale, cool, clammy skin; the pulse becomes weak and rapid; the respiratory rate becomes increased and shallow; blood pressure decreases; and in severe situations there is urinary retention and fecal incontinence. If conscious, the athlete may display a disinterest in his or her surroundings or may display irritability, restlessness, or excitement. There may also be extreme thirst.[15]

Management

Depending on the causative factor for the shock, the following emergency care should be given:

1. Maintain body temperature as close to normal as possible.
2. Elevate the feet and legs 8 to 12 inches for most situations. However, shock positioning varies according to the type of injury.[15] For example, for a neck injury, the athlete should be immobilized as found; for a head injury, his or her head and shoulders should be elevated; and for a leg fracture, his or her legs should be kept level and should be raised after splinting.

Shock can also be compounded or initially produced by the psychological reaction of the athlete to an injury situation. Fear or the sudden realization that a serious situation has occurred can result in shock. In the case of a psychological reaction to an injury, the athlete should be instructed to lie down and avoid viewing the injury. The athlete should be handled with patience and gentleness, but firmness as well. Spectators should be kept away from the injured athlete. Reassurance is of vital concern to the injured individual. The person should be given immediate comfort through the loosening of clothing. Nothing should be given by mouth until a physician has determined that no surgical procedures are indicated.

Secondary Survey

Once the life-threatening injuries have been dealt with, the athletic trainer should conduct a secondary survey to assess the existing injury more precisely.

Recognizing Vital Signs

The ability to recognize physiological signs of injury is essential to the proper handling of potentially critical injuries. When evaluating the seriously ill or injured athlete, the coach, athletic trainer, or physician must be aware of nine response areas: heart rate, breathing rate, blood pressure, temperature, skin color, pupils of the eye, movement, the presence of pain, and unconsciousness.

Pulse

The pulse is the direct extension of the functioning heart. In emergency situations it is usually determined at the carotid artery at the neck or the radial artery in the wrist (Figure 8-11). A normal pulse rate per minute for adults ranges between 60 and 80

Signs of shock:
Blood pressure is low.
Systolic pressure is usually below 90 mm Hg.
Pulse is rapid and weak.
Athlete may be drowsy and appear sluggish.
Respiration is shallow and extremely rapid.
Skin is pale, cool, and clammy.

Vital signs to observe:
Pulse
Respiration
Blood pressure
Temperature
Skin color
Pupils
State of consciousness
Movement
Abnormal nerve response

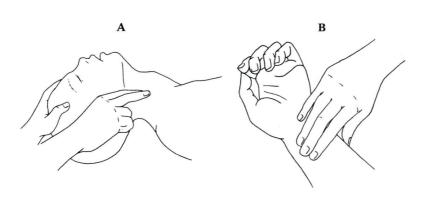

A   B

Figure 8-11

Pulse rate taken at the carotid artery, **A,** and radial artery, **B.**

beats and in children from 80 to 100 beats; however, it should be noted that trained athletes usually have slower pulses than the typical population.

An alteration of a pulse from the normal may indicate the presence of a pathological condition. For example, a rapid but weak pulse could mean shock, bleeding, diabetic coma, or heat exhaustion. A rapid and strong pulse may mean heatstroke or severe fright, a strong but slow pulse could indicate a skull fracture or stroke, and no pulse means cardiac arrest or death.[4]

Respiration

The normal breathing rate per minute is approximately 12 breaths in adults and 20 to 25 breaths in children. Breathing may be shallow (indicating shock), irregular, or gasping (indicating cardiac involvement). Frothy blood being coughed up indicates a chest injury, such as a fractured rib, that has affected a lung. Look, listen, and feel: look to ascertain whether the chest is rising or falling; listen for air passing in and out of the mouth, nose, or both; and feel where the chest is moving.

Blood Pressure

systolic blood pressure
The pressure caused by the heart's pumping.

diastolic blood pressure
The residual pressure when the heart is between beats.

Blood pressure, as measured by the sphygmomanometer, indicates the amount of pressure exerted against the arterial walls. It is indicated at two pressure levels: systolic and diastolic. **Systolic blood pressure** occurs when the left ventricle contracts pumping blood, and **diastolic blood pressure** is the residual pressure present in the arteries when the heart is between beats. The normal systolic pressure for 15- to 20-year-old males ranges from 115 to 120 mm Hg. The diastolic pressure usually ranges from 75 to 80 mm Hg. The normal blood pressure of females is usually 8 to 10 mm Hg lower than in males for both systolic and diastolic pressures. Between the ages of 15 and 20, a systolic pressure of 135 mm Hg and above may be excessive; 110 mm Hg and below may be considered too low. The outer ranges for diastolic pressure should not exceed 60 and 85 mm Hg, respectively. A lowered blood pressure could indicate hemorrhage, shock, heart attack, or internal organ injury.

Blood pressure is measured by applying the cuff circumferentially around the upper arm just proximal to the elbow (Figure 8-12). The cuff should be inflated to 200 mm Hg, which occludes blood flow in the brachial artery distal to the cuff in the cubital fossa. The cuff should be slowly deflated with the stethoscope in place; the first beating sound is recorded as systolic pressure. Continue deflating the cuff until the beating sound disappears; diastolic pressure is then recorded.

Temperature

To convert Fahrenheit to centigrade (Celsius): °C = (°F − 32) ÷ 1.8.
To convert centigrade to Fahrenheit: °F = (1.8 × °C) + 32.

Body temperature is maintained by water evaporation and heat radiation. It is normally 98.6° F (37° C). Temperature is measured with a thermometer, which is placed under the tongue, in the armpit, against the tympanic membrane in the ear, or in case of unconsciousness in the rectum. Core temperature is most accurately measured in the rectum or at the tympanic membrane in the ear (Figure 8-13). Changes in body temperature can be reflected in the skin. For example, hot, dry skin might indicate disease, infection, or overexposure to environmental heat. Cool, clammy skin could reflect trauma, shock, or heat exhaustion; cool, dry skin is possibly the result of overexposure to cold.

A rise or fall of internal temperature may be caused by a variety of circumstances such as the onset of a communicable disease, cold exposure, pain, fear, or nervousness. Characteristically, with lowered temperature there may be chills with chattering teeth, blue lips, goose bumps, and pale skin.

Skin Color

For individuals who are lightly pigmented, the skin can be a good indicator of the state of health. In this instance, three colors are commonly identified in medical emergencies: red, white, and blue. A red skin color may indicate heatstroke, high blood

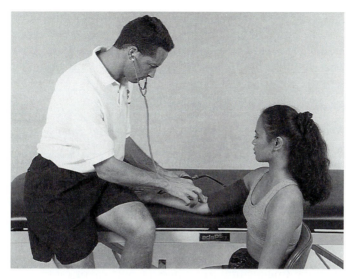

Figure 8-12

Blood pressure is measured using a sphygmomanometer and a stethoscope.

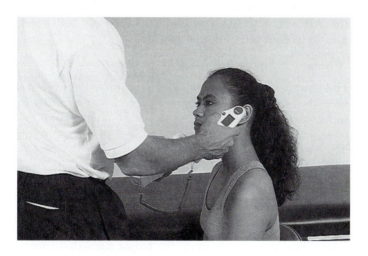

Figure 8-13

Thermometer for measuring tympanic membrane temperature.

pressure, or elevated temperature. A pale, ashen, or white skin can mean insufficient circulation, shock, fright, hemorrhage, heat exhaustion, or insulin shock. Skin that is bluish in color (cyanotic), primarily noted in lips and fingernails, usually means there is an airway obstruction or respiratory insufficiency.

Assessing skin color in a dark-skinned athlete is more difficult than in a light-skinned athlete. These individuals normally have pink coloration of the nail beds and inside the lips, mouth, and tongue. When a dark-skinned person goes into shock, the skin around the mouth and nose will often have a grayish cast, and the tongue, the inside of the mouth, the lips, and the nail beds will have a bluish cast. Shock resulting from hemorrhage will cause the tongue and inside of the mouth to become a pale, grayish color instead of blue. Fever in these athletes can be noted by a red flush at the tips of the ears.[4]

Pupils

The pupils are extremely sensitive to situations affecting the nervous system. Although most persons have pupils of regular outline and equal size, some individuals normally have pupils that may be irregular and unequal. This disparity requires the coach or athletic trainer to know which athletes deviate from the norm.

A constricted pupil may indicate that the athlete is using a central nervous system–depressant drug. If one or both pupils are dilated, the athlete may have sustained a head injury; may be experiencing shock, heatstroke, or hemorrhage; or may

Some athletes normally have irregular and unequal pupils.

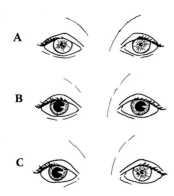

Figure 8-14

The pupils of the eyes are extremely sensitive to situations affecting the nervous system. **A,** Normal pupils. **B,** Dilated pupils. **C,** Irregular pupils.

have ingested a stimulant drug (Figure 8-14). The pupils' response to light should also be noted. If one or both pupils fail to accommodate to light, there may be brain injury or alcohol or drug poisoning. When examining an athlete's pupils, the examiner should note the presence of contact lenses. Pupil response is more critical in evaluation than pupil size.

State of Consciousness

When recognizing vital signs, the examiner must always note the athlete's state of consciousness. Normally the athlete is alert, is aware of the environment, and responds quickly to vocal stimulation. Head injury, heatstroke, and diabetic coma can alter the athlete's level of conscious awareness.

Movement

The inability to move a body part can indicate a serious central nervous system injury that has involved the motor system. An inability to move one side of the body (hemiplegia) could be caused by a head injury or cerebrovascular accident (stroke). Bilateral tingling and numbness or sensory or motor deficits of the upper extremity may indicate a cervical spine injury. Weakness or inability to move the lower extremities could mean an injury below the neck, and pressure on the spinal cord could lead to limited use of the limbs.[4,13]

Abnormal Nerve Response

The injured athlete's pain or other reactions to adverse stimuli can provide valuable clues to the coach or athletic trainer. Numbness or tingling in a limb with or without movement can indicate nerve or cold damage. Blocking of a main artery can produce severe pain, loss of sensation, or lack of a pulse in a limb. A complete lack of pain or of awareness of serious but obvious injury may be caused by shock, hysteria, drug usage, or a spinal cord injury. Generalized or localized pain in the injured region probably means there is no injury to the spinal cord.[2]

Musculoskeletal Assessment

A logical process must be used to evaluate accurately the extent of a musculoskeletal injury. One must be aware of the major signs that reveal the site, nature, and above all severity of the injury. Detection of these signs can be facilitated, as is true with all trauma, by understanding the mechanism or traumatic sequence and methodically inspecting the injury. Knowledge of the mechanism of an injury is extremely important in determining which area of the body is most affected. When the injury mechanism has been determined, the examiner proceeds to the next phase: physical inspection of the affected region. At this point information is gathered by what is seen, heard, and felt.

In an attempt to understand the mechanism of injury, a brief history of the complaint must be taken. The athlete is asked, if possible, about the events leading up to the injury and how it occurred. The athlete is further asked what was heard or felt when the injury took place. Sounds occurring at the time of injury or during manual inspection yield pertinent information about the type and extent of pathology present. Such uncommon sounds as grating or harsh rubbing may indicate fracture. Joint sounds may be detected when either arthritis or internal derangement is present. Areas of the body that have abnormal amounts of fluid may produce crepitus when palpated or moved. Such sounds as a snap, crack, or pop at the moment of injury often indicate bone fracture or injury to ligaments or tendon.

The athletic trainer makes a visual observation of the injured site, comparing it to the uninjured body part. The initial visual examination can disclose obvious deformity, swelling, and skin discoloration.

Finally, the region of the injury is gently palpated. Feeling, or palpating, a part with trained fingers can, in conjunction with visual and audible signs, indicate the nature of the injury. Palpation is started away from the injury and gradually moves toward it. As the examiner gently feels the injury and surrounding structures with the fingertips, several factors can be revealed: the extent of point tenderness, the extent of irritation (whether it is confined to soft tissue alone or extends to the bony tissue), and deformities that may not be detected by visual examination alone.

Assessment Decisions

After a quick on-site injury inspection and evaluation, the athletic trainer makes the following decisions:
1. The seriousness of the injury.
2. The type of first aid and immobilization necessary.
3. Whether the injury warrants immediate referral to a physician for further assessment.
4. The manner of transportation from the injury site to the sidelines, training room, or hospital.

All information about the initial history, signs, and symptoms of the injury must be documented, if possible, so that they may be described in detail to the physician.

Decisions that can be made from the secondary survey:
Seriousness of injury
Type of first aid required
Whether injury warrants physical referral
Type of transportation needed

Immediate Treatment

Musculoskeletal injuries are extremely common in sports. The athletic trainer must be prepared to provide appropriate first aid immediately to control hemorrhage and associated swelling. Every first aid effort should be directed toward one primary goal—reducing the amount of swelling resulting from the injury. There is little question that if swelling can be controlled initially, the amount of time required for injury rehabilitation will be significantly reduced. Initial management of musculoskeletal injuries should include rest, ice, compression, and elevation (RICE).

Rest, ice, compression, and elevation (RICE) are essential in the emergency care of musculoskeletal injuries.

Rest   Rest after any type of injury is an extremely important component of any treatment program. Once a body part is injured, it immediately begins the healing process. If the injured part is not rested and is subjected to external stresses and strains, the healing process never gets a chance to do what it is supposed to do. Consequently, the injured part does not heal, and the time required for rehabilitation is greatly increased. The number of days necessary for resting varies with the severity of the injury. Parts of the body that have experienced minor injury should rest for approximately 72 hours before a rehabilitation program is begun.

Ice (cold application)   The initial treatment of acute injuries should use cold.[5] Therefore ice is used for most conditions involving strains, sprains, and contusions.[14] It is most commonly used immediately after injury to decrease pain and promote local constriction of the vessels (vasoconstriction), thus controlling hemorrhage and edema. Cold applied to an acute injury will lower metabolism and the tissue demands for oxygen and reduce hypoxia.[6] This benefit extends to uninjured tissue, preventing injury-related tissue death from spreading to adjacent normal cellular structures. It is also used in the acute phase of inflammatory conditions such as bursitis, tenosynovitis, and tendinitis conditions in which heat may cause additional pain and swelling. Cold is also used to reduce the muscle guarding that accompanies pain. Its pain-reducing (analgesic) effect is probably one of its greatest benefits. One explanation of the analgesic effect is that cold slows the speed of nerve transmission, so the pain sensation is reduced. It is also possible that cold bombards pain receptors with so many cold impulses that pain impulses are lost. With ice treatments, the athlete usually reports an uncomfortable sensation of cold, followed by burning, then an aching sensation, and finally complete numbness.

Because the subcutaneous (under the skin) fat slowly conducts the cold temperature, applications of cold for short periods of time will be ineffective in cooling deeper tissues. For this reason, longer treatments of at least 20 minutes are recommended. It should be noted, however, that prolonged application of cold can cause tissue damage.[5]

It is generally believed that cold treatments are more effective in reaching deep tissues than most forms of heat. Cold applied to the skin is capable of significantly lowering the temperature of tissues at a considerable depth. The temperature to which the deeper tissues can be lowered depends on the type of cold that is applied to the skin, the duration of its application, the thickness of the subcutaneous fat, and the region of the body to which it is applied.[16] Ice packs should be applied to the area for at least 72 hours after an acute injury. With many injuries, regular ice treatments may be continued for several weeks.

For best results, ice packs (crushed ice and towel) should be applied over a compression wrap. Frozen gel packs should not be used directly against the skin, because they reach much lower temperatures than ice packs. A good rule of thumb is to apply a cold pack to a recent injury for a 20-minute period and repeat every 1 to 1½ hours throughout the waking day. Depending on the severity and site of the injury, cold may be applied intermittently for 1 to 72 hours. For example, a mild strain will probably require 1 day of 20-minute periods of cold application, whereas a severe knee or ankle sprain might need 3 to 7 days of intermittent cold. If in doubt about the severity of an injury, it is best to extend the time ice is applied.

Compression In most cases immediate compression of an acute injury is considered an important adjunct to cold and elevation and in some cases may be superior to them. Placing external pressure on an injury assists in decreasing hemorrhage and hematoma formation by mechanically reducing the space available for swelling to accumulate.[17] Fluid seepage into interstitial spaces is retarded by compression, and absorption is facilitated. However, application of compression to an anterior compartment syndrome or to certain injuries involving the head and neck is contraindicated.

Many types of compression are available. An elastic wrap that has been soaked in water and frozen in a refrigerator can provide both compression and cold when applied to a recent injury. Pads can be cut from felt or foam rubber to fit difficult-to-compress body areas. For example, a horseshoe-shaped pad placed around the malleolus in combination with an elastic wrap and tape provides an excellent way to prevent or reduce ankle edema (Figure 8-15). Although cold is applied intermittently, compression should be maintained throughout the day and if possible throughout the night. Because of the pressure buildup in the tissues, it may become painful to leave a compression wrap in place for a long time. However, there is no question that it is essential to leave the wrap in place even though there may be significant pain because it is so important in the control of swelling. The compression wrap should be left in place for at least 72 hours after an acute injury. In many chronic overuse problems, such as tendinitis, tenosynovitis, and particularly bursitis, the compression wrap should be worn until all swelling is almost entirely gone.

Elevation Along with cold and compression, elevation reduces internal bleeding. The injured part, particularly an extremity, should be elevated to eliminate the effects of gravity on blood pooling in the extremities. Elevation assists the veins, which drain blood and other fluids from the injured area, returning them to the central circulatory system. The greater the degree of elevation, the more effective the reduction in swelling. For example, in an ankle sprain the leg should be placed in a position so that the ankle is virtually straight up in the air. The injured part should be elevated as much as possible during the first 72 hours.

The appropriate technique for initial management of the acute musculoskeletal injuries, regardless of where they occur, is the following:

1. Apply a compression wrap directly over the injury. Wrapping should start distally and continue proximally. Tension should be firm and consistent. It may be helpful to wet the elastic wrap to facilitate the passage of cold from ice packs. A dry compression wrap should be left in place for at least 72 hours or until there is little chance of continued swelling.

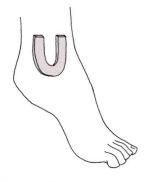

Figure 8-15

A horseshoe-shaped pad can be placed around the malleolus to reduce edema.

2. Surround the injured area entirely with ice packs or bags, and secure them in place. The ice should be left on for 20 minutes initially and then 1 hour off and 30 minutes on as much as possible over the next 24 hours. During the following 48-hour period, ice should again be applied as often as possible.

3. The injured part should be elevated for most of the initial 72-hour period after injury. It is particularly important to keep the injury elevated while sleeping. This also allows the damaged part to rest after the injury. The initial management of an injury is extremely important to reduce the length of time required for rehabilitation.

Emergency Splinting

Any suspected fracture should always be splinted before the athlete is moved. Transporting a person with a fracture without proper immobilization can result in increased tissue damage, hemorrhage, and shock. Conceivably, a mishandled fracture could cause death. Therefore a thorough knowledge of splinting techniques is important. The application of splints should be a simple process through the use of commercial emergency splints. In most instances the coach or athletic trainer does not have to improvise a splint because such devices are readily available in most sports settings.

Rapid form vacuum immobilizers   The rapid form vacuum immobilizer is a relatively new type of splint that is widely used by both EMTs and athletic trainers. It consists of styrofoam chips contained inside an air-tight cloth sleeve that is pliable. It can be molded to the shape of any joint or angulated fracture using Velcro straps. A handheld pump sucks the air out of the sleeve, giving it a cardboardlike rigidity. This splint is most useful for injuries that are angulated and must be splinted in the position in which they are found (Figure 8-16, *A*).

Air splints   An air splint is a clear plastic splint that is inflated with air around the affected part and can be used for extremity splinting, but its use requires some special training. This splint provides support and moderate pressure to the body part and affords a clear view of the site for x-ray examination. The inflatable splint should not be used if it will alter a fracture deformity (Figure 8-16, *B*).

Half-ring splint   For fractures of the femur the half-ring type of traction splint offers the best support and immobilization but takes considerable practice to master. An open fracture must be carefully dressed to avoid additional contamination.

Whatever the material used, the principles of good splinting remain the same. Two major concepts of splinting are to splint from one joint above the fracture to one joint below the fracture and to splint where the athlete lies. If at all possible, do not move the athlete until he or she has been splinted.

Splinting of lower-limb fractures   Fractures of the ankle or leg require immobilization of the foot and knee. Any fracture involving the knee, thigh, or hip needs splinting of all the lower-limb joints and one side of the trunk.

Splinting of upper-limb fractures   Fractures around the shoulder complex are immobilized by a sling and swathe bandage, with the upper limb bound to the body securely. Upper-arm and elbow fractures must be splinted, with immobilization effected in a straight-arm position to lessen bone override. Lower-arm and wrist fractures should be splinted in a position of forearm flexion and should be supported by a sling. Hand and finger dislocations and fractures should be splinted with tongue depressors, gauze rolls, or aluminum splints.

Splinting of the spine and pelvis   Injuries involving a possible spine or pelvic fracture are best splinted and moved using a spine board. Recently, a total body rapid form vacuum immobilizer has been developed for dealing with spinal injuries (Figure 8-17). The effectiveness of this piece of equipment as an immobilization device has yet to be determined.

A suspected fracture must be splinted before the athlete is moved.

8-4

Critical Thinking Exercise

A field hockey player trips over an opponent's stick, planterflexing and inverting her ankle, and falls to the turf sustaining a grade 2 ankle sprain. She has immediate effusion and significant pain. On examination there appears to be some laxity in the ankle joint. The athletic trainer transports the athlete to the training room so that the ankle sprain can be managed properly.

? What specifically should the athletic trainer do to most effectively control the initial swelling associated with this injury?

Figure 8-16

Examples of splints. **A,** Rapid form vacuum immobilizer. **B,** Air splint.

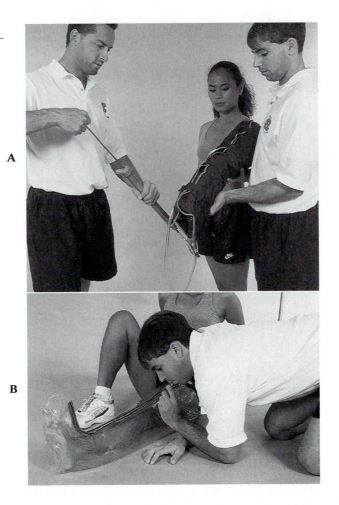

A

B

Figure 8-17

Athletic mattress total body immobilizer.

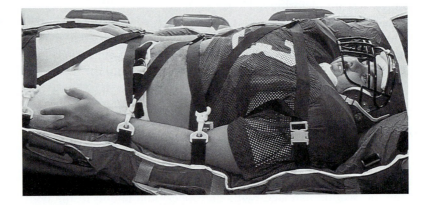

Great caution must be taken when transporting the injured athlete.

MOVING AND TRANSPORTING THE INJURED ATHLETE

Moving, lifting, and transporting the injured athlete must be executed using techniques that will prevent further injury. It has been suggested that moving or transporting the athlete improperly causes more additional injuries than any other emergency procedure.[4,9] There is no excuse for poor handling of the injured athlete. Planning should take into consideration all the possible transportation methods and the necessary equipment to execute them. Capable and well-trained personnel, spine boards, stretchers, and a rescue vehicle may be needed to transport the injured athlete. Special consideration must be given to extracting the injured athlete from a pool.

Suspected Spinal Injury

When such injuries are suspected, the coach or athletic trainer should access the Emergency Medical System and wait until the rescue squad arrives before attempting to move the athlete. The only exception would be in cases where the athlete is not breathing and logrolling the athlete onto the back is required for CPR.

A suspected spinal injury requires extremely careful handling and is best left to properly trained paramedics, EMTs, or athletic trainers who are more skilled and have the proper equipment for such transport. If such personnel are not available, moving should be done under the express direction of a physician, and a spine board should be used (Figure 8-18). One danger inherent in moving an athlete with a suspected spinal injury, in particular a cervical injury, is the tendency of the neck and head to turn because of the victim's inability to control his or her movements. Torque so induced creates considerable possibility of spinal cord or root damage when small fractures are present. The most important principle in transporting an individual on a spine board is to keep the head and neck in alignment with the long axis of the body. In such cases it is best to have one individual whose sole responsibility is to ensure and maintain proper positioning of the head and neck until the head is secured to a spine board.

Placing the Athlete on a Spine Board

Once an injury to the neck has been recognized as severe, a physician and a rescue squad should be summoned immediately. Primary emergency care involves maintaining normal breathing, treating for shock, and keeping the athlete quiet and in the position found until medical assistance arrives. Ideally, transportation should not be attempted until the physician has examined the athlete and has given permission to move him or her. The athlete should be transported while lying on the back with the curve of the neck supported by a rolled-up towel or pad or encased in a stabilization collar. Neck stabilization must be maintained throughout transportation, first to the emergency vehicle, then to the hospital, and throughout the hospital procedure. If stabilization is not continued, additional cord damage and paralysis may ensue.

These steps should be followed when moving an athlete with suspected neck injury:
1. Establish whether the athlete is breathing and has a pulse.
2. Plan to move the athlete on a spine board.
3. If the athlete is lying prone, he or she must be logrolled onto the back for CPR or to be secured to the spine board. An athlete with a possible cervical fracture is transported face up. An athlete with a spinal fracture in the lower trunk area may be transported face down.[2]
    a. Place all extremities in an axial alignment (see Figure 8-18, A).
    b. To roll the athlete over requires four or five persons, with the "captain" of the team protecting the athlete's head and neck. The neck must be stabilized and must not be moved from its original position, no matter how distorted it may appear.
    c. The spine board is placed close to the side of the athlete (see Figure 8-18, B).
    d. Each assistant is responsible for one of the athlete's body segments. One assistant is responsible for turning the trunk, another the hips, another the thighs, and the last the lower legs.
4. With the spine board close to the athlete's side, the captain gives the command to logroll him or her onto the board as one unit (see Figure 8-18, C).
5. On the board, the athlete's head and neck continue to be stabilized by the captain (see Figure 8-18, D).
6. If the athlete is a football player, the helmet is not removed; however, the face guard is removed or lifted away from the face for possible CPR. NOTE: To remove the face guard, the plastic fasteners holding it to the helmet should be cut.
7. The head and neck are next stabilized on the spine board by a chin strap secured

Figure 8-18

A, When moving an unconscious athlete, first establish whether the athlete is breathing and has a pulse. An unconscious athlete must always be treated as having a serious neck injury. If lying prone, the athlete must be turned over for CPR or be secured to a spine board for possible cervical fracture. One coach or athletic trainer (the "captain") stabilizes the athlete's neck and head. **B,** The spine board is placed as close to the athlete as possible. **C,** Each assistant is responsible for one of the athlete's segments. When the coach or athletic trainer (captain) gives the command "roll," the athlete is moved as a unit onto the spine board. *(continued)*

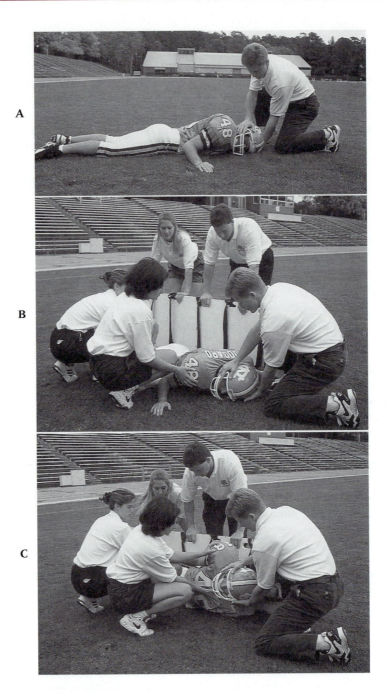

to metal loops. Finally, the trunk and lower limbs are secured to the spine board by straps (see Figure 8-18, *E* and *F*).

An alternative method of moving the athlete onto a spine board, if he or she is face up, is the straddle slide method. Four or five persons are used—a captain stationed at the athlete's head and three or four assistants. One assistant is in charge of lifting the athlete's trunk, one the hips, and one the legs. On the command "lift" by the captain, the athlete is lifted while the fourth assistant slides a spine board under the athlete between the feet of the captain and the assistants (Figure 8-19).

Ambulatory Aid

Ambulatory aid is that support or assistance given to an injured athlete who is able to walk (Figure 8-20). Before the athlete is allowed to walk, he or she should be

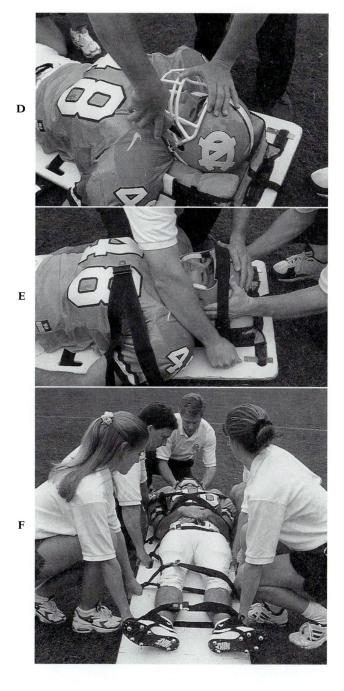

Figure 8-18—cont'd

D, The face mask is cut away while the captain continues to stabilize the athlete's neck. **E,** The head and neck are stabilized onto the spine board by means of a chin strap secured to metal loops. **F,** The trunk and lower limbs are secured to the spine board by straps. *(continued)*

carefully scrutinized to make sure that the injuries are minor. Whenever serious injuries are suspected, walking should be prohibited. Complete support should be given on both sides of the athlete by two individuals who are approximately the same height. The athlete's arms are draped over the assistants' shoulders, and their arms encircle his or her back.

Manual Conveyance

Manual conveyance may be used to move a mildly injured individual a greater distance than could be walked with ease (Figure 8-21). As with the use of ambulatory aid, any decision to carry the athlete must be made only after a complete examination to determine the existence of potentially serious conditions. The most convenient carry is performed by two assistants.

Figure 8-18—cont'd

G, All carriers assume a position to stand. **H,** Once the carriers are standing, the athlete may be transported.

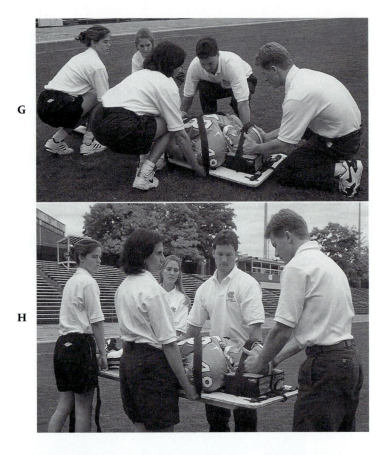

Figure 8-19

An alternative method of placing the athlete on a spine board is the straddle slide method.

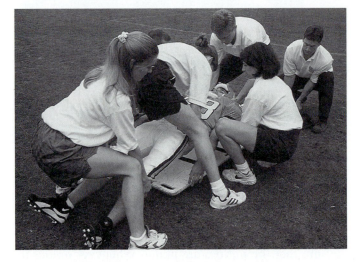

Stretcher Carrying

Whenever a serious injury is suspected, the best and safest mode of transportation for a short distance is by stretcher. With each segment of the body supported, the athlete is gently lifted and placed on the stretcher, which is carried adequately by four assistants, two supporting the ends of the stretcher and two supporting either side (Figure 8-22). Any person with an injury serious enough to require the use of a stretcher must be carefully examined before being moved.

When transporting a person with a limb injury, be certain the injury is splinted properly before transport. Athletes with shoulder injuries are more comfortably moved in a semisitting position, unless other injuries preclude such positioning. If

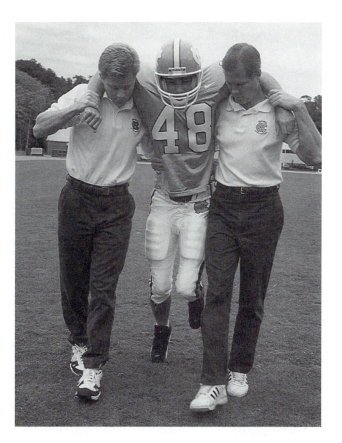

Figure 8-20

The ambulatory aid method of transporting a mildly injured athlete.

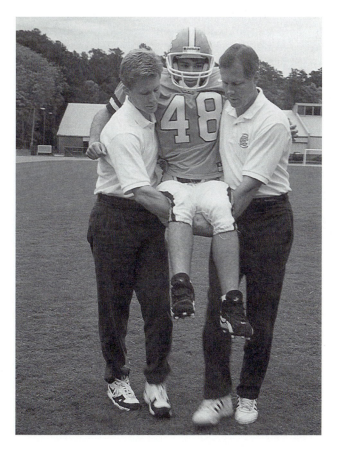

Figure 8-21

Manual conveyance method for transporting a mildly injured athlete.

Figure 8-22

Whenever a serious injury is suspected, a stretcher is the safest method for transporting the athlete.

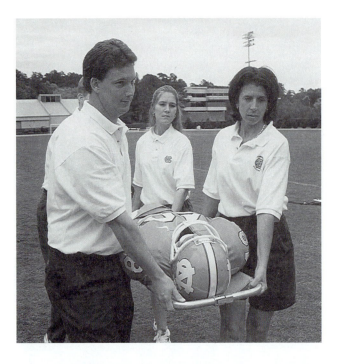

injury to the upper extremity is such that flexion of the elbow is not possible, the individual should be transported on a stretcher with the limb properly splinted and carried at the side, with adequate padding placed between the arm and the body.

Pool Extraction

Removing an injured athlete from a swimming pool requires some special consideration on the part of the athletic trainer.

1. The injured athlete who has not sustained a head or neck injury should be told to roll onto his or her back in the water and then towed to the edge of the pool using a cross-chest technique (Figure 8-23).
2. If the athlete is not breathing, a single rescuer should get the athlete out of the water and onto the deck as quickly as possible to perform CPR. If two rescuers

Figure 8-23

Cross-chest technique for towing an injured athlete.

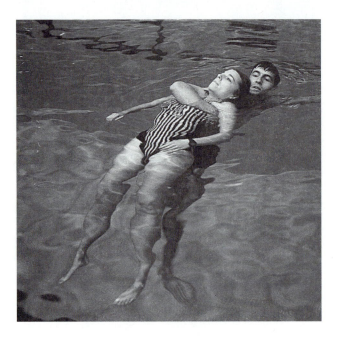

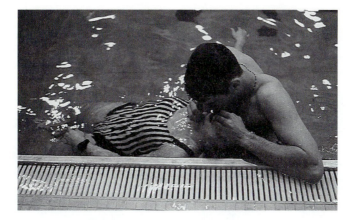

Figure 8-24

Rescue breathing should begin in the water.

are present resuscitation should begin immediately while still in the water. With the athlete supine in the water, one rescuer supports the shoulders and head while the other performs a jaw thrust to open the airway and begins rescue breathing if necessary. The athlete should be moved onto the deck where CPR is continued as rapidly as possible (Figure 8-24).

3. Athletes with a suspected head or cervical neck injury and who are unconscious require special precaution. The athletic trainer should approach the athlete in the water carefully to minimize wave action, which causes unnecessary movement of the head and neck. Using a head-chin support technique, which uses the forearms to splint the chest and upper back and the hands to stabilize the head and neck, the athlete should be rolled onto his or her back and maintained in a horizontal position until help arrives (Figure 8-25, *A*). NOTE: If nec-

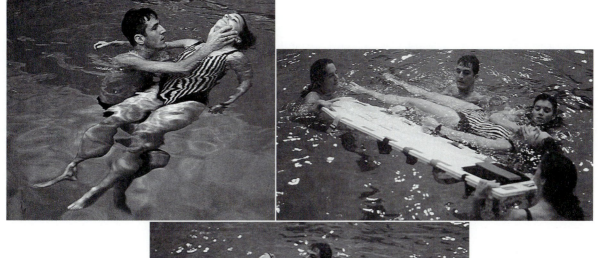

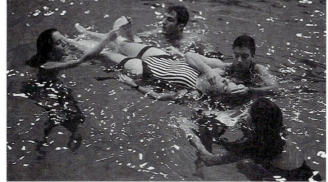

Figure 8-25

In suspected head or cervical neck injury, **A,** use a head-chin support technique; **B,** place the spine board under the athlete; **C,** secure the athlete to the board.
(continued)

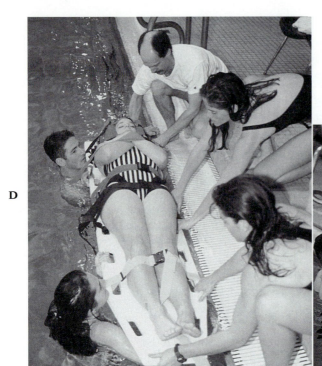

D

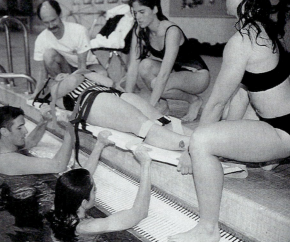

E

Figure 8-25—cont'd
In suspected head or cervical neck injury, **D** and **E,** lift the spine board out of the water.

essary, a second rescuer can provide CPR in this position. The athlete should be secured to the spine board while still in the water. The spine board should be placed diagonally under the victim from the side with the foot end of the board going down into the water first. Slide the board under the victim and allow it to rise directly under the victim (Figure 8-25, *B*). Once on the spine board the athlete's head should be stabilized by one rescuer while the others strap the athlete onto the board, securing the victim's head (Figure 8-25, *C*). When lifting the spine board out of the water, the rescuer at the head should be in charge and the spine board should be removed head first (Figure 8-25, *D*).

FITTING AND USING THE CRUTCH OR CANE

When an athlete has a lower-limb injury, weight bearing may be contraindicated. Situations of this type call for the use of a crutch or cane. Often, the athlete is assigned one of these aids without proper fitting or instruction in its use. Improper fit and usage can place abnormal stresses on various body parts. Constant pressure of the body weight on the crutch's axillary pads can cause crutch palsy. This pressure on the axillary radial nerves and blood vessels can lead to temporary or even permanent numbness in the hands. Faulty mechanics in the use of crutches or canes could produce chronic low back or hip strain.

Fitting the Athlete

The adjustable wooden crutch is well suited to the athlete. For a correct fit the athlete should wear low-heeled shoes and stand with good posture and the feet close together. The crutch length is determined first by placing the tip 6 inches (15 cm) from the outer margin of the shoe and 2 inches (5 cm) in front of the shoe. The underarm crutch brace is positioned 1 inch (2.5 cm) below the anterior fold of the axilla. Next, the hand brace is adjusted so that it is even with the athlete's hand and the elbow is flexed at approximately a 30-degree angle (Figure 8-26).

Fitting a cane to the athlete is relatively easy. Measurement is taken from the superior aspect of the greater trochanter of the femur to the floor while the athlete is wearing street shoes.

Properly fitting a crutch or cane is essential to avoid placing abnormal stresses on the body.

Walking with the Crutch or Cane

Many elements of crutch walking correspond with walking. The technique commonly used in sports injuries is the tripod method. In this method, the athlete swings through the crutches without making any surface contact with the injured limb or by partially bearing weight with the injured limb. The following sequence is performed:

1. The athlete stands on one foot with the affected foot completely elevated or partially bearing weight.
2. Placing the crutch tips 12 to 15 inches (30 to 37.5 cm) ahead of the feet, the athlete leans forward, straightens the elbows, pulls the upper crosspiece firmly against the side of the chest, and swings or steps between the stationary crutches (Figure 8-27). The athlete should avoid placing the major support in the axilla.
3. After moving through, the athlete recovers the crutches and again places the tips forward.

An alternative method is the four-point crutch gait. In this method, the athlete stands on both feet. One crutch is moved forward, and the opposite foot is stepped forward. The crutch on the same side as the foot that moved forward moves just ahead of the foot. The opposite foot steps forward, followed by the crutch on the same side, and so on.

Once the athlete is able to move effectively on a level surface, negotiating stairs should be taught. As with level crutch walking, a tripod is maintained on stairs. In going up stairs, the unaffected support leg moves up one step while the body weight is supported by the hands. The full weight of the body is transferred to the support leg, followed by moving the crutch tips and affected leg to the step. In going down stairs, the crutch tips and the affected leg move down one step followed by the support leg. If a handrail is available, both crutches are held by the outside hand, and a similar pattern is followed as with the crutch on each side.

Emergency Emotional Care

Besides responding to the emergency physical requirements of an injury, the coach and the athletic trainer must respond appropriately to the emotions engendered by

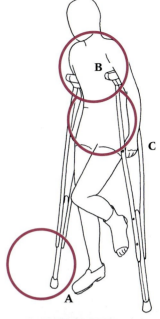

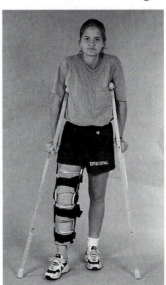

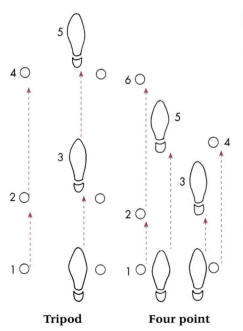

Figure 8-27

Crutch gait. **A,** Tripod method. **B,** Four-point gait.

Tripod

A

Four point

B

Figure 8-26

The crutch must be properly fitted to the athlete. **A,** The crutch tips are placed 6 inches (15 cm) from the outer margin of the shoe and 2 inches (5 cm) in front of the shoe. **B,** The underarm crutch brace is positioned 1 inch (2.5 cm) below the anterior fold of the axilla. **C,** The hand brace is placed even with the athlete's hand, with the elbow flexed approximately 30 degrees.

the situation. The American Psychiatric Association has set forth major principles for the emergency care of emotional reactions to trauma.[4] They are as follows:

1. Accept everyone's right to personal feelings, because everyone comes from a unique background and has had different emotional experiences. Do not tell the injured person how he or she should feel. Show empathy, not pity.

2. Accept the injured person's limitations as real.

3. Athletic trainers must accept their own limitations as providers of first aid.

In general, the athletic trainer dealing with injured athletes' emotions should be empathetic and calm, making it obvious that their feelings are understood and accepted.

SUMMARY

- An emergency is defined as "an unforeseen combination of circumstances and the resulting state that calls for immediate action."[7] The primary concern of emergency aid is to maintain cardiovascular function and, indirectly, central nervous system function. All sports programs should have an emergency system that is activated whenever an athlete is seriously injured.

- The athletic trainer must make a systematic assessment of the injured athlete to determine appropriate emergency care. A primary survey assesses and deals with life-threatening situations. Once stabilized, the secondary survey makes a more detailed assessment of the injury.

- The mnemonic for cardiopulmonary resuscitation is ABC: A—airway opened; B—breathing restored; C—circulation restored. In adult CPR the ratio of compression to breaths is 15:2, with 80 to 100 compressions per minute. To relieve an obstructed airway the Heimlich maneuver, the finger sweep of the throat, or both should be performed.

- Hemorrhage can occur externally and internally. External bleeding can be controlled by direct pressure, applying press at pressure points, and by elevation. Internal hemorrhage can occur subcutaneously, intramuscularly, or within a body cavity.

- Shock can occur from a variety of situations. Shock can be hypovolemic, respiratory, neurogenic, psychogenic, cardiogenic, septic, anaphylactic, and metabolic. Symptoms include skin paleness, dilated eyes, weak and rapid pulse, and rapid, shallow breathing. Management includes maintaining normal body temperature and slightly elevating the feet.

- Rest, ice, compression, and elevation (RICE) should be used for the immediate care of a musculoskeletal injury. Ice should be applied for at least 20 minutes every 1 to 1½ hours, and compression and elevation should be continuous for at least 72 hours after injury.

- Any suspected fracture should be splinted before the athlete is moved. Commercial rapid form vacuum immobilizers and air splints are most often used in an athletic training setting.

- Great care must be taken in moving the seriously injured athlete. The unconscious athlete must be handled as though he or she has a cervical fracture. Moving an athlete with a suspected serious neck injury must be performed only by persons specifically trained to do so. A spine board should be used, avoiding any movement of the cervical region.

- When removing an injured athlete from a swimming pool, the athletic trainer should make every effort to minimize movement of the head and cervical spine while placing the athlete on a spine board in the water.

- The athletic trainer should be responsible for the proper fitting and instruction in the use of crutches or a cane by an athlete with an injury to the lower extremity.

- Athletes who are injured will respond emotionally to the situation. Their feelings must be understood and fully accepted by the coach and the athletic trainer.

....

Solutions to Critical Thinking EXERCISES

8-1 Because of the mechanism of injury, it should be suspected that the athlete has a cervical neck injury. The head should be stabilized throughout. If the athlete is prone and breathing, do nothing until consciousness returns. An on-field exam should determine the athlete's neurological status. Then carefully log-roll him onto a spine board because CPR could be necessary at any time. The face mask should be removed in case CPR is required. The helmet and shoulder pads should be left in place. The athlete should then be transported to the emergency facility. Remember, in this situation the worst mistake the athletic trainer can make is not exercising enough caution.

8-2 The athletic trainer must first take precautions to protect against the transmission of bloodborne pathogens. The wound should be cleaned with soap and water. Direct pressure using a gauze pad should be applied along with cold. If the athlete is not dizzy he should remain in a sitting position. The athlete should be referred to a physician for suturing. Sterile strips or a butterfly bandage may also be applied, although sutures will generally leave a smaller scar. All blood-contaminated supplies should be disposed of in a clearly marked biohazard bag.

8-3 The athlete may be going into hypovolemic shock secondary to hemorrhage and trauma, which can potentially be a life-threatening situation. The athletic trainer should first direct someone to dial 911 to access the emergency medical system. Next it is essential to control the bleeding by using direct pressure, elevation, and pressure points. If bleeding is controlled and the rescue squad has not arrived, the forearm should be immobilized in a vacuum immobilizer. With the athlete supine the feet should be elevated in the shock position. Body temperature should be maintained.

8-4 The ankle should be wrapped with a wet elastic compression wrap. Ice should be applied to both sides of the joint over the compression wrap and secured. The ankle should be elevated such that the leg is above 45 degrees at a minimum. The compression wrap, ice, and elevation should be maintained initially for at least 30 minutes but not longer than an hour. The athletic trainer should also make some determination as to whether a fracture is suspected and make the appropriate referral.

8-5 The athletic trainer should most likely place the athlete on a spine board and secure her before extracting her from the pool. Several people may be required to get the athlete appropriately positioned on the spine board while still in the water. The athlete should be given a brief neurological exam to determine the extent of the injury. The athlete should then be transported to an emergency facility in a rescue vehicle.

REVIEW QUESTIONS AND CLASS ACTIVITIES

1. What considerations are important in a well-planned system for handling emergency situations?
2. Discuss the rules for managing and moving an unconscious athlete.
3. What are the life-threatening conditions that should be evaluated in the primary survey?
4. What are the ABCs of life support?
5. Identify the major steps in giving CPR and managing an obstructed airway. When may these procedures be used in a sports setting?
6. List the basic steps in assessing a musculoskeletal injury.
7. What techniques should be used to stop external hemorrhage?
8. There are numerous types of shock that can occur from a sports injury or illness; list them and their management.
9. What first aid procedures are used to decrease hemorrhage, inflammation, muscle spasm, and pain from a musculoskeletal injury?
10. Describe the basic concepts of emergency splinting.
11. How should an athlete with a suspected spinal injury be transported?
12. What techniques can be used when transporting an athlete with a suspected musculoskeletal injury?
13. Discuss the methods for extracting an injured athlete from a swimming pool.
14. Explain how to properly fit crutches.
15. Describe methods that should be used when dealing with an injured athlete's emotional response to the injury.

REFERENCES

1. American Red Cross: *First aid: responding to emergencies,* St Louis, 1991, Mosby.
2. American Academy of Orthopaedic Surgeons: *Athletic training and sports medicine,* Park Ridge, Ill, 1991, AAOS.
3. Feld F: Management of the critically injured football player, *J Ath Train* 28(3):206, 1993.
4. Hafen BQ: *First aid for health emergencies,* ed 4, St Paul, Minn, 1988, West Publishing.
5. Knight K: *Cryotherapy in sport injury management,* Champaign, Ill, 1995, Human Kinetics.
6. Knight KL: ICE for immediate care of injuries, *Phys Sportsmed* 10:137, 1982.
7. National Safety Council: *First aid and CPR,* Boston, 1991, Jones & Bartlett.
8. Ortolani A: Helmets and face masks, *J Ath Train* 27(4):294, 1992 (letter).
9. Parcel GS: *Basic emergency care of the sick and injured,* ed 4, St Louis, 1990, Mosby.
10. Putman L: Alternative methods for football helmet fask mask removal, *J Ath Train* 27(2):107, 1992.
11. Ray R: Helmets and face masks, *J Ath Train* 27(4):294, 1992 (letter).
12. Standards and guidelines for cardiopulmonary resuscitation (CPR) and emergency cardiac care (ECC), *JAMA* 255:2841, 1986.
13. Stephenson HE Jr, editor: *Immediate care of the acutely ill and injured,* ed 2, St Louis, 1978, Mosby.

14. Thorsson O et al: The effect of local cold application on intramuscular blood flow at rest and after running, *Med Sci Sports Exerc* 17:710, 1985.

15. Thygerson AL: *First aid and emergency care workbook, National Safety Council*, Boston, 1989, Jones & Bartlett.

16. Walton M et al: Effects of ice packs on tissue temperatures at various depths before and after quadriceps hematoma: studies using sheep, *J Orthop Sports Phys Ther* 8:294, 1986.

17. Wilkerson GB: External compression for controlling traumatic edema, *Phys Sportsmed* 13:96, 1985.

ANNOTATED BIBLIOGRAPHY

American Red Cross: *First aid: responding to emergencies*, St Louis, 1991, Mosby.

A well-illustrated, simple approach to the treatment of emergency illness and injury.

doCarmo PB: *Basic EMT skills and equipment*, St Louis, 1988, Mosby.

Contains information about the skills required for basic emergency medical techniques.

Hafen BQ: *First aid for health emergencies*, ed 4, St Paul, Minn, 1988, West Publishing.

Presents in-depth coverage of emergency care. Of particular interest are chapters on shock, psychological first aid, and bone, joint, and muscle injuries.

Judd RL, Ponsell DD: *Mosby's first responder: the critical first minutes*, St Louis, 1988, Mosby.

A complete guide to emergency care.

Parcel GS: *Basic emergency care of the sick and injured*, ed 4, St Louis, 1990, Mosby.

Presents wide coverage of emergency care. Of special interest are Chapter 2, Legal Considerations Involved in Emergency Care by Nonmedical Personnel, and Section III, Trauma Emergencies.

Bloodborne Pathogens

When you finish this chapter, you should be able to

- Explain what bloodborne pathogens are and how they can infect athletes and athletic trainers.
- Describe the transmission, symptoms, signs, and treatment of hepatitis B virus.
- Describe the transmission, symptoms, and signs of human immunodeficiency virus.
- Explain how human immunodeficiency virus is most often transmitted.
- List the pros and cons of sports participation of athletes with hepatitis B virus or human immunodeficiency virus.
- Discuss universal precautions as mandated by the Occupational Safety and Health Administration and how they apply to the athletic trainer.

Bloodborne pathogens are transmitted through contact with blood or other bodily fluids. Hepatitis, especially the hepatitis B virus (HBV), and human immunodeficiency virus (HIV) are of special concern.[3]

It has always been important for the athletic trainer as a health care provider to be concerned with maintaining an environment in the athletic training room that is as clean and sterile as possible.[1,9] In our society of the 1990s it has become critical for everyone in the population to take measures to prevent the spread of infectious diseases.[8] Failure to do so may predispose any individual to life-threatening situations. The athletic trainer must take every precaution to minimize the potential for exposure to blood or other infectious materials (Figure 9-1).

VIRUS REPRODUCTION

A virus is a submicroscopic parasitic organism that is dependent on the nutrients within cells. A virus consists of a strand of either deoxyribonucleic acid (DNA) or ribonuleic acid (RNA). A virus contains one or the other, but not both. A virus consists of a shell of proteins surrounding genetic material. It is a parasite dependent on a host cell for metabolic and reproductive requirements. In general, viruses make their cell hosts ill by redirecting cellular activity to create more viruses (Figure 9-2).

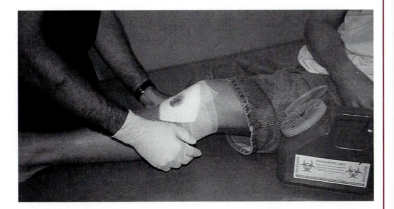
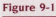

Figure 9-1

The athletic trainer must take precautions to prevent exposure to and transmission of bloodborne pathogens.

Figure 9-2

The reproducing virus.

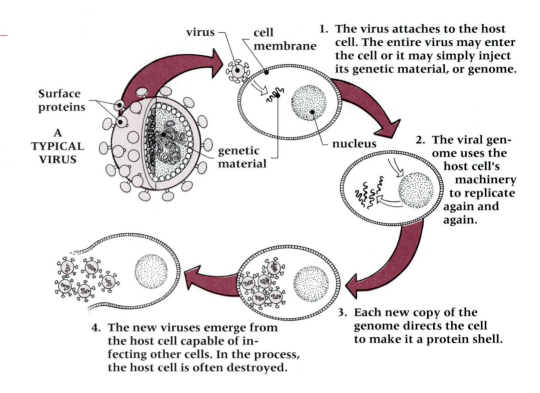

virus — cell membrane

1. The virus attaches to the host cell. The entire virus may enter the cell or it may simply inject its genetic material, or genome.

Surface proteins

A TYPICAL VIRUS

genetic material

nucleus

2. The viral genome uses the host cell's machinery to replicate again and again.

4. The new viruses emerge from the host cell capable of infecting other cells. In the process, the host cell is often destroyed.

3. Each new copy of the genome directs the cell to make it a protein shell.

Mode of transmission includes
   Human blood
   Semen
   Vaginal secretions
   Cerebrospinal fluid
   Synovial fluid

Bloodborne pathogens include
   Hepatitis B virus
   Human immunodeficiency
      virus

9-1

Critical Thinking Exercise

The athletic trainer is responsible for taking every precaution in preventing infection by bloodborne pathogens.

? How are bloodborne pathogen infections prevented from spreading from one athlete to another?

BLOODBORNE PATHOGENS

In 1991 the Occupational Safety and Health Administration (OSHA) established standards for an employer to follow that govern occupational exposure to bloodborne pathogens.[20] Bloodborne pathogens are pathogenic microorganisms that can potentially cause disease and are present in human blood and other body fluids, including semen, vaginal secretions, cerebrospinal fluid, synovial fluid, and any other fluid contaminated with blood. The two most significant bloodborne pathogens are HBV and HIV. A number of other bloodborne diseases exist, including hepatitis C, hepatitis D, and syphilis. Hepatitis A virus (HAV) is spread by lack of personal hygiene and can be transmitted during unprotected sexual intercourse, from contact with feces of infected persons, and from shellfish taken from contaminated water.[11] Good sanitation, personal hygiene, and properly cooking shellfish at high temperatures are essential for prevention.

Although HIV has been widely addressed in the media, HBV has a higher possibility for spread than HIV.[12] Hepatitis B virus is stronger and more durable than HIV and can be spread more easily via sharp objects, open wounds, and bodily fluids.[13]

Hepatitis B Virus

Hepatitis B virus is a major cause of viral infection; it results in swelling, soreness, and loss of normal function in the liver. The number of cases of HBV has risen dramatically during the last 10 years. It has been estimated that as many as 1.25 million people in the United States have chronic hepatitis, which can potentially infect others. New cases are occuring at rates as high as 300,000 per year.[18]

Symptoms and Signs

The symptoms and signs in a person infected with HBV include flulike symptoms such as fatigue, weakness, nausea, abdominal pain, headache, fever, and possibly jaundice. It is possible that an individual infected with HBV will exhibit no signs or symptoms, and the virus may go undetected. In these individuals, the HBV antigen will always be present. Thus the disease may be unknowingly transmitted to others through exposure to blood or other body fluids or through intimate contact. Cases of chronic active hepatitis may occur because of a problem with the immune system that prevents the complete destruction of virus-infected liver cells.

An infected person's blood may test positive for the HBV antigen within 2 to 6 weeks after the symptoms develop. Approximately 85% of those infected recover within 6 to 8 weeks.

Prevention

Good personal hygiene and avoiding high-risk activities is the best way to avoid HBV.[9] Hepatitis B virus can survive for at least 1 week in dried blood or on contaminated surfaces and may be transmitted through contact with these surfaces. Caution must be taken to avoid contact with any blood or other fluid that potentially contains a bloodborne pathogen.

Management

Vaccination against HBV must be made available by the employer at no cost to any individual who may be exposed to blood or other body fluids and may thus be at risk of contracting HBV. It is recommended that all athletic trainers, as well as any individual working in an allied health care profession, receive immunization. It is estimated that 8700 health care workers contract HBV each year, and as many as 200 of these cases may end in death.[18] The vaccine is given in three doses over a 6-month period. Approximately 87% will be immune after the second dose, and 96% develop immunity after the third dose. Postexposure vaccination is available when individuals have come into direct contact with bodily fluids of an infected person.[7]

Human Immunodeficiency Virus

Human immunodeficiency virus is a **retrovirus** that combines with a host cell. A number of cells in the immune system may be infected, such as T_4 blood cells, B cells, and monocytes (macrophages), decreasing their effectiveness in preventing disease. It has been estimated that 1 in 250 people in the United States is infected with HIV.[18] Approximately 1 of every 100 adults males between the ages of 20 and 49 is HIV positive. There are 40,000 to 50,000 new cases each year.[16] The World Health Organization estimates that worldwide there are 10 to 12 million adult carriers of the virus with 40 million estimated by the year 2000.[24]

Symptoms and Signs

As is the case with HBV, HIV is transmitted by exposure to infected blood or other body fluids or by intimate sexual contact.[23] Symptoms of HIV include fatigue, weight loss, muscle or joint pain, painful or swollen glands, night sweats, and fever. Antibodies to HIV can be detected in a blood test within 1 year after exposure. As with HBV, people with HIV may be unaware that they have contracted the virus and may go as long as 8 to 10 years before developing any signs or symptoms. Unfortunately most individuals who test positive for HIV will ultimately develop acquired immunodeficiency syndrome (AIDS). Table 9-1 summarizes information on HBV and HIV.

Acquired Immunodeficiency Syndrome

A syndrome is a collection of signs and symptoms that are recognized as the effects of an infection. An individual with AIDS has no protection against even the simplest infections and thus is extremely vulnerable to developing a variety of illnesses, opportunistic infections, and cancers (such as Kaposi's sarcoma and non-Hodgkin's lymphoma) that cannot be stopped.[7]

Acquired immunodeficiency syndrome is the disease of the 1990s. Since it was first identified in 1981, more than 500,000 Americans have been reported as having AIDS, and about two thirds of those patients had died through 1995.[25]

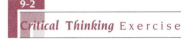

9-2

Critical Thinking Exercise

A wrestler has been diagnosed with hepatitis B virus.

? What are the symptoms and signs of HBV infection?

retrovirus

A virus that enters a host cell and changes its RNA to a proviral DNA replica.

TABLE 9-1 Transmission of Hepatitis B Virus and Human Immunodeficiency Virus

Disease	Symptoms and Signs	Mode of Transmission	Infectious Materials
Hepatitis B virus	Flulike symptoms, jaundice	Direct and indirect contact	Blood, saliva, semen, feces, food, water, and other products
Human immuno-deficiency virus/ acquired im-munodeficiency syndrome	Fever, night sweats, weight loss, diarrhea, severe fatigue, swollen lymph nodes, lesions	Direct and indirect contact	Blood, semen, vaginal fluid

A positive HIV test cannot predict when the individual will show the symptoms of AIDS. About 50% develop AIDS within 10 years of becoming HIV infected. Those individuals who develop AIDS generally die within 2 years after the symptoms appear.

Management

Unlike HBV, there is no vaccine for HIV. Even though some drug therapy may extend their lives, there is likewise currently no available treatment to cure patients with AIDS. Much research is being done to find a preventive vaccine and an effective treatment. Presently, antiviral drugs such as AZT have slowed replication of the virus and improved survival prospects.

Prevention

Human immunodeficiency virus is most often transmitted through intimate sexual contact.

Athletes must understand that their greatest risk for contracting HIV is through intimate sexual contact with an infected partner.[14] Practicing safe sex is of major importance. The athlete must choose nonpromiscuous sex partners and use condoms for vaginal or anal intercourse. Latex condoms provides a barrier against both HBV and HIV. Male condoms should have reservoir tips to reduce the chance of ejaculate being released from the sides of the condom. Condoms that are prelubricated are less likely to tear. Water-based, greaseless spermicides or lubricants should be avoided.[24] If the condom tears, a vaginal spermicide should be used immediately. The condom should carefully be removed and discarded.[24] Additional ways to reduce risk of HIV infection can be found in the Focus box.

The use of latex condoms can reduce the chances of contracting HIV.

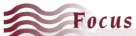

Focus

HIV risk reduction
- Avoid contact with others' bodily fluids, feces, and semen.
- Avoid sharing needles (e.g., when injecting anabolic steroids or human growth hormones).
- Choose nonpromiscuous sex partners.
- Limit sex partners.
- Consistently use condoms.
- Avoid drugs that impair judgment.
- Avoid sex with known HIV carriers.
- Get regular tests for sexually transmitted diseases.
- Practice good hygiene before and after sex.

BLOODBORNE PATHOGENS IN ATHLETICS

In general the chances of transmitting HIV among athletes is low.[22] There is minimal risk of on-field transmission of HIV from one player to another in sports.[22] One study involving professional football estimated the risk of transmission from player to player was less than 1 per 1 million games. At this writing there have been no validated reports of HIV transmission in sports.[16]

Some sports may have a potentially higher risk for transmission where there is close contact and possibility of passing blood on to the other person.[10] Sports such as the martial arts, wrestling, and boxing have more theoretical potential for transmission (see the Focus box below).[16]

Policy Regulation

Athletes participating in organized sports are subject to procedures and policies relative to transmission of bloodborne pathogens. The U.S. Olympic Committee (USOC), the National Collegiate Athletic Association (NCAA), the National Federation of State High School Athletic Associations, the National Basketball Association, the National Hockey League, the National Football League, and Major League Baseball have established policies to help prevent the transmission of bloodborne pathogens. They have also initiated programs to help educate athletes under their control.

All institutions should take the responsibility for educating their student athletes about how bloodborne pathogens are transmitted. In the case of a high school athlete, efforts should also be made to educate the parents.[6] Professional, collegiate, and high school athletes should be made to understand that the greatest risk of contracting HBV or HIV is through their off-the-field activities, which may include unsafe sexual practices and sharing of needles, particularly in the use of steroids. Athletes, perhaps more than other individuals in the population, think that they are immune and that infection will always happen to someone else. The athletic trainer should also assume the responsibility of educating and informing student trainers of exposure control policies.

Each institution should implement policies and procedures concerning bloodborne pathogens.[22] A recent survey of NCAA institutions found that a large number of athletic trainers and other health care providers at many colleges and universities demonstrated significant deficits in following the universal guidelines mandated by **OSHA.** It was suggested that following universal precautions in a sports medicine or other health care setting would protect both the athlete and the health care provider.[15]

Human Immunodeficiency Virus and Athletic Participation

There is no definitive answer as to whether asymptomatic HIV carriers should participate in sports.[12] It is reasonable that bodily fluid contact should be avoided and

9-3

Critical Thinking Exercise

The World Health Organization estimates that there will be 10 to 12 million adult carriers of HIV by the year 2000.

? How may an infected athlete transmit HIV to another athlete?

OSHA
Occupational Safety and Health Administration.

Focus

Risk catagories for HIV transmission in sports[10]

- Highest Risk: boxing, martial arts, wrestling, rugby.
- Moderate Risk: basketball, field hockey, football, ice hockey, judo, soccer, team handball.
- Lowest Risk: archery, badminton, baseball, bowling, canoeing/kayaking, cycling, diving, equestrianism, fencing, figure skating, gymnastics, modern pentathalon, racquetball, rhythmic gymnastics, roller skating, rowing, shooting, softball, speed skating, skiing, swimming, synchronized swimming, table tennis, volleyball, water polo, weight lifting, yachting.

that the participant should also avoid engaging in exhaustive exercise that may led to an increased susceptibility to infection.[12]

The Americans with Disabilities Act of 1991 says that athletes infected with HIV cannot be discriminated against and may be excluded from participation only with a medically sound basis.[16] Exclusion must be based on objective medical evidence taking into consideration the extent of risk of infection to others and potential harm to self and what means can be taken to reduce this risk.[23]

Testing Athletes for Human Immunodeficiency Virus

Testing for HIV should not be used as a screening tool to determine if an athlete can participate in sports.[22] Mandatory testing for HIV may not be allowed because of legal reasons related to the Americans with Disabilities Act.[22] In terms of importance, mandatory testing should be secondary to education to prevent transmission of HIV.[15] Neither the NCAA nor the Centers for Disease Control and Prevention (CDC) recommends mandatory HIV testing for athletes.[22]

Athletes who engage in high-risk activities should be encouraged to seek voluntary anonymous testing for HIV. A blood test analyzes serum using enzyme-linked immunosorbent assay (ELISA). The ELISA test detects antibodies to HIV proteins. Positive ELISA tests should be repeated to rule out false-positive results. A second positive test requires the Western blot examination, which is a more sensitive test.[7] Detectable antibodies may appear from 3 months to 1 year after exposure. Testing therefore should occur at 6 weeks, 3 months, and 1 year.[24]

Many states have enacted laws that protect the confidentiality of the HIV-infected person. The athletic trainer should be familiar with state law and make every effort to guard the confidentiality and anonymity of HIV testing for athletes.

UNIVERSAL PRECAUTIONS IN AN ATHLETIC ENVIRONMENT

The guidelines instituted by OSHA were developed to protect the health care provider and the patient against bloodborne pathogens.[18] It is essential that every sports program develop and carry out a bloodborne pathogen exposure control plan. This plan should include counseling, education, volunteer testing, and the management of bodily fluids.[22]

These guidelines should be followed by anyone coming into contact with blood or other body fluids. The following should be considerations specifically in the sports arena.

Preparing the Athlete

Before an athlete participates in practice or competition all open skin wounds and lesions must be covered with a dressing that is fixed in place and does not allow for transmission to or from an athlete.[21] An occlusive dressing lessens the chances of cross-contamination. One example is the hydrocolloid dressing, which is considered a superior barrier. Wearing this type of dressing also reduces chances of the wound reopening by keeping it moist and pliable.[21]

When Bleeding Occurs

As mandated by the NCAA and the USOC, open wounds or other skin lesions considered a risk for disease transmission should be provided with aggressive treatment. Athletes with active bleeding must be removed from participation as soon as possible and returned only when it is deemed safe by the medical staff.[17] Uniforms containing blood must be evaluated for infectivity. A uniform that is saturated with blood must be removed and changed before the athlete can return to competition. All personnel managing potential infective wound exposure must follow universal precautions.[18]

For additional information on HIV and AIDS care, contact the Centers for Disease Control and Prevention (CDC) National AIDS Hotline: 1 (800) 342-2437.

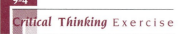

9-4

Critical Thinking Exercise

A sports program must initiate and carry out a bloodborne pathogen exposure control plan.

? What should be the universal precautions in an athletic environment as proposed by OSHA?

Personal Precautions

The health care personnel working directly with bodily fluids on the field or in the athletic training facility must make use of the appropriate protective equipment in all cases in which there is potential contact with bloodborne pathogens. Protective equipment includes disposable latex gloves, gowns or aprons, masks and shields, eye protection, nonabsorbant gowns, and disposable mouthpieces for resuscitation devices.[5] One-time-use latex gloves are used when handling any potentially infectious material. Double gloving is suggested when there is heavy bleeding or sharp instruments are used. Gloves are always carefully removed after use. In cases of emergency, heavy toweling may be used until gloves can be obtained.[1] (See the Focus box below.)

Hands and all skin surfaces that come in contact with blood or other body fluids should be washed immediately with soap and water or other antigermicidal agents. Also, it is recommended that hands be washed between each patient treatment.

If there is the possibility of bodily fluids becoming splashed, spurted, or sprayed, the mouth, nose, and eyes should be protected. Aprons or nonabsorbant gowns should be worn to avoid clothing contamination.

First aid kits must have protection for hands, face, and eyes and resuscitation mouthpieces. Kits should also make towelettes available for cleaning skin surfaces.[3]

Availability of Supplies and Equipment

In keeping with universal precautions the sports program must also have available chlorine bleach, antiseptics, proper receptacles for soiled equipment and uniforms, wound care bandages, and a designated container for sharps disposal such as needles, syringes, and scalpels.[17]

Biohazard warning labels should be fixed to regulated wastes, refrigerators containing blood, and other containers used to store or ship potentially infectious materials (Figure 9-3). The labels are fluorescent orange or red and should be affixed to containers. Red bags or containers should be used for disposal of potentially infected materials.

Disinfectants

All contaminated surfaces such as treatment tables, taping tables, work areas, and floors should be cleaned immediately with a solution consisting of 1 part bleach to 10 parts water (1:10) or a disinfectant approved by the Environmental Protection Agency.[6] Disinfectants should inactivate the virus. Towels or other linens that have been contaminated should be bagged and separated from other laundry. Soiled linen is to be transported in red containers or bags that prevent soaking or leaking and labeled with biohazard warning labels (Figure 9-3). Contaminated laundry should be washed in hot water (71°C for 25 minutes) using a detergent that deactivates the virus. Laundry done outside of the institution should use a facility that follows OSHA standards. Gloves must be worn during bagging and cleaning of contaminated laundry.

Latex gloves should be worn whenever the athletic trainer handles blood or body fluids.

9-5

Critical Thinking Exercise

An athletic trainer manages a facial laceration.

? What personal precautions must be taken by the athletic trainer when managing a facial laceration?

Universal precautions minimize the risk of exposure and transmission.

Focus

Glove use and removal
1. Avoid touching personal items when wearing contaminated gloves.
2. Remove first glove and turn inside out beginning at wrist to peel off without touching skin.
3. Remove second glove making sure not to touch ungloved hand to soiled surfaces.
4. Discard gloves that have been used, discolored, torn, or punctured.
5. Wash hands immediately after glove removal.

Figure 9-3

Soiled linens should be placed in a leakproof bag marked as a biohazard.

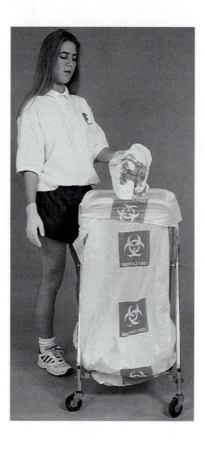

Sharps

Sharps include:
    Scalpels
    Razor blades
    Needles

Sharps refers to sharp objects used in athletic training such as needles, razor blades, and scalpels. Extreme care should be taken when handling and disposing of sharps to minimize risk of puncturing or cutting the skin. Athletic trainers rarely use needles, but it is not unusual for them to use scalpels or razor blades. Whenever needles are used, they should not be recapped, bent, or removed from a syringe. Sharps should be disposed of in a leakproof and puncture-resistant container.[6] The container should be red and labeled as a biohazard (Figure 9-4). Although they are not as likely to injure as sharps, scissors and tweezers should be sterilized with a disinfecting agent and stored in a clean place after use.

Protecting the Coach and Athletic Trainer

It must be pointed out that OSHA guidelines for bloodborne pathogens are intended to protect the coach, athletic trainer, and other employees and not the athlete.[20] Coaches do not usually come in contact with blood or other bodily fluids from an injured athlete, so their risk is considerably reduced. It is the responsibility of the high school, college, professional team, or clinic to ensure the safety of the athletic trainer as a health care provider by instituting and annually updating policies for education on the prevention of transmission of bloodborne pathogens through contact with athletes. The institution must provide the necessary supplies and equipment to carry out these recommendations.

The athletic trainer has the personal responsibility of adhering to these policies and guidelines and enforcing them in the training room. Athletic trainers may further minimize risk of exposure in the athletic training setting by avoiding eating, drinking, applying cosmetics or lip balm, handling contact lenses, and touching the face before washing hands. Never place food products in a refrigerator containing contaminated blood.[2]

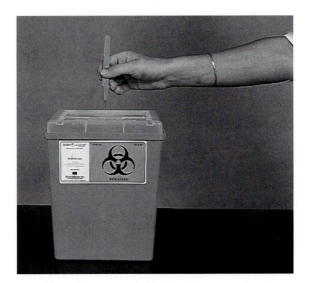

Figure 9-4
Sharps should be disposed of in a red puncture-resistant plastic container marked as a biohazard.

Protecting the Athlete from Exposure

Several additional recommendations may further help protect the athlete. The USOC supports the required use of mouthpieces in high-risk sports. It is also recommended that all athletes shower immediately after practice or competition. Athletes who may be exposed to HIV or HBV should also be evaluated for immunization against HBV.

POSTEXPOSURE PROCEDURES

After a report of an exposure incident, the athletic trainer should have a confidential medical evaluation that includes documentation of the exposure route, identification of the source individual, a blood test, counseling, and an evaluation of reported illness. Again, the laws that pertain to reporting and notification of the test results relative to confidentiality vary from state to state.[20]

SUMMARY

- Bloodborne pathogens are microorganisms that can potentially cause disease and are present in human blood and other body fluids, including semen, vaginal secretions, cerebrospinal fluid, synovial fluid, and any other fluid contaminated with blood. Hepatitis B virus and HIV are bloodborne pathogens.
- A virus is a submicroscopic parasitic organism that contains DNA or RNA, but not both. It is dependent on the host cell to function and reproduce.
- A vaccine is available to prevent HBV. Currently no effective vaccine exists for treating HIV.
- An individual infected with HIV may develop AIDS, which is fatal.
- The risks of contracting HBV or HIV may be minimized by avoiding exposure to blood and other body fluids and practicing safe sex.
- The risk of an athlete being exposed to bloodborne pathogens on the field is minimal. Off-field activities involving risky sexual behaviors pose the greatest threat for transmission.
- Various national medical and sports organizations have established policies and procedures for dealing with bloodborne pathogens in the athletic population.
- The Occupational Safety and Health Administration has established rules and regulations that protect the health care employee.

■ Universal precautions must be taken to avoid bloodborne pathogen exposure. All sports programs must carry out a plan for counseling, education, volunteer testing, and the management of exposure.

....

Solutions to Critical Thinking EXERCISES

9-1 To prevent the spread of bloodborne pathogens the athletic trainer must follow the standards established by the Occupational Safety and Health Administration.

9-2 The wrestler complained of flulike symptoms such as headache, fever, fatigue, weakness, nausea, and some abdominal pain. A blood test reveals the presence of the HBV antigen.

9-3 The greatest risk of contracting HIV is through intimate sexual contact with an infected partner. There is little chance of HIV transmission among athletes. There is a theoretical potential risk of transmission among athletes in close contact who pass blood from one to the other.

9-4 Universal precautions should be practiced by anyone coming in contact with blood or other body fluids. This plan must include counseling, education, volunteer testing, and management of bodily fluids.

9-5 The athletic trainer wears one-time-use latex gloves. All materials used in cleaning and managing the laceration are disposed of in a red biohazard container.

REVIEW QUESTIONS AND CLASS ACTIVITIES

1. Define and identify the bloodborne pathogens.
2. Describe HBV transmission, symptoms, signs, prevention, and treatment.
3. Explain the pros and cons of allowing an athlete to participate who is an HBV carrier.
4. Describe HIV transmission, symptoms, signs, prevention, and treatment.
5. How is HIV transmitted, and why is it eventually fatal at this time?
6. Should an athlete who tests positive for HBV or HIV be allowed to participate in sports? Why or why not?
7. How can an athlete reduce the risk of HIV infection?
8. Define OSHA universal precautions in dealing with preventing bloodborne pathogen exposure.
9. What precautions would you, as an athletic trainer, take when caring for a bleeding wound on the field?

REFERENCES

1. American Academy of Pediatrics: Human immunodeficiency virus [acquired immunodeficiency syndrome (AIDS) virus] in athletic settings, *Pediatrics* 88:640, 1991.
2. American College Health Association: *General statement of institutional response to aids*, Rockville, Md, 1988, Task Force on Aids, American College Health Association.
3. American Medical Association Department of HIV, Division of Health Science: *Digest of HIV/AIDS policy*, Chicago, 1993, American Medical Association.
4. American Red Cross: *Emergency response*, St Louis, 1993, Mosby.
5. American Red Cross: *First aid: responding to emergencies*, St Louis, 1991, Mosby.
6. Arnold BL: A review of selected blood-borne pathogen position statements and federal regulations, *J Ath Train* 30(2):171, 1995.
7. Berkow R, editor: *The Merck manual diagnosis of therapy*, ed 16, Raway, NJ, 1992, Merck Sharp and Dohne Research Laboratories.
8. Brown L, Dortman P: What is the risk of HIV infection in athletic competition? International Conference on AIDS 19939:PO-C21-3102, 1993.
9. Buxton BP et al: Prevention of hepatitis B virus in athletic training, *J Ath Train* 29(2):107, 1994.
10. Garl T, Hrisomalos T, Rink R: *Transmission of infectious agents during athletic competition*, Colorado Springs, 1991, USOC Sports Medicine and Science Committee.
11. Hamann B: *Disease: identification, prevention, and control*, St Louis, 1994, Mosby.
12. Howe WB: The athlete with chronic illness. In Birrer RB, editor: *Sports medicine for the primary care physician*, ed 2, Boca Raton, Fla, 1994, CRC Press.
13. Hunt BP, Pujol TJ: Athletic trainers as HIV/AIDS educators, *J Ath Train* 29(2):102, 1994.
14. Landry GL: HIV infection and athletes, *Sports Med Digest* 15(4):1, 1993.
15. McGrew C, Dick R, Schneidewind K: Survey of NCAA institutions concerning HIV/AIDS policies and universal precautions, *Med Sci Sport Exerc* 25:917, 1993.
16. Mitten MJ: HIV-positive athletes, *Phys Sportsmed* 22(10):63, 1994.
17. Benson MT, editor: *1994-95 NCAA sports medicine handbook*, Overland Park, Kans, 1994, National Collegiate Athletic Association.
18. National Safety Council: *Bloodborne pathogens*, Boston, 1993, Jones & Bartlett.
19. National Safety Council: *First aid and CPR*, Boston, 1991, Jones & Bartlett.
20. OSHA: The OSHA bloodborne pathogens standard, *Federal Register* 55(235):64175, 1991.
21. Rheinecker SB: Wound management: the occlusive dressing, *J Ath Train* 30(2):143, 1995.
22. Rogers KJ: Human immunodeficiency virus in sports. In Torg JS, Shephard RJ, editors: *Current therapy in sports medicine*, St Louis, 1995, Mosby.
23. School Board of Nassau County, Fla, J Arlene, 480 US 273 (1987).
24. Seltzer DG: Educating athletes on HIV disease and AIDS, *Phys Sportsmed* 21(1):109, 1993.
25. First 500,000 AIDS cases: United States, 1995, *MMWR* 44(46):850, 1995.

ANNOTATED BIBLIOGRAPHY

Benson MA, editor: *National Collegiate Athletic Association 1994-95 sports medicine handbook*, Overland Park, Kans, 1994, National Collegiate Athletic Association.

A complete discussion of bloodborne pathogens and intercollegiate athletic policies and administration.

Berkow R, editor: *The Merck manual of diagnosis and therapy*, ed 16, Rahway, NJ, 1992, Merck Sharp and Dohne Research Laboratories.

An excellent guide to discussing diagnosis, symptoms, signs, and treatment of bloodborne pathogens.

Bradley-Springer L, Fendrick RA: *AIDS/HIV instant instructor,* El Paso, Tex, 1994, Skidmore-Roth.

An excellent card system covering transmission, transmission prevention, occupational exposure prevention, testing, counseling, disease progression, and treatment of HIV and AIDS.

Hall K et al: *Bloodborne pathogens,* Boston, 1993, Jones & Bartlett.

A manual dedicated to presenting OSHA regulations specific to bloodborne pathogens.

Hamann B: *Disease: identification, prevention, and control,* St Louis, 1994, Mosby.

A text designed for health educators; AIDS and hepatitis are covered in detail.

Injury Assessment and Evaluation

When you finish this chapter, you should be able to

- Differentiate between evaluation and diagnosis.
- Define terminology used in injury evaluation.
- Discuss the importance of the off-the-field secondary evaluation.
- Identify the aspects of the musculoskeletal evaluation sequence.
- Discuss additional diagnostic techniques available to the athletic trainer through the team physician.

T he evaluation of sports injuries is a proficiency that all athletic trainers and sports physicians must have. As one of the most important members of the sports medicine team, the athletic trainer is charged with performing accurate and detailed assessments under a number of specific circumstances. As discussed in Chapter 8, the athletic trainer often performs primary or on-site injury assessment. In other words, the athletic trainer is often the first person to inspect and evaluate the athlete's injury, usually almost immediately after it has occurred. Under circumstances that do not require first aid or emergency care, assessment is often performed at a place other than where the injury occurred and has generally been called secondary assessment.

INJURY EVALUATION VERSUS DIAGNOSIS

> Athletic trainers recognize and evaluate sports injuries, but by law they cannot make diagnoses.

Although athletic trainers and coaches recognize and evaluate sports injuries, by law they cannot make a diagnosis. A diagnosis denotes what disease, injury, or syndrome a person has or is believed to have. Making a diagnosis is usually reserved for individuals specifically licensed by a state to do so. Health professionals such as physicians are generally permitted to diagnose. Health professionals restricted to diagnosing one body area are dentists, who are limited to diagnosing mouth disorders; podiatrists, who are limited to diagnosing foot disorders; and optometrists, who are limited to determining refractory problems of the eyes and prescribing lenses to increase the efficiency of vision. Chiropractors usually base their diagnoses on the relationship of the body's structure to its overall function. In some states, nurse practitioners may make limited diagnoses.

There is a fine line between the evaluation of an injury and its diagnosis. Debating this difference serves no useful purpose other than to confound the distinction further. In situations in which time is of the essence, as is often the case in sports injuries, the ability to evaluate quickly, accurately, and decisively is vitally important. In such situations the coach or the athletic trainer must remain within the limits of his or her ability and training and must act in full accord with professional ethics.

BASIC KNOWLEDGE REQUIREMENTS

> The examiner of sports injuries must have a thorough knowledge of human anatomy and its function and of the hazards inherent in sports.

The athletic trainer or coach who is examining an athlete with a sports injury must have a general knowledge of normal human anatomy and biomechanics and an understanding of the major hazards inherent in a particular sport. Without this information, accurate assessment becomes impossible.

Normal Human Anatomy

Surface Anatomy

Understanding typical surface or topographical anatomy is essential when evaluating a possible injury. Key surface landmarks provide the examiner with indications of the normal or injured anatomical structures lying underneath the skin.[7]

Body planes and anatomical directions   Associated with surface anatomy is the understanding of body planes and anatomical directions. Body planes are used as points of reference from which positions of body parts are indicated. The three most commonly mentioned planes are the midsagittal, transverse, and frontal (or coronal) planes (Figure 10-1). Anatomical directions refer to the relative position of one part to another (Figure 10-2).

Abdominopelvic quadrants   The abdominopelvic quadrants are the four corresponding regions of the abdomen that are divided for evaluative and diagnostic purposes (Figure 10-3).

Musculoskeletal System

Anyone examining the musculoskeletal system for sports injuries must have an in-depth knowledge of both structural and functional anatomy. This knowledge encompasses the major joints and bony structures, as well as skeletal musculature. A knowledge of neural anatomy is also of major importance, particularly that which is involved in movement control and sensation, along with the neural factors that influence superficial and deep pain.

Standard musculoskeletal terminology for bodily positions and deviations   When assessing the musculoskeletal system, a standard terminology must be used to convey more precisely information to others who may become professionally involved with the athlete. These terms are found in Table 10-1.

Biomechanics   The understanding of biomechanics is the foundation for the assessment of musculoskeletal sports injuries. **Biomechanics** is the application of mechanical forces, which may stem from within or outside of the body, to living organ-

biomechanics
Application of mechanical forces to living organisms.

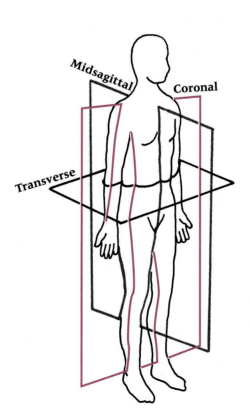

Figure 10-1

Knowledge of body planes helps provide points of reference.

Figure 10-2

Anatomical directions refer to the relative position of one body part to another.

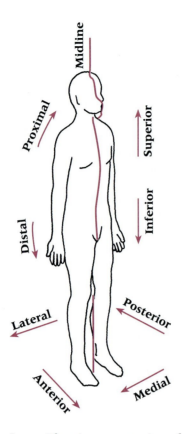

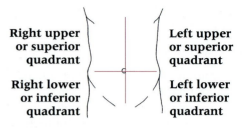

Figure 10-3

Knowledge about the four abdominopelvic quadrants helps in injury assessment.

pathomechanics

Mechanical forces that are applied to a living organism and adversely change the body's structure and function.

etiology

Cause of disease.

pathology

Structural and functional changes that result from injury.

symptom

Change that indicates injury or disease.

sign

Indicator of a disease.

isms. Of major concern is pathomechanics, which may precede an injury. **Pathomechanics** refers to mechanical forces that are applied to the body because of a structural body deviation, leading to faulty alignment. Pathomechanics often cause overuse syndromes.

Knowing sport hazards The more the examiner of sports injuries knows about how a sport is performed and its potential for trauma, the better an injury assessment can be. To fully understand injuries that occur in a sport, a detailed knowledge of the correct kinesiological and biomechanical principles that should be applied is necessary. Violation of these principles can lead to repetitive and overuse syndromes. Understanding how an acute or chronic injury might occur helps the examiner "zero in" more directly on tissues that have been affected.

Descriptive Assessment Terms

When evaluating sports injuries, selected terms are used to describe and characterize what is being learned about the condition. The student should become familiar with these terms.

Etiology refers to the cause of an injury or disease. In sports medicine, the term *mechanism* is often exchanged for etiology. **Pathology** refers to the structural and functional changes that result from the injury process.

After understanding of an injury's etiology, symptoms and signs are ascertained. **Symptom** refers to a perceptible change in an athlete's body or its functions that indicates an injury or disease. Symptoms are subjective and are described by the athlete to the coach, athletic trainer, or physician. In comparison, a **sign** is objective, being definitive and obvious as an indicator for a specific condition. Signs are often determined when the athlete is examined.

After it is inspected, an injury may be assigned a degree or grade. First, second, or third degree corresponds to an injury that is mild, moderate, or severe, respectively. Sometimes grade is used in place of degree, depending on the examiner's preference. To add to this confusion, grades may be combined with degrees. For example, the

TABLE 10-1 Standard Orthopedic Definitions for Positions and Deviations

Term	Definition
Abduction	To draw away or deviate from the midline of the body
Adduction	To deviate toward or draw toward the midline of the body
Eversion	Turning outward
Extension	To straighten; when the part distal to a joint extends, it straightens; joint angle decreases toward 0 degrees
External rotation	Rotary motion in the transverse plane away from the midline
Flexion	To bend; when a joint is flexed, the part distal to the joint bends; joint angle increases toward 180 degrees
Internal rotation	Rotary motion in the transverse plane toward the midline
Inversion	Turning inward
Kyphosis	An increased rounding of the normal thoracic curve of the spine
Lordosis	The anterior concavity in the curvature of the lumbar and cervical spines when viewed from the side
Pronation	Assuming the foot is in a prone position, a combination of eversion and abduction movements, resulting in a lowering of the medial margin of the foot; when applied to the hand, it means the palm is turned downward
Supination	To assume a supine position; applied to the foot, it refers to raising the medial margin of the foot; applied to the palm of the hand, it refers to turning the palm upward
Valgus	Deviation of a part or portion of the extremity distal to a joint toward the midline of the body
Varus	Deviation of a part or portion of an extremity distal to a joint away from the midline of the body

first degree may be divided into two grades. Thus a first degree–grade one injury would be very mild, whereas a first degree–grade two injury would be more serious; however, it would be less serious than a second-degree, or moderate, injury. In most cases, a grade-three condition corresponds with moderate injury, and a grade-four condition corresponds with severe injury. To avoid confusion, students must carefully read, in detail, the description of the injury and make their own logical designation.

Diagnosis denotes the name of a specific condition. To establish the diagnosis of an athlete's injury or illness, all aspects of the condition must be studied. Once all the possible information has been gathered about the athlete's condition, a prognosis is made. This is a prediction of the course of the condition. In other words, the athlete is told what is to be expected as the injury heals. The amount of pain, swelling, or loss of function is discussed. **Prognosis** also refers to the projected outcome of an illness or injury and to the length of time predicted for complete recovery. For the athlete, prognosis translates into "the length of time before I can compete."

Sequela refers to a condition following and resulting from a disease or injury. It refers to the development of an additional condition as a complication of an existing disease or injury. For example, pneumonia might result from a bout with the flu, or osteoarthritis might follow a severe joint sprain.

The term **syndrome** is used throughout the text and refers to a group of symptoms and signs that, together, indicate a particular injury or disease.

EVALUATION OF SPORTS INJURIES

Injury evaluation is an essential part of athletic training. Each examiner must develop his or her own systematic approach to injury evaluation. Three distinct evaluations are commonly conducted: the primary, or on-site, injury inspection and evalu-

diagnosis
Name of a specific condition.

prognosis
Predicted outcome of an injury.

sequela
Condition resulting from disease or injury.

syndrome
Group of symptoms that indicate a condition or disease.

Focus

Musculoskeletal evaluation sequence

1. History
   a. Past
   b. Present
2. Observation
   a. General
   b. Specific
3. Physical examination
   a. Palpation
      (1) Bony
      (2) Soft tissue
   b. Movement
      (1) Active
      (2) Passive
      (3) Resistive
   c. Manual muscle test
   d. Neurological examination
      (1) Cerebral function
      (2) Cranial nerves
      (3) Cerebellar function
      (4) Sensory tests
      (5) Reflex tests
   e. Special tests
   f. Testing joint play
   g. Functional evaluation
   h. Postural evaluation

ation; the secondary, or off-site, injury evaluation; and the evaluation for determining the progress of a specific treatment regimen.

Primary Assessment or Survey

The primary assessment or survey, as discussed in Chapter 8, involves the determination of serious, life-threatening injuries and the proper disposition of the injured athlete. The secondary assessment or survey concerns the detailed sequence of evaluative procedures that determine specifically the nature, site, and severity of injury. A secondary assessment is done on the field immediately after injury to rule out those injuries that may potentially become life-threatening, to assess musculoskeletal injuries, and to determine how the athlete should be transported from the field. Once

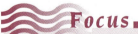

Focus

History of musculoskeletal injuries

Information to obtain:
- Chief complaints and present problems.
- If pain is present, its location, character, duration, variation, aggravation, distribution or radiation, intensity, and course.
- Is the pain increased or decreased by specific activities or stresses?
- What situation or trauma caused the problem?
- Has the problem occurred before? If so, when, and how was it treated? Was treatment successful?

the athlete is off the field, a more detailed secondary evaluation is performed according to the procedures described in this chapter.

Secondary Assessment

A secondary evaluation is more thoroughly performed once the athlete has been removed from the site of initial injury to a place of comfort and safety. This detailed assessment may be performed on the sidelines, in an emergency room, in the training room, or in a sports medicine clinic. Further inspection and evaluation may be performed when the injury is still in an acute phase or has become chronic or recurrent. The evaluation scheme is divided into three broad categories: history, general observation, and physical examination (see the Focus box, opposite). There are numerous special tests that provide additional information about the extent of injuries. The following discussion provides the student with a brief overview of some of the steps and techniques that can be used in a secondary evaluation. (Chapters 17 through 27 provide the reader with specific injury assessment procedures.)

History

Obtaining as much information as possible about the injury is of major importance to the examiner. Understanding how the injury may have occurred and listening to the complaints of the athlete and how key questions are answered can provide important clues to the exact nature of the injury. The examiner becomes a detective in pursuit of as much accurate information as possible, which will lead to a determination of the true nature of the injury (see the Focus box, opposite below). From the history, the examiner develops strategies for further examination and possible immediate and follow-up management.[3]

When obtaining a history, the examiner should do the following:
- Be calm and reassuring.
- Express questions that are simple, not leading.
- Listen carefully to the athlete's complaints.
- Maintain eye contact to try and see what the athlete is feeling.
- Record exactly what the athlete said without interpretation.

Questions might be stated under specific headings in an attempt to get as complete a historical picture as possible. In many cases, a history becomes clear-cut because the mechanism, trauma, and pathology are obvious; in other situations, symptoms and signs may be obscured.

Primary complaint If conscious and coherent, the athlete is encouraged to describe the injury in detail. If the athletic trainer or coach did not see the injury happen, try to get the athlete to describe in detail the mechanism of the injury. What is the problem? How did it occur? Did you fall? How did you land? Which direction did your joint move? When did it occur? Has this happened before? If so, when? Was something heard or felt when it occurred? If the athlete is unable to describe accurately how the injury occurred, perhaps a teammate or someone who observed the event can do so.

Injury location Ask the athlete to locate the area of complaint by pointing to it with one finger only. If the athlete can point to a specific pain site, it is probably a localized injury. If the exact pain site cannot be indicated, the injury may be generalized and nonspecific.

Pain characteristics What type of pain is it? Nerve pain is sharp, bright, or burning. Bone pain tends to be localized and piercing. Pain in the vascular system tends to be poorly localized, aching, and referred from another area. Muscle pain is often dull, aching, and referred to another area.[15] Determining pain origin makes the evaluation of musculoskeletal injuries difficult. The deeper the injury site, the more difficult it is to match the pain with the site of trauma. This factor often causes treatment to be performed at the wrong site. Conversely, the closer the injury is to the body surface, the better the elicited pain corresponds with the site of pain stimulation.[14]

Secondary assessment consists of:
History
Observation
Physical examination

10-1
Critical Thinking Exercise

A soccer player is taken down and lies on the field holding her knee. The athletic trainer comes onto the field and quickly examines the knee. There does not appear to be any major instability so the athlete is moved to the sideline where the trainer does a more careful evaluation. The athletic trainer is fairly certain that the soccer player has sustained a minor grade 1 MCL sprain and elects not to refer the athlete to the physician. The next day the athlete comes into the training room with a very swollen knee. The athletic trainer now decides to refer the athlete to the physician.

? On examination, the physician determines that the athlete does have an MCL sprain but has also sustained a tear of the medial meniscus. How could the athletic trainer have done a better job in handling this situation?

Does the pain change at different times? Pain that subsides during activity usually indicates a chronic inflammation. Pain that increases in a joint throughout the day indicates a progressive increase in edema.

Does the athlete feel sensations other than pain? Pressure on nerve roots can produce pain or a sensation of "pins and needles" (paresthesia). What movement, if any, causes pain or other sensations?

Joint responses   If the injury is related to a joint, is there instability? Does the joint feel as though it will give way? Does the joint lock and unlock? Positive responses may indicate that the joint has a loose body that is catching or that is inhibiting the normal muscular support in the area.

Determining whether the injury is acute or chronic   Ask the athlete how long he or she has had the symptoms and how frequently they appear.

General Observation

Along with gaining knowledge and understanding of the athlete's major complaint from a history, general observation is also performed, often at the same time the history is taken (see the Focus box below). What is observed is commonly modified by the athlete's major complaints. The following are suggested as specific points to observe:

1. How does the athlete move? Is there a limp? Are movements abnormally slow, jerky, and asynchronous? Is movement not possible in a body part?
2. Is the body held stiffly to protect against pain? Does the athlete's facial expression indicate pain or lack of sleep?
3. Are there any obvious body asymmetries? Is there an obvious deformity? Does soft tissue appear swollen or wasted as a result of atrophy? Are there unnatural protrusions or lumps such as occur with a dislocation or fracture? Is there a postural malalignment?
4. Are there abnormal sounds such as crepitus when the athlete moves?
5. Does a body area appear inflamed? Are there swelling, heat, and redness?

Physical Examination

In performing a more detailed examination of the musculoskeletal system, the examiner engages in palpation, movement assessment, neurological assessment, and special tests of specific body areas, such as testing joint play and posture when called for. At certain times functional tests are also given.

Palpation   Some examiners use palpation in the beginning of the examination procedure, whereas others use it only when they believe they have identified the specific injury site by other assessment means.[5,15] In some cases, palpation would be beneficial at both the beginning and the end of the examination. The two areas of palpation are bony and soft tissue. As with all examination procedures, palpation must be performed systematically, starting with very light pressure followed by gradu-

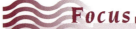

Focus

Observation of musculoskeletal injuries

Concerns During Observation:
- Is there obvious soft-tissue or bone deformity?
- Are limb positions symmetrical?
- How do the limbs' size, shape, color, temperature, and muscle tone compare?
- Are there trophic changes of the skin?
- Are there skin sites in which there is heat, swelling, or redness?
- Is the athlete willing to move a body part?
- Does the athlete display facial expressions indicating pain?

ally deeper pressure, usually beginning away from the site of complaint and then gradually moving toward it.

Bony palpation   Both the injured and noninjured sites should be palpated and compared. The sense of touch might reveal an abnormal gap at a joint, swelling on a bone, joints that are misaligned, or abnormal protuberances associated with a joint or a bone.

Soft-tissue palpation   Through palpation, with the athlete as relaxed as possible, normal soft-tissue relationships can be ascertained. Tissue deviations such as swellings, lumps, gaps, and abnormal muscle tensions and temperature variations can be detected. The palpation of soft tissue can detect where ligaments or tendons have torn. Variations in the shape of structures, differences in tissue tightness and textures, differentiation of tissue that is pliable and soft from tissue that is more resilient, and pulsations, tremors, and other involuntary muscle twitching can be discerned. Excessive skin dryness and moisture can also be noted. Abnormal skin sensations such as diminished sensation (dysesthesia), numbness (anesthesia), or increased sensation (hyperesthesia) can be noted. Like bony palpation, soft-tissue palpation must be performed on both sides of the body for comparison.

Movement assessment   If a joint or soft-tissue lesion exists, the athlete is likely to complain of pain on movement. Cyriax has developed a method for locating and identifying a lesion by applying tension selectively to each of the structures that might produce this pain.[5] Tissues are classified as being either contractile or inert. Contractile tissues include muscles and their tendons; inert tissues include bones, ligaments, joint capsules, fascia, bursae, nerve roots, and dura mater.

Movement examination includes:
Active movement
Passive movement
Resisted isometric movement

If a lesion is present in contractile tissue, pain will occur on active motion in one direction and on passive motion in the opposite direction. Thus a muscle strain would cause pain both on active contraction and passive stretch. Contractile tissues are tested through the midrange by an isometric contraction against maximum resistance. The specific location of the lesion within the musculotendinous unit cannot be specifically identified by the isometric contraction.[17]

A lesion of inert tissue will elicit pain on active and passive movement in the same direction. A sprain of a ligament will result in pain whenever that ligament is stretched either through active contraction or passive stretching. It is not possible to identify a specific lesion of inert tissue by looking at movement patterns alone; other special tests must be done to identify injured structures.[3]

Active movement   Movement assessment should begin with active range of motion (AROM). The athletic trainer should evaluate the quality of movement, range of movement, motion in other planes, movement at varying speeds, and strength throughout the range but in particular at the endpoint. A complaint of pain on active motion will not distinguish contractile pain from inert pain, so the athletic trainer must proceed with an evaluation of both passive and resistive motion. An athlete who seems to be pain free in each of these tests throughout a full range should be tested by applying passive pressure at the endpoint.

Active movement refers to joint motion that occurs because of muscle contraction.

Passive movement   When assessing passive range of motion (PROM) the athlete must relax completely and allow the athletic trainer to move the extremity to reduce the influence of the contractile elements. Particular attention should be directed toward the sensation of the athlete at the end of the passive range. The athletic trainer should categorize the "feel" of the endpoints as follows.[4]

NORMAL ENDPOINTS   Normal endpoints include the following:

- Soft-tissue approximation—soft and spongy, a gradual painless stop (e.g., knee flexion).
- Capsular feel—an abrupt, hard, firm endpoint with only a little give (e.g., endpoint of hip rotation).
- Bone to bone—a distinct and abrupt endpoint when two hard surfaces come in contact with one another (e.g., elbow in full extension).

Passive movement refers to movement that is performed completely by the examiner.

- Muscular—springy feel with some associated discomfort (e.g., end of shoulder abduction).

ABNORMAL ENDPOINTS   Abnormal endpoints include the following:

- Empty feel—movement is definitely beyond the anatomical limit, and pain occurs before the end of the range (e.g., a complete ligament rupture).
- Spasm—involuntary muscle contraction that prevents motion because of pain; should also be called guarding (e.g., back spasms).
- Loose—occurs in extreme hypermobility (e.g., previously sprained ankle).[15]
- Springy block—a rebound at the endpoint (e.g., meniscus tear).

Throughout the passive range of movement, the athletic trainer is looking for limitation in movement and the presence of pain. If the athlete reports pain before the end of the available range, this probably indicates acute inflammation in which stretching and manipulation are both contraindicated as treatments. Pain occuring synchronous with the end of the range indicates that the condition is subacute and has progressed to some inert tissue fibrosis. If no pain occurs at the end of the range, the condition is chronic and contractures have replaced inflammation.[21]

Resisted motions   The purpose of resisting movement is to evaluate the status of the contractile tissues. The athlete is asked to perform an isometric contraction near the midrange of movement to avoid a position in which there is pinching of other inert structures around the joint. It should also be mentioned that muscular contraction is under neural control; thus lesions of the nervous system may affect the strength of muscular contraction. Cyriax has designed the following system for differentiating lesions through assessment of muscular contraction.[4]

1. Strong and painless—normal muscle.
2. Strong and painful—minor lesion in some part of the muscle or tendon.
3. Weak and painless—complete rupture of muscle or tendon or some nervous system disorder.
4. Weak and painful—a gross lesion of contractile tissue.
5. Pain on repetition—a single contraction is strong and painless, but repetition produces pain as would exist in some vascular disorder.
6. All muscles painful—may indicate a serious emotional or psychological problem.

Goniometric measurement of joint range   Goniometry, which measures joint range of motion, is an essential procedure during the early, intermediate, and late stages of injury. Full range of motion of an affected body part is a major criterion for the return of the athlete to participation. Active and passive joint range of motion can be measured using goniometry (Figure 10-4).

Although a number of different types of goniometers are on the market, the most commonly used are ones that measure 0 to 180 degrees in each direction. The arms of the instrument are usually 12 to 16 inches (30 to 40 cm) long, with one arm stationary and the other fully movable.[4,8]

When measuring joint range of motion, the goniometer should generally be placed along the lateral surface of the extremity being measured. The 0, or starting, position for any movement is identical to the standard anatomical position. The athlete should move the joint either actively or passively through the available range to the endpoint. The stationary arm of the goniometer should be placed parallel with the longitudinal axis of the fixed reference part. The movable arm should be placed along the longitudinal axis of the movable segment. (NOTE: The axis of rotation will change throughout the range as movement occurs. Thus the axis of rotation is located at the intersection of the stationary and movable arms.) A reading in degrees of motion should be taken and recorded as either active or passive range of motion for that specific movement. Accuracy and consistency in goniometric measurement require practice and repetition.

Resisted movement requires an isometric contraction at the midpoint in the range.

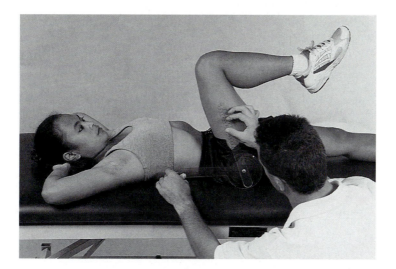

Figure 10-4
Goniometric measurement of
hip joint flexion.

The normal available range of motion for specific movements at individual joints is indicated in Table 10-2. Specific goniometric measurement techniques for each joint are described in Chapters 17 through 26.

Manual muscle testing   Manual muscle testing is an integral part of the physical examination process.[10] The ability of the injured athlete to tolerate varying levels of resistance can indicate a great deal about the extent of the injury to the contractile units. For the athlete, the limitation in muscular strength is generally caused by pain. As pain diminishes and the healing process progresses, levels of muscular strength gradually return to normal. The development of isokinetic testing devices has enabled the athletic trainer to test levels of muscular strength objectively within the limitations of those devices.[6]

Manual muscle testing is usually performed with the athlete positioned such that individual muscles or muscle groups can be isolated and tested through a full range of motion through the application of manual resistance. The ability of the athlete to move through a full range of motion or to offer resistance to movement is subjectively graded by the athletic trainer according to various classification systems and grading criteria that have been developed. Table 10-3 indicates a commonly used grading system for manual muscle testing.

Neurological examination   The neurological examination usually follows manual muscle testing. It consists of five major areas: cerebral function, cranial nerve function, cerebellar function, sensory testing, and reflex testing. In cases of musculoskeletal injury that does not involve head injury, it is generally not necessary to assess cerebral function, cranial nerve function, and cerebellar function. The athletic trainer should concentrate instead on sensation testing and reflex testing to determine involvement of the peripheral nervous system after injury.

Cerebral function   Tests for general cerebral function include questions that assess general affect, level of consciousness, intellectual performance, emotional status, thought content, sensory interpretation (visual, auditory, tactile), and language skills.

Cranial nerve function   The function of the twelve cranial nerves can be quickly determined by assessing the quality of the following: sense of smell, eye tracking, imitation of facial expressions, biting down, balance, swallowing, tongue protrusion, and strength of shoulder shrugs.

Cerebellar function   Because the cerebellum controls purposeful coordinated movement, tests such as touching finger to nose, finger to finger of examiner, drawing alphabets in the air with the foot, heel-toe walking, and others will determine dysfunction.

10-2

Critical Thinking Exercise

An athletic trainer is evaluating a volleyball player who complains of pain in her elbow. During the evaluation, manual muscle testing and active and passive range of motion tests reveal pain when the elbow is moved into extension both actively and passively. However, there is no pain when the elbow is moved actively into flexion.

? Is it more likely that the injury involves the ligament or the musculotendinous unit?

Neurological examination: cerebral function, cranial nerve function, cerebellar function, sensory testing, reflex testing.

TABLE 10-2   **Range of Joint Motion**

Joint	Action	Degrees of Motion
Shoulder	Flexion	180
	Extension	50
	Adduction	40
	Abduction	180
	Medial rotation	90
	Lateral rotation	90
Elbow	Flexion	145
Forearm	Pronation	80
	Supination	85
Wrist	Flexion	80
	Extension	70
	Abduction	20
	Adduction	45
Hip	Flexion	125
	Extension	10
	Abduction	45
	Adduction	40
	Medial rotation	45
	Lateral rotation	45
Knee	Flexion	140
Ankle	Flexion	45
	Extension	20
Foot	Inversion	40
	Eversion	20

TABLE 10-3   **Manual Muscle Strength Grading**

Grade	Percentage (%)	Value of Concentration	Muscle Strength
5	100	Normal	Complete range of motion (ROM) against gravity, with full resistance
4	75	Good	Complete ROM against gravity, with some resistance
3	50	Fair	Complete ROM against gravity, with no resistance
2	25	Poor	Complete ROM, with gravity omitted
1	10	Trace	Evidence of slight contractility, with no joint motion
0	0	Zero	No evidence of muscle contractility

Sensory testing   A major component of musculoskeletal assessment is determining the distribution of peripheral nerves and dermatomes. Although peripheral nerve distribution varies with individuals, it is more predictable than dermatome distribution.[6] As the examination progresses, the examiner scrutinizes the variance, if any, in sensation from one side of the body to the other or on the same side. Superficial sensation is commonly tested with a pin, and deep pain may be elicited by squeezing the muscle of the specific body part.[11] In testing for altered sensation, referred pain should be considered a possibility (Figure 10-5).

Reflex testing   The term *reflex* refers to an involuntary response to a stimulus. In terms of the neurological examination there are three types of reflexes: deep tendon reflexes, superficial reflexes, and pathological reflexes.

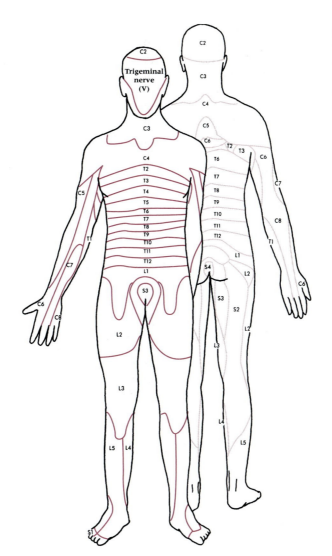

Figure 10-5

Numbness, referred pain, or other nerve involvements often follow the segmental distribution of spinal nerves on the skin's surface.

A deep tendon reflex is caused by stimulation of the stretch reflex (Chapter 3) and results in an involuntary contraction of a muscle because of stretch of its tendon. Deep tendon reflexes can be elicited at the tendons of the biceps, brachioradialis, triceps, patella, and Achilles. Table 10-4 shows a grading system for deep reflexes.[9]

Superficial reflexes are elicited by stimulation of the skin at specific sites, which produces a reflex muscle contraction. Superficial reflexes include abdominal, cremasteric, plantar, and anal. An absence of a superficial reflex is indicative of some lesion in the cerebral cortex of the brain.[9]

Pathological reflexes are also superficial reflexes. The presence of a pathological reflex indicates a lesion in the cerebral cortex; an absence indicates integrity. Babinski's sign, in which stroking of the lateral plantar surface produces extension and splaying of the toes, is an example of a pathological reflex.[9]

Determining projected referred pain   As discussed in Chapter 7, a complaint of deep, burning pain or of an ache that is diffused or of a painful area with no signs of disorder or malfunctioning is most likely referred pain.[4] Cyriax considers that the common sites for pain referral are, in order of importance, joint capsule, tendon, muscle, ligament, and bursa.[4] Pressures from the dura mater or nerve sheath can also produce referred pain or other sensory responses. Palpation of what is thought to be the area at fault often is misleading. Detecting the selective tension of the tissue at fault is one of the best means for gathering correct data. Some musculoskel-

TABLE 10-4 Reflex Grading

	Grade	Definition
Absence of a reflex	0	Areflexia
Diminished reflex	1	Hyporeflexia
Average reflex	2	
Exaggerated reflex	3	Hyperreflexia
Clonus	4	Spasmodic alteration of muscle contraction and relaxation, indicating a nerve irritation

joint play
Movement that is not voluntary but accessory.

Functional examination determines if there is full strength, joint stability, and coordination and if the part is pain free.

etal pain is caused by myofascial trigger points, which are not related to deeper, referred-type pain. Palpation is used to determine the presence or absence of tense tissue bands and tender trigger points.

Special tests Special tests have been designed for almost every body region as means for detecting specific pathologies. They are often used to substantiate what has been learned from other testing. For example, special tests are commonly used to determine ligament stability, impingement signs, tightness of specific structures, blood circulation, muscle imbalance, and body alignment discrepancies. (See Chapters 17 through 25.)

Testing joint play Joint play refers to that movement, found in diathroidial joints, that is not voluntary but accessory, being revealed by specific stresses applied by the examiner. A joint that has lost its joint play is dysfunctional, leading to pathology. Techniques of joint mobilization are designed to free these joints.[12] To be tested, the joint is positioned in the position of least strain, which is often called the loose-pack position.[11,15] Joint mobilization is discussed in detail in Chapter 15.

Functional evaluation The functional evaluation of an athlete may be performed early in the initial examination or be made to determine whether or not rehabilitation has been successful. It is an important factor that precedes the return to full sports participation. A functional evaluation proceeds gradually from little stress to one that mimics the actual stress that would normally come from full sports participation. The major concern is whether the athlete has regained full strength, joint stability, and coordination and is pain free. A lack of any one of these abilities may be a factor in excluding the athlete from his or her sport.

Postural examination As discussed in Chapter 24, many cases of injuries in athletes can be attributed to body malalignments. Musculoskeletal assessment might be one area of a postural examination. It is designed to test for malalignments and asymmetries by viewing the body in comparison to a grid or plumb line (see Figures 24-23 through 24-25).

SOAP Notes

Documentation of acute athletic injury can be effectively accomplished through a system designed to record subjective and objective findings and to document the immediate and future treatment plan for the athlete (subjective, objective, assessment, and plan, or SOAP).[20] This method combines information provided by the athlete and the observations of the examiner.[13] Figure 10-6 presents a recommended injury report form that includes these components of documentation. This form also includes a provision to document findings arising from more definitive evaluation or from the examiner's subsequent day evaluation.

S (Subjective)

This component includes the subjective statements provided by the injured athlete. History taking is designed to elicit the subjective impressions of the athlete relative to time, mechanism, and site of injury. The type and course of the pain and the degree of disability experienced by the athlete are also noteworthy.

10-3

Critical Thinking Exercise

A fencer comes into the training room complaining of pain in his shoulder that he has had for about a week. He indicates that he first hurt the shoulder when lifting weights but did not think it was a bad injury. During the past week he has not been able to lift because of pain. He has continued to fence during practice, but his shoulder seems to be getting worse instead of better.

? When doing a standard evaluation, what would be a normal evaluation scheme that an athletic trainer might use?

O (Objective)

Objective findings result from the athletic trainer's visual inspection, palpation, and assessment of active, passive, and resistive motion. Findings of special testing should also be noted here. Thus the objective report would include assessment of posture, presence of deformity or swelling, and location of point tenderness. Also, limitations of active motion and pain arising or disappearing during passive and resistive motion should be noted. Finally, the results of special tests relative to joint stability or apprehension are also included.

A (Assessment)

Assessment of the injury is the athletic trainer's professional judgment with regard to impression and nature of injury. Although the exact nature of the injury will not always be known initially, information pertaining to suspected site and anatomical structures involved is appropriate. A judgment of severity may be included but is not essential at the time of acute injury evaluation.

P (Plan)

The plan should include the first aid treatment rendered to the athlete and the sports therapist's intentions relative to disposition. Disposition may include referral for more definitive evaluation or simply application of splint, wrap, or crutches and a request to report for reevaluation the next day. If the injury is of a more chronic nature, the examiner's plan for treatment and therapeutic exercise would be appropriate.

Additional Diagnostic Tests

The physician, as does the athletic trainer, often performs a detailed musculoskeletal examination. Often, the physician and the athletic trainer will discuss and compare their individual findings. Because the physician is legally charged with the diagnosis and course of treatment, he or she may have to acquire and compare additional information, which may come from roentgenograms (x-rays), arthrography, arthroscopy, or myelography or through newer imaging techniques such as computed tomography (CT), bone scanning, magnetic resonance imaging (MRI), and sonography. Other tests might include electromyography, determining nerve conduction velocity, synovial fluid analysis, blood testing, and urinalysis.

Blood Testing

The physician may decide to run a complete blood count (CBC) on the athlete for many different reasons. The most common reasons are to screen for anemia (too few red cells) or infection (too many white cells).[22] Samples may be taken in a syringe from a vein in the arm or from a needle stick in the finger. A routine CBC addresses the following:

- Red blood cell count looks at the number of cells per unit volume to detect anemias, prolonged infections, iron deficiencies, internal bleeding, and certain types of cancers.
- Hemoglobin levels are closely associated with red blood cell count and tend to reflect overall blood volume.
- Hematocrit measures how much of the total blood volume is made up of red blood cells. A low hematocrit indicates certain types of anemias.
- White blood cell count is used to determine the presence of bacteria. Differentiation of white cell types microscopically can identify specific types of infection.
- A deficiency in the platelet count can lead to dangerous internal bleeding.

Normal laboratory values for the CBC are summarized in Table 10-5.

Urinalysis

Urinalysis is a common test that can yield a large quantity of information.[18] In most cases a sample of urine in a small dry container is all that is needed. If the urine will

---

SOAP note:
  Subjective
  Objective
  Assessment
  Plan

10-4

Critical Thinking Exercise

A receiver in football has his feet taken out from under him by a tackler and lands flat on his low back with his legs above him. An on-the-field evaluation reveals that there is unilateral decreased muscle strength, decreased sensation, and a decreased patellar tendon reflex in the right lower extremity.

? Based on the findings of the evaluation, how should the athletic trainer manage this injury?

INJURY REPORT FORM

ATHLETE'S NAME _____ DATE OF INJURY _____

INJURY SITE: R L _____ TODAY'S DATE _____

SPORT _____

Subjective findings (history):

Objective findings (inspection, palpation, mobility, and special tests):

Assessment (impression):

Plan (treatment administered and disposition):

Follow-up notes: Date _____

EVALUATED BY _____

RECORDED BY _____

Figure 10-6

SOAP note form.

not be analyzed within 1 hour the sample should be refrigerated. A routine urinalysis addresses the following[22]:

- Specific gravity indicates the ability of the kidney to concentrate and dilute fluids.
- The pH refers to how acid or alkaline the urine is. It may be acidic in cases of diabetes or dehydration. Alkaline urine is present in urinary tract infections and kidney disease.
- Presence of glucose in the urine may indicate diabetes.
- Presence of ketones, a by-product of fat metabolism, may also indicate diabetes.
- Presence of hemoglobin may appear in urine after intense exercise or from kidney disease.
- Presence of protein indicates kidney disease.
- Presence of nitrate indicates infection.
- A small amount of urine is examined under a microscope to find red blood cells, white blood cells, and bacteria.
- If bacteria are present, a urine culture may be necessary to determine the specific bacteria causing an infection.

TABLE 10-5 Normal Laboratory Values of a Complete Blood Count

Test	Normal Values
Red blood cell count	Males 5.4 million/mm^3
	Females 4.8 million/mm^3
White blood cell count	5000-9000/mm^3
Platelet count	250,000-400,000/mm^3
Hematocrit	Male 40%-54%
	Female 38%-47%
Hemoglobin	Male 14-16.5 g/100 ml
	Female 12-15 g/100ml

■ Many additional tests may also be done on urine, including electrolytes, hormones, and drug levels.

Normal laboratory values for a standard urinalysis are listed in Table 10-6.

Roentgenograms (X-rays)

An x-ray examination is designed to rule out serious disease such as an infection or neoplasm. It assists the physician in determining fractures and dislocations or any bone abnormality that may be present. An experienced physician can detect some soft-tissue factors, such as joint swelling and ectopic bone development in ligaments and tendons[2] (Figure 10-7, *A*).

Arthrography

Arthrography is the visual study of a joint through x-ray study after injection of an opaque dye, air, or a combination of air and opaque dye into the joint space. This procedure can show the disruption of soft tissue and loose bodies in the joint.

Arthroscopy

The fiberoptic arthroscope is widely used by orthopedists in surgery. It is considered more accurate than the arthrogram but is more invasive, requiring anesthesia and a small incision for the introduction of the arthroscope (endoscope) into the joint space. While the arthroscope is in the joint, the surgeon can perform surgical procedures such as removing loose bodies and, in some cases, suturing torn tissues.[16]

Arthroscopy uses a fiberoptic arthroscope to view the inside of a joint.

Myelography

During myelography an opaque dye is introduced into the spinal canal (epidural space) through a lumbar puncture. While the patient is tilted, the dye is allowed to flow to different levels of the spinal cord. Using this contrast medium, physicians can detect conditions such as tumors, nerve root compression, and disk disease, as well as other diseases within the spinal cord.

Computed Tomography

Computed tomography penetrates the body with a thin fan-shaped x-ray beam, producing a cross-sectional view of tissues. Unlike x-ray studies, this viewing can be performed from many angles. As the machine scans, a computer compares the many views; these electrical signals are then processed by a computer into a visual image (Figure 10-7, *B*).

Bone Scanning

A bone scan involves the introduction of a radioactive tracer such as technetium-99 intravenously. By imaging the entire skeleton or part of a skeleton, bony lesions in which there is some inflammation, such as stress fractures, can be detected (Figure 10-7, *C*).

TABLE 10-6 **Normal Laboratory Values of a Urinalysis**

Test	Normal Values
Output	1000-1500 ml
Color	Yellow to amber and clear
Specific gravity	1.010-1.025
Osmolality	500-800 mosm/kg water
pH	4.6-4.8
Uric acid	0.6-1 g/24 hr
Urea	23-25 g/24 hr
Creatine	1-2g/24 hr

Figure 10-7

Figure 10-7

Examination of the knee. **A,** X-ray. **B,** CT scan. **C,** Bone scan. *(continued)*

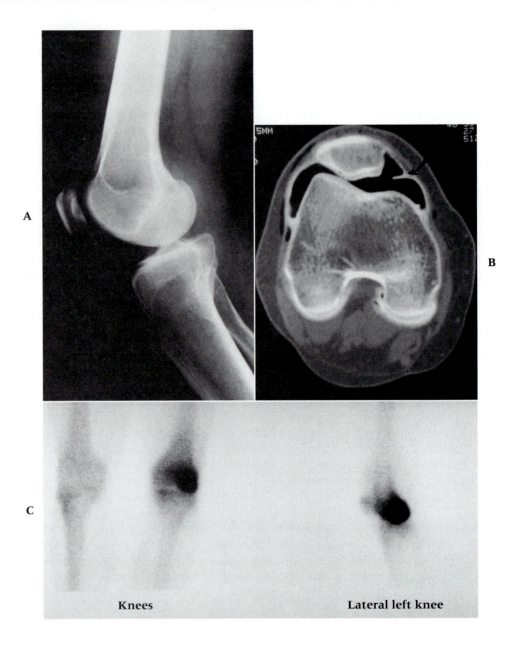

Knees   **Lateral left knee**

10-5

Critical Thinking Exercise

A field hockey player is tripped, twists her knee, and falls hard on artificial turf on that same knee. There is immediate swelling and pain. After evaluation the athletic trainer is not sure what the injury is and sends the athlete directly to the physician for diagnosis. The physician decides that additional diagnostic tests are necessary to determine the exact pathology.

? What diagnostic tests is the physician likely to order to determine the exact nature and extent of the knee injury?

Magnetic Resonance Imaging

Magnetic resonance imaging surrounds the body with powerful electromagnets, creating a field as much as 600,000 times as strong as that of the earth.[2] The magnetic current focuses on hydrogen atoms in water molecules and aligns them; when the current is shut off, the atoms continue to spin, emitting an energy that is detected by the computer. The hydrogen atoms in different tissue spin at different rates, thus producing different images. In many ways MRI provides clearer images than CT scanning. Despite its expense it is currently the test of choice by physicians for detecting soft-tissue lesions (Figure 10-7, *D*).

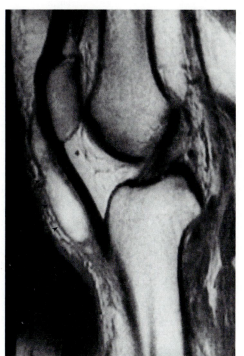

Figure 10-7—cont'd
D, MRI.

D

Sonography

Sonography is the use of sound waves to view the interior of the body. It uses a piezoelectric crystal that converts electrical pulses into vibrations that can penetrate the body. The sound waves reflect back to the crystal, which reconverts them into electrical signals and forms a picture.

Electromyography

Various muscular conditions can be detected by using electromyography. Electromyography refers to a muscular contraction that follows an electrical stimulation. The procedure consists of inserting a thin electrode needle into the muscle to be studied. Motor unit potentials can be observed on an oscilloscope screen or from a graphic recording called an electromyogram. Denervated muscles, as well as nerve root compression or other nerve compression sites, can be detected by electromyography.[2] Other muscle disease can be confirmed through this method.

Nerve Conduction Velocity

Determining the conduction velocity of a nerve may provide key information to the physician about a number of neuromuscular conditions. After a stimulus is applied to a peripheral nerve, the speed with which a muscle action occurs is measured. Delays in conduction might indicate nerve compression or other muscular or nerve disease.

Synovial Fluid Analysis

On occasion, the physician will opt to make an analysis of an athlete's synovial fluid. The purpose of this test is to detect whether an infection is present. The test also confirms the diagnosis of gout and differentiates noninflammatory joint disease such as degenerative arthritis from inflammatory conditions such as rheumatoid arthritis.[2]

Analysis of synovial fluid and blood can be used to detect musculoskeletal infections.

SUMMARY

- Injury evaluation is a proficiency needed by all athletic trainers and sports physicians. In sports medicine, assessment is used in first aid and under secondary circumstances.
- Athletic trainers recognize and evaluate, whereas physicians, according to the law, diagnose sports injuries. Diagnosis refers to identifying a disease, injury, or syndrome.
- To assess effectively, an examiner of athletes with sports injuries must have a foundation in a number of areas. This foundation consists of a thorough background in human anatomy, including surface anatomy, body planes, and anatomical directions. Of particular importance is an in-depth understanding of the musculoskeletal system, with special focus on adverse biomechanical forces, which become pathomechanical. Every examiner of sports trauma must have a clear knowledge of injuries that can be sustained in a particular sport.
- After they are assessed, sports injuries must be described in a similar manner, using the following terms: etiology or mechanism, symptoms and signs, and the degree of trauma that is considered to have occurred. A diagnosis is made by a physician, who then establishes a prognosis for the condition.
- Assessment may be categorized into the primary emergency or first aid type and the secondary, more detailed, follow-up type. Secondary assessment consists of a more detailed procedure. It consists of three major areas: history, general observation, and the actual physical examination. The physical examination includes palpation, movement assessment, and the neurological examination. Special tests may also be warranted, depending on the body site. Joint play testing, a postural examination, and a functional evaluation are other possible assessments that may be used by an examiner.
- Besides the assessment procedures mentioned, a physical examination may require additional information before an accurate diagnosis can be made. This information may include a variety of diagnostic tests such as blood test, urinalysis, x-ray, arthrograms, arthroscopy, computed tomography scans, bone scans, magnetic resonance imaging, or sonography. When there is muscle injury, electromyography or determining nerve conduction velocity may be used. In cases of suspected infection, a synovial fluid analysis may be required.

Solutions to Critical Thinking EXERCISES

10-1 The athletic trainer must realize that the physician has more training and is usually more skilled in injury diagnosis. Although the athletic trainer correctly identified the MCL sprain, the meniscus tear was completely overlooked. The athletic trainer should routinely refer an injured athlete to the physician for diagnosis. The injury evaluation done by the athletic trainer should reveal the same results as the physician diagnosis.

10-2 In this case a ligamentous injury is more likely. A lesion of inert tissue will elicit pain on active and passive movement in the same direction. If a lesion is present in contractile tissue, pain will occur on active motion in one direction and on passive motion in the opposite direction. A sprain of a ligament will result in pain whenever that ligament is stretched either through active contraction or passive stretching.

10-3 The athletic trainer should first take a subjective history from the injured athlete, followed by an objective examination that includes observation, palpation, range-of-motion testing, manual muscle testing, a neurological examination, special tests, tests for joint stability, and a functional performance evaluation.

10-4 Generally, injury to the spinal cord would result in bilateral symptoms. Unilateral changes are more indicative of peripheral nerve injury. However, any change in the neurological status of the athlete is cause for great concern. The athletic trainer should remove the athlete from the playing field using a stretcher or preferably a spine board.

10-5 Initially it is likely that standard knee radiographs (x-rays) would be used to determine the presence of a fracture. An MRI is widely used by sports medicine physicians to determine injury to ligamentous, meniscal, or other soft tissues. On occasion a diagnostic arthroscopy might be done to allow direct observation of the injured structures.

REVIEW QUESTIONS AND CLASS ACTIVITIES

1. Differentiate between injury evaluation and diagnosis.
2. What basic knowledge must the examiner have before making an injury assessment?

3. Explain the key terminology necessary to communicate the results of an assessment.
4. Identify the various descriptive assessment terms.
5. How should an examiner take a history? What questions should be asked?
6. Describe palpation and when and how it should be performed.
7. What can be ascertained from active, passive, and resisted isometric movement?
8. Explain how muscle testing, reflex testing, and sensation testing are performed.
9. What part do special tests, testing joint play, and postural examination play in injury assessment?
10. When should a functional evaluation be given?
11. What information should be included in a SOAP note?
12. What insights can a physician gain by having special laboratory tests performed? Describe each test in detail.

REFERENCES

1. Barak T, Rosen E, Sofer R: Mobility: passive orthopedic manual therapy. In Gould J, Davies G, editors: *Orthopedic and sports physical therapy,* St Louis, 1994, Mosby.
2. Birnbaum JS: *The musculoskeletal manual,* Orlando, 1986, Grune & Stratton.
3. Bates B: *A guide to physical examination and history taking,* Philadelphia, 1991, Lippincott.
4. Clarkson H, Gilewich G: *Musculoskeletal assessment: joint range of motion and manual muscle strength,* Baltimore, 1989, Williams & Wilkins.
5. Cyriax J: *Textbook of orthopaedic medicine,* ed 8, London, 1982, Bailliere Tindale.
6. Daniels L, Worthingham C: *Muscle testing: techniques of manual examination,* Philadelphia, 1989, Saunders.
7. Ellison AE, chairman, editorial board: *Athletic training and sports medicine,* Chicago, 1984, American Academy of Orthopaedic Surgeons.
8. Gehring P: Physical assessment begins with a history, *RN* 54(11):27, 1991.
9. Hartley A: *Practical joint assessment,* St Louis, 1991, Mosby.
10. Hoppenfeld S: *Physical examination of the spine and extremities,* New York, 1976, Appleton-Century-Crofts.
11. Kaltenborn FM: *Mobilization of the extremity joints: examination and basic treatments,* Oslo, 1980, Olaf Norlis Bokhandel.
12. Kendall F, Kendall E: *Muscles testing and function,* Baltimore, 1983, Williams & Wilkins.
13. Kettenbach G: *Writing SOAP notes,* Philadelphia, 1990, Davis.
14. Lynch MK, Kessler RM: Pain. In Kessler RM, Hertling D, editors: *Management of common musculoskeletal disorders,* Philadelphia, 1983, Harper & Row.
15. Magee DL: *Orthopedic physical assessment,* Philadelphia, 1992, Saunders.
16. Minkoff J, Putterman E: The unheralded value of arthroscopy using local anesthetic for diagnostic specificity and intraoperative corroboration of therapeutic achievement. In Minkoff J, Sherman OH, editors: *Clinics in sports medicine,* vol 6, no 3, Philadelphia, 1987, Saunders.
17. Moore ML: Clinical assessment of joint motion. In Basmajian JF, editor: *Therapeutic exercise,* ed 3, Baltimore, 1978, Williams & Wilkins.
18. Peterson M, Holbrook J, Von-Hales D: Contributions of the history, physical examination, and laboratory investigation in making medical diagnosis, *West J Med* 156(2): 163, 1992.
19. Post M: *Physical examination of the musculoskeletal system,* Chicago, 1987, Year Book.
20. Prentice W: *Rehabilitation techniques in sports medicine,* St Louis, 1994, Mosby.
21. Wadsworth C: *Manual examination and treatment of the spine and extremities,* Baltimore, 1988, Williams & Wilkins.
22. Wurman R: *Medical access,* Los Angeles, 1985, Access Press.

ANNOTATED BIBLIOGRAPHY

Birnbaum JS: *The musculoskeletal manual,* Orlando, 1986, Grune & Stratton.

Written for medical professionals who require a direct and simple approach for recognizing and managing musculoskeletal problems. A great number of the conditions discussed relate to sports trauma.

Booher JM, Thibodeau GA: *Athletic injury assessment,* ed 3, St Louis, 1994, Mosby.

An outstanding text addressed directly to the practitioner in sports medicine or athletic training. All aspects of musculoskeletal and internal sports injuries are considered.

Cyriax J, Cyriax P: *Illustrated manual of orthopaedic medicine,* London, 1983, Butterworth.

A beautifully color-illustrated text designed for diagnosing and providing Cyriax management to musculoskeletal conditions.

Gross J, Fetto J, Rosen E: *Musculoskeletal examination,* Cambridge, Mass, 1996, Blackwell Scientific.

An evaluation text written primarily for physicians.

Hoppenfeld S: Physical examination of the spine and extremities, New York, 1976, Appleton-Century-Crofts.

Presents an easy-to-follow, methodical, and in-depth procedure for examining musculoskeletal conditions.

Magee DJ: *Orthopedic physical assessment,* Philadelphia, 1987, Saunders.

An extremely well-illustrated book, with excellent depth of coverage. Its strength lies in its coverage of injuries commonly found during athletic training.

Post M: *Physical examination of the musculoskeletal system,* Chicago, 1987, Year Book.

A text that has been contributed to by many experts in the field of orthopedic examination. Each major joint is covered in detail.

Starkey C, Ryan J: *Evaluation of orthopedic and athletic injuries,* Philadelphia, 1996, FA Davis.

A detailed, well-illustrated text that addresses all aspects of injury assessment for the athletic trainer.

Psychology of Sport Injury and Illness

When you finish this chapter, you should be able to

- Describe why and under what circumstances sports participation is a psychological stressor.
- Explain all the aspects of overtraining and staleness that stem from sports.
- Define the conflict adjustments that may occur as a result of becoming over-stressed in sports.
- Identify physiological responses to stress.
- Describe how an athlete may respond psychologically to injuries or illnesses.
- Describe the roles of coaches, athletic trainers, and physicians when working with an overly stressed athlete.

The injured or ill athlete experiences not only physical disability but also major psychological reactions. The sports medicine team and the coach must understand how feelings and emotions enter into an athlete's reaction to serious injury or illness and the rehabilitation process[21] (Figure 11-1).

STRESS IN SPORT

stress

The positive and negative forces than can disrupt the body's equilibrium.

Sports participation is both a physical and an emotional stressor.

Stress is not something that an athlete can do to his or her body, but it is something that the brain tells the athlete is happening.[17] When change occurs, the brain interprets that change and tells the body how to react to it. Selye[22] also considers stress as not necessarily implying a morbid change, but a change that could also be associated with intense pleasure.

Sports participation serves as both a physical and an emotional stressor. Stress can be a positive or negative influence. All living organisms are endowed with the ability to cope effectively with stressful situations. Pelletier[17] stated that "without stress, there would be very little constructive activity or positive change." Negative stress can contribute to poor health, whereas positive stress produces growth and development. A healthy life must have a balance of stress; too little causes a "rusting out," and too much stress can cause "burnout."

Athletes place their bodies in countless daily stress situations. Their bodies undergo numerous "fight-or-flight" reactions to avoid injury or other threatening situations.[20]

Physiological Responses to Stress

Stress is a psychophysiological phenomenon. A serious sports injury is a major stressor for the athlete. Three phases characterize this stressor: alarm, resistance, and exhaustion.[22]

Alarm

In the alarm stage, secretions from the adrenal gland sharply increase, creating the well-known flight-or-fight response. With adrenaline in the bloodstream, pupils dilate, hearing becomes more acute, muscles become more responsive, and blood pressure increases to facilitate the absorption of oxygen. In addition to these responses, respiration and heart rate increase to further prepare the body for action.

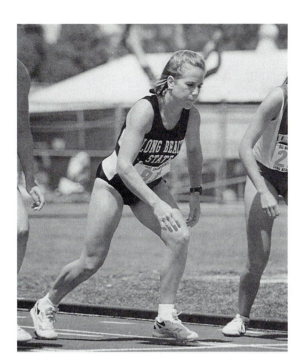

Figure 11-1

Sports participation can cause the athlete to experience either negative or positive stress.

Resistance

After the alarm stage, the body gradually changes to the resistance stage. During this stage, the body prepares itself for coping by diminishing the adrenocortical secretions and directing stress to a particular body site. This stage is the body's way of resisting the stressor. Physiological response may remain high and could eventually lead to the final stage, exhaustion.

Exhaustion

The exhaustion stage refers to an entire organ system, or a single organ, becoming dysfunctional and diseased as a result of chronic stress. It is generally accepted that chronic stress can adversely affect brain function, the autonomic nervous system, the endocrine system, and the immune system, eventually leading to a psychosomatic illness.[2]

Thus it is concluded that there are two kinds of stress—acute and chronic. During acute stress, the threat is immediate, and response is instantaneous. Physiologically, the body remains in the alarm stage. The primary reaction of the alarm stage is produced by the epinephrine and norepinephrine of the adrenal medulla. Chronic stress primarily involves the stages of resistance and exhaustion. During chronic stress, there is an increase of blood corticoids from the adrenal cortex.

An athlete who is taken out of a sport because of an injury or illness reacts in a personal way. The athlete who has trained diligently, has looked forward to a successful season, and is suddenly thwarted in that goal by an injury or illness can be emotionally devastated.

At the time of serious injury or illness the athlete may normally fear the experience of pain or possible disability. There may be a sense of anxiety about suddenly becoming disabled and unable to continue sport participation.[14] An injury or illness is a stressor that results from an external or internal sensory stimulus. Coping with the stressor depends on the athlete's cognitive appraisal.

The Psychology of Loss

The athlete who has suddenly sustained an injury of such intensity that he or she is unable to perform for a long period will generally experience five reactions: denial

11-1

Critical Thinking Exercise

A world-class sprinter tears his left hamstring muscle, which eliminates him from the Olympic trials.

? What could be the psychological ramifications to this athlete?

or disbelief, anger, bargaining, depression, and acceptance of the situation. (See the Focus box below.) These reactions are typical for anyone who has experienced a sudden serious loss. The injured athlete initially may be in shock and unable to grasp the full consequences of the injury.[14] The athlete may not believe that he or she is vulnerable and not impervious to injury. There may be a loss of self-esteem, a sense of worthlessness, and self-reproach.[8] Often an athlete who has sustained a serious disability will undergo reactions characteristic of a sudden loss (Figure 11-2).

In general the injured athlete experiences a number of personal reactions besides a sense of loss. These include physical, emotional, and social reactions. (See the Focus box on p. 250.)[23]

Although some athletes experience minimal mood disturbances after a serious sports injury, others experience depression.[24] Deep depression may become a risk for suicide.[25] The profile of at-risk athletes is as follows:

- The athlete belongs to the high-risk age group of between 15 and 24 years of age.
- The athlete sustains a serious injury requiring surgery.
- The athlete is faced with a long rehabilitation period.
- The athlete is faced with being replaced by a teammate.

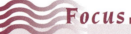

Focus

Psychological reactions to loss

Denial or disbelief

When suddenly becoming disabled and unable to perform, the athlete will commonly deny the seriousness of the condition. When indications are that the injury is serious and will not heal before the end of the season, the athlete might respond by saying, "Not so, I'll be back in 2 weeks." This irrational thinking indicates denial of the true seriousness of the injury.

Anger

Anger commonly follows disbelief. As the athlete slowly becomes aware of the seriousness of the injury, a sense of anger develops. The athlete begins to ask, "Why me?" "What did I do wrong?" "Why am I being punished?" "It's not fair." Commonly, this anger becomes displaced toward other people. The athletic trainer may be blamed for not providing a good enough tape job, or another player may be blamed for causing the situation that set up the injury.

Bargaining

As anger becomes less intense, the athlete gradually becomes aware of the real nature of the injury and, with this awareness, begins to have doubts and fears about the situation, which leads to a need to bargain. Bargaining may be reflected in prayer: "God, if you will heal this injury in 3 weeks instead of 6, I'll go to church every Sunday." Or it may be reflected by pressure being put on the athletic trainer or physician to do his or her best for a fast healing.

Depression

As the athlete becomes increasingly aware of the nature of the injury and that healing will take a specific length of time, depression can set in. Crying episodes may occur; there may be periods of insomnia, and the athlete may lose the desire for food.

Acceptance

Gradually, the athlete begins to feel less dejected and isolated and becomes resigned to the situation.

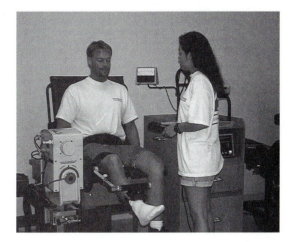

Figure 11-2

A sports injury can cause the athlete psychological reactions characteristic of a sudden loss.

Athletes facing a severe injury that requires surgery with a long period of rehabilitation and an uncertainty of returning to competition may also experience a number of behavioral signs, such as exaggerated pain complaints, sleep disturbances, feelings of fatigue, and moodiness.[18] The injured athlete often becomes anxious and loses his or her dedication to the rehabilitation process.[10]

Personality Factors Leading to Injury

Ruling out high-risk situations, some athletes seem to receive more than their share of injuries. Athletes who are anxious, tense, restless, and nervous may be more prone to some injuries.[7] A sense of insecurity reflected in a low self-confidence and low self-esteem may predispose an athlete to injury.[7] The athlete who is undisciplined in developing skills in his or her sport and who lacks structure in his or her personal and social life may be accident prone.[7]

Overtraining and Staleness

Where there is an imbalance between a physical load placed on an athlete and his or her coping capacity the state of overtraining and staleness can occur.[1] This condition is also known as burnout, overreaching, overwork, or an overtraining syndrome.[6]

Both physiological and psychological factors underlie overtraining and staleness. There are countless reasons why some athletes become stale. In fact, the athlete could be training too hard and long without proper rest. Often staleness is attributed to emotional problems stemming from daily worries, fears, and anxieties. **Anxiety** is one of the most common mental and emotional stress producers. It is reflected by a nondescript fear, a sense of apprehension, and restlessness. Typically the anxious athlete is unable to describe the problem. The athlete feels inadequate in a certain situation but is unable to say why. Heart palpitations, shortness of breath, sweaty palms, constriction in the throat, and headaches may accompany anxiety. Children who are pushed too hard by parents may acquire a number of psychological problems. They may even fail purposely in their sport just to rid themselves of the painful stress of achieving. A coach who acts like a drill sergeant—one who continually gives negative reinforcements—will more than likely cause the athlete to develop symptoms of overstress.

Athletes are much more prone to staleness if the rewards of their efforts are minimal. A losing season commonly causes many athletes to become stale.[2]

Symptoms of Staleness

Staleness is evidenced by a wide variety of symptoms, among which are a deterioration in the usual standard of performance, chronic fatigue, apathy, loss of appetite,

11-2

Critical Thinking Exercise

A 17-year-old world-class gymnast sustains a major knee injury after a horizontal bar dismount. The injury may end the athlete's career. As a result of this injury the athlete becomes very depressed.

? What should the athletic trainer be concerned with in terms of this athlete's emotional stability?

anxiety
A feeling of uncertainty or apprehension.

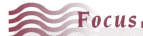

Athlete's reactions to serious injury[8]

Physical reactions

- Pain (range of motion, muscle weakness)
- Physical disability (temporary, permanent)

Emotional reactions

- Loss and grief
- Fear of surgery (pain and outcome)
- A fear of performing in the future
- A fear of treatment and rehabilitation

Social well-being

- Separation from teammates, friends, and family
- Dependency on others

Self-concept

- Loss of self-control
- Altered self-image
- Threat to goals and personal values

catecholamine
Active amines, epinephrine and norepinephrine, that affect the nervous and cardiovascular systems.

indigestion, weight loss, and inability to sleep or rest properly.[7] Often athletes will exhibit higher blood pressure or an increased pulse rate, both at rest and during activity, as well as increased **catecholamine** excretions. All these signs indicate adrenal exhaustion. The athlete becomes irritable and restless, has to force himself or herself to practice, and exhibits signs of boredom and lassitude in respect to everything connected with the activity[4] (see the Focus box below).

When an athlete shows signs of staleness there also can occur increased potential for both acute and overuse injuries and infections.[7] Stress fractures and tendinitis are typical injuries that can occur during a time of staleness.

OVERTRAINING

It is generally accepted that sports are stressors to the athlete. There is often a fine line between the athlete's reaching and maintaining peak performance and overtraining. Besides performance concerns, many peripheral stressors can be imposed on the athlete, such as unreasonable expectations by the athlete, the coaches, or the parents. Worries that stem from school, work, and family can also be major causes of emotional stress.

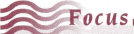

Recognizing signs of staleness in athletes

An athlete who is becoming stale will often display some or most of the following signs. He or she may

- Show a decrease in performance level.
- Have difficulty falling asleep.
- Be awakened from sleep for no apparent reason.
- Experience a loss of appetite and a loss of weight; conversely, the athlete may overeat because of chronic worry.
- Have indigestion.
- Have difficulty concentrating.
- Have difficulty enjoying sex.
- Experience nausea for no apparent reason.
- Be prone to head colds or allergic reactions.
- Show behavioral signs of restlessness, irritability, anxiety, or depression.
- Have an elevated resting heart rate and elevated blood pressure.
- Display psychosomatic episodes of perceiving bodily pains such as sore muscles, especially before competing.

The Coach

The coach is often the first person to notice that an athlete is overstressed. The athlete whose performance is declining and whose personality is changing may need a training program that is less demanding. A good talk with the athlete by the coach might reveal emotional and physical problems that need to be dealt with by a counselor, psychologist, or physician.

The Athletic Trainer

Injury prevention is both *psychological* and *physiological*. The athlete who enters a contest while angry, frustrated, or discouraged or while undergoing some other disturbing emotional state is more prone to injury than is the individual who is better adjusted emotionally. The angry player, for example, wants to vent ire in some way and therefore often loses perspective of desirable and approved conduct. In the grip of emotion, skill and coordination are sacrificed, resulting in an injury that otherwise would have been avoided.

Although athletic trainers are typically not educated as professional counselors or psychologists, they must nevertheless be concerned with the feelings of the athletes they work with. No one can work closely with human beings without becoming involved with their emotions and, at times, their personal problems. The athletic trainer is usually a caring person and, as such, is placed in numerous daily situations in which close interpersonal relationships are important. The athletic trainer must have appropriate counseling skills to confront an athlete's fears, frustrations, and daily crises and to refer individuals with serious emotional problems to the proper professionals. To help reduce the athlete's muscle tension caused by stress, the athletic trainer is in a position to provide education in relaxation techniques.

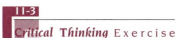

The athletic trainer must have some counseling skills.

It is important that overtraining be recognized early and dealt with immediately. A short interruption of training should be carried out over a 3- to 5-day period.[6] A lower amount of work but with the same intensity should be carried out.[6]

When the athlete shows signs of a full recovery a gradual return to the same workload can be initiated. Competition must be stopped. It should be noted that an abrupt cessation of training can produce a serious physiological and psychological condition known as sudden exercise abstinence syndrome (see the Focus box below).

The Physician

The team physician, as do the coach and the athletic trainer, plays an integral part with the athlete who is overly stressed. Many of the psychophysiological responses thought to be emotional are in fact caused by some undetected physical dysfunction. Therefore referral to the physician must be routine.

REACTING TO ATHLETES WITH INJURIES

No matter what reaction the injured athlete displays, he or she must be responded to as a person, not an injury. Sometimes an athlete can be difficult to be around, especially in the early stages of a serious injury. The athlete may be suddenly forced to be dependent and helpless.[16] During this time the athlete may regress to a

11-3

Critical Thinking Exercise

A football player is forced to stop playing at midseason because of a shoulder injury.

? What psychological and physiological problems might this athlete experience by suddenly stopping his participation?

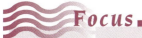

Focus

Sudden exercise abstinence syndrome[6]
Symptoms include the following:
- Heart palpitations
- Irregular heartbeat
- Chest pain
- Disturbed appetite and digestion
- Sleep disorders
- Increased sweating
- Depression
- Emotional instability

TABLE 11-1 Emotional First Aid

Type of Emotional Reaction	Outward Signs	Trainer's Reactions	
		Yes	No
Normal	Weakness, trembling Nausea, vomiting Perspiration Diarrhea Fear, anxiety Heart pounding	Be calm and reassuring	Avoid pity
Overreaction	Excessive talking Argumentativeness Inappropriate joke telling Hyperactivity	Allow athlete to vent emotions	Avoid telling athlete he or she is acting abnormally
Underreaction	Depression; sitting or standing numbly Little talking if any Emotionless Confusion Failure to respond to questions	Be empathetic; encourage talking to express feelings	Avoid being abrupt; avoid pity

childlike behavior, crying or displacing anger toward the person administering first aid. Table 11-1 provides some suggestions on rendering emotional first aid. During the period of emotional first aid, comfort, care, and communication should be given freely.[16]

It is important that the sports medicine team be honest, supporting, and respectful of the injured athlete during the time of disability. It is important that the athlete is understood at a deeper level and how he or she is coping with this major stress event.[18]

A number of questions should be asked. Is there a good doctor-patient relationship stemming from confidence, trust, and optimism?[16] Does the athlete have a fear of a pending surgery in terms of more pain or inability to continue in his or her sport?[16] How long is the recovery? What is the possibility of reinjury?[16] Is there a possibility of a forced retirement, and if so how well is the athlete's adjustment? What are the athlete's attitudes toward rehabilitation?

THE REHABILITATION PROCESS

If a program of rehabilitation is to be successful the athlete's psyche must be taken into consideration. Success in treatment involving therapeutic modalities and exercise rehabilitation depends on rapport, cooperation, and learning[4] (Figure 11-3).

Rapport

The term *rapport* means a relationship of mutual trust and understanding. The athlete must thoroughly trust the athletic trainer or therapist to achieve maximum rehabilitation, and he or she must believe that at all times his or her best interests are being considered.[12]

Cooperation

A highly motivated athlete begrudges every moment spent out of action and can become somewhat difficult to handle if the rehabilitative process moves slowly. Often the athlete blames the physician or the athletic trainer for not doing all that he or she can. To avoid this situation, early in the rehabilitative process the athlete must be taught that healing is a cooperative undertaking. It must be

---

11-4

Critical Thinking Exercise

A seriously injured athlete displays outward signs of being depressed. He talks little and displays mental confusion. He refuses to respond to the athletic trainer's questions.

? How should the athletic trainer respond to this athlete? What should the athletic trainer avoid?

The psychology of sports rehabilitation must include establishing all of the following:
Rapport
A sense of cooperation
Exercise rehabilitation as an educational process
Competitive confidence

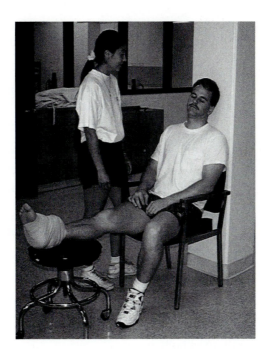

Figure 11-3

Treatment success requires rapport, cooperation, and learning.

established that the athlete, physician, and athletic trainer are a team, all working toward the same end—the return of the athlete to full function as soon as physiologically possible. To ensure this atmosphere the athlete must feel free to vent frustrations, to ask questions, and to expect clear answers about any aspect of the rehabilitative process. The athlete must feel a major responsibility to come into the training room on time and not skip appointments. He or she must be motivated to perform all exercises correctly and to perform all home assignments on a regular basis.

Many injured athletes lack patience. Nevertheless, patience and desire are necessary adjuncts in securing a reasonable rate of recovery.

Sports Rehabilitation as an Educational Process

To ensure maximum positive responses from the athlete in all aspects of rehabilitation, continual education must occur. All education is provided in layman's language or is commensurate with the athlete's background and education. The following is a list of educational matters to address carefully:

1. Describe the nature of the injury clearly, using anatomy charts or other visual aids. The athlete must fully understand the nature of his or her injury and its prognosis based on similar cases. A false hope for a fast "comeback" should not be engendered if a full recovery is doubtful.
2. Explain how the healing process occurs, and estimate the time needed for such healing.
3. Describe in detail the consequences of not following proper procedures.
4. Describe an overall rehabilitative plan, including progressive steps or phases within the plan.
5. Explain each physical modality or exercise, how it works, and its specific purpose.
6. Make the athlete aware that his or her recovery depends as much on his or her attitude toward the rehabilitative process as on what therapy is being given. A positive attitude leads to a conscientious and persistent effort to speed recovery.
7. The athlete needs to see immediate results.[5]
8. Rehabilitation is planned around the athlete's schedule.[5]

9. The rehabilitation facility must be convenient to the athlete.

10. The athlete must be regularly monitored.

Phases of Rehabilitation

The rehabilitation process incorporates both therapeutic modalities and exercise rehabilitation. During each phase of rehabilitation the athletic trainer or therapist must address specific psychological issues of the athlete.

11-5

Critical Thinking Exercise

A football athlete is undergoing physical rehabilitation after major knee surgery. The process of rehabilitation will take 12 to 18 months.

? What psychological aspects of the rehabilitation process must be considered by the athletic trainer?

Immediate Postinjury Period

The immediate postinjury period is a time of fear and denial often with severe pain and disability. Emotional first aid must be given. An accurate diagnosis must be given by the physician with a full explanation given to the athlete and family members. As much as possible the athlete needs to know the course of treatment, prognosis, and plan to attain goals. The athlete must know from the beginning that he or she is an integral part of rehabilitation.[26]

Early Postoperative Period

When surgery is performed the athlete becomes a disabled patient. The athlete is educated to each phase of the healing process and the purpose of each treatment procedure. The athlete is encouraged to maintain aerobic conditioning by exercising the noninjured body parts.

Advanced Postoperative or Rehabilitation Period

While the athlete rehabilitates the injured body part, he or she continues to condition unaffected body regions both aerobically and anaerobically. The athlete must feel that he or she is in control and can make choices. Increasing the athlete's confidence is built on small successes. Milestones must be kept realistic with positive verbal reinforcement given by the coach, peers, and sports medicine team.[26]

This period has greater emphasis on movement patterns that mimic a specific sport. Athletes need reassurance that they will be able to return to their sport and once again achieve success. Their fear of failure and anxiety is dealt with by positive reinforcement.[26]

Overrehabilitation Compliance

Athletic trainers or therapists are often faced with an athlete who overcomplies with the rehabilitation process. Such overcompliance produces treatment setbacks and possible reinjury[10] (see the Focus box below).

Poor Rehabilitation Compliance

The opposite extreme of overrehabilitation is found among athletes who comply poorly with the rehabilitation process.[10] Poor adherence could be indicative of a number of factors (see the box on the next page).

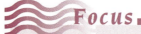

Focus

Factors indicating overcompliance
- Mild degree of denial
- Obsessive-compulsive and impulsive tendencies
- Excessive risk taking
- Behavior masking an underlying fear
- Proving worthiness

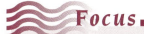

Focus

Factors that cause poor compliance[11]
- Scheduling problems
- School, financial, or family concerns
- Unclear on treatment rationale
- Mistrust of treatment choices
- Mistrust of rehabilitation specialists
- Fear of pain or reinjury

INITIAL SPORTS REENTRY PERIOD

Often an athlete returns to participation physically ready but psychologically ill prepared. Although few athletes will admit it, when returning to participation they often feel anxious about getting hurt again. This feeling may, in some ways, be a self-fulfilling prophecy. In other words, anxiety can lead to muscle tension, which in turn can lead to disruption of normal coordination, thus producing conditions that are favorable for reinjury or for injury to another body part.[18] The following are suggestions for helping an athlete regain competitive confidence:

1. Allow the athlete to regain full performance by progressing in small increments. Return might include, first, performing all the necessary skills away from the team. This action may be followed by engaging in a highly controlled, small-group practice and then attempting participation in full-team noncontact practice. The athlete should be encouraged to express freely any anxiety that may be felt and to engage in full contact only when anxiety is at a minimum.

2. One technique that an athletic trainer might teach the athlete is systematic desensitization. The athlete first learns to consciously relax as much as possible through the Jacobson progressive relaxation method.[13] When relaxation can be achieved at will, the athlete, with the help of the athletic trainer, develops a fear hierarchy related to returning to the sport and going "all out." Each progressive step is imagined and the athlete is fully relaxed. As the progressive steps are imagined and fear is experienced at a specific step, the thought processes are halted. When coming to a point of anxiety, the athlete is taught to relax even more until the anxiety has passed. The athlete then goes on to the next, more anxiety-producing event, with the relaxation process being repeated until no anxiety is felt. When the athlete is able to complete the entire list of events without anxiety and has also completed the proper physical rehabilitation, he or she should be ready for competition.

Mental Training

Mental training techniques have long been used to enhance sports skills. Many of these techniques are appropriate for athletes in the process of healing and rehabilitating a serious injury or illness.

Athletic trainers and therapists can assist athletes to positively respond to their injuries via specific mental training techniques. It should be noted that serious emotional instabilities must be referred to a professional psychologist. Some techniques that are available are quieting the anxious mind, mental and emotional assessment, pain control, and healing approaches.

Quieting the Anxious Mind

Fear and anxiety are always present to some degree in a serious sport injury or illness. Fear of pain, loss of control, and unknown consequences of disability can create physical and emotional tensions. Two techniques to deal with anxiety and tension that can be taught to the athlete are meditation and progressive relaxation.

Meditation

Meditators focus on a constant mental stimulus such as a phrase repeated silently or audibly or a sound or a single word, or they gaze steadily at some object. In the passive attitude of meditation, a "don't work at it" approach is taken. As thoughts come into the consciousness, they are quietly turned away, and the individual returns to the focus of attention. For decreased muscle tone, a comfortable position is taken with the various major body areas relaxed and placed in as comfortable a position as possible. To effectively conduct a meditation session, a quiet environment is essential. Normally, the eyes are closed unless the meditator is focusing on some external object[2] (see the Focus box below).

Progressive Relaxation

Progressive muscle relaxation is probably the most extensively used technique for relaxation today.[13] It can be considered intense training in the awareness of tension and its release. Progressive relaxation may be practiced in a reclining position or while seated in a chair. Each muscle group is tensed from 5 to 7 seconds, then relaxed for 20 to 30 seconds. In most cases, one repetition of the procedure is sufficient; however, if tension remains in the area, repeated contraction and relaxation is permitted. The sequence of tensing and releasing is systematically applied to the following body areas: the dominant hand and forearm; dominant upper arm; nondominant hand and forearm; nondominant upper arm; forehead; eyes and nose; cheeks and mouth; neck and throat; chest; back; respiratory muscles; abdomen; dominant upper leg, calf, and foot; and nondominant upper leg, calf, and foot. Throughout the session, a num-

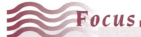

Focus

The meditation technique

Quieting the body

The athlete sits comfortably in a position that maintains a straight back; the head is erect and the hands are placed loosely on each leg or on the arm of a chair with both feet firmly planted on the floor. To ensure a relaxed state, the meditator should mentally relax each body part, starting at the feet. If a great deal of tension is present, Jacobson's relaxation exercise might be appropriate, or several deep breaths are taken in and exhaled slowly and completely, allowing the body to settle more and more into a relaxed state after each emptying of the lungs.

The meditative technique

Once the athlete is in a quiet environment and fully physically relaxed, the meditative process can begin. With each exhalation the athlete emits a repetitive self-talk of a short word such as "one" or "peace." It is repeated over and over for 10 to 20 minutes. Such words as "peace" or "relaxed" are excellent relaxers; however, Benson[2] has suggested that the word "one" produces the same physiological responses as any other word. If extraneous thoughts occur the athlete just returns to the meditation process.

After meditating

After repeating the special word the athlete comes back to physical reality slowly and gently. As awareness increases, physical activity should also increase. Moving too quickly or standing up suddenly might produce light-headedness or dizziness.

ber of expressions for relaxing may be used: "Let the tension dissolve. Let go of the tension. I am bringing my muscles to zero. Let the tension flow out of my body."

After the athlete has become highly aware of the tension in the body, the contraction is gradually decreased until little remains. At this point, the athlete focuses on one area and mentally wills the tension to decrease to zero, or complete relaxation. Jacobson's progressive relaxation normally takes longer than the time allowed in a typical session or than the individual would want to spend. A short form can be developed that, although not as satisfactory, helps the individual become better aware of the body. (See the Focus box on the next page.) *The essence of Jacobson's method is recognizing muscular tension and the conscious release of that tension.*

Cognitive Restructuring

Some injured athletes practice irrational thinking and negative self-talk. This can hinder the treatment progress. An important approach to negative thoughts is cognitive restructuring. Two successful methods to thought restructuring are *refuting irrational thoughts* and *thought stopping.*[3]

Refuting Irrational Thoughts

This method is designed to deal with a person's internal dialogue. Psychologist Albert Ellis[3] developed a system to change irrational ideas and beliefs. His system is called rational emotive therapy. The basic premise is that actual events do not create emotions but, rather, it is the self-talk after the event that does. In other words, irrational self-talk causes anxiety, anger, and depression.

Athletes who are under severe stress should explore their self-talk. The following is an example:

Facts and events: A tennis player, after surgical repair of his shoulder, is impatient about the speed of recovery. Emotions of anger and depression are present.

Negative self-talk:
  "I was stupid to get hurt."
  "Why me? Why did I have to get hurt?"
  "I have never been laid up before. It's not fair!"

Positive self-talk:
  "I was hurt and now I am doing my best to get well."
  "Every day I am getting better."
  "The athletic trainers are doing their best for me."

Another example is as follows:

Facts and events: A football player "blows a knee out" and requires surgery. Emotions of anger and denial are present.

Negative self-talk:
  "I was blindsided and no penalty was called."
  "I could have avoided such a serious injury if the coaches coached better."

Positive self-talk:
  "I am hurt, but because of my good fitness level I will recover quickly."
  "I plan to do everything I am told to recover quickly."

Thought Stopping

Thought stopping is an excellent cognitive technique for helping the athlete overcome worries and doubts. The anxious athlete, especially one that is hurt, will often repeat negative, unproductive, and unrealistic statements during self-talk, such as "I am no good to anyone now that I am hurt" or "Everyone on the team is going to pass me by while I am recovering."

Thought stopping consists of focusing on the undesired thoughts and stopping them with the command "stop" or a loud noise. After the thought interruption, a positive statement is inserted, such as "My shoulder is getting healed and I'll play as well as, if not better than, before."[15]

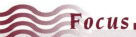

Focus

Jacobson's progressive relaxation

Beginning instructions

1. Get into a position that is relaxed and comfortable.
2. Breathe in and out easily and allow yourself to relax as much as possible.
3. Make yourself aware of your total body and the tensions that your muscles might have within them.

Arm relaxation

1. Clench your right fist. Increase the grip more and more until you feel the tension created in your hand and forearm.
2. Slowly open your fist and allow the tension to flow out slowly until there is no tension left in your hand and forearm.
3. Feel how soft and relaxed the hand and forearm are, and contrast this feeling with the left hand.
4. Repeat this procedure with the left hand, gripping hard and bringing the tension into the fist and forearm.
5. Bend your right elbow and bring tension into the right biceps, tensing it as hard as you possibly can and observing the tightness of the muscle.
6. Relax and straighten the arm, allowing the tension to flow out.
7. Repeat the tension and relaxation technique with the left biceps.

The head

1. Wrinkle your forehead as hard as you can and hold that tension for 5 seconds or longer.
2. Relax and allow the forehead and face to completely smooth out.
3. Frown and feel the tension that comes in between the eyes and eyebrows.
4. Let go to a completely blank expression. Feel the tension flow out of your face.
5. Squint your eyes tighter and tighter, feeling the tension creep into the eyes.
6. Relax and gently allow your eyes to be closed without tension.
7. Clench your jaw, bite down hard, harder. Notice the tension in your jaw.
8. Relax. When you are relaxed, allow your lips to be slightly parted and your face to be completely without expression, without wrinkles or tension.
9. Stick your tongue up against the roof of your mouth as hard as possible, feeling the tension in the tongue and the mouth. Hold that tension.
10. Relax, allowing the face and the mouth to be completely relaxed. Allow the tongue to be suspended lightly in the mouth. Relax.
11. Form an O with your lips. Purse the lips hard together so that you feel the tension around the lips only.
12. Relax, allowing the tension to leave around the lips. Allow your lips to be slightly parted, and allow tension to be completely gone from the face.

The neck and shoulders

1. Press your head back against the mat or chair and feel the tension come into the neck region. Hold that tension. Be aware of it, sense it.
2. Slowly allow the tension to leave, decreasing the amount of pressure applied until the tension has completely gone and there is as much relaxation as possible.
3. Bring your head forward so that your chin is pressing against your chest and tension is brought into the throat and back of the neck. Hold that tension.
4. Slowly return to the beginning position and feel the tension leave the neck. Relax completely.
5. Shrug your shoulders upward, raising your shoulders as far as you can toward your ears, hunching your head between your shoulders. Feel the tension creep into your shoulders. Hold that tension.
6. Slowly let the tension leave by returning the shoulders to their original position. Allow the tension to completely leave the neck and shoulder region. Have a sense of bringing the muscles to zero, where they are completely at ease and without strain.

Respiration and the trunk

1. When the body is completely relaxed and you have a sense of heaviness, allow tension to move to your respiration. Fill the lungs completely and hold your breath for 5 seconds, feeling the tension come into the chest and upper back muscles.
2. Exhale slowly, allowing the air to go out slowly as you feel the tension being released slowly.
3. While your breath is coming slowly and easily, sense the contrast of the breath holding to the breath that is coming freely and gently.

Continued

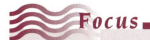

Focus

Jacobson's progressive relaxation—cont'd

4. Tighten the abdominal muscles by pressing downward on the stomach. Note the tension that comes into the abdominal region, the respiratory center, and the back region.
5. Relax the abdominal area and feel the tension leave the trunk region.
6. Slightly arch the back against the mat or back of the chair. This should be done without hyperextending or straining. Feel the tension that creeps into and along the spine. Hold that tension.
7. Gradually allow the body to sink back into its original position. Feel the tension leave the long muscles of the back.
8. Flatten the lower back by rolling the hips forward. Feel the tension come into the lower back by rolling the hips forward. Hold that tension. Try to isolate that tension from all the other parts of your body.
9. Gradually return to the original position, and feel the tension leave the body. Be aware of any tension that might have crept into body regions that you have already relaxed. Allow your mind to scan your body; go back over the areas that you have released from tension and become aware of whether any tension has returned.

The buttocks and thighs

1. Tense your buttocks for 5 seconds. Try to isolate just the contraction of the buttocks region.
2. Slowly allow the buttocks to return to their normal state, relaxing completely.
3. Contract your thighs by straightening your knees. Hold that contraction, feeling the tension, isolating the tension just to that region, focusing just on the thigh region.
4. Slowly allow the tension to leave the region, bringing the entire body to a relaxed state, especially the thighs.
5. To bring the tension to the back of the thighs, press your heels as hard as you can against the floor or mat, slightly bending the knees; bring the tension to the hamstring region and the back of the thighs. Hold this tension, study it, concentrate on it. Try to isolate the tension from other tensions that might have crept into the body.
6. Relax. Allow the tension to flow out. Return your legs to the original position, and let go of all the tensions of the body.

The lower legs and feet

1. With the legs fully extended, point your feet downward as hard as possible, bringing tension into both calves. Hold that tension. Hold it as hard as you can without cramping.
2. Slowly allow the foot to return to a neutral position, and allow relaxation to occur within the calf muscle. Bring it to zero, if possible—no tension.
3. Curl the toes of the feet downward as hard as you can without pointing the foot downward, isolating the tension just in the bottoms of the feet and toes. Hold that tension. Isolate the tension, if possible, from the calves. Hold it, feel the tension on the bottoms of your feet.
4. Slowly relax and allow the tension to release from the foot as the toes straighten out.
5. Curl the toes backward toward the kneecaps and bring the foot back into dorsiflexion so that you feel the tension in the tops of the toes, the tops of the feet, and the shin. Hold that tension. Be aware of it, study the tension.
6. After 5 seconds or longer, return to a neutral state where the foot is completely relaxed and the toes have returned to their normal position. Feel the tension leave your body.

Therapeutic Imagery

Imagery, or visualization, can be beneficial tool in the rehabilitation process. Imagery, or seeing with the "mind's eye," encourages the athlete to focus on a goal such as rehearsal of rehabilitation, pain control, and stimulating the healing process.[9,19]

Rehearsing the Rehabilitation Process

The athlete starts becoming as relaxed as possible and then proceeds to imagine with eyes closed important events in the rehabilitation process. All senses of the imagination are used: sight, sound, touch, and kinesthesia.[19] An example might be imagining success

- After leaving the hospital.
- When starting and carrying out active rehabilitation.
- During the healing process.

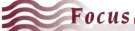

Focus

Healing images

Treatment Modalities
- Ultrasound increases circulation, bringing healthy new tissue to the area.
- Cold application inhibits pain.

Exercise rehabilitation
- Muscle fibers increase in number and become stronger.
- Joint range of motion—joints become fully functional.

Medications
- Antiinflammatories decrease inflammation and swelling.
- Pain medication inhibits pain.

- When returning to practice.
- When in full practice without fear.
- When competing without fear.

Imagery and visualization can be used specifically to enhance each treatment approach. A foundation to imagery is the education that the athletic trainer or therapist provides the athlete as treatment is given.[9] The athlete imagines treatment positively affecting the body (see the Focus box above).[9]

HEALING PROCESS AND PAIN CONTROL
Improving the Healing Process

It is important that the athlete be educated about the physiological process of healing (Figure 11-4). Once the healing process is understood, the athlete is instructed to imagine it taking place during therapy and throughout the day. If an infection is being fought, the body's phagocytes can be imagined as "Pac Men" gobbling up infectious material. When tissue is torn, clot formation and organization can be imagined, followed by tissue regeneration and healing.

Techniques for Coping with Pain

The injured athlete can be taught relatively simple techniques to inhibit pain and discomfort. At no time should pain be completely inhibited because pain is a protective mechanism. The athlete can reduce pain in three ways: reducing muscle tension, diverting attention away from the pain, or changing the pain sensation to another sensation.[2]

Tension Reduction

The pain response can be associated with general muscular tension stemming from anxiety and the pain-spasm-pain cycle of the specific injury. In both of these situations muscle tension increases the sensation of pain. Conversely, relaxation methods that reduce muscle tension can also decrease the awareness of pain. Both the Benson[2] and Jacobson[13] techniques of stress reduction can be advantageous in pain reduction.

Attention Diversion

A positive method for decreasing pain perception is to divert attention from the injury. This can be performed in a painful injury and can be beneficial. An example might be to engage in mental problem solving, such as adding or subtracting a column of numbers or counting spots on the floor. Pain also can be diverted by fantasizing about pleasant events, such as sunbathing at the beach, sailing, or skiing.

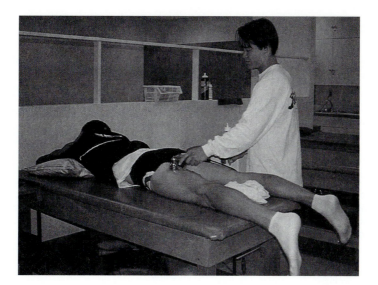

Figure 11-4

Educating the athlete about pain is a major goal in the healing process.

Altering the Pain Sensation

Imagination is one of the most powerful forces available to human beings. Negative imagination can be a major cause of illness, stress, and muscular tension, whereas positive imagination can produce wellness and counteract stress.

Through imagination the athlete can alter pain sensation to another sensation. For example, a body part immersed in ice-cold water can change the pain to a sensation of cold dampness. The injured part might be imagined to be relaxed and comfortable instead of painful. Imagining a peaceful scene at a pleasant spot such as the beach or mountains can both relax the athlete and divert attention from the pain.

SUMMARY

- The injured or ill athlete not only experiences physical disability but major psychological reactions. Sport can be a major psychophysiological stressor.
- The athlete who sustains a serious injury may experience psychological characteristics of sudden loss including denial, anger, bargaining, depression, and acceptance. Injury can cause physical, emotional, social, and self-concept reactions by the athlete.
- Some athletes, because of personality factors, receive more than their share of injuries and illness. Anxiety, low self-esteem, and poor discipline may lead one to be accident prone.
- Overtraining and staleness result in a physical load being placed on the athlete's ability to cope. An athlete who is pushed or who pushes himself or herself too hard may experience burnout. Under these conditions overuse injuries have a higher incidence.
- At all times the injured or ill athlete must be treated as a person, not a condition. Comfort, care, and good communication should be the approach of the health care providers.
- During the rehabilitation process there must be mutual trust, understanding, and cooperation. Rehabilitation must be an educational process. Education is carried out through each phase of rehabilitation. The health care personnel are continually aware of athletes who overcomply or poorly comply.
- There are many mental training aids that can help the injured athlete through the rehabilitation process and reentry to competition. Some of these are systematic desensitization, mental and emotional assessment, refuting irrational thoughts, and thought stopping.

Solutions to Critical Thinking Exercises

11-1 This athlete experiences the psychological reaction to a sudden loss: disbelief, anger, bargaining, depression, and finally resignation.

11-2 This athlete has the profile that may be a risk for suicide. He is in a high-risk age group. He has been a successful athlete who now faces surgery and a period of long rehabilitation. He is also faced with the possible ending of his career or, if he is able to return, being replaced by another athlete.

11-3 The athletic trainer should be aware of the possibility of the sudden exercise abstinence syndrome. In this syndrome the athlete may experience heart palpitations, irregular heartbeat, chest pain, problems with appetite and digestion, sleep disorders, increased sweating, depression, and in some cases emotional instability.

11-4 The athletic trainer should be empathetic and encourage the athlete to talk and express his feelings. The athletic trainer should avoid being abrupt and avoid showing pity.

11-5 The athletic trainer must develop a mutual trust and understanding with the athlete. The athlete must realize that rehabilitation is a cooperative undertaking. Continual education must occur throughout the rehabilitation process.

REVIEW QUESTIONS AND CLASS ACTIVITIES

1. What is the importance of psychology to sports injuries?
2. How does stress relate to athlete injuries and illness?
3. Discuss the psychology of loss in sports injuries.
4. Describe the physical, emotional, social, and self-concept factors in sports injuries.
5. As an athletic trainer, how would you psychologically assist the athlete about to undergo major knee surgery?
6. Discuss overtraining, staleness, and overuse injuries.
7. What actions would you take with an athlete who is stale?
8. Psychologically, how should an athletic trainer react to serious injury immediately after injury and during the disability?
9. Psychologically, what makes for a successful rehabilitation climate?
10. Discuss psychological problems common to the rehabilitation process and possible ways of intervening.
11. What mental training techniques might be employed to assist the athlete who is fearful and anxious?
12. Practice teaching mental training techniques.

REFERENCES

1. Anderson MB, Williams JM: Psychological risk factors and injury prevention. In Heil J, editor: *Psychology of sports injury*, Champaign, Ill, 1993, Human Kinetics.
2. Benson HH: *Beyond the relaxation response*, New York, 1984, Times.
3. Ellis A: *A new guide to rational living*, North Hollywood, Calif, 1975, Wilshire.
4. Faris GJ: Psychological aspects of athletic rehabilitation. In Harvey JS, editor: *Symposium on rehabilitation of the injured athlete. Clinics in sports medicine*, vol 4, no 3, Philadelphia, 1988, Saunders.
5. Fisher AC: Athletic trainer's attitudes and judgements of injured athletes' rehabilitation adherence, *J Ath Train* 28(1):43, 1993.
6. Froehlich J: Overtraining. In Heil J, editor: *Psychology of sport injury*, Champaign, Ill, 1993, Human Kinetics.
7. Graham DJ: Personality traits relevant to the cause and treatment of athletic injuries, *Sports Med Digest* 15(2):1, 1993.
8. Heil J: A psychologist's view of the personal challenge of injury. In Heil J, editor: *Psychology of sport injury*, Champaign, Ill, 1993, Human Kinetics.
9. Heil J: Mental training in injury management. In Heil J, editor: *Psychology of sport injury*, Champaign, Ill, 1993, Human Kinetics.
10. Heil J: Sport psychology, the athlete at risk, and the sports medicine team. In Heil J, editor: *Psychology of sport injury*, Champaign, Ill, 1993, Human Kinetics.
11. Heil J: Specialized treatment approaches: problems in rehabilitation. In Heil J, editor: *Psychology of sport injury*, Champaign, Ill, 1993, Human Kinetics.
12. Heil J: Specialized treatment approaches: severe injury. In Heil J, editor: *Psychology of sport injury*, Champaign, Ill, 1993, Human Kinetics.
13. Jacobson E: *Progressive relaxation*, ed 2, Chicago, 1938, University of Chicago Press.
14. Mary JR: Psychological sequelae and rehabilitation of the injured athlete, *Sports Med Digest* 12(11):1, 1990.
15. McKay M et al: *Thoughts and feelings*, Richmond, Calif, 1981, New Harbinger Publications.
16. McGuire R: Emotional healing, training and conditioning, *J Ath Train* 4(4):4, 1994.
17. Pelletier KR: *Mind as healer, mind as slayer*, New York, 1977, Dell.
18. Petrie G: Injury from the athlete's point of view. In Heil J, editor: *Psychology of sport injury*, Champaign, Ill, 1993, Human Kinetics.
19. Richardson PA, Latuda LM: Therapeutic imagery and athletic injuries, *J Ath Train* 30(1):10, 1995.
20. Rotella RJ, Heyman SR: Stress, injury and the psychological rehabilitation of athletes. In Williams JM, editor: *Applied sports psychology*, Palo Alto, Calif, 1986, Mayfield.
21. Rotella RJ: Psychological care of the injured athlete. In Kulund DN, editor: *The injured athlete*, Philadelphia, 1988, Lippincott.
22. Selye H: *Stress without distress*, New York, 1974, Lippincott.
23. Smith AM et al: Emotional responses of athletes to injury, *Mayo Clin Proc* 65:38, 1990.
24. Smith AM, Milliner EK: Injured athletes and the risk of suicide, *J Athl Train* 29(4):337, 1994.
25. Steadman J: A physician's approach to the psychology of injury. In Heil J, editor: *Psychology of sport injury*, Champaign, Ill, 1993, Human Kinetics.
26. Weiss MR, Troxel RK: Psychology of the injured athlete, *Ath Train* 21:104, 1986.

ANNOTATED BIBLIOGRAPHY

Heil J, editor: *Psychology of sport injury*, Champaign, Ill, 1993, Human Kinetics.

An in-depth look at the psychology of sport injury for sports psychologists.

Pelletier KR: *Mind as healer, mind as slayer*, New York, 1977, Dell.

Provides an in-depth discussion of the relationship of the mind to the cause and healing of disease.

Selye H: *Stress without distress*, New York, 1974, Lippincott.

A practical guide to understanding the role of stress in life.

Environmental Considerations

When you finish this chapter, you should be able to

- Describe the physiology of hyperthermia and the clinical signs of heat stress and how they can be prevented.
- Identify the causes of hypothermia and the major cold disorders and how they can be prevented.
- Describe the problems that high altitude might present to the athlete and how they can be managed.
- Explain how an athlete should be protected from exposure to the sun.
- Describe precautions that should be taken in an electrical storm.
- List the problems that are presented to the athlete by air pollution and how they can be avoided.
- Discuss what effect circadian dysrhythmia can have on athletes and the best procedures for handling any problems that arise.
- Discuss the effect of artificial versus natural turf on the incidence of injury.

Environmental stress can adversely affect an athlete's performance and in some instances can pose a serious health threat. The environmental categories that are of major concern to the coach, athletic trainer, and sports physician include hyperthermia, hypothermia, altitude, exposure to the sun, electrical storms, air pollution, and circadian dysrhythmia (jet lag).

HYPERTHERMIA

hyperthemia
Elevated body temperature.

A major concern in sports is the problem of hyperthermia. Among football players and distance runners in high school and college there have been a number of deaths caused by hyperthermia.[1,26]

It is vitally important that the coaching staff and athletic trainer have knowledge about temperature and humidity factors to assist them in planning practice. The coach or athletic trainer must clearly understand when environmental heat and humidity are at a dangerous level and act accordingly. In addition, the clinical symptoms and signs of heat stress must be recognized and managed properly.

Heat Stress

Regardless of the level of physical conditioning, extreme caution must be taken when exercising in hot, humid weather. Prolonged exposure to extreme heat can result in heat illness.[25] Heat stress is preventable, but each year many athletes suffer illness and even death from some heat-related cause. Athletes who exercise in hot, humid environments are particularly vulnerable to heat stress.[35]

Heat can be gained or lost through
  Metabolic heat production
  Conductive heat exchange
  Convective heat exchange
  Radiant heat exchange
  Evaporative heat loss

The physiological processes in the body will continue to function only as long as body temperature is maintained within a normal range.[17] Maintenance of normal temperature in a hot environment depends on the ability of the body to dissipate heat. Body temperature can be affected by five factors.

Metabolic Heat Production

Normal metabolic function in the body results in the production and radiation of heat. Consequently, metabolism will always cause an increase in body heat depending on the intensity of the physical activity. The higher the metabolic rate, the more the heat produced.

Conductive Heat Exchange

Physical contact with other objects can result in either a heat loss or heat gain. A football player competing on AstroTurf on a sunny August afternoon will experience an increase in body temperature simply by standing on the turf.

Convective Heat Exchange

Body heat can be either lost or gained depending on the temperature of the circulating medium. A cool breeze will always tend to cool the body by removing heat from the body surface. Conversely, if the temperature of the circulating air is higher than the temperature of the skin, there will be a gain in body heat.

Radiant Heat Exchange

Radiant heat from sunshine causes an increase in body temperature. Obviously, the effects of radiation are much greater in the sunshine than in the shade. However, on a cloudy day the body also emits radiant heat energy, and thus radiation may also result in either heat loss or heat gain. During exercise the body attempts to dissipate heat produced by metabolism by dilating superficial arterial and venous vessels, thus channeling blood to the superficial capillaries in the skin.

Evaporative Heat Loss

Sweat glands in the skin allow water to be transported to the surface, where it evaporates, taking large quantities of heat with it. When the temperature and radiant heat of the environment become higher than body temperature, loss of body heat becomes highly dependent on the process of sweat evaporation.

A normal person can sweat off about 1 quart of water per hour for about 2 hours. Sweating does not cause heat loss. The sweat must evaporate for heat to be dissipated. But the air must be relatively free of water for evaporation to occur. Heat loss through evaporation is severely impaired when the relative humidity reaches 65% and virtually stops when the humidity reaches 75%.

It should be obvious that heat-related problems have the greatest chance of occurring on days when the sun is bright and the temperature and relative humidity are high. However, cramps, heat exhaustion, and heatstroke can occur whenever the body's ability to dissipate heat is impaired.

Monitoring the Heat Index

The WBGT index measures heat and humidity.

The athletic trainer must exercise common sense when overseeing the health care of athletes training or competing in the heat. Obviously, when the combination of heat, humidity, and bright sunshine is present, extra caution is warranted. The universal wet bulb globe temperature (WBGT) index provides the athletic trainer with an objective means for determining necessary precautions for practice and competition in hot weather.[22] The index incorporates readings from several different thermometers. The dry bulb temperature (DBT) is recorded from a standard mercury thermometer. The wet bulb temperature (WBT) uses a wet wick or piece of gauze wrapped around the end of a thermometer that is swung around in the air. Globe temperature (GT) measures the sun's radiation and has a black metal casing around the end of the thermometer. Once the three readings have been taken, the following formula is used to calculate the WBGT index:

$$WBGT = 0.1 \times DBT + 0.7 \times WBT + GT \times 0.2$$

Using this formula yields an index on which recommendations relative to outdoor activity are based (Table 12-1).

The DBT and WBT are easily measured using an instrument called a physio-dyne (Figure 12-1). This instrument contains a scale to calculate the difference between DBT and WBT, which is relative humidity. This instrument is relatively inexpensive

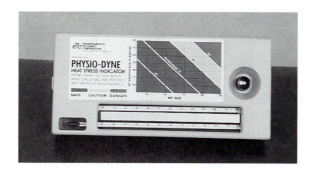

Figure 12-1

An instrument called a physio-dyne may be used to determine the heat index.

and easy to use. The following suggestions regarding temperature and humidity will serve as a guide (Table 12-2).

Heat Illnesses

Exercising in a hot, humid environment can cause various forms of heat illness, including heat rash, heat syncope, heat cramps, heat exhaustion, and heatstroke (heat hyperexia).

Heat Rash

A heat rash, also called prickly heat, is a benign condition associated with a red, raised rash accompanied by sensations of prickling and tingling during sweating. It usually occurs when the skin is continuously wet with unevaporated sweat. The rash is generally localized to areas of the body covered with clothing. Continually toweling the body can help prevent the rash from developing.[30]

Heat Syncope

Heat syncope, or heat collapse, is associated with rapid physical fatigue during overexposure to heat. It is usually caused by standing in heat for long periods or by not being accustomed to exercising in the heat. It is caused by peripheral vasodilation of superficial vessels, hypotension, or a pooling of blood in the extremities, which re-

TABLE 12-1 Universal WBGT Index

WBGT Index for Outdoor Activities (Wet Bulb Global Temperature)		
Range	**Signal Flag**	**Activity**
82-84.9	Green	Alert for possible increase in index
85-87.9	Yellow	Active practice curtailed (unacclimated athletes)
88-89.9	Red	Active practice curtailed (all athletes—except most acclimated)
90+		All training stopped, skull session—demonstrations

TABLE 12-2 Procedures for Dealing with Heat and Humidity

Temperature (° F)	Humidity	Procedure
80°-90° (26.7° C-32.2° C)	Under 70%	Watch those athletes who tend toward obesity.
80°-90° (26.7° C-32.2° C)	Over 70%	Athletes should take a 10-minute rest every hour, and tee shirts should be changed when wet. All athletes should be under constant and careful supervision.
90°-100° (32.2° C-37.8° C)	Under 70%	
90°-100° (32.2° C-37.8° C)	Over 70%	Under these conditions it would be well to suspend practice. A shortened program conducted in shorts and tee shirts could be established.
Over 100° (37.8° C)		

sults in dizziness, fainting, and nausea. It is quickly relieved by laying the athlete down in a cool environment and replacing fluids.[30]

Heat Cramps

Heat cramps are extremely painful muscle spasms that occur most commonly in the calf and abdomen, although any muscle can be involved (Table 12-3). The occurrence of heat cramps is related to excessive loss of water and several electrolytes or ions (sodium, chloride, potassium, magnesium, and calcium), which are each essential elements in muscle contraction.

Profuse sweating involves losses of large amounts of water and small quantities of sodium, potassium, magnesium, and calcium, thus destroying the balance in concentration of these elements within the body. This imbalance will ultimately result in painful muscle contractions and cramps. The person most likely to get heat cramps is one who is in fairly good condition but who simply overexerts in the heat.

Heat cramps may be prevented by adequate replacement of sodium, potassium, magnesium, calcium, and, most importantly, water. Ingestion of salt tablets is not recommended. Simply salting food a bit more heavily can replace sodium; bananas are particularly high in potassium; and calcium is present in milk, cheese, and dairy products. The immediate treatment for heat cramps is ingestion of large quantities of water and mild stretching with ice massage of the muscle in spasm. An athlete who experiences heat cramps will generally not be able to return to practice or competition for the remainder of the day because cramping is likely to reoccur.

Heat Exhaustion

Heat exhaustion results from inadequate replacement of fluids lost through sweating (Table 12-3). Clinically, the victim of heat exhaustion will collapse and manifest profuse sweating, pale skin, mildly elevated temperature (102° F), dizziness, hyperventilation, and rapid pulse.

It is sometimes possible to spot athletes who are having problems with heat exhaustion. They may begin to develop heat cramps. They may become disoriented and light-headed, and their physical performance will not be up to their usual standards when fluid replacement has not been adequate. In general, persons in poor physical condition who attempt to exercise in the heat are most likely to get heat exhaustion.

Immediate treatment of heat exhaustion requires ingestion and eventually intravenous replacement of large quantities of water. It is essential for the athletic trainer to obtain a rectal temperature to differentiate heat exhaustion from heatstroke. In heat exhaustion the rectal temperature will be around 102° F. If possible, the athlete should be placed in a cool environment, although it is more critical to replace fluids.

Heatstroke

Unlike heat cramps and heat exhaustion, heatstroke is a serious, life-threatening emergency (Table 12-3). The specific cause of heatstroke is unknown; however, it is clinically characterized by sudden collapse with loss of consciousness; flushed, hot skin with less sweating than would be seen with heat exhaustion; shallow breathing; a rapid, strong pulse; and, most important, a core temperature of 106° F or higher. Basically there is a breakdown of the thermoregulatory mechanism, caused by excessively high body temperature; the body loses the ability to dissipate heat through sweating.

Heatstroke can occur suddenly and without warning. The athlete will not usually experience signs of heat cramps or heat exhaustion. The possibility of death from heatstroke can be significantly reduced if body temperature is lowered to normal within 45 minutes. The longer body temperature is elevated to 106° F or higher, the higher the mortality rate.

Every first aid effort should be directed to lowering body temperature. Get the athlete into a cool environment. Strip all clothing off the athlete, sponge him or her

12-1

Critical Thinking Exercise

A wrestler collapses during a match and exhibits signs of profuse sweating, pale skin, mildly elevated temperature (102° F), dizziness, hyperventilation, and rapid pulse. When questioned by the athletic trainer the athlete indicates that earlier in the day he took diuretic medication to facilitate water loss in an effort to help him make weight.

? What type of heat illness is the athlete experiencing, and what does the athletic trainer need to do to manage this situation appropriately?

TABLE 12-3 Heat Disorders: Treatment and Prevention

Disorders	Cause	Clinical Features and Diagnosis	Treatment	Prevention
Heat cramps	Hard work in heat; sweating heavily; imbalance between water and electrolytes	Muscle twitching and cramps, usually after midday; spasms in arms, legs, abdomen	Ingesting large amounts of water, mild stretching, and ice massage of affected muscle	Acclimatize athlete properly; provide large quantities of water; increase intake of calcium, sodium, and potassium slightly
Heat exhaustion	Prolonged sweating; inadequate replacement of body fluid losses; diarrhea; intestinal infection	Excessive thirst, dry tongue and mouth; weight loss; fatigue; weakness; incoordination; mental dullness; small urine volume; slightly elevated body temperature; high serum protein and sodium; reduced swelling	Bed rest in cool room, IV fluids if drinking is impaired; increase fluid intake to 6 to 8 L/day; sponge with cool water; keep record of body weight; keep fluid balance record; provide semiliquid food until salination is normal	Supply adequate water and other liquids Provide adequate rest and opportunity for cooling
Heatstroke	Thermoregulatory failure of sudden onset	Abrupt onset, preceded by headache, vertigo, and fatigue, flushed skin; relatively less sweating than seen with heat exhaustion; pulse rate increases rapidly and may reach 160 to 180; respiration increases; blood pressure seldom rises; temperature rises rapidly to 105° or 106° F (40° to 41° C); athlete feels as if he or she is burning up; diarrhea, vomiting; circulatory collapse may produce death; could lead to permanent brain damage	Heroic measures to reduce temperature must be taken immediately (e.g., sponge cool water and air fan over body, massage limbs); remove to hospital as soon as possible	Ensure proper acclimatization, proper hydration Educate those supervising activities conducted in the heat Adapt activities to environment Screen participants with past history of heat illness for malignant hyperthermia

ad libitum
To the amount desired.

down with cool water, and fan with a towel. Do not immerse the athlete in cold water. It is imperative that the victim be transported to a hospital as quickly as possible. Do not wait for an ambulance; transport the victim in whatever vehicle happens to be available. The replacement of fluid is not critical in initial first aid.

Malignant hyperthermia Malignant hyperthermia is a rare muscle disorder that causes hypersensitivity to anesthesia and hot environments. This disorder causes muscle temperatures to increase faster than core temperatures, and its symptoms are similar to those of heatstroke. The athlete complains of muscle pain after exercise, and rectal temperature remains elevated for 10 to 15 minutes after exercise. Muscle biopsy is necessary for diagnosis. Athletes with malignant hyperthermia should be disqualified from competing in hot, humid environments.[20]

Preventing Heat Illness

The coach and athletic trainer should understand that heat illness is preventable. By exercising some common sense and caution there is little reason for heat illnesses to occur. The following should be considered when planning a training-competitive program that is likely to take place during hot weather.

Fluid and Electrolyte Replacement

During hot weather it is essential to continually replace fluids lost through evaporation by drinking large quantities of water.[7] An average runner may lose from 1.5 to 2.5 L of water per hour through active sweating; much greater amounts can be lost by football players in warm-weather activity.[3] Seldom is more than 50% of this fluid loss replaced, even though replacement fluids are taken **ad libitum,** because athletes usually find it uncomfortable to exercise vigorously on a full stomach, which could interfere with respiration. The problem in fluid replacement is how rapidly the fluid can be eliminated from the stomach into the intestine, from which it can enter the bloodstream. Cold drinks (45° to 55° F [7.2° to 12.8° C]) tend to empty more rapidly from the stomach than do warmer drinks; they are not more likely to induce cramps, nor do they offer any particular threat to a normal heart.

Sweating occurs whether or not the athlete drinks water, and if the sweat losses are not replaced by fluid intake over a period of several hours, dehydration results. Sweat is always hypotonic; that is, it contains a lower concentration of salt than does the blood, and its loss establishes a deficit of water in excess of the salt deficit. This is reflected in several physiological changes, which may manifest themselves in peripheral vascular collapse, renal decompensation, and uremia.[12]

Athletes must have unlimited access to water. Failure to permit ad libitum access will not only undermine their playing potentialities, but also may be responsible for permitting a dangerous situation to develop that could conceivably have fatal consequences (Figure 12-2).

Commercially prepared drinks A number of commercially prepared drinks may be used in fluid replacement.[18] It has been documented that ingestion of hypertonic solutions containing simple sugars and electrolyes tends to slow gastric emptying, thus depriving the working cell of much-needed fluid.[24] A cell needs water to be able to function normally and may be damaged if sufficient amounts of water are not available. A solution that contains only 5% glucose will significantly retard the replacement of lost fluids.[7] Thus ingestion of drinks containing simple sugars and electrolytes during activity is not recommended, although they may be useful for replenishing fluids and electrolytes before and after activity in the heat.[28] It may be necessary to replace glucose in activities lasting longer than 1 hour, and in this case the drinks may be beneficial.

The new generation of commercially manufactured drinks has reduced the negative effects of simple sugar solutions on gastric emptying by using a polymerized form of glucose. This process maximizes carbohydrate content while making the solution

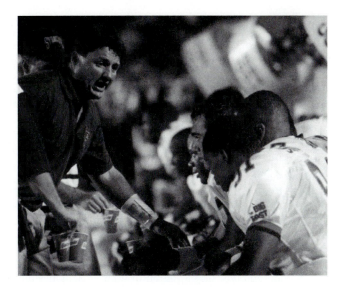

Figure 12-2

Athletes must have unlimited access to water, especially in hot weather.

less hypertonic. Thus a 5% solution of polymerized glucose provides the athlete with more water and carbohydrate compared with a drink containing simple sugars.[24]

Gradual Acclimatization

Gradual acclimatization is probably the single most effective method of avoiding heat stress. Acclimatization should involve not only becoming accustomed to heat but also becoming acclimatized to exercising in hot temperatures.[21] A good preseason conditioning program, started well before the advent of the competitive season and carefully graded as to intensity, is recommended.[3] During the first 5 or 6 days an 80% acclimatization can be achieved on the basis of a 2-hour practice period in the morning and a 2-hour practice period in the afternoon. Each should be broken down into 20 minutes of work alternated with 20 minutes of rest in the shade.

Identifying Susceptible Individuals

Athletes with a large muscle mass are particularly prone to heat illness.[27] Most deaths that occur among American football players are to interior linemen.[27] It must also be noted that fat produces more body heat than proteins or carbohydrates.[39] In addition, a considerable loss of fluid makes the athlete highly susceptible to heat illness. Women are apparently more physiologically efficient in body temperature regulation than men; although they possess as many heat-activated sweat glands as men, they sweat less and manifest a higher heart rate when working in heat. Although slight differences exist, the same precautionary measures apply to both genders. Body build must be considered when determining individual susceptibility to heat stress. Overweight individuals may have as much as 18% greater heat production than underweight individuals because metabolic heat is produced proportionately to surface area. It has been found that heat victims tend to be overweight. Death from heatstroke increases at a ratio of approximately 4 to 1 as body weight increases.

Uniforms

Uniforms should be selected on the basis of temperature and humidity. Initial practices should be conducted in short-sleeved tee shirts, shorts, and socks, moving gradually into short-sleeved net jerseys, lightweight pants, and socks as acclimatization proceeds. All early-season practices and games should be conducted in lightweight uniforms with short-sleeved net jerseys and socks. Long sleeves and full stockings are indicated only when the temperature is low.

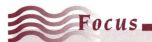

Environmental conduct of sports, particularly football

I. General warning
   A. Most adverse reactions to environmental heat and humidity occur during the first few days of training.
   B. It is necessary to become thoroughly acclimatized to heat to successfully compete in hot or humid environments.
   C. Occurrence of a heat injury indicates poor supervision of the sports program.

II. Athletes who are most susceptible to heat injury
   A. Individuals unaccustomed to working in the heat.
   B. Overweight individuals, particularly large linemen.
   C. Eager athletes who constantly compete at capacity.
   D. Ill athletes who have an infection, fever, or gastrointestinal disturbance.
   E. Athletes who receive immunization injections and subsequently develop temperature elevations.

III. Prevention of heat injury
   A. Take complete medical history and provide physical examination.
      1. Include history of previous heat illnesses or fainting in the heat.
      2. Include inquiry about sweating and peripheral vascular defects.
   B. Evaluate general physical condition and type and duration of training activities for previous month.
      1. Extent of work in the heat.
      2. General training activities.
   C. Measure temperature and humidity on the practice or playing fields.
      1. Make measurements before and during training or competitive sessions.
      2. Adjust activity level to environmental conditions.
         a. Decrease activity if hot or humid.
         b. Eliminate unnecessary clothing when hot or humid.
   D. Acclimatize athletes to heat gradually.
      1. Acclimatization to heat requires work in the heat.
         a. Use recommended type and variety of warm weather workouts for preseason training.
         b. Provide graduated training program for first 7 to 10 days and other abnormally hot or humid days.
      2. Provide adequate rest intervals and water replacement during the acclimatization period.
   E. Monitor body weight loss during activity in the heat.
      1. Body water should be replaced as it is lost.
         a. Allow additional water as desired by player.
         b. Provide salt on training tables (no salt tablets should be taken).
         c. Weigh each day before and after training or competition.
            (1) Treat athlete who loses excessive weight each day.
            (2) Treat well-conditioned athlete who continues to lose weight for several days.
   F. Monitor clothing and uniforms.
      1. Provide lightweight clothing that is loose fitting at the neck, waist, and sleeves; use shorts and tee shirt at beginning of training.
      2. Avoid excessive padding and taping.
      3. Avoid use of long stockings, long sleeves, double jerseys, and other excess clothing.
      4. Avoid use of rubberized clothing or sweatsuits.
      5. Provide clean clothing daily—all items.
   G. Provide rest periods to dissipate accumulated body heat.
      1. Rest in cool, shaded area with some air movement.
      2. Avoid hot brick walls or hot benches.
      3. Loosen or remove jerseys or other garments.
      4. Take water during the rest period.

IV. Trouble signs: stop activity!

Headache	
Nausea	Diarrhea
Mental slowness	Cramps
Incoherence	Seizures
Visual disturbance	Rigidity
Fatigue	Weak, rapid pulse
Weakness	Pallor
Unsteadiness	Flush
Collapse	Faintness
Unconsciousness	Chill
Vomiting	Cyanotic appearance

Weight Records

Careful weight records of all players must be kept. Weights should be measured both before and after practice for at least the first 2 weeks of practice. If a sudden increase in temperature or humidity occurs during the season, weight should be recorded again for a period of time. A loss of 3% to 5% of body weight will reduce blood volume and could lead to a health threat.[41]

Temperature and Humidity Readings

Dry-bulb and wet-bulb readings should be taken on the field before practice to monitor the heat index. Modifications to the practice schedule should be made according to the severity of existing environmental conditions. The purchase of a physio-dyne for this purpose is recommended (see Figure 12-1).

Clinical Indications and Treatment

The Focus box (opposite) and Table 12-3 list the clinical symptoms of the various hyperthermal conditions and the indications for treatment. Although the box calls particular attention to some of the procedures for football, the precautions, in general, apply to all sports. Because of the specialized equipment worn by the players, football requires special consideration. To a degree, many uniforms are heat traps and serve to compound the environmental heat problem, which is not the case with the lighter uniforms.

HYPOTHERMIA

Cold weather is a frequent adjunct to many outdoor sports in which the sport itself does not require heavy protective clothing; consequently, the weather becomes a pertinent factor in injury susceptibility.[43] In most instances, the activity itself enables the athlete to increase the metabolic rate sufficiently to be able to function physically in a normal manner and dissipate the resulting heat and perspiration through the usual physiological mechanisms. An athlete may fail to warm up sufficiently or may become chilled because of relative inactivity for varying periods of time demanded by the particular sport either during competition or training; consequently, the athlete is exceedingly prone to injury. Low temperatures alone can pose some problems, but when such temperatures are further accentuated by wind, the chill factor becomes critical[31] (Figure 12-3). For example, a runner proceeding at a pace of 10 mph directly into a wind of 5 mph creates a chill factor equivalent to a 15-mph headwind.

A third factor, dampness or wetness, further increases the risk of hypothermia. Air at a temperature of 50° F is relatively comfortable, but water at the same temperature is intolerable. The combination of cold, wind, and dampness creates an environment that easily predisposes the athlete to hypothermia.

Sixty-five percent of heat that is produced by the body is lost through radiation. This loss occurs most often from the warm vascular areas of the head and neck.[4] Twenty percent of heat loss is through evaporation, of which two thirds is through the skin and one third is through the respiratory tract.[4]

During strenuous physical activity in cold weather, as muscular fatigue builds up the rate of exercise begins to drop and may reach a level wherein the body heat loss to the environment exceeds the metabolic heat protection, resulting in definite impairment of neuromuscular responses and exhaustion. A relatively small drop in body core temperature can induce shivering sufficient to materially affect one's neuromuscular coordination. Shivering ceases below a body temperature of 85° to 90° F (29.4° to 32.2° C). Death is imminent if the core temperature rises to 107° F (41.6° C) or drops to between 77° and 85° F (25° and 29° C).

12-2

Critical Thinking E x e r c i s e

A high school football coach in southern Louisiana is concerned about the likelihood that several of his players will suffer heat-related illness during preseason football practice in the first 2 weeks of August. The school has recently hired an athletic trainer, and the coach has come to the athletic trainer to ask what can be done to minimize the risk of heat-related illnesses.

? What recommendations or intervention strategies can the athletic trainer implement to help the athletes avoid heat-related illnesses?

Many sports played in cold weather do not require heavy protective clothing; thus weather becomes a factor in injury susceptibility.

Low temperatures accentuated by wind and dampness can pose major problems for athletes.

Figure 12-3

Low temperatures can pose serious problems for the athlete, but wind chill could be a critical factor.

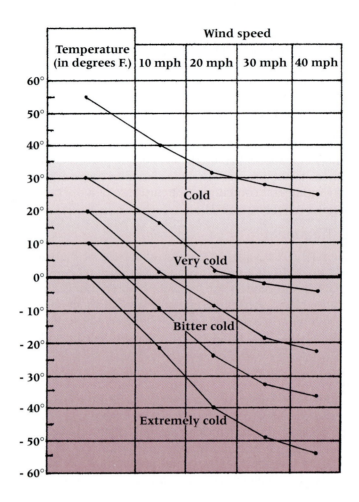

Prevention

Apparel for competitors must be geared to the weather.[15] The function of such apparel is to provide a semitropical microclimate for the body and to prevent chilling. There are several fabrics available on the market that are waterproof and windproof but permit the passage of heat and allow sweat to evaporate. The clothing should not restrict movement, should be as lightweight as possible, and should consist of material that will permit the free passage of sweat and body heat that would otherwise accumulate on the skin or the clothing and provide a chilling factor when activity ceases. The athlete should routinely dress in thin layers of clothing that can easily be added or removed as the temperature decreases or increases. Continuous adjustment of these layers will reduce sweating and the likelihood that clothing will become damp or wet. Again, wetness or dampness plays a critical role in the development of hypothermia. Preliminary to exercise, during activity breaks or rest periods, and at the termination of exercise, a warm-up suit should be worn to prevent chilling. Activity in cold, wet, and windy weather poses some problem because such weather reduces the insulating value of clothing; consequently the individual may be unable to achieve energy levels equal to the subsequent body heat losses. Runners who wish to continue outdoor work in cold weather should use lightweight insulating clothing and, if breathing cold air seems distressful, should use ski goggles and a ski face mask or should cover the mouth and nose with a free-hanging cloth.

Inadequate clothing, improper warm-up, and a high chill factor form a triad that can lead to musculoskeletal injury, chilblains, frostbite, or the minor respiratory disorders associated with lower tissue temperatures. For work or sports in temperatures below 32° F (0° C), it is advisable to add a layer of protective clothing for every 5 mph of wind.

Cold Disorders

As is true in a hot environment, there is need of fluid replacement in a cold environment. With reduced blood volume because of dehydration, there is less fluid available for warming the tissues.[33] Athletes performing in a cold environment should be weighed before and after practice, especially in the first 2 weeks of the season.[6] Severe overexposure to a cold climate occurs less often than hyperthermia does in a warm climate; however, it is still a major risk of winter sports, long-distance running in cold weather, and swimming in cold water.[16]

Common Cold Injuries

Local cooling of the body can result in tissue damage ranging from superficial to deep. Exposure to a damp, freezing cold can cause frostnip. In contrast, exposure to dry temperatures well below freezing more commonly produces a deep freezing type of frostbite.

Below-freezing temperatures may cause ice crystals to form between or within the cells and may eventually destroy the cell. Local capillaries can be injured, blood clots may form, and blood may be shunted away from the injury site to ensure the survival of the nonaffected tissue.

Cold injuries in sports include:
  Frostnip
  Frostbite

Frostnip

Frostnip involves ears, nose, cheeks, chin, fingers, and toes. It commonly occurs when there is a high wind, severe cold, or both. The skin initially appears very firm, with cold, painless areas that may peel or blister in 24 to 72 hours. Affected areas can be treated early by firm, sustained pressure of the hand (without rubbing), blowing hot breath on the spot, or, if the injury is to the fingertips, by placing them in the armpits.

Frostbite

Chilblains result from prolonged and constant exposure to cold for many hours. In time there is skin redness, swelling, tingling, and pain in the toes and fingers. This adverse response is caused by problems of peripheral circulation and can be avoided by preventing further cold exposure.

Superficial frostbite involves only the skin and subcutaneous tissue. The skin appears pale, hard, cold, and waxy. Palpating the injured area will reveal a sense of hardness but with yielding of the underlying deeper tissue structures. When rewarming, the superficial frostbite will at first feel numb, then will sting and burn. Later the area may produce blisters and be painful for a number of weeks.[29]

Deep frostbite is a serious injury indicating tissues that are frozen. This is a medical emergency requiring immediate hospitalization. As with frostnip and superficial frostbite, the tissue is initially cold, hard, pale or white, and numb. Rapid rewarming is required, including hot drinks, heating pads, or hot water bottles that are 100° to 110° F (38° to 43° C). During rewarming, the tissue will become blotchy red, swollen, and extremely painful. Later the injury may become gangrenous, causing a loss of tissue.

ALTITUDE

Most athletic events are not conducted at extreme altitudes. For example, Mexico City's elevation, which is 7600 feet high, is considered moderate, yet at this height there is a 7% to 8% decrease in maximum oxygen uptake.[38] This loss in maximum oxygen uptake represents a 4% to 8% deterioration in an athlete's performance in

Most athletic events are not conducted at high altitudes.

endurance events, depending on the duration of effort and lack of wind resistance. Often, the athlete's body compensates for this decrease in maximum oxygen uptake with corresponding tachycardia.[38] When the body is suddenly without its usual oxygen supply, hyperventilation can occur. Many of these responses are results of having fewer red blood cells than necessary to adequately capture the available oxygen in the air.[40]

Acclimatization to Altitude

A major factor in altitude adaptation is the problem of oxygen deficiency. With a reduction in barometric pressure the partial pressure of oxygen in inspired air is also low. Under these circumstances the existing circulating red blood cells become less saturated, depriving tissue of needed oxygen.[23]

An individual's acclimatization to high altitude depends on whether he or she is a native, resident, or visitor to the area. Natives of areas with high altitudes (e.g., the Andes and Nepal) have a larger chest capacity, more alveoli, more capillaries that transport blood to tissue, and a higher red blood cell level.[14] In contrast, the resident or individual who stays at a high altitude for months or years makes a partial acclimatization. His or her later adaptation includes the conservation of glucose, an increased number of mitochondria (the sources of energy in a cell), and increased formation of hemoglobin. In the visitor or person who is in an early stage of adaptation to high altitude, a number of responses represent a physiological struggle. The responses include increased breathing, increased heart action, increased hemoglobin in circulating blood, increased blood alkalinity, and increased myoglobin, as well as changes in the distribution of blood flow and cell enzyme activity.

There are many uncertainties about when to have an athlete go to an area of high altitude to compete. Some believe that 2 to 3 weeks before competition provides the best adjustment period, whereas others believe that, for psychological as well as physiological reasons, 3 days before competition is enough time.[38] This shorter time allows time for the recovery of the acid-base balance in the blood but does not provide enough time for achieving a significant adjustment in blood volume and maximum cardiac output.[38]

Altitude Illness

Coaches and athletic trainers must be apprised that some of their athletes may become ill when suddenly subjected to high altitudes.[45] These illnesses might include acute mountain sickness, pulmonary edema, and, when present in some athletes, an adverse reaction to the sickle cell trait.

Acute Mountain Sickness

One out of three individuals who go from a low to a moderate altitude of 7000 to 8000 feet will experience mild to moderate symptoms of acute mountain sickness. Symptoms include headache, nausea, vomiting, sleep disturbance, and dyspnea, which may last up to 3 days.[38] These symptoms have been attributed by some to a tissue disruption in the brain affecting the sodium and potassium balance. This imbalance can cause excess fluid retention within the cells and the subsequent occurrence of abnormal pressure.[38]

Pulmonary Edema

At an altitude of 9000 to 10,000 feet, high-altitude pulmonary edema may occur. Characteristically, lungs at this altitude will accumulate a small amount of fluid within the alveolar walls.[38] In most individuals this fluid is absorbed in a few days, but in some it continues to collect and forms pulmonary edema. Symptoms of high-altitude pulmonary edema are dyspnea, cough, headache, weakness, and in some cases unconsciousness.[38] The treatment of choice is to get the athlete to a lower altitude as soon as possible and give oxygen. When he or she is at a lower altitude, the condition rapidly resolves.[36]

Sickle Cell Trait Reaction

Approximately 8% to 10% of American blacks (approximately 2 million persons) have the sickle cell trait. In most of them the trait is benign. The sickle cell trait relates to an abnormality of the structure of the red blood cell and its hemoglobin content.[11] When the abnormal hemoglobin molecules become deoxygenated as a result of exercise at a high altitude, the cells tend to clump together. This process causes an abnormal "sickle" shape to the red blood cell, which can be easily destroyed. This condition can cause an enlarged spleen, which, in some cases, has been known to rupture at high altitudes.[38] (See Chapter 27.)

OVEREXPOSURE TO SUN

Athletes, along with coaches, athletic trainers, and other support staff, frequently spend a great deal of time outdoors in direct sunlight. Precautions to protect these individuals from overexposure to ultraviolet light by applying sunscreens are often totally ignored.

Long-Term Effects on Skin

The most serious effects of long-term exposure to ultraviolet light are premature aging of the skin and skin cancer.[9] Lightly pigmented individuals are more susceptible to these maladies. Premature aging of the skin is characterized by dryness, cracking, and a decrease in the elasticity of the skin. Skin cancer is the most common malignant tumor found in humans and has been epidemiologically and clinically associated with exposure to ultraviolet radiation. Damage to DNA is suspected as the cause of skin cancer, but the exact cause is unknown. The major types of skin cancer are basal cell carcinoma, squamous cell carcinoma, and malignant melanoma. Fortunately, the rate of cure exceeds 95% with early detection and treatment.[9]

Sunscreens

Sunscreens applied to the skin can help prevent many of the damaging effects of ultraviolet radiation. A sunscreen's effectiveness in absorbing the sunburn-inducing radiation is expressed as the sun protection factor (**SPF**). An SPF of 6 indicates that an athlete can be exposed to ultraviolet light six times longer than without a sunscreen before the skin will begin to turn red. Higher numbers provide greater protection. However, athletes who have a family or personal history of skin cancer may experience significant damage to the skin even when wearing an SPF-15 sunscreen. Therefore these individuals should wear an SPF-30 sunscreen.

Sunscreen should be worn regularly by athletes, coaches, and athletic trainers who spend time outside. This is particularly true for individuals with fair complexions, light hair, blue eyes, or those whose skin burns easily. People with dark complexions should also wear sunscreens to prevent sun damage.

It has been clearly shown that sun exposure causes a premature aging of skin (wrinkling, freckling, prominent blood vessels, coarsening of skin texture), induces the formation of precancerous growths, and increases the risk of developing basal and squamous cell skin cancers. Because 60% to 80% of our lifetime sun exposure is often obtained by age 20, everyone over 6 months of age should use sunscreens.

Sunscreens are needed most during March to November but should preferably be used year-round. They are needed most between 10 AM and 4 PM and should be applied 15 to 30 minutes before sun exposure. Although clothing and hats provide some protection from the sun, they are not a substitute for sunscreens (a typical white cotton tee shirt provides an SPF of only 5). Reflected sunlight from water, sand, and snow may effectively increase sun exposure and risk of burning.

12-3

Critical Thinking Exercise

A track athlete is competing in a day-long outdoor track meet. She is extremely concerned about getting sunburned and has liberally applied sunscreen with an SPF of 30 during the early morning. It is a hot, sunny day and she is sweating heavily. She is worried that her sunscreen has worn off and asks the athletic trainer for more sunscreen. The athletic trainer hands her sunscreen with an SPF of 15 and she complains that it is not strong enough to protect her.

? What can the athletic trainer tell the athlete to assure her that she will be well protected by the sunscreen she has been given?

SPF
Sun protection factor.

ELECTRICAL STORMS

Research indicates that lightning is the number two cause of death by weather phenomena, accounting for 110 deaths per year.[44] If you hear thunder or see lightning, you are in immediate danger and should seek protective shelter in an indoor facility at once. An indoor facility is recommended as the safest protective shelter. However, if an indoor facility is not available, an automobile is a relatively safe alternative. If neither of these is available, the following guidelines are recommended. Avoid standing under large trees and telephone poles. If the only alternative is a tree, choose a small tree in a wooded area that is not on a hill. As a last alternative, find a ravine or valley. In all instances outdoors, assume a crouched position. Avoid standing water and metal objects at all times (metal bleachers, metal cleats, umbrellas, etc.).

The most dangerous storms give little or no warning; thunder and lightning are not heard or seen. Up to 40% of all lightning is not accompanied by thunder, and 20% to 40% of thunder cannot be heard because of atmospheric disturbances. At times, the only natural forewarning that might precede a strike is feeling your hair stand on end and skin tingle. At this point, you are in imminent danger of being struck by lightning and should drop to the ground and assume a crouched position immediately. Do not lie flat. Should a ground strike occur near you, lying flat increases the body's surface area that is exposed to the current traveling through the ground.[44]

The National Weather Service recommends that 30 minutes should pass after the last sound of thunder is heard or lightning strike is seen before resuming play. This is sufficient time to allow the storm to pass and move out of lightning strike range. The perilous misconception that it is possible to see lightning coming and have time to act before it strikes could prove to be fatal. In reality, the lightning that we see flashing is actually the return stroke flashing upward from the ground to the cloud, not downward. When you see the lightning strike, it already has hit.[44]

The following basic guidelines on thunder and lightning should be followed[44]:

- If thunder or lightning can be heard or seen, stop activity and seek protective shelter immediately.
- In situations where thunder or lightning may or may not be present and you feel your hair stand on end and skin tingle, immediately assume the following crouched position: drop to your knees, place your arms on your legs, and lower your head. Do not lie flat.
- In the event that either situation should occur, allow 30 minutes to pass after the last sound of thunder or lightning strike before resuming play.

AIR POLLUTION

Air pollution is a major problem common in urban areas with large industries and heavy automobile traffic. There are two types of pollution: photochemical "haze" and smog. Photochemical haze consists of nitrogen dioxide and stagnant air that are acted on by sunlight to produce ozone.[40] Smog is produced by the combination of carbon monoxide and sulphur dioxide, which emanates from the combustion of a fossil fuel such as coal.

Ozone

Ozone is a form of oxygen in which three atoms of the element combine to form the molecule O_3. It is produced by a reaction of oxygen (O_2), nitrogen oxides, and hydrocarbon, plus sunlight.[37]

When individuals are engaged in physical tasks requiring minimum effort, an increase in ozone in the air does not usually reduce functional capacity in normal work output. However, when there is an increase in work output (e.g., during exercise), the work capacity is decreased. The athlete may experience shortness of breath, coughing, chest tightness, pain during deep breathing, nausea, eye irritation, fatigue,

---

The most dangerous storms give little or no warning.

12-4

Critical Thinking Exercise

A lacrosse team is practicing on a remote field with no indoor facility in close proximity. The weather is rapidly worsening with the sky becoming dark and the wind blowing harder. There are 20 minutes left in the practice session, and the coach is hoping to finish practice before it begins to rain. Suddenly, there is a bolt of lightening and an immediate burst of thunder.

? How should the athletic trainer manage this extremely dangerous situation?

Air pollution is a major problem common in urban areas with large industries and heavy automobile traffic.

lung irritation, and a lowered resistance to lung infections. Over a period of time, individuals may, to some degree, become desensitized to ozone. Asthmatics are at greater risk when ozone levels increase.

Sulfur Dioxide

Sulfur dioxide (SO_2) is a colorless gas that is a component of burning coal or petroleum. As an air contaminant it causes an increased resistance to air movement in and out of the lungs, a decreased ability of the lungs to rid themselves of foreign matter, shortness of breath, coughing, fatigue, and increased susceptibility to lung diseases. Sulfur dioxide causes an adverse effect mostly on asthmatics and other sensitive individuals. Nose breathing lessens the effects of sulfur dioxide because the nasal mucosa acts as a sulfur dioxide scrubber.[12]

Carbon Monoxide

Carbon monoxide (CO) is a colorless, odorless gas. In general, it reduces hemoglobin's ability to transport oxygen and restricts the release of oxygen to the tissue. Besides interfering in performance during exercise, carbon monoxide exposure interferes with various psychomotor, behavioral, and attention-related activities.[12]

Carbon monoxide (CO) reduces hemoglobin's ability to transport and release oxygen in the body.

Prevention

To avoid problems created by air pollution the athlete must stop or significantly decrease physical activity during periods of high pollution. If activity is conducted, it should be performed when commuter traffic has lessened and when ambient temperature has lowered. Ozone levels rise during dawn, peak at midday, and are much reduced after the late-afternoon rush hour. Running should be avoided on roads where there is a concentration of auto emission and carbon monoxide.

CIRCADIAN DYSRHYTHMIA (JET LAG)

Jet power has made it possible to travel thousands of miles in just a few hours. Athletes and athletic teams are now quickly transported from one end of the country to the other and to foreign lands. For some, such travel induces a particular physiological stress, resulting in a syndrome that is identified as a circadian dysrhythmia and that reflects a desynchronization of the athlete's biological and biophysical time clock.[13]

The term *circadian* (from the Latin *circa dies,* "about a day") implies a period of time of approximately 24 hours. The body maintains many cyclical mechanisms (circadian rhythms) that follow a pattern (e.g., the daily rise and fall of body temperature or the tidal ebb and flow of the cortical steroid secretion, which produces other effects on the metabolic system that are in themselves cyclical in nature). Body mechanisms adapt at varying rates to time changes. Some (e.g., protein metabolism) adjust immediately, whereas others take time (e.g., the rise and fall of body temperature, which takes approximately 8 days). Others, such as the adrenal hormones, which regulate metabolism and other body functions, may take as long as 3 weeks. Even intellectual proficiency, or the ability to think, clearly is cyclical.

The term *jet lag* refers to the physical and mental effects caused by traveling rapidly across several time zones. It results from disruption of both circadian rhythms and the sleep-wake cycle. As the length of travel increases over several time zones, the effects of jet lag become more profound.

Disruption of circadian rhythms has been shown to cause fatigue, headache, problems with the digestive system, and changes in blood pressure, heart rate, hormonal release, endocrine secretions, and bowel habits. Any of these changes may have a negative effect on athletic performance and may predispose the athlete to injury.[8]

Younger individuals adjust more rapidly to time zone changes than do older people, although the differences are not great. The stress induced in jet travel occurs only when flying either east or west at high speed. There is 30% to 50% faster adaptation in individuals flying westward than in individuals flying eastward.[19] Travel north or south has no effect on the body unless several time zones are crossed in an east or west progression. The changes in time zones, illumination, and environment prove somewhat disruptive to the human physiological mechanisms, particularly when one flies through five or more time zones, as occurs in some international travel.[34] Some people are much more susceptible to the syndrome than are others, but the symptoms can be sufficiently disruptive to interfere with one's ability to perform maximally in a competitive event. In some cases, an athlete will become ill for a short period of time with anorexia, severe headache, blurred vision, dizziness, insomnia, or extreme fatigue.

Minimizing the Effects of Jet Lag

The negative effects of jet lag can be reduced by paying attention to the following guidelines:

- Depart for a trip well rested.
- Preadjust circadian rhythms by getting up and going to bed 1 hour later for each time zone crossed when traveling west and 1 hour earlier for each time zone when traveling east.
- When traveling west, eat light meals early and heavy meals late in the day. When traveling east, eat a heavy meal earlier in the day.
- Drink plenty of fluids to avoid dehydration, which occurs because of dry, high-altitude, low-humidity cabin air.
- Consume caffeine in coffee, tea, or soda when traveling west. Caffeine should be avoided when traveling east.
- Exercise or training should be done later in the day if traveling west and earlier in the day if traveling east.
- Reset watches according to the new time zone time after boarding the plane.
- If traveling west, get as much sunlight as possible on arrival.
- On arrival, immediately adopt the local time schedule for training, eating, and sleeping. Forget about what the time is where you came from.
- Avoid using alcohol before, during, and after travel.

ARTIFICIAL TURF

Artificial turf was first used in the Houston Astrodome in 1966, and was first marketed under the trade name AstroTurf. The artificial surface was said to be more durable, offer greater consistency, require less maintenance, be more "playable" during inclement weather, and offer greater performance characteristics such as increased speed and resiliency. Since the late 1960s, a number of companies have manufactured synthetic surfaces that are variations of AstroTurf. Today artificial turfs being manufactured include Southwest Resources (AstroTurf, Polypro, Polyknit, Omniturf), Eidelgras, Desso, Kony Green, and Ssupergrass.

There has been an ongoing debate over the advantages and disadvantages of artificial surfaces as compared with natural surfaces.[17] From an injury perspective, there is not enough conclusive evidence in the literature to indicate that an artificial surface is more likely to cause injury than a natural surface.[10,32] Empirically, it seems that most athletes, coaches, and athletic trainers agree that injuries are more likely to occur on artificial surfaces than on natural grass, and most of these individuals would rather practice and play on natural grass. In recent years the trend in many colleges, universities, and arenas has been to move away from artificial surfaces, replacing them with natural grass. New hybrid grasses are now available that are more durable.

It has been argued that synthetic surfaces lose their inherent shock absorption capability as they age.[5] Higher speeds are said to be possible on artificial surfaces, thus injuries involving collision can potentially be more severe because of increased force on impact.[10] A shoe that does not "stick" to the artificial

12-5

Critical Thinking Exercise

A college tennis team from the west coast must travel to the east coast to play a scheduled match. The coach has done a lot of traveling and knows that traveling from west to east seems to be more difficult than traveling east to west. This is an important match, and the tennis coach asks the athletic trainer what the athletes can do to minimize the effects of jet lag.

? What things can the athletic trainer recommend to help the athletes adjust to the new time zone in as short a time as possible?

surface while providing solid footing will significantly reduce the likelihood of injury.[42]

Two injuries that seem to occur more frequently in athletes competing on an artificial surface are abrasions and turf toe (a hyperextension of the great toe). The incidence of abrasions can be greatly reduced by wearing pads on the elbows and knees. Turf toe is less likely to occur if the shoe has a stiff, firm sole.

SUMMARY

- Environmental stress can adversely affect an athlete's performance, as well as pose a serious health problem. Hyperthermia is one of sport's major concerns. In times of high temperatures and humidity, the wet bulb globe temperature index should be routinely determined using the sling psychrometer. Losing 3% or more of body weight because of fluid loss could pose a potential health problem.

- Cold weather requires athletes to wear the correct apparel and to warm up properly before engaging in sports activities. The wind chill factor must always be considered when performing. As is true in a hot environment, the athlete must ingest adequate fluids when in cold conditions. Alcohol must be avoided at all times. Extreme cold exposure can cause conditions such as frost nip, chilblains, and frostbite.

- An athlete going from a low to a high altitude in a short time may encounter problems with performance and perhaps experience some health problems. Because it takes time for acclimatization to occur, there is a question as to when to bring the athlete to the higher altitude, especially for an endurance event. Many coaches and athletic trainers believe that 3 days at the higher altitude will provide enough time for acclimatization to occur. Others believe a much longer time period is needed. If an athlete experiences a serious illness because of his or her presence at a particular altitude, he or she must be returned to a lower altitude as soon as possible.

- Air pollution can produce a major decrement to performance and, in some cases, can cause illness. Increased ozone levels can cause respiratory distress, nausea, eye irritation, and fatigue. Sulfur dioxide, a colorless gas, can also cause physical reactions in some athletes and can be a serious problem for asthmatics. Carbon monoxide, a colorless and odorless gas, reduces hemoglobin's ability to use oxygen and, as a result, adversely affects performance.

- Travel through different time zones can place a serious physiological stress on the athlete. This stress is called circadian dysrhythmia, or jet lag. This disruption of biological rhythm can adversely affect performance and may even produce health problems. The coach or athletic trainer must pay careful attention to helping the athlete acclimatize to time-zone shifting.

- There is inconclusive evidence that the incidence of injury on artificial surfaces is higher than on natural surfaces, although most coaches, athletes, and athletic trainers seem to prefer practicing and playing on natural grass. Two frequently seen injuries that occur on artificial turf are turf toe and abrasions.

· ·

▌Solutions to Critical Thinking Exercises

12-1 The wrestler is experiencing heat exhaustion, which results from inadequate fluid replacement or dehydration. If conscious, the athlete should be forced to drink large quantities of water. By far the most rapid method of fluid replacement is for a physician to use an IV (fluids administered intravenously). It is desirable but not necessary to move the athlete to a cooler environment. The athlete should be counseled relative to the dangers of using diuretic medication.

12-2 The coach should understand that heat-related illnesses are for the most part totally preventable. The athletes should come into preseason practice at least partially acclimatized to working in a hot, humid environment and during the first week of practice should become fully acclimatized. Temperature and humidity readings should be monitored and practice modified according to conditions. Practice uniforms should maximize evaporation and minimize heat absorption to the greatest extent possible. Weight records should be maintained to identify individuals who are becoming dehydrated. Most important, the athletes must keep themselves hydrated by constantly drinking large quantities of water both during and between practice sessions.

12-3 The sun protection factor (SPF) indicates the sunscreen's effectiveness in absorbing the sunburn-inducing radiation. An SPF of 15 indicates that an athlete can be exposed to ultraviolet light 15 times longer than without a sunscreen before the skin will begin to turn red. Therefore the athlete needs to understand that a higher SPF does not indicate a greater degree of protection. She must simply apply the sunscreen with an SPF of 15 twice as often as would be necessary with an SPF of 30.

12-4 As soon as lightening is observed, the athletic trainer should immediately end practice and get the athletes under cover. If an indoor facility is not available, an automobile is a relatively safe alternative. The athletes should avoid standing under large trees or telephone poles. As a last alternative, find a ditch or ravine and assume a crouched position. If possible, avoid any standing water or metal objects around the fields.

12-5 Most important, the athletes should leave for the trip well rested. The day before leaving, the athletes should go to bed and get up 3 hours earlier than normal. Watches should be reset according to the new time zone time on boarding the plane. During the trip they should drink plenty of fluids to prevent dehydration but avoid caffeine. The largest meal should be eaten earlier in the day. On arrival, they should immediately adopt the local time schedule for training, eating, and sleeping. Get as much sunlight as possible on arrival. Training sessions should be done earlier in the day.

REVIEW QUESTIONS AND CLASS ACTIVITIES

1. How do temperature and humidity cause heat disorders?
2. What steps should be taken to avoid heat disorders?
3. Describe the symptoms and signs of the most common heat disorders.
4. How is heat lost from the body to produce hypothermia?
5. What should an athlete do to prevent heat loss?
6. Identify the physiological basis for the body's susceptibility to a cold disorder.
7. Describe the symptoms and signs of the major cold disorders affecting athletes.
8. How should athletes protect themselves from the effects of ultraviolet radiation from the sun?
9. What precautions can be taken to minimize the possibility of injury during an electrical storm?
10. What concerns should a coach or athletic trainer have when athletes are to perform an endurance sport at high altitudes?
11. What altitude illnesses might be expected among some athletes, and how should they be managed?
12. What adverse effects could high air concentrations of ozone, sulfur dioxide, and carbon monoxide have on the athlete? How should they be dealt with?
13. How can the adverse effects of circadian dysrhythmia be avoided or lessened?
14. What are two common injuries in athletes who compete on artificial turf?

REFERENCES

1. ACSM position statement on prevention of thermal injuries during distance running, *Med Sci Sport Exer* 19(5):529, 1987.
2. Appenzeller O, Atkinson R: Temperature regulation and sports. In Appenzeller O, Atkinson R, editors: *Sports medicine,* Baltimore, 1981, Urban & Schwarzenberg.
3. Armstrong LE et al: Heat acclimatization during summer running in the northeastern United States, *Med Sci Sports Exerc* 19(2):131, 1987.
4. Bangs CC: Cold injuries. In Strauss RH, editor: *Sports medicine,* Philadelphia, 1984, Saunders.
5. Bowers KD Jr, Martin RB: Impact absorption, new and old Astro-Turf at West Virginia University, *Med Sci Sports* 6:217, 1974.
6. Brotherhood JR: Snow, cold and energy expenditure: a basis for fatigue and skiing accidents, *Aust J Sci Med Sports* 17:3, 1985.
7. Coyle E: Fluid and carbohydrate replacement during exercise: how much and why? *Sports Science Exchange* 7(50):1, 1994.
8. Davis JO et al: *Jet lag and athletic performance,* Colorado Springs, 1986, United States Olympic Committee Sports Medicine Council.
9. Davis M: Ultraviolet therapy. In Prentice W, editor: *Therapeutic modalities in sports medicine,* St Louis, 1994, Mosby.
10. Duda M: More grid injuries on grass, *Phy Sportsmed* 16(4):41, 1988.
11. Eichner ER: Sickle cell trait, exercise, and altitude, *Phys Sportsmed* 14(11):144, 1986.
12. Folinsbee LJ: Air pollution and exercise. In Welsh RP, Shephard RJ, editors: *Current therapy in sports medicine 1985-1986,* Philadelphia, 1985, Decker.
13. French J: Circadian rhythms, jet lag, and the athlete. In Torg J, Shepard R, editors: *Current therapy in sports medicine,* St Louis, 1995, Mosby.
14. Frim JJ: Hazards of cold air. In Welsh RP, Shephard RJ, editors: *Current therapy in sports medicine 1985-1986,* Philadelphia, 1985, Decker.
15. Fritz R, Perrin D: Cold exposure injuries: prevention and treatment. In Ray R, editor: *Clinics in sports medicine,* Philadelphia, 1989, Saunders.
16. Gutmann L: Temperature-related problems in athletic and recreational activities, *Semin Neurol* 1(4):242, 1981.
17. Hammer DA: Artificial playing surfaces, *Ath Train* 16:240, 1981.
18. Harrelson G: Factors affecting the gastric emptying of athletic drinks, *J Ath Train* 21(1):20, 1986.
19. Houston CS: Man at altitude. In Strauss RH, editor: *Sports medicine,* Philadelphia, 1984, Saunders.
20. Hunter SL et al: Malignant hyperthermia in a college football player, *Phys Sportsmed* 15(12):77, 1987.
21. Inbar O: Exercise and heat. In Welsh RP, Shephard RJ, editors: *Current therapy in sports medicine 1985-1986,* Philadelphia, 1985, Decker.
22. Kulund DN: *The injured athlete,* Philadelphia, 1988, Lippincott.
23. Levine B, Stray-Gundersen J: Exercise at high altitudes. In Torg J, Shepard R, editors: *Current therapy in sports medicine,* St Louis, 1995, Mosby.
24. McArdle WD, Katch FI, Katch VL: *Exercise physiology,* Philadelphia, 1994, Lea & Febiger.
25. Micheli LJ, Puffer JC, Yocum L: Mixed heat injury syndrome, *Sports Med Dig* 9(7):7, 1987.
26. Moore M: What are we learning from road races? *Phys Sportsmed* 10:151, 1982.
27. Murphy RJ: Heat illness in the athlete, *Ath Train* 19:1, 1984.
28. Nadel ER: *Sports science exchange—new ideas for rehydration during and after exercise in hot weather,* Chicago, 1988, Gatorade Sports Science Institute.
29. Nelson WE, Gieck J II, Kolb P: Treatment and prevention of hypothermia and frostbite, *Ath Train* 18:330, 1983.
30. Pandolf K: Avoiding heat illness during exercise. In Torg J, Shepard R, editors: *Current therapy in sports medicine,* St Louis, 1995, Mosby.

31. Pate RR: *Sports science exchange—special considerations for exercise in cold weather,* Chicago, 1988, Gatorade Sports Science Institute.
32. Powell JW: Incidence of injury associated with playing surfaces in the National Football League 1980-1985, *Ath Train* 22:202, 1987.
33. Replacing body fluids is vital during winter, *First Aider* 56(4):1, 1987.
34. Rietveld WJ: Time-zone shifts and international competition. In Welsh RP, Shephard, RJ, editors: *Current therapy in sports medicine 1985-1986,* Philadelphia, 1985, Decker.
35. Ryan A: Heat stress. In Mueller F, Ryan A, editors: *Prevention of athletic injuries: the role of the sports medicine team,* Philadelphia, 1991, Davis.
36. Schoene RB, Bracker MD: High altitude pulmonary edema: the disguised killer, *Phys Sportsmed* 16(8):103, 1988.
37. Schonfeld SA, Dixon GF: The respiratory system. In Strauss RH, editor: *Sports medicine,* Philadelphia, 1984, Saunders.
38. Shephard RJ: Adjustment to high altitude. In Welsh RP, Shephard RJ, editors: *Current therapy in sports medicine 1985-1986,* Philadelphia, 1985, Decker.
39. Sinclair RE: Be serious about siriasis: guidelines for avoiding heat injury during "dog days," *Postgrad Med* 5:261, 1985.
40. Stanitski CL: Environmental problems of runners. In Drez D Jr, editor: *Symposium on running. Clinics in sports medicine,* vol 4, no 4, Philadelphia, 1985, Saunders.
41. Thein L: Environmental conditions affecting the athlete, *J Orthop Sports Phys Ther* 21(3):158, 1995.
42. Torg JS: Football shoes and playing surfaces: from safe to unsafe, *Phys Sportsmed* 1(3):51, 1973.
43. Vellerand A: Exercise in the cold. In Torg J, Shepard R, editors: *Current therapy in sports medicine,* St Louis, 1995, Mosby.
44. Walters F: Position stand on lightning and thunder: the Athletic Health Care Services of the District of Columbia Public Schools, *J Ath Train* 28(3):201, 1993.
45. White-Clergerie AM: Mountaineering without oxygen: courting death? *Phys Sportsmed* 15(3):38, 1987.

ANNOTATED BIBLIOGRAPHY

Haymes EM, Wells CL: *Environment and human performance,* Champaign, Ill, 1986, Human Kinetics.

Examines sports performance during a variety of environmental conditions. Two hundred and fifty references are reported.

Strauss RH, editor: *Sports medicine,* Philadelphia, 1984, Saunders.

Provides four pertinent chapters on the subject of environmental disorders that could affect the athlete.

Wilkerson JA, editor: *Hypothermia, frostbite and other cold injuries,* Seattle, 1986, Mountaineers Books.

Provides a nontechnical approach to hypothermia and explains the importance of preparing for cold and how to recognize and manage cold injuries.

Bandaging and Taping

When you finish this chapter, you should be able to

- Explain the need for and demonstrate the application of roller bandages.
- Explain the need for and demonstrate the application of triangular and cravat bandages.
- Demonstrate site preparation for taping.
- Demonstrate basic skill in the use of taping in sports.
- Demonstrate the skillful application of tape for a variety of musculoskeletal problems.

Bandaging and taping are major skills used in the protection and management of the injured athlete. Each of these skill areas requires a great deal of practice before a high level of proficiency can be attained.

BANDAGING

bandage
Strip of cloth or other material used to cover a wound.

dressing
Covering, protective or supportive, that is applied to an injury or wound.

A **bandage,** when properly applied, can contribute decidedly to recovery from sports injuries. Bandages carelessly or improperly applied may cause discomfort, allow wound contamination, and hamper repair and healing. In all cases bandages must be firmly applied—neither so tight that circulation is impaired nor so loose that the **dressing** is allowed to slip.

Bandage Materials

Bandages used on sports injuries consist essentially of gauze, cotton cloth, and elastic wrapping.

Gauze materials are used in three forms: as sterile pads for wounds, as padding in the prevention of blisters on a taped ankle, and as a roller bandage for holding dressings and compresses in place.

Cotton Cloth is used primarily for cloth ankle wraps and for triangular and cravat bandages. It is soft, is easily obtained, and can be washed many times without deterioration.

The *elastic roller bandage* is extremely popular in sports because of its extensibility, which allows it to conform to most parts of the body. Elastic wraps are active bandages; they let the athlete move without restriction. They act as controlled compression bandages where hemorrhage or swelling must be prevented and can also help support soft tissue.

A *cohesive elastic bandage* exerts constant, even pressure. It is lightweight and contours easily to the body part. The bandage is composed of two layers of nonwoven rayon, which are separated by strands of spandex material. The cohesive elastic bandage is coated with a substance that makes the material adhere to itself, eliminating the need for metal clips or adhesive tape for holding it in place.

Roller Bandages

Roller bandages are made of many materials; gauze, cotton cloth, and elastic wrapping are predominantly used in the training room. The width and length vary according to the body part to be bandaged. The sizes most frequently used are the 2-inch (5 cm) width by 6-yard (5.5 m) length for hand, finger, toe, and head bandages; the 3-inch (7.5 cm) width by 10-yard (9 m) length for the extremities; and the 4-inch (10 cm) or 6-inch (15 cm) width by 10-yard length for thigh, groin, and trunk. For ease and convenience in the application of the roller bandage, the strips of material are first rolled into a cylinder. When a bandage is selected, it should be a single piece that is free from wrinkles, seams, and any other imperfections that may cause skin irritation.[4]

Wrinkles or seams in roller bandages may irritate skin.

Application

Application of the roller bandage must be executed in a specific manner to achieve the purpose of the wrap. When a roller bandage is about to be placed on a body part, the roll should be held in the preferred hand with the loose end extending from the bottom of the roll. The back surface of the loose end is placed on the part and held in position by the other hand. The bandage cylinder is then unrolled and passed around the injured area. As the hand pulls the material from the roll, it also standardizes the bandage pressure and guides the bandage in the proper direction. To anchor and stabilize the bandage, a number of turns, one on top of the other, are made. Circling a body part requires the operator to alternate the bandage roll from one hand to the other and back again.

To apply a roller bandage, hold it in the preferred hand with the loose end extending from the bottom of the roll.

To acquire maximum benefit from a roller bandage, it should be applied uniformly and firmly but not too tightly. Excessive or unequal pressure can hinder the normal blood flow within the part. The following points should be considered when using the roller bandage:

1. A body part should be wrapped in the position of maximum muscle contraction to ensure unhampered movement or circulation.
2. It is better to use a large number of turns with moderate tension than a limited number of turns applied too tightly.
3. Each turn of the bandage should be overlapped by at least one half of the overlying wrap to prevent the separation of the material while engaged in activity. Separation of the bandage turns tends to pinch and irritate the skin.
4. When limbs are wrapped, fingers and toes should be scrutinized often for signs of circulation impairment. Abnormally cold or cyanotic phalanges are signs of excessive bandage pressure.

The usual anchoring of roller bandages consists of several circular wraps directly overlying each other. Whenever possible, anchoring is commenced at the smallest circumference of a limb and is then moved upward. Wrists and ankles are the usual sites for anchoring bandages of the limbs. Bandages are applied to these areas in the following manner:

Begin anchoring bandages at the smallest part of the limb.

1. The loose end of the roller bandage is laid obliquely on the anterior aspects of the wrist or ankle and held in this position. The roll is then carried posteriorly under and completely around the limb and back to the starting point.
2. The triangular portion of the uncovered oblique end is folded over the second turn.
3. The folded triangle is covered by a third turn, which finishes a secure anchor.

After a roller bandage has been applied, it is held in place by a *locking technique.* The method most often used to finish a wrap is that of firmly tying or pinning the bandage or placing adhesive tape over several overlying turns.

Once a bandage has been put on and has served its purpose, removal can be performed either by unwrapping or by carefully cutting with bandage scissors. Whatever method of bandage removal is used, extreme caution must be taken to avoid additional injury.

Cloth ankle wrap   Because tape is so expensive, the ankle wrap is an inexpensive and expedient means of mildly protecting ankles (Figure 13-1).

Materials needed   Each muslin wrap should be 1½ to 2 inches (3.8 to 5 cm) wide and 72 to 96 inches (180 to 240 cm) long to ensure complete coverage and protection. The purpose of this wrap is to give mild support against lateral and medial motion of the ankle. It is applied over a sock.

Figure 13-1

Ankle wrap.

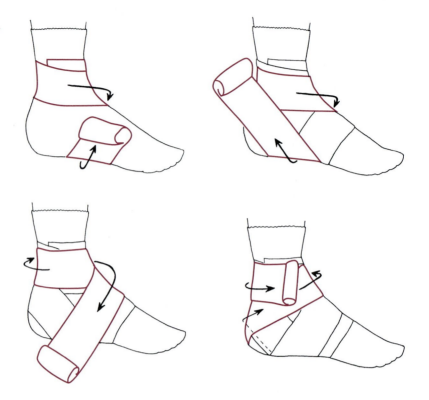

Figure 13-2

Ankle and foot spica.

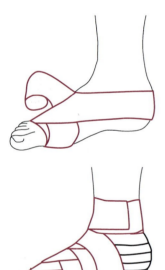

Check circulation after applying an elastic wrap.

Position of the athlete   The athlete sits on a table, extending the leg and positioning the foot at a 90-degree angle. To avoid any distortion, it is important that the ankle be neither overflexed nor overextended.

   Procedure

   1. Start the wrap above the instep around the ankle, circle the ankle, and move it at an acute angle to the inside of the foot.
   2. From the inside of the foot, move the wrap under the arch, coming up on the outside and crossing at the beginning point, where it continues around the ankle, hooking the heel.
   3. Move the wrap up, inside, over the instep, and around the ankle, hooking the opposite side of the heel. This completes one series of the ankle wrap.
   4. Complete a second series with the remaining material.
   5. For additional support, two heel locks with adhesive tape may be applied over the ankle wrap.

Elastic Wrap Techniques

Any time an elastic wrap is applied to the athlete always check for and avoid decreased circulation and blueness of the extremity, and check for a blood capillary refill.

   Ankle and foot spica   The ankle and foot spica bandage (Figure 13-2) is primarily used in sports for the compression of new injuries and for holding wound dressings in place.

   Materials needed   Depending on the size of the ankle and foot, a 2- or 3-inch wrap is used.

   Position of the athlete   The athlete sits with ankle and foot extended over a table.

   Procedure

   1. An anchor is placed around the foot near the metatarsal arch.
   2. The elastic bandage is brought across the instep and around the heel and returned to the starting point.
   3. The procedure is repeated several times, with each succeeding revolution progressing upward on the foot and the ankle.

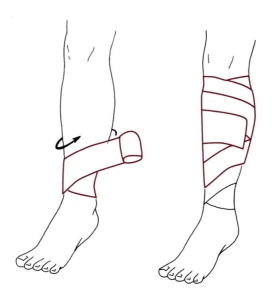

Figure 13-3

Spiral bandage.

4. Each **spica** overlaps approximately three fourths of the preceding layer.

Spiral bandage   The spiral bandage (Figure 13-3) is widely used in sports for covering a large area of a cylindrical part.

Materials needed   Depending on the size of the area, a 3- or 4-inch wrap is required.

Position of the athlete   If the wrap is for the lower limb, the athlete bears weight on the opposite leg.

Procedure

1. The elastic spiral bandage is anchored at the smallest circumference of the limb and is wrapped upward in a spiral against gravity.
2. To prevent the bandage from slipping down on a moving extremity, two pieces of tape should be folded lengthwise and placed on the bandage at either side of the limb, or tape adherent can be sprayed on the part.
3. After the bandage is anchored, it is carried upward in consecutive spiral turns, each overlapping the other by at least ½ inch.
4. The bandage is terminated by locking it with circular turns, which are then firmly secured by tape.

Groin support   The following procedure is used to support a groin strain and hip adductor strains (Figure 13-4).

spica
A figure-8 bandage, with one of the two loops larger than the other.

13-1

Critical Thinking Exercise

A baseball player strains his right groin while running the bases.

? Which elastic wrap should be applied when the athlete returns to his sport and why?

Figure 13-4

Elastic groin support.

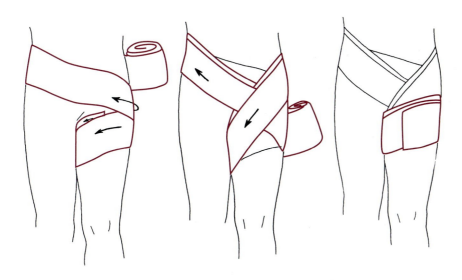

Materials needed   One roll of extra-long 6-inch (15 cm) elastic bandage, a roll of 1½-inch (3.8 cm) adhesive tape, and nonsterile cotton.

Position of the athlete   The athlete stands on a table with weight placed on the uninjured leg. The affected limb is relaxed and internally rotated. This procedure is different from that described earlier, in which the wrap was used for pressure only.

Procedure

1. A piece of nonsterile cotton or a felt pad may be placed over the injured site to provide additional compression and support.
2. The end of the elastic bandage is started at the upper part of the inner aspect of the thigh and is carried posteriorly around the thigh. It is then brought across the lower abdomen and over the crest of the ilium on the opposite side of the body.

Figure 13-5

Hip spica for hip flexors.

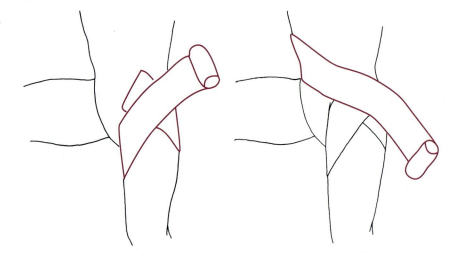

Figure 13-6

Method used to limit movement of bottocks.

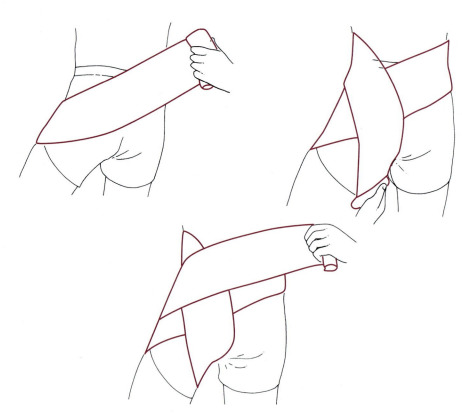

3. The wrap is continued around the back, repeating the same pattern and securing the wrap end with a 1½-inch (3.8 cm) adhesive tape.

Variations of this method can be seen in Figure 13-5 (to support injured hip flexors) and Figure 13-6 (to limit the movement of the buttocks).

Shoulder spica   The shoulder spica (Figure 13-7) is used mainly for the retention of wound dressings and for moderate muscular support.

Materials needed   One roll of extra-long 4- to 6-inch elastic wrap, 1½-inch adhesive tape, and padding for axilla.

Position of the athlete   The athlete stands with his or her side toward the operator.

Procedure

1. The axilla must be well padded to prevent skin irritation and constriction of blood vessels.
2. The bandage is anchored by one turn around the affected upper arm.
3. After anchoring the bandage around the arm on the injured side, the wrap is carried around the back under the unaffected arm and across the chest to the injured shoulder.
4. The affected arm is again encircled by the bandage, which continues around the back. Every figure-8 pattern moves progressively upward with an overlap of at least half of the previous underlying wrap.

Elbow figure-8 bandage   The elbow figure-8 bandage (Figure 13-8) can be used to secure a dressing in the antecubital fossa or to restrain full extension in hyperextension injuries. When it is reversed, it can be used on the posterior aspect of the elbow.

Materials needed   One 3-inch elastic roll and 1½-inch adhesive tape.

Position of the athlete   The athlete flexes his or her elbow between 45 degrees and 90 degrees, depending on the restriction of movement required.

Procedure

1. Anchor the bandage by encircling the lower arm.
2. Bring the roll obliquely upward over the posterior aspect of the elbow.
3. Carry the roll obliquely upward, crossing the antecubital fossa; then pass once again completely around the upper arm and return to the beginning position by again crossing the antecubital fossa.
4. Continue the procedure as described, but for every new sequence move upward toward the elbow one half the width of the underlying wrap.

Gauze hand and wrist figure-8   A figure-8 bandage (Figure 13-9) can be used for mild wrist and hand support and for holding dressings in place.

Materials needed   One roll of ½-inch gauze, ½-inch tape, and scissors.

Position of the athlete   The athlete positions his or her elbow at a 45-degree angle.

Procedure

1. The anchor is executed with one or two turns around the palm of the hand.
2. The roll is then carried obliquely across the anterior or posterior portion of the hand, depending on the position of the wound, to the wrist, which it circles once; then it is returned to the primary anchor.
3. As many figures as needed are applied.

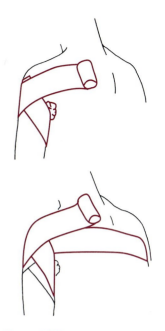

Figure 13-7

Elastic shoulder spica.

13-2

Critical Thinking Exercise

A wrestler sustains a left shoulder point injury.

? The athletic trainer cuts a sponge rubber doughnut to protect the shoulder point from further injury. How is the doughnut held in place?

Figure 13-8

Elastic elbow figure-8 bandage.

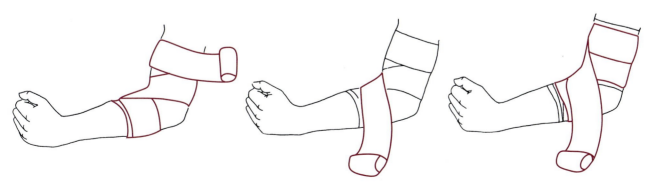

Figure 13-9

Hand and wrist figure-8 bandage.

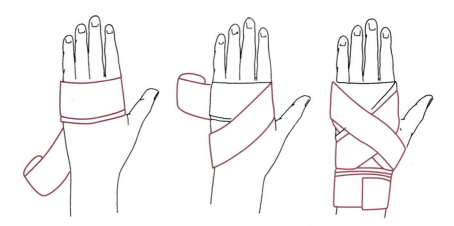

Triangular and Cravat Bandages

Triangular and cravat bandages allow ease and speed of application.

Triangular and cravat bandages, usually made of cotton cloth, may be used if roller types are not applicable or available. The triangular and cravat bandages are primarily used as first aid devices. They are valuable in emergency bandaging because of their ease and speed of application. In sports the more diversified roller bandages are usually available and lend themselves more to the needs of the athlete. The principal use of the triangular bandage in athletic training is for arm slings. There are two basic kinds of slings, the cervical arm sling and the shoulder arm sling, and each has a specific purpose.

Cervical arm sling   The cervical arm sling (Figure 13-10) is designed to support the forearm, wrist, and hand. A triangular bandage is placed around the neck and under the bent arm that is to be supported.

Materials needed   One triangular bandage.

Position of the athlete   The athlete stands with the affected arm bent at approximately a 70-degree angle.

Procedure

1. The triangular bandage is positioned by the operator under the injured arm with the apex facing the elbow.
2. The end of the triangle nearest the body is carried over the shoulder of the uninjured arm. The other end is allowed to hang down loosely.
3. The loose end is pulled over the shoulder of the injured side.
4. The two ends of the bandage are tied in a square knot behind the neck. For the sake of comfort, the knot should be on either side of the neck, not directly in the middle.

Figure 13-10

Cervical arm sling.

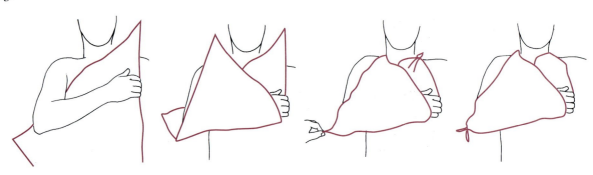

5. The apex of the triangle is brought around to the front of the elbow and fastened by twisting the end, then tying in a knot.

In cases in which greater arm stabilization is required than that afforded by a sling, an additional bandage can be swathed about the upper arm and body.

Shoulder arm sling   The shoulder arm sling (Figure 13-11) is suggested for forearm support when there is an injury to the shoulder girdle or when the cervical arm sling is irritating to the athlete.

Materials needed   One triangular bandage and one safety pin.

Position of the athlete   The athlete stands with his or her injured arm bent at approximately a 70-degree angle.

Procedure

1. The upper end of the shoulder sling is placed over the *uninjured* shoulder side.
2. The lower end of the triangle is brought over the forearm and drawn between the upper arm and the body, swinging around the athlete's back and then upward to meet the other end, where a square knot is tied.
3. The apex end of the triangle is brought around to the front of the elbow and fastened with a safety pin.

Sling and swathe   The sling and swathe combination is designed to stabilize the arm securely in cases of shoulder dislocation or fracture (Figure 13-12).

TAPING

Historically, taping has been an important part of athletic training. It is one area of proficiency that the athletic trainer must have.

Tape Usage

Injury Care

When used for sports injuries, adhesive tape offers a number of possibilities:

- Retention of wound dressings.
- Stabilization of compression-type bandages that control external and internal hemorrhaging.
- Support of recent injuries to prevent additional insult that might result from the activities of the athlete.

Injury Protection

Protecting against acute injuries is another major use of tape support. This protection can be achieved by limiting the motion of a body part or by securing some special device.

Linen Adhesive Tape

Modern adhesive tape has great adaptability for use in sports because of its uniform adhesive mass, adhering qualities, lightness, and the relative strength of the backing materials. All of these qualities are of value in holding wound dressings in place and in supporting and protecting injured areas. This tape comes in a variety of sizes; 1-, 1½-, and 2-inch (2.5, 3.75, and 5 cm) widths are commonly used in sports medicine. When linen tape is purchased, factors such as cost, grade of backing, quality of adhesive mass, and properties of unwinding should be considered.

Tape Grade

Linen-backed tape is most often graded according to the number of longitudinal and vertical fibers per inch of backing material. The heavier and more costly backing contains 85 or more longitudinal fibers and 65 vertical fibers per square inch. The lighter, less expensive grade has 65 or fewer longitudinal fibers and 45 vertical fibers.

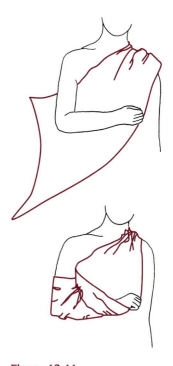

Figure 13-11

Shoulder arm sling.

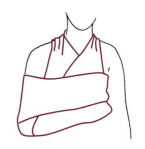

Figure 13-12

Sling and swathe.

When purchasing linen tape, consider:

Grade of backing

Quality of adhesive mass

Winding tension

13-3

Critical Thinking Exercise

An athlete falls and sustains a dislocated right shoulder.

? How should the athlete be transported safely to the hospital?

Adhesive Mass

As a result of improvements in adhesive mass, certain essentials should be expected from tape. It should adhere readily when applied and should maintain this adherence in the presence of profuse perspiration and activity. Besides sticking well, the mass must contain as few skin irritants as possible and must be able to be removed easily without leaving a mass residue or pulling away the superficial skin.

Winding Tension

The winding tension of a tape roll is important to the operator. Sports place a unique demand on the unwinding quality of tape; if tape is to be applied for protection and support, there must be even and constant unwinding tension. In most cases a proper wind needs little additional tension to provide sufficient tightness.

Stretch Tape

Increasingly, tape with varying elasticity is being used in sports medicine.

Increasingly, tape with varying elasticity is being used in sports medicine, often in combination with linen tape. Because of its conforming qualities, stretch tape is used for small, angular body parts, such as the feet, wrist, hands, and fingers. As with linen tape, stretch tape comes in a variety of widths.

Tape Storage

Store tape in a cool place, and stack it flat.

When storing tape, take the following steps:
1. Store in a cool place such as in a low cupboard.
2. Stack so that the tape rests on its flat top or bottom to avoid distortion.

Using Adhesive Tape in Sports

Preparation for Taping

Skin should be cleansed and hair should be shaved before applying tape.

Special attention must be given when applying tape directly to the skin. Perspiration and dirt collected during sport activities will prevent tape from properly sticking to the skin. Whenever tape is used, the skin surface should be cleansed with soap and water to remove all dirt and oil. Also, hair should be shaved to prevent additional irritation when the tape is removed. If additional adherence or protection from irritation is needed, a preparation containing rosin and a skin toughener offer astringent action and dry readily, leaving a tacky residue to which tape will adhere firmly.

Taping directly on skin provides maximum support. However, applying tape day after day can lead to skin irritation. To overcome this problem many athletic trainers sacrifice some support by using a protective covering on the skin. The most popular is a moderately elastic commercial underwrap material that is extremely thin and fits snugly to the contours of the part to be taped. One commonly used underwrap material is polyester and urethane foam, which is fine, porous, extremely lightweight, and resilient. Proper use of an underwrap requires the part to be shaved and sprayed with a tape adherent. Underwrap material should be applied only one layer thick.

Proper Taping Technique

The correct tape width depends on the area to be covered. The more acute the angles, the narrower the tape must be to fit the many contours. For example, the fingers and toes usually require ½- or 1-inch (1.25 or 2.5 cm) tape; the ankles require 1½-inch (3.75 cm) tape; and the larger skin areas such as thighs and back can accommodate 2- to 3-inch (5 to 7.5 cm) tape with ease.

NOTE: *Supportive tape improperly applied can aggravate an existing injury or disrupt the mechanics of a body part, causing an initial injury to occur.*

Tearing Tape

Coaches and athletic trainers use various techniques in tearing tape (Figure 13-13). A method should permit the operator to keep the tape roll in hand most of the time. The following is a suggested procedure:

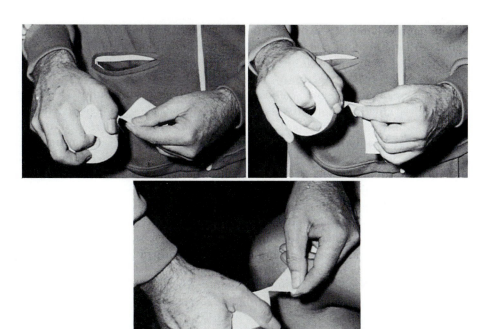

Figure 13-13

Methods of tearing linen-backed tape.

1. Hold the tape roll in the preferred hand with the index finger hooked through the center of the tape roll and the thumb pressing its outer edge.
2. With the other hand, grasp the loose end between the thumb and index finger.
3. With both hands in place, pull both ends of the tape so that it is tight. Next, make a quick, scissorslike move to tear the tape. In tearing tape the movement of one hand is away from the body and the other hand toward the body. Remember, do not try to bend or twist the tape to tear it.

To tear tape, move hands quickly in opposite directions.

When tearing is properly executed, the torn edges of the linen-backed tape are relatively straight, without curves, twists, or loose threads sticking out. Once the first thread is torn, the rest of the tape tears easily. Learning to tear tape effectively from many different positions is essential for speed and efficiency. Many tapes other than the linen-backed type cannot be torn manually but require a knife, scissors, or razor blade.

Rules for Tape Application

The following are a few of the important rules to be observed in the use of adhesive tape. In practice the athletic trainer will identify others.

1. *If the part to be taped is a joint, place it in the position in which it is to be stabilized.* If the part is musculature, make the necessary allowance for contraction and expansion.
2. *Overlap the tape at least half the width of the tape below.* Unless tape is overlapped sufficiently, the active athlete will separate it, exposing the underlying skin to irritation.
3. *Avoid continuous taping.* Tape continuously wrapped around a part may cause constriction. It is suggested that one turn be made at a time and that each encirclement be torn to overlap the starting end by approximately 1 inch. This rule is particularly true of the nonyielding linen-backed tape.
4. *Keep the tape roll in the hand whenever possible.* By learning to keep the tape roll in the hand, seldom putting it down, and by learning to tear the tape, an operator can develop taping speed and accuracy.
5. *Smooth and mold the tape as it is laid on the skin.* To save additional time, tape

strips should be smoothed and molded to the body part as they are put in place; this is done by stroking the top with the fingers, palms, and heels of both hands.

6. *Allow tape to fit the natural contour of the skin.* Each strip of tape must be placed with a particular purpose in mind. Linen-backed tape is not sufficiently elastic to bend around acute angles but must be allowed to fall as it may, fitting naturally to the body contours. Failing to allow this fit creates wrinkles and gaps that can result in skin irritations.

7. *Start taping with an anchor piece and finish by applying a lock strip.* Commence taping, if possible, by sticking the tape to an anchor piece that encircles the part. This placement affords a good medium for the stabilization of succeeding tape strips so that they will not be affected by the movement of the part.

8. *Where maximum support is desired, tape directly over skin.* In cases of sensitive skin, other mediums may be used as tape bases. With artificial bases, some movement can be expected between the skin and the base.

9. *Do not apply tape if skin is hot or cold from a therapeutic treatment.*

Removing Adhesive Tape

Tape usually can be removed from the skin by hand, by tape scissors or tape cutters, or by chemical solvents.

Manual removal   When pulling tape from the body, be careful not to tear or irritate the skin. Tape must not be wrenched in an outward direction from the skin but should be pulled in a direct line with the body (Figure 13-14). Remember to remove the skin carefully from the tape and not to peel the tape from the skin. One hand gently pulls the tape in one direction, and the opposite hand gently presses the skin away from the tape.

Use of tape scissors or cutters   The characteristic tape scissors have a blunt nose that slips underneath the tape smoothly without gouging the skin. Take care to avoid cutting the tape too near the site of the injury, lest the scissors aggravate the condition. Cut on the uninjured side.

Taping Supplies

Effective taping requires the availability of numerous supplies:

1. Razor—hair removal.
2. Soap—cleaning skin.
3. Alcohol—oil removal from skin.
4. Adhesive spray—tape adherent.
5. Underwrap material—skin protection.

Peel the skin from the tape, not the tape from the skin.

Figure 13-14

Removing tape by pulling in a direct line with the body.

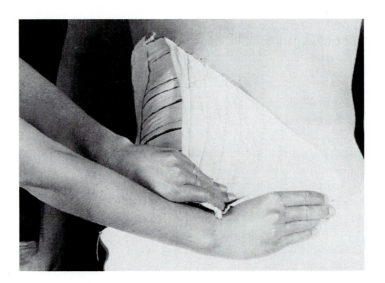

6. Heel and lace pads.
7. White zinc oxide tape (linen-backed tape) (½ inch, 1 inch, 1½-inch, and 2 inch).
8. Adhesive and stretch tape (1 inch, 2 inch, and 3 inch).
9. Felt and foam padding material.
10. Tape scissors.
11. Tape cutters.
12. Elastic bandages (2 inch, 3 inch, 4 inch, and 6 inch).

Common Taping Procedures

The Arch

Arch technique no. 1: with pad support   Arch taping with pad support uses the following procedures to strengthen weakened arches (Figure 13-15). NOTE: The longitudinal arch should be lifted.

Site preparation   Clean foot of dirt and oil; if hairy, shave dorsum of foot. Spray area with tape adherent.

Materials needed   One roll of 1½-inch (3.8 cm) tape, tape adherent, and a ⅛- or ¼-inch (0.3 or 0.6 cm) adhesive foam rubber pad or wool felt pad, cut to fit the longitudinal arch.

Position of the athlete   The athlete lies face down on the table with the foot that is to be taped extending approximately 6 inches (15 cm) over the edge of the table. To ensure proper position, allow the foot to hang in a relaxed position.

Procedure
1. Place a series of strips of tape directly around the arch or, if added support is required, around an arch pad and the arch. The first strip should go just above the metatarsal arch (1).
2. Each successive strip overlaps the preceding piece about half the width of the tape (2 through 4).

CAUTION: Avoid putting on so many strips of tape as to hamper the action of the ankle.

Arch technique no. 2: the X for the longitudinal arch   When using the figure-8 method for taping the longitudinal arch, execute the following steps (Figure 13-16).

Site preparation   Same as for arch technique no. 1.

Materials needed   One roll of 1-inch tape and tape adherent.

Position of the athlete   The athlete lies face down on the table with the affected foot extending approximately 6 inches (15 cm) over the edge of the table. To ensure proper position, allow the foot to hang in a relaxed position.

Procedure
1. Lightly place an anchor strip around the ball of the foot, making certain not to constrict the action of the toes (1).
2. Start tape strip 2 from the lateral edge of the anchor. Move it upward at an acute angle, cross the center of the longitudinal arch, encircle the heel, and descend. Then cross the arch again and end at the medial aspect of the anchor (2). Repeat three or four times (3 and 4).
3. Lock the taped Xs with a single piece of tape placed around the ball of foot.

After all the X strips are applied, cover the entire arch with 1½-inch circular tape strips.

Arch technique no. 3: the X teardrop arch and forefoot support   As its name implies, this taping both supports the longitudinal arch and stabilizes the forefoot into good alignment (Figure 13-17).

Materials needed   One roll of 1-inch (2.5 cm) tape and tape adherent.

Position of the athlete   The athlete lies face down on the table with the foot to be taped extending approximately 6 inches (15 cm) over the edge of the table.

Procedure
1. Place an anchor strip around the ball of the foot (1).
2. Start tape strip 2 on the side of the foot, beginning at the base of the great toe.

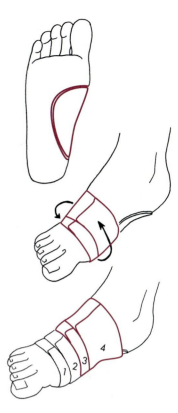

Figure 13-15

Arch taping technique no. 1, including an arch pad and circular tape strips.

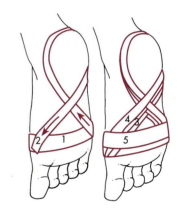

Figure 13-16

Arch taping technique no. 2 (X taping).

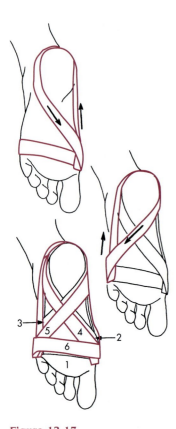

Figure 13-17

Teardrop arch taping technique no. 3 with double X and forefoot support.

Take the tape around the heel, crossing the arch and returning to the starting point (2).

3. The pattern of the third strip of tape is the same as the second strip except that it is started on the little toe side of the foot (3). Repeat two or three times (4 through 6).

4. Lock each series of strips by placing tape around the ball joint. A completed procedure usually consists of a series of three strips.

Arch technique no. 4: fan arch support   The fan arch technique supports the entire plantar aspect of the foot (Figure 13-18).

Materials needed   One roll of 1-inch (2.5 cm) tape and tape adherent. One roll of 1½-inch tape.

Position of athlete   The athlete lies face down on the table with the foot to be taped extending approximately 6 inches (15 cm) over the edge of the table.

Procedure

1. Place an anchor strip around the ball of the foot (1).

2. Starting at the third metatarsal head, take the tape around the heel from the lateral side and meet the strip where it began (2 and 3).

3. The next strip starts near the second metatarsal head and finishes on the fourth metatarsal head (4).

LowDye technique   The LowDye technique is an excellent method for managing the fallen medial longitudinal arch, foot pronation, arch strains, and plantar fasciitis. Moleskin is cut in 3-inch (7.5 cm) strips to the shape of the sole of the foot. It should cover the head of the metatarsal bones and the clacaneus bone (Figure 13-19).

Materials needed   One roll of 1-inch (2.5 cm) and one roll of 2-inch (5 cm) tape and moleskin.

Position of the athlete   The athlete sits with the foot in a neutral position with the great toe and medial aspect of the foot in plantar flexion.

Procedure

1. Apply the moleskin to the sole of the foot, pulling it slightly downward before attaching it to the clacaneus.

2. Grasp the forefoot with the thumb under the distal 2 to 5 metatarsal heads, pushing slightly upward, with the tips of the second and third fingers pushing downward on the first metatarsal head. Apply two or three 1-inch (2.5 cm) tape strips laterally, starting from the distal head of the first metatarsal bone (1 through 3). Keep these lateral strips below the outer malleolus.

3. Secure the moleskin and lateral tape strip by circling the forefoot with four

Figure 13-18

Fan arch taping technique.

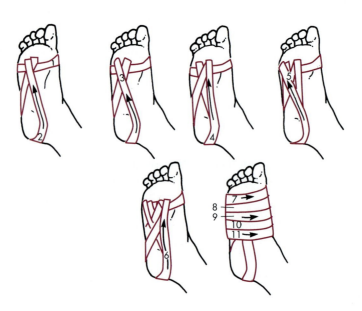

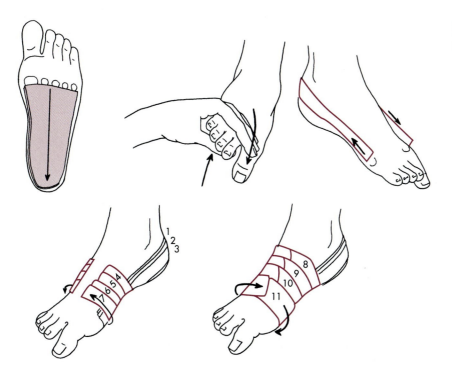

Figure 13-19

LowDye taping technique.

2-inch (5 cm) strips (4 through 7). Start at the lateral dorsum of the foot, circle under the plantar aspect, and finish at the medial dorsum of the foot. Apply four strips of 2-inch stretch-tape strips that encircle the arch (8 through 11).

A variation of this method is to use two 2-inch (5 cm) moleskin strips, one at the ball of the foot and the other at the base of the fifth metatarsal. Cross the strips and extend them along the plantar surface of the foot. For anchors, apply 2-inch (5 cm) elastic tape around the forefoot, lateral to medial, giving additional support.

The Toes

The sprained great toe   This procedure is used for taping a sprained great toe (Figure 13-20).

Materials needed   One roll of 1-inch (2.5 cm) tape and tape adherent.

Site preparation   Clean foot of dirt and oil, shave hair from toes, and spray area with tape adherent.

Position of the athlete   The athlete assumes a sitting position.

Procedure

1. The greatest support is given to the joint by a half–figure-8 taping (1 through 3). Start the series at an acute angle on the top of the foot and swing down between the great and first toes, first encircling the great toe and then coming up, over, and across the starting point. Repeat this process, starting each series separately.

2. After the required number of half–figure-8 strips are in position, place one lock piece around the ball of the foot (4).

Bunions

Materials needed   One roll of 1-inch (2.5 cm) tape, tape adherent, and ¼-inch (0.62 cm) sponge rubber or felt (Figure 13-21).

Position of the athlete   The athlete assumes a sitting position.

Procedure

1. Cut the ¼-inch sponge rubber to form a wedge between the great and second toes.

2. Place anchor strips to encircle the midfoot and distal aspect of the great toe (Figure 13-21, 1 and 2).

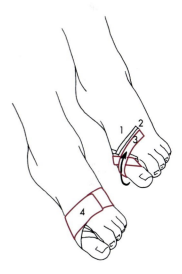

Figure 13-20

Taping for a sprained great toe.

· 13-4

Critical Thinking Exercise

A football lineman has a severe right foot pronation with a fallen medial longitudinal arch. He is subject to arch strains.

? What taping technique is designed for this situation?

Figure 13-21

Bunion taping.

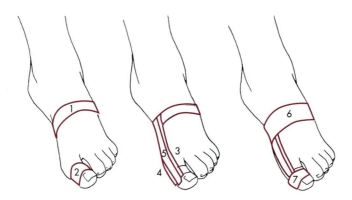

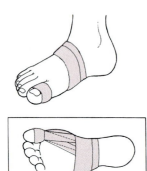

Bottom view

Figure 13-22

Turf toe taping.

3. Place two or three strips on the medial aspect of the great toe to hold the toe in proper alignment (3 through 5).
4. Lock the ends of the strips with tape (6 and 7).

Turf toe   Turf toe taping is designed to prevent excessive hyperextension of the metatarsophalangeal joint (Figure 13-22).

Materials needed   One roll of 1½-inch adhesive tape, 1-inch adhesive tape adherent.

Skin preparation   Hair is shaved off of the top of the forefoot and great toe. Spray the area with tape adherent.

Position of the athlete   The great toe is placed into a neutral position.

Procedure   Apply one 1-inch tape strip around the great toe. Using 1½-inch tape apply two arch anchors to the midarch area. On the middle of the great toe, anchor attach three 1-inch tape strips to create a checkrein. Attach the checkrein to the arch anchor tape trip crossing the MP joint line. Lock both of the checkrein in place.

Hammer, or clawed, toes   This technique is designed to reduce the pressure of the bent toes against the shoe (Figure 13-23).

Materials needed   One roll of ½- or 1-inch (1.25 or 2.5 cm) adhesive tape and tape adherent.

Position of the athlete   The athlete sits on the table with the affected leg extended over the edge.

Procedure
1. Tape one affected toe; then lace under the adjacent toe and over the next toe.
2. Tape can be attached to the next toe or can be continued and attached to the fifth toe.

Fractured toes

Materials needed   One roll of ½- or 1-inch (1.25 to 2.5 cm) tape, ⅛-inch (0.82 cm) sponge rubber, and tape adherent.

Position of the athlete   The athlete assumes a sitting position.

Procedure
1. Cut a ⅛-inch sponge rubber wedge and place it between the affected toe and a healthy one.
2. Wrap two or three strips of tape around the toes (Figure 13-24). This technique splints the fractured toe with a nonfractured one.

The Ankle Joint

Routine noninjury taping

Site preparation   Ankle taping applied directly to the athlete's skin affords the greatest support; however, when applied and removed daily, skin irritation will occur. To avoid this problem apply an underwrap material. Before taping, follow these procedures:
1. Clean foot and ankle thoroughly.
2. Shave all the hair off the foot and ankle.

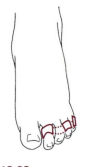

Figure 13-23

Hammer, or clawed, toe taping.

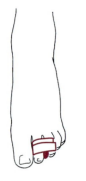

Figure 13-24

Fractured toe taping.

3. Apply a coating of a tape adherent to protect the skin and offer an adhering base. NOTE: It may be advisable to avoid the use of a tape adherent, especially if the athlete has a history of developing tape blisters. In cases of skin sensitivity the ankle surface should be thoroughly cleansed of dirt and oil and an underwrap material applied; alternatively, one can tape directly to the skin.

4. Apply a gauze pad coated with friction-reducing material such as grease over the instep and to the back of the heel.

5. If underwrap is used, apply a single layer. The tape anchors extend beyond the underwrap and adhere directly to the skin.

6. Do not apply tape if skin is cold or hot from a therapeutic treatment.

Materials needed   One roll of 1½-inch (3.8 cm) tape, tape adherent, and underwrap.

Position of the athlete   The athlete sits on the table with the leg extended and the foot held at a 90-degree angle.

Procedure

1. Place an anchor around the ankle approximately 5 or 6 inches (12.7 or 15.2 cm) above the malleolus (Figure 13-25).

2. Apply two strips in consecutive order, starting behind the outer, adjoining piece of tape (2 and 3).

3. After applying the strips, wrap seven or eight circular strips around the ankle, from the point of the anchor downward until the malleolus is completely covered (4 through 12).

4. Apply two or three arch strips from lateral to medial, giving additional support to the arch (13 through 15).

5. Additional support is given by a heel lock. Starting high on the instep, bring the tape along the ankle at a slight angle, hooking the heel, leading under the arch, then coming up on the opposite side, and finishing at the starting point.

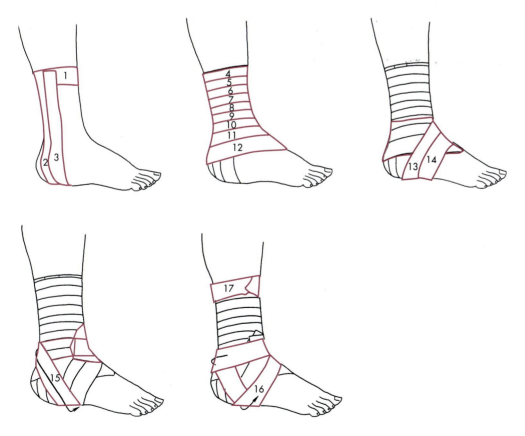

Figure 13-25

Routine noninjury ankle taping.

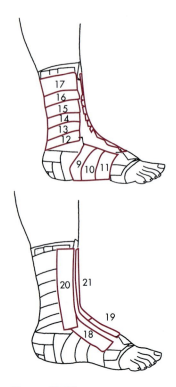

Figure 13-26

Open basket weave ankle taping.

Critical Thinking Exercise

A cross-country runner steps in a hole and suffers a lateral sprain to the right ankle.

? What taping technique should be selected to provide ankle joint support while still allowing for swelling?

Tear the tape to complete half of the heel lock (16). Repeat on the opposite side of the ankle. Finish with a band of tape around the ankle (17).

Closed basket weave (Gibney) technique   The closed basket weave technique (Figure 13-26) offers strong tape support and is primarily used in athletic training for newly sprained or chronically weak ankles.

Materials needed   One roll of 1½-inch (3.8 cm) tape and underwrap, tape adherent.

Position of the athlete   The athlete sits on the table with the leg extended and the foot at a 90-degree angle.

Procedure

1. Place one anchor piece around the ankle approximately 5 or 6 inches (12.7 or 15.2 cm) above the malleolus just below the belly of the gastrocremius muscle. Place a second anchor around the instep directly over the styloid process of the fifth metatarsal (1 and 2).
2. Apply the first strips posteriorly to the malleolus and attach it to the ankle strips (3). NOTE: When applying strips, pull the foot into eversion for an inversion strain and into a neutral position for an eversion strain.
3. Start the first Gibney directly under the malleolus and attach it to the foot anchor (4).
4. In an alternating series, place three strips and three Gibneys on the ankle with each piece of tape overlapping at least half of the preceding strip (5 through 8).
5. After applying the basket weave series, continue the Gibney strips up the ankle, thus giving circular support (9 through 15).
6. For arch support, apply two or three circular strips laterally to medially (16 and 17).
7. After completing the conventional basket weave, apply two or three heel locks to ensure maximum stability (18 and 19).

Open basket weave   This modification of the closed basket weave, or Gibney, technique is designed to give freedom of movement in dorsiflexion and plantar flexion while providing lateral and medial support and giving swelling room. Taping in this pattern (Figure 13-26) may be used immediately after an acute sprain in conjunction with a pressure bandage and cold applications because it allows for swelling.

Materials needed   One roll of 1½-inch (3.8 cm) tape and tape adherent.

Position of the athlete   The athlete sits on the table with the leg extended and the foot held at a 90-degree angle.

Procedure

1. The procedures are the same as for the closed basket weave (Figure 13-27) with the exception of incomplete closures of the Gibney strips.
2. Lock the gap between the Gibney ends with two pieces of tape running on either side of the instep (1 through 21). NOTE: Application of a 1½-inch (3.8 cm) elastic bandage over the open basket weave affords added control of swelling; however, the athlete should remove it before going to bed. Apply the elastic bandage distal to proximal to assist in preventing swelling from moving into the toes.

Of the many ankle-taping techniques in use today, those using combinations of strip, basket weave pattern, and heel lock have been determined to offer the best support.

Continuous stretch tape technique   This technique provides a fast alternative to other taping methods for the ankle (Figure 13-28).[3]

Materials needed   One roll of 1½-inch (3.75 cm) linen tape, one roll of 2-inch (5 cm) stretch tape, tape adherent, and underwrap.

Position of the athlete   The athlete sits on the table with the leg extended and the foot at a 90-degree angle.

Figure 13-27

Closed basket weave ankle taping.

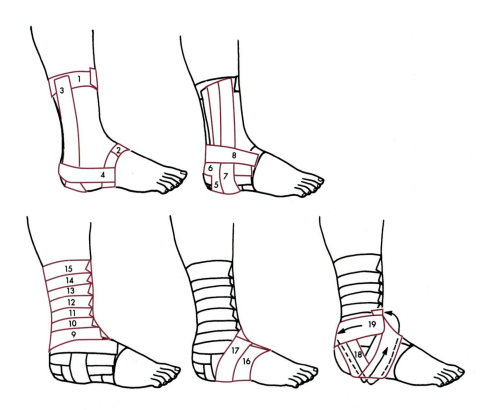

Procedure

1. Place one anchor strip around the ankle approximately 5 to 6 inches (12.5 cm to 15 cm) above the malleolus (1).
2. Apply three strips, covering the malleolli (2 through 4).
3. Start the stretch tape in a medial-to-lateral direction around the midfoot and continue it in a figure-8 pattern to above the lateral malleolus (5).
4. Continue to stretch tape across the midfoot, then across the heel.
5. Apply two heel locks, one in one direction and one in the reverse direction.
6. Next, repeat a figure-8 pattern followed by a spiral pattern, filling the space up to the anchor.
7. Use the lock technique at the top with a linen tape strip.

The Lower Leg

Achilles tendon   Achilles tendon taping (Figure 13-29) is designed to prevent the Achilles tendon from overstretching.

Site preparation   Clean and shave the area, spray with tape adherent, and apply underwrap to the lower one third of the calf.

Materials needed   One roll of 3-inch (7.5 cm) elastic tape, one roll of 1½-inch (3.8 cm) linen tape, and tape adherent.

Position of the athlete   The athlete kneels or lies face down with the affected foot hanging relaxed over the edge of the table.

Procedure

1. Apply two anchors with 1½-inch (3.8 cm) tape, one circling the leg loosely approximately 7 to 9 inches (17.8 to 22.9 cm) above the malleoli, and the other encircling the ball of the foot (1 and 2).
2. Cut two strips of 3-inch (7.5 cm) elastic tape approximately 8 to 10 inches (20 to 25 cm) long. Moderately stretch the first strip from the ball of the athlete's foot along its plantar aspect up to the leg anchor (3). The second elastic strip (4) follows the course of the first, but cut it and split it down the middle length-

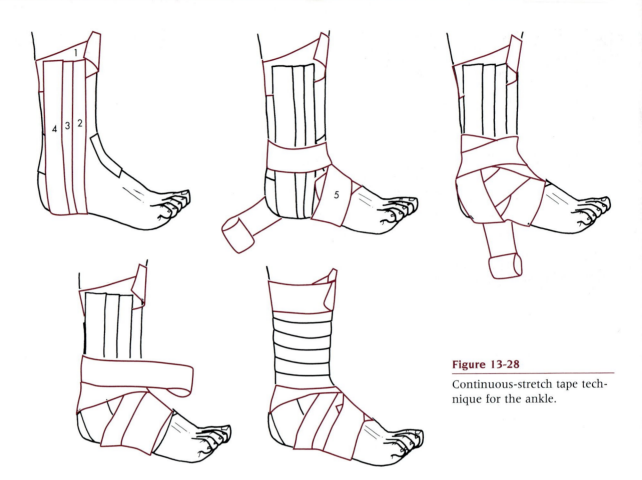

Figure 13-28

Continuous-stretch tape technique for the ankle.

Figure 13-29

Achilles tendon taping.

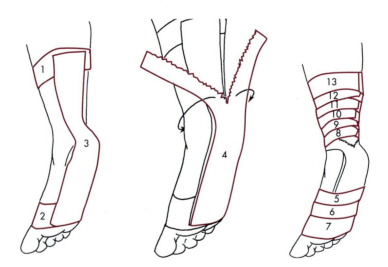

wise. Wrap the cut ends around the lower leg to form a lock. CAUTION: Keep the wrapped ends above the level of the strain.

3. Complete the series by placing two or three lock strips of elastic tape (5 through 7) loosely around the arch and five or six strips (8 through 13) around the athlete's lower leg.

Note that locking too tightly around the lower leg and foot will tend to restrict the normal action of the Achilles tendon and create more tissue irritation.

A variation on this method is to use three 2-inch (5 cm) elastic strips in place of strips 3 and 4. Apply the first strip at the plantar surface of the first metatarsal head and end it on the lateral side of the leg anchor. Apply the second strip at the plantar surface of the fifth metatarsal head and end it on the medial side of the leg anchor. Center the third strip between the other two strips and end it at the posterior aspect of the calf. Wrap strips of 3-inch elastic tape around the forefoot and lower calf to close them off.[1]

The Knee

Medial collateral ligament   As with ankle instabilities, the athlete with an unstable knee should never use tape and bracing as a replacement for proper exercise rehabilitation. If properly applied, taping can help protect the knee and aid in the rehabilitation process[3] (Figure 13-30).

Site preparation   Clean, shave, and dry skin to be taped. Cover skin wounds. Lubricate the hamstring and popliteal areas and apply tape adherent.

Materials needed   One roll of 2-inch (5 cm) linen tape, one roll of 3-inch (7.5 cm) elastic tape, a 1-inch (2.5 cm) heel lift lubricant, gauze pad, tape adherent, and underwrap.

Position of the athlete   The athlete stands on a 3-foot (90 cm) table with the injured knee held in a moderately relaxed position by a 1-inch (2.5 cm) heel lift. The hair is completely removed from an area 6 inches (15 cm) above to 6 inches (15 cm) below the patella.

Procedure
1. Lightly encircle the thigh and leg at the hairline with a 3-inch (7.5 cm) elastic anchor strip (1 and 2).
2. Precut 12 elastic tape strips, each approximately 9 inches (22.5 cm) long. Stretching them to their utmost, apply them to the knee as indicated in Figure 13-30 (3 through 14).
3. Apply a series of three strips of 2-inch (5 cm) linen tape (15 through 22). Some individuals find it advantageous to complete a knee taping by wrapping loosely with an elastic wrap, thus providing an added precaution against the tape's coming loose from perspiration.

NOTE: Tape must *not* constrict the patella.

Rotary taping for instability of an injured knee   The rotary taping method is designed to provide the knee with support when it is unstable from injury to the medial collateral and anterior cruciate ligaments (Figure 13-31).

Materials needed   One roll of 3-inch (7.5 cm) elastic tape, tape adherent, 4-inch (10 cm) gauze pad, lubricant, scissors, and underwrap.

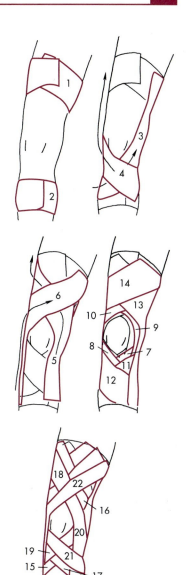

Figure 13-30

Collateral ligament knee taping.

Figure 13-31

Rotary taping.

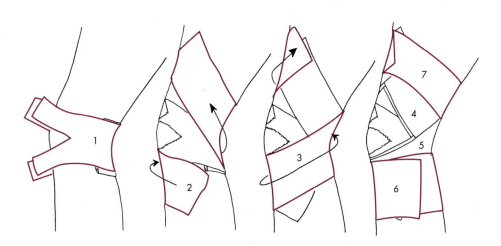

Position of the athlete   The athlete sits on the table with the affected knee flexed 15 degrees.

Procedure

1. Cut a 10-inch (25 cm) piece of elastic tape with both the ends snipped. Place the gauze pad in the center of the 10-inch (25 cm) piece of elastic tape to limit skin irritation and protect the popliteal nerves and blood vessels.
2. Put the gauze with the elastic tape backing on the popliteal fossa of the athlete's knee. Stretch both ends of the tape to the fullest extent and tear them. Place the divided ends firmly around the patella and interlock them (1).
3. Starting at a midpoint on the gastrocremius muscle, spiral a 3-inch (7.5 cm) elastic tape strip to the front of the leg, then behind, crossing the popliteal fossa, and around the thigh, finishing anteriorly (2).
4. Repeat procedure 3 on the opposite side (3).
5. You may apply three or four spiral strips for added strength (4 and 5).
6. Once they are in place, lock the spiral strips by the application of two strips around the thigh and two around the calf (6 and 7).

NOTE: Tracing the spiral pattern with linen tape yields more rigidity.

Hyperextension   Hyperextension taping (Figure 13-32) is designed to prevent the knee from hyperextending and also may be used for a strained hamstring muscle or slackened cruciate ligaments.

Materials needed   One roll of 2½-inch (5.5 cm) tape or 2-inch (5 cm) elastic tape, cotton or a 4-inch (10 cm) gauze pad, tape adherent, underwrap, and a 2-inch (5 cm) heel lift.

Procedure

1. Place two anchor strips at the hairlines, two around the thigh, and two around the leg (1 through 4). They should be loose enough to allow for muscle expansion during exercise.

Figure 13-32

Hyperextension taping.

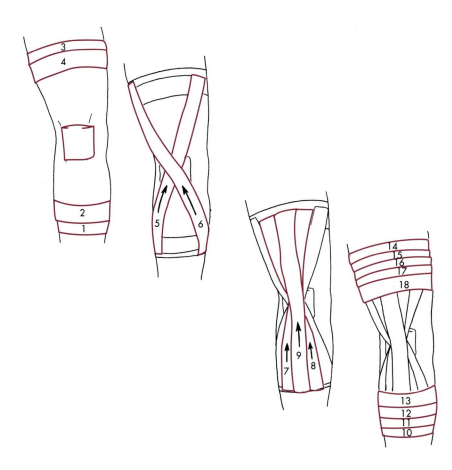

2. Place a gauze pad at the popliteal space to protect the popliteal nerves and blood vessels from constriction by the tape.

3. Start the supporting tape strips by forming an X over the popliteal space (5 and 6).

4. Cross the tape again with two more strips and one up the middle of the leg (7 through 9).

5. Complete the technique by applying four or five locking strips around the thigh and calf (10 through 18).

6. Apply an additional series of strips if the athlete is heavily muscled.

7. Lock the supporting strips in place by applying two or three overlapping circles around the thigh and leg.

Patellofemoral taping (McConnell technique)   Patellofemoral orientation may be corrected to some degree by using tape. The McConnell technique evaluates four components of patellar orientation: glide, tilt, rotation, and anteroposterior (AP) orientation.

The glide component looks at side-to-side movement of the patella in the groove. The tile component assesses the height of the lateral patellar border relative to the medial border. Patellar rotation is determined by looking for deviation of the long axis of the patella from the long axis of the femur. Anteroposterior alignment evaluates whether the inferior pole of the patella is tilted either anteriorly or posteriorly relative to the superior pole. Correction of patellar position and tracking is accomplished by passive taping of the patella in a more biomechanically correct position. In addition to correcting the orientation of the patella, the tape provides a prolonged gentle stretch to soft-tissue structure that affects patellar movement.[6]

Site preparation   Clean and shape, and apply tape adherent.

Materials needed   Two special types of extremely sticky tape are required. Fixomull and Leuko Sportape are manufactured by Biersdorf Australia, Ltd.

Position of the athlete   The athlete should be seated with the knee in full extension.

Procedure

1. Two strips of Fixomull are extended from the lateral femoral condyle just posterior to the medial femoral condyle around the front of the knee. This tape is used as a base to which the other tape may be adhered. Leuko Sportape is used from this point on the correct patellar alignment (Figure 13-33).

2. To correct a lateral glide, attach a short strip of tape one thumb's width from the lateral patellar border, pushing the patella medially in the frontal plane. Crease the skin between the lateral patellar border and the medial femoral condyle and secure the tape on the medial side of the joint (Figure 13-34).

3. To correct a lateral tilt, flex the knee to 30 degrees, adhere a short strip of tape beginning at the middle of the patella, and pull medially to lift the lateral border. Again, crease the skin underneath and adhere it to the medial side of the knee (Figure 13-35).

4. To correct an external rotation of the inferior pole relative to the superior pole, adhere a strip of tape to the middle of the inferior pole, pulling upward and medially while internally rotating the patella with the free hand. The tape is attached to the medial side of the knee (Figure 13-36).

5. For correcting AP alignment in which there is an inferior tilt, take a 6-inch piece of tape, place the middle of the strip over the upper one half of the patella, and attach it equally on both sides to lift the inferior pole (Figure 13-37).

6. Once patellar taping is completed, the athlete should be instructed to wear the tape all day during all activities. The athlete should periodically tighten the strips as they loosen.

NOTE: The McConnell technique for treating patellofemoral pain also stresses the importance of more symmetrical loading of the patella through reeducation and strengthening of the vastus medialis.[1]

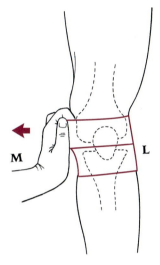

Figure 13-33

The McConnell patellar technique uses a base to which additional tape is adhered.

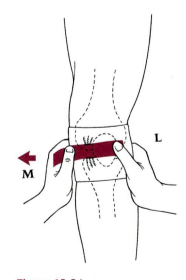

Figure 13-34

McConnell patellar technique to correct a lateral glide.

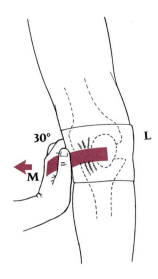

Figure 13-35

McConnell patellar technique to correct a lateral tilt.

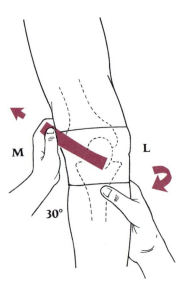

Figure 13-36

McConnell patellar technique to correct external rotation of the inferior pole.

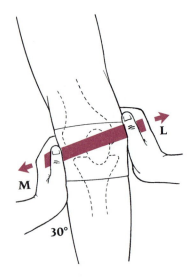

Figure 13-37

McConnell patellar technique to correct AP alignment with an inferior tilt.

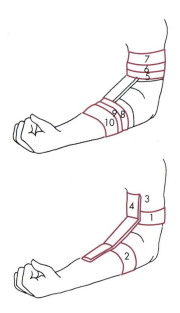

Figure 13-38

Elbow restriction taping.

The Elbow

Elbow restriction   The procedure for taping the elbow to prevent hyperextension follows (Figure 13-38).

Site preparation   Clean and shave area and apply adherent.

Materials needed   One roll of 1½-inch (3.8 cm) tape, tape adherent, and 2-inch (5 cm) elastic bandage.

Position of the athlete   The athlete stands with the affected elbow flexed at 90 degrees.

Procedure

1. Apply two anchor strips loosely around the arm using a 2-inch (5 cm) elastic bandage.
2. Construct a checkrein by cutting a 10-inch (25 cm) and a 4-inch (10 cm) strip of tape and placing the 4-inch (10 cm) strip against the center of the 10-inch (25 cm) strip, blanking out that portion. Next place the checkrein so that it spans the two anchor strips with the blanked-out side facing downward. Leave the checkrein extended 1 to 2 inches past the anchor strips on both ends. This allows anchoring of the checkreins with circular strips to secure against slippage (3 and 4).
3. Place five additional 10-inch (25 cm) strips of tape over the basic checkrein.
4. Finish the procedure by securing the checkrein with three lock strips on each end (5 through 10). A figure-8 elastic wrap applied over the taping will prevent the tape from slipping because of perspiration.

NOTE: A variation of this method is to fan the checkreins, dispersing the force over a wider area (Figure 13-39).

The Wrist and Hand

Wrist technique no. 1   This wrist-taping technique (Figure 13-40) is designed for mild wrist strains and sprains.

Site preparation   Clean, shave, and apply adherent.

Materials needed   One roll of 1-inch (2.5 cm) tape and tape adherent.

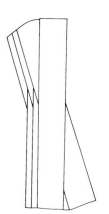
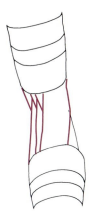

Figure 13-39

Fanned checkrein technique.

Position of the athlete   The athlete stands with the affected hand flexed toward the injured side and the fingers moderately spread to increase the breadth of the wrist for the protection of nerves and blood vessels.

Procedure

1. Starting at the base of the wrist, bring a strip of 1-inch (2.5 cm) tape from the palmar side upward and around both sides of the wrist (1).
2. In the same pattern, with each strip overlapping the preceding one by at least half its width, lay two additional strips in place (2 and 3).

Wrist technique no. 2   This wrist-taping technique (Figure 13-41) stabilizes and protects badly injured wrists. The materials and positioning are the same as in technique 1.

Materials needed   One roll of 1-inch tape and tape adherent.

Position of the athlete   The athlete stands with the affected hand flexed toward the injured side and the fingers moderately spread to increase the breadth of the wrist for the protection of nerves and blood vessels.

Procedure

1. Apply one anchor strip around the wrist approximately 3 inches (7.5 cm) from the hand (1); wrap another anchor strip around the spread hand (2).
2. With the wrist bent toward the side of the injury, run a strip of tape from the anchor strip near the little finger obliquely across the wrist joint to the wrist anchor strip. Run another strip from the anchor strip and the index finger side across the wrist joint to the wrist anchor. This forms a crisscross over the wrist joint (3 and 4). Apply a series of four or five crisscrosses, depending on the extent of splinting needed (5 through 8).

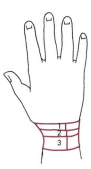

Figure 13-40

Wrist-taping technique no. 1.

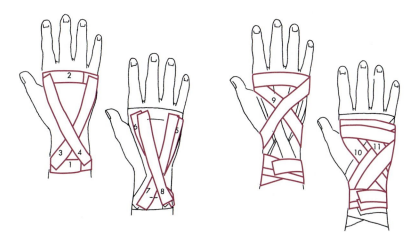

Figure 13-41

Wrist-taping technique no. 2.

3. Apply two or three series of figure-8 tapings over the crisscross taping (9 through 11). Starting by encircling the wrist once, carry a strip over the back of the hand obliquely upward across the back of the hand to where the figure-8 started. Repeat this procedure to ensure a strong, stabilizing taping.

Bruised hand   The following method is used to tape a bruised hand (Figure 13-42).

Materials needed   One roll of 1-inch (2.5 cm) adhesive tape, one roll of ½-inch (1.3 cm) tape, ¼-inch (0.63 cm) thick sponge rubber pad, and tape adherent.

Position of the athlete   The fingers are spread moderately.

Procedure

1. Lay the protective pad over the bruise and hold it in place with three strips of ½-inch (1.3 cm) tape laced through the webbing of the fingers.
2. Apply a basic figure-8 bandage made of 1-inch (2.5 cm) tape.

Sprained thumb   Sprained thumb taping (Figure 13-43) is designed to give both protection to the muscle and joint and support to the thumb.

Materials needed   One roll of 1-inch (2.5 cm) tape and tape adherent.

Position of the athlete   The athlete should hold the injured thumb in a relaxed, neutral position.

Procedure

1. Place an anchor strip loosely around the wrist and another around the distal end of the thumb (1 and 2).
2. From the anchor at the tip of the thumb to the anchor around the wrist apply four splint strips in a series on the side of greater injury (dorsal or palmar side) (3 through 5) and hold them in place with one lock strip around the wrist and one encircling the tip of the thumb (6 and 7).
3. Add three thumb spicas. Start the first spica on the radial side at the base of the thumb and carry it under the thumb, completely encircling it, and then cross the starting point. The strip should continue around the wrist and finish at the preceding strip by at least 2.3 inches (1.7 cm) and move downward on the thumb (8 and 9). The thumb spica with tape provides an excellent means of protection during recovery from an injury (Figure 13-44).

Finger and thumb checkreins   The sprained finger or thumb may require the additional protection afforded by a restraining checkrein (Figure 13-45).

Materials needed   One roll of 1-inch (2.5 cm) tape.

Position of the athlete   The athlete spreads the injured fingers widely but within a range free of pain.

Procedure

1. Bring a strip of 1-inch (2.5 cm) tape around the middle phalanx of the injured finger over to the adjacent finger and around it also. The tape left between the two fingers, which are spread apart, is called the checkrein.
2. Add strength with a lock strip around the center of the checkrein.

SUMMARY

- Common types of bandages used in sports are roller, triangular, and cravat for wrist aid and arm slings, of which the cervical and shoulder types are the most common.
- Common roller bandages are gauze for wounds, cotton cloth ankle wraps, and elastic wraps.
- As with taping, roller bandages must be applied uniformly, firmly but not so tightly as to impede circulation.
- Historically, taping has been an important aspect of athletic training. Sports tape is used in a variety of ways—as a means of holding a wound dressing in place, as support, and as protection against musculoskeletal injuries.
- For supporting and protecting musculoskeletal injuries, two types of tape are currently used—linen and stretch.

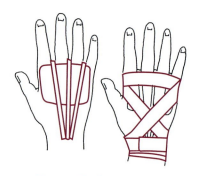

Figure 13-42

Bruised hand taping.

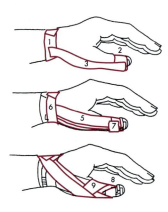

Figure 13-43

Sprained thumb taping.

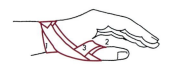

Figure 13-44

Thumb spica.

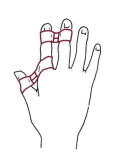

Figure 13-45

Finger and thumb checkreins.

- Sports tape must be stored in a cool place and must be stacked on the flat side of each roll.
- The skin of the athlete must be carefully prepared before tape is applied. The skin should first be carefully cleaned; then all hair should be removed. An adherent may be applied, followed by an underwrap material, if necessary, to help prevent skin irritation.
- When tape is applied, it must be done in a manner that provides the least amount of irritation and the maximum support. All tape applications require great care that the proper materials are used, that the proper position of the athlete is ensured, and that procedures are carefully followed.

Solutions to Critical Thinking EXERCISES

13-1 The athletic trainer applies a 6-inch elastic wrap as a hip adductor restraint. This technique is designed to prevent the groin from being overstretched and the hip adductors reinjured.

13-2 The athletic trainer applies tape and a 4-inch elastic shoulder spica to hold the doughnut in place.

13-3 The athletic trainer applies a sling and swathe combination. This combination stabilizes the shoulder joint and upper arm.

13-4 The LowDye technique is designed to assist in the management of foot pronation and fallen medial longitudinal arch, which predisposes the athlete to arch strain.

13-5 Initially in a sprained ankle the open basket weave taping technique is selected. This technique in conjunction with a pressure bandage and cold application can also control swelling.

REVIEW QUESTIONS AND CLASS ACTIVITIES

1. What are some common types of bandages used in sports medicine today?
2. Observe the athletic trainer when he or she is dressing wounds in the training room.
3. Demonstrate proper use of the roller, triangular, and cravat bandages.
4. What types of tape are available? What is the purpose of each type? What qualities should you look for in selecting tape?
5. How should you prepare an area to be taped?
6. How should you tear tape?
7. How should you remove tape from an area? Demonstrate the various methods and cutters that can be used to remove tape.
8. Bring the different types of tape to class. Discuss their uses and the qualities to look for in purchasing tape. Have the class practice tearing tape and preparing an area for taping.
9. Take each joint or body part and demonstrate the common taping procedures used to give support to that area. Have the students pair up and practice these tapings on each other. Discuss the advantages and disadvantages of using tape as a supportive device.

REFERENCES

1. Austin K et al: *Taping techniques,* Chicago, 1994, Mosby-Wolfe.
2. Hafen BQ: *First aid for health emergencies,* ed 4, St Paul, Minn, 1994, West Publishing.
3. Handling KA: Taping procedure for an unstable knee, *Ath Train* 16:371, 1984.
4. Parcel GS: *Basic emergency care of the sick and injured,* ed 5, St Louis, 1994, Mosby.
5. The continuous technique of ankle support, *Sports Med Guide* 3:14, 1984.
6. McConnell J: The management of chondro-malacia patella: a long term solution, *Aust J Physiother* 32:215, 1986.

ANNOTATED BIBLIOGRAPHY

Athletic training, National Athletic Training Association, PO Box 1865, Greenville, NC 27835-1865.

Each issue of this quarterly journal contains practical procedures for bandaging and taping, as well as for orthotic application.

Austin K et al: *Taping techniques,* Chicago, 1994, Mosby-Wolfe.

An illustrated atlas of taping.

Beuersdors's Medical Program: *Manuals of taping and strapping technique,* Agoura, Calif, 1988, Macmillan.

A complete, detailed guide to various taping and strapping techniques.

First aider, Gardner, Kan, Gramer Products.

Published seven times throughout the school year, this periodical contains useful taping and bandaging techniques that have been submitted by readers.

Kenney R, Berry R: *Sports therapy guide,* Ontario, 1991, Sports Medix.

A well-illustrated guide to taping for the athletic trainer.

National Safety Council: *First aid and CPR,* Boston, 1993, Jones & Bartlett.

Chapter 5 provides an excellent discussion on wound care.

Perrin D: *Athletic taping,* Champaign, Ill, 1995, Human Kinetics.

Complete book of athletic taping for the practitioner.

Sports Medicine Guide, Mueller Sports Medicine, 1 Quench Dr, Prairie du Sac, Wisc 53578.

Published four times a year, this quarterly often presents, along with discussions on specific injuries, many innovative taping and bandaging techniques.

Manual of athletic taping, Philadelphia, 1995, FA Davis.

In-depth text on the skill of athletic taping.

Therapeutic Modalities

When you finish this chapter, you should be able to

- Discuss the legal ramifications of treating the athlete with therapeutic modalities.
- Explain the relationship of most therapeutic modalities relative to electromagnetic energy.
- Describe the theoretical uses of the various types of modalities.
- Correctly demonstrate a variety of thermotherapy and cryotherapy techniques.
- Discuss the use of ultrasound in an athletic training setting.
- Discuss the physiological basis and therapeutic uses of electrical stimulating currents.
- Describe how massage, traction, and intermittent compression can be used as therapeutic agents.

Most athletic trainers routinely incorporate the use of therapeutic modalities into their rehabilitation programs. When used appropriately, therapeutic modalities can be an effective adjunct to various techniques of therapeutic exercise. This chapter is an introduction to the therapeutic modalities most commonly used by an athletic trainer, including cryotherapy, thermotherapy, diathermy, ultrasound, electrotherapy, lasers, massage, traction, and intermittent compression.

LEGAL CONCERNS

Therapeutic modalities must be used in sports medicine with the greatest care possible. At no time should there be an indiscriminate use of any therapeutic modality. Specific laws governing the use of therapeutic modalities vary considerably from state to state. The athletic trainer must follow laws that specifically dictate how athletic trainers can use certain therapeutic modalities. An athletic trainer who uses any type of therapeutic modality must have a thorough understanding of the functions and the indications or contraindications for its use.[33]

The athletic trainer should avoid using a "shotgun" approach when deciding to incorporate therapeutic modalities into a treatment program. Selection of the appropriate modality should be based on an accurate evaluation of the injury and a decision about which modality can most effectively reach the desired target tissue to achieve specific results. If used appropriately, modalities can be an integral part of a treatment and rehabilitation program.[33]

HOW ARE THE MODALITIES RELATED?

Electrical stimulating currents, shortwave and microwave diathermy, the infrared modalities (e.g., hot packs, cold packs), ultraviolet therapy, and the low-powered laser are all therapeutic agents that emit or produce similar types of radiation and can be classified as electromagnetic energy. Ultrasound is a form of radiation that must be classified as acoustic energy rather than electromagnetic energy.[33]

The common characteristics of electromagnetic energy are as follows: it can be transmitted without a medium for support; all forms of electromagnetic energy travel at 300 million meters per second in a vacuum; energy waveforms travel in a straight line; and depending on the medium with which the waveform comes into contact, it may be reflected, refracted, absorbed, or transmitted. The electromagnetic radiation spectrum represents various regions classified according to specific wavelengths and

The athletic trainer must carefully follow laws that prohibit him or her from use of certain therapeutic modalities.

frequencies. The lower the frequency, the longer the wavelength, and vice versa. Generally the longer the wavelength of the radiation, the greater the depth of penetration. In human tissue, the energy must be absorbed before any physiological changes can take place.[33]

TRANSMISSION OF THERMAL ENERGY

The transmission of thermal energy is through **conduction, convection, radiation,** and **conversion.**

Conduction

Conduction occurs when heat is transferred from a warmer object to a cooler one. The ratio of this heat exchange is dependent on the temperature and the exposure time. Skin temperatures are basically influenced by the type of heat or cold medium, the conductivity of the tissue, the quantity of blood flow in the area, and the speed at which heat is being dissipated.[22] To avoid tissue damage the temperature should never exceed 116.6° F (47° C). An exposure that includes close contact with a hot medium that has a temperature of 113° F (45° C) should not exceed 30 minutes. Examples of conductive therapeutic modalities are moist hot packs, paraffin baths, electric heating pads, ice packs, and cold packs.

Convection

Convection refers to the transference of heat through the movement of fluids or gases. Factors that influence convection heating are temperature, speed of movement, and the conductivity of the part.[36] The best example of a modality that uses convection is the whirlpool bath.

Radiation

Radiation is the process whereby heat energy is transferred from one object through space to another object. Shortwave and microwave diathermy, infrared heating, and ultraviolet therapy all rely on the process of radiation for energy transfer.

Conversion

Conversion refers to the generation of heat from another energy form such as sound, electricity, and chemical agents. The mechanical energy produced by high-frequency sound waves changes to heat energy at tissue interfaces (ultrasound therapy).[36] The deep heat of diathermy can be produced by applying electrical currents of specific wavelengths to the skin. Chemical agents such as liniments and balms create a heat type of energy through counterirritation of sensory nerve endings.[36]

CRYOTHERAPY

Application of cold for the first aid of trauma to the musculoskeletal system is a widely used practice in sports medicine. When applied intermittently after injury, along with compression, elevation, and rest, it reduces many of the adverse conditions related to the inflammatory or reactive phase of an acute injury.[21,26] Depending on the severity of the injury, rest, ice, compression, and elevation may be used from day 1 to as long as 2 weeks after injury.

Physical Principles

Cold as a therapeutic agent is a type of electromagnetic energy classified specifically as infrared radiation. When a cold object is applied to a warmer object, heat is abstracted. In terms of cryotherapy, the most common method for cold transfer to tissue is through conduction. The extent to which tissue is cooled depends on the cold medium that is being applied, the length of cold exposure, and the conductivity of the area being cooled.[29] In most cases the longer the cold exposure, the deeper the cooling. At a temperature of 38.3° F (3.5° C), muscle temperatures can be reduced as

conduction
Heating through direct contact with a hot medium.

convection
Heating indirectly through another medium such as air or liquid.

radiation
Transfer of heat through space from one object to another.

conversion
Heating through other forms of energy.

The major therapeutic value of cold is its ability to produce anesthesia, allowing pain-free exercise.

deep as 4 cm. Cooling is dependent on the type of tissue. For example, tissue with a high water content, such as muscle, is an excellent cold conductor, whereas fat is a poor conductor. Because of fat's low cold conductivity, it acts as the body's insulator.[29] Tissue that has previously been cooled takes longer to return to a normal temperature than tissue that has been heated.

The two most common means used to deliver cold as therapy to the body is through ice or cold packs or immersion in cool or cold water. The most effective type of pack contains wet ice, as compared with ice in a plastic container or commercial Cryogen pack.[3] Wet ice is a more effective coolant because of the extent of internal energy needed to melt the ice.[36]

Physiological Effects of Cold

When cold is applied to skin for 15 minutes or less at a temperature of 50° F (10° C) or less, vasoconstriction of the arterioles and venules in the area occurs. This vasoconstriction is caused in part by the reflex action of the smooth muscles, which can result from stimulation of the sympathetic nervous system and adrenal medulla, causing a secretion of norepinephrine and epinephrine.[36] Also causing vasoconstriction is cooled blood circulating to the anterior hypothalamus. If cold is continuously applied for 15 to 30 minutes, an intermittent period of vasodilation occurs for 4 to 6 minutes. This period is known as the **hunting response,** a reaction against tissue damage from too much cold exposure.[21] When the hunting response occurs, the tissue temperature does not return to preapplication levels. This response has primarily been observed in the appendages. Cold during this period also causes an increase in blood viscosity and a decrease in vasodilator metabolites.[36]

hunting response
Causes a slight temperature increase during cooling.

Much of the damage done to cells after trauma occurs as a result of compromised circulation, which decreases the amount of oxygen being delivered to the cells in the area of injury. The immediate use of ice after injury decreases the extent of hypoxic injury to those cells on the periphery of the primary injury by slowing their metabolic rate. This results in less damage to the tissues, thus decreasing rehabilitation time.[21]

Because cold lowers the metabolic rate and produces vasoconstriction, swelling will be reduced in an acute inflammatory response. It should be emphasized that cold does not reduce swelling that is already present.[21]

Cooling tissues can directly decrease a muscle spasm by slowing metabolism in the area, thus decreasing the waste products, which act as a muscle irritant and thus cause spasm, that may have accumulated in the area. A muscle spasm can also be decreased when cold is applied to decrease the muscle spindle's threshold and its myotactic reflex response and when cold increases the muscle's viscosity, slowing its ability to contract.[18]

Because the local application of cold can decrease an acute muscle spasm, the muscle becomes more amenable to stretch. A gentle stretch of a spastic muscle after an acute injury may be indicated; however, the stretching of long-standing contractures is contraindicated. Cold tends to cause collagen stiffness.[23]

Cold decreases free nerve-ending excitability, as well as the excitability of peripheral nerves. Analgesia is caused by raising the nerve's threshold.[18,45] Nerve fiber re-

TABLE 14-1   Skin Response to Cold

Stage	Response	Estimated Time after Initiation
1	Cold sensation	0 to 3 minutes
2	Mild burning, aching	2 to 7 minutes
3	Relative cutaneous anesthesia	5 to 12 minutes

sponse to cold depends mainly on the presence of myelination and the diameter of the fiber. For example, most sensitive to cold are the small light-touch, cold, and gamma efferent myelinated fibers to the muscle spindles.[18] The next most sensitive to cold are the large myelinated fibers of the proprioceptors and alpha motor nerves.[18] The least sensitive to cold are the unmyelinated pain fibers and postganglionic sympathetic nerves.[18] Table 14-1 indicates the usual outward sequential response to cold application.

Cold, in general, is more penetrating than heat. Once a muscle has been cooled through the subcutaneous fat layer, cold's effects last longer than heat because fat acts as an insulator against rewarming.[24] The major problem is to penetrate the fat layer initially so that muscle cooling occurs. In individuals with less than ½ inch (1.25 cm) of subcutaneous fat, significant muscle cooling can occur after 10 minutes of cold application. In persons with more than ⅘ inch (2 cm) of subcutaneous fat, muscle temperatures barely drop after 10 minutes[18] (Table 14-2).

> The extent of cooling depends on the thickness of the subcutaneous fat layer.

Another unique quality of cooling is its ability to decrease muscle fatigue and increase and maintain muscular contraction. This ability is attributed to decreasing the local metabolic rate and the tissue temperature.[24]

Special Considerations

Although adverse reactions to therapeutic cold application are uncommon, they do happen and are described as follows:
- Cooling for an hour at 30.2° to 15.8° F (−1° to −9° C) produces redness and edema that lasts for 20 hours after exposure.[17] Frostbite has been known to occur in subfreezing temperatures of 26.6° to 24.8° F (−3° to −4° C).[21]
- Immersion at 41° F (5° C) increases limb fluid volume by 15%.
- Exposure for 90 minutes at 57.2° to 60.8° F (14° to 16° C) can delay resolution of swelling up to 1 week.[21]
- Some individuals are allergic to cold, reacting with hives and joint pain and swelling.[36]
- **Raynaud's phenomenon** is a condition that causes vasospasm of digital arteries lasting for minutes to hours, which could lead to tissue death. The early signs of Raynaud's phenomenon are attacks of intermittent skin blanching or cyanosis of the fingers or toes, skin pallor followed by redness, and finally a return to normal color. Pain is uncommon, but numbness, tingling, or burning may occur during and shortly after an attack.
- Paroxysmal cold hemoglobinuria is a rare disease that occurs minutes after cold exposure and may lead to renal dysfunction, secondary hypertension, and coma. Early symptoms are severe pain in the back and legs, headache, vomiting, diarrhea, and dark brown urine.
- Although it is relatively uncommon, application of ice can cause nerve palsy. Nerve palsy occurs when cold is applied to a part that has motor nerves close to the skin surface, such as the peroneal nerve at the fibular head. Usually the con-

> **Raynaud's phenomenon**
> Condition in which cold exposure causes vasospasm of digital arteries.

TABLE 14-2 **Physiological Variables of Cryotherapy**

Variable	Effect
Muscle spasm	Decreases
Pain perception	Decreases
Blood flow	Decreases up to 10 minutes
Metabolic rate	Decreases
Collagen elasticity	Decreases
Joint stiffness	Increases
Capillary permeability	Increases
Edema	Controversial

dition resolves spontaneously with no significant problem. As a general rule, ice should not be applied longer than 20 to 30 minutes at any one time.

Cryotherapeutic Methods

A number of methods of cold applications can be used therapeutically. The ones most commonly used in sports medicine are ice massage, cold or ice water immersion, ice packs, and vapocoolant sprays.

Ice Massage

Ice massage is a cryotherapeutic method that is performed on a small body area. It can be applied by the athletic trainer and the athlete alike.

Equipment   Water is frozen in a Styrofoam cup, which forms a cylinder of ice. When using this method, the Styrofoam is removed approximately an inch from the top of the cup. The remaining Styrofoam provides a handle to grasp while massaging. Another method is to fill a paper cup with water, with a tongue depressor added to act as a handle when the water is frozen. A towel should be present to absorb the water that is collected.

Indications   Ice massage is commonly used over a small muscle area such as the tendons, the belly of the muscle, the bursa, or over myofascial trigger points.

Application   Grasping the ice cylinder, the athletic trainer rubs the ice over the athlete's skin in overlapping circles, ranging in a 10 to 15 cm area for a period of 5 to 10 minutes. The athlete should experience the sensations of cold, burning, aching, and numbness. When analgesia has been reached, the athlete can engage in stretching or exercise (Figure 14-1).

Special considerations   In an athlete with normal circulation, tissue damage seldom occurs from cold application. The temperature of the tissue seldom goes below 59° F (15° C). The comfort of the athlete must be considered at all times.

Cold or Ice Water Immersion

Cold water immersion is a relatively simple means for treating a distal body part.

Equipment   Depending on the body part to be immersed, a variety of containers or basins can be used. In some cases, a small whirlpool can be used. Water and crushed ice are mixed together to reach a temperature of 50° F (10° C) to 60° F (15° C). Towels must be available for drying.

Indications   Where circumferential cooling of a body part is desired, cold or ice water immersion is preferred.

Application   The athlete immerses the body part in the water and proceeds through the four stages of cold response. This process may take 10 to 15 minutes. When the pain cycle has been interrupted, the part is removed from the water, and normal movement patterns are conducted. When pain returns, the part is reimmersed. This procedure may be repeated three times.

Special considerations   Because cold makes collagen tissue brittle, caution should be taken in allowing the athlete to return to full sports performance after receiving cold treatment. Overcooling can lead to frostbite. Any allergic response to cold should also be noted.

Ice Packs

The use of ice packs is another way to apply cryotherapy.

Equipment   There are a number of types of ice packs. As discussed previously, wet ice packs provide the best cooling properties. Flaked or crushed ice can be encased in a wet towel and placed on the part to be treated. Although not as efficient but less messy, a pack made by placing crushed or chipped ice in a self-sealing plastic bag may be used. If isopropyl alcohol is added at a 2:1 ratio, the packs can be put into a freezer and not completely frozen. When they are removed from the freezer, the packs easily fit the contour of the part. These packs are

Cold therapy can begin 1 to 3 days after injury.

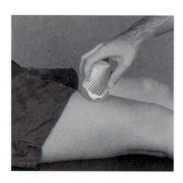

Figure 14-1

Ice massage can lead to an analgesia that can be followed by gentle muscle stretching.

useful for approximately 15 or 20 minutes.[36] When the plastic packs are used, a wet towel should be placed between the skin and the pack. Besides toweling, an elastic wrap should be available and should be used to hold the pack firmly in place.

There are two different types of chemical cold packs available. One is a gel pack that may be refrozen after use and is hypoallergenic. These are commonly used in many athletic training settings. The other type is a liquid bag within a bag of crystals. When the inner bag is ruptured the chemicals mix, causing an endothermic reaction. If allowed contact with the skin these chemicals can cause a chemical burn and a liability problem.[3]

Indications As with the other cryotherapeutic modalities, the four stages of cold are experienced, followed by normal movement patterns (Figure 14-2).

Special considerations As with other modalities, excessive cold exposure must be avoided. With any indication of allergy to cold or of abnormal pain, the therapy should be discontinued.

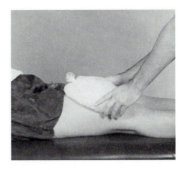

Figure 14-2

Ice packs can be another way to apply cryotherapy.

Vapocoolant Sprays

Increasingly, vapocoolant sprays are being used for treatment of musculoskeletal conditions attributed to sports activity.

Equipment Currently the vapocoolant of choice is Fluori-methane, a nonflammable, nontoxic substance. Under pressure in a bottle, it gives off a fine spray when it is inverted and an emitter is pressed.

Indications The major value of a vapocoolant spray is its ability to reduce muscle spasm and increase range of motion. It is also a major treatment for myofascial pain and trigger points.[32] Care must be taken, however, to avoid frostbite.

Application When spraying vapocoolant spray to increase the athlete's range of motion in an area in which there is no trigger point, the following procedure is performed:

1. The vapocoolant is held at a 30-degree angle, 12 to 18 inches (30 to 47 cm) from the skin.
2. The entire length of the muscle is sprayed from its proximal attachment to its distal attachment.
3. The skin is covered at a rate of approximately 10 cm per second, and the spray is applied two or three times as a gradual stretch is applied.

When dealing with a possible trigger point, the procedure is first to determine its presence, then to alleviate it.

One method of determining an active trigger point is to reproduce the injured athlete's major pain complaint by pressing firmly on the site for 5 to 10 seconds. Another assessment technique is to elicit a jump response by placing the athlete's muscle under moderate tension, applying firm pressure, and briskly pulling a finger across the tight band of muscle. This procedure causes the tight band of muscle to contract and the athlete to wince or cry out.[30] The spray and stretch method[29] for treating trigger points and myofascial pain has become a major approach (Figure 14-3) and is performed as follows:

1. Position the athlete in a relaxed but well-supported position. The muscle that contains the trigger point is stretched (an exception to this is the sternocleidomastoid muscle).
2. Alert the athlete that the spray will feel cool.
3. Hold the Fluori-Methane bottle approximately 12 inches (30 cm) away from the skin to be sprayed.
4. Direct the spray at an acute angle in one direction toward the reference zone of pain.
5. Direct the spray to the full length of the muscle, including the reference zone of pain.
6. Begin firm stretching that is within the athlete's pain tolerance.

Fluori-methane spray is used in the spray and stretch technique.

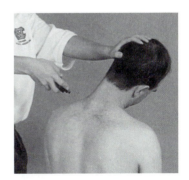

Figure 14-3

A vapocoolant spray such as Fluori-methane can assist in reducing muscle spasm.

7. Continue spraying in parallel sweeps that are approximately ¼ inch (0.6 cm) apart at a speed of approximately 4 inches (10 cm) every second.
8. Cover the skin area one or two times.
9. Continue passive stretching while spraying (do not force the stretch; allow time for the muscle to "let go").
10. After the first session of spraying and stretching, warm the muscle with a hot pack or by vigorous massage.
11. A second session may be necessary after step 10.
12. When a stretch has been completed, have the athlete actively but gently move the part in a full range of motion.
13. Do not overload a muscle with strenuous exercise immediately after a stretch.
14. After an initial spraying and stretching session, instruct the athlete about stretch exercises that should be performed at home on a daily basis.

Cryokinetics

cryokinetics
Combines cryotherapy with exercise.

Cryokinetics is a technique that combines cryotherapy, or the application of cold, with exercise.[21] The goal of cryokinetics is to numb the injured part to the point of analgesia and then work toward achieving normal range of motion through progressive active exercise.

The technique begins by numbing the body part via ice immersion, cold packs, or ice massage. Most athletes report a feeling of numbness within 12 to 20 minutes. If numbness is not perceived within 20 minutes, the athletic trainer should proceed with exercise regardless. The numbness usually lasts for 3 to 5 minutes, at which point ice should be reapplied for an additional 3 to 5 minutes until numbness returns. This sequence should be repeated five times (see the Focus box below).

Exercises are performed during the periods of numbness. The exercises selected should be pain free and progressive in intensity, concentrating on both flexibility and strength. Changes in the intensity of the activity should be limited by both the nature of the healing process and by individual patient differences in perception of pain. However, progression always should be encouraged within the framework of those limiting factors, the ultimate goal being a return to full sport-type activities.[21]

THERMOTHERAPY

The application of heat to treat disease and traumatic injuries has been used for centuries. Recently, however, its use in the immediate treatment phase of musculoskeletal injury has been replaced with cold application. Heat is an energy form that in-

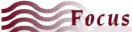 *Focus*

Summary of cryokinetics
1. Immerse ankle in ice water until numb (12 to 20 min).
2. Exercise within limits of pain (see progression below) (3 to 5 min).
3. Renumb ankle by immersion (3 to 5 min).
4. Exercise within limits of pain (3 to 5 min).
5. Repeat steps 3 and 4 three more times.
6. Principles of exercising:
   a. All exercise should be active, that is, performed totally by the patient.
   b. All exercise must be pain free.
   c. All exercise must be performed smoothly, without limping, twitching, or any other abnormal motion.
   d. The exercise must be aggressively progressive, that is, progress to more complex and difficult levels as quickly as possible (remember—*no pain*).

creases molecular activity by conduction, convection, conversion, and radiation.[36] Thermotherapy modes are moist, dry, superficial, and deep.

Physiological Effects of Heat

The body's response to heat depends on the type of heat energy applied, the intensity of the heat energy, the duration of application, and the unique tissue response to heat. For a physiological response to occur, heat must be absorbed into the tissue, causing an increase in molecular activity. After the tissue's absorption of heat energy, heat is spread to adjacent tissue. To effect a therapeutic change that results in normal function of the absorbing tissue, the correct amount of heat must be applied. With too little, no change occurs; with too much, the tissue is damaged further.

There are still many unanswered questions about how heat produces therapeutic responses and what types of thermotherapy are most appropriate for a given condition. The desirable therapeutic effects of heat include increasing the extensibility of collagen tissues; decreasing joint stiffness; reducing pain; relieving muscle spasm; reducing inflammation, edema, and exudates in the postacute phase of healing; and increasing blood flow.[36]

Heat affects the extensibility of collagen tissue by increasing the viscous flow of collagen fibers and subsequently relaxing the tension. From a therapeutic point of view, heating contracted connective tissue permits an increase in extensibility through stretching. Muscle fibrosis, a contracted joint capsule, and scars can be effectively stretched while being heated or just after the heat is removed.[36] An increase in extensibility does not occur unless heat treatment is associated with stretching exercises.

> Heat has the capacity to increase the extensibility of collagen tissue.

Both heat and cold relieve pain, stimulating the free nerve endings and peripheral nerves by a gating mechanism or secretion of endorphins. (See Chapter 7.) Muscle spasm caused by **ischemia** can be relieved by heat, which increases blood flow to the area of injury. Heat is also believed to assist inflammation and swelling by a number of related factors such as raising temperature, increasing metabolism, reducing oxygen tension, lowering the pH level, increasing capillary permeability, and releasing histamine and bradykinin, which cause vasodilation. Histamine and bradykinin are released from some cells during acute and chronic inflammation. Heat is also produced by axon reflexes and vasomotor reflex change. Parasympathetic impulses stimulated by heat are believed to be one reason for vasodilation[24] (Table 14-3).

> **ischemia**
> Lack of blood supply to a body part.

Superficial Heat

The superficial heating modalities, along with the cold modalities discussed previously, are all considered to be forms of electromagnetic energy whose wavelengths and frequencies are classified in the infrared region of the electromagnetic spectrum. Heat applied superficially to the skin directly increases the subcutaneous temperature and indirectly spreads to the deeper tissues. Muscle temperature increases through a reflexive effect on circulation and through conduction.[36] Comparatively,

TABLE 14-3 Physiological Variables of Thermotherapy

Condition	Response to Therapy
Muscle spasm	Decreases
Pain perception	Decreases
Blood flow	Increases
Metabolic rate	Increases
Collagen elasticity	Increases
Joint stiffness	Decreases
Capillary permeability	Increases
Edema	Increases

when heat is applied at the same temperature, moist heat causes a greater indirect increase in the deep-tissue temperature than does dry. Dry heat, in contrast to moist heat, can be tolerated at higher temperatures. Superficial heat application causes vasodilation that continues for up to 1 hour after its removal.[6]

Special Considerations in the Use of Superficial Heat

In general, superficial heating of the skin is a safe therapeutic medium, assuming of course that the heat is kept at a reasonable intensity and that application does not occur for too long a period. The following are important contraindications and precautions to be taken when using superficial heat:

- Never apply heat when there is a loss of sensation.
- Never apply heat immediately after an injury.
- Never apply heat when there is decreased arterial circulation.
- Never apply heat directly to the eyes or the genitals.
- Never heat the abdomen during pregnancy.
- Never apply heat to a body part that exhibits signs of acute inflammation.

Moist Heat Therapies

Heated water is one of the most widely used therapeutic modalities in sports medicine. It is readily available for use in any sports medicine program. The greatest disadvantage of hydrotherapy is the difficulty in controlling the therapeutic effects, primarily as a result of the rapid dissipation of heat, which makes maintaining a constant tissue temperature difficult.

For the most part moist heat aids the healing process in some local conditions by causing higher superficial tissue temperatures; however, joint and muscle circulation increase little in temperature. Superficial tissue is a poor thermal conductor, and temperature rises quickly on the skin surface as compared with the underlying tissues.

Superficial tissue is a poor thermal conductor.

Moist Heat Packs

Commercial moist heat packs, sometimes called Hydrocollator packs, heat by conduction.

Equipment Moist heat packs contain silicate gel in a cotton pad, which is immersed in thermostatically controlled hot water at a temperature of 160° F (71.1° C) to 170° F (76.7° C). Each pad retains water and a constant heat level for 20 to 30 minutes. Six layers of toweling or commercial terry cloth are used between the packs and the skin (Figure 14-4).

Figure 14-4

At least two protective layers of toweling must be applied between the skin and a moist heat pack.

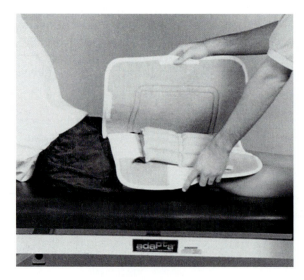

Indications   The major value of the moist heat pack is that its use results in general relaxation and reduction of the pain-spasm-ischemia-hypoxia-pain cycle. There are limitations of the moist heat pack and all other superficial heating modalities: "the deeper tissues, including the musculature, are usually not significantly heated because the heat transfer from the skin surface into deeper tissues is inhibited by the subcutaneous fat, which acts as a thermal insulator, and by the increased skin flow, which cools and carries away the heat externally applied."[24]

Application
1. Remove pack from water and allow to drain for a few seconds.
2. Cover pack with six layers of dry toweling or commercial cover.
3. Treat the area for 15 to 20 minutes.
4. As pack cools, remove layers of toweling to continue the heating.

Special considerations
- The athlete should not be lying on packs.
- Be sure the athlete is comfortable at all times.

Whirlpool Bath

Whirlpool therapy is a combination of massage and water immersion. It has become one of the most popular thermotherapies used in sports medicine.

Equipment   There are generally three types of whirlpools: the extremity tank, which is used for treating legs and arms and is 15 inches wide, 28 to 32 inches long, and 18 to 25 inches deep; the low boy tank, which is approximately 24 inches wide, 52 to 62 inches long, and approximately 18 inches deep and used for full-body immersion; and the high boy tank, which is designed for the hip or the leg and is 20 to 24 inches wide, 36 to 48 inches long, and 28 inches deep.[50]

The whirlpool is essentially a tank and a turbine motor, which regulates the movement of water and air. The amount of movement (agitation) is controlled by the amount of air that is emitted. The more air there is, the more water movement.[50]

The turbine motor can be moved up and down on a tubular column. It can also be rotated on the column and locked in place at a specific angle.

Indications   The whirlpool provides both conduction and convection. Conduction is achieved by the skin's contacting the higher water temperature. As the water swirls around the skin surface, convection occurs (Figure 14-5).

This medium assists the body part in reducing swelling, muscle spasm, and pain. Because of the buoyancy of the water, active movement of the part is also assisted.

14-1

Critical Thinking Exercise

A volleyball player has an elbow sprain that occurred 5 days ago. To this point he has been using cryotherapy as exclusive treatment. His elbow is still tender with some minimal swelling. He says that he really hates the ice and wants to know if he can switch over to some form of heat, which he feels will be more comfortable.

? In the course of an injury rehabilitation program, when should the athletic trainer decide to change from using cold to using heat?

The whirlpool bath combines heated water and massaging action.

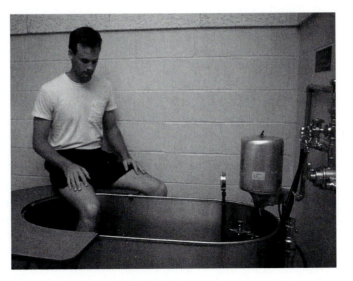

Figure 14-5

A whirlpool bath provides therapy through heat conduction and convection.

TABLE 14-4 Whirlpool Temperatures

Descriptive Terms	Temperature
Very cold	>55° F (12.8° C)
Cold	55°-65° F (12.8°-18.3° C)
Tepid	80°-90° F (27°-33.5° C)
Neutral	92°-96° F (33.5°-35.5° C)
Warm	96°-98° F (35.5°-36.5° C)
Hot	98°-104° F (36.5°-40° C)

Application

1. Set water temperature according to Table 14-4. Some athletic trainers prefer to perform only cold water treatments, whereas others prefer to increase the temperature according to the healing phase of an acute injury. Chronic conditions normally require a higher water temperature.
2. Once the tank has been filled with water at the desired temperature, the athlete is comfortably positioned so that the part to be treated can be easily reached by the agitated water. In many cases it is best that the water jet is not placed directly on the part but to the side of the tank. This is particularly true in the early stages of the acute injury. In cases in which the stream is concentrated directly toward the injury site, the site should be at least 8 to 10 inches from the jet.
3. The duration of treatment is of major concern for the athletic trainer. The maximum length of treatment time for acute injuries should not exceed 20 minutes. In the early stages of treating an acute injury, a graduated program should be implemented, increasing slowly on a daily basis—to 5 minutes, 10 minutes, 15 minutes, and finally to 20 minutes. A duration of 20 minutes is usually recommended for treatment of chronic injuries.

Special considerations

1. Great caution should be taken when an athlete undergoes full-body immersion because of the possibility of his or her experiencing light-headedness.[4]
2. Whirlpool care is of major importance to avoid infection. The following procedures should be adhered to:
   a. Empty tank after use.
   b. Scrub inside of tank with a commercial disinfectant, rinse with clean water, and dry.
   c. Polish external surface of tank with a commercial stainless steel polish.
3. Safety is of major importance in the use of the whirlpool. All electrical outlets should have a ground fault circuit interrupter. At no time should the athlete turn the motor on or off. Ideally, the on/off switch should be a considerable distance from the machine.[50]

Paraffin Bath

Paraffin bath therapy is particularly effective for injuries to the more angular body areas.

Paraffin is a popular method for applying heat to the distal extremities.

Equipment The commercial paraffin bath is a thermostatically controlled unit that maintains a temperature of 126° to 130° F (52° to 54° C). The paraffin mixture consists of a ratio of 25 kg of paraffin wax to 1 L of mineral oil. Slats at the bottom of the container protect the athlete from burns and collect the settling dirt. Also required for treatment are plastic bags, paper towels, and towels.

Indications The mineral oil acts to lower the melting point of the paraffin and thus the specific heat. Consequently, the ability to tolerate the heat from the paraffin is greater than it would be from water at the same temperature.

This therapy is especially effective in treating chronic injuries occurring to the more angular areas of the body such as the hands, wrists, elbows, ankles, and feet.

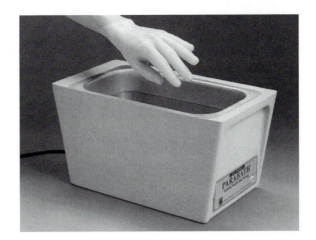

Figure 14-6

A paraffin bath is an excellent form of therapeutic heat for the distal extremities. After paraffin coating has been accomplished, the part is covered by a plastic material. When heat is no longer generated, the paraffin is scraped back into the container.

Application   Therapy by means of the paraffin bath can be delivered in several ways. It can be dipped and wrapped in a plastic bag, dipped and reimmersed forming 8 to 10 layers, painted on in several layers, or soaked.

Before therapy, the part to be treated is thoroughly cleaned and dried. Then the athlete dips the affected part into the paraffin bath and quickly pulls it out, allowing the accumulated wax to dry and form a solid covering. The process of dipping and withdrawing is repeated 6 to 12 times until the wax coating is ¼ to ½ inch (0.62 to 1.3 cm) thick.

If the dip and wrap technique is to be employed, the accumulated wax is allowed to solidify on the last withdrawal; then it is completely wrapped in a plastic material that in turn is wrapped with a towel. The packed body part is placed in a position of rest for approximately 30 minutes or until heat is no longer generated. The covering is then removed and the paraffin is scraped back into the container.

If the soak technique is selected, the athlete is instructed to soak the wax-coated part in the hot wax container for 20 to 30 minutes without moving it, after which the part is removed from the container and the paraffin on it is allowed to solidify. The pack procedure can follow the soak, or the paraffin coating can be scraped back into the container immediately after it hardens. Once the paraffin has been removed from the part, an oily residue remains that provides an excellent surface for massage (Figure 14-6).

Special considerations   Avoid paraffin bath therapy in areas where there is hemorrhaging or a decrease in normal circulation.

It is essential that the athlete clean the part thoroughly before therapy to avoid contaminating the mixture. In most cases, if this rule is closely adhered to, the mixture will only have to be replaced approximately every 6 months.[36]

Fluidotherapy

Fluidotherapy creates a therapeutic environment through dry heat and forced convection through a suspended airstream.

Equipment   Fluidotherapy units come in a variety of sizes, ranging from ones that treat distal extremities to ones that treat large body areas. The unit contains fine cellulose particles in which warm air is circulated. As the air is circulated, the cellulose particles become suspended, giving properties that are similar to liquid.[36] Fluidotherapy allows the athlete to tolerate much greater temperatures than would be possible using water or paraffin heat (Figure 14-7).

Indications   Fluidotherapy is successful, resulting in decreased pain, increased joint range of motion, and decreased spasm and swelling.

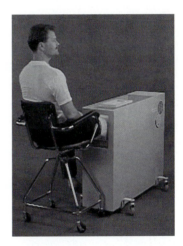

Figure 14-7

Fluidotherapy units contain five cellulose particles in which warm air is circulated.

Fluidotherapy consists of cellulose particles in which warm air is circulated.

Application

- Treatment temperature usually ranges from 100° to 113° F (37.8° to 45° C).
- Particle agitation should be controlled for comfort.
- Exercise can be performed while the athlete is in the cabinet.
- The athlete should be positioned for comfort.
- Treatment duration is 15 to 20 minutes.

Contrast Bath

Contrasting hot and cold water is a popular therapy in sports medicine. It is primarily used in the treatment of the extremities.

Equipment   The contrast bath technique requires the use of two containers, one to hold hot water at 105° to 110° F (40.6° to 43.3° C) and one to hold cold water at 50° to 65° F (10° to 18° C). A whirlpool can be used for the hot container, and a basin or bucket can be used for the cold.

Indications   Contrast baths are used when changing the treatment modality from cold to heat to facilitate a mild tissue temperature increase. The use of contrast baths allows for a transitional period during which a slight rise in temperature may be effective for increasing blood flow to an injured area without causing accumulation of additional edema. It has been demonstrated that only a slight temperature change occurs superficially using the contrast technique.[27] The theory that contrast baths induce a type of pumping action by alternating vasoconstriction with vasodilation has little or no credibility.[36]

Application   During the initial stages of contrast bath treatment, the ratio of heat to cold treatment begins with a relatively brief exposure to heat; this exposure is gradually increased in subsequent treatments. Recommendations as to specific ratios are extremely variable. However, it appears that a 3:1 ratio (3 minutes in heat, 1 minute in cold) or 4:1 for 19 or 20 minutes is fairly well accepted[36] (Figure 14-8). The ratio may be modified as the transition from cold to heat progresses.

Special considerations

- Care must be taken to keep the water temperature constant.
- The athlete should be kept as comfortable as possible throughout the procedure.

Alternative method   A second method of contrast that has become popular in sports medicine uses the concept of alternatively submerging the limb in an ice slush bath for 2 minutes and then in tepid water at 93° to 98° F (33.9° to 37.7° C) for 30 seconds. The baths are alternated for 15 minutes, beginning and ending with cold immersion.

SHORTWAVE AND MICROWAVE DIATHERMY

Shortwave and microwave diathermy are two modalities that emit electromagnetic energy that is capable of producing temperature increases in the deeper tissues. Tissues with a higher water content (e.g., muscle) selectively absorb the heat delivered by shortwave and microwave diathermies.[18] The extent of muscle heating is dependent on the thickness of the subcutaneous fat layer. Both shortwave and microwave diathermies provide less heat penetration than ultrasound. In contrast to shortwave and microwave diathermies, ultrasonic vibration is not absorbed by fat and is therefore not influenced by its thickness.[18]

Shortwave Diathermy

Shortwave diathermy heats deeper tissues by introducing a high-frequency electrical current. Shortwave diathermy is in essence a radio transmitter; the Federal Communications Commission (FCC) has assigned a wavelength of 7.5 to 22 meters and a frequency of 13.56 or 27.12 megacycles per second for therapeutic purposes.[37]

There are two ways that shortwave diathermy can be used: through a condenser that uses electrostatic field heating or through electromagnetic or induction field heating.[16] In electrostatic field heating, the patient is a part of the circuit.[37] Heating is

---

contrast bath procedure
Two minutes of immersion in ice slush, followed by 30 seconds in tepid water (93° to 98° F [33.9° to 37.7° C]).

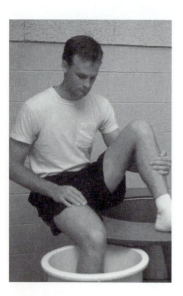

Figure 14-8

A contrast bath, which uses alternating cold water immersion and hot water immersion, is a popular therapy with many athletic trainers.

uneven because of different tissue resistance to energy flow, an application of Joule's law, which states that the greater the resistance or impedance, the more the heat that will be developed. In electromagnetic field heating the patient is not part of the circuit but is heated by an electromagnetic field.[37]

Pulsed Shortwave Diathermy

Pulsed shortwave diathermy is a relatively new form of diathermy.[28] Pulsed diathermy is created by simply interrupting the output of continuous shortwave diathermy at consistant intervals. This reduces the likelihood of any significant tissue temperature increase and reduces the patient's perception of heat. Generators that deliver pulsed shortwave diathermy typically use a drum type of electrode.

Pulsed diathermy is claimed to have therapeutic value and to produce nonthermal effects with minimal thermal physiological effects, depending on the intensity of the application. When pulsed diathermy is used in intensities that create an increase in tissue temperature, its effects are no different from those of continuous shortwave diathermy.

Equipment

In general, the shortwave diathermy unit consists of a power supply to a power amplifier and a frequency generator. It has an oscillator that produces high frequency (either 13.56 or 27.12 megacycles) and a power amplifier that converts alternating current (AC) to direct current (DC).[22] It also has a circuit that tunes in the patient automatically or manually as part of the circuitry (Figure 14-9).

The shortwave diathermy treatment applicators are either condensor or inductive types.[37] With the condensor, or field heating, the patient is a natural part of the circuit. The condensor applicator consists of electrodes that are formed by sheets of flexible or rigid metal covered by heavy insulation.

There are two types of inductive electrodes—the coil and the single drum unit. The inductive coil is a cable electrode, which ranges from 2 to 5 meters long and is wound around the patient's injured part. Whereas the coil can heat generally, the

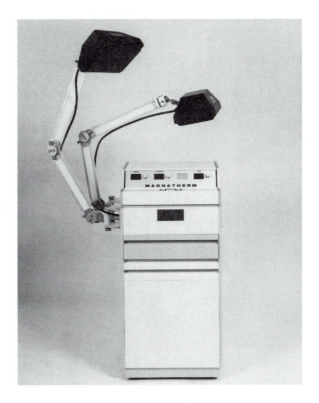

Figure 14-9

The Magnatherm is an example of a currently used Shortwave diathermy unit.

single drum type is designed to treat a more specific area.[20] Tissues with high water content such as blood and muscle are the most easily heated.

Indications

Shortwave diathermy is highly effective in cases of bursitis, capsulitis, osteoarthritis, deep muscle spasm, and strains. The depth of the inductive technique can be as much as 2 inches (5 cm). The condensor technique penetrates from 1 to 2 inches (2.5 to 5 cm). Tissue temperature can reach 107° F (41.7° C).

Application

If more superficial heating is desired, a condensor plate is used; when deeper therapy is desired, the induction coil should be used. A double-layered towel is placed between the applicator and the skin. When the patient is as comfortable as possible, he or she is tuned in with the oscillating circuit of the unit. In most cases the treatment times range from 20 to 30 minutes.

Special Considerations

- It is difficult to treat localized body areas.
- Dosage is subjective.
- There is less heating of skin and more chance for deep tissue burns.
- Towels must be placed between the applicator and the skin. Towels absorb perspiration during treatment.
- When there is loss of sensation, shortwave diathermy should not be used.
- When metal objects such as implants, pacemakers, jewelry, a metal table, intrauterine devices (IUDs), zippers on clothing, or glasses are present, shortwave diathermy should not be administered.
- Avoid use when the athlete is hemorrhaging, is pregnant, or has open wounds or contact lenses.
- Diathermy cables or coils must not touch one another or any metal.
- Avoid heating eyes, testicles, ovaries, bony prominences, and bone-growth areas.
- A deep, aching sensation during treatment may indicate overheating.

Microwave Diathermy

Clinical microwave diathermy generally has a wavelength of 12 cm to 33 cm and an FCC-assigned frequency of 915 to 2450 megacycles. Lower microwave frequencies (e.g., 915 megacycles per second) cause less conversion of energy into the subcutaneous tissue and, as a result, produce more uniform muscle heating.[28] Microwave diathermy heats deeper tissue by conversion. It is more easily absorbed in tissue with higher water content such as muscle and blood when compared with shortwave diathermy.[20]

Equipment

In the microwave diathermy unit AC is changed into DC. The unit consists of a magnetron oscillator, which is a tube that incorporates a complete oscillator circuit capable of generating a radio frequency. A **coaxial cable** transports the energy from the magnetron oscillator to the applicator head. Within the delivery head is an antenna that radiates energy to the athlete. A commonly used spaced applicator is contained within a rectangular metallic reflector. It is suggested for use on flat or concave body surfaces.[20] The further away the reflector is from the skin, the greater the body coverage will be with a proportional increase in wattage.

A coaxial cable consists of an insulated central conductor with tubular stranded conductors, which are separated by layers of insulation laid over it concentrically.

Indications

Microwave diathermy is highly effective in treating conditions such as fibrositis, myositis, osteoarthritis, bursitis, calcific tendinitis, sprains, strains, and posttraumatic joint

TABLE 14-5 Sample Shortwave Diathermy and Microwave Diathenny Dosage

Dosage	Effect	Application
Lowest dose (I)	Just below the point of any sensation of heat (acute inflammatory process)	2 to 5 minutes daily for 2 weeks
Low dose (II)	Mild heat sensation, barely felt (subacute, resolving inflammatory process)	2 to 5 minutes daily for 2 weeks
Medium dose (III)	Moderate but pleasant heat sensation (subacute, resolving inflammatory process)	2 to 30 minutes from 2 to 3 times weekly for 1 to 4 weeks
Heavy dose (IV)	Vigorous heating that causes a sensation that is well tolerated (chronic conditions); pain threshold should not be exceeded	5 to 30 minutes for 2 to 3 times weekly for 1 to 4 weeks.

stiffness.[22] In an athlete with a subcutaneous fat thickness of 0.5 cm or less, microwave diathermy can penetrate tissue as much as 5 cm thick.[37]

Application

The athlete is made comfortable, and the microwave diathermy director is positioned at right angles to the part to be treated. The athlete's subjective heat sensation is the major guide to dosage. As with shortwave diathermy, the microwave diathermy's therapeutic heat range is 104° to 113° F (40° to 45° C).[16] The length of treatment does not usually exceed 30 minutes. A dosage scheme has been suggested that can be used for both shortwave diathermy and microwave diathermy (Table 14-5).[20,25,44] A towel must be placed over the skin to absorb any perspiration that accumulates.

Special Considerations

The same considerations must be given to microwave diathermy as are given to shortwave diathermy. The applicator should never come in contact with the skin. At no time should heating exceed the athlete's pain threshold.[37]

Comparing Microwave Diathermy and Shortwave Diathermy

In general, shortwave and microwave diathermies penetrate the body to approximately the same depth; however, with microwave diathermy, there is deeper muscle heating and comparatively more skin heating with shortwave diathermy.[22] Microwave diathermy heating is more localized than heating with shortwave diathermy.

ULTRASOUND THERAPY

In athletic training, ultrasound is one of the most widely used modalities in addition to superficial heat and cold and electrical stimulating currents. It has been used for therapeutic purposes as a valuable tool in the rehabilitation of many different injuries for the purpose of stimulating the repair of soft tissue injuries and for relief of pain.[10] It has traditionally been classified as a deep-heating modality and used primarily for the purpose of elevating tissue temperatures. Ultrasound is a form of acoustic rather than electromagnetic energy. Ultrasound is defined as inaudible, acoustic vibrations of high frequency that may produce either thermal or nonthermal physiological effects.[35] The use of ultrasound as a therapeutic agent may be extremely effective if the athletic trainer has an adequate understanding of its effects on biological tissues and of the physical mechanisms by which these effects are produced.[10]

Ultrasound can be applied either to the skin or through a water medium.

attenuation
A decrease in intensity as the sound enters deeper tissues.

The number of movements, or oscillations, in 1 second is referred to as the frequency of a sound wave. The number of oscillations occurring in 1 second is known as a hertz (Hz) unit. More commonly, 1 Hz equals 1 cycle per second, 1 kHz equals 1000 cycles per second, and 1 MHz equals 1 million cycles per second.[12] The human ear cannot detect sound greater than 20,000 Hz; therefore inaudible sound is considered ultrasound. When sound scatters and absorbs as it penetrates tissue, its energy is decreased **(attenuation).** Absorption of sound increases with an increase in frequency.

Tissue penetration depends on impedance or acoustical properties of the media that are proportional to tissue density.[9] Sound reflection occurs when adjacent tissues have different impedance. The greater the impedance, the greater the reflection, and more heat is produced. The greatest heat is developed between bone and the adjacent soft-tissue interface.

Equipment

piezoelectric effect
Electrical current produced by applying pressure to certain crystals such as quartz.

The main piece of equipment for delivering therapeutic ultrasound is a high-frequency generator, which provides an electrical current through a coaxial cable to a transducer contained within an applicator. In the applicator or transducer are synthetic crystals such as barium titanate or lead zirconate titanate that possess the property of piezoelectricity. These crystals are in disks 2 to 3 mm thick and 1 to 3 cm in diameter.[48] The **piezoelectric effect** causes expansion and contraction of the crystals, which produce oscillation voltage at the same frequency as the sound wave.[35]

Therapeutic ultrasound has a frequency range between 0.75 and 3.0 MHz (megahertz). The majority of ultrasound generators are set at a frequency of 1 MHz, although there are ultrasound units that are set at a frequency of 3 MHz. A generator that can be set between 1 and 3 MHz affords the athletic trainer the greatest treatment flexibility. Ultrasound energy generated at 1 MHz is transmitted through the more superficial tissues and absorbed primarily in the deeper tissues at depths of 3 to 5 cm. A 1 MHz frequency is most useful in individuals with high percent body fat cutaneously and whenever the desired effects are in the deeper structures.[35] At 3 MHz the energy is absorbed in the more superficial tissues with a depth of penetration between 1 and 2 cm.

Ultrasound Beam

effective radiating area
That portion of the transducer that produces sound energy.

The portion of the surface of the ultrasound transducer that produces the sound wave is referred to as the **effective radiating area.** Energy is delivered to the tissues in a collimated cylindrical beam. The beam from ultrasound generated at 1 MHz is more divergent than at 3 MHz. Within this beam, the distribution of ultrasound energy is nonuniform. The amount of variability of intensity in the beam is indicated by the **beam nonuniformity ratio (BNR).** The lower the BNR, the more uniform the energy output. Optimally the BNR would be 1:1.

beam nonuniformity ratio (BNR)
The amount of variability in intensity of the ultrasound beam.

Intensity

The intensity of the ultrasound beam is determined by the amount of energy delivered to the sound head (applicator). It is expressed in the number of watts per square centimeter (W/cm^2). As a therapeutic modality used in sports medicine, it ranges from 0.1 to 3 W/cm^2.

Pulsed Versus Continuous Ultrasound

Ultrasound can be pulsed or continuous.

Virtually all therapeutic ultrasound generators can emit either continuous or pulsed ultrasound waves. If continuous ultrasound is used, the sound intensity remains constant throughout the treatment and the ultrasound energy is being produced 100% of the time. With pulsed ultrasound the intensity is periodically interrupted with no ultrasound energy being produced during the off period. The percentage of time that ultrasound is being generated is referred to as the **duty cycle.** If the pulse duration is 1 ms and the total pulse period is 5 ms the duty cycle would be 20%. Therefore the

Duty cycle indicates the percentage of time ultrasound is being generated.

total amount of energy being delivered to the tissues would be only 20% of the energy delivered if a continuous wave were being used.

Continuous ultrasound is most commonly used when the desired effect is to produce thermal effects. The use of pulsed ultrasound results in a reduced average heating of the tissues. Pulsed ultrasound or continuous ultrasound at a low intensity will produce nonthermal or mechanical effects, which may be associated with soft-tissue healing.[35]

Indications

Therapeutic ultrasound produces both thermal and nonthermal effects.[10] Traditionally, ultrasound has been used primarily to produce a tissue temperature increase. The clinical effects of using ultrasound to heat the tissues are similar to other forms of superficial heat, which have already been discussed. For the majority of these effects to occur the tissue temperature must be raised to a level of 40° to 45° C for a minimum of 5 minutes. Temperatures below this range will be ineffective, and temperatures above 45° C may be potentially damaging.[35] Ultrasound at 1 MHz with an intensity of 1 W/cm^2 can raise soft-tissue temperature by as much as 0.86° C per minute.

> Ultrasound produces effects that are thermal or nonthermal.

Whenever ultrasound is used to produce thermal changes, nonthermal changes also occur. However, if appropriate treatment parameters are selected, nonthermal effects can occur with minimal thermal effects. The nonthermal effects of therapeutic ultrasound include cavitation and acoustic microstreaming. Cavitation is the formation of gas-filled bubbles that expand and compress because of ultrasonically induced pressure changes in tissue fluids.[10] Cavitation results in an increased flow in the fluid around these vibrating bubbles. Microstreaming is the unidirectional movement of fluids along the boundaries of cell membranes resulting from the mechanical pressure wave in an ultrasonic field.[10] Microstreaming can alter cell membrane structure and function because of changes in cell membrane permeability to sodium and calcium ions important in the healing process. As long as the cell membrane is not damaged, microstreaming can be of therapeutic value in accelerating the healing process.[10]

> Nonthermal effects include: Cavitation and microstreaming

The nonthermal effects of therapeutic ultrasound in the treatment of injured tissues may be as important as if not more important than the thermal effects. The nonthermal effects of cavitation and microstreaming can be maximized while the thermal effects are minimized by using an intensity of 0.1 to 0.2 W/cm^2 with continuous ultrasound, or 1.0 W/cm^2 at a duty cycle of 20%.

It is generally accepted that acute conditions require more frequent treatments over a shorter period of time, whereas more chronic conditions require fewer treatments over a longer period of time.[35] Ultrasound treatments should begin as soon as possible after injury, ideally within hours but definitely within 48 hours to maximize effects on the healing process.[35] Acute conditions may be treated using low-intensity ultrasound once or twice daily for 6 to 8 days until acute symptoms such as pain and swelling subside. In chronic conditions, when acute symptoms have subsided, treatment may be done on alternating days for a total of 10 to 12 treatments.

Application

As mentioned previously, there are a number of options for using ultrasound in sports medicine.

Direct Skin Application

Because acoustic energy cannot travel through air and is reflected by the skin, there must be a **coupling medium** applied to the skin.[35] Coupling mediums can include a variety of materials, such as mineral oil or water-soluble creams or gels. The purpose of a coupling medium is to provide an air-tight contact with the skin and a slick, low-friction surface to glide over. When a water-soluble material is used, the skin

> **coupling medium**
> Used to facilitate the transmission of ultrasound into the tissues.

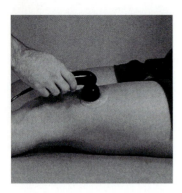

Figure 14-10

Ultrasound therapy, when applied directly to the skin, must be performed over a coupling medium because acoustical energy cannot travel through air.

should first be washed and dried to prevent air bubbles from hampering the flow of mechanical energy into the skin (Figure 14-10).

Underwater Application

Underwater ultrasound is suggested for such irregular body parts as the wrist, hand, elbow, knee, ankle, and foot. The part is fully submerged in water, and then the ultrasound head is submerged and positioned approximately 1 inch (2.5 cm) from the body part to be treated. The water medium provides an air-tight coupling, allowing sound waves to travel at a constant velocity. To ensure uninterrupted therapy, air bubbles that form on the skin must be continually wiped away. The sound head is moved slowly in a circular or longitudinal pattern.[35]

Underwater application should be done in a plastic or rubber nonmetal container to avoid reflection of energy off the metal walls. Another technique for treating irregular surfaces has been recommended in which a water-filled balloon is placed between the transducer and the treatment area with sufficient amounts of coupling gel to ensure good contact.

Bladder Technique

If for some reason the treatment area cannot be immersed in water, a bladder technique can be used in which a balloon is filled with water and the ultrasound energy is transmitted from the transducer to the treatment surface through this bladder. Both sides of the balloon should be coated with gel to ensure good contact.[35]

Moving the Transducer

Moving the transducer during treatment leads to a more even distribution of energy within the treatment area and can reduce the likelihood of developing hot spots. The transducer should be moved slowly at approximately 4 cm per second. The transducer should be kept in maximum contact with the skin via some coupling agent throughout the treatment.

Movement of the transducer can be in a circular pattern or a stroking pattern. In the circular pattern the transducer is applied in small overlapping circles. In the stroking pattern the transducer is moved back and forth, overlapping the preceding stroke by half. Both techniques are performed slowly and deliberately. The field covered should not exceed 3 to 4 inches (7.5 to 10 cm). The pattern is determined mainly by the skin area to be treated. For example, the circular pattern is best for highly localized areas such as the shoulder, whereas in larger, more diffuse injury areas, the stroking pattern is best used. When a highly irregular surface area is to be given therapy, the underwater method should be used.[51]

Dosage and Treatment Time

Dosage of ultrasound varies according to the depth of the tissue treated and the state of injury, such as subacute or chronic.[5] Basically, 0.1 to 0.3 W/cm^2 is regarded as low intensity, 0.4 to 1.5 W/cm^2 is medium intensity, and 1.5 to 3 W/cm^2 is high intensity. The duration of treatment ranges from 5 to 10 minutes.

Special Considerations

Although ultrasound is a relatively safe modality, certain precautions must be taken, and in some situations ultrasound should never be used. Great care must be taken when treating anesthetized areas because the sensation of pain is one of the best indicators of overdosage. Great precautions must be used in areas that have reduced circulation. In general, ultrasound must not be applied to highly fluid areas of the body such as the eyes, ears, testes, brain, spinal cord, and heart. Reproductive organs and women who are pregnant must not receive ultrasound. Acute injuries should not be treated with ultrasound. Epiphyseal areas in children should have only minimum ultrasound exposure.[51]

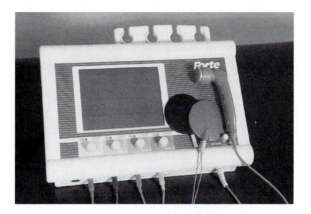

Figure 14-11

Combination ultrasound and electrical stimulator unit.

Ultrasound in Combination with Other Modalities

In an athletic training environment, it is not uncommon to combine modalities to accomplish a specific treatment goal. Ultrasound is frequently used with other modalities, including hot packs, cold packs, and electrical stimulating currents.

Hot packs and ultrasound are a useful combination because of the relaxing effects of hot packs in muscle spasm or muscle guarding. Hot packs produce more superficial heating while ultrasound produces heating in the deeper tissues. The application of a hot pack before ultrasound has no effect on increasing temperature.[14]

The use of cold packs before ultrasound application is done frequently. However, if the treatment goal is an increase in deep tissue temperature the use of a cold pack before ultrasound interferes with heating and is not recommended.[8,40]

Ultrasound is often used with electrical stimulating currents and is thought to be particularly effective in treating trigger points and acupuncture points. Ultrasound increases the blood flow to the deep tissues while the electrical currents produce a muscle contraction or modulate pain associated with an injury[35] (Figure 14-11).

> Ultrasound is commonly used in conjunction with other modalities.

Phonophoresis

Phonophoresis is a method of driving molecules through the skin by ion transfer or by the mechanical vibration of the ultrasound.[42] Like iontophoresis, it is designed to move medication into injured tissues. Some sports medicine personnel prefer this to iontophoresis, indicating that it is less hazardous to the skin and that there is greater penetration.[39] As with iontophoresis, phonophoresis is predominantly used to introduce hydrocortisone and an anesthetic into the tissues. This method has been successful in treating painful trigger points, tendinitis, and bursitis.[39]

Many clinicians prefer to use a 10% hydrocortisone ointment.[39] Sometimes lidocaine is added to the cortisone to provide a local anesthetic effect. This medicine is massaged into the skin over an area of tendinitis, bursitis, or other chronic soft-tissue condition. The coupling gel is then spread over the medication, and the ultrasound is applied.

Chem-pads are commercially produced pads that are impregnated with medication; they may be used instead of the traditional medicated ointment application.

> Phonophoresis is a method of driving molecules through the skin through ultrasound.

ELECTROTHERAPY

The use of electrotherapy is commonplace in the athletic training setting.

Physical Principles

In general, electricity is a form of energy that displays magnetic, chemical, mechanical, and thermal effects on tissue. It implies a flow of electrons between two points. Electrons are particles of matter that have a negative electrical charge and revolve around the core, or nucleus, of an atom.

14-2

Critical **Thinking** E x e r c i s e

A field hockey player has a 3-week-old deep quadriceps contusion. She has returned to full practice. There is still a palpable swollen area present and some remaining purplish-yellow discoloration. She is no longer tender to touch but does not have full range of motion in flexion.

? At this point in the process of healing, what modalities would be most appropriate?

ampere
Volume or amount.

ohm
Resistance.

voltage
Force.

watt
Power.

Current parameters:
  Waveform
  Modulation
  Intensity
  Duration
  Frequency
  Polarity
  Electrode setup

Electrical currents include:
  AC, DC, pulsed

An electrical current refers to a string of electrons that pass along a conductor such as a nerve or wire. The volume or amount of the current is measured in **amperes** (A); 1 A equals the rate of flow of 1 coulomb (C) per second. A coulomb is a unit of electrical charge and is defined as the quantity of an electrical charge that can be transferred by 1 A in 1 second.

Resistance to the passing of an electrical current along a conductor is measured in **ohms** (Ω), and the force that moves the current along is called **voltage (V).** One volt is the amount of electrical force required to send a current of 1 A through a resistance of 1 Ω. In terms of electrotherapy, currents of 0 to 150 V are considered low-voltage currents, and currents above 150 V are considered high voltage. The intensity of a current varies directly with the voltage and inversely with the resistance. Electrical power is measured in **watts** (amps × volts).[46]

An electrical current applied to nerve tissue at a sufficient intensity and duration to reach that tissue's excitability threshold will result in a membrane depolarization or firing of that nerve. There are three major types of nerve fibers: sensory, motor, and pain. As current intensity or duration is increased, the threshold for depolarization will be reached first for sensory fibers, then for motor fibers, and then for pain fibers. Thus it is possible to produce different physiological responses by adjusting the treatment parameters.[15]

Electrical Stimulating Units

Electrotherapeutic devices generate three different types of current, which when introduced into biological tissue are capable of producing specific physiological changes. These three types of current are AC, DC, and pulsed.[34]

A great deal of confusion has developed relative to the terminology used to describe electrotherapeutic currents. All therapeutic electrical generators, regardless of whether they deliver AC, DC, or pulsed currents through electrodes attached to the skin, are *transcutaneous electrical stimulators*. The majority of these are used to stimulate peripheral nerves and are correctly called *transcutaneous electrical nerve stimulators (TENS)* (Figure 14-12). Occasionally the terms *neuromuscular electrical stimualtor (NMES)* or *electrical muscle stimulator (EMS)* are used; however, these terms are appropriate only when the electrical current is being used to stimulate muscle directly, as would be the case with denervated muscle where peripheral nerves are not functioning. In recent years, a new type of transcutaneous electrical stimulator has gained popularity that uses current intensities too small to excite peripheral nerves. In the past they have been called *microcurrent electrical nerve stimulators (MENS)*, although they are currently being referred to as *low-intensity stimulators (LIS).*[34]

Direct Current

Direct current, or galvanic current, flows in one direction only from the positive pole to the negative pole. Direct current may be used for pain modulation, for muscle

Figure 14-12

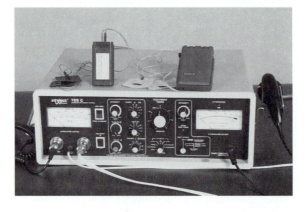

Many therapeutic electrical generators are transcutaneous electrical nerve stimulators (TENS) units.

contraction, or to produce ion movement. Specific physiological effects are determined by how the treatment parameters are set on the stimulating unit. The majority of the electrical stimulators being used currently in athletic training settings are DC units.

Alternating Current

With AC, the direction of current flow reverses itself once during each cycle. Alternating current may be used for pain modulation or muscle contraction.

Pulsed Current

Pulsed currents usually contain three or more pulses grouped together. These groups of pulses are interrupted for short periods of time and repeat themselves at regular intervals. Pulsed currents are used in interferential and so-called Russian currents.

Current Parameters

Waveforms

Electrical stimulating units can take on various waveforms depending on the capability of the generator. A waveform is a graphic representation of the shape, direction, amplitude, and direction of a particular electrical current. Both AC and DC units can produce currents with waveforms that are either sine, square, or triangular in shape (Figure 14-13).

Modulation

Current modulation refers to the ability of the electrical stimulating unit to change or alter the magnitude or duration of a waveform. Modulation may be continuous, interrupted, or surged for both AC and DC currents (Figure 14-14).

Current Intensity

Intensity refers to the voltage output of the stimulating unit. Generators that produce voltage outputs of up to 150 V are referred to as low-voltage generators. Those that produce up to 500 V are called high-voltage generators. Low-voltage generators are almost always DC; high-voltage generators may be either AC or DC. The majority of the electrical stimulators used in athletic training settings are high-voltage DC generators.

Current Duration

Duration refers to the length of time that current is flowing. It is also referred to as pulse width or pulse duration. Duration is preset on most of the high-voltage DC stimulators.

Frequency

Frequency refers to the number of waveforms being emitted by the electrical stimulating unit in 1 second. Frequency is identified in pulses per second (PPS), cycles per second (CPS), or hertz. Frequencies may range from 1 PPS to several thousand PPS.

Polarity

Polarity refers to the direction of current flow. It may move toward either a positive or a negative pole.

Electrode Setup

In electrotherapy, moist electrode pads are fixed directly to the skin. The smaller active pad, which brings the current to the body, can range from very small to 4 inches (10 cm) square; the larger dispersal pad, from which electrons leave the body, should be as large as possible. Because the current flows between the two pads, the distance between the pads depends on the type of muscle contraction desired. The closer the

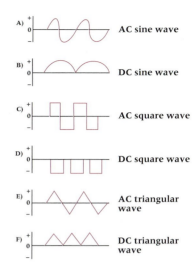

Figure 14-13

Waveforms can be either sine, square, or triangular for both AC and DC.

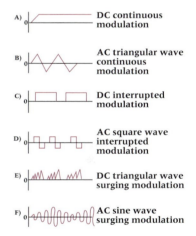

Figure 14-14

Modulation may be continuous, surged, or interrupted for either AC or DC.

pads are, the shallower and more isolated the contraction; the farther apart the pads are, the deeper and more generalized the contraction. The physiological effects can occur anywhere between the two pads, but they usually occur at the active electrode, because current density is greater at this point.[15]

Indications

Alternating, direct, and pulsed currents can be used to modulate pain and to induce muscle contraction.[19] Direct current may also be used to produce ion movement (iontophoresis).[15]

Pain Modulation

It is well documented that electrical stimulating currents can reduce pain associated with injury.[49] The neurophysiological mechanisms associated with pain modulation include gate control, central biasing, and endogenous opiates.[2] (See Chapter 7.)

Muscle Contraction

A muscle contraction can be used for:
Muscle pumping
Muscle strengthening
Retardation of atrophy
Muscle reeducation

The quality of a muscle contraction will change according to the changes in current parameters. As the frequency of stimulation increases, the muscle will develop more tension because of progressive shortening of the muscle until a tetanic contraction is achieved. Tetany will occur for virtually all muscles at approximately 50 PPS. Increases in intensity spread the current over a larger area and increase the number of motor units activated by the current. Increases in current duration also cause more motor units to be activated. A variety of therapeutic gains can be made by electrically stimulating a muscle contraction; these include muscle pumping contractions, muscle strengthening, retardation of atrophy, and muscle reeducation.

Muscle Pumping

This type of contraction is used to help stimulate circulation by pumping fluid and blood through the venous and lymphatic channels back to the heart. High-voltage DC is recommended. Intensity should be increased to elicit a muscle contraction at a frequency of 20 to 40 PPS, using a surged mode with on/off times at 5 seconds each. The injured part should be elevated, and active contraction should be encouraged. Treatment time is 20 to 30 minutes.[15]

Muscle Strengthening

Electrical stimulation can be used to facilitate strength gains. High-frequency AC is recommended (e.g., Electrostim 380). Intensity should be increased at a frequency of 50 to 60 PPS to elicit a tetanic muscle contraction using surging current set at 15 seconds on and 50 seconds off. Treatment should include 10 repetitions three times per week. For best results, the athlete should combine this electrically induced tetanic contraction with maximal active contraction against some resistance.[15]

Retardation of Atrophy

Electrically induced muscle contraction can be used to minimize atrophy and loss of muscle function that typically occurs with immobilization after injury. High-frequency AC is recommended. Intensity should be increased to 30 to 60 PPS to elicit a tetanic contraction using interrupted current mode. The athlete should incorporate voluntary isometric contraction. Treatment time should be 15 to 20 minutes.[15]

Muscle Reeducation

Muscular inhibition after surgery or injury can be reduced by electrically stimulating a muscle. Intensity should be increased to a level necessary for a comfortable contraction at 30 to 50 PPS using either interrupted or surged current. The athlete should watch and feel the contraction and attempt to initiate a voluntary contraction. Treatment time is 15 to 20 minutes; treatment is repeated several times daily.[15]

Iontophoresis

Iontophoresis is a technique whereby chemical ions are transported through the intact skin using electrical current for the purpose of treating skin infections or for a counterirritating effect.[13] The type of current used is always a low-voltage direct current set on a continuous mode because the pulse duration must be long enough to allow for migration of ions.

There are three techniques of application: an active pad is applied over gauze that is saturated with a solution containing the ions (this is positioned as close as possible to the involved tissue); the active electrode is suspended in a container of the ion solution, and then the part to be treated is immersed in the container; or a special stimulator with a specially adapted electrode containing the treatment ions is positioned as close to the involved tissue as possible. In all cases, a large dispersive pad is applied to the patient and the proper polarity of the active electrode is selected based on the polarity of the ions in the solution.

Positive ions require an active electrode that is positive; negative ions require an active electrode that is negative. Treatment time will vary. A more comprehensive source dealing with iontophoresis should be consulted before using this technique.[13]

Iontophoresis uses electrical current to drive ions.

Interferential Currents

Interferential currents make use of two separate electrical generators that emit currents at two slightly different frequencies. Two pairs of electrodes are arranged in a square pattern such that the currents cross one another, creating an interference pattern at a central point of stimulation. The interference pattern creates a broader area of stimulation[31] (Figure 14-15).

LOW-INTENSITY STIMULATORS

Low-intensity stimulators are among the newest of the electrical stimulators available to the athletic trainer. Low-intensity stimulator is the latest term for what used to be called microcurrent electrical nerve stimulator, or MENS. Low-intensity stimulators deliver current to the athlete at very low frequencies (1 PPS) and at extremely low intensities that are subsensory. This type of current is being used to stimulate the healing process in both soft tissue and bone by altering the electrical activity of individual cells. The effectiveness of LIS therapy is currently based primarily on theory; there is little research information to support its use.[15]

LOW-POWER LASER

Laser is an acronym that stands for light amplification by stimulated emission of radiation.[11] The low-power laser is a relatively new device whose proposed applications in an athletic training setting include acceleration of collagen synthesis, control

laser
Light amplification by stimulated emission of radiation.

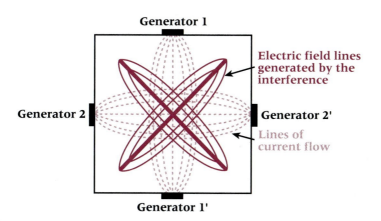

Figure 14-15

Pattern created by interferential current.

of microorganisms, increased vascularization, and reduction of pain and inflammation.[43]

The helium-neon (HeNe) and the gallium-arsenide (GaAs) lasers are two low-power lasers currently being investigated by the Food and Drug Administration (FDA) for potential use in physical medicine. Currently the FDA has not approved the use of the the low-power laser except in laboratory and experimental settings.[11]

ADDITIONAL TREATMENT MODALITIES

Several additional treatment modalities are available to the athletic trainer, including massage, traction, and intermittent compression.

Massage

Massage is defined as the systematic manipulation of the soft tissues of the body. The movements of gliding, compressing, stretching, percussing, and vibrating are regulated to produce specific responses in the athlete.[47]

Primarily, massage is separated into five basic categories: effleurage, pétrissage, friction, tapotement, and vibration.

Therapeutic Effects of Massage

Historically, wherever sports have been seriously undertaken, massage has been used in some form. Today sports massage seems to be regaining popularity among athletic trainers as a treatment modality. Manipulation of soft tissue by massage is a useful adjunct to other modalities. Sports massage causes mechanical, physiological, and psychological responses.

Mechanical responses   Mechanical responses to massage occur as a direct result of the graded pressures and movements of the hand on the body. Such actions encourage venous and lymphatic drainage and mildly stretch superficial and scar tissue. Connective tissue can be effectively stretched by friction massage, which helps prevent rigidity in scar formation. When enforced inactivity is imposed on the athlete as the aftermath of an injury or when edema surrounds a joint, the stagnation of circulation may be prevented by using certain massage techniques.

Physiological responses   Massage can increase circulation and, as a result, increase metabolism to the musculature and aid in the removal of metabolites such as lactic acid.[47] It also helps overcome venostasis and edema by increasing circulation at and around the injury site, assisting in the normal venous blood return to the heart.

The reflex effects of massage are processes that, in response to nerve impulses initiated through rubbing the body, are transmitted to one organ by afferent nerve fibers and then back to another organ by efferent fibers. Reflex responses elicit a variety of organ reactions such as body relaxation, stimulation, and increased circulation.[38]

Relaxation can be induced by slow, superficial stroking of the skin. It is a type of massage that is beneficial for tense, anxious athletes who may require gentle treatment.

Stimulation is attained by quick, brisk action that causes a contraction of superficial tissue. The benefits derived by the athlete are predominantly psychological. He or she feels invigorated after intense manipulation of the tissue. In the early days of American sports, stimulation massage was given as a warm-up procedure, but it has gradually lost popularity because of the time involved and the recognition that it is relatively ineffectual physiologically.[38]

Increased circulation is accomplished by mechanical and reflex stimuli. Together they cause the capillaries to dilate and be drained of fluid as a result of firm outside pressure, thus stimulating cell metabolism, eliminating toxins, and increasing lymphatic and venous circulation. In this way the healing process is aided.

Possible physiological responses of massage include:
Reflex effects
Relaxation
Stimulation
Increased circulation

Psychological responses   The tactile system is one of the most sensitive systems in the human organism. From earliest infancy humans respond psychologically to being touched. Because massage is the act of laying on of hands, it can be an important means for creating a bond of confidence between the athletic trainer and the athlete.

Sports Massage

Massage in sports is usually confined to a specific area and is seldom given to the full body. The time required for giving an adequate and complete body massage is excessive in athletics. It is not usually feasible to devote this much time to one athlete; 5 minutes is usually all that is required for massaging a given area.

Massage lubricants   To enable the hands to slide easily over the body, a friction-reducing medium must be used. Rubbing the dry body can cause gross skin irritation by tearing and breaking off the hair. Many mediums (e.g., fine powders, oil liniments, or almost any substance having a petroleum base) can be used to advantage as lubricants.

Positioning of the athlete   Proper positioning for massage is of great importance. The injured part must be made easily accessible; the athlete must be comfortable, and the part to be massaged must be relaxed.

Confidence   Lack of confidence on the part of the person doing the massage is easily transmitted through inexperienced hands. Every effort should be made to think out the procedure to be used and to present a confident appearance to the athlete.

Massage Procedures

Effleurage   Effleurage, or stroking (Figure 14-16), is divided into light and deep methods. Light stroking is designed primarily to be sedative. It is also used in the early stages of injury treatment. Deep stroking is a therapeutic compression of soft tissue, which encourages venous and lymphatic drainage. A different application of effleurage may be used for a specific body part.

Stroking variations   There are many variations in effleurage massage; some that are of particular value to sports injuries are pressure variations, the hand-over-hand method, and the cross-body method.[47] Pressure variations range from very light to deep and vigorous stroking. Light stroking, as discussed previously, can induce relaxation or may be used when an area is especially sensitive to touch; on the other hand, deep massage is designed to bring about definite physiological responses. Light and deep effleurage can be used alternately when both features are desired. The hand-over-hand stroking method is of special benefit to those surface areas that are particularly unyielding. It is performed by an alternate stroke in which one hand strokes, followed immediately by the other hand, somewhat like shingles on a roof (Figure 14-17). The cross-body effleurage technique is an excellent massage for the low back region. The operator places a hand on each side of the athlete's spine. Both hands

14-3
Critical Thinking Exercise

A javelin thrower has a muscle strain in his back. He comes into the training room on the sixth day after the initial injury complaining of pain. He asks the athletic trainer if there is anything that can be done to help modulate his pain.

? What modalities does the athletic trainer have available that can be used to modulate pain?

effleurage
Stroking.

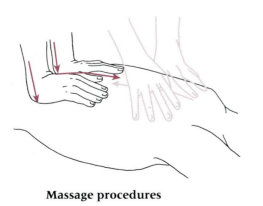

Massage procedures

Figure 14-16

Effleurage.

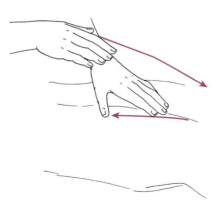

Figure 14-17

Hand-over-hand effleurage.

pétrissage
Kneading.

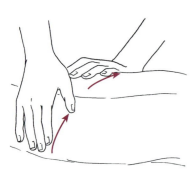

Figure 14-18

Cross-body effleurage.

friction
Heat producing.

tapotement
Percussion.

vibration
Rapid shaking.

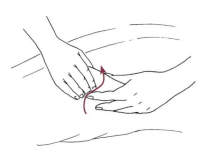

Figure 14-19

Pétrissage.

first stroke simultaneously away from the spine, then both hands at the same time stroke toward the spine (Figure 14-18).

Pétrissage   Kneading, or **pétrissage** (Figure 14-19), is a technique adaptable primarily to loose and heavy tissue areas such as the trapezius, the latissimus dorsi, or the triceps muscles. The procedure consists of picking up the muscle and skin tissue between the thumb and forefinger of each hand and rolling and twisting it in opposite directions. As one hand is rolling and twisting, the other begins to pick up the adjacent tissue. The kneading action wrings out the muscle, thus loosening adhesions and squeezing congestive materials into the general circulation. Picking up skin may cause an irritating pinch. Whenever possible, deep muscle tissue should be gathered and lifted.

Friction   The **friction** massage (Figure 14-20) is used often around joints and other areas where tissue is thin, as well as on tissues that are especially unyielding such as scars, adhesions, muscle spasms, and fascia. The action is initiated by bracing with the heels of the hands, then either holding the thumbs steady and moving the fingers in a circular motion or holding the fingers steady and moving the thumbs in a circular motion. Each method is adaptable to the type of area or articulation that is being massaged. The motion is started at a central point, and then a circular movement is initiated, with the hands moving in opposite directions away from the center point. The purpose is to stretch the underlying tissue, develop friction in the area, and increase circulation around the joint.

Tapotement   The most popular methods of **tapotement,** or percussion, are the cupping, hacking, and pincerlike or pincing movements.

Cupping   The cupping action produces an invigorating and stimulating sensation. It is a series of percussion movements rapidly duplicated at a constant tempo. One's hands are cupped to such an extent that the beat emits a dull and hollow sound, unlike the sound of the slap of the open hand. The hands move alternately, from the wrist, with the elbow flexed and the upper arm stabilized (Figure 14-21, *A*). The cupping action should be executed until the skin in the area develops a pinkish coloration.

Hacking   Hacking can be used in conjunction with cupping to bring about a varied stimulation of the sensory nerves (Figure 14-21, *B*). It is similar to cupping, except the hands are rotated externally and the ulnar, or little finger, border of the hand is the striking surface. Only the heavy muscle areas should be treated in this manner.

Pincing   Although pincing is not in the strictest sense percussive, it is categorized under tapotement because of the vigor with which it is applied. Alternating hands lift small amounts of tissue between the first finger and thumb in quick, gentle pinching movements (Figure 14-21, *C*).

Vibration   Vibration is rapid movement that produces a quivering or trembling effect. It is mainly used in sports for its ability to relax and soothe. Although vibration can be done manually, the machine vibrator is usually the preferred modality.

Effective Massaging

Besides knowing the different kinds of massage, one should understand how to give the most effective massage. The following rules should be used whenever possible:
1. Make the athlete comfortable.
    a. Place the body in the proper position on the table.
    b. Place a pad under the areas of the body that are to be massaged.
    c. Keep the training room at a constant 72° F (22.2° C) temperature.
    d. Respect the athlete's privacy by draping him or her with a blanket or towel, exposing only the body parts to be massaged.
2. Develop a confident, gentle approach when massaging.
    a. Assume a position that is easy both on you and on the athlete.
    b. Avoid using too harsh a stroke, or further injury may result.

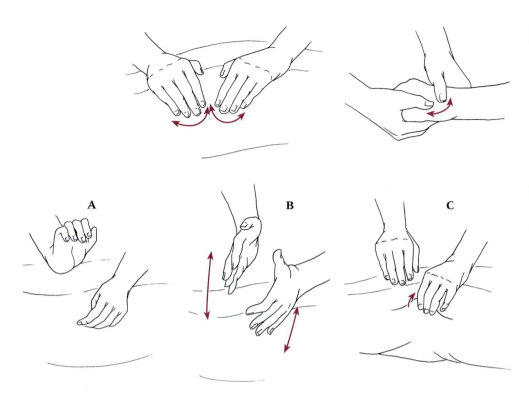

Figure 14-20

Friction massage.

Figure 14-21

Tapotement. **A,** Cupping. **B,** Hacking. **C,** Pincing.

3. To ensure proper lymphatic and venous drainage, stroke toward the heart whenever possible.
4. Know when not to use massage.
   a. Never give a massage when there may be a local or general infection. To do so may encourage its spread or may aggravate the condition.
   b. Never apply massage directly over a recent injury; limit stroking to the periphery. Massaging over recent injuries may dislodge the clot organization and start bleeding.

Deep Transverse Friction Massage

The transverse, or Cyriax, method of deep friction massage is increasingly being used in sports medicine. It is a specific technique for treating muscles, tendons, ligaments, and joint capsules. The major goal of transverse massage is to move transversely across a ligament or tendon to mobilize it as much as possible. This technique often precedes active exercise. Deep transverse friction massage restores mobility to a muscle in the same way that mobilization frees a joint.[7]

The position of the athletic trainer's hands is important in gaining maximum strength and control. Four positions are suggested: index finger crossed over the middle finger, middle finger crossed over the index finger, two fingers side by side, and an opposed finger and thumb (Figure 14-22).

The massage must be directly over the site of lesion and pain. The fingers move with the skin and do not slide over it. Massage must be across the grain of the affected tissue. The thicker the structure, the more friction is given.[47] The technique is to sweep back and forth over the full width of the tissue. Massage should not be given to acute injuries or over highly swollen tissues. A few minutes of this method will produce a numbness in the area, and exercise or mobilization can be instituted.

Acupressure Massage

Acupressure is a type of massage based on the ancient Chinese art of acupuncture. Acupuncture, along with herbal medicine, composes traditional Chinese medicine.

Transverse massage is a method of deep transverse friction massage.

Traction is commonly used in the cervical and lumbar spine.

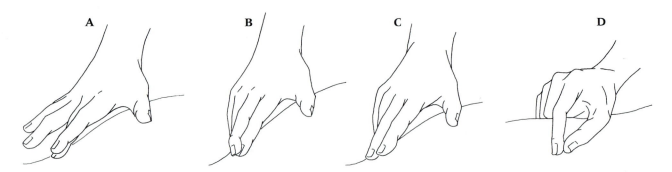

Figure 14-22

Cyriax massage is a specific technique for muscle, tendons, ligaments, and joint capsules using a variety of hand positions. **A,** Index finger crossed over the middle finger. **B,** Middle finger crossed over the index finger. **C,** Two fingers side by side. **D,** Opposed finger and thumb.

Only recently has the amount of research, publication, and interest in acupuncture in Western medical literature increased dramatically.

Acupuncture points lie along a series of meridians that run throughout the body. These points are named according to the meridian on which they lie. Whenever there is pain or illness, certain points on the surface of the body become tender. When pain is eliminated or the disease is cured, these tender points seem to disappear. According to acupuncture theory, stimulation of specific points through needling can dramatically reduce pain in areas of the body known to be associated with a particular point. Thousands of acupuncture points have been identified by the Chinese.

There is some evidence for the physical existence of these points. The electrical resistance of the skin at certain points corresponding to the acupuncture points is lower than that of the surrounding skin, especially when a disease state is present. Examining acupuncture points by sectioning indicates increased nerve endings at these points. Russian investigators have reportedly discovered differences in skin temperature at these points. Despite this evidence, there is no definite physical attribute of all acupuncture points, nor is there a thoroughly demonstrated mode of action for the technique. Whatever the explanation, it appears that the locations and effects of stimulating specific acupuncture points for the relief of pain have been determined empirically.

In Western medicine, the counterpart of the acupuncture point is the trigger point. Trigger points, like acupuncture points, are associated with visceral structures; stimulation of these points has also been proved to relieve pain.

Physiological explanations of the effectiveness of acupressure massage may likely be attributed to some interaction of the various mechanisms of pain modulation discussed in Chapter 7.

By using acupuncture charts specific points are selected, which are described in the literature as having some relationship to the area of pain. The charts provide the athletic trainer with a general idea of where these points are located. Two techniques may be used to specifically locate acupressure points. Because it is known that electrical impedance is reduced at acupuncture points, an ohmmeter may be used to locate the points. Perhaps the easiest technique is simply to palpate the area until either a small fibrous nodule or a strip of tense muscle tissue that is tender to the touch is felt.

Once the point is located, massage is begun using the index or middle fingers, the thumb, or the elbow. Small circular motions are used on the point. The amount of pressure applied to these acupressure points should be determined by patient tolerance; however, it must be intense and will likely be painful to the patient. Generally, the more pressure the patient can tolerate, the more effective the treatment.

Effective treatment times range from 1 to 5 minutes at a single point per treatment. It may be necessary to massage several points during the treatment to obtain the greatest effects. If this is the case, it is best to work distal points first and to move proximally.

During the massage, the patient will report a dulling or numbing effect and will frequently indicate that the pain has diminished or subsided totally during the massage. The lingering effects of acupressure massage vary tremendously from patient to patient. The effects may last for only a few minutes in some but may persist in others for several hours.

Traction

Traction can be defined as a drawing tension applied to a body segment. It is most commonly used in the cervical and lumbar regions of the spine.[17]

Physiological Effects

Traction is used to produce separation of the vertebral bodies and in so doing can effect stretching of the ligaments and joint capsules of the spine, stretching of spinal and paraspinal muscles, increased separation of the articular facet joints, relief in pressure on nerves and nerve roots, decrease in the central pressure of the intervertebral disks allowing for the movement of herniated disk material back into the center of the disk, increases of and changes in joint proprioception, and relief of the compressive effects of normal posture.[17]

Indications

Traction is most commonly used for the treatment of spinal nerve root impingement, which may result from many causes, including vertebral disk herniation or prolapse and spondylolisthesis. It may also be used to decrease muscle guarding, to treat muscle strain, to treat sprain of the spinal ligaments, and to relax discomfort resulting from normal spinal compression.

Application

Traction may be applied to the spine through the use of manual techniques or traction machines, including table traction units, wall-mounted traction units, and inverted traction techniques.

Manual techniques Manual traction is infinitely more adaptable and offers greater flexibility than mechanical traction. Changes in force, direction, duration, and patient position can be made instantaneously as the athletic trainer senses relaxation or resistance (Figure 14-23).

Table traction units For lumbar traction, a split table with a movable section to eliminate friction must be used to allow for smooth nonrestricted traction. A nonslip traction harness applied directly to the skin is needed to transfer the traction force comfortably to the athlete and to stabilize the trunk while the lumbar spine is placed under traction (Figure 14-24). For cervical traction, the athlete may be either in the supine or sitting position. A nonslip cervical harness should be secured under the chin and back of the head.

Wall-mounted traction Cervical traction can be accomplished using a wall-mounted system. Weight application can be accomplished with plates, sand bags,

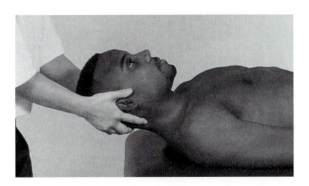

Figure 14-23

Manual cervical traction.

Figure 14-24

Lumbar traction using a split table and a traction machine.

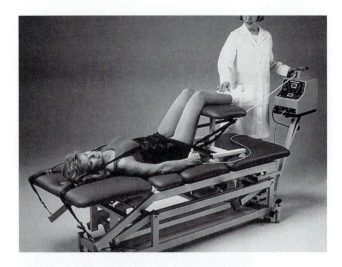

Figure 14-25

Cervical traction using a wall-mounted unit.

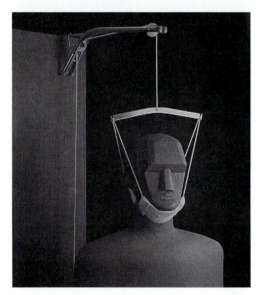

14-4

Critical Thinking Exercise

A gymnast has been told by a physician that she has a sprain of a ligament between two lumbar vertebrae in her low back. He tells her that it is important to stretch her low back. Because she was extremely flexible before her injury, she does not feel that the stretching she has been doing is effectively stretching the injured ligament.

? The gymnast comes to the athletic trainer and asks if there is any other therapeutic technique that she can use to help stretch the injured ligament.

or water bags. These units are relatively inexpensive and effective (Figure 14-25).

Inverted traction Specialized equipment or simply hanging upside down will place the person in an inverted position. The spine is lengthened because of the stretch provided by the weight of the trunk (Figure 14-26).

Special Considerations

- Good results have been achieved using both intermittent and sustained traction. In most cases of lumbar disk problems, sustained traction seems to be the treatment of choice. Intermittent traction is considered to be more comfortable.[17]
- Progressive traction increases the traction force gradually in a preselected number of steps. This allows the athlete to adapt slowly to the traction and helps him or her to stay relaxed.
- Recommendations on length of treatment and on/off times are extremely variable depending on the specific problem to be treated.
- For the lumbar spine a traction force equal to one half the athlete's body weight is a good guideline to use in selecting a force high enough to cause vertebral separation. Cervical traction forces can be adjusted from between 20 to 50 pounds depending on patient comfort and response.

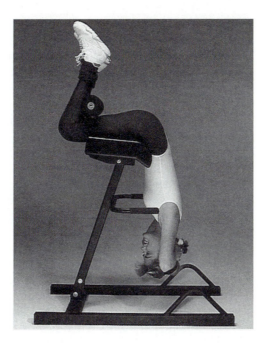

Figure 14-26

Inversion traction apparatus.

Intermittent Compression Devices

Intermittent compression units are used for the purpose of controlling or reducing swelling after acute injury or for pitting edema, which tends to develop in the injured area several hours after injury.[16]

Equipment

Intermittent compression makes use of a nylon pneumatic inflatable sleeve applied around the injured extremity (Figure 14-27). The sleeve can be inflated to a specific pressure that forces excessive fluid accumulated in the interstitial spaces into vascular and lymphatic channels through which it is removed from the area of injury. Compression facilitates the movement of lymphatic fluid, which helps eliminate the byproducts of the injury process.[41] The extremity should be elevated during treatment.

Intermittent compression devices have three parameters that may be adjusted: on/off time, inflation pressures, and treatment time. Recommended treatment protocols have been established through clinical trial and error with little experimental data currently available to support any protocol.[16]

On/off times are variable, including 1 minute on, 2 minutes off; 2 minutes on, 1 minute off; and 4 minutes on, 1 minute off. Again, these recommendations are not research based. Thus patient comfort should be the primary guide.

14-5

Critical Thinking Exercise

A basketball player has a 2-day-old postacute ankle sprain. The initial injury was not managed appropriately and as a result there is a considerable amount of swelling. He has little range of motion and is capable of only touchdown weight bearing.

? The athlete will have a difficult time regaining function until the swelling is reduced. What therapeutic modalities can be used to help get rid of this postacute lymphedema?

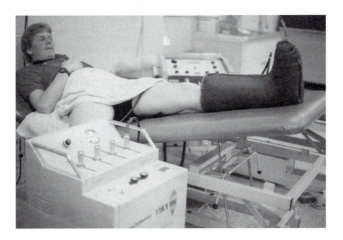

Figure 14-27

Intermittent compressive devices are designed to reduce edema after injury.

Recommended inflation pressures have been loosely correlated with blood pressures. The Jobst Institute recommends that pressure be set at 30 to 50 mm Hg for the upper extremity and at 30 to 60 mm Hg for the lower extremity. Because arterial capillary pressures are approximately 30 mm Hg, any pressure that exceeds this should encourage the absorption of edema and the flow of lymphatic fluid.[41]

Clinical studies have demonstrated a significant reduction in limb volume after 30 minutes of compression.[1,41] Thus a 30-minute treatment time seems to be efficient in reducing edema.

Some intermittent compression units have the capability of combining cold along with compression. It has been demonstrated that compression when combined with cold is more effective in reducing edema.[1,41] It is also common to use electrical stimulating currents to produce muscle pumping, thus facilitating lymphatic flow.

SUMMARY

■ To avoid legal problems, therapeutic modalities must be used with extreme care. Athletic trainers must be familiar with the laws of their state regarding therapeutic modality use. Before any modality is used, there must be a thorough understanding of its function and when it should and should not be used.

■ Heat energy is transmitted through conduction, convection, radiation, and conversion. Conduction occurs when heat is transferred from a warmer object to a cooler one. Convection heating occurs by means of fluid or gas movement. Radiation is heat energy that is transmitted through empty space. Conversion is heat that is generated when one type of energy is changed to another.

■ Cold used for therapeutic purposes and as part of an emergency procedure is extremely popular in sports medicine. Cold penetrates deeper than superficial heat. Therapy is usually performed when the tissue has reached a state of relative anesthesia. Cryotherapy decreases muscle spasm, pain perception, and blood flow. It increases the inelasticity of collagen fibers, joint stiffness, and capillary permeability. Common cryotherapy procedures are cold water immersion, ice massage, ice packs, and the use of vapocoolant sprays.

■ Thermotherapy increases blood flow, increases collagen viscosity, decreases joint stiffness, and reduces pain and muscle spasm. When the body's temperature is raised, tissue metabolism is increased, vascular permeability is increased, and chemicals such as histamine, bradykinin, and serotonin are released.

■ Superficial therapeutic heat should not be applied when there is a loss of sensation, immediately after an acute injury, when there is decreased arterial bleeding, over the eyes or genitals, or over the abdomen of a pregnant woman. Types of superficial heat are moist heat packs, whirlpool baths, paraffin baths, fluidotherapy, and contrast baths.

■ Both shortwave and microwave diathermies produce heat through the production of electromagnetic energy, whereas ultrasound produces heat through acoustical energy. The contraindications for use of shortwave diathermy and microwave diathermy are basically the same as for superficial heating, with the additional restrictions of no implants, jewelry, or intrauterine devices. Care must be taken not to cross the cables.

■ Ultrasound is a form of acoustic energy. It creates a mechanical vibration that is converted to heat energy within the body. Heating occurs in the denser tissues such as bone and connective tissue. More heat is built up at tissue interfaces. Ultrasound has both thermal and nonthermal physiological effects. It can be combined with electrical stimulation or used to drive molecules through the skin with the method known as phonophoresis.

■ The use of electrical stimulating currents is popular in sports medicine. Electrical stimulating units produce either alternating current (AC), direct current (DC), or pulsed current. Both AC and DC can be used for pain modulation and muscle contraction. Direct current can also be used for iontophoresis. The physiological effects of electrical current are determined by the treatment parameters and equipment selected, including waveforms, modulation, intensity, duration, frequency, polarity, and electrode placement. Interferential currents and LIS are two of the newest electrical stimulating currents available to the athletic trainer.

- The low-power laser may be used to stimulate the healing process or to modulate pain. Currently it has not been approved as a treatment modality.
- Massage is a useful modality for many sport-related injuries. Techniques include effleurage, pétrissage, friction, tapotement, and vibration. Deep transverse massage is used on connective tissue.
- Traction is used to produce separation of the vertebrae, most commonly for the treatment of spinal nerve root impingement and associated abnormalities. It is typically used in the cervical and lumbar spine and may involve either manual or machine-assisted traction.
- Intermittent compression devices are used for the purpose of controlling swelling after acute injury or for reducing pitting edema.

Solutions to Critical Thinking EXERCISES

14-1 The decision is to some extent subjective. It is essential to understand what is going on with the healing process. At day 5 the inflammatory process is ending and the fibroblastic stage is establishing itself. At this point it is still advisable to avoid any treatment that can potentially increase swelling, which can interfere with healing. Heat would be used to increase circulation, which might increase swelling. The athletic trainer would not likely exacerbate the injury by using heat, but it is recommended that cold be used during this time. A rule of thumb is that when tenderness is gone it will generally be safe to change to some form of heat.

14-2 At this point some form of heat to increase blood and lymphatic flow to the injured area is warranted. Increased blood flow will help facilitate the process of healing, and an increased lymphatic flow will help remove the by-products of the inflammatory process. Hot packs provide superficial heat and would not be effective in this case. Both the diathermics and ultrasound would be recommended because they have a depth of penetration great enough to affect the injured area, with ultrasound being somewhat more effective. Remember, modalities should always be used along with stretching and strengthening exercises for best results.

14-3 The athletic trainer can use cryotherapy, heat, or electrical stimulating currents to help reduce pain. Electrical stimulating currents may be the most useful if the athletic trainer wants to also elicit a muscle contraction to help decrease muscle guarding. Massage is also useful for modulating pain and for relaxing muscle. Regardless of the modality chosen, the athlete should engage in some stretching and strengthening exercises after the modality treatment.

14-4 The athletic trainer should try using manual lumbar traction techniques, which if done properly can be effective in isolating a specific ligament between two lumbar vertebrae. If the athletic trainer cannot manually generate enough traction force to stretch the ligament, a table traction unit or an inverted traction technique may prove to be more useful.

14-5 Proper initial management of the injury could have prevented a great deal of the swelling that has occurred. At this point the athletic trainer should make use of ice to modulate pain, intermittent compression and electrical stimulating current to induce a muscle pumping contraction (both of which can help the lymphatic system remove the swelling), and low-intensity ultrasound (>0.2 W/cm^2), which can help facilitate the healing process. In addition, the athlete should continually wear a compressive elastic wrap. He must also progress to full weight bearing, concentrating on regaining a normal gate as soon as tolerated.

REVIEW QUESTIONS AND CLASS ACTIVITIES

1. Explain the legal factors that a coach or athletic trainer should consider before using a therapeutic modality.
2. Give an example of modalities that heat through conduction, convection, radiation, and conversion.
3. What physiological changes occur when heat is applied to the body?
4. Discuss the physiological effects of using cryotherapy.
5. Demonstrate the proper technique in using a variety of cryotherapeutic approaches.
6. Compare therapy delivered through heat to that through cold. When would you use each?
7. What are shortwave and microwave diathermy used for?
8. Discuss how ultrasound can be used during a rehabilitation program.
9. Compare phonophoresis with iontophoresis.
10. What is a TENS unit?
11. Identify potential treatment goals of using an electrically stimulated muscle contraction.
12. How is massage best used in a sports medicine setting?
13. List the mechanical effects of using cervical and lumbar traction.
14. Explain when and how intermittent compression can best be used as a treatment modality.

REFERENCES

1. Angus J, Prentice W, Hooker D: A comparison of two external intermittent compression devices and their effect on post acute ankle edema, *J Ath Train* 29(2):178, 1994.
2. Barr J: Transcutaneous electrical nerve stimulation characteristics for altering pain perception, *Phys Ther* 66(10):1037, 1987.
3. Belitsky RB et al: Evaluation of the effectiveness of wet ice, dry ice, and Crogen packs in reducing skin temperature, *Phys Ther* 67(7):1080, 1987.
4. Bell AT, Horton PG: The use and abuse of hydrotherapy in athletics: a review, *Ath Train* 22:115, 1987.
5. Castel C, Draper D, Castel D: Rate of temperature increase during ultrasound treatments: are traditional times long enough? *J Ath Train* 29(2):156, 1994.
6. Dalzell M: The physiotherapist's armamentarium. In Welsh RP, Shephard RJ, editors: *Current therapy in sports medicine, 1985-1986,* Philadelphia, 1985, Brian C Decker.
7. deBruijn R: Deep transverse friction: its analgesic effect, *Int J Sports Med* 5:35, 1984.
8. Draper D, Schulthies S, Sorvisto P: The effect of cooling the tissue prior to ultrasound treatment, *J Ath Train* 29(2):154, 1994.
9. Draper D, Sunderland S: Examination of the law of Grotthus-Draper: does ultrasound penetrate subcutaneous fat? *J Ath Train* 28(3):246, 1993.
10. Dyson M: The use of ultrasound in sports physiotherapy. In Grisogono V, editor: *Sports injuries: international perspectives in physiotherapy,* Edinburgh, 1989, Churchill Livingstone.
11. Enwemeka C: Laser biostimulation of healing wounds: specific effects and mechanisms of action, *J Orthop Sports Phys Ther* 9:333, 1988.
12. Geick J et al: Therapeutic ultrasound: technology, performance standards, biological effect, and clinical application, HSH Publication, FOA 84-XXXX, August, 1984.
13. Harris PR: Iontophoresis: clinical research in musculoskeletal inflammatory conditions, *J Orthop Sports Phys Ther* 4:109, 1982.
14. Harris S, Draper D, Schulthies S: The effect of ultrasound on temperature rise in preheated human muscle, *J Ath Train* 30(2):S-42, 1995.
15. Hooker D: Electrical stimulating currents. In Prentice W, editor: *Therapeutic modalities in sports medicine,* St Louis, 1994, Mosby.
16. Hooker D: Intermittent compression devices. In Prentice W, editor: *Therapeutic modalities in sports medicine,* St Louis, 1994, Mosby.
17. Hooker D: Traction as a specialized modality. In Prentice W, editor: *Therapeutic modalities in sports medicine,* St Louis, 1994, Mosby.
18. Hunter LY: Physical therapy modalities. In Hunter LY, Funk FJ, editors: *Rehabilitation of the injured knee,* St Louis, 1984, Mosby.
19. Jacobs SR et al: Electrical stimulation of muscle. In Stillwell GK, editor: *Therapeutic electricity and ultraviolet radiation,* ed 3, Baltimore, 1983, Williams & Wilkins.
20. Kloth L: Shortwave and microwave diathermy. In Michlovitz SL, editor: *Thermal agents in rehabilitation,* Philadelphia, 1990, Davis.
21. Knight K: *Cryotherapy in sport injury management,* Champaign, Ill, 1995, Human Kinetics.
22. Krumholz A, Gelfand B, O'Conner P: Therapeutic modalities. In Nicholas J, Hershman EB, editors: *The lower extremity and spine in sports medicine,* vol 1, St Louis, 1995, Mosby.
23. Lehmann JF, DeLateur BJ: Cryotherapy. In Lehmann JF, editor: *Therapeutic heat and cold,* ed 3, Baltimore, 1982, Williams & Wilkins.
24. Lehmann JF, DeLateur BJ: Therapeutic heat. In Lehmann JF, editor: *Therapeutic heat and cold,* ed 3, Baltimore, 1982, Williams & Wilkins.
25. Lehmann JF et al: Comparison of relative heating patterns produced in tissues by exposure to microwave energy at frequencies of 2450 to 900 megacycles, *Arch Phys Med Rehabil* 46:307, 1965.
26. McMaster WC: Cryotherapy, *Phys Sportsmed* 10:112, 1982.
27. Meyer J, Draper D, Durrant E: Contrast therapy and intramuscular temperature in the leg, *J Ath Train* 29(4):318, 1994.
28. Michlovitz SL: Biophysical principles of heating and superficial heat agents. In Michlovitz SL, editor: *Thermal agents in rehabilitation,* Philadelphia, 1990, Davis.
29. Michlovitz SL: Cryotherapy: the use of cold as a therapeutic agent. In Michlovitz SL, editor: *Thermal agents in rehabilitation,* Philadelphia, 1990, Davis.
30. Nielsen AJ: Case study: myofascial pain of posterior shoulder relieved by spray and stretch, *J Orthop Sports Phys Ther* 3:21, 1981.
31. Patterson RP: Instrumentation for electrotherapy. In Stillwell GK, editor: *Therapeutic electricity and ultraviolet radiation,* ed 3, Baltimore, 1983, Williams & Wilkins.
32. Peppard A, Riegter HF: Trigger point therapy for myofascial pain, *Phys Sportsmed* 9:161, 1981.
33. Prentice, W: Preface. In Prentice W, editor: *Therapeutic modalities in sports medicine,* St Louis, 1994, Mosby.
34. Prentice W: Basic principles of electricity. In Prentice W, editor: *Therapeutic modalities in sports medicine,* St Louis, 1994, Mosby.
35. Prentice W: Therapeutic ultrasound. In Prentice W, editor: *Therapeutic modalities in sports medicine,* St Louis, 1994, Mosby.
36. Prentice W, Bell G: Infrared modalities. In Prentice W, editor: *Therapeutic modalities in sports medicine,* St Louis, 1994, Mosby.
37. Prentice W, Donley P: Shortwave and microwave diathermy. In Prentice W, editor: *Therapeutic modalities in sports medicine,* St Louis, 1994, Mosby.
38. Prentice W, Lehn C: Therapeutic massage. In Prentice W, editor: *Therapeutic modalities in sports medicine,* St Louis, 1994, Mosby.
39. Quillin WS: Ultrasonic phonophoresis, *Phys Sportsmed* 10:211, 1982.
40. Rimington S, Draper D, Durrant E: Temperature changes during therapeutic ultrasound in the precooled human gastrocnemius muscle, *J Ath Train* 29(4):325, 1994.
41. Rucinski T et al: The effects of intermittent compression on edema in postacute ankle sprains, *J Orthop Sports Phys Ther* 13(8):65-69, 1991.
42. Rusk HA: *Rehabilitation medicine,* ed 4, St Louis, 1977, Mosby.
43. Saliba E: Low-power laser. In Prentice W, editor: *Therapeutic modalities in sports medicine,* St Louis, 1994, Mosby.
44. Schliephakle E: Carrying out treatment. In Throm H, editor: *Introduction to shortwave and microwave therapy,* ed 3, Springfield, Ill, 1966, Charles C Thomas.
45. Sherman M: Which treatment to recommend? Hot or cold? *Am Pharm* NS20:46, 1980.
46. Snyder-Mackler L, Robinson A: *Clinical electrophysiology: electrotherapy and electrophysiology,* Baltimore, 1989, Williams & Wilkins.
47. Tappan FM: *Massage techniques,* New York, 1964, Macmillan.
48. ter Harr C: Basic physics of therapeutic ultrasound, *Physiotherapy* 73(3):110, 1987.
49. Thorsteinsson G: Electrical stimulation for analgesia. In Stillwell GK, editor: *Therapeutic electricity and ultraviolet radiation,* ed 7, Baltimore, 1983, Williams & Wilkins.
50. Walsh M: Hydrotherapy: the use of water as a therapeutic agent. In Michlovitz SL, editor: *Thermal agents in rehabilitation,* Philadelphia, 1990, Davis.
51. Ziskin MC, Michlovitz SL: Therapeutic ultrasound. In Michlovitz SL, editor: *Thermal agents in rehabilitation,* Philadelphia, 1990, Davis.

ANNOTATED BIBLIOGRAPHY

Knight KL: *Cryotherapy in sports injury management,* Champaign, Ill, 1995, Human Kinetics.

Presents excellent coverage, both theoretical and practical, of one of the most widely used therapeutic approaches in sports medicine and athletic training—cryotherapy. It is clearly written and easily applied.

Michlovitz SL, editor: *Thermal agents in rehabilitation*, Philadelphia, 1990, Davis.

An excellent text about understanding of the foundations and use of thermal agents in sports medicine and athletic training. It provides detailed discussions of inflammation, pain, superficial heat and cold, and the therapeutic use of ultrasound, shortwave, and microwave diathermies.

Prentice WE: *Therapeutic modalities in sports medicine*, ed 3, St Louis, 1994, Mosby.

A complete and comprehensive guide about the use of therapeutic modalities in the sports medicine setting. Addresses all aspects of modality use, including massage traction and intermittent compression. An excellent blend of theory and practical application.

Snyder-Mackler L, Robinson A: *Clinical electrophysiology: electrotherapy and electrophysiology*, Baltimore, 1989, Williams & Wilkins.

Addresses all aspects of electrical stimulation as a therapeutic technique, as well as techniques for testing nerve and muscle responses.

Starkey C: *Therapeutic modalities for athletic trainers*, Philadelphia, 1993, Davis.

Discusses many of the modalities used by athletic trainers in a clinical setting.

Travell JG, Simons DG: *Myofascial pain and dysfunction*, Baltimore, 1983, Williams & Wilkins.

A valuable text about myofascial trigger points. It provides a clear understanding of trigger-point evaluation in the upper body and the treatment of choice, as well as muscle stretch after the application of a vapocoolant.

Rehabilitation Techniques

When you finish this chapter, you should be able to

- Describe the consequences of sudden inactivity and injury immobilization.
- Explain the importance of early injury mobility.
- Describe how exercise may be coordinated with other therapeutic modalities.
- Compare therapeutic and conditioning exercises.
- Describe the primary components of an exercise rehabilitation program.
- Describe the value of aquatic exercise in rehabilitation.
- Discuss the techniques and principles of proprioceptive neuromuscular facilitation.
- Demonstrate mobilization techniques for improving accessory joint motions.

The athletic trainer is responsible for design, implementation, and supervision of the rehabilitation program.

The long-term goal is to return the injured athlete to practice or competition as quickly and safely as possible.

Therapeutic exercises are concerned with restoring normal body function after injury.

O ne of the primary goals of coach and athletic trainer is to create a playing environment for the athlete that is as safe as it can possibly be. Regardless of that effort, the nature of athletic participation dictates that injuries will eventually occur. When injuries do occur the focus of the athletic trainer shifts from injury prevention to injury treatment and rehabilitation.

The process of rehabilitation begins immediately after injury. Initial first aid and management techniques can have a substantial impact on the course and ultimate outcome of the rehabilitative process. Thus, in addition to possessing sound understanding of how injuries can be prevented, the athletic trainer must also be competent in providing correct and appropriate initial care when injury occurs. In a sports medicine setting, the athletic trainer generally assumes the primary responsibility for design, implementation, and supervision of the rehabilitation program for the injured athlete.

Designing programs for rehabilitation is relatively simple and involves several basic short-term goals: controlling pain, maintaining or improving flexibility, restoring or increasing strength, reestablishing neuromuscular control, and maintaining levels of cardiorespiratory fitness. The long-term goal is to return the injured athlete to practice or competition as quickly and safely as possible. This is the easy part of supervising a rehabilitation program. The difficult part comes in knowing exactly when and how to change or alter the rehabilitation protocols to most effectively accomplish both long- and short-term goals.

The approach to rehabilitation in an athletic training environment is considerably different than in most other rehabilitation settings. The competitive nature of athletics necessitates an aggressive approach to rehabilitation. Because the competitive season in most sports is relatively short, the athlete does not have the luxury of being able to simply sit around and do nothing until the injury heals. The goal is to return to activity as soon as safely possible. Thus the athletic trainer who is supervising the rehabilitation program must perform a balancing act between not pushing the athlete hard enough and being overly aggressive. In either case, a mistake in judgment on the part of the athletic trainer may hinder the athlete's return to activity.

Decisions as to when and how to alter and progress a rehabilitation program should be based within the framework of the healing process. The athletic trainer must possess a sound understanding of both the sequence and time frames for the various phases of healing and must realize that certain physiological events must occur during each of the phases. Anything that is done during a rehabilitation program that interferes with this healing process will likely increase the length of time required for rehabilitation and slow return to full activity. The healing process must have an opportunity to accomplish what it is supposed to. At best the athletic trainer can only try to create an environment that is conducive to the healing process. Little can be done to speed up the process physiologically, but many things can be done during rehabilitation to impede healing.

The athletic trainer has many tools at his or her disposal that can facilitate the rehabilitative process. How the athletic trainer chooses to use those tools is often a matter of individual preference and experience. Additionally, each individual patient is different, and the responses to various treatment protocols are variable. Thus it is impossible to "cookbook" specific protocols that can be followed like a recipe. In fact, use of rehabilitation "recipes" should be strongly discouraged. Instead the athletic trainer must develop a broad theoretical knowledge base from which specific techniques of rehabilitation may be selected and applied to each individual athlete.

SUDDEN PHYSICAL INACTIVITY AND INJURY IMMOBILIZATION

The human body is a dynamic moving entity that requires physical activity to maintain proper physical function. When an injury occurs, two problems immediately arise that must be addressed. First is the generalized loss of physical fitness that occurs when activity is stopped, and second is the specific inactivity of the injured part, resulting from protective splinting of the soft tissue and, in some cases, immobilization by some external means.

Effects of General Inactivity

An athlete who is highly conditioned will experience a rapid generalized loss of fitness when exercise is suddenly stopped.[11] With this sudden lack of activity, loss of muscle strength, endurance, and coordination occurs. Whenever possible, the athlete, without aggravating the injury, must continue to exercise the entire body.

A sudden loss of physical activity leads to a generalized loss of physical fitness.

Effects of Immobilization

When an injured body part is immobilized for a period of time, a number of disuse problems adversely affect muscle, joints, ligaments, bone, neuromuscular efficiency, and the cardiorespiratory system.

Muscle and Immobilization

When a body part is immobilized for as short a period as 24 hours, definite adverse muscular changes occur.

Atrophy and fiber-type conversion   Disuse of a body part quickly leads to a loss of muscle mass. The greatest atrophy occurs in the type I (slow-twitch) fibers. Over time, the slow-twitch fibers develop fast-twitch characteristics. Slow-twitch fibers also diminish in number without type II (fast-twitch) fibers lessening in number.[28] A muscle that is immobilized in a lengthened or neutral position tends to atrophy less. In contrast, immobilizing a muscle in a shortened position encourages atrophy and greater loss of contractile function.[15] In addition to maintaining an immobilized muscle in a lengthened position, atrophy can also be prevented through isometric contraction and electrical stimulation of the muscles. As the unused muscle decreases in size because of atrophy, protein is also lost. When activity is resumed, normal protein synthesis is reestablished.

Immobilization of a part causes atrophy of slow-twitch muscle fibers.

Decreased neuromuscular efficiency   Immobilization causes motor nerves to become less efficient in recruiting and stimulating individual muscle fibers within a given motor unit.[2] Once immobilization ends, the original motor neuron discharge returns within about 1 week.

Joints and Immobilization

Immobilization of joints causes loss of normal compression, which in turn leads to a decrease in lubrication within the joint that subsequently causes degeneration. This

Joint immobilization decreases normal lubrication.

degeneration occurs because the articular cartilage is deprived of its normal nutrition. The use of continuous passive motion, electrical muscle stimulation, or hinged casts has in some cases retarded loss of articular cartilage.[2]

Ligament and Bone and Immobilization

Both ligaments and bones adapt to normal stress by maintaining their strength or becoming stronger. However, when stress is eliminated or decreased, ligament and bone become weaker.[15] Once immobilization has been removed, high-frequency, low-duration endurance exercise positively enhances the mechanical properties of ligaments. Endurance activities tend to increase both the production and the hypertrophy of the collagen fibers. Full remodeling of ligaments after immobilization may take as long as 12 months or more.

Cardiorespiratory System and Immobilization

As with other structures, the cardiorespiratory system is adversely affected by immobilization. The resting heart rate increases approximately one-half beat per minute each day of immobilization. The stroke volume, maximum oxygen uptake, and vital capacity decrease concurrently with the increase in heart rate.

THERAPEUTIC EXERCISE VERSUS CONDITIONING EXERCISE

Exercise is an essential factor in sports conditioning, injury prevention, and injury rehabilitation. Chapter 3 describes in some detail exercises used for physical conditioning and training that are also important in injury prevention. Techniques of therapeutic exercise are specifically concerned with restoring normal body function after injury.

MAJOR COMPONENTS OF A REHABILITATION PROGRAM

Components of a rehabilitation program include:
  General body conditioning
  Controlling pain
  Maintaining cardiorespiratory fitness
  Restoring full range of motion
  Restoring muscle strength and endurance
  Reestablishing neuromuscular control
  Functional progressions

A well-designed rehabilitation program should routinely address several key components before an injured athlete can return to preinjury competitive levels. They include controlling pain, maintaining levels of cardiorespiratory fitness, restoring full range of motion, restoring or increasing strength, reestablishing neuromuscular control, and functional progressions.[22]

General Body Conditioning

It is essential that an injured athlete maintain the conditioning level of the unaffected parts of the body during a period of relative inactivity. There are two reasons for this: when the injured body part is rehabilitated, the rest of the body must be ready to compete; and there is some indication that conditioning of the body in general, in addition to reconditioning of a specific injured part, assists in the rehabilitation of the injured part through some neural irradiation.

Controlling Pain

When an injury occurs, the athletic trainer must realize that the athlete will experience some degree of pain. (See Chapter 6.) The extent of the pain will be determined to some degree by the severity of the injury, the athlete's individual response to and perception of pain, and the circumstances under which the injury occurred. The athletic trainer can modulate acute pain by using the RICE technique immediately after injury.[22] A physician may also make use of various medications to help ease pain.

Persistent pain can make strengthening or flexibility exercises more difficult, thus interfering with the rehabilitation process. The athletic trainer should routinely address pain during each individual treatment session. Making use of appropriate therapeutic modalities, including various techniques of cryotherapy, thermotherapy, and electrical stimulating currents, will help modulate pain throughout the rehabilitation process.[24]

Maintaining Cardiorespiratory Fitness

Although strength and flexibility are commonly regarded as essential components in any injury rehabilitation program, relatively little consideration is given toward maintaining levels of cardiorespiratory fitness. An athlete spends a considerable amount of time preparing the cardiorespiratory system to be able to handle the increased demands made on it during a competitive season. When injury occurs and the athlete is forced to miss training time, levels of cardiorespiratory endurance may decrease rapidly. Thus the athletic trainer must design or substitute alternative activities that allow the individual to maintain existing levels of cardiorespiratory fitness during the rehabilitation period.

Depending on the nature of the injury, there are a number of possible activities open to the athlete. When there is a lower-extremity injury, non–weight-bearing activities should be incorporated. Pool activities provide an excellent means for injury rehabilitation. Cycling also can positively stress the cardiorespiratory system (Figure 15-1).

Restoring Range of Motion

After injury to a joint, there will always be some associated loss of motion. That loss of movement may be attributed to a number of pathological factors, including contracture of connective tissue (i.e., ligaments, joint capsules); resistance of the musculotendinous unit (i.e., muscle, tendon, and fascia) to stretch; or some combination of the two.

Physiological versus Accessory Movements

Two types of movement govern range of motion about a joint. Physiological movements result from an active muscle contraction that moves an extremity through flexion, extension, abduction, adduction, and rotation. Accessory motions refer to the manner in which one articulating joint surface moves relative to another and include spin, roll, and glide.[10]

Physiological movement is voluntary, and accessory movements normally accompany physiological movement. The two occur simultaneously. Normal accessory motions must occur for full-range physiological movement to take place. If any of the accessory component motions are restricted, normal physiological cardinal plane movement will not occur.[33]

Traditionally, rehabilitation programs tend to concentrate more on passive physiological movements without paying much attention to accessory motions. It is critical for the athletic trainer to closely evaluate the injured joint to determine whether motion is limited because of physiological movement constraints involving musculotendinous units or because of limitation in accessory motion involving the joint capsule and ligaments. If physiological movement is restricted, the athlete should engage in stretching activities designed to improve flexibility. Stretching exercises should be used whenever there is musculotendinous resistance to stretch. If accessory motion is limited because of some restriction of the joint capsule or the ligaments, the athletic trainer should incorporate mobilization techniques into the treatment program. Mobilization techniques should be used whenever there are tight articular structures.[21]

Restoring Muscular Strength and Endurance

Muscular strength is one of the most essential factors in restoring the function of a body part to preinjury status. Isometric, isotonic, isokinetic, and plyometric exercises can benefit rehabilitation. Whatever type of strength exercise is used, the pain it may produce should be carefully monitored. A major goal in performing strengthening exercises is to work through a full pain-free range of motion.

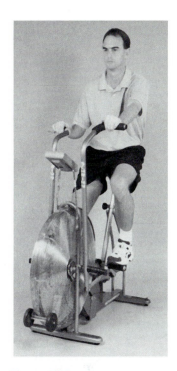

Figure 15-1

Stationary cycling provides a means of maintaining cardiorespiratory fitness during rehabilitation.

Accessory motions:
  Spin
  Roll
  Glide

Restricted physiologic movement = stretching.
Restricted accessory motion = joint mobilization.

Isometric Exercise

Isometric exercises are commonly performed in the early phase of rehabilitation when a joint is immobilized for a period of time. They are useful when using resistance training through a full range of motion may make the injury worse. Isometrics increase static strength and assist in decreasing the amount of atrophy. Isometrics also can lessen swelling by causing a muscle pumping action to remove fluid and edema.

Strength gains are limited primarily to the angle at which the joint is exercised. No functional force or eccentric work is developed. Other major difficulties are motivation and measuring the force that is being applied.

Progressive Resistive Exercise

Progressive resistive exercise is the most commonly used strengthening technique in a reconditioning program. It may be done using free weights, exercise machines, or rubber tubing (Figure 15-2). Progressive resistive exercise uses isotonic contractions in which force is generated while the muscle is changing in length.

Concentric and eccentric muscle contractions   Isotonic contractions may be either concentric or eccentric. Traditionally, progressive resistive exercise has concentrated primarily on the concentric component without paying much attention to the importance of the eccentric component. The use of eccentric contractions particularly in rehabilitation of various injuries related to sport has received considerable emphasis in recent years.[18] Eccentric contractions are critical for deceleration of limb motion, especially during high-velocity dynamic activities. For example, a baseball pitcher relies on an eccentric contraction of the external rotators at the glenohumeral joint to decelerate the humerus, which may be internally rotating at speeds as high as 8000 degrees per second. Strength deficits or an inability of a muscle to tolerate these eccentric forces can predispose to injury. Eccentric contractions are used to facilitate concentric contractions in plyometric exercises and may also be incorporated with functional proprioceptive neuromuscular facilitation strengthening exercises. Thus in a rehabilitation program the athletic trainer should incorporate both eccentric and concentric strengthening exercises.

Both concentric and eccentric contractions are possible with free weights, with the majority of isotonic exercise machines, and with rubber tubing or theraband. A disadvantage of machines and free weights is that they do not allow exercises to be performed in diagonal or functional planes. It is also difficult to exercise at functional velocities without producing additional injuries. Conversely, resistive exercise using rubber tubing allows both concentric and eccentric resistance and is not encumbered by the design of an exercise machine. It offers a wide range of usefulness at an extremely low cost.

Isokinetic Exercise

Isokinetic exercise is commonly used in the rehabilitative process.[18] It most often is incorporated during the later phases of a rehabilitation program. Isokinetics uses a fixed speed with accommodating resistance to provide maximal resistance throughout the range of motion (Figure 15-3). Isokinetic devices are generally capable of calculating measures of torque, average power, total work, and torque–to–body weight ratios, each of which may be used diagnostically by the athletic trainer. Isokinetic measures are commonly used as a criterion for return of the athlete to functional activity after injury.

The speed of movement can be altered in isokinetic exercise. Gains in strength from training at slower speeds are fairly specific to the angular velocity used in training. Isokinetic machines allow the athlete to exercise at speeds that are somewhat more functional. Training at faster speeds seems to produce more general improvement because increases in torque values can be seen at both fast and slow speeds. Isokinetic exercise performed at high speeds tends to decrease the joint's compressive forces. Comparatively, fast-speed exercises produce fewer negative effects on

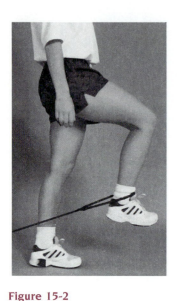

Figure 15-2

Exercises using rubber tubing are used for strengthening.

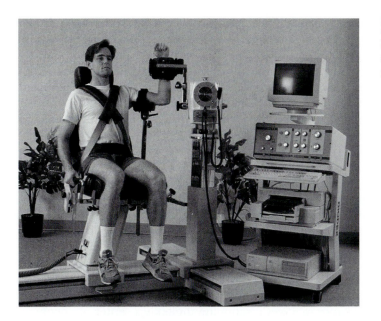

Figure 15-3

Isokinetics are primarily used as a diagnostic tool to determine levels of strength.

joints than do slow-speed exercises. Short-arc submaximal isokinetics spreads out synovial fluid that helps to nourish the articular cartilage and therefore to prevent deterioration.[18] It also develops neuromuscular "patterning" for functional speed and movements demanded by specific sports.

Reestablishing Proprioception, Kinesthesia, and Neuromuscular Control

Reestablishing proprioception, kinesthesia, and neuromuscular control should be of primary concern to the athletic trainer in all rehabilitation programs.[14] **Proprioception** is the ability to determine the position of a joint in space; **kinesthesia** refers to the ability to detect movement.[6]

The ability to sense the position of a joint in space is mediated by mechanoreceptors found in both muscle and joints, in addition to cutaneous, visual, and vestibular input. Neuromuscular control relies on the central nervous system to interpret and integrate proprioceptive and kinesthetic information and then to control individual muscles and joints to produce coordinated movement.[32]

Joint Mechanoreceptors

Joint mechanoreceptors are found in ligaments, capsules, menisci, labra, and fat pads. They include Ruffini's endings, pacinian corpuscles, and free nerve endings. These receptors are sensitive to changes in the shape of various joint structures and to the rate and direction of movement of the joint. They are most active in the end ranges of motion.[26]

Muscle Mechanoreceptors

The receptors found in muscles and tendons are the muscle spindles and the Golgi tendon organs. The muscle spindles are sensitive to changes in length of the muscle, and Golgi tendon organs are sensitive to changes in tension. The actions of these receptors are discussed in detail in Chapter 3.[26]

Neuromuscular Control in Rehabilitation

After injury and subsequent rest and immobilization, the central nervous system "forgets" how to put together information coming from muscle and joint mechanoreceptors and from cutaneous, visual, and vestibular input. Regaining neuromuscular control means regaining the ability to follow some previously established sensory pat-

proprioception
The ability to determine the position of a joint in space.

kinesthesia
The ability to detect movement.

Neuromuscular control produces coordinated movements.

Joint mechanoreceptors include Ruffini's endings, pacinian corpuscles, and free nerve endings.

Muscle mechanoreceptors include muscle spindles and Golgi tendon organs.

tern. The central nervous system compares the intent and production of a specific movement with stored information, continually adjusting until any discrepancy in movement is corrected.[32]

Neuromuscular control is the mind's attempt to teach the body conscious control of a specific movement. Successful repetition of a patterned movement makes its performance progressively less difficult, thus requiring less concentration, until the movement becomes automatic. This requires many repetitions of the same movement progressing step-by-step from simple to more complex movements. Strengthening exercises, particularly those that tend to be more functional, such as closed kinetic chain exercises, are essential for reestablishing neuromuscular control.[32]

Relearning normal functional movement and timing after injury to a joint may require several months. Addressing neuromuscular control is critical throughout the recovery process but may be most critical during the early stages of rehabilitation to avoid reinjury.[32]

Balance

Balance involves the complex integration of muscular forces, neurological sensory information received from the mechanoreceptors, and biomechanical information.[9] Balance involves positioning the body's center of gravity within the base of support. When the center of gravity extends beyond the base of support, the limits of stability have been exceeded even though the base of support has not changed, and a corrective step or stumble is necessary to prevent a fall. Even when an individual appears to be motionless, the body is undergoing constant postural sway caused by reflexive muscle contractions, which correct and maintain dynamic equilibrium in an upright posture.[4] When balance is disrupted the response to correct it is primarily reflexive and automatic. The primary mechanisms for controlling balance occur in the joints of the lower extremity.[32]

The ability to balance and maintain postural stability is essential to acquiring or reacquiring complex motor skills.[32] Athletes who show a decreased sense of balance or lack of postural stability after injury may lack sufficient proprioceptive and kinesthetic information or muscular strength, either of which may limit the ability to generate an effective correction response when there is not equilibrium. A rehabilitation program must include functional exercises that incorporate balance and proprioceptive training to prepare the athlete for return to activity. Failure to address balance problems may predispose the athlete to reinjury (Figure 15-4).

Open versus Closed Kinetic Chain Exercises

The concept of the kinetic chain deals with the anatomical functional relationships that exist in the upper and lower extremities. In a weight-bearing position, the lower extremity kinetic chain involves the transmission of forces among the foot, ankle, lower leg, knee, thigh, and hip. In the upper extremity, when the hand is a weight-bearing surface, forces are transmitted to the wrist, forearm, elbow, upper arm, and shoulder girdle.[20]

An open kinetic chain exists when the foot or hand is not in contact with the ground or some other surface.[19] In a closed kinetic chain, the foot or hand is weight bearing. Movements of the more proximal anatomical segments are affected by open and closed kinetic chain positions.[3] For example, the rotational components of the ankle, knee, and hip reverse direction when changing from an open to closed kinetic chain activity. In a closed kinetic chain the forces begin at the ground and work their way up through each joint. In a closed kinetic chain forces must be absorbed by various tissues and anatomical structures rather than simply dissipating as would occur in an open chain.[25]

In rehabilitation, the use of closed-chain strengthening techniques has become the treatment of choice for many athletic trainers.[13] Because most sport activities involve some aspect of weight bearing with the foot in contact with the ground or the hand

Balance involves the integration of muscular, neurological, and biomechanical information.

A closed kinetic chain occurs when the foot or hand is on the ground.

An open kinetic chain occurs when the foot or hand is off the ground.

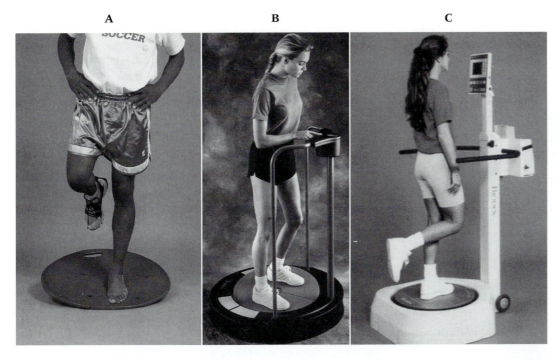

Figure 15-4

Balance training is essential in the rehabilitation program. **A,** BAPS Board. **B,** Kinesthetic Awareness Trainer. **C,** Biodex Balance System.

in a weight-bearing position, closed kinetic chain strengthening activities are more functional than are open-chain activities. Closed kinetic chain exercises are more sport or activity specific, involving exercise that more closely approximates the desired activity. For athletes, specificity of training must be emphasized to maximize carryover to functional activities on the playing field.[20] Therefore rehabilitative exercises should be incorporated that emphasize strengthening the entire kinetic chain rather than an isolated body segment.

Closed kinetic chain exercises use varying combinations of isometric, concentric, and eccentric contractions, which must occur simultaneously in different muscle groups within the chain. Isolation exercises typically make use of one specific type of muscular contraction to produce or control movement.[7] Consequently there must be some neuromuscular adaptation to this type of strengthening exercise.

In the athletic training setting, a number of different closed kinetic chain exercises have gained popularity and have been incorporated into rehabilitation protocols. Exercises commonly used for the lower extremity are minisquats, leg presses, stair climbing or stepping machines, forward and lateral step-ups, slide boards, terminal knee extensions using tubing, and stationary bicycling.[5] Push-ups and weight-shifting exercises on a medicine ball are two of the more typically used upper extremity exercises[29,30] (Figure 15-5).

Functional Progressions

The purpose of any program of rehabilitation is to restore normal function after injury. Functional progressions involve a series of gradually progressive activities designed to prepare the individual for return to a specific sport.[32] Functional progressions should be incorporated into the treatment program as early as possible. Well-

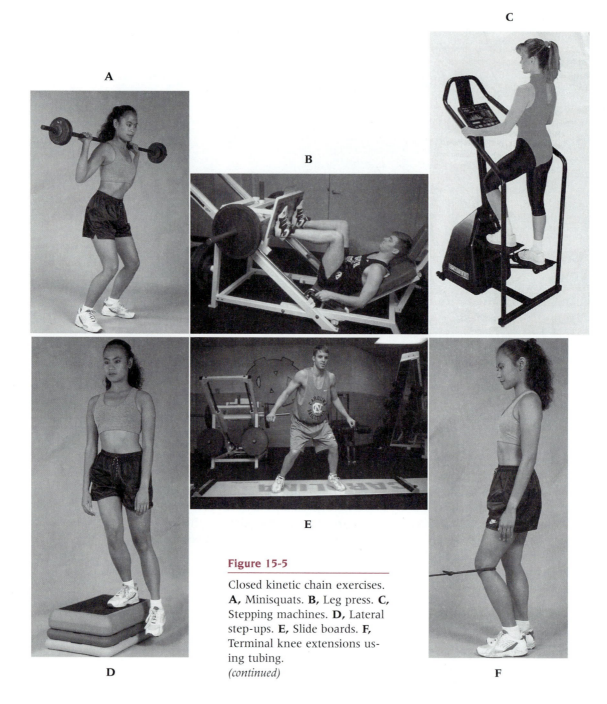

Figure 15-5

Closed kinetic chain exercises. **A,** Minisquats. **B,** Leg press. **C,** Stepping machines. **D,** Lateral step-ups. **E,** Slide boards. **F,** Terminal knee extensions using tubing. *(continued)*

designed functional progressions will gradually assist the injured athlete in achieving normal pain-free range of motion, restoring adequate strength levels, and regaining neuromuscular control throughout the rehabilitation program (Figure 15-6). Ultimately, the focus becomes a safe return to competition. Those skills necessary for successful participation in a given sport are broken down into component parts, and the athlete gradually reacquires those skills within the limitations of his or her own individual progress.[32]

G   H   I

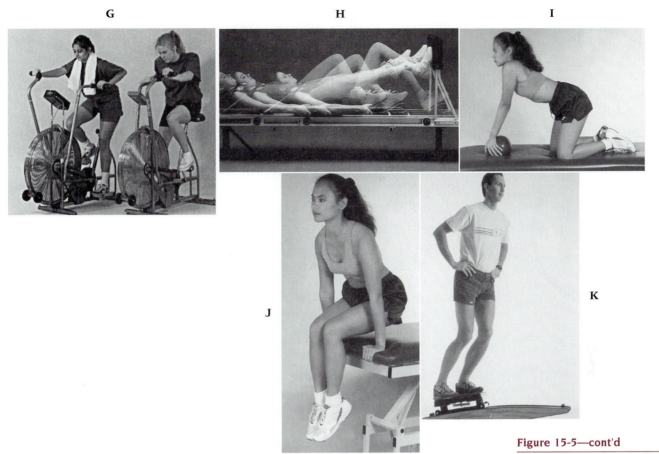

J   K

Figure 15-5—cont'd

Closed kinetic chain exercises.
G, Stationary bicycling. **H,**
Shuttle 2000. **I,** Weight shift-
ing. **J,** Push-ups. **K,** Fitter.

Functional activities follow a consistent progression from simple to complex skills, slow to fast speeds, short to longer distances, or light to heavy activities. Every new activity introduced must be carefully monitored by the athletic trainer to determine the athlete's ability to perform and his or her physical tolerance. If an activity does not produce additional pain or swelling, the level should be advanced; new activities should be introduced as quickly as possible. Thus the injured athlete would be gradually introduced to the stresses imposed by a particular demand until function is adequate for the athlete to return to sport-specific activity.[32]

The optimal functional progression program would be designed such that the athlete would have an opportunity to practice every possible skill that is required in a sport before returning to competition. This would certainly minimize the normal anxiety and apprehension experienced by the athlete on return to a competitive environment.[17]

Supervised functional progression activities can be done during team practice sessions. This allows athletes to be around teammates and coaches, which should help them to feel more accepted as team members.[17]

Functional Testing

Functional testing uses functional progression drills for the purpose of assessing the athlete's ability to perform a specific activity. Functional testing involves a single maximal effort performed to get some idea of how close the athlete is to full return to activity. For years athletic trainers have used a variety of functional tests to assess

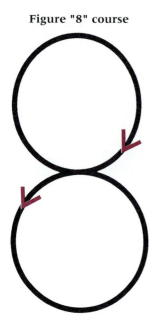

Figure "8" course

Figure 15-6

A figure-8 run is an example of a functional progression test.

All exercise rehabilitation must be conducted as part of a carefully designed plan.

15-2

Critical Thinking Exercise

A runner complains of anterior knee pain. She has greatly cut back on the distance of her training runs and indicates that she has been taking antiin-flammatory medication to help her continue to train. However, she is frustrated because her knee seems to be getting worse instead of better.

? What can the athletic trainer recommend to most effectively help the athlete deal with her knee pain?

Exercise performed during the presurgical phase can often assist recovery after surgery.

the athlete's progress, including agility runs (figure-8, shuttle run, carioca), side stepping, vertical jump, hopping for time or distance, and cocontraction tests.[32]

DEVELOPING AN EXERCISE REHABILITATION PLAN

No exercise rehabilitation program can be properly undertaken without a carefully designed plan. The plan must consider as many variables as possible, including the injury situation and the actual management plan.

Injury Situation

Athletic trainers responsible for overseeing an exercise rehabilitation program must have as complete an understanding of the injury as possible, including knowledge of how the injury was sustained, the major anatomical structures affected, the degree or grade of trauma, and the stage or phase of the injury's healing.

Management Plan

Often the management plan follows the phases of the healing process and the functional capacity that is present in a part. Great care should be taken to coordinate exercise with other therapeutic modalities such as heat, cold, and electrical muscle stimulation. Swelling and muscle spasm limit movement and should always be considered when an exercise program is undertaken. Another major consideration in exercise therapy is to recognize exercise overdosage and to respond appropriately.

Exercise Overdosage

Engaging in exercise that is too intense or too prolonged can be detrimental to the progress of rehabilitation. Indications that the intensity of the exercises being incorporated into the rehabilitation program exceed the limits of the healing process include an increase in the amount of swelling, an increase in pain, a loss or a plateau in strength, a loss or a plateau in range of motion, or an increase in the laxity of a healing ligament.[32] If an exercise or activity causes any of these signs the athletic trainer must back off and become less aggressive in the rehabilitation program.

Exercise Intensity

In most injury situations, early exercise rehabilitation involves submaximal exercise performed in short bouts that are repeated several times daily. Exercise intensity must be commensurate with healing. As recovery increases, the intensity of exercise also increases, with the exercise performed less often. Finally, the athlete returns to a conditioning mode of exercise, which often includes high-intensity exercise three or four times per week.

Exercise Phases

Rehabilitation exercise progressions in sports medicine can generally be subdivided into three phases based primarily on the three stages of the healing process: phase 1, the acute phase; phase 2, the repair phase; and phase 3, the remodeling phase. (See Chapter 7.) Depending on the type and extent of injury and the individual response to healing, phases will usually overlap. Each phase must include carefully considered goals and criteria for advancing from one phase to another.

Presurgical Exercise Phase

The presurgical exercise phase applies only to those athletes who sustain injuries that require surgery. If surgery can be postponed, exercise may be used as a means to improve its outcome. By allowing the initial inflammatory response phase to resolve and by maintaining or increasing muscle strength and flexibility, cardiorespiratory fitness, and neuromuscular control, the athlete may be better prepared to continue the exercise rehabilitative program after surgery.

Phase 1, the Acute Injury Phase

Phase 1 begins immediately when injury occurs and may last as long as 4 days. During this phase, the inflammatory stage of the healing process is attempting to "clean up the mess," thus creating an environment that is conducive to the fibroblastic stage. The primary focus of rehabilitation during this stage is to control swelling and to modulate pain by using rest, ice, compression, and elevation (RICE) immediately after injury. Ice, compression, and elevation should be used as much as possible during this phase.[22]

Rest of the injured part is critical during this phase. It is widely accepted that early mobility during rehabilitation is essential. However, if the athletic trainer becomes overly aggressive during the first 48 hours after injury and does not allow the injured part to be rested during the inflammatory stage of healing, the inflammatory process never gets a chance to accomplish its purpose. Consequently, the length of time required for inflammation may be extended. Therefore immobility during the first 2 days after injury is necessary to control inflammation.

It must be emphasized that rest does not mean that the athlete does nothing. The term *rest* applies only to the injured body part. During this period, the athlete should continue to work on cardiorespiratory fitness and strengthening and flexibility exercises for the parts of the body not affected by the injury. When immobilized, muscle tensing or isometrics may be used to maintain muscle strength.

By day 3 or 4 swelling begins to subside and eventually stops altogether. The injured area may feel warm to the touch, and some discoloration is usually apparent. The injury is still painful to the touch, and some pain is elicited on movement of the injured part. At this point the athlete may begin active mobility exercises working through a pain-free range of motion. If the injury involves the lower extremity, the athlete should be encouraged to progressively bear more weight.

The team physician may choose to have the athlete take nonsteroidal antiinflammatory drugs (NSAIDs) to help control swelling and inflammation. It is usually helpful to continue this medication throughout the rehabilitative process.

Phase 2, the Repair Phase

Once the inflammatory response has subsided the repair phase begins. During this stage of the healing process, fibroblastic cells are laying down a matrix of collagen fibers and forming scar tissue. This stage may begin as early as 4 days after the injury and may last for several weeks. At this point, swelling has stopped completely. The injury is still tender to the touch but is not as painful as during the last stage. Pain is also less on active and passive motion.[22]

As soon as inflammation is controlled the athletic trainer should immediately begin to incorporate activities into the rehabilitation program that can maintain levels of cardiorespiratory fitness, restore full range of motion, restore or increase strength, and reestablish neuromuscular control.

As in the acute phase, modalities should be used to control pain and swelling. Cryotherapy should be used during the early portion of this phase to reduce the likelihood of swelling. Electrical stimulating currents can help with controlling pain and improving strength and range of motion.[24]

Phase 3, the Remodeling Phase

The remodeling phase is the longest of the three phases and may last for several years, depending on the severity of the injury. The ultimate goal during this maturation stage of the healing process is return to activity. The injury is no longer painful to the touch, although some progressively decreasing pain may still be felt on motion. The collagen fibers must be realigned according to tensile stresses and strains placed on them during functional sport-specific exercises.[22]

Phases of rehabilitation:
  Phase 1—acute phase
  Phase 2—repair phase
  Phase 3—remodeling

The postsurgical exercise phase should start 24 hours after surgery.

Functional progressions incorporate sport-specific skills into the rehabilitation program.

The focus during this phase should be on regaining sport-specific skills. Dynamic functional activities related to individual sport performance should be incorporated into the rehabilitation program. Functional training involves the repeated performance of an athletic skill for the purpose of perfecting that skill. Strengthening exercises should progressively place stresses and strains on the injured structures that would normally be encountered during that sport. Plyometric strengthening exercises can be used to improve muscle power and explosiveness.[31] Functional testing should be done to determine specific skill weaknesses that need to be addressed before full return.

At this point some type of heating modality is beneficial to the healing process. The deep-heating modalities, ultrasound, or the diathermies should be used to increase circulation to the deeper tissues. Massage and gentle mobilization may also be used to reduce spasm, increase circulation, and reduce pain. Increased blood flow delivers the essential nutrients to the injured area to promote healing, and increased lymphatic flow assists in breakdown and removal of waste products.[24]

Controlled Mobility during Rehabilitation

Wolff's law states that after injury both bone and soft tissue will respond to the physical demands placed on them, causing them to remodel or realign along lines of tensile force.[22] Therefore it is critical that injured structures be exposed to progressively increasing loads throughout the rehabilitation process.

Controlled mobilization has been shown to be superior to immobilization for scar formation, revascularization, muscle regeneration, and reorientation of muscle fibers and tensile properties.[22] However, immobilization of the injured tissue during the acute, inflammatory response phase will likely facilitate the process of healing by controlling inflammation, thus reducing clinical symptoms. As healing progresses to the repair phase, controlled activity directed toward return to normal flexibility and strength should be combined with protective support or bracing. Generally, clinical signs and symptoms disappear at the end of this phase. As the remodeling phase begins, aggressive, active range-of-motion and strengthening exercises should be incorporated to facilitate tissue remodeling and realignment.

To a great extent, pain will dictate rate of progression. With initial injury, pain is intense and tends to decrease and eventually subside altogether as healing progresses. Any exacerbation of pain, swelling, or other clinical symptoms during or after a particular exercise or activity indicates that the load is too great for the level of tissue repair or remodeling. The athletic trainer must be aware of the timelines required for the process of healing and realize that being overly aggressive can interfere with that process.

Criteria for Full Recovery

All exercise rehabilitation plans must determine what is meant by complete recovery from an injury. Often it means that the athlete is fully reconditioned and has achieved full range of movement, strength, neuromuscular control, cardiovascular fitness, and sport-specific functional skills. Besides physical well-being, the athlete must also have regained full confidence to return to his or her sport.

The decision to release an athlete recovering from injury to a full return to athletic activity is the final stage of the rehabilitation and recovery process. The decision should be carefully considered by each member of the sports medicine team involved in the rehabilitation process. The team physician should be ultimately responsible for deciding that the athlete is ready to return to practice or competition. In considering the athlete's return to activity, the following concerns should be addressed:

- Physiological healing constraints
- Pain status
- Swelling

- Range of motion
- Strength
- Proprioception, kinesthesia, and neuromuscular control
- Cardiorespiratory fitness
- Sport-specific demands
- Functional testing
- Prophylactic strapping, bracing, or padding
- Responsibility of the athlete
- Predisposition to injury
- Psychological factors
- Gradual, progressive return to activity
- Athlete education and preventive maintenance program

ADDITIONAL APPROACHES TO EXERCISE REHABILITATION
Aquatic Exercise

Aquatic exercise has become popular as a rehabilitative tool in sports medicine.[1] An athletic trainer who has access to a swimming pool is fortunate. Water submersion offers an excellent environment for beginning a program of exercise therapy, or it can complement all phases of rehabilitation.

Because of buoyancy and hydrostatic pressure, submersion in a pool presents a versatile exercise environment that can be easily varied according to individual needs.[27] With the proper technique, the athlete can reduce muscle spasm, relax tense muscles, increase the range of joint motion, reestablish correct movement patterns, and, above all, increase strength, power, and muscular endurance.[2]

Using the water's buoyancy and pressure, aquatic exercise can be described as assistive, supportive, and resistive. As an assistive medium, the water's buoyancy can increase range of motion, strength, and control. Starting below the water level, the athlete first allows the part to be carried passively upward, keeping within pain-free limits. As the athlete gains strength, movement is actively engaged in, and the buoyancy of the water becomes assistive. Progression of the movement can be initiated by increasing speed and making the water above the body part become a resistive medium (Figure 15-7).

A second use of water buoyancy is support. The limb normally will float just below the water's surface. In this position the limb is parallel to the surface of the water. As with the assistive technique, increasing the speed will make the movement more difficult. Progression also can be accomplished by making the part less streamlined. In exercising the arm, the athlete can increase the difficulty by moving across the water with the flat of the hand or by using a hand paddle or webbed glove. Flippers can increase resistance to the leg.

A third use of water buoyance is resistance. The injured body part is moved downward against the upward thrust of the water. Maximum resistance is attained by keeping the limb at a right angle to the water's surface. As with the supportive technique, the resistive technique can be made progressively more difficult by using different devices. Extra resistance is added by pushing or dragging flotation devices down into the water.

Besides specific exercises, the athlete can practice sports skills, using the water's buoyancy and resistance to advantage. For example, locomotor or throwing skills can be practiced to regain normal movement patterns. The swimming pool can also be an excellent medium for retaining or restoring functional capacities, as well as restoring cardiovascular endurance. Wearing a flotation device around the waist, the athlete performs a variety of upper- and lower-limb movement patterns (Figure 15-8). While the athlete is in 3 to 5 feet of water, movements of straight-ahead running, backward running, side stepping, figure-8s, and carioca can be performed bearing full weight.

15-3

Critical Thinking Exercise

After an ankle sprain a basketball player is placed in an ankle immobilizer and given crutches with instructions to begin totally non–weight bearing and progress to full weight bearing without crutches as soon as possible. After 4 days the athlete is out of the immobilizer and can walk without crutches but still has a significant limp.

? What should the athletic trainer do to help the athlete regain a normal gait pattern, and why is it important to do so as soon as possible?

Aquatic exercise provides an excellent means for rehabilitation.

A   B   C

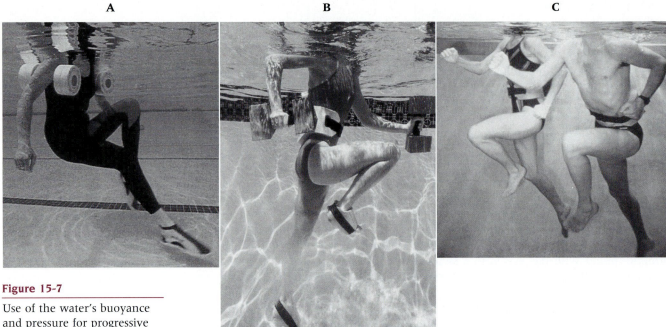

Figure 15-7

Use of the water's buoyance and pressure for progressive exercise. **A,** Several buoyancy and resistive devices may be used in aquatic exercise. **B,** Using the water for buoyancy. **C,** Using the water for resistance.

PNF strengthening techniques:
  Rhythmic initiation
  Repeated contraction
  Slow reversal
  Slow-reversal-hold
  Rhythmic stabilization

PNF stretching techniques:
  Contract-relax
  Hold-relax
  Slow-reversal hold-relax

Proprioceptive Neuromuscular Facilitation Techniques

Proprioceptive neuromuscular facilitation (PNF) is an approach to therapeutic exercise that uses proprioceptive, cutaneous, and auditory input to produce functional improvement in motor output and can be a vital element in the rehabilitation process of many sports-related injuries.[12] These techniques have been recommended for increasing strength, flexibility, and coordination in response to demands placed on the neuromuscular system. The principles and techniques of PNF are based primarily on the neurophysiological mechanisms involving the stretch reflex.[19] (See Chapter 3.)

Techniques of Proprioceptive Neuromuscular Facilitation

The PNF techniques are generally used in rehabilitation for the purposes of facilitating strength and increasing range of motion. Flexibility is increased by the techniques of contract-relax, hold-relax, and slow-reversal-hold-relax. In contrast, strength can be facilitated by repeated contraction and the slow-reversal, rhythmic initiation, and rhythmic stabilization techniques.[23]

Strengthening techniques To assist the athlete in developing muscle strength, muscle endurance, and coordination, the following techniques are used.

Rhythmic initiation Rhythmic initiation consists of a progressive series, first of passive movement, then of active assistive movement, followed by an active movement through an agonist pattern. The purpose of this approach is for athletes who have limited movement to regain strength through the range of motion progressively.

Repeated contraction Repeated contraction of a muscle or a muscle group is used when there is general weakness or weakness at one specific point. The athlete moves isotonically against the maximum resistance of the athletic trainer until fatigue is experienced. At the time fatigue is felt, stretch is applied to the muscle at that point in the range to facilitate greater strength production. All resistance must be carefully accommodated to the strength of the athlete. Because the athlete is resisting as much as possible, this technique may be contraindicated for some injuries.

Slow reversal The athlete moves through a complete range of motion against maximum resistance. Resistance is applied to facilitate antagonist and agonist muscle

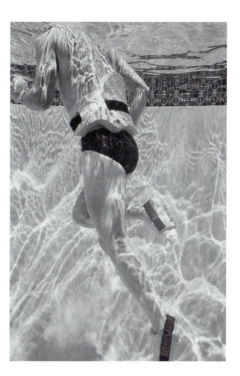

Figure 15-8

A wet vest can facilitate exercise programs in the water by making the athlete more buoyant.

groups and to ensure smooth and rhythmic movement. It is important that reversals of the movement pattern be instituted before the previous pattern has been fully completed. The major benefits of this PNF technique is that it promotes normal reciprocal coordination of agonist and antagonist muscles.

Slow-reversal-hold   In this technique the athlete moves a body part isotonically using agonist muscles, followed immediately by an isometric contraction. The athlete is instructed to hold at the end of each isotonic movement. The primary purpose of this technique is to develop strength at a specific point in the range of movement.

Rhythmic stabilization   Rhythmic stabilization uses an isometric contraction of the agonists, followed by an isometric contraction of the antagonist muscles. With repeated cocontraction of these muscles, strength is maximum at this point.

Stretching techniques   To produce muscle relaxation through an inhibitory response for purposes of increasing range of motion, the following PNF techniques may be used.

Contract-relax   The affected body part is passively moved until resistance is felt. The athlete is then told to contract the antagonistic muscle isotonically. The movement is resisted by the athletic trainer for 10 seconds or until fatigue is felt. The athlete is instructed to relax for 10 seconds. The athletic trainer passively moves the limb to a new stretch position. The exercise is repeated three times.

Hold-relax   The hold-relax technique is similar to contract-relax except that an isometric contraction is used. The athlete moves the body part to the point of resistance and is told to hold. The muscles are isometrically resisted by the athletic trainer for 10 seconds. The athlete is then told to relax for 10 seconds, and the body part is moved to a new range either actively by the athlete or passively by the athletic trainer. This exercise is repeated three times.

Slow-reversal-hold-relax   The athlete moves the body part to the point of resistance and is told to hold. The muscles are isometrically resisted by the athletic trainer for 10 seconds. The athlete is then told to relax for 10 seconds, thus relaxing the antagonist while the agonist is contracted, moving the part to a new limited range (Figure 15-9).

15-4

Critical Thinking Exercise

A racquetball player twists his knee during a match and sprains his ACL. Knee movement is limited because of the pain, and full weight bearing is extremely painful. He has a weekend-long racquetball tournament in 2 weeks and is concerned about regaining his knee motion while being able to maintain the fitness levels necessary to compete for 2 consecutive days.

? What type of rehabilitative technique could the athletic trainer recommend that would allow the athlete to address both his range of motion and fitness concerns even though he is unable to bear weight?

Figure 15-9

The slow-reversal-hold-relax stretching technique for the hamstring muscle.

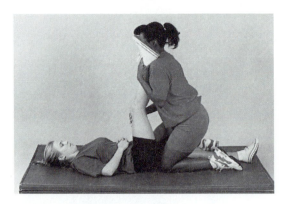

Basic Principles for Using Proprioceptive Neuromuscular Facilitation Techniques

These principles are the basis of PNF that must be used with any specific techniques. Application of the following principles may assist in promoting a desired response in the individual being treated.[12]

1. The athlete must be taught the PNF patterns regarding the sequential movements from starting position to terminal positions using brief, simple descriptions.
2. When learning the patterns, the athlete should look at the moving limb for feedback on directional and positional control.
3. Verbal commands should be firm and simple—push, pull, or hold.
4. Manual contact with the hands can facilitate a movement response.
5. The athletic trainer must use correct body mechanics when providing resistance.
6. The amount of resistance given should facilitate a maximal response that allows smooth, coordinated motion.
7. Rotational movement is a critical component in all of the PNF patterns.
8. The distal movements of the patterns should occur first and should be completed by no later than halfway through the pattern.
9. The stronger components are emphasized to facilitate the weaker components of a movement pattern.
10. Pressing the joint together causes increased stability, whereas traction pulls the joint apart and facilitates movement.
11. Giving a quick stretch causes a reflex contraction of that muscle.

Proprioceptive Neuromuscular Facilitation

The exercise patterns involve three component movements: flexion-extension, abduction-adduction, and internal-external rotation. Human movement is patterned and rarely involves straight motion because all muscles are spiral in nature and lie in diagonal directions.[12]

The PNF patterns involve distinct diagonal and rotational movements of upper extremity, lower extremity, upper trunk, lower trunk, and neck. The exercise pattern is initiated with the muscle groups in the lengthened or stretched position. The muscle group is then contracted, moving the body part through the range of motion to a shortened position.

The upper and lower extremities each have two separate patterns of diagonal movement for each part of the body, which are referred to as the diagonal 1 (D1) and diagonal 2 (D2) patterns. These two diagonal patterns are subdivided into D1 moving into flexion, D1 moving into extension, D2 moving into flexion, and D2 moving into extension. The patterns are named according to the movement occurring at either the shoulder or the hip.

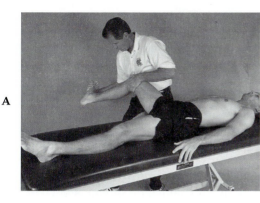
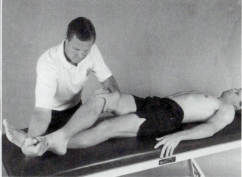

Figure 15-10

The D2 lower-extremity pattern moving into hip extension. **A,** Starting position. **B,** Terminal position.

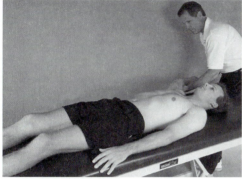
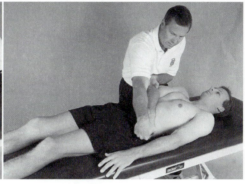

Figure 15-11

The D2 upper-extremity pattern moving into shoulder extension. **A,** Starting position. **B,** Terminal position.

Figures 15-10 and 15-11 are examples of PNF patterns that may be used for rehabilitating some sports injuries.

Joint Mobilization

The techniques of joint mobilization are used to improve joint mobility or to decrease joint pain by restoring accessory movements to the joint, thus allowing for full, nonrestricted, pain-free range of motion.[21] Mobilization techniques may be used to attain a variety of treatment goals, including reducing pain; decreasing muscle guarding; stretching or lengthening tissue surrounding a joint, especially capsular and ligamentous tissue; reflexogenic effects that either inhibit or facilitate muscle tone or the stretch reflex; and proprioceptive effects that improve postural and kinesthetic awareness.

Mobilization Techniques

Mobilization techniques are used to increase the accessory motions about a joint.[10] Treatment techniques designed to improve accessory motion involve small-amplitude oscillating movements within a specific part of the range.[9] Mobilization should be done with both the athlete and the athletic trainer in comfortable and relaxed positions. The athletic trainer should mobilize one joint at a time. The joint should be stabilized as near one articulating surface as possible; the other surface should be held with a firm, confident grasp.[21]

Maitland[16] has categorized mobilization techniques into five grades as follows:
- Grade I—a small-amplitude movement at the beginning of the range of movement. Used when pain and spasm limit movement early in the range of motion.
- Grade II—a large-amplitude movement within the midrange of movement. Used

Mobilization works to improve accessory motions.

when spasm limits movement sooner with a quick oscillation than with a slow one, or when slowly increasing pain restricts movement halfway into the range.

■ Grade III—a large-amplitude movement up to the pathological limit in the range of movement. Used when pain and resistance from spasm, inert tissue tension, or tissue compression limit movement near the end of the range.

■ Grade IV—a small-amplitude movement at the end of the range of movement. Used when resistance limits movement in the absence of pain and spasm.

■ Grade V—a small-amplitude, quick thrust delivered at the end of the range of movement, usually accompanied by a popping sound that is called a manipulation. Used when minimal resistance limits the end of the range. Manipulation is most effectively accomplished by the velocity of the thrust rather than by the force of the thrust. Most authorities agree that manipulation should be used only by individuals trained specifically in these techniques because a great deal of skill and judgment is necessary for safe and effective treatment.

In Maitland's system, grades I and II are used primarily for treatment of pain, and grades III and IV are used for treating stiffness. It is necessary to treat pain first and stiffness second. Figure 15-12 shows the various grades of oscillation that are used in a joint with some limitation of motion.

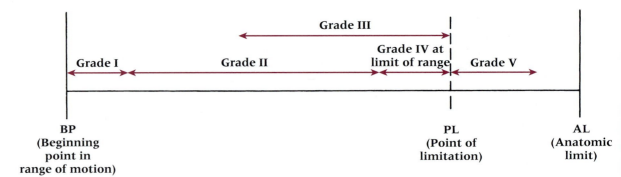

Figure 15-12

Maitland's five grades of motion. *PL,* Point of limitation; *AL,* anatomic limit.

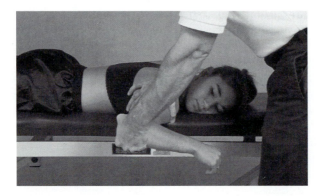

Figure 15-13

Anterior humeral glide (for increasing extension and lateral rotation).

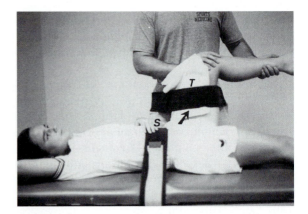

Figure 15-14

Inferior femoral glide (for increasing abduction and flexion).

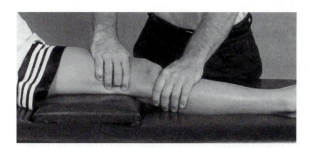

Figure 15-15

Posterior tibial glide (for increasing flexion).

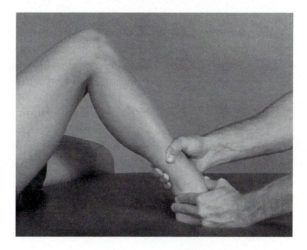

Figure 15-16

Posterior tibial glide (for increasing plantar flexion).

The shape of the articulating surfaces usually dictates the direction of the mobilization being performed.[21] Generally one articulating surface may be considered to be concave and the other to be convex. When the concave surface is stationary and the convex surface is moving, mobilization should be done in the opposite direction of the bone movement. If the convex surface is stationary and the concave surface is moving, mobilization should be done in the same direction as the bone movement. If mobilization in the appropriate direction exacerbates complaints of pain or stiffness, the athletic trainer should apply the technique in the opposite direction until the patient can tolerate application of the technique in the appropriate direction.

Figures 15-13 through 15-16 demonstrate mobilization techniques for the various joints and body segments.

SUMMARY

- When injuries occur in sports medicine the focus of the athletic trainer shifts from injury prevention to injury treatment and rehabilitation. The athletic trainer generally assumes the primary responsibility for design, implementation, and supervision of the rehabilitation program for the injured athlete. Two major goals of rehabilitation are to prevent deconditioning and to restore the injured part to a preinjury state. Besides the physical aspect, the mental and emotional aspects of rehabilitation must always be considered.
- When an injured body part is immobilized for a period of time, a number of disuse problems adversely affect muscle, joints, ligaments, bone, cartilage, neuromuscular efficiency, and the cardiorespiratory system.
- Designing programs for rehabilitation is relatively simple and involves several basic short-term goals: controlling pain, maintaining or improving flexibility, restoring or increasing strength, reestablishing neuromuscular control, and maintaining levels of cardiorespiratory fitness. The long-term goal is to return the injured athlete to practice or competition as quickly and safely as possible.
- An open kinetic chain exists when the foot or hand is not in contact with the ground or some other surface. In a closed kinetic chain, the foot or hand is weight bearing. In rehabilitation, the use of closed-chain strengthening techniques has become the treatment of choice for many athletic trainers. Closed kinetic chain strengthening activities are more functional than are open kinetic chain activities.
- Functional progressions involve a series of gradually progressive activities designed to prepare the athlete for return to a specific sport. Functional progressions should be incorporated into the treatment program as early as possible.
- Rehabilitation exercise progressions in sports medicine can generally be subdivided into three phases based primarily on the three stages of the healing process: phase 1, the acute phase; phase 2, the repair phase; and phase 3, the remodeling phase.

- The decision to release an athlete recovering from injury to a full return to athletic activity is the final stage of the rehabilitation and recovery process. The decision should be carefully considered by each member of the sports medicine team involved in the rehabilitation process.
- Aquatic exercises can be an important rehabilitative tool for the athletic trainer, particularly with injuries involving the lower extremity. Aquatic exercises allow for resistance with motion without weight bearing.
- Proprioceptive neuromuscular facilitation is a manual therapy technique that can be used for strengthening muscle or increasing range of motion. The PNF movement patterns involve a sequential series of specific movements for the lower extremity, lower trunk, upper trunk, and upper extremity.
- Mobilization is another manual therapy technique that is used to improve joint mobility or to decrease joint pain by restoring accessory movements to the injured joint, thus allowing full, pain-free range of motion.

Solutions to Critical Thinking EXERCISES

15-1 In sports medicine, the short-term goals in any rehabilitation program should include controlling pain, regaining range of motion, regaining strength, reestablishing neuromuscular control, and maintaining levels of cardiorespiratory fitness. The approach to rehabilitation should be aggressive, and decisions as to when and how to alter and progress specific components within a rehabilitation program should be based on and are limited by the healing process. The long-term goal is to return the athlete to full activity as soon as safely possible.

15-2 Anterior knee pain can result from many different causes. Strengthening of the quadriceps can be helpful. If full range of motion strengthening exercises increase pain, the athlete should begin with positional isometric exercises done at different points in the range, progressing to full-range concentric and eccentric exercise as tolerated. Closed-kinetic chain exercises such as minisquats, stepping exercises, or leg presses are excellent quadriceps-strengthening exercises and tend to be more functional in nature than traditional open kinetic chain exercises done on an exercise machine.

15-3 After injury and subsequent rest and immobilization, it is not unusual for the athlete to "forget" how to walk. The athletic trainer must help the athlete relearn neuromuscular control, which means regaining the ability to follow some previously established motor and sensory pattern by regaining conscious control of a specific movement until that movement becomes automatic. Strengthening exercises, particularly those that tend to be more functional, such as closed kinetic chain exercises, are essential for reestablishing neuromuscular control. Addressing neuromuscular control is critical throughout the recovery process but may be most critical during the early stages of rehabilitation to avoid reinjury or overuse injuries to additional structures.

15-4 Perhaps the best recommendation would be to have the athlete engage in an aquatic exercise program. In the water, the athlete would not be weight bearing and could exercise the injured knee through a pain-free range of motion while simultaneously working on maintaining levels of fitness by engaging in water-resisted conditioning exercises.

15-5 Remember that to achieve a full physiological range of movement the joint must have normal accessory motions. Stretching techniques address motion restriction caused by tightness of the musculotendinous unit. The athletic trainer should incorporate joint mobilization techniques that address restriction of motion caused by some tightness of capsular and ligamentous structures that surround the affected joint.

REVIEW QUESTIONS AND CLASS ACTIVITIES

1. What occurs physiologically when an athlete is suddenly forced to stop physical activity?
2. Discuss the physiological effects of immobilization on muscles, ligaments, joints, neuromuscular efficiency, and the cardiovascular system.
3. Discuss similarities and differences between training and conditioning exercises and therapeutic exercise.
4. Why must an athlete condition the entire body while an injury heals?
5. Why is it important to modulate pain during a rehabilitation program?
6. How is range of motion restored after an injury?
7. Critically compare the use of isometric, isotonic, and isokinetic exercises in rehabilitation.
8. Discuss the difference between proprioception and kinesthesia, and explain how they are related to neuromuscular control.
9. Why are closed kinetic chain exercises more useful than open kinetic chain exercises in the rehabilitation of sports injuries?
10. How and when should functional progressions be incorporated into the rehabilitation program?
11. Describe how to determine if an athlete is ready to return to activity after injury.
12. What is the importance of developing an exercise rehabilitation plan? Include the criteria for moving to various phases.
13. What are the important considerations during each of the three phases of rehabilitation?
14. How may aquatic exercise be incorporated into a rehabilitation program?
15. Proprioceptive neuromuscular facilitation (PNF) includes stretching, strengthening, and movement-patterning techniques. How can these techniques apply to sports injuries?

16. Explain why it is necessary to use stretching techniques to increase physiological movement and mobilization techniques to improve accessory motions.

REFERENCES

1. Arrigo C: Aquatic rehabilitation, *Sports Med Update* 7(2):1, 1992.
2. Barak T, Rosen E, Sofer R: Mobility: passive orthopedic manual therapy. In Gould J, Davies G, editors: *Orthopedic and sports physical therapy,* St Louis, 1990, Mosby.
3. Bunton E, Pitney W, Kane A: The role of limb torque muscle action and proprioception during closed kinetic chain rehabilitation of the lower extremity, *J Ath Train* 28(1):11, 1993.
4. Cox E, Lephart S, Irrgang J: Unilateral balance training of noninjured individuals and the effects on postural sway, *J Sport Rehab* 2(2):87, 1993.
5. Graham V, Gelhsen G, Edwards J: Electromyographic evaluation of closed and open kinetic chain rehab exercises, *J Ath Train* 28(1):23, 1993.
6. Grigg P: Peripheral neural mechanisms in proprioception, *J Sport Rehab* 3(1):2, 1994.
7. Hillman S: Principles and techniques of open kinetic chain rehabilitation, *J Sport Rehab* 3(4):319, 1994.
9. Irrgang J, Whitney S, Cox E: Balance and proprioceptive training for rehabilitation of the lower extremity, *J Sport Rehab* 3(1):68, 1994.
10. Kaltenborn F: *Mobilization of the extremity joints: examination and basic treatment techniques,* Norway, 1980, Olaf Norlis Bokhandel.
11. Knight KJ: Guidelines for rehabilitation of sports injuries. In Harvey JS, editor: *Rehabilitation of the injured athlete. Clinics in sports medicine,* vol 4, no 3, Philadelphia, 1985, Saunders.
12. Knott M, Voss EE: *Proprioceptive neuromuscular facilitation: patterns and techniques,* ed 2, Philadelphia, 1968, Harper & Row.
13. Lafree J, Mozingo A, Worrell T: Comparison of open kinetic chain knee and hip extension to closed kinetic chain leg performance, *J Sport Rehab* 4(2):99, 1995.
14. Lephart S: Reestablishing proprioception, kinesthesia, joint position sense, and neuromuscular control in rehabilitation. In Prentice W, editor: *Rehabilitation techniques in sports medicine,* ed 2, St Louis, 1994, Mosby.
15. Magnusson P, McHugh M: Current concepts on rehabilitation in sports medicine. In Nicholas J, Hirschman E, editor: *The lower extremity and spine in sports medicine,* St Louis, 1995, Mosby.
16. Maitland G: *Extremity manipulation,* London, 1977, Butterworth.
17. McGee M: Functional progression in rehabilitation. In Prentice W, editor: *Rehabilitation techniques in sports medicine,* ed 2, St Louis, 1994, Mosby.
18. Perrin D: *Isokinetic exercise and assessment,* Champaign, Ill, 1993, Human Kinetics.
19. Prentice W, Kooima E: The use of proprioceptive neuromuscular facilitation techniques in the rehabilitation of sport-related injuries, *Ath Train* 21:26, 1986.
20. Prentice W: Closed-kinetic chain exercise. In Prentice W, editor: *Rehabilitation techniques in sports medicine,* ed 2, St Louis, 1994, Mosby.
21. Prentice W: Mobilization and traction techniques in rehabilitation. In Prentice W, editor: *Rehabilitation techniques in sports medicine,* ed 2, St Louis, 1994, Mosby.
22. Prentice W: The healing process and pathophysiology of musculoskeletal injury. In Prentice W, editor: *Rehabilitation techniques in sports medicine,* ed 2, St Louis, 1994, Mosby.
23. Prentice W: Proprioceptive neuromuscular facilitation techniques. In Prentice W, editor: *Rehabilitation techniques in sports medicine,* ed 2, St Louis, 1994, Mosby.
24. Prentice W: *Therapeutic modalities in sports medicine,* St Louis, 1994, Mosby.
25. Rivera J: Open vs closed kinetic chain rehabilitation of the lower extremity, *J Sport Rehab* 3(2):154, 1994.
26. Rowinski M: Afferent neurobiology of the joint. In Gould J, Davies G: *Orthopedic and sports physical therapy,* St Louis, 1990, Mosby.
27. Selepak G: Aquatic therapy in rehabilitation. In Prentice W, editor: *Rehabilitation techniques in sports medicine,* ed 2, St Louis, 1994, Mosby.
28. Smith MJ: Muscle fiber types: their relationship to athletic training and rehabilitation. In Garron GW, editor: *Gymnastics. Clinics in sports medicine,* vol 4, no 1, Philadelphia, 1985, Saunders.
29. Stone J, Lueken J, Partin N: Closed kinetic chain rehabilitation of the glenohumeral joint, *J Ath Train* 28(1):34, 1993.
30. Stone J, Partin N, Lueken J: Upper extremity proprioceptive training, *J Ath Train* 2(1):15, 1994.
31. Tippett S: Sports rehabilitation concepts. In Saunders B: *Sports physical therapy,* Norwalk, Conn, 1990, Appleton & Lange.
32. Tippett S, Voight M: *Functional progressions for sport rehabilitation,* Champaign, Ill, 1995, Human Kinetics.
33. Wadsworth C: *Manual examination and treatment of the spine and extremities,* Baltimore, 1988, Williams & Wilkins.

ANNOTATED BIBLIOGRAPHY

Buschbacher R, Braddom R: *Sports medicine and rehabilitation: a sport specific approach,* Philadelphia, 1994, Hanley & Belfus.

Discusses the rehabilitation of injuries that occur in specific sports.

Edmond S: *Manipulation and mobilization: extremity and spinal techniques,* St Louis, 1993, Mosby.

Provides the entry-level student and the practicing clinician with a comprehensive text on mobilization and manipulation techniques.

Kisner C, Colby A: *Therapeutic exercise: foundations and techniques,* Philadelphia, 1986, Davis.

Provides a clear, concise presentation of the field of therapeutic exercise. It is well suited to sports medicine and covers exercise for increasing range of motion and for treating soft tissue, bone, and postsurgical problems extremely well.

Prentice W: *Mobilization and traction: principles and techniques,* video, 33 minutes, St Louis, 1993, Mosby.

This videotape presents a thorough overview of mobilization and traction and includes detailed demonstrations of various techniques.

Prentice W: *Proprioceptive neuromuscular facilitation: principles and techniques,* video, 26 minutes, St Louis, 1993, Mosby.

This videotape presents an introduction to PNF stretching and strengthening exercises complete with detailed hands-on demonstration of specific techniques.

Prentice W: *Rehabilitation techniques in sports medicine,* ed 2, St Louis, 1994, Mosby.

A comprehensive text dealing with all aspects of rehabilitation used in a sports medicine setting.

Tippett S, Voight M: *Functional progressions for sport rehabilitation,* Champaign, Ill, 1995, Human Kinetics.

Presents scientific principles and practical applications for using functional exercise to rehabilitate athletic injuries.

Zachazewski J, Magee D, Quillen W: *Athletic entries and rehabilitation,* Philadelphia, 1996, Saunders.

An extremely detailed scientifically-based advanced text dealing with athletic injury rehabilitation.

Drugs and Sports

When you finish this chapter, you should be able to

- Define drugs and list some of the more common drug vehicles.
- Discuss the various methods by which drugs can be administered.
- Explain the difference between administering and dispensing medications.
- Discuss legal ramification for dispensing and purchasing medications.
- Describe the various protocols that the athletic trainer should follow for administering over-the-counter medications to athletes.
- Discuss the various drugs that can be used to treat infection, reduce pain and inflammation, relax muscle, treat gastrointestinal disorders, treat colds and congestion, and control bleeding.
- Discuss the problem of substance abuse in the athletic population.
- Describe the ergogenic aids used by athletes to improve performance.
- Discuss the use of alcohol, drugs, and tobacco by athletes.
- Explain the drug testing policies and procedures, and list the different types of banned drugs.

pharmacology
The study of drugs and their origin, nature, properties, and effects on living organisms.

Pharmacology is the branch of science that deals with the actions of drugs on biological systems, especially drugs that are used in medicine for diagnostic and therapeutic purposes. Pharmaceutical care is the direct provision of medication-related care for the purpose of achieving definite outcomes that improve quality of life. Medications of all types, both prescription and over-the-counter, are commonly used by athletes as they are by other individuals in the population[1] (Figure 16-1).

Unfortunately, the abuse of various drugs and other substances for performance enhancement or for "recreational" mood alteration is also widespread among athletes. Thus the athletic trainer must be knowledgeable about all aspects of drug use and abuse within the athletic population.

WHAT IS A DRUG?

The use of substances for the express purpose of treating some infirmity or disease dates back to early history. The ancient Egyptians were highly skilled in making and using medications, treating a wide range of external and internal conditions.

Many of our common drugs such as aspirin and penicillin are derived from natural sources. Historically, medications were composed of roots, herbs, leaves, or other natural materials when they were identified or believed to have medicinal properties. Today many medications that originally came from nature are produced synthetically.

drug
Any chemical substance that affects living matter.

A **drug** is any chemical agent that affects living matter. Used in the treatment of disease, drugs may either be applied directly to a specific tissue or organ or be administered internally to affect the body systemically. When a drug enters the bloodstream by absorption through the gastrointestinal tract or through direct injection, it can affect specific tissues and organs far from the site of introduction.

Drug Vehicles

Although athletic trainers and coaches cannot dispense a prescription drug, they should have a basic comprehension of why, how, and by what means a drug is being delivered to the athlete's body. This section provides the reader with an understand-

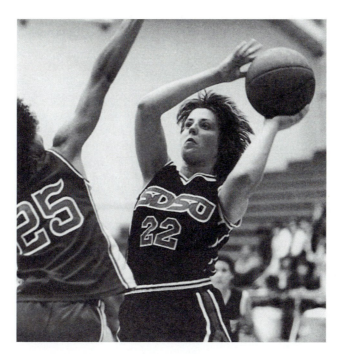

Figure 16-1

Medications of all types are commonly taken by athletes.

ing of the vehicles in which a drug may be housed, how it may be administered, and the response it may have, both positive and negative.

A drug **vehicle** is a therapeutically inactive substance that transports a drug. A drug is housed in a vehicle that may be either a solid or a liquid. Some of the more common drug vehicles are listed in Table 16-1.

vehicle
The substance in which a drug is transported.

DRUG ADMINISTRATION VERSUS DISPENSING

Administering a drug is defined as providing a single dose of medication for immediate use by the patient. Dispensing refers to providing the patient with a drug in a quantity sufficient to be used for multiple doses. The administration of medications in athletes, as in any individual, can be either internal or external and is based on the type of local or general response desired.

Drugs can be administered internally or externally.

Internal Administration

Drugs and medications can be taken internally through inhalation, or they may be administered intradermally, intramuscularly, intranasally, intraspinally, intravenously, orally, rectally, or sublingually.

Inhalation is a means of bringing medication or substances to the respiratory tract. This method is most often used in sports to relieve the athlete of the symptoms of respiratory illness such as asthma. The vehicle for inhalation is normally water vapor, oxygen, or highly aromatic medications.

Intradermal (into the skin) or subcutaneous (under the cutaneous tissues) administration is usually accomplished through a hypodermic needle injection. Such introduction of medication is initiated when a rapid response is needed, but it does not produce as rapid a response as that after intravenous injection.

Intramuscular injection means that the medication is given directly into the muscle tissue. The site for such an injection is usually the gluteal area or the deltoid muscle of the upper arm.

Intranasal application is varied according to the condition that is to be treated. The introduction of a decongestant intranasal solution by using a dropper or an atomizer may relieve the discomfort of head colds and allergies.

Intraspinal injection may be indicated for any of the following purposes: introduction of drugs to combat specific organisms that have entered the spinal cord, injec-

TABLE 16-1 Drug Vehicles

Liquid preparations

Aqueous solution	Sterile water containing a drug substance
Elixir	Alcohol, sugar, and flavoring with a drug dissolved in solution, designed for internal consumption
Liniment	Alcohol or oil containing a dissolved drug, designed for external massage
Spirit	A drug dissolved in water and alcohol or in alcohol alone
Suspension	Undissolved powder in a fluid medium; must be mixed well by shaking before use
Syrup	A mixture of sugar and water containing a drug

Solid preparations

Ampule	A closed glass receptacle containing a drug
Capsule	A gelatin receptacle containing a drug
Ointment (emollient)	A semisolid preparation for external application of such consistency that it may be applied to the skin by inunction
Paste	An inert powder combined with water
Tablet	A solid pharmaceutical dosage compressed into a small oval, circle, square, or other form
Plaster	A substance intended for external application, made of such materials and of such consistency as to adhere to the skin and thereby attach a dressing
Powder	Finely ground drug plus vehicle or effervescent granules
Suppository	A medicated gelatin molded into a cone for placement in a body orifice (e.g., the anal canal)

tion of a substance such as procaine to anesthetize the lower limbs, or withdrawal of spinal fluid to be studied.

Intravenous injection (into a vein) is given when an immediate reaction to the medication is desired. The drug enters the venous circulation and is spread rapidly throughout the body.

Oral administration of medicines is the most common method of all. Forms such as tablets, capsules, powders, and liquids are easily administered orally.

Rectal administration of drugs is limited. In the past some medications have been introduced through the rectum to be absorbed by its mucous lining. Such methods have proved undesirable because of difficulties in regulating dosage.

Sublingual and *buccal* introductions of medicines usually consist of placing easily dissolved agents such as troches (or lozenges), or tablets, under the tongue. They dissolve slowly and are absorbed by the mucous lining.

External Administration

Medications administered externally include inunctions, ointments, pastes, plasters, and solutions.

Inunctions are oily or medicated substances that are rubbed into the skin and result in a local or systemic reaction. Oil-based liniments and petroleum analgesic balms used as massage lubricants are examples of inunctions.

Ointments consisting of oil, petroleum jelly, or lanolin combined with drugs are applied for long-lasting topical medication.

Pastes are ointments with a nonfat base. They are spread on cloth and usually produce a cooling effect on the skin.

Plasters are thicker than ointments and are spread either on cloth or paper or directly on the skin. They usually contain an irritant, are applied as a counterirritant, and are used for relieving pain, increasing circulation, and decreasing inflammation.

Transdermal patches are Band-Aid–like patches that contain various types of slow-release medications. They may be left in place for several days.

Solutions can be administered externally and are extremely varied, consisting principally of bacteriostatics. Antiseptics, disinfectants, vasoconstrictors, and liquid rubefacients are examples.

Legal Concerns

Dispensing Prescription Drugs

The dispensing of drugs to the athlete by a member of the coaching staff or an athletic trainer, in a legal sense, is both clear and concise. *At no time can anyone other than a person licensed by law legally prescribe or dispense drugs for an athlete.* An athletic trainer, unless specifically allowed by state licensure, is not permitted to dispense a prescription drug. Failure to heed this fact can be a violation of the federal Food, Drug, and Cosmetic Act and state statutes. A violation of these laws could mean legal problems for the physician, athletic trainer, school, school district, or even the league.

At no time can anyone other than a person licensed by law legally prescribe or dispense drugs for an athlete.

Dispensing Over-the-Counter Drugs

The situation is not so clear-cut for nonprescription drugs. Basically, the athletic trainer may be allowed to administer a single dose of a nonprescription medication. For example, most secondary schools do not allow the athletic trainer or coach to dispense nonprescription (over-the-counter [OTC]) drugs that are to be taken internally by the athlete, including aspirin and OTC cold remedies. The application of nonprescription wound medications is allowed by some secondary schools under the category of first aid. On the other hand, some high school athletic trainers in the United States are not allowed to apply even a wound medication in the name of first aid but can only clean the wound with soap and water. The athlete must then be sent to the school nurse for medication. The dispensing of vitamins and even dextrose may be specifically disallowed by some school districts. At the college or professional level, minors are not usually involved, and the administration of nonprescription medications may be less restrictive. It is assumed that athletes who are of legal age have the right to use whatever nonprescription drugs they choose. However, this right does not preclude the fact that the athletic trainer or coach must be reasonable and prudent about the types of nonprescription drugs offered to the athlete.

Generally, the administration of single doses of nonprescription medicines by a member of the athletic staff to any athlete depends on the philosophy of the school district and must be under the direction of the team physician. As in all other areas of sports medicine and athletic training, one is obligated to act reasonably and prudently.

Record Keeping

Those involved in any health care profession are acutely aware of the necessity of maintaining complete, up-to-date medical records. The sports medicine setting is no exception. If medications are administered by an athletic trainer, maintaining accurate records of the types of medications administered is just as important as recording progress notes, treatments given, and rehabilitation plans. The athletic trainer may be dealing with a number of different patients simultaneously while trying to get a team ready for practice or competition. At times things become hectic, and stopping to record each time a medication is administered is difficult. Nevertheless, the athletic trainer should include the following information on the medication administration log: name of the athlete, complaint or symptoms, name of medication given, quantity of medication given, method of administration, and date and time of administration.[32]

Each athletic trainer should be aware of state regulations and laws that pertain to the ordering, prescribing, distributing, storing, and dispensing or administering of medications. Obtaining legal counsel, working with the state board of pharmacy or a student health clinic, working in cooperation with a team physician, and establishing strict written policies can all minimize the chances of violating state laws that regulate the use of medications.[32]

The Safety of Pharmaceutical Drugs

As stated many times before, no drug can be considered completely safe and harmless. If a drug is potent enough to effect some physiological action, it is also strong enough, under some conditions, to be dangerous. All persons react individually to any drug. A given amount of a specific medication may result in no adverse reaction in one athlete, whereas another athlete may experience a pronounced adverse response. Both the athlete and the athletic trainer should be fully aware of any untoward effect a drug may have. It is essential that the athlete be instructed clearly about when specifically to take medications, with meals or not, and what not to combine with the drug, such as other drugs or specific foods. Some drugs can nullify the effect of another drug or can cause a serious antagonistic reaction. For example, calcium, which is found in a variety of foods and in some medications, can nullify the effects of the antibiotic tetracycline (Figure 16-2).

Drug Responses

Individuals react differently to the same medication, and different conditions may alter the effect of a drug on the athlete. Drugs themselves can be changed through age or improper preservation, as well as through the manner in which they are administered. Response variations also result from differences in each individual's size or age.

Alcohol should not be ingested with a wide variety of drugs, both prescription and nonprescription. A fatty diet may decrease a drug's effectiveness by interfering with its absorption. Excessively acid foods such as fruits, carbonated drinks, or vegetable juice may cause adverse drug reactions.[3] Athletic trainers and coaches must thor-

16-1

Critical Thinking Exercise

A college-age softball player comes into the training room complaining of a sore throat and stuffy head and asks the athletic trainer to give her some "drugs" to get rid of her problem.

? Is the athletic trainer legally allowed to give her any type of medication, and if so how should the athletic trainer give it to the athlete?

Figure 16-2

It must be remembered that all persons react individually to any drug.

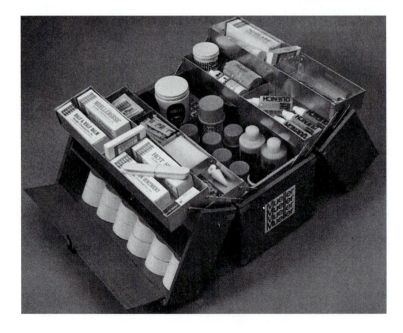

TABLE 16-2   **General Responses Produced by Drugs and Medication**

Addiction	Body response to certain types of drugs that produces both a physiological need and a psychological craving for the substance
Antagonistic action	Result observed when medications, used together, have adverse effects or counteract one another
Cumulative effect	Exaggerated drug effects, which occur when the body is unable to metabolize a drug as rapidly as it is administered; the accumulated, unmetabolized drug may cause unfavorable reactions
Depressive action	Effect from drugs that slow down cell function
Habituation	Individual's development of a psychological need for a specific medication
Hypersensitivity	Allergic response to a specific drug; such allergies may be demonstrated by a mild skin irritation, itching, a rash, or a severe anaphylactic reaction, which could be fatal
Idiosyncrasy	Unusual reaction to a drug; a distinctive response
Irritation	Process, as well as effect, caused by substances that result in a cellular change; mild irritation may stimulate cell activity, whereas moderate or severe irritation by a drug may decrease cell activity
Paradoxical reaction	A drug-induced effect that is the exact opposite of that which is therapeutically intended
Potentiating agent	A pharmaceutical that increases the effect of another; for example, codeine is potentiated by aspirin, and therefore less of it is required to relieve pain
Specific effect	Action usually produced by a drug in a select tissue or organ system
Side effect	The result of a medication that is given for a particular condition but affects other body areas or has effects other than those sought
Stimulation	Effect caused by drugs that speed up cell activity
Synergistic effect	Result that occurs when drugs given together produce a greater reaction than when given alone
Tolerance	Condition existing when a certain drug dosage is no longer able to give a therapeutic action and must therefore be increased

oughly know the athletes with whom they work. The possibility of an adverse drug reaction is ever present and requires continual education and vigilance.

Table 16-2 is a list of general body responses sometimes produced by drugs and medications.

Buying Medications

One of the athletic department's best friends is the local pharmacist. The pharmacist can assist in the selection and purchase of nonprescription drugs, can save money by suggesting the lower-priced generic drugs, and can act as a general advisor on what drugs are most effective, the dose of a medicine, and even the inherent dangers in a specific drug.

All pharmaceuticals must be properly labeled, indicating clearly the content, expiration date, and any dangers or contraindications for use. Pharmaceutical manufacturers place the expiration date on drugs, and it is up to the athletic trainer or coach to locate this date on the package. Individuals buying medications should always learn the best ways to store them, including the correct temperature and moisture and the amount of light that may be tolerated.[32]

PROTOCOLS FOR USING OVER-THE-COUNTER MEDICATIONS

In most cases, the athletic trainer will be concerned only with nonprescription medications. A nonprescription drug is also called an over-the-counter drug; it is one that can be bought without a prescription.

There is a major difference between prescription and nonprescription drugs. A prescription drug is designed to relieve symptoms or cure a disease or injury. The OTC drug is not curative but is generally designed to relieve pain or inflammation. As with prescription drugs, great caution must be taken with OTC drugs.

The Protocols for the Use of Over-the-Counter Drugs for Athletic Trainers presented on pages 373-379 are guidelines for treating a number of minor illnesses or conditions seen frequently in the athletic population. The authors and publisher have exerted every effort to ensure that drug selection and dosage set forth in this text are in accord with current recommendations and practice at the time of publication. However, in view of ongoing research, changes in government regulations, and the constant flow of information relating to drug therapy and drug reactions, the reader is urged to check the package insert for each drug for any change in indications and dosage and for added warnings and precautions. This is especially important when the recommended agent is a new or infrequently employed drug.

SELECTED THERAPEUTIC DRUGS USED TO TREAT THE ATHLETE

In sports the use of drugs and medicine is widespread, as in society in general, but it also is unique to the special needs of the athlete (Figure 16-3). Table 16-3 (see p. 380) summarizes the various classifications of drugs available.

This section discusses the most common pharmaceutical practices in athletic training to date and the specific drugs that are in use. The discussion includes both prescription and nonprescription drugs, with emphasis on what should most concern the coach or athletic trainer and what the medications or materials are designed to accomplish. *(Text continues on page 380.)*

Figure 16-3

Athletic trainers and coaches must understand the health belief systems of the athletes with whom they work.

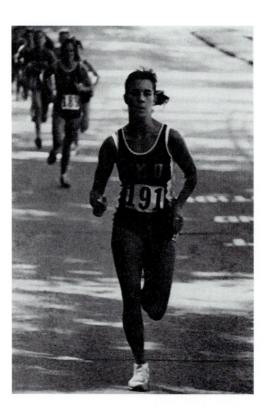

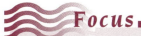

Focus

Protocols for the use of over-the-counter drugs for athletic trainers

The athletic trainer is often responsible for initial screening of athletes who have various illnesses or injuries. Frequently, the athletic trainer must make decisions regarding the appropriate use of over-the-counter medications for athletes. Subjective findings such as onset, duration, medication taken, and known allergies must be included in the screening evaluation.

The following protocols should be viewed as guidelines to the disposition of the athlete. The protocols are aimed at clarifying the use of over-the-counter drugs in the treatment of common problems encountered by the sports therapist while covering or traveling with a particular team. These guidelines do not cover every situation the sports therapist encounters in assessing and managing the athlete's physical problems. Therefore physician consultation is recommended wherever there is uncertainty in making a decision regarding the appropriate care of the athlete.

Existing Illness or Injury	Appropriate Treatment Protocol
Temperature	
Greater than or equal to 102° F orally	Consult physician ASAP.
Less than 102° F but more than 99.5° F	Patient may be given acetaminophen. See the section on acetaminophen administration later in this box.
	Limit exercise of athlete. Do not allow participation in practice.
	If fever decreases to less than 99.5° F the athlete may participate in practice.
	If athlete is to be involved in an intercollegiate event, consult with a physician concerning participation.
Less than or equal to 99.5° F orally	Follow management guidelines for fever less than 102° F, but allow athlete to practice or compete.
Throat	
History	Advise saline gargles (½ tsp salt in a glass of warm water).
Sore throat	Patient may also be given Cepastat/Chloraseptic throat lozenges. Before administering determine the following:
No fever	
No chills	Is the patient allergic to Cepastat/Chloraseptic (phenol containing) lozenges? If yes, do not administer.
Sore throat, fever	Determine temperature. If fever, manage as outlined in temperature protocol and consult physician ASAP.
Sore throat, fever, or swollen glands	Consult physician ASAP.
Nose	
Watery discharge	Patient may be given pseudoephedrine (Sudafed) tablets. See pseudoephedrine administration protocols.
Nasal congestion	Patient may be given oxymetazoline HCl (Afrin) nasal spray. See oxymetazoline administration protocol.
Chest	
Cough	Patient may be administered Robitussin DM (generic guaifenesin with dextromethorphan). Before administering determine the following:
Dry hacking	
Clear mucoid sputum	Is the patient going to be involved in practice or game within 4 hours of administration of medication? If yes, do not give Robitussin DM
	If indicated, administer one dose, 10 ml (2 tsp). Inform the patient that drowsiness may occur. Repeat doses may be administered every 6 hours. Push fluids, encourage patient to drink as much as possible.

Continued

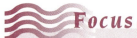

Focus

Protocols for the use of over-the-counter drugs for athletic trainers—cont'd

Chest—cont'd

Green or rusty sputum	Consult physician ASAP.
Severe, persistent cough	Consult physician ASAP.

Ears

Discomfort due to ears popping	Patient may be given pseudoephedrine (Sudafed) tablets or oxymetazoline HCl (Afrin) nasal spray. See pseudoephedrine administration protocol, oxymetazoline protocol.
Earache (or external otitis)	Patient may be given acetaminophen. Consult physician ASAP. See acetaminophen administration protocol.
Recurrent earache	Consult physician ASAP.

Prevention of motion sickness

Complaint: history of nausea, dizziness, or vomiting associated with travel	Patient may be given dimenhydrinate (Dramamine) or diphenhydramine (Benadryl).
	Before administering determine the following:
	Is the patient sensitive or allergic to Dramamine, Benadryl, or any other antihistamine? If yes, do not administer.
	Has the patient taken any other antihistamines (e.g., Actifed, Chlor-Trimeton, various cold medications) or other medications that cause sedation within the last 6 hours? If yes, do not administer.
	Does the patient have asthma, glaucoma, or enlargement of the prostate gland? If yes, do not administer.
	Is the patient going to be involved in practice or game within 4 hours after administration of medication? If yes, do not administer.
	Administer Dramamine or Benadryl dose based on body weight, 30 to 60 minutes before departure time. Dramamine: under 125 lb, one 50 mg tablet; over 125 lb, two 50 mg tablets. Benadryl: under 125 lb, one 25 mg capsule; over 125 lb, two 25 mg capsules.
	Inform the patient that drowsiness may occur for 4-6 hours after taking these medications. Avoid alcoholic beverages. Avoid driving for 6 hours after taking. If traveling time is extended, another dose may be administered 6 hours after the first dose.

Nausea, vomiting

Prolonged, severe	Consult physician ASAP.

Nausea, gastric upset, heartburn, butterflies in the stomach

Associated with dietary indiscretion or tension	Administer an antacid as a single dose, as defined by label of particular antacid (e.g., Riopan, Gelusil, Maalox, Pepto Bismol, Titralac).
Associated with abdominal or chest pain	Consult physician ASAP.
Vomiting, nausea—no severe distress	Monitor symptoms. Patient may be given dimenhydrinate (Dramamine) or diphenhydramine (Benadryl) orally.
	Same as instructions and precautions under motion sickness prevention.

Continued

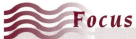

Focus

Protocols for the use of over-the-counter drugs for athletic trainers—cont'd

Nausea, gastric upset, heartburn, butterflies in the stomach—cont'd

Vomiting: projectile, coffee ground, febrile	Consult physician ASAP.

Diarrhea

Associated with abdominal pain or tenderness or dehydration, bloody stools, febrile, recurrent diarrhea	Consult physician ASAP.
Frequent loose stools not associated with any of the above signs or symptoms	Encourage clear liquid diet. Encourage avoidance of dairy products and high-fat foods for 24 hours. If diarrhea persists consult physician ASAP.

Patient may be given kaolin-pectin (Kaopectate) or loperamide (Imodium A-D). Before administering determine the following:

How long has patient had diarrhea? If longer than 24 hours, see physician.

Is patient taking any digitalis medication (e.g., digoxin, lanoxin, Lanoxicaps)? If yes, see physician.

Patient may be administered one dose of kaolin-pectin (Kaopectate) (6-8 tsp). Shake well. Repeat dose after each loose bowel movement until diarrhea is controlled. Should not be used for more than 2 days. Discontinue use if fever develops or if diarrhea is not controlled within 24 hours of treatment, and consult physician. **OR:** Administer one dose (2 caplets) of loperamide (Imodium A-D 2 mg per caplet). One caplet may be administered after each loose stool not to exceed 8 mg (4 caplets) per 24 hours. Inform the patient that dizziness or drowsiness may occur within 12 hours after taking this medication. Avoid alcoholic beverages. Use caution while driving or performing tasks requiring alertness.

Constipation

Prolonged or severe abdominal pain or tenderness, nausea, or vomiting	Consult physician ASAP.
Discomfort associated with dietary change or decreased fluid intake	Patient may be administered milk of magnesia 30 ml as a single dose. Before administering determine the following: Does the patient have chronic renal disease? If yes, do not administer.

Recommend increased fluid intake, increased intake of fruits, bulk vegetables, or cereals.

Headache

Pain associated with elevated blood pressure, temperature elevation, blurred vision, nausea, vomiting, or history of migraine.	Consult physician ASAP.

Continued

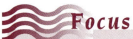

Focus

Protocols for the use of over-the-counter drugs for athletic trainers—cont'd

Headache—cont'd

Pain across forehead (mild headache)	Patient may be given acetaminophen. See acetaminophen administration protocol.
Tension headache, occipital pain	Patient may be given acetaminophen. See acetaminophen administration protocol.
Pain in antrum or forehead associated with sinus or nasal congestion	Patient may be given pseudoephedrine (Sudafed) tablets and acetaminophen. See protocols for pseudoephedrine and acetaminophen administration.

Musculoskeletal injuries

Deformity	Consult physician ASAP.

Localized pain and tenderness, impaired range of motion	First aid to part as soon as possible:
	  Ice
	  Compression—Ace bandage
	  Elevation
	  Protection—crutches, sling, or splint

Pain with swelling, discoloration, no impaired movement or localized tenderness	If injury interferes with patient's normal activities, consult physician within 24 hours. Patient may be given acetaminophen. See acetaminophen administration protocol.

Skin

Localized or generalized rash accompanied by elevated temperature, enlarged lymph nodes, sore throat, stiff neck, infected skin lesion, dyspnea, wheezing	Consult physician ASAP.

Mild, localized, nonvesicular skin eruptions accompanied by pruritis	Hydrocortisone 0.5% cream may be applied.
	Before administering determine the following:
	  Is the patient taking any medication? If yes, do not administer. Refer to physician.
	  Are eyes or any large area of the body involved? If yes, do not administer. Refer to physician.
	  Is there any evidence of lice infestation? If yes, do not administer. Refer to physician.
	The cream may be repeated every 6 hours if needed. Do not use more than 3 times daily.

Abrasions	Control bleeding. Clean with antibacterial soap and water. Apply appropriate dressing and antibiotic ointment. Monitor for signs of infection. Dressing may be changed 2-3 times a day if needed.
Localized erythema caused by ultraviolet rays	Advise application of compresses soaked in a solution of cold water.

Continued

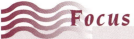

Focus

Protocols for the use of over-the-counter drugs for athletic trainers—cont'd

Skin—cont'd

Jock itch or athlete's foot	Advise 10-15 minute application of compresses soaked in cool water to relieve intense itching. Patient may be given miconazole (Micatin) cream topically. Before administering determine the following: Is the patient sensitive or allergic to miconazole? If yes, do not administer. Consult physician ASAP. Is the patient receiving other types of treatment for rash in same area? If yes, do not administer. Consult physician ASAP. Instruct patient to wash and dry area of rash and then apply ¼-½ inch ribbon of cream (give patient the cream on a clean gauze pad) and rub gently on the infected area. Spread evenly and thinly over rash. The dose may be repeated in 8-12 hours (twice a day). Consult physician within 24 hours.

Skin wounds

Lacerations	Control bleeding. Cleanse area with antibacterial soap and water. Apply sterile strips. Consult physician immediately if there is any question about the necessity for suturing.
Extensive lacerations or other severe skin wounds	Control bleeding. Protect area with dressing. Refer to physician immediately.

Wound infection

Febrile, marked cellulitis, red streaks, tender or enlarged nodes	Consult physician ASAP.
Localized inflammation, afebrile, absence of nodes and streaks	Warm soaks to affected area. Consult physician ASAP.

Burns

Grade 1—erythema of skin, limited area	Apply cold compresses to affected area. Dressing is not necessary on grade 1 burns. If less than 45 minutes have elapsed since burn injury, clean gently with soap and water. Patient may be given acetaminophen. See acetaminophen administration protocol.
Grade 1 with extensive involvement over body	Consult physician ASAP.
Grade 2—erythema with blistering	Consult physician ASAP.
Grade 3—pearly white appearance of affected area, no pain	Consult physician ASAP.

Continued

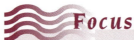

Focus

Protocols for the use of over-the-counter drugs for athletic trainers—cont'd

Allergies

Athlete with known seasonal allergies who forgot to bring own medication

Patient may be given chlorpheniramine (Chlor-Trimeton) 4 mg tablets. Before administering determine the following:

Is the patient sensitive to chlorpheniramine? If yes, do not administer. Consult physician ASAP.

Does the patient have asthma, urinary retention, or glaucoma? If yes, do not administer. Consult physician ASAP.

Is patient going to be involved in training or game within 4 hours of administration of medication? If yes, do not administer. Consult physician ASAP.

Has the patient taken any other antihistamines (e.g., Actifed, Dramamine, various cold medications) or other medications that cause drowsiness within the last 6 hours? If yes, do not administer. Consult physician ASAP.

Patient may be administered one dose of chlorpheniramine 4 mg, ½ or 1 tablet. Repeat doses may be administered every 4 hours. Inform the patient that drowsiness may occur for 4-6 hours after taking this medication. Avoid alcoholic beverages. Avoid driving or operation of machinery for 6 hours after taking. Contact physician if symptoms do not abate.

Contact lens care

NOTE: There are three types of contact lenses:
   Hard
   Gas permeable
   Soft

Solutions are labeled for use with a *particular* type of lens and should not be used for any other type of lens.

Do not use solutions preserved with thimersol or chlorhexidine because of possible allergy or irritation.

Lens needs rinsing/wetting before insertion

Hard lens: use all-purpose wetting/soaking solution (e.g., Wet-N-Soak).

Gas-permeable lens: use all-purpose wetting/soaking solution (e.g., Wet-N-Soak).

Soft lens: use rinsing/soaking solution (e.g., Soft Mate ps).

Lens needs soaking/storage

Hard lens: use all-purpose wetting/soaking solution (e.g., Wet-N-Soak).

Gas-permeable lens: use all-purpose wetting/soaking solution (e.g., Wet-N-Soak).

Soft lens: use rinsing/soaking solution (e.g., Soft Mate ps).

Lens needs cleaning

Hard lens: use cleaning solution (e.g., EasyClean).

Gas-permeable lens: use cleaning solution (e.g., EasyClean).

Soft lens: use cleaning solution (e.g., Lens Plus Daily Cleaner).

Eye care

Foreign body—minor: sand, eyelash, etc.

Use eye wash irrigation solution (Dacriose).

Irritation—minor

Use artificial tears. Do not use with contact lens in eye.

Severe irritation, foreign body not easily removed, trauma

Consult physician ASAP.

Continued

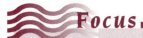

Focus

Protocols for the use of over-the-counter drugs for athletic trainers—cont'd

Administration protocols for common over-the-counter drugs used in sports medicine

Acetaminophen protocol (Tylenol)

Before *administering* determine the following:

Is the patient allergic to acetaminophen? If yes, do not give acetaminophen.

Administer acetaminophen 325 mg, two tablets. Repeat doses may be *administered* every 6 hours if needed. If *dispensing* occurs, use labeled package only. Patient instructions must accompany *dispensing*.

Ibuprofen (Advil) or naproxin sodium (Aleve) protocol

Before *administering* determine the following:

Is the patient allergic to aspirin (e.g., asthma, swelling, shock, or hives associated with aspirin use)? If yes, do not give ibuprofen or naproxin sodium because even though they contain no aspirin or salicylates, cross-reactions may occur in patients allergic to aspirin.

Does the patient have renal disease or gastrointestinal ulcerations? If yes, do not administer ibuprofen or naproxin sodium.

Administer ibuprofen 200 mg (Advil) or naproxin sodium 200 mg (Aleve). Repeat doses may be *administered* every 4 to 6 hours if needed. Do not exceed 6 tablets in a 24-hour period without consulting physician.

The patient should take ibuprofen with food if occasional and mild heartburn, upset stomach, or mild stomach pain occurs. Consult physician if these symptoms are more than mild or persist.

Pseudoephedrine protocol (Sudafed)

Before *administering* determine the following:

Is the patient allergic or sensitive to pseudoephedrine? If yes, do not administer.

Does the patient have high blood pressure, heart disease, diabetes, urinary retention, glaucoma, or thyroid disease? If yes, do not administer.

Does the patient have problems with sweating? If yes, do not administer.

Do not administer 4 hours before practice or game.

Do not administer if patient is involved in postseason play.

Administer pseudoephedrine (Sudafed) 30 mg, two tablets. Repeat doses may be *administered* every 6 hours up to 4 times a day. If *dispensing* occurs use labeled package only. Patient instructions must accompany *dispensing*.

Oxymetazoline protocol (Afrin)

Before *administering* determine the following:

Is the patient allergic or sensitive to Afrin or Otrivin? If yes, do not administer.

Does the patient react unusually to nose sprays or drops? If yes, do not administer.

Administer 2-3 sprays of oxymetazoline (Afrin) 0.05% nasal spray into each nostril. Repeat doses may be administered every 12 hours. (The container can be marked with the patient's name and maintained by the trainer for repeat *administration*, or it can be *dispensed* to the patient. Patient instructions must accompany *dispensing*.)

Do not use the same container for different patients.

Do not use for more than 3 days without physician supervision.

Use small package sizes to reduce risk of overuse or rebound congestion.

The information in this box is based on the most up-to-date research and suggestions made by individuals in the field of athletic training. The authors and publisher disclaim any responsibility for any adverse effects or consequences from the misapplication or injudicious use of information within this box. It is also accepted as judicious that the athletic trainer performing his or her duties is, at all times, working under the guidance of a licensed physician.

TABLE 16-3 Pharmaceutical Classifications

Analgesics (anodynes)	Pain-relieving drugs
Anesthetics	Agents that produce local or general numbness to touch, pain, or stimulation
Antacids	Substances that neutralize acidity; commonly used in the digestive tract
Anticoagulants	Agents that prevent coagulation of blood
Antidotes	Substances that prevent or counteract the action of a poison
Antipruritics	Agents that relieve itching
Antiseptics	Agents that kill bacteria or inhibit their growth and can be applied to living tissue
Antispasmodics	Agents that relieve muscle spasm
Antitussives	Agents that inhibit or prevent coughing
Astringents	Agents that cause contraction or puckering action
Bacteriostatics and fungistatics	Agents that retard or inhibit the growth of bacteria or fungi
Carminatives	Agents that relieve flatulence (caused by gases) in the intestinal tract
Cathartics	Agents used to evacuate substances from the bowels; active purgatives
Caustics	Burning agents, capable of destroying living tissue
Counterirritants	Agents applied locally to produce an inflammatory reaction for the relief of a deeper inflammation
Depressants	Agents that diminish body functions or nerve activity
Disinfectants	Agents that kill or inhibit the growth of microorganisms; should be applied only to nonliving materials
Diuretics	Agents that increase the secretion of urine
Emetics	Agents that cause vomiting
Expectorants	Agents that suppress coughing
Hemostatics	Substances that either slow down or stop bleeding or hemorrhage
Irritants	Agents that cause irritation
Narcotics	Drugs that produce analgesic and hypnotic effects
Sedatives	Agents that relieve anxiety
Skeletal muscle relaxants	Drugs that depress neural activity within skeletal muscles
Stimulants	Agents that excite the central nervous system
Vasoconstrictors and vasodilators	Drugs that, respectively, constrict or dilate blood vessels

Drugs to Combat Infection

Combating infection, especially skin infection; is of major importance in sports. Serious infection can cause countless hours of lost time and has even been the indirect cause of death.

> Drugs used to combat infection include local antiseptics and disinfectants, antifungal agents, and antibiotics.

Local Antiseptics and Disinfectants

Antiseptics are substances that can be placed on living tissue for the express purpose of either killing bacteria or inhibiting their growth. Disinfectants are substances that combat microorganisms but should be applied only to nonliving objects. Other general names given to antiseptics and disinfectants are germicides, which are designed to destroy bacteria; fungicides, which kill fungi; sporicides, which destroy spores; and sanitizers, which minimize contamination by microorganisms.

> Antiseptics and disinfectants include alcohol, phenol, halogens, and oxidizing agents.

In sports many agents are used to combat infection. It is critical that agents have a broad spectrum of activity against infective organisms, including the human immunodeficiency virus (HIV).

Alcohol   Alcohol is one of the most widely used skin disinfectants. Ethyl alcohol (70% by weight) and isopropyl alcohol (70%) are equally effective. They are inexpensive and nonirritating; they kill bacteria immediately, with the exception of spores. However, they have no long-lasting germicidal action. Besides being directly combined with other agents to form tinctures, alcohol acts independently on the skin as an antiseptic and astringent. In a 70% solution it can be used for disinfecting instruments. Because of alcohol's rapid rate of evaporation, it produces a mild anesthetic action. Combined with 20% benzoin, it is used in athletics as a topical skin dressing to provide a protective skin coating and astringent action.

Phenol   Phenol was one of the earliest antiseptics and disinfectants used by the medical profession. From its inception to the present it has been used to control disease organisms, both as an antiseptic and as a disinfectant. It is available in liquids of varying concentrations and emollients. Substances that are derived from phenol and that cause less irritation are now used more extensively. Some of these derivatives are resorcinol, thymol, and the common household disinfectant Lysol.

Halogens   Halogens are chemical substances (chlorine, fluoride, and bromine) that are used for their antiseptic and disinfectant qualities. Iodophors, or halogenated compounds, a combination of iodine and a carrier, create a much less irritating preparation than tincture of iodine. A popular iodophor is povidone-iodine complex (Betadine), which is an excellent germicide commonly used as a surgical scrub by surgeons. Betadine as an antiseptic and germicide in athletic training has proved extremely effective on skin lesions such as lacerations, abrasions, and floor burns.

Oxidizing agents   Oxidizing agents, as represented by hydrogen peroxide (3%), are commonly used in athletic training. Hydrogen peroxide is an antiseptic that, because of its oxidation, affects bacteria but readily decomposes in the presence of organic substances such as blood and pus. For this reason it has little effect as an antiseptic. Contact with organic material produces an effervescence, during which no great destruction of bacteria takes place. The chief value of hydrogen peroxide in the care of wounds is its ability to cleanse the infected cutaneous and mucous membranes. Application of hydrogen peroxide to wounds results in the formation of an active effervescent gas that dislodges particles of wound material and debris and, by removing degenerated tissue, eliminates the wound as a likely environment for bacterial breeding. Hydrogen peroxide also possesses compounds that are widely used as antiseptics. Because it is nontoxic, hydrogen peroxide may be used for cleansing mucous membranes. A diluted solution (50% water and 50% hydrogen peroxide) can be used for treating inflammatory conditions of the mouth and throat.

Antifungal Agents

Many medicinal agents on the market are designed to treat fungi, which are commonly found in and around athletic facilities. The three most common fungi are *Epidermophyton*, *Trichophyton*, and *Candida albicans*.

In recent years there has been successful development and use of antifungal agents such as ketoconazole (Nizoral), amphotericin B (Fungizone), and griseofulvin. Both ketoconazole and amphotericin B seem to be effective against deep-seated fungus infections such as those caused by *Candida albicans*. Ketoconazole, fluconazole, and griseofulvin, all of which can be administered orally, produce an effective fungistatic action against the specific fungus species of *Microsporum*, *Trichophyton*, and *Epidermophyton*, all of which are associated with common athlete's foot.[3] Given over a long period of time griseofulvin becomes a functioning part of the cutaneous tissues, especially the skin, hair, and nails, producing a prolonged and continuous fungistatic action. Miconazole (Micatin), clotrimazole (Lotrimin), and tolnaftate (Tinactin, which does not treat *Candida* infections) are topical medications for a superficial fungus infection caused by *Trichophyton* and other fungi.

Mechanical antiseptics, usually soaps that provide a cleansing and detergent action, remove pathogens from the skin.

Antibiotics

Antibiotics include penicillin, bacitracin, tetracycline, erythromycin, sulfonamides, and quinolones.

Antibiotics are chemical agents that are produced by microorganisms. Their useful action is primarily a result of their interfering with the necessary metabolic processes of pathogenic microorganisms. In sports they are used by the physician as either topical dressings or systemic medications. The indiscriminate use of antibiotics can produce extreme hypersensitivity or idiosyncrasies and can prevent the development of natural immunity or resistance to subsequent infections. The use of any antibiotic must be carefully controlled by the physician, who selects the drug on the basis of the most desirable type of administration and the least amount of toxicity to the patient.

The antibiotics mentioned here are just a few of the many available. New types continue to be developed, mainly because, over a period of time, microorganisms often become resistant to a particular antibiotic, especially if it is indiscriminately used. Some of the more common antibiotics are penicillin, streptomycin, bacitracin, tetracycline, erythromycin, and the sulfonamides.[3]

Penicillin   Penicillin as a prescription medication is probably the most important of the antibiotics; it is useful in a variety of skin and systemic infections. In general, penicillin interferes with the metabolism of the bacteria.

Bacitracin   Bacitracin has a broad spectrum of effectiveness as an antibacterial agent. Bacitracin plus polymixin (Polysporin) also has a broad spectrum of effectiveness as an antibacterial agent. Adding neomycin to the product (Neosporin) does not increase effectiveness, and some individuals are allergic to neomycin.

Tetracycline   Tetracyclines consist of a wide group of antibiotics that have a broad antibacterial spectrum. Their application, which is usually oral, modifies the infection rather than eradicating it completely.

Erythromycin   Erythromycin is most often used for streptococcal infection and *Mycoplasma pneumoniae*. It has the same general spectrum as penicillin and is a useful alternative in the penicillin-allergic patient.

Sulfonamides   Sulfonamides are a group of synthetic antibiotics. In general, sulfonamides make pathogens vulnerable to phagocytes by inhibiting certain enzymatic actions.

Quinolones   Quinolones are a relatively new group of antibiotics. They have a broad spectrum of activity. Patients taking these must be carefully monitored for adverse effects.

Drugs that Inhibit Pain and Inflammation

Pain Relievers

Drugs used to inhibit pain or inflammation include counterirritants and local anesthetics, narcotic analgesics, and nonnarcotic analgesics and antipyretics.

Controlling pain in an athlete can involve innumerable drugs and procedures, depending on the beliefs of the athletic trainer, coach, or physician. As discussed in Chapter 7, why pain is positively affected by certain methods is not clearly understood; however, some of the possible reasons are as follows:

- The excitatory effect of an individual impulse is depressed.
- An individual impulse is inhibited.
- The perceived impulse is decreased.
- Anxiety created by the pain or impending pain is decreased.

Counterirritants and Local Anesthetics

Analgesics give relief by causing a systemic and topical analgesia. Many chemical reactions on the skin can inhibit pain sensations through rapid evaporation, which causes a cooling action, or by counterirritating the skin. Irritating and counterirritating substances used in sports act as rubefacients (skin reddeners) and skin stimulants, although their popularity has decreased in recent years. Their application causes a local increase in blood circulation, redness, and a rise in skin temperature. Frequently mild pain can be reduced by a counterirritant, which produces a stimulus to the skin of such intensity that the athlete is no longer aware of the pain. Some examples of counterirritants include liniments, analgesic balms, heat, and cold.

Spray coolants   Spray coolants, because of their rapid evaporation, act as topical anesthetics to the skin. Several commercial coolants are presently on the market. Chloromethane is one of the most popular spray coolants currently used in sports. Cooling results so quickly that superficial freezing takes place, inhibiting pain impulses for a short time. Athletic trainers disagree on the effectiveness of spray coolants. Some athletic trainers use them extensively for strains, sprains, and contusions. In most cases, spray coolants are useful only when other analgesics are not available.

Alcohol   Alcohol evaporates rapidly when applied to the skin, causing a refreshingly cool effect that gives a temporary analgesia.

Cold   Cold applications also immediately act to constrict blood vessels and to numb sensory nerve endings. Applications of ice packs or submersion of a part in ice water may completely anesthetize an area. If extreme cold is used, caution must be taken that tissue damage does not result.

Menthol   Menthol is an alcohol taken from mint oils and is principally used as a local analgesic, counterirritant, and antiseptic. Most often in sports it is used with a petroleum base for treating cold symptoms and in analgesic balms.

Local anesthetics   Local anesthetics are usually injected by the physician in and around injury sites for minor surgical procedures or to alleviate the pain of movement. Lydocaine hydrochloride is used extensively as a local anesthetic.

> Counterirritants include spray coolants, alcohol, cold, menthol, and local anesthetics.

Narcotic Analgesics

Most narcotics used in medicine are derived directly from opium or are synthetic opiates. They depress pain impulses and the individual's respiratory center. The two most often used derivatives are codeine and morphine.

Codeine   Codeine resembles morphine in its action but is less potent. Codeine is effective in combination with nonnarcotic analgesics. In small doses it is a cough suppressant found in many cough medicines.

Propoxyphene hydrochloride   Propoxyphene hydrochloride (Darvon) is a mild analgesic narcotic that is slightly stronger than aspirin in its pain relief. It is not an antiinflammatory drug. It is addictive, and when combined with alcohol, tranquilizers, or other sedatives or depressants, it can be fatal.

Morphine   Morphine depresses pain sensations to a greater extent than any other drug. It is also the most dangerous drug because of its ability to depress respiration and because of its habit-forming qualities. Morphine is never used in the following situations: before a diagnosis has been made by the physician; when the subject is unconscious; when there is a head injury; or when there is a decreased rate of breathing. It is never repeated within 2 hours.

Meperidine   Meperidine (Demerol) is used as a substitute for morphine for the relief of mild or moderate pain and is effective only when given intravenously or intramuscularly.

> Narcotic analgesics include codeine, propoxyphene hydrochloride, morphine, and meperidine.

Nonnarcotic Analgesics and Antipyretics

Nonnarcotic analgesics are those drugs designed to suppress all but the most severe pain, without the patient's losing consciousness. In most cases these drugs also act as antipyretics, regulating the temperature control centers.

Acetaminophen   Acetaminophen (Tylenol) is an effective analgesic and antipyretic but has no antiinflammatory activity. Because it does not irritate the gastroin-

> Nonnarcotic analgesics include acetaminophen.

testinal system, it is often a replacement for aspirin in noninflammatory conditions. Overingestion could lead to liver damage.

Drugs to Reduce Inflammation

Sports physicians have a wide choice of drugs at their disposal for treatment of inflammation. There is also a great variety of over-the-counter drugs that claim to deal effectively with inflammation of the musculoskeletal system. The problem of proper drug selection is tenuous, even for a physician, because of new drugs continually coming to the forefront. The situation is compounded by highly advertised over-the-counter preparations. Any drug selection, especially drugs designed to treat the inflammatory process, must be effective, must be appropriate for the highly physical athlete, and must not create any adverse reactions. With these points in mind, the more generally accepted antiinflammatory drugs are discussed.

Acetylsalicylic acid (aspirin)   Aspirin is one of the most widely used analgesics, antiinflammatories, and antipyretics. It is also one of the most abused drugs in use today. A number of medications that have salicylates act in reducing pain, fever, and inflammation. Aspirin has been associated with various adverse reactions that are primarily centered in the gastrointestinal region. They include difficulty in food digestion (dyspepsia), nausea, vomiting, and gastric bleeding.

Overingestion of aspirin can lead to serious side effects. Adverse reactions to aspirin, especially in high doses, are ear ringing or buzzing (tinnitus) and dizziness. A major problem that can arise in individuals under 18 years of age is Reye's syndrome. The administration of aspirin to a child during chickenpox or influenza can induce Reye's syndrome. Its etiology is unknown.

Severe allergic response resulting in an anaphylactic reaction can occur in individuals who have an intolerance to aspirin. Asthmatic patients may be at greater risk for allergic reactions to aspirin. Aspirin use should be avoided by athletes in contact sports since it prolongs blood clotting time.

Nonsteroidal Antiinflammatory Drugs

Nonsteroidal drugs have antiinflammatory, antipyretic, and analgesic properties. They are strong inhibitors of prostaglandin synthesis and are effective for such chronic problems as rheumatoid arthritis and osteoarthritis.[3] Nonsteroidal antiinflammatory drugs (NSAIDs) are used primarily for reducing the pain, stiffness, swelling, redness, and fever associated with localized inflammation. Their antiinflammatory capabilities are thought to be equal to those of aspirin, their advantages being that NSAIDs have fewer side effects and relatively longer duration of action. They are effective for patients who cannot tolerate aspirin because of gastrointestinal distress associated with aspirin use. Even though NSAIDs have analgesic and antipyretic capabilities, they should not be used in cases of mild headache or increased body temperature in place of aspirin or acetaminophen. However, they can be used to relieve many other mild to moderately painful somatic conditions such as menstrual cramps and soft-tissue injury. Table 16-4 lists the NSAIDs commonly used in treating athletes.

The NSAIDs can produce adverse reactions and should be used cautiously. Athletes who have aspirin allergy triad of nasal polyps, associated bronchospasm or asthma, and history of anaphylaxis should not receive any NSAID. The NSAIDs can cause gastrointestinal tract reactions, headache, dizziness, depression, tinnitus, and a variety of other systemic reactions.

Corticosteroids

Corticosteroids, of which cortisone is the most common, are used primarily for chronic inflammation of musculoskeletal and joint regions. Cortisone is a synthetic glucocorticoid that is usually given orally or by injection. Increasingly, more caution is taken in the use of corticosteroids than was practiced in the past. Prolonged use of corticosteroids can produce the following serious complications:

Antiinflammatories include acetylsalicylic acid (aspirin), NSAIDs, and corticosteroids.

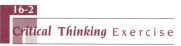

16-2

Critical Thinking Exercise

A college-age softball player comes into the training room complaining of a headache and asks the athletic trainer to give her some ibuprofin to get rid of her headache.

? Is ibuprofin the most appropriate medication to use in this case?

TABLE 16-4 Commonly Used NSAIDs among Athletes

Drug	Initial Dosage	Maximum Daily Dose (mg)
Over-the-counter drugs		
Aspirin	325-650 mg every 4 hours	4000
Advil	200-400 mg 3 times a day	1200
Aleve	200 mg 2-3 times a day	600
Prescription drugs		
Voltaren	50-75 mg twice a day	200
Dolobid	500-1000 mg followed by 250-300 mg 2-3 times a day	1500
Nalfon	400-800 mg 3-4 times a day	3200
Motrin, Rufin	400-800 mg 3-4 times a day	3200
Indocin	75-150 mg a day in 3-4 divided doses	200
Orudis	75 mg 3 times a day or 50 mg 4 times a day	300
Ponstel	500 mg followed by 250 mg every 6 hours	1000
Naprosyn	500 mg followed by 250 mg every 6-8 hours	1250
Anaprox	550 mg followed by 275-550 mg 3 times a day	1650
Feldene	20 mg a day	20
Clinoril	200 mg twice a day	400
Tolectin	400 mg 3-4 times a day	1800
Ansaid	50-100 mg 2-3 times a day	300
Toradol	10 mg every 4-6 hours for pain	40
Lodine	400 mg 2-3 times a day	1200

- Fluid and electrolyte disturbances (e.g., water retention caused by excess sodium levels)
- Musculoskeletal and joint impairments (e.g., bone thinning and muscle and tendon weakness)
- Dermatological problems (e.g., delayed wound healing)
- Neurological impairments (e.g., vertigo, headache, convulsions)
- Endocrine dysfunctions (e.g., menstrual irregularities)
- Ophthalmic conditions (e.g., glaucoma)
- Metabolic impairments (e.g., negative nitrogen balance, muscle wasting)

Cortisone is primarily administered by injection. Other ways are iontophoresis and phonophoresis. (See Chapter 14.) Studies have indicated that cortisone injected directly into tendons, ligaments, and joint spaces can lead to weakness and degeneration. Strenuous activity may predispose the treated part to rupturing. Tennis elbow and plantar fasciitis have benefitted from corticosteroid treatment.

Drugs that Produce Skeletal Muscle Relaxation

Drugs that produce skeletal muscle relaxation include methocarbamol (Robaxin), and carisoprodol (Soma). Because centrally acting muscle relaxants also act as sedatives or tranquilizers on the higher brain centers, there is growing speculation among physicians that these drugs are less specific to muscle relaxation than was once believed. Another major side effect is that they cause drowsiness.

Muscle spasm and guarding accompany many musculoskeletal injuries. Elimination of spasm and guarding should facilitate programs of rehabilitation. In many situations, centrally acting oral muscle relaxants are used to reduce spasm and guarding. However, to date the efficacy of using muscle relaxants has not been substantiated, and they do not appear to be superior to analgesics or sedatives in either acute or chronic conditions.

Drugs Used to Treat Gastrointestinal Disorders

Drugs used to treat gastrointestinal disorders include antacids, antiemetics, carminatives, cathartics or laxatives, histamine-2 blockers, and antidiarrheals.

Disorders of the gastrointestinal tract include upset stomach or formation of gas because of food incompatibilities and acute or chronic hyperacidity, which leads to inflammation of the mucous membrane of the intestinal tract. Poor eating habits may lead to digestive tract problems such as diarrhea or constipation. Drugs that elicit responses within the gastrointestinal tract include antacids, antiemetics, carminatives, cathartics and laxatives, and antidiarrheals.

Antacids

The primary function of an antacid is to neutralize acidity in the upper gastrointestinal tract by raising the pH, inhibiting the activity of the digestive enzyme pepsin, and thus reducing its action on the gastric mucosal nerve endings. Antacids are effective not only for relief of acid indigestion and heartburn but also in the treatment of peptic ulcer. Antacids available in the market possess a wide range of acid-neutralizing capabilities and side effects.

One of the most commonly used antacid preparations is sodium bicarbonate, or baking soda. Other antacids include alkaline salts, which again neutralize hyperacidity but are not easily absorbed in the blood. Ingestion of antacids containing magnesium tends to have a laxative effect. Those containing aluminum or calcium seem to cause constipation. Consequently, many antacid liquids or tablets are combinations of magnesium and either aluminum or calcium hydroxides. Overuse can cause electrolyte imbalance and other adverse effects.

Antiemetics

Antiemetics are used to treat the nausea and vomiting that may result from a variety of causes. Antiemetics are classified as acting either locally or centrally. The locally acting drugs, such as most over-the-counter medications (e.g., Pepto-Bismol), reportedly affect the mucosal lining of the stomach. However, the effects of soothing an upset stomach may be more of a placebo effect. The centrally acting drugs affect the brain by making it less sensitive to irritating nerve impulses from the inner ear or stomach. A variety of prescription antiemetics can be used for controlling nausea and vomiting, including phenothiazines (Phenegran), antihistamines, anticholinergic drugs for preventing motion sickness, and sedative drugs. The primary side effect of these medications is drowsiness.

Carminatives

Carminatives are drugs that give relief from flatulence (gas). Their action on the digestive canal is to inhibit gas formation and aid in its expulsion. Simethicone is the most commonly used carminative.

Cathartics (Laxatives)

The use of laxatives in sports should always be under the direction of a physician. Constipation may be symptomatic of a serious disease condition. Indiscriminant use of laxatives may render the athlete unable to have normal bowel movements. It may also lead to electrolyte imbalance. There is little need for healthy, active individuals to rely on artificial means for stool evacuation.

Antidiarrheals

Diarrhea may result from many causes, but it is generally considered to be a symptom rather than a disease. It can occur as a result of emotional stress, allergies to food or drugs, or many different types of intestinal problems. Diarrhea may be acute or chronic. Acute diarrhea, the most common, comes on suddenly and may be accompanied by nausea, vomiting, chills, and intense abdominal pain. It typically runs its course rapidly, and symptoms subside once the irritating agent is removed from the system. Chronic diarrhea, which may last for weeks, may result from more serious disease states.

Medications used for control of diarrhea are either locally acting or systemic. The locally acting medications most typically contain kaolin, which absorbs other chemicals, and pectin, which sooths irritated bowel. Some contain substances that add bulk to the stool. The systemic agents, which are generally antiperistaltic or antispasmodic medications, are considered to be much more effective in relieving symptoms of diarrhea, but most, except loperamide (Imodium AD), are prescription drugs. The systemic medications are either opiate derivatives or anticholinergic agents, both of which reduce peristalsis. Common side effects of the systemic antidiarrheals include drowsiness, nausea, dry mouth, and constipation.

Histamine-2 Blockers (H$_2$ Blockers)

The H$_2$ blockers reduce stomach acid output by blocking the action of histamine on certain cells in the stomach. They are used to treat peptic and gastric ulcers and other gastrointestinal hypersecretory conditions. Cimetidine (Tagamet) and ranitidine (Zantac) are examples.

Drugs Used to Treat Colds and Allergies

Drugs on the market designed to affect colds and allergies are almost too numerous to count. In general, they fall into three basic categories, all of which deal with the symptoms of the condition and not the cause. They are drugs dealing with nasal congestion, histamine reactions, and cough.

Drugs used to treat colds and allergies include nasal decongestants, antihistamines, cough suppressants, and sympathomimetics.

Nasal Decongestants

Topical nasal decongestants that contain mild vasoconstricting agents such as oxymetazoline (Afrin) and xylometazoline (Otivin) are on the market. These agents are relatively safe. However, prolonged use can cause rebound congestion and dependency.

An effective oral decongestant is psuedoephedrine hydrochloride (Sudafed). Repeated dosing does not lead to rebound congestion.

Antihistamines

Antihistamines are often added to nasal decongestants. Histamine is a protein substance contained in animal tissues that, when released into the general circulation, causes the reactions of an allergy. Histamine causes dilation of arteries and capillaries, skin flushing, and a rise in temperature. An antihistamine is a substance that opposes histamine action. Antihistamines offer little benefit in treating the common cold. They are beneficial in allergies. Examples are terfenadine (Seldane), diphenhydramine hydrochloride (Benadryl), and chlorphenerimine (Chlor-Trimeton).

Cough Medicines

Cough medicines either suppress the cough (antitussives) or increase the fluid content to increase the production of fluid in the respiratory system (expectorants). Antitussives are available in liquid, capsule, troche, or spray form. Narcotic antitussives contain codeine (Robitussin AC); nonnarcotic antitussives contain diphenhydramine (Benylin Cough Syrup), dextromethorphan (Benylin DM, Sucrets), or benzonatate (Tessalon). The advantage of nonnarcotic antitussives is that they have few side effects and are not addictive. There is little evidence that expectorants (guaifenesin) are any more effective in controlling coughing than simply drinking water.

Sympathomimetics

Exercise-induced bronchospasm involves spasm of smooth muscle in the bronchioles and shortness of breath. Drugs used to treat exercise-induced bronchospasm are called sympathomimetics. An example is albuterol (Proventil, Ventolin). Bronchodilators generally reverse the symptoms. Sympathomimetics may cause heat-related problems if used in a hot environment.

Drugs Used to Control Bleeding

Various drugs and medicines cause selective actions on the circulatory system, including vasoconstrictors and anticoagulants.

Drugs used to control bleeding include vasoconstrictors, hemostatic agents, and anticoagulants.

Vasoconstrictors

In sports vasoconstrictors are most often administered externally to sites of profuse bleeding. The drug most commonly used for this purpose is epinephrine (adrenaline), which is applied directly to a hemorrhaging area. It acts immediately to constrict damaged blood vessels and is extremely valuable in cases of epistaxis (nosebleed) in which normal procedures are inadequate.

Hemostatic Agents

Drugs that immediately inhibit bleeding are currently being investigated. Hemostatic agents such as thrombin may prove to be useful; however, specific drug recommendations are not available at this time.

Anticoagulants

The most common anticoagulants used by physicians in sports are heparin and coumarin derivatives. Heparin prolongs the clotting time of blood but will not dissolve a clot once it has developed. Heparin is used primarily to control extension of a thrombus that is already present. Coumarin derivatives act by suppressing the formation of prothrombin in the liver. Given orally, they are used to slow clotting time in certain vascular disorders.

SUBSTANCE ABUSE AMONG ATHLETES

Perhaps no other topic related to pharmacology has received more attention from the media during recent years than the use and abuse of drugs by athletes. Much has been written regarding the use of performance-enhancing drugs among Olympic athletes and the widespread use of "street drugs" by collegiate and professional athletes. Clearly, substance abuse has no place in the athletic population.[2]

Although much of the information being disseminated to the public by the media may be based on hearsay and innuendo, the use and abuse of many different types of drugs can have a profound impact on athletic performance. To say that many experts in the field of sports medicine regard drug abuse among athletes with growing concern is a gross understatement. The athletic trainer must be knowledgeable about substance abuse in the athletic population and should be able to recognize signs that may indicate when an athlete is engaging in substance abuse (see the Focus box on the next page).

Performance-Enhancing Substances (Ergogenic Aids)

Ergogenic aid is a term used to describe any method, legal or illegal, used to enhance athletic performance.[31] The use of various pharmacological agents by athletes for enhancing performance should be of primary concern to the athletic trainer.

Common ergogenic aids include stimulants, beta blockers, narcotic analgesics, diuretics, anabolic steroids, human growth hormone, and blood doping.

Stimulants

The intention of the athlete when he or she ingests a stimulant may be to increase alertness, reduce fatigue, or in some instances increase competitiveness and even hostility.[13] Some athletes respond to stimulants with a loss of judgment that may lead to personal injury or injury to others.

Two major categories of stimulants are psychomotor-stimulant drugs and adrenergic (sympathomimetic) drugs. Psychomotor stimulants are of two general types: am-

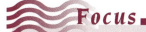

phetamines (e.g., methamphetamine) and nonamphetamines (e.g., methylphenidate and cocaine). The major actions of psychomotor stimulants result from the rapid turnover of catecholamines, which have a strong effect on the nervous and cardiovascular systems, metabolic rates, temperature, and smooth muscle.

Sympathomimetic drugs act directly on adrenergic receptors, or those that release catecholamines (i.e., epinephrine and norepinephrine) from nerve endings, and thus act indirectly on catecholamines. Ephedrine is an example of this type, and can, in high doses, cause mental stimulation and increased blood flow. As a result, it may also cause elevated blood pressure and headache, increased and irregular heartbeat, anxiety, and tremor.

Amphetamines and cocaine are the psychomotor drugs most commonly used in sports. Cocaine is discussed in the section on recreational drug abuse. Sympathomimetic drugs present an extremely difficult problem in sports medicine because they are commonly found in cold remedies.[13] The U.S. Olympic Committee (USOC) has approved some substances to be used by asthmatics who develop exercise-induced bronchospasms. These substances are selective B_2 agonists and consist of albuterol (Proventil), salbutamol (Serevent), and terbutaline (in its aerosol form). Before an athlete engages in Olympic competition, his or her team physician must notify the USOC Medical Subcommission in writing concerning their usage.[13]

Amphetamines   Amphetamines are synthetic alkaloids that are extremely powerful and dangerous drugs. They may be injected, inhaled, or taken as tablets. Amphetamines are among the most abused drugs used with the goal of enhancing sports performance. In ordinary doses, amphetamines can produce euphoria, with an increased sense of well-being and heightened mental activity, until fatigue sets in (from lack of sleep), accompanied by nervousness, insomnia, and anorexia. In high doses, amphetamines reduce mental activity and impair performance of complicated motor skills. The athlete's behavior may become irrational. The chronic user may be "hung up," that is, stuck in a repetitive behavioral sequence. This perseveration may last for hours, becoming increasingly more irrational. The long-term or even short-term use of amphetamines can lead to amphetamine psychosis, manifested by auditory and visual hallucinations and paranoid delusions. Physiologically, high doses of amphetamines can cause mydriasis (abnormal pupillary dilation), increased blood pressure, hyperreflexia (increased reflect action), and hyperthermia.

In terms of their sports performance, athletes believe that amphetamines promote quickness and endurance, delay fatigue, and increase confidence, thereby causing increased aggressiveness. Studies indicate that there is no improvement in performance, but there is an increased risk of injury, exhaustion, and circulatory collapse.[9]

Caffeine   Caffeine is found in coffee, tea, cocoa, and cola and is readily absorbed into the body[22] (Table 16-5). It is a central nervous system stimulant and diuretic and also stimulates gastric secretion. One cup of coffee can contain from 100 to 150 mg of caffeine. In moderation, caffeine causes stimulation of the cerebral cortex and medullar centers, resulting in wakefulness and mental alertness. In larger amounts and in individuals who ingest caffeine daily, it raises blood pressure, decreases and then increases the heart rate, and increases plasma levels of epinephrine, norepinephrine, and renin. It affects coordination, sleep, mood, behavior, and thinking processes.[22]

In terms of exercise and sports performance, caffeine is controversial. Like amphetamines, caffeine can affect some athletes by acting as an ergogenic aid during prolonged exercise. The USOC considers caffeine a stimulant if the concentration in the athlete's urine exceeds 12 μg/ml. Some adverse effects of caffeine ingestion are tremors, nervousness, headaches, diuresis, arrhythmias, restlessness, hyperactivity, irritability, dry mouth, tinnitus, ocular dyskinesia, scotomata, insomnia, headaches, and depression.[9] A habitual user of caffeine who suddenly stops may experience withdrawal, including headache, drowsiness, lethargy, rhinorrhea, irritability, nervousness, depression, and loss of interest in work. Caffeine also acts as a diuretic when hydration may be important.[22]

Narcotic Analgesic Drugs

Narcotic analgesic drugs are derived directly from opium or are synthetic opiates. Morphine and codeine (methylmorphine) are examples of substances made from the alkaloid of opium. Narcotic analgesics are used for the management of moderate to severe pain. They have a high risk of physical and psychological dependency, as well as many other problems stemming from their use. It is believed that slight to moderate pain can be effectively dealt with by drugs other than narcotics.

TABLE 16-5   Examples of Caffeine-Containing Products

Product	Dose
Coffee (1 cup)	100.0 mg
Diet Coke (12 oz)	45.6 mg
Diet Pepsi (12 oz)	36.0 mg
No-Doz (1)	100.0 mg
Anacin (1)	32.0 mg
Excedrin (1)	65.0 mg
Midol (1)	32.4 mg

Beta Blockers

The "beta" in beta blockers refers to the type of sympathetic nerve ending receptor that is blocked.[12] Medically, beta blockers are used primarily for hypertension and heart disease. Beta blockers have been used in sports that require steadiness, such as marksmanship, sailing, archery, fencing, ski jumping, and luge.[12] Beta blockers are one class of adrenergic agents that inhibit the action of catecholamines released from sympathetic nerve endings. Beta blockers produce relaxation of blood vessels. This relaxation in turn slows heart rate and decreases contractility of heart muscle, thus decreasing cardiac output.

Diuretics

Diuretic drugs increase kidney excretion by decreasing the kidney's resorption of sodium. The excretion of potassium and bicarbonate may also be increased. Therapeutically, diuretics are used for a variety of cardiovascular and respiratory conditions (e.g., hypertension) in which elimination of fluids from tissues is necessary. Sports participants have misused diuretics mainly in two ways: to reduce body weight quickly or to decrease a drug's concentration in the urine (increasing its excretion to avoid the detection of drug misuse). In both cases, there are ethical and health grounds for banning certain classes of diuretics from use during competition.

Anabolic Steroids

Anabolic steroids are synthetically created chemical compounds whose structure closely resembles naturally occurring sex hormones—in particular the male hormone testosterone.[8,15] Anabolic steroids have both androgenic and anabolic effects. Androgenic effects include growth development and maintenance of reproductive tissues and masculinization in males. Anabolic effects promote nitrogen retention, which leads to protein synthesis in skeletal muscles and other tissues, resulting in increased muscle mass and weight, general growth, and bone maturation.[18]

Athletes who choose to take anabolic steroids are seeking to maximize the anabolic effects while minimizing the androgenic side effects. The problem is that no steroids exist that have only anabolic effects; they also have androgenic effects.

In 1984 the American College of Sports Medicine (ACSM) reported that anabolic steroids taken with an adequate diet could contribute to an increase in body weight, and with a heavy resistance program there could be a significant gain in strength.[27] However, when used in mass quantities, as is typically done by individual athletes, they can have many deleterious and irreversible side effects that constitute a major threat to the health of the athlete.[23] (See the Focus box on the next page.)

Anabolic steroids present an ethical dilemma for the sport world.[15] It is estimated that over a million young male and female athletes are taking or have taken them, with most being purchased through the black market.[33] Approximately 6.5% of male and 1.9% female athletes are taking anabolic steroids.[5] An estimated 2.5% of intercollegiate athletes take anabolic steroids.[19] The more commonly used anabolic steroids include Anavar, Dianabol, Anadrol, and Finajet.[9]

Usage of anabolic steroids is a major problem in sports that involve strength.[34] Powerlifting, the throwing events in track and field, and American football are some of the sports in which the use of anabolic steroids is a serious problem.

Human Growth Hormone

Human growth hormone (HGH) is produced by the somatotropic cells of the anterior region of the pituitary gland from which it is released into the circulatory system. The amount released varies with age and the developmental periods of a person's life. A lack of HGH can result in dwarfism. In the past, HGH was in limited supply because it was extracted from cadavers. Now, however, it can be made synthetically and is more readily available.[17,29]

16-3

Critical Thinking Exercise

A football linebacker returns to school for preseason practice and to the shock of both his teammates and the coaches he has gained 30 pounds and greatly increased his muscle bulk since leaving for the summer in June. Even though this athlete is known to be "religious" about his weight training, the coaches are fairly certain that he has engaged in steroid abuse. The athlete vehemently denies taking steroids and is willing to take a drug test to prove it.

? One of the coaches approaches the athletic trainer and asks if the athlete is using steroids. Without subjecting the athlete to a definitive drug test, what physical signs are indicative of steroid abuse?

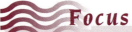

Experiments indicate that HGH can increase muscle mass, skin thickness, connective tissues in muscle, and organ weight and can produce lax muscles and ligaments during rapid growth phases. It also increases body length and weight and decreases body fat percentage.[29]

The use of HGH by athletes throughout the world is on the increase because it is more difficult to detect in urine than anabolic steroids.[16] There is currently a lack of concrete information about the effects of HGH on the athlete who does not have a growth problem. It is known that an overabundance of HGH in the body can lead to premature closure of long-bone growth sites or, conversely, can cause acromegaly, a condition that produces elongation and enlargement of bones of the extremities and thickening of bones and soft tissues of the face. Also associated with acromegaly is diabetes mellitus, cardiovascular disease, goiter, menstrual disorders, decreased sexual desire, and impotence. It decreases the life span by up to 20 years. As with anabolic steroids, HGH presents a serious problem for the sports world. At this time there is no proof that an increase of HGH combined with weight training contributes to strength and muscle hypertrophy.[16]

Blood Reinjection (Blood Doping, Blood Packing, and Blood Boosting)

Endurance, acclimatization, and altitude make increased metabolic demands on the body, which responds by increasing blood volume and the number of red blood cells to meet the increased aerobic demands.

Recently, researchers have replicated these physiological responses by removing 900 ml of blood, storing it, and reinfusing it after 6 weeks. The reason for waiting at least 6 weeks before reinfusion is that it takes that long for the athlete's body to re-establish a normal hemoglobin and red blood cell concentration. Using this method, endurance performance has been significantly improved. From the standpoint of scientific research such experimentation has merit and is of interest. However, not only is use of such methods in competition unethical, but use by nonmedical personnel could prove to be dangerous, especially when a matched donor is used.[13]

There are serious risks with transfusing blood and related blood products. The risks include allergic reactions, kidney damage (if the wrong type of blood is used), fever, jaundice, the possibility of transmitting infectious diseases (hepatitis B or HIV), or a blood overload, resulting in circulatory and metabolic shock.[10]

Recreational Substance Abuse among Athletes

Recreational drugs include tobacco, alcohol, cocaine, and marijuana.

As is true with the general public, recreational substance use is a part of the world of sports. Reasons for using these substances may include desire to experiment, temporarily to escape from problems, or just to be part of a group (peer pressure). For some, recreational drug use leads to abuse and dependence. Drug abuse may be defined as the use of drugs for nonmedical reasons, that is, with the intent of getting "high"—altering mood or behavior

Psychological versus Physical Dependence

There are two general aspects of dependence—psychological and physical. Psychological dependence is the drive to repeat the ingestion of a drug to produce pleasure or to avoid discomfort. Physical dependence is the state of drug adaptation that manifests as the development of tolerance and, when the drug is removed, causes a withdrawal syndrome. Tolerance of a drug is the need to increase the dosage to create the effect that was obtained previously by smaller amounts.

Withdrawal   The withdrawal syndrome consists of an unpleasant physiological reaction when the drug is abruptly stopped. Some drugs that are abused by the athlete overlap with those thought to enhance performance. Examples include amphetamines and cocaine. Tobacco (nicotine), alcohol, cocaine, and marijuana are the most abused recreational drugs. The athletic trainer and coach might also come in contact with abuse by athletes of barbiturates, nonbarbiturate sedatives, psychotomimetic drugs, or different inhalants.

Tobacco Use

Although smoking cigarettes, cigars, and pipes is becoming increasingly rare in the athletic population, the use of smokeless tobacco and the passive exposure to others who are smoking are ongoing problems for athletes.

Cigarette smoking   On the basis of various investigations into the relationship between smoking and performance, the following conclusions can be drawn:
1. There is individual sensitivity to tobacco that may seriously affect performance in instances of relatively high sensitivity. Because more than one third of the men studied indicated tobacco sensitivity, it may be wise to prohibit smoking by athletes.
2. Tobacco smoke has been associated with as many as 4700 different chemicals, many of which are toxic.
3. As few as 10 inhalations of cigarette smoke cause an average maximum decrease in airway conductance of 50%. This occurs in nonsmokers who inhale smoke secondhand as well.
4. Smoking reduces the oxygen-carrying capacity of the blood. A smoker's blood carries from 5 to as much as 10 times more carbon monoxide than normal. Carbon monoxide inhibits the capability of oxygen molecules binding to the hemoglobin molecule. Thus the red blood cells are prevented from picking up sufficient oxygen to meet the demands of the body's tissues. The carbon monoxide also tends to make arterial walls more permeable to fatty substances, a factor in atherosclerosis.
5. Smoking aggravates and accelerates the heart muscle cells through overstimulation of the sympathetic nervous system.
6. Total lung capacity and maximum breathing capacity are significantly decreased in heavy smokers; this is important to the athlete, because both changes would impair the capacity to take in oxygen and make it readily available for body use.
7. Smoking decreases pulmonary diffusing capacity.
8. After smoking, an accelerated thrombolic tendency is evidenced.
9. Smoking is a carcinogenic factor in lung cancer and is a contributing factor to heart disease.

The addictive chemical of tobacco is nicotine, which is one of the most toxic drugs. When inhaled, it causes blood pressure elevation, increased bowel activity, and an antidiuretic action. Moderate tolerance and strong physical dependence occur.

Use of smokeless tobacco   It is estimated that over 7 million individuals use smokeless tobacco, which comes in three forms: loose-leaf, moist or dry powder (snuff), and compressed. The tobacco is placed between the cheek and the gum. Then it is sucked and chewed. Aesthetically, this is an unsavory habit during which an athlete is continually spitting into a container. Besides the unpleasant appearance, the use of smokeless tobacco proposes an extremely serious health risk.[4] Smokeless tobacco causes bad breath, stained teeth, tooth sensitivity to heat and cold, cavities, gum recession, tooth bone loss, leukoplakia, and oral and throat cancer. Aggressive oral and throat cancer and periodontal destruction (with tooth loss) have been associated with this habit.[6]

The major substance ingested is nitrosonornicotine, which is the drug responsible for this habit's addictiveness. It is absorbed through the mucous membranes, and within a short period of time the level of nicotine in the blood is equivalent to that of a cigarette smoker. This chemical makes smokeless tobacco a more addictive habit than smoking. The user of chewing tobacco experiences the nicotine effects without exposure to the tar and carbon monoxide associated with a burning cigarette. Smokeless tobacco increases heart rate but does not affect reaction time, movement time, or total response time among athletes or nonathletes.[11]

Passive smoke   There are dangers associated with the passive inhalation of smoke (second hand) by nonsmokers. Both smokers and nonsmokers are exposed to smoke containing carbon monoxide, nicotine, ammonia, and cyanide. Obviously smokers inhale the greater quantity of contaminated air. However, it has been estimated that for each pack of cigarettes smoked, the nonsmoker, sharing a common air supply, will inhale the equivalent of 3 to 5 cigarettes. Significant numbers of individuals exposed to passive smoke develop nasal symptoms, eye irritation, headaches, cough, and in some cases allergies to smoke. For these reasons and others, many state, local, and private sector policies have been established that restrict or ban smoking in public areas. There is little doubt that passive smoking poses a significant health threat to the nonsmoker.

Alcohol Use

Alcohol is the most widely used and abused substance among athletes.[21] Alcohol is a drug that depresses the central nervous system. Alcohol is absorbed from the digestive system into the bloodstream very rapidly. Factors that affect how rapidly absorption takes place include the number of drinks consumed, the rate of consumption, alcohol concentration of the beverage, and the amount of food in the stomach. Some alcohol is absorbed into the blood through the stomach, but the greater part is absorbed through the small intestine. Alcohol is transported through the blood to the liver, where it can be oxidized at a rate of ⅔ oz per hour. An excess causes an increase in the level of alcohol circulating in the blood. As blood alcohol levels continue to increase, predictable signs of intoxication appear. At 0.1% the person loses motor coordination; from 0.2% to 0.5% the symptoms become progressively more profound and perhaps even life threatening. Intoxication persists until the remainder of the alcohol can be metabolized by the liver. There is no way to accelerate the liver's metabolism of alcohol ("sober up"); it just takes time. Alcohol has no place in sports participation.

Approximately 20% of cases of alcoholism are associated with genetic reasons and 80% with overindulgence. The athlete who is suffering from alcohol abuse may display the following characteristics: mood changes, missed practices, isolation, attitude changes, fighting or inappropriate outbursts of violence, changes in appearance, hostility toward authority figures, complaints from family, and changes in peer group.[25]

Drug Use

Cocaine   Cocaine, also known as coke, snow, toot, happy dust, and white girl, is a powerful central nervous system stimulant with effects of very short duration. Cocaine use produces immediate feelings of euphoria, excitement, decreased sense of

16-4

Critical Thinking Exercise

The baseball team has a number of players who routinely chew tobacco or use "dip." The athletic trainer is extremely concerned about the possible long-term effects of using smokeless tobacco and has convinced the coach that banning "chewing" is in the players' best interest.

? Because many of the players know that using smokeless tobacco is a long-standing practice among players and a part of the baseball "cult," what can the athletic trainer do to help the players accept this new rule?

fatigue, and heightened sexual drive. Cocaine may be snorted, taken intravenously, or smoked (freebased). The initial effects are extremely intense, and because they are pleasurable, strong psychological dependence is developed rapidly by users who can or cannot afford to support this expensive habit.

Habitual use of cocaine will not lead to physical tolerance or dependence but will cause psychological dependence and addiction. Long-term effects include nasal congestion and damage to the membranes and cartilage of the nose if snorted, bronchitis, loss of appetite leading to nutritional deficiencies, convulsions, impotence, and cocaine psychosis with paranoia, depression, hallucinations, and disorganized mental function. An overdose can lead to overstimulation of the sympathetic nervous system and can cause tachycardia, hypertension, extra heartbeats, coronary vasoconstriction, strokes, pulmonary edema, aortic rupture, and sudden death.[24]

Crack Crack is a rocklike crystalline form of cocaine that is heated in a small pipe and then inhaled, producing an immediate rush. The effects last for only a matter of minutes and are frequently followed by a state of depression. This sudden intense stimulation of the nervous system predisposes the user to cardiac failure or respiratory failure and makes this commonly available drug extremely dangerous.

Marijuana Marijuana is one of the most abused drugs in Western society. It is more commonly called grass, weed, pot, dope, or hemp. The marijuana cigarette is called a joint, jay, number, reefer, or root.

Marijuana is not a harmless drug. The components of marijuana smoke are similar to those of tobacco smoke, and the same cellular changes are observed in the user.

Continued use leads to respiratory diseases such as asthma and bronchitis and a decrease in vital capacity of 15% to as much as 40% (certainly detrimental to physical performance). Among other deleterious effects are lowered sperm counts and testosterone levels. Evidence of interference with the functioning of the immune system and cellular metabolism has also been found. The most consistent sign is the increase in pulse rate, which averages close to 20% higher during exercise and is a definite factor in limiting performance. Some decrease in leg, hand, and finger strength has been found at higher dosages. Like tobacco, marijuana must be considered carcinogenic.

Psychological effects such as a diminution of self-awareness and judgment, a slowdown of thinking, and a shorter attention span appear early in the use of the drug. Postmortem examinations of habitual users reveal not only cerebral atrophy but alterations of anatomical structures, which suggest irreversible brain damage. Marijuana also contains unique substances (cannabinoids) that are stored, in much the same manner as are fat cells, throughout the body and in the brain tissues for weeks and even months. These stored quantities result in a cumulative deleterious effect on the habitual user.

A drug such as marijuana has no place in sports. Claims for its use are unsubstantiated, and the harmful effects, both immediate and long-term, are too significant to permit indulgence at any time.

DRUG TESTING IN ATHLETES

Drug testing of athletes for the purpose of identifying individuals who may have some problems with drug abuse is commonplace.[14] Both the National Collegiate Athletic Association (NCAA) and the USOC routinely conduct drug testing.[20,30] The legality and ethics of testing only those individuals involved with sports are still open to debate. The pattern of drug usage among athletes may simply reflect that of our society in general. Great care must be taken that an athlete's personal rights are not violated.[28]

Drug testing began with the 1968 Olympic games. In 1985 the USOC began drug testing athletes involved in both national and international competitions. In January 1986 the member institutions of the NCAA voted overwhelmingly to expand the

Both the NCAA and the USOC conduct drug testing programs.

16-5

Critical Thinking E x e r c i s e

A university has recently implemented a drug testing program for athletes in all sports. In deciding how the program should be conducted, the athletic director has decided that the athletic trainer is perhaps the best individual to supervise the program.

? Should the athletic trainer be willing to take on the additional responsibilities of overseeing the drug testing program for the athletes?

NCAA drug education program to include mandatory random drug testing in specific sports throughout the year and during and after NCAA championship events.[20] The major goals of both organizations are to protect the health of athletes and to help ensure that competition is fair and equitable.[9]

Most professional teams and many individual colleges and universities have initiated drug testing programs for their athletes.[26] Unfortunately, drug testing is rarely done at the high school level because of cost constraints.

The Drug Test

There are some slight differences between NCAA and USOC drug testing procedures and protocols. Most of these differences have to do with how the athletes are selected for random tests. The NCAA requires all athletes to sign a consent form agreeing to participate in the drug testing program throughout the year. The USOC tests athletes on a random basis throughout the year and all athletes before a USOC-sanctioned competition.[9]

During the drug test, the athlete must first provide positive identification. Then, under direct observation, the athlete must urinate into two separate specimen bottles (labeled A and B), which are sealed and submitted to an official NCAA or USOC testing laboratory for analysis. In the laboratory, specimen A is used for both screening and confirmation tests. A confirmation test uses analysis techniques that are more sensitive and accurate should a positive test result occur during the screening test. Specimen B is used only when a reconfirmation is needed for a positive test of speci-

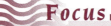

Focus

Banned drugs

Drugs banned by both NCAA and USOC

Anabolic steroids

Diuretics

Beta blockers (used to lower blood pressure, decrease heart rate, decrease cardiac arrythmias)

Peptide hormones (human growth hormone, corticotropin, erythropoeitin, human chorionic gonadotropin, etc.)

Stimulants* (amphetamines, cocaine, and anorexians)

Caffeine (limited ingestion permits up to 12 μg/ml USOC and 15 μg/ml NCAA)

Blood doping

Drugs banned by USOC only

Narcotic analgesics (codeine is permitted)

Skeletal muscle relaxants (banned for modern pentathlon and biathlon events only)

Cough and cold decongestants (sympathomimetic drugs)

Injectable anesthetics (acceptable with prior written permission)

Corticosteroids (intramuscular, intravenous, rectal, and oral use is banned; most topical and inhaled use is permitted with written permission)

Drugs banned by NCAA only†

Substances that contain alcohol (banned for riflery)

Street drugs (heroin and marijuana)

Modified from Fuentes R, Rosenberg J, Davis A: *Allen and Hanbury's athletic drug reference,* Durham, NC, 1996, Galaxo.

*USOC permits inhaled albuterol and terbutaline with prior written permission; NCAA permits all inhalants.

†USOC reserves the right to test for alcohol and street drugs with possible sanctions for positive tests.

men A. The athlete is then notified of a positive test result and becomes subject to sanctions from either the NCAA or the USOC.[9]

Sanctions for Positive Tests

For a first-time positive test, the NCAA will declare the athlete ineligible for all regular and postseason competitions for a minimum of 1 year. During that year the athlete may be retested at any time. The athlete must be retested with a negative result and have eligibility restored before he or she may return to competition. Additional positive tests can result in a lifetime disqualification from NCAA competition.[20]

The USOC sanctions range from 3 to 24 months of disqualification depending on the drug, for a first-time violation, and a minimum of 2 years to a lifetime ban for subsequent positive tests.[30]

Banned Substances

Both the NCAA and the USOC have established lists of substances that are banned from use by athletes. The lists include performance-enhancing drugs and "street" or "recreational" drugs, as well as many over-the-counter and prescription drugs.

The list of drugs banned by either the NCAA or the USOC or both is extensive and includes approximately 4600 separate medications.[9] The list of drugs banned by the USOC is considerably more extensive than the NCAA list because the USOC is subject to internationally used drugs banned by the International Olympic Committee (IOC). The Focus box on the previous page summarizes the various categories of drugs that appear on the banned lists for the NCAA and the USOC.[9]

Some drugs appear on the banned list for both the NCAA and the USOC.

The athletic trainer who is working with an athlete who may be tested for drugs by the NCAA, or with world-class or Olympic athletes governed by the USOC, should be thoroughly familiar with the list of banned drugs.[7] Having an athlete disqualified because of the indiscriminate use of some perscription or over-the-counter medication would be most unfortunate.

SUMMARY

- A drug is any chemical agent used in the treatment of disease that may either be applied directly to a specific tissue or organ or be administered internally to affect the body systemically. It is transported in an inactive substance called a vehicle.
- Administering a drug is defined as providing a single dose of medication for immediate use by the athlete. Dispensing refers to providing the athlete with a drug in a quantity sufficient to be used for multiple doses. At no time can anyone other than a person licensed by law legally prescribe or dispense drugs for an athlete. In certain situations, the athletic trainer may be allowed to administer a single dose of a nonprescription medication.
- The athletic trainer is often responsible for initial screening of athletes who have various illnesses or injuries. Frequently, the athletic trainer must make decisions regarding the appropriate use of over-the-counter medications for athletes. Specific protocols have been established that can serve as a guide for the use of these medications by the athletic trainer.
- Drugs used to combat infection include local antiseptics and disinfectants, antifungal agents, and antibiotics.
- Drugs used to inhibit pain or inflammation include counterirritants and local anesthetics, narcotic analgesics, nonnarcotic analgesics and antipyretics, acetylsalicylic acid (aspirin), nonsteroidal antiinflammatory drugs, and corticosteroids.
- Drugs used to treat gastrointestinal disorders include antacids, antiemetics, carminatives, carthartics or laxatives, and antidiarrheals.
- Drugs used to treat colds and allergies include nasal decongestants, antihistamines, cough suppressants, and asthma drugs.
- Drugs used to control bleeding include vasoconstrictors, hemostatic agents, and anticoagulants.

- Substance abuse involves the use of performance-enhancing drugs and the widespread use of recreational drugs, or "street drugs." The athletic trainer must be knowledgeable about substance abuse in the athletic population and should be able to recognize signs that may indicate when an athlete is engaging in substance abuse. Substance abuse has no place in the athletic population.

- The use of performance-enhancing drugs (ergogenic aids) by athletes must be discouraged because of potential health risks and to ensure equal competition. Among the more common ergogenic aids used by athletes are stimulants, beta blockers, narcotic analgesics, diuretics, anabolic steroids, human growth hormone, and blood doping.

- Recreational drug abuse among athletes is of major concern. It can potentially lead to serious psychological and physical health problems. The most prevalent substances that are abused are tobacco, alcohol, cocaine, and marijuana.

- Drug testing of athletes for the purpose of identifying individuals who may have some problems with drug abuse is done routinely by the NCAA and the USOC. The major goals are to protect the health of athletes and to help ensure that competition is fair and equitable. Most professional teams and many individual colleges and universities have initiated drug testing programs for their athletes. Unfortunately, drug testing is rarely done at the high school level because of cost constraints.

- Both the NCAA and USOC have established lists of drugs that are banned for use by athletes competing in either NCAA- or USOC-sanctioned events.

Solutions to Critical Thinking EXERCISES

16-1 Remember, at no time can anyone other than a person licensed by law legally prescribe or dispense drugs for an athlete. An athletic trainer is not permitted to administer or dispense a prescription drug. However, the athletic trainer may be allowed to administer a single dose of a nonprescription medication. The athletic trainer or coach must be reasonable and prudent about the types of nonprescription drugs offered to the athlete. If medications are administered by an athletic trainer, maintaining accurate records of the types of medications administered is essential. Each athletic trainer should be aware of state regulations and laws that pertain to the use of medications.

16-2 Ibuprofin is an NSAID. The NSAIDs are most effective for reducing pain, stiffness, swelling, redness, and fever associated with localized inflammation. Even though NSAIDs have analgesic and antipyretic capabilities, they should not be used in cases of mild headache or increased body temperature in place of aspirin or acetaminophen. However, they can be used to relieve many other mild to moderately painful somatic conditions, such as menstrual cramps and soft-tissue injury.

16-3 The visible signs of steroid abuse include male pattern baldness, acne, voice deepening, mood swings, aggressive behavior, gynecomastia, reduction in the size of a testicle, and changes in libido. Because the athlete denies steroid abuse the athletic trainer might suspect that human growth hormone has been used to achieve similar results.

16-4 The athletic trainer should first point out the potential long-term effects of using smokeless tobacco, which include bad breath, stained teeth, tooth sensitivity to heat and cold, cavities (with tooth loss), gum recession, periodontal destruction, and oral and throat cancer. The trainer may also try to substitute for the tobacco by giving the players chewing gum or sunflower seeds so

that their habitual need to chew on something and spit while playing baseball is satisfied.

16-5 In this particular case, the issue of added responsibility is irrelevant. The athletic trainer should be more concerned with the potential effects that assuming this responsibility would have on his or her ability to perform normal job functions. The athletic trainer must work hard to develop a sense of trust in the athletes for whom he must provide health care. Being forced to assume a role as a "policeman" or "enforcer" can only serve to undermine that trust. Thus the athletic trainer should be adamant in recommending to the athletic director that some other individual assume that responsibility.

REVIEW QUESTIONS AND CLASS ACTIVITIES

1. What is the branch of science known as pharmacology, and what is the difference between a prescription and a nonprescription drug?
2. What is a drug vehicle? Give some examples of drug vehicles.
3. How can drugs be administered to an individual?
4. List procedures that should be followed in the selection, purchase, storage, record keeping, and safety precautions of over-the-counter drugs.
5. What are the legal implications if an athletic trainer administers prescription and nonprescription drugs?
6. List the responses to a drug that an athlete may experience.
7. Describe the specific protocols for administering over-the-counter medications to athletes.
8. List examples of common drugs used by athletes to combat infection, for reducing pain and inflammation, for treating colds and allergies, for treating gastrointestinal disorders, for treating muscle dysfunctions, and for controlling bleeding.
9. Discuss the use of performance-enhancing drugs by athletes.

10. How do stimulants enhance an athlete's performance?

11. What are the purposes of narcotic analgesic drugs in sports? How do they affect performance?

12. What type of athlete would use beta blockers? Why are they used?

13. Describe why anabolic steroids, diuretics, and growth hormones are used by athletes. What are their physiological effects on the athlete?

14. Describe blood doping in sports. Why is it used? What are its dangers?

15. Contrast psychological and physical dependence, tolerance, and withdrawal syndromes.

16. List the dangers of smokeless tobacco. List the effects of nicotine on the body.

17. Why is cocaine use a danger to the athlete?

18. Select a recreational drug to research. What are the physiological responses to it, and what dangers does it pose to the athlete?

19. How can an athlete who is abusing drugs be identified? Describe behavioral identification, as well as drug testing.

20. Debate the issue of drug testing in athletics.

REFERENCES

1. Almekinders L: Athletic injuries and the use of medication. In Torg J, Shepard R, editors: *Current therapy in sports medicine,* St Louis, 1995, Mosby.

2. Blood K: Nonmedical substance use among athletes at a small liberal arts college, *Ath Train* 25(4):335, 1990.

3. Clark W: *Goth's medical pharmacology,* ed 13, St Louis, 1992, Mosby.

4. Connolly G: Use of smokeless tobacco in major league baseball, *N Engl J Med* 318:1281, 1988.

5. DuRant R: Use of multiple drugs among adolescents who use anabolic steroids, *N Engl J Med* 328:922, 1993.

6. Edwards S et al: The effects of smokeless tobacco on heart rates and neuromuscular reactivity, *Phys Sportsmed* 15(7):141, 1987.

7. Erlich N: The athletic trainer's role in drug testing, *Ath Train* 21:225, 1986.

8. Frankel M, Leffers D: Athletes on anabolic-androgenic steroids, *Phys Sportsmed* 20(6):75, 1992.

9. Fuentes R, Rosenberg J, Davis A: *Allen and Hanbury's athletic drug reference,* Durham, NC, 1995, Galaxo.

10. Gledhill N: Control of drug abuse in sports. In Torg J, Shephard R, editors: *Current therapy in sports medicine,* St Louis, 1995, Mosby.

11. Glover ED et al: Smokeless tobacco: questions and answers, *Ath Train* 25(1):10, 1990.

12. Gordon NF et al: Effect of beta-blockers on exercise physiology: implication for exercise training, *Med Sci Sports Exerc* 23(6):668, 1991.

13. *Guide to banned medications,* United States Olympic Committee, Division of Sports Medicine, Drug Education, and Doping Control Program, Nov 1, 1990.

14. Heck J: Drug testing, *J Ath Train* 28(3):197, 1993.

15. Izumi H: Anabolic steroid use among athletes and the future, *Ath Train* 25(1):58, 1990.

16. Jacobson B: Effect of amino acids on growth hormone release, *Phys Sportsmed* 18(1):63, 1990.

17. Murray T: Human growth hormone in sports, *Phys Sportsmed* 14(5):29, 1986.

18. Laster J, Russell J: Anabolic steroid–induced tendon pathology: a review of literature, *Med Sci Sports Exerc* 23(1):81, 1991.

19. National Collegiate Athletic Association: Ergogenic drug use down: binge-drinking on the rise according to a national study, *NCAA Sport Sciences Education Newsletter,* Winter 4:1, 1993.

20. National Collegiate Athletic Association: *1994-95 NCAA drug testing: education programs,* Overland Park, KS, 1994, NCAA.

21. O'Brien C: Alcohol and sport: impact of social drinking on recreational and competitive sports performance, *Sports Med* 15:71, 1993.

22. Partin P: Effects of caffeine on athletes, *Ath Train* 23(4):12, 1988.

23. Potteiger J, Stilger V: Anabolic steroid use in the adolescent athlete, *J Ath Train* 29(1):60, 1994.

24. Randall T: Cocaine and alcohol mix in the body to form even longer lasting more lethal drug, *JAMA* 267:1943, 1992.

25. Samples P: Alcoholism in athletes: new directions for treatment, *Phys Sportsmed* 17(4):192, 1989.

26. Schneider D, Morris J: College athletes and drug testing: attitudes and behaviors, by gender and sport, *J Ath Train* 28(2):146, 1993.

27. Shroyer J: Getting tough on anabolic steroids: can we win the battle? *Phys Sportsmed* 18(2):106, 1990.

28. Starkey C, Abdenour T, Finnane D: Athletic trainers' attitudes toward drug screening of intercollegiate athletes, *J Ath Train* 29(2):120, 1994.

29. Terney R, McLain L: The use of anabolic steroids in high school students, *Am J Dis Child* 144:99, 1990.

30. US Olympic Committee: *Drug education handbook 1993-1996,* Colorado Springs, Colo, 1993, USOC.

31. Wagner J: Enhancement of sport performance with drugs: an overview, *Sports Ed* 12:250, 1991.

32. Whitehill W, Wright K, Robinson J: Guidelines for dispensing medications, *J Ath Train* 27(1):20, 1992.

33. Windsor R, Dumitru D: Prevalence of anabolic steroid use by male and female adolescents, *Med Sci Sports Exerc* 21(5):494, 1989.

34. Yesalis C: Anabolic-androgenic steroid use in the United States, *JAMA* 270:1217, 1993.

ANNOTATED BIBLIOGRAPHY

Bolling LE, editor: *1994/1995 NCAA drug testing/education programs,* Overland Park, Kans, 1994, National Collegiate Athletic Association.

An NCAA manual presenting publications and educational materials, drug education program, NCAA drug testing legislation, and suggested forms and testing protocol.

Clark WG: *Goth's medical pharmacology,* ed 13, St Louis, 1992, Mosby.

Presents modern pharmacology in a readable and easily understood manner.

Fuentes R, Rosenberg J, Davis A: *Allen and Hanbury's athletic drug reference,* Durham, NC, 1996, Galaxo.

Provides what is perhaps the most complete resource for the use of medications, substance abuse, and drug testing in the athletic population. It has a comprehensive listing of all drugs banned by the NCAA and USOC.

US Olympic Committee: *Drug education handbook 1993-1996,* Colorado Springs, 1993, USOC.

A handbook providing in a well-written and succinct manner the goals of the U.S. Olympic Committee's drug education program.

US Pharmacological Convention Inc.: *The complete drug reference,* New York, 1991, Consumer Reports.

A comprehensive book including current information on both prescription and nonprescription drugs.

Specific Sports Conditions

The Foot

When you finish this chapter, you should be able to

- Identify the major anatomical components of the foot that are commonly injured in sports.
- Evaluate the foot after injury.
- Describe the etiological factors, symptoms and signs, and management procedures for the major injuries of the foot.

The foot has one of the highest incidences of sports injuries. Because of this and the complicated nature of the anatomical structures of this body part, injuries to the foot represent a major challenge to the coach and athletic trainer.

FOOT ANATOMY
Bones

The foot is designed basically for strength, flexibility, and coordinated movement. It also transmits throughout the body the stresses that create the locomotor activities of walking and running. It consists of 26 bones: 14 phalangeal, 5 metatarsal, and 7 tarsal (Figure 17-1). The tarsal bones, which form the instep or ankle portion of the foot, consist of the talus, the calcaneus (os calcis), the navicular, cuboid, and the first, second, and third cuneiform bones.

Toes

The toes are somewhat similar to the fingers in appearance but are much shorter and serve a different function. The toes are designed to give a wider base both for balance and for propelling the body forward. The first toe, or hallux, has two phalanges, and the other toes consist of three phalanges.

The two sesamoid bones are located beneath the first matatarsophalangeal joint. Their functions are to assist in reducing pressure in weight bearing, to increase the mechanical advantage of the flexor tendons of the great toe, and to act as sliding pulleys for tendons.

Metatarsus

The metatarsus consists of five bones that lie between and articulate with the tarsals and the phalanges, thus forming the semimovable tarsometatarsal and metatarsophalangeal joints. Although there is little movement permitted, the ligamentous arrangement gives elasticity to the foot in weight bearing. The metatarsophalangeal joints permit hinge action of the phalanges, which is similar to the action found between the hand fingers. The first metatarsal is the largest and strongest and functions as the main body support during walking and running.

Tarsal Bones

The tarsus consists of seven bones (tarsal bones), which are located between the bones of the lower leg and the metatarsus. These bones are important for support of the body and its locomotion. They consist of the calcaneus (os calis), talus (astralgus), cuboid (os cuboideum), navicular (scaphoid), and the first, second, and third cuneiform bones.

Calcaneus The calcaneus is the largest tarsal bone. It supports the talus and shapes the heel; its main functions are to convey the body weight to the ground and to act as a level attachment for the calf muscles.

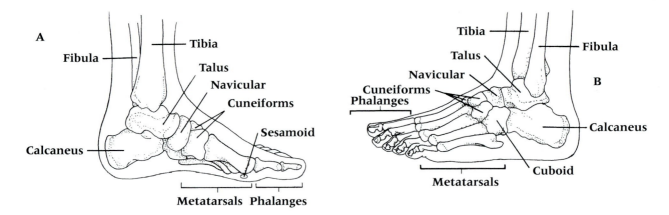

Figure 17-1

Bony structure of the foot. **A,** Medial aspect. **B,** Lateral aspect.

The wider portion of the posterior extremity is called the *tuberosity* of the calcaneus. The medial and lateral tubercles are located on the inferior lateral and medial aspects, which are the only parts that normally touch the ground.

Talus   The irregularly shaped talus is the most superior of the tarsal bones. It is situated on the calcaneus over a bony projection called the *sustentaculum tali*. The talus consists of a body, neck, and head. Uppermost is the trochlea, which articulates with the end of the tibia's medial and lateral malleoli. The trochlea is broader anteriorly than posteriorly, thus preventing forward slipping of the tibia during locomotion.

Because the talus fits principally into the space formed by the malleoli, little lateral movement is present unless the restrictive ligaments have been stretched. Because the uppermost articular surface of the talus is narrower posteriorly than anteriorly, dorsiflexion is limited. At a position of full dorsiflexion the anterior aspect of the medial collateral ligaments is taut, whereas in plantar flexion internal rotation occurs because of the shape of the talus. The average range of motion is 10 degrees in dorsiflexion and 23 degrees in plantar flexion.

Navicular and cuboid bones   The navicular bone is positioned anterior to the talus on the medial aspect of the foot. Anteriorly the navicular bone articulates with the three cuneiform bones. The cuboid is positioned on the lateral aspect of the foot. It articulates posteriorly with the calcaneus and anteriorly with the fourth and fifth metatarsals.

Cuneiform bones   The three cuneiform bones are located between the navicular and the base of the three metatarsals on the medial aspect of the foot.

Arches of the Foot

The foot is structured, by means of ligamentous and bony arrangements, to form several arches. The arches assist the foot in supporting the body weight in an economical fashion, in absorbing the shock of weight bearing, and in providing a space on the plantar aspect of the foot for the blood vessels, nerves, and muscles.[5] The arches' presence aids in giving the foot mobility and a small amount of prehensility. There are four arches: the medial longitudinal, the lateral longitudinal, the anterior metatarsal, and the transverse (Figure 17-2).

Medial Longitudinal Arch

The medial longitudinal arch originates along the medial border of the calcaneus and extends forward to the distal head of the first metatarsal. It is composed of the calcaneus, talus, navicular, first cuneiform, and first metatarsal. The main supporting ligament of the longitudinal arch is the plantar calcaneonavicular ligament, which acts as a "spring" by returning the arch to its normal position after it has been

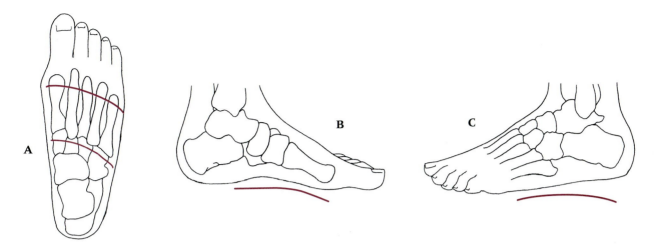

Figure 17-2

The arches of the foot **A,** Anterior metatarsal and transverse arches. **B,** Medial longitudinal arch. **C,** Lateral longitudinal arch.

stretched. The tendon of the posterior tibialis muscle helps to reinforce the plantar calcaneonavicular ligament.

Lateral Longitudinal Arch

The outer longitudinal arch is on the lateral aspect of the foot and follows the same pattern as that of the inner longitudinal arch. It is formed by the calcaneus, cuboid, and fifth metatarsal bones. It is much lower and less flexible than the inner longitudinal arch.

Anterior Metatarsal Arch

The anterior metatarsal arch is shaped by the distal heads of the metatarsals. The arch has a semiovoid appearance, stretching from the first to the fifth metatarsal.

Transverse Arch

The transverse arch extends across the transverse tarsal bones, primarily the cuboid and the internal cuneiform, and forms a half dome. It gives protection to soft tissue and increases the foot's mobility.

Plantar Fascia (Plantar Aponeurosis)

The plantar fascia is a thick white band of fibrous tissue originating from the medial tuberosity of the calcaneus and ending at the proximal heads of the metatarsals. Along with ligaments, the plantar fascia supports the foot against downward forces (Figure 17-3).

Articulations

Joints of the foot are categorized into five regions: interphalangeal, metatarsophalangeal, intermetatarsal, tarsometatarsal, and intertarsal.

Interphalangeal Articulations

The interphalangeal joints are located at the distal extremities of the proximal and middle phalanges at the bases of the adjacent middle and terminal phalanges. These joints are designed only for flexion and extension. All interphalangeal joints have reinforcing collateral ligaments on their medial and lateral sides. Also located between the collateral ligaments on the plantar and dorsal surface are interphalangeal ligaments (Figure 17-4).

Metatarsophalangeal Articulations

The metatarsophalangeal joints are the condyloid type, which is permitted all forms of angular movement, with the exception of axial rotation; allowable movements in-

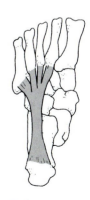

Figure 17-3

Plantar aponeurosis.

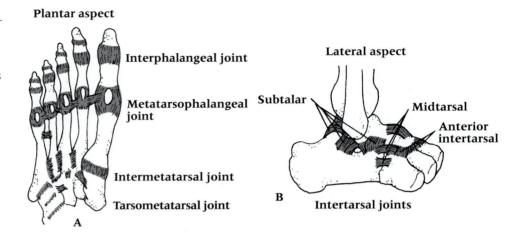

clude flexion, extension, adduction, and abduction. Each of these joints has collateral ligaments, as well as plantar and dorsal metatarsophalangeal ligaments.

Intermetatarsal Articulations

The intermetatarsal joints are sliding joints. They include two sets of articulations. One set consists of an articulation on each side of the base of the metatarsal bones, and the second articulations are on each side of the heads of the metatarsal bone. Each of these articulations permits only slight gliding movements. Shafts of the metatarsals are connected by interosseous ligaments. The bases are connected by plantar and dorsal ligaments, and the heads are attached by transverse metatarsal ligaments.

Tarsometatarsal Articulations

The tarsometatarsal joints are formed by the junction of the bases of the metatarsal bones with the tarsal bones. Their slight saddle shape allows some gliding and thus a restricted amount of flexion, extension, adduction, and abduction. Metatarsal bones are attached to the tarsal bones by the dorsal and plantar tarsometatarsal ligaments. Interosseous ligaments connect the first cuneiform to the second metatarsal, the third cuneiform to the second metatarsal, and the fourth cuneiform to the third metatarsal.

Intertarsal Articulations

The intertarsal joints include the subtalar, midtarsal (transverse tarsal), and anterior intertarsal (cuneonavicular) joints. In general, they are sliding joints. The subtalar joint is the articulation between the talus and the calcaneus. The midtarsal joint's articulation on the medial aspect is the talonavicular joint and on the lateral aspect is the articulation between the navicular and the cuneiform bones. Movements of the intertarsal articulations are gliding, flexion, extension, abduction, adduction, inversion, and eversion. Gliding occurs primarily at the anterior intertarsal joint and provides shock absorption for the weight of the body. Slight flexion and extension occur at the midtarsal region. Slight abduction and adduction of the forefoot also occur at the talonavicular joint. Inversion and eversion occur at the subtalar joint. *Inversion* refers to the sole of the foot turning medially, and *eversion* refers to its turning laterally. Foot *pronation* refers to the combined movements of talar plantar flexion and adduction and calcaneal eversion. In contrast, foot *supination* is the combined movements of talar dorsiflexion and abduction and calcaneal inversion.

Ligaments

The subtalar ligaments are the talocalcaneal interosseus and the anterior, posterior, lateral, and medial talocalcaneal (Figure 17-5). A major ligament is the plantar cal-

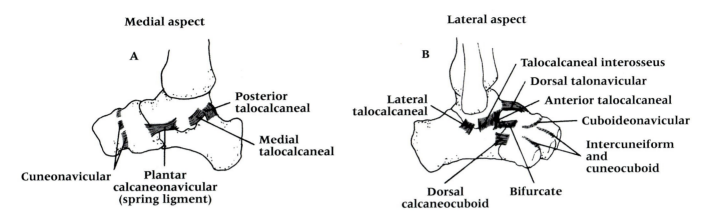

Medial aspect

A

Posterior
talocalcaneal

Medial
talocalcaneal

Cuneonavicular   Plantar
calcaneonavicular
(spring ligment)

Lateral aspect

B

Talocalcaneal interosseus

Dorsal talonavicular

Lateral
talocalcaneal

Anterior talocalcaneal

Cuboideonavicular

Intercuneiform
and
cuneocuboid

Dorsal
calcaneocuboid   Bifurcate

Figure 17-5

Ligaments of the subtalar joint. **A,** Medial aspect. **B,** Lateral aspect.

caneonavicular. It passes from the medial longitudinal arch. Because of its relatively large number of elastic fibers and its primary purpose of providing shock absorption, it is commonly called the *spring ligament.*

The primary ligaments of the midtarsal joint are the dorsal talonavicular, bifurcate, and dorsal calcaneocuboid. The midtarsal joint is given added strength in its plantar aspect by the long and plantar ligaments.

Ligaments of the anterior tarsal joints are divided into those of the cuneonavicular, cuboideonavicular, intercuneiform, and cuneocuboid joints. Each of these joints has both dorsal and plantar ligaments. The intercuneiform ligaments have three transverse bands, with one band connecting the first with the second and the second with the third cuneiform. A ligament also connects the third cuneiform with the cuboid bone.

Muscles and Movement

The movements of the foot are accomplished by numerous muscles (Figures 17-6 and 17-7; Table 17-1).

TABLE 17-1 Actions of the Intrinsic Foot Muscles

Location	Muscle	Action
Dorsal surface	Extensor digitorum brevis	Extension of first through fourth toes
First layer, plantar aspect	Abductor hallucis	Abduction and flexion of big toe
	Abductor digiti minimi pedis	Abduction and flexion of little toe
	Flexor digitorum brevis	Flexion of second through fifth toes
Second layer, plantar aspect	Quadratus plantae	Flexion of second through fifth toes
	Flexor digiti minimi brevis pedis	Flexion and abduction of little toe
	Lumbricalis pedis	Flexion of proximal phalanges and extension of distal phalanges of second through fifth toes; abduction of second toe; adduction of third, fourth, and fifth toes
Third layer, plantar aspect	Adductor hallucis	Adduction and flexion of big toe
	Flexor hallucis brevis	Flexion of big toe
Fourth layer, plantar aspect	Interosseus plantaris	Adduction of third, fourth, and fifth toes; flexion of these toes when acting with dorsal interossei
	Interosseus dorsalis pedis	When acting alone, first interosseus pulls second toe toward the big toe and pulls second, third, and fourth toes away from the big toe
		When acting with plantar interossei, flexion of second, third, and fourth toes

Figure 17-6

Muscles and tendons of the anterior aspect of the ankle and foot.

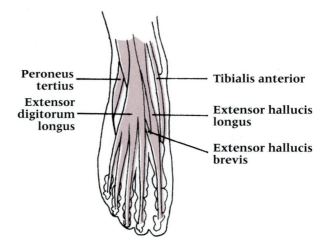

Peroneus tertius

Extensor digitorum longus

Tibialis anterior

Extensor hallucis longus

Extensor hallucis brevis

Figure 17-7

The movements of the foot are accomplished by a complex of many muscles.

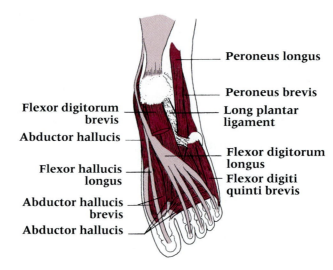

Peroneus longus

Peroneus brevis

Long plantar ligament

Flexor digitorum brevis

Abductor hallucis

Flexor hallucis longus

Flexor digitorum longus

Flexor digiti quinti brevis

Abductor hallucis brevis

Abductor hallucis

Dorsiflexion and Plantar Flexion

Dorsiflexion and plantar flexion of the foot take place at the ankle joint and will be discussed in greater detail in Chapter 18. The gastrocnemius, soleus, plantaris, peroneus longus, peroneus brevis, and tibialis posterior muscles are the plantar flexors. Dorsiflexion is accomplished by the tibialis anterior, extensor digitorum longus, extensor hallucis longus and brevis, and peroneus tertius muscles (see Figure 17-6).

Inversion, Adduction, and Supination

The medial movements of the foot are produced by the same muscles as inversion, adduction (medial movement of the forefoot), and supination (a combination of inversion and adduction). Muscles that produce these movements pass behind and in front of the medial malleolus. Muscles passing behind are the tibialis posterior, flexor digitorum longus, and flexor hallucis longus (see Figure 18-23, *D*). Muscles passing in front of the medial malleolus are the tibialis anterior and the extensor hallucis longus (see Figure 18-23, *A*).

Eversion, Abduction, and Pronation

The lateral movements of the foot are caused by the same muscles that produce eversion, abduction (lateral movement of the forefoot), and pronation (a combination of eversion and abduction). Muscles passing behind the lateral malleolus are the peroneus longus and the peroneus brevis. Muscles passing in front of the lateral malleolus are the peroneus tertius and extensor digitorum longus (see Figure 18-23, *B*).

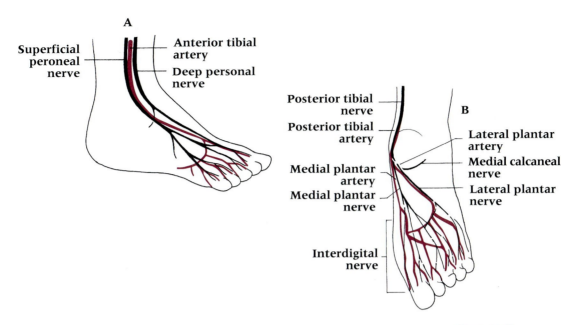

Figure 17-8

The major nerves of the foot. **A,** Dorsal aspect. **B,** Plantar aspect.

Movement of the Phalanges

The movements of the phalanges are flexion, extension, abduction, and adduction. Flexion of the second, third, fourth, and fifth distal digitus is executed by the flexor digitorum longus and the quadratus plantar. Flexion of the middle phalanges is performed by the flexor digitorum brevis, and flexion of the proximal phalanges is by the lumbricales and the interossei. The great toe is flexed by the flexor hallucis longus. The extension of all the middle phalanges is done by the abductor hallucis and abductor digiti quanti, the lumbricales, and the interossei. Extension of all distal phalanges is effected by the extensor digitorus longus, the extensor hallucis longus, and the extensor digitorum brevis. The adduction of the foot is performed by the interossei plantares and adductor hallucis; abduction is by the interossei dorsalis, the abductor hallucis, and the abductor digiti quanti.

Nerve Supply and Blood Supply

Nerve Supply

The tibial nerve, largest division of the sciatic nerve, supplies the muscles of the back of the leg and the plantar aspect of the foot. The common peroneal nerve is a smaller division of the sciatic nerve and, with its branches, supplies the front of the leg and the foot (Figure 17-8).

Blood Supply

The major portion of the blood is supplied to the foot by the anterior and posterior tibial arteries. The dorsal venous arch and digital veins and the dorsal digital vein stem from the short and long saphenous veins.

FOOT BIOMECHANICS

A study of lower-extremity chronic and overuse injuries related to sports participation must include some understanding of biomechanics of the foot, especially in the act of walking and running (Figure 17-9).

The action of the lower extremity during a complete stride in running can be divided into two phases (Figure 17-10). The first is the stance, or support, phase, which starts with initial contact at heel strike and ends at toe-off. The second is the swing or recovery phase. This represents the time immediately after toe-off in which the

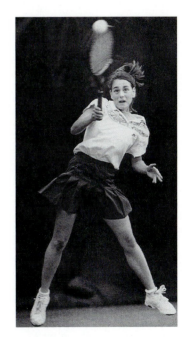

Figure 17-9

Chronic and overuse foot injuries are on the increase.

Figure 17-10

Walking gait cycle.

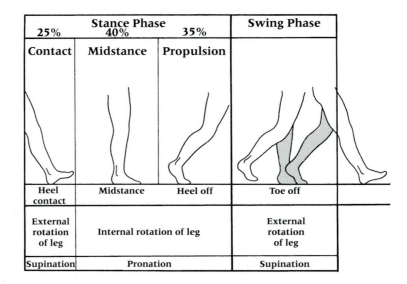

Stance Phase			Swing Phase
25%	40%	35%	
Contact	**Midstance**	**Propulsion**	
Heel contact	Midstance	Heel off	Toe off
External rotation of leg	**Internal rotation of leg**		**External rotation of leg**
Supination	**Pronation**		**Supination**

leg is moved from behind the body to a position in front of the body in preparation for heel strike.[1]

The foot's function during the support phase of running is twofold. At heel strike, the foot acts as a shock absorber to the impact forces and then adapts to the uneven surfaces. At push-off, the foot functions as a rigid lever to transmit the explosive force from the lower extremity to the running surface.[1] In a heel-strike running gait, initial contact of the foot is on the lateral aspect of the calcaneus with the subtalar joint in supination (Figure 17-11). It is estimated that 80% of distance runners use this heel-strike pattern and the remainder are either midfoot or forefoot strikers. In running, both feet are off the surface at the same time (Figure 17-12). Sprinters tend to be forefoot strikers, whereas a number of joggers are midfoot strikers.

At initial contact, the subtalar joint is supinated. Associated with this supination of the subtalar joint is an obligatory external rotation of the tibia.[1] As the foot is loaded, the subtalar joint moves into a pronated position until the forefoot is in contact with the running surface. The change in subtalar motion occurs between initial heel strike and 20% into the support phase of running.[1] As pronation occurs at the subtalar joint, there is obligatory internal rotation of the tibia. Transverse plane rotation occurs at the knee joint because of this tibial rotation. Pronation of the foot unlocks the midtarsal joint and allows the foot to assist in shock absorption and to adapt to uneven surfaces. It is important during initial impact to reduce the ground reaction forces and to distribute the load evenly on many different anatomical structures throughout the foot and leg. Pronation is normal and allows for this distribution of forces on as many structures as possible to avoid excessive loading on just a few structures. The subtalar joint remains in a pronated position until 55% to 85% of the support phase with maximum pronation is concurrent with the body's center of gravity passing over the base of support.

The foot begins to resupinate and will approach the neutral subtalar position at 70% to 90% of the support phase. In supination the midtarsal joints are locked and the foot becomes stable and rigid to prepare for push-off. This rigid position allows the foot to exert a great amount of force from the lower extremity to the running surface.

Subtalar Joint Pronation and Supination

It must be emphasized that pronation and supination of the foot and subtalar joint are normal during the support phase of running. However, excessive or prolonged

Figure 17-11

Foot bearing weight in walking as it moves from heel-strike to toe-off.

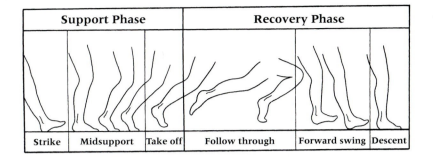

Support Phase			Recovery Phase		
Strike	Midsupport	Take off	Follow through	Forward swing	Descent

Figure 17-12

Running gait cycle.

pronation or supination will often cause or contribute to overuse injuries. When structural or functional deformities exist in the foot or leg, compensation is likely to occur at the subtalar joint. The subtalar joint compensates in a manner that allows the foot to make stable contact with the ground and get into a weight-bearing position (Figure 17-13, *B*). This excessive motion compensates for an existing structure deformity.

The most typical structural deformities of the foot that produce excessive pronation or supination include forefoot varus, forefoot valgus, and rearfoot varus (Figure 17-13, *A*). Structural forefoot varus and structural rearfoot varus deformities are usually associated with excessive pronation. A structural forefoot valgus causes excessive supination. The deformities usually exist in one plane, but the subtalar joint will interfere with the normal functions of the foot and make it more difficult for it to act as a shock absorber, to adapt to uneven surfaces, and to act as a rigid lever for push-off. The compensation rather than the deformity itself usually causes overuse injuries.[14]

Excessive or prolonged pronation of the subtalar joint during the support phase of running is one of the major causes of stress injuries. Overload of specific structures

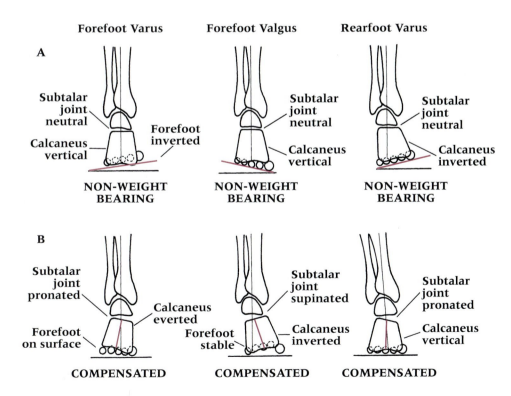

Forefoot Varus

A

Subtalar joint neutral

Calcaneus vertical

Forefoot inverted

NON-WEIGHT BEARING

B

Subtalar joint pronated

Forefoot on surface

Calcaneus everted

COMPENSATED

Forefoot Valgus

Subtalar joint neutral

Calcaneus vertical

NON-WEIGHT BEARING

Subtalar joint supinated

Forefoot stable

Calcaneus inverted

COMPENSATED

Rearfoot Varus

Subtalar joint neutral

Calcaneus inverted

NON-WEIGHT BEARING

Subtalar joint pronated

Calcaneus vertical

COMPENSATED

Figure 17-13

Structural foot deformities (posterior view). **A,** Bony alignment in a non–weight-bearing position. **B,** Compensated bony alignment in a weight-bearing position.

results when excessive pronation is produced in the support phase or when pronation is prolonged into the propulsive phase of running. Excessive pronation during the support phase will cause compensatory subtalar joint motion such that the midtarsal joint remains unlocked, resulting in an excessively loose foot. There is also an increase in tibial rotation, which forces the knee joint to absorb more transverse rotation motion. Prolonged pronation of the subtalar joint will not allow the foot to resupinate in time to provide a rigid lever for push-off, resulting in a less powerful and efficient force. Thus various foot and leg problems will occur with excessive or prolonged pronation during the support phase; these include stress fractures of the second metatarsal, plantar fasciitis, posterior tibial tendinitis, Achilles tendinitis, tibial stress syndrome, and medial knee pain.

At heel strike in prolonged or excessive supination, compensatory movement at the subtalar joint will not allow the midtarsal joint to unlock, causing the foot to remain excessively rigid. Thus the foot cannot absorb the ground reaction forces as efficiently. Excessive supination limits tibial internal rotation. Injuries typically associated with excessive supination include inversion ankle sprains, tibial stress syndrome, peroneal tendinitis, iliotibial band friction syndrome, and trochanteric bursitis.[8]

SPECIFIC JOINT SEGMENTS RELATED TO AMBULATION

Many foot segments are interdependent on one another; if one segment is weak, it adversely affects all other segments.

The Subtalar Joint

The subtalar joint must lock completely during the toe-off phase of locomotion and unlock in the support phase, allowing pronation to occur. The position of the calcaneus during ambulation and stance is a good indicator of the habitual movement of the subtalar joint. At all times it should remain in a straight-line or vertical position.

The Talonavicular Joint

The talonavicular joint moves independently from the hindfoot. In relation to the hindfoot it can dorsiflex and move in eversion and inversion. The talonavicular joint, like the subtalar joint, locks and unlocks. It has mobility during the first part of surface contact and should become highly stable before toe-off. Normally the talonavicular joint is positioned higher than the calcaneocuboid joint. If the subtalar joint is hypermobile, the talonavicular and calcaneocuboid joints become parallel and weakened, making them susceptible to surface forces. Another factor is that the surface stresses cause dorsiflexion of the forefoot on the hindfoot, thereby increasing hypermobility (Figure 17-14).

Figure 17-14

Stress sites in the hypermobile foot.

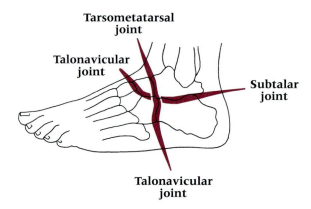

Tarsometatarsal joint

Talonavicular joint

Subtalar joint

Talonavicular joint

The Tarsometatarsal Joint

The tarsometatarsal joint comprises the cuboid; first, second, and third cuneiform; and bases of the metatarsal bones. These bones allow for great rotational forces when engaged in weight-bearing activities. They move as a unit, depending on the functioning of the talonavicular and subtalar joints. Also known as the Lisfranc joint, the tarsometatarsal joint is a locking device that provides foot stability. As the talonavicular joint becomes neutral or supinated, the tarsometatarsal joint becomes dorsally convex to resist the surface stress on the foot. In pronation the tarsometatarsal joint loses its convexity, and the bones becomes more parallel to one another, thus causing the forefoot to become hypermobile. The primary muscle support in the region is produced by the posterior tibial muscle pulling medially and the long and short peroneal muscles pulling laterally.

THE METATARSAL REGION

Together with subtalar, talonavicular, and tarsometatarsal interrelationships, foot stabilization depends on the functioning of the metatarsal joints.

The first metatarsal bone, along with the first cuneiform (first ray) bone, moves independently from the other metatarsal bones. As a main weight bearer, the first ray is concerned with body propulsion. Instability of the first ray occurs with forefoot varus. Stabilization depends on the long peroneal muscle that attached on the medial aspect of the first ray. The long peroneal muscle allows both plantar flexion of the first ray and foot abduction. When there is excessive subtalar pronation, the long peroneal muscle loses its ability to pull the first ray into plantar flexion effectively and tends to adduct the foot. For mechanically effective toe-off to occur, the proximal head of the first ray must be lifted above the cuboid bone by the foot's moving into a position of supination. Inadequate supination causes forefoot instability.

The fifth metatarsal bone, like the first metatarsal bone, moves independently. In plantar flexion it moves into adduction and inversion; conversely, in dorsiflexion it moves the foot into abduction and eversion. As with the other segments of the foot, stability of the fifth metatarsal bone depends on the relative position of the subtalar and talonavicular joints.

THE FOOT, ANKLE, AND LOWER LEG AS A KINETIC CHAIN

As discussed earlier in this chapter, there are a number of biomechanical factors that may be related to injuries of the lower leg region. It is important to realize when considering foot, ankle, and leg injuries that these segments are joined together to form a kinetic chain. With each movement of a body segment there is a direct effect on adjoining and distant body segments.[8] Each motion of the foot, ankle, and lower leg is closely linked with a proximal segment of the kinetic chain and can produce problems in other segments within the chain.[8]

Prevention of Foot Injuries

As with all body regions, preventing foot injuries is complex. Of major importance is the understanding of the foot's structural strength, weaknesses and mechanics, physical conditioning, footwear, and surface concerns.

Physical Conditioning

Feet are often neglected when physical conditioning for the prevention of injury is considered. Strengthening, stretching, and mobility exercises should be performed routinely by athletes whose sport places a great deal of emphasis on feet.

Most people will at some time in their lives develop foot problems.

Structural Concerns

Each athlete has feet that are individual and unique based on genetics and habitual usage. Athletic trainers and coaches must note athletes who may be predisposed to injuries caused by muscular or tendinous tightness or, conversely, weakness or hypermobility. Such situations, when recognized early, can possibly be remediated by exercise and mechanical intervention or by selecting appropriate shoes.

Footwear

Proper footwear is essential for the athlete in the prevention of injury, including shoes and socks. Chapter 5 discusses footwear in detail.

Surface Concerns

Athletes who propel themselves by means of their feet must continually adapt to the contact surface. Surfaces that are irregular and vary in resistance can serve to strengthen the foot over time. On the other hand, a nonyielding surface may in some cases overtax joints and soft tissue, eventually leading to an acute or chronic pathological condition in the foot or the entire kinetic chain. In contrast, a surface that is too resilient and absorbs too much of the impact energy may lead to early fatigue in sports such as basketball and indoor tennis.

FOOT ASSESSMENT

When assessing foot injuries, there must be a clear understanding that the foot is part of a kinetic chain that includes both the ankle and the lower leg. Acute injuries must be differentiated from those that had a relatively slow onset.[12]

History

When making a decision about how to manage a foot injury, a quick assessment must be performed to determine the type of injury and its history. The following questions should be asked[2]:

- How did the injury occur? Did it occur suddenly or come on slowly? Was the mechanism a sudden strain, twist, or blow to the foot?
- What type of pain is there? Is there muscle weakness? Are there noises such as crepitation during movement? Is there any alteration in sensation?
- Can the athlete point to the exact site of pain?
- When is the pain or other symptoms more or less severe?
- On what type of surface has the athlete been training?
- What type of footwear was being used during training? Is it appropriate for the type of training? Is discomfort increased when footwear is worn?
- Is this the first time this condition has occurred, or has it happened before? When, how often, and under what circumstances?

Observation

The athlete should be observed to determine the following:

- Whether he or she is favoring the foot, walking with a limp, or is unable to bear weight.
- Whether the injured part is deformed, swollen, or discolored.
- Whether the foot changes color when weight bearing and non–weight bearing (changing rapidly from a darker to lighter pink when not weight bearing).
- Whether the foot is well aligned and whether it maintains its shape on weight bearing.

Shoe Wear

The athletic trainer examines a well-worn pair of athlete's shoes. They are examined inside and outside for weight-bearing and wear patterns. Both shoes are compared for symmetry of wear. The greatest wear, in a normal foot, is beneath the ball of the foot and slightly to the lateral side. Shoes with excessive bulging on the medial side of the shoe suggest a valgus or everted heel; bulging on the lateral side indicates an

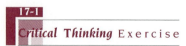

17-1

Critical Thinking Exercise

A sprinter is experiencing low back pain. Examination by the athletic trainer reveals that the athlete's right leg is three fourths of an inch shorter than his left leg.

? What street shoe wear patterns would the athletic trainer expect to observe?

inverted foot. Shoe soles with opposite wear patterns may be indicative of a short leg.

Palpation

Besides determining pain sites, swelling, and deformities, palpation is used to determine and evaluate circulation.

Bony Palpation

If the site of the injury is uncertain, palpate the following bony sites for point tenderness:

Medial Aspect	Lateral Aspect
Medial calcaneus	Lateral calcaneus
Medial malleolus	Lateral malleolus
Sustentaculum tali	Sinus tarsi
Talar head	Peroneal tubercle
Navicular tubercle	Cuboid bone
First cuneiform	Styloid process (proximal head of the fifth metatarsal)
First metatarsal	Fifth metatarsal
First metatarsophalangeal joint	Fifth metatarsophalangeal joint
First phalanx	Fifth phalanx

Dorsal Aspect	Plantar Aspect
Fourth, third, second metatarsals	Metatarsal heads
Fourth, third, second metatarsophalangeal joints	Medial calcaneal tubercle
Fourth, third, second phalanges	
Third and fourth cuneiform bones	

Soft-Tissue Palpation

Palpate the following soft-tissue sites:

Medial and Plantar Aspect	Lateral and Dorsal Aspect
Tibialis posterior tendon	Anterior talofibular ligament
Deltoid ligament	Calcaneofibular ligament
Calcaneonavicular ligament (spring ligament)	Posterior talofibular ligament
Medial longitudinal arch	Peroneal tendon
Plantar fascia	Extensor tendons of toes
Bursal head of the first metatarsal bone	Tibialis anterior tendon
Transverse arch	

Special Tests

Movement and Neurological Assessment

Both the extrinsic and the intrinsic foot muscles should be assessed for pain and range of motion during active, passive, and resistive isometric movement. Reflexes and cutaneous distribution should also be tested. Skin sensation should be noted for any alteration.

Tendon reflexes such as in the Achilles tendon (S_1 nerve root) should elicit a response when gently tapped. Sensation is tested by running the hands over the anterior, lateral, medial, and posterior surfaces of the foot and toes.

Pulses

To ensure that there is proper blood circulation to the foot, the pulse is measured at the posterior tibial and dorsalis pedis arteries (Figure 17-15). Pulsation in the dorsalis pedis artery is normally felt between the tendons of the extensor hallucis longus and extensor digitorum longus, on a line from the midpoint between the medial and lateral malleoli to the proximal end of the first intermetatarsal space.

Pulsation in the posterior tibial artery is normally palpable behind the medial malleolus, 2.5 cm in front of the medial border of the Achilles tendon.

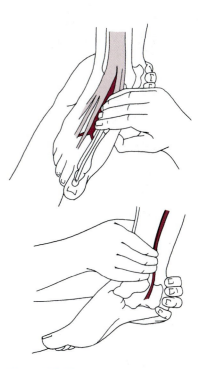

Figure 17-15

An ankle injury may impede blood flow, making routine measurement of the pulse extremely important.

Functional Examination

Passive, active, and resistive movement is performed in the numerous joints of the foot and adjacent ankle. Inspection is first performed while the athlete is on a table and then during weight bearing. Movement is performed in the following joints:

- Ankle mortice
- Subtalar
- Midtarsal
- Metatarsophalangeal
- Interphalangeal

The foot is then inspected while the athlete stands and walks. The posture of the foot and whether it maintains the same shape in weight bearing as in non–weight bearing are noted.[12]

Test for flexible and rigid flatfeet   The athlete is observed as full weight is borne on a foot and then is removed. A flexible flatfoot is one in which the medial longitudinal arch becomes flattened during weight bearing and produces an obvious arch after removal of the weight. Conversely, a rigid arch remains flat during both weight bearing and non–weight bearing. Care includes the use of properly fitting shoes that give sufficient support to the arch or permit the normal anatomy of the foot to function, exercise, arch supports, and protective taping. In addition, when there is chronic pain, care should include daily hydrotherapy and friction massage until the inflammation has subsided.

RECOGNITION AND MANAGEMENT OF FOOT INJURIES

Most people will at some time develop foot problems. This development is attributed to the use of improper footwear, poor foot hygiene, or anatomical structural deviations that result from faulty postural alignments or abnormal stresses.

Many sports place exceptional demands on the feet—far beyond the normal daily requirements. The coach and the athletic trainer should be well aware of potential foot problems and should be capable of identifying, ameliorating, or preventing them whenever possible.

Acute Conditions of the Foot

Contusions

Two common contusions of the foot are the heel bruise and the instep bruise. Each can cause the athlete a great deal of discomfort and disability.

Heel bruise   Of the many contusions and bruises that an athlete may receive, there is no bruise more disabling than the heel bruise.

Etiology   Sport activities that demand a sudden stop-and-go response or a sudden change from a horizontal to a vertical movement (e.g., basketball, jumping, or the landing action in long jumping) are particularly likely to cause heel bruises. The heel has a thick, cornified skin layer and a heavy fat pad covering, but even this thick padding cannot always protect against a sudden abnormal force directed to this area.[10]

The major purpose of the tissue heel pad is to sustain hydraulic pressure through fat columns. Tissue compression is monitored by pressure nerve endings from the skin and plantar aponeurosis. Often the irritation is on the lateral aspect of the heel because of the heel strike in walking or running.

Symptoms and signs   When injury occurs, the athlete complains of severe pain in the heel and is unable to withstand the stress of weight bearing. Often there is warmth and redness over the tender area.

Management   A bruise of the heel usually develops into chronic inflammation of the periosteum. Follow-up management of this condition should be started 2 to 3 days after insult, involving a variety of superficial and deep-heat therapies. If the athlete recognizes the problem in its acute stage, he or she should adhere to the following precedures:

- If possible, the athlete should not step on the heel for a period of at least 24 hours.
- Initially, rest, ice, compression, and elevation (RICE) are applied, and a nonsteroidal antiinflammatory drug (NSAID) is administered.[9]
- On the third and subsequent days the athlete can receive warm whirlpool and ultrasound or cold therapy.
- If pain when walking has subsided by the third day, the athlete may resume moderate activity with the protection of a heel cup or protective doughnut. The athlete should wear shock-absorbent footwear (Figure 17-16).

Note that because of the nature of this condition, it may recur throughout the entire season.

An athlete who is prone to or who needs protection from a heel bruise should routinely wear a heel cup with a foam rubber pad as a preventive aid. By surrounding the heel with a firm heel cup, traumatic forces are diffused.

The bruised instep   The bruised instep, like the bruised heel, can cause disability.

Etiology   It commonly occurs from the athlete being stepped on or from being hit with a fast-moving hard projectile such as a baseball or hockey puck.

Symptoms and signs   Irritation of the synovial sheaths covering the extensor tendon can make wearing a shoe difficult. If the force is of great intensity, there is a good chance of fracture, requiring an x-ray.

Management   Immediate application of cold compresses must be performed to control inflammation and to prevent swelling. Once inflammation is reduced and the athlete returns to competition, a ⅛-inch (0.3 cm) pad protection should be worn on the skin directly over the bruise, as well as a rigid instep guard that is worn external to the shoe.

Foot Strain

Insufficient conditioning of musculature, structural imbalance, or incorrect mechanics can cause the foot to become prone to strain. Common strains occur to the metatarsal arch, the longitudinal arch, and the plantar fascia (Figure 17-17). See the Focus box on the following page for the management of arch problems.

Metatarsal arch strain

Etiology   The athlete who has a fallen metatarsal arch or who has a pes cavus (high arch) is susceptible to strain (Figure 17-18). In both cases, malalignment of the forefoot subjects the flexor tendons to increased tension.

Symptoms and signs   The athlete has pain or cramping in the metatarsal region. There is point tenderness and weakness in the area.

Management   Treatment of acute metatarsalgia usually consists of applying a pad to elevate the depressed metatarsal heads. The pad is placed in the center and just behind the ball of the foot (metatarsal heads) (Figure 17-19).

Longitudinal arch strain

Etiology   Longitudinal arch strain is usually an early-season injury caused by subjecting the musculature of the foot to unaccustomed, severe exercise and forceful contact with hard playing surfaces. In this condition there is a flattening or depression of the longitudinal arch while the foot is in the midsupport phase, resulting in a strain to the arch. Such a strain may appear suddenly, or it may develop slowly over a considerable length of time.

Symptoms and signs   As a rule, pain is experienced only when running is attempted and usually appears just below the medial malleolus and the posterior tibial tendon, accompanied by swelling and tenderness along the medial aspects of the foot. Prolonged strain will also involve the calcaneonavicular ligament and first cuneiform with the navicular. The flexor muscle of the great toe (flexor hallucis longus) often develops tenderness as a result of overuse in compensating for the stress on the arch ligaments.

Management   The management of a longitudinal arch stain involves immediate care, consisting of RICE followed by appropriate therapy and reduction of weight

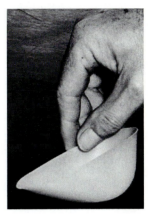
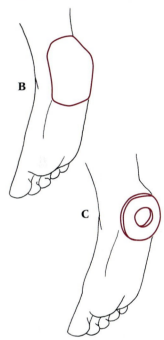

Figure 17-16

A and **B,** Heel protection achieved through the use of a heel cup. **C,** Protective heel doughnut.

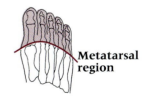

Metatarsal region

Figure 17-17

Bones of the metatarsal region.

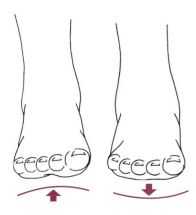

Figure 17-18

Normal and fallen metatarsal arch.

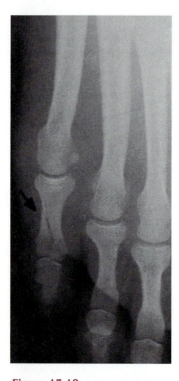

Figure 17-19

Fracture of the fifth phalanx.

point tenderness
Pain is produced when an injury site is palpated.

Focus

Management of arch problems

1. Shoes should fit properly.
2. Hydrotherapy, especially a whirlpool, should be given three or four times daily at a temperature of 105° F (40.6° C) until the initial inflammation has subsided.
3. Deep therapy, such as ultrasound, can be used when prescribed by a physician.
4. Arch orthoses may ameliorate irritation of the weakened ligaments. If a pathological condition of the arch can be detected in the first or second degree, arch supports may be needed.
5. Weakened arches, if detected early, can be aided by an exercise program. If the arch is allowed to drop and the condition becomes chronic, exercising can offer little relief other than palliation.

bearing. Weight bearing must be performed pain free. Arch taping technique no. 1 or 2 might be used to allow earlier pain-free weight bearing (see Figures 13-15 through 13-18).

Plantar fascia strain   Running the length of the sole of the foot is a broad band of dense connective tissue called the *plantar aponeurosis.* It is attached to the under surface of the calcaneus at the back and fans out toward the front, with fibers and their various small branches attaching to the metatarsophalangeal articulations and merging into the capsular ligaments. Other fibers, arising from well within the aponeurosis, pass between the intrinsic muscles of the foot and the long flexor tendons of the sole and attach themselves to the deep fascia below the bones. The function of the plantar aponeurosis is to assist in maintaining the stability of the foot and in securing or bracing the longitudinal arch.

Etiology   Strains to the fascia commonly occur during the early season among tennis and basketball players and runners. The fascia is placed under strain either by extension of the toes or by depression of the longitudinal arch as the result of weight bearing. When the weight is principally on the heel, as in ordinary standing, the tension exerted on the fascia is negligible. However, when the weight is shifted to the ball of the foot (on the heads of the metatarsals), fascial tension is so increased that it equals approximately twice the body weight. In running, because the push-off phase involves both a forceful extension of the toes and a powerful thrust by the ball of the foot (on the heads of the metatarsals), fascial tension is so increased that it equals approximately twice the body weight. In running, because the push-off phase involves both a forceful extension of the toes and a powerful thrust by the ball of the foot against a relatively unyielding surface, the degree of fascial tension is greatly increased.

Athletes who have a mild pes cavus are particularly prone to fascial strain. Modern street shoes, by nature of their design, take on the characteristics of splints and tend to restrict foot action to such an extent that the arch may become somewhat rigid because of shortening of the ligaments and other mild abnormalities. The athlete, when changing from such footwear into a flexible gymnastic slipper or soft track shoe, often experiences trauma when the foot is subject to stresses. Trauma may also result from running improperly, either as the result of poor technique or because of lordosis, a condition in which the increased forward tilt of the pelvis produces an unfavorable angle of foot-strike when there is considerable force exerted on the ball of the foot.

Symptoms and signs   The athlete complains of having a sudden pain in the arch region that is relieved by becoming non–weight bearing. There is great difficulty in walking and an inability to run. During inspection there is **point tenderness** in the plantar aponeurosis, expecially in the region of the epicondyle of the calcaneus. Swelling and later ecchymosis may be associated with this problem.

Management   Management is symptomatic. A heel doughnut may relieve some of the irritation, along with a heel lift, and a stiff shank will distribute the body weight more effectively. Also, performing a gradual stretch of the plantar muscle and the gastrocnemius-soleus complex will help relieve tension in that region. A gradual program of arch exercises should be performed. If the condition is associated with pronation, taping with the LowDye technique may be helpful (see Figure 13-19).

Foot Sprain

Two sites where foot sprain may occur are the midfoot or forefoot and the phalanges.

Midfoot or forefoot sprain   Although not common, sprains of the midfoot and forefoot do occur.

Etiology   The most frequent mechanism is excessive dorsiflexion or plantar flexion of the toes or forefoot. Supportive ligaments are injured along with tendons. A common foot sprain among gymnasts and dancers occurs to the midtarsal ligament, caused by forced dorsiflexion and plantar flexion of the midfoot.

Symptoms and signs   Acute response pain and swelling over the involved area occur. If chronic there is a dull pain in the forefoot.

Management   Management usually consists of RICE and limitation in weight bearing. Use RICE and NSAIDs as needed.[9] Tape support (see Chapter 13) helps relieve pain during weight bearing; and placing the foot into a firm, solid shoe with a rocker-bottom sole often prevents pain.

The sprained toe   Sprains of the phalangeal joint of the foot are caused most often by kicking some nonyielding object. Sprains result from a considerable force applied in such a manner as to extend the joint beyond its normal range of motion (jamming it) or to impart a twisting motion to the toe, thereby twisting and tearing the supporting tissues. Symptoms of an acute injury appear.

Turf toe   Turf toe is the sprain of the metatarsophalangeal joint of the great toe.

Etiology   This injury results from the combination of artifical playing surfaces and flexible types of sport footwear.

Symptoms and signs   Turf toe is an acute injury stemming from a sudden hyperextension of the first metatarsophalangeal joint. The trauma causes the joint capsule to be torn from the metatarsal head.

Management   This condition is handled as an acute sprain. Fracture must be ruled out by x-ray. Wearing stiff-soled shoes and taping can serve to restrict motion. Taping provides restraint (see Figure 13-22).

Fractures and Dislocations

Because of the foot's susceptibility to trauma in sports, fractures and dislocations can occur. Any moderate to severe contusion or twisting force must be suspected as a fracture. X-ray examination should be routine in these situations.

Fractures and dislocations of the foot phalanges

Etiology   Fractures of the phalanges (see Figure 17-19) are usually the bone-crushing type such as may be incurred by kicking an object or stubbing a toe.

Symptoms and signs   Generally they are accompanied by swelling and discoloration. If the fracture is to the proximal phalanx of the great toe or of the distal phalanx and also involves the interphalangeal joint, it should be referred to an orthopedist (see Figure 17-19).[2]

Management   If the break is in the bone shaft, adhesive tape is applied. (See Chapter 13.) However, if more than one toe is involved, a cast may be applied for a few days. As a rule 3 or 4 weeks of inactivity permit healing, although tenderness may persist for some time. A shoe with a wide toe box should be worn; in cases of great toe fracture, a stiff sole should be worn.

17-2

Critical Thinking Exercise

A distance runner with lordosis is experiencing pain in his left arch. There is palpable tenderness in the left foot's aponeurosis primarily in the epicondyle region of the calcaneus.

? What condition does this scenario describe, and how should it be managed?

17-3

Critical Thinking Exercise

A football player who commonly plays on artificial turf complains of pain in his right great toe.

? What type of injury frequently occurs to the great toe while playing on artificial turf?

Fractures and dislocations of the foot phalanges can be caused by kicking an object or by stubbing a toe.

17-4

Critical Thinking Exercise

While roughhousing in the locker room, an athlete inadvertently kicks a locker and injures his right great toe.

? What should the athletic trainer be concerned with in this type of injury mechanism?

Dislocations of the phalanges are less common than fractures. If one occurs, it is a dorsal dislocation of the middle phalanx proximal joint. The mechanism of injury is the same as for fractures. Reduction is usually performed easily without anesthesia by the physician.

Fractures of the metatarsals

Etiology   Fractures of the metatarsals can be caused by direct force, such as being stepped on by another player, or by abnormal stress. The most common acute fracture is to the base of the fifth metatarsal (Jones fracture).

Symptoms and signs   Fractures of the metatarsals are characterized by swelling and pain. They have the appearance of a severe sprain and are usually caused by sharp inversion and plantar flexion of the foot.

Management   Treatment is usually symptomatic, with RICE used to control swelling. Once swelling has subsided, a short leg walking cast is applied for 3 to 6 weeks. Ambulation is usually possible by the second week. A shoe with a large toe box should be worn. The injured toe should be taped to an adjacent toe in the same manner as for fractures of the other phalanges.

Fractures and dislocations of the talus

Etiology   Fracture or dislocation of the talus usually results from a severe ankle twist or being hit behind the leg while the foot is firmly planted on the ground.

Symptoms and signs   There is extreme pain and point tenderness at the distal end of the tibia.

Management   For accurate diagnosis an x-ray is essential. If the fracture is severe, there could be a severance of the blood supply to the area, resulting in bone necrosis. If present, the athlete's future in sports participation may be jeopardized. The following procedures should be used:

- The foot and ankle should be immobilized, and the athlete should be transported for medical care.
- After the fracture has been reduced, the physician will usually cast the foot in a plaster boot for approximately 6 weeks and then allow only limited weight bearing on the injured leg for at least another 8 weeks.

Fracture of the os calis

Etiology   The os calis fracture is the most common fracture of the tarsus bone and is usually caused by a jump or fall from a height.

Symptoms and signs   There is usually extreme swelling and pain. This condition may eventually predispose the athlete to arthritis of the articulating surface.

Management   Reduction may be delayed for as much as 24 to 48 hours or until swelling has been reduced. In the interval the following steps should be initiated:

17-5

Critical Thinking Exercise

A basketball player sustains a second-degree lateral sprain of the left ankle.

? What metatarsal fracture may be associated with this type of sprain?

Figure 17-20

Fallen medial longitudinal arch.

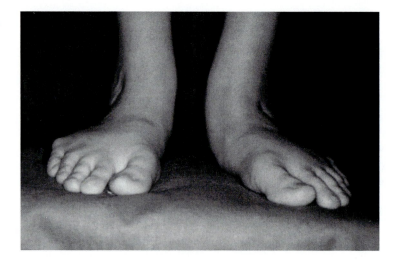

1. Cold and a pressure bandage should be applied intermittently for 24 to 48 hours.
2. The foot should be elevated immediately after the injury and maintained in this postion for at least 24 hours or until medical treatment has been instituted.

Fallen Medial Longitudinal Arch (Flatfoot)

Etiology   Various stresses weaken ligaments and muscles that support the arch, thus forcing the navicular bone downward (Figure 17-20). Ankle sprains frequently result from weakened arches, and abnormal friction sites may develop within the shoe because of changes in weight distribution. This condition may be the result of several factors: shoes that cramp and deform the feet, weakened supportive tissues, overweight, postural anomalies that subject the arches to unaccustomed or unnatural strain, or overuse, which may be the result of repeatedly subjecting the arch to severe pounding through participation on an unyielding surface. Commonly, the fallen medial longitudinal arch is associated with foot pronation (see Figure 17-20).

Symptoms and signs   The athlete may complain of tiredness and tenderness in the arch and heel, along with point tenderness.

Management   Unless flatfeet are painful or associated with conditions such as foot pronation, treatment is unnecessary. Taping provides some support (see Figures 13-15 through 13-18). Where there is a potential for abnormal lower-limb stress orthoses may be warranted.

Pes Cavus

Pes cavus (Figure 17-21), common called *clawfoot, hollow foot,* or an *abnormally high arch,* is not as common as pes planus, or flatfeet. In the rigid type of pes cavus, shock absorption is poor and can lead to problems such as general foot pain, metatarsalgia, and clawed or hammer toes. Pes cavus also may be asymptomatic.

The accentuated high medial longitudinal arch may be congenital or indicate a neurological disorder. Commonly associated with this condition are clawed toes and abnormal shortening of the Achilles tendon. The Achilles tendon is directly linked with the plantar fascia (Figure 17-22). Also, because of the abnormal distribution of body weight, heavy calluses develop on the ball and heel of the foot.

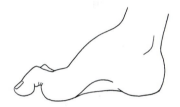

Figure 17-21

Pes cavus.

Figure 17-22

The achilles tendon is directly linked with the plantar fascia. Achilles tendon stretching releases a tight medial longitudinal arch.

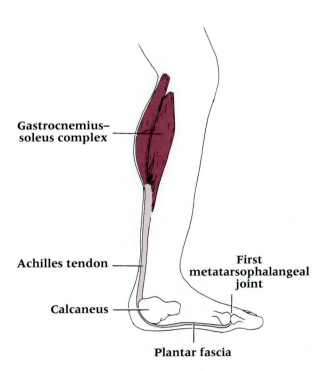

Gastrocnemius–soleus complex

Achilles tendon

First metatarsophalangeal joint

Calcaneus

Plantar fascia

Conditions of the Forefoot, Ball of the Foot, and Toe

A number of deformities and structural deviations affect the forefoot and the ball of the foot. Conditions commonly seen in sports include bunions, hallux valgus, bunionettes, sesamoiditis, metatarsalgia, interdigital neuroma, and Morton's syndrome.

Bunion (Hallux Valgus) and Bunionettes (Tailor's Bunions)

A bunion is one of the most frequent painful deformities of the great toe (Figure 17-23).

Etiology   The reasons why a bunion develops are complex. It is generally believed that women's shoes play a predominant role in the development of a hallux valgus deformity.[7]

Commonly it is associated with a structural forefoot varus in which the first ray tends to splay outward, putting pressure on the first metatarsal head caused by wearing shoes that are pointed, too narrow, too short, or have high heels. The bursa over the first metatarsophalangeal joint becomes inflamed and eventually thickens. The joint becomes enlarged and the great toe becomes malaligned, moving laterally toward the second toe, sometimes to such an extent that it eventually overlaps the second toe. This type of bunion is also associated with a depressed or flattened transverse arch and a pronated foot.

The bunionette, or tailor's bunion, is much less common than hallux valgus and affects the fifth metatarsophalangeal joint. In this case, the little toe angulates toward the fourth toe, causing an enlarged metatarsal head.[3]

In all bunions, both the flexor and extensor tendons are malpositioned, creating more angular stress on the joint. NOTE: Sesamoid fractures and sesamoiditis could be secondary to hallux valgus.

Symptoms and signs   In the beginning of bunion formation there is tenderness, swelling, and enlargement of the joint (see Figure 17-23). Poorly fitting shoes increase the irritation and pain. As the inflammation continues, angulation of the toe progresses, eventually leading to instability in the forefoot.

Figure 17-23

Mild bunion deformity of the left great toe.

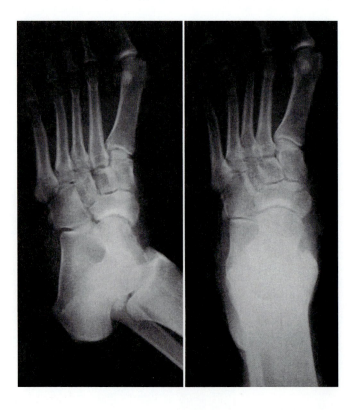

Management   Each bunion has unique characteristics. Early recognition and care can often prevent increased irritation and deformity. Following are some management procedures:

1. Wear correctly fitting shoes with a wide toe box.
2. Place a felt or sponge rubber doughnut pad or lamb's wool over the first and/or fifth metatarsophalangeal joint.
3. Wear a tape splint along with a resilient wedge placed between the great toe and the second toe (see Figure 13-21).
4. Apply thermal therapy or cryotherapy to reduce the inflammation.
5. Engage in daily foot exercise to strengthen the extensor and flexor muscles.

If the condition progresses, a special orthotic device may help normalize foot mechanics. Surgery might be required in the later stages of this condition.

Sesamoid Injuries of the First Toe

Sesamoiditis is most common in dancing and basketball. It is estimated that 40% of sesamoid injuries are fractures and 30% are sesamoiditis.[9]

Etiology   Sesamoid injuries are caused by repetitive microtrauma primarily in athletes with a pes cavus foot or having a hallux valgus.

Symptoms and signs   The athlete complains of pain under the great toe, especially during a push-off. There is palpable tenderness, medial and lateral to the first metatarsal head.

Management   Treatment usually requires x-ray to determine a fracture. Sesamoiditis is treated with a semirigid orthotic device with a metatarsal bar (see Figure 17-27).

Metatarsalgia

Although **metatarsalgia** is a general term used to describe pain in the ball of the foot, it is more commonly associated with pain under the second and sometimes the third metatarsal head. A heavy callus often forms in the area of pain. Figure 17-24 shows some of the more common pain sites in the foot.

17-6

Critical Thinking Exercise

A field hockey player complains to the athletic trainer of swelling, tenderness, and aching in the head of the first metatarsophalangeal joint of her left foot. On inspection it is observed that the great toe is deviated laterally.

? What is this condition commonly called, and why does it occur?

metatarsalgia
A general term used to describe pain in the ball of the foot.

Figure 17-24

Common pain sites in the foot.

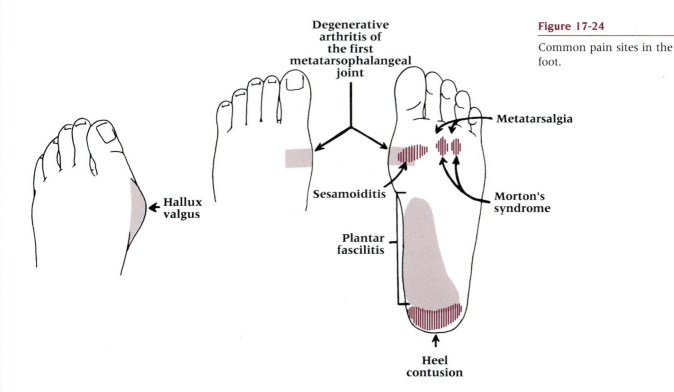

Figure 17-25

Normal weight bearing of the forefoot and abnormal spread (splayed foot).

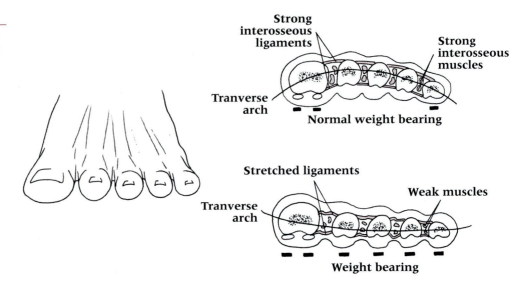

Figure 17-26

Metatarsal pad.

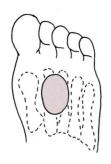

Figure 17-27

Metatarsal bar to release severe metatarsalgia.

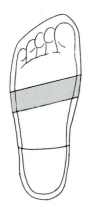

neuroma

A tumor that emanates from a nerve.

Etiology   One of the causes of metatarsalgia is restricted extensibility of the gastrocnemius-soleus system. Because of this restriction, the athlete shortens the mid-stance phase of the gait and emphasizes the toe-off phase, causing excessive pressure under the forefoot. This excess pressure over time causes a heavy callus to form in this region. As the forefoot bears weight, normal skin becomes pinched against the inelastic callus and produces pain.

Another cause of matatarsalgia is a fallen metatarsal arch. Normally the heads of the first and fifth metatarsal bones bear slightly more weight than the heads of the second, third, and fourth metatarsal bones. The first metatarsal head bears two sixths of the body weight, the fifth bears slightly more than one sixth, and the second, third, and fourth each bear approximately one sixth. If the foot tends toward pronation or if the intermetatarsal ligaments are weak, allowing the foot to spread abnormally (splayed foot), occurrence of a fallen metatarsal arch is probable (Figure 17-25).

Symptoms and signs   As the transverse arch becomes flattened and the heads of the second, third, and fourth metatarsal bones become depressed, pain can result. A cavus deformity can also cause metatarsalgia.

Management   Management of metatarsalgia usually consists of applying a pad to elevate the depressed metatarsal heads. See the accompanying Focus box. NOTE: The pad is placed *behind* and not *under* the metatarsal heads (Figure 17-26). In severe cases a metatarsal bar may be applied (Figure 17-27). Abnormal callus buildup should be removed by paring or filing. In an athlete in whom the etiology of metatarsalgia is primarily a gastrocnemius-soleus contracture, a regimen of static stretching should be performed several times per day. If the athlete's metatarsal arch is depressed as a result of weakness, a daily regimen of exercise should be practiced, concentrating on strengthening flexor and intrinsic muscles and stretching the Achilles tendon. A Thomas heel (Figure 17-28), which elevates the medial aspect of the heel from 1/8 to 3/16 inch (0.3 to 0.47 cm), also could prove beneficial.

Interdigital Neuroma

Interdigital nerves travel between the metatarsal bones to innervate the toes.

Etiology   An interdigital **neuroma** emanates from and entraps the nerves. It usually involves the third plantar inderdigital nerve, which innervates the third and fourth toes (Figure 17-29).

Symptoms and signs   The athlete complains of severe intermittent pain in the region of the nerve impingement. The pain radiates from the distal metatarsal heads to the tips of the toes and is often relieved when no weight is borne. The pain may be

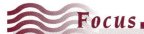

Focus

Metatarsal pad support

The purpose of the metatarsal pad is to reestablish the normal relationships of the metatarsal bones. It can be purchased commercially or constructed out of felt or sponge rubber (see Figure 17-26).

Materials needed

One roll of 1-inch tape (2.5 cm), a ⅛-inch (0.3 cm) adhesive felt oval cut to a 2-inch (5 cm) circumference, and tape adherent.

Position of the athlete

The athlete sits on a table or chair with the plantar surface of the affected foot turned upward.

Position of the operator

The operator stands facing the plantar aspect of the athlete's foot.

Procedure

1. The circular pad is placed just behind the metatarsal heads.
2. Approximately two or three circular strips of tape are placed loosely around the pad and foot.

duplicated, and the tumor may be felt. Sometimes the skin between the metatarsal heads is numb.[13]

Management   Conservative treatment of an interdigital neuroma includes the following:

- Broad-toed shoe
- Transverse arch support
- Metatarsal bar
- Injection of lidocaine and steroids

If conservative treatment is ineffective, surgical excision may provide complete relief.[13]

Morton's Toe

Another foot deformity causing major forefoot pain is Morton's toe. Metatarsalgia is produced by an abnormally short first metatarsal bone. Weight is borne mainly by the second proximal metatarsal joints (Figure 17-30). The management is the same as that for foot pronation.

Toe Deformities

Hallux Rigidus

Etiology   Hallus rigidus is a painful condition caused by fusion or partial fusion of the first metatarsophalangeal joint.[7]

Symptoms and signs   The great toe is unable to dorsiflex, causing the athlete to toe-off on the second, third, fourth, and fifth toes. Walking becomes awkward. Often, with complete fusion, pain disappears.

Management   Management usually includes placing a pad under the first metatarsal bone to prevent great toe dorsiflexion. A metatarsal bar on the shoe may help to avoid increasing the joint's irritation. Surgery may be the only means of recovering function.[16]

Hammer or clawed toes

Etiology   Hammer or clawed toes may be congenital, but more often the conditions are caused by wearing shoes that are too short over a long period of time, thus

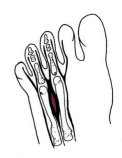

Figure 17-28

The Thomas heel elevates the medial aspect of the calcaneus ⅛ to ³⁄₁₆ inch (0.3 to 0.47 cm), which can help relieve pronation and metatarsalgia.

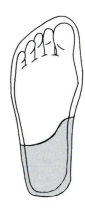

Figure 17-29

Interdigital neuroma.

Figure 17-30

Morton's syndrome with an abnormally short first metatarsal bone.

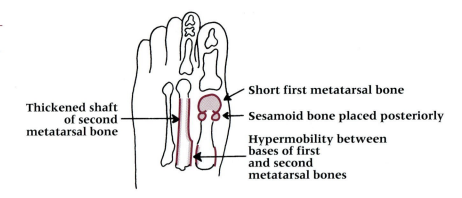

Thickened shaft of second metatarsal bone

Short first metatarsal bone

Sesamoid bone placed posteriorly

Hypermobility between bases of first and second metatarsal bones

cramping the toes. Hammer toe usually involves the second or third toe; clawed toes involve more than one toe.

Symptoms and signs   In both conditions the metatarsophalangeal and proximal interphalangeal joints become malaligned, along with overly contracted flexor tendons and overly stretched extensor tendons. Such deformities eventually result in the formation of hard corns or calluses on the exposed joints.

Management   Often surgery is the only cure. However, wearing proper shoes and using protective taping (see Figure 13-24) can help prevent irritation.

Overlapping Toes

Etiology   Overlapping of the toes (Figure 17-31) may be congenital or may be brought about by improperly fitting footwear, particularly shoes that are too narrow.

Symptoms and signs   At times the condition indicates an outward projection of the great toe articulation or a drop in the longitudinal or metatarsal arch.

Management   As in the case of hammer toes, surgery is the only cure, but some therapeutic modalities such as a whirlpool bath can assist in alleviating inflammation. Taping may prevent some of the contractural tension within the sport shoe.

CHRONIC AND OVERUSE SYNDROMES

Because of the hard use that feet receive in many sports, they are prone to chronic and overuse syndromes. This is especially true if weight-transmission or biomechanical problems exist. Because distance running is becoming increasingly popular, musculoskeletal problems of the feet are becoming more prevalent.

Exostoses

Exostoses are benign bony outgrowths that protrude from the surface of a bone and are usually capped by cartilage. Sometimes called *spurs,* such outgrowths occur principally at the head of the first metatarsal bone on the dorsum of the foot (Figure 17-32). In certain instances, what may at first appear to be an exostosis actually may be a subluxation of the joints between the metatarsal and cuneiform bones. The causes of exostoses are highly variable, including heredity influences, faulty patterns of walking and running, excessive weight, joint impingements, and continual use of ill-fitting footwear.

Impingement Exostoses

Etiology   Impingement, one of the causes of exostoses, occurs when a joint is continually forced beyond the ranges of normal motion so that contact is effected by the bones of the joint. Continual contact creates inflammation and irritation, eventually activating the formation of new bone, which builds up to such a degree that the bones contact each other. Extreme dorsiflexion, such as when the foot is at the end of the support period immediately before the forward-carry, may cause exostoses to form on the anterior articular lip of the tibia and top of the talus as a consequence of the impingement.

Symptoms and signs Pain and tenderness are usually present, and performance is impaired, especially when the foot is in extreme dorsiflexion. This pain is usually apparent at the anterior aspect of the joint and may be severe enough to weaken the drive from the foot as it thrusts against the ground in the push-off, resulting in a loss of drive and speed.

Management Some impingement spurring conditions are asymptomatic and require no treatment. For cases of impingement that are symptomatic, surgery may be warranted to allow continued sports participation.

Chronic Irritation Exostoses

Poorly fitting shoes or a chronic irritation may also predispose an area to exostoses, which usually appear either at the head of the fifth metatarsal bone or as a calcaneal spur. If an exostosis becomes chronically irritated or disabling, surgery may be necessary. Sometimes protective doughnuts and custom-made pads provide relief.

Retrocalcaneal Bursitis

A common bursitis of the foot is retrocalcaneal bursitis, which is located between the calcaneous and the Achilles tendon, just above the attachment of the Achilles tendon (Figure 17-33). It is also referred to as a "pump."

Etiology Retrocalcaneal bursitis often occurs because of pressure and rubbing by the upper edge of a sports shoe. This condition is chronic, developing gradually over a long period of time, and takes many days—sometimes weeks or months—to heal properly.

Symptoms and signs Irritation produces an inflamed, swollen area.

Management Initially use RICE plus NSAIDs and analgesics as needed. Often use of ultrasound can reduce the inflammation. All activity should be held to a minimum. Padded heel counters and heel lifts should be placed in the shoes to relieve the Achilles tendon of as much tension as possible. If necessary, larger shoes with softer heel contours should be worn. After a workout, the tendon should be cooled with ice packs or ice massage.

Apophysitis of the Calcaneus (Sever's Disease)

Calcaneal **apophysitis,** or *Sever's disease,* is one of the many osteochondroses that physically active athletes who are physically immature suffer from.

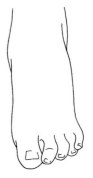

Figure 17-31

Overlapping toes.

apophysitis
Inflammation of an apophysis.

Figure 17-32

Exostoses (bony overgrowths). X-ray film of a large plantar calcaneal exostotic spur.

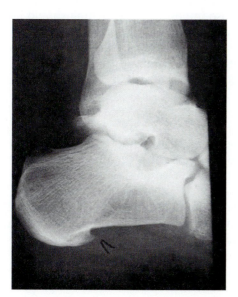

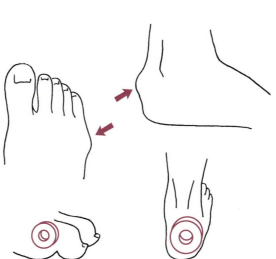

apophysis
Bony outgrowth such as a tubercle or tuberosity.

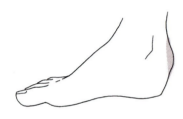

Figure 17-33

Retrocalcaneal bursitis.

Etiology   This condition can be compared to Osgood-Schlatter disease (see Chapter 19). Instead of the tibial tubercle, Sever's disease is a traction-type injury at the epiphysis of an **apophysis** (bone protrusion) where the Achilles tendon attaches to the calcaneus. As with other such conditions, circulation to the ephiphysis is disrupted, causing degeneration and sometimes fragmentation.

Symptoms and signs   Pain occurs at the posterior heel below the attachment of the Achilles tendon insertion of the child or adolescent athlete. Pain occurs during vigorous activity and does not continue at rest.

Management   This condition is usually completely resolved when the apophysis closes. Until such time, relief can be provided by restricting dorsiflexion of the foot, which can be accomplished by elevating both heels with a ¼-inch (0.6 cm) lift. Commonly, rest for several weeks will relieve the symptoms. If the symptoms do not resolve, a walking cast may be needed for 6 to 8 weeks.

Plantar Fasciitis (Heel Spur Syndrome)

As a major support of the longitudinal arch, the plantar fascia biomechanically acts as a "bowstring." Another chronic problem commonly associated with a resistance to stretch of the gastrocnemius–soleus–Achilles tendon–plantar fascial system is plantar fasciitis. This condition is the most frequent hindfoot problem among distance runners.[15]

Etiology   A number of anatomical and biomechanical conditions have been studied as possible causes of plantar fasciitis. They include leg length inequality, greater pronation of the subtalar joint, inflexibility of the longitudinal arch, and tightness of the gastrocnemius-soleus unit.[9] Athletic shoes, stride length, and running surfaces have also been linked to this condition. To date, no one factor has been clearly delineated as a cause of plantar fasciitis.

Symptoms and signs   The athlete complains of anterior medial heel pain, usually at the attachment of the plantar fascia to the calcaneus. During palpation the pain is usually localized on the plantar medial tuberosity of the calcaneus, radiating toward the sole of the foot. Often the pain intensifies when the athlete gets out of bed in the morning and first puts weight on the foot; however, the pain lessens after a few steps. Pain also will be intensified when the toes and forefoot are forcibly dorsiflexed.

Management   Management of this condition follows the same procedures as for a chronic foot strain, including longitudinal arch support or LowDye arch support (see Figure 13-19). Stretching the plantar fascia by passively hyperextending the great toe and Achilles tendon stretching, especially if the athlete's ankle cannot dorsiflex 10 to 15 degrees from a neutral position, are also important.[15] Stretching should be conducted at least three times a day in the positions of straight-ahead, toe-in, and toe-out. Techniques for stretching should follow the procedures discussed in Chapter 15. The athlete should wear a stiff shoe with a firm arch support. Antiinflammatory drugs are suggested. Steroidal injection may be warranted along with Indocin or Motrin.

Cuboid Subluxation

Approximately 4% of athletes with plantar foot pain have a cuboid syndrome.

Etiology   It is associated with a pronated foot, which causes a subluxation of the cuboid bone. The problem usually occurs in the early season after training on uneven surfaces or after a sudden twist of the foot.

Symptoms and signs   The pain is localized on the lateral side of the foot in the region of the cuboid bone. The primary reason for pain is the stress placed on the long peroneal muscle when the foot is in pronation. In this position, the long peroneal muscle allows the cuboid bone to move downward medially.

Management   Management of the cuboid syndrome involves manipulating the bone into a correct position, rest, and application of an arch pad and tape support or

Plantar Fasciitis

Injury Situation A male cross-country runner injured the proximal arch and his heel when stepping into a hole during a meet. The athlete continued to run and work out for a week before reporting to the athletic trainer.

Symptoms and Signs The athlete complained of early pain in the medial arch and medial distal heel that tended to move centrally as the week progressed. He complained of severe pain when rising in the morning and after sitting for a long period. The area appeared slightly swollen with a severe sharp pain on palpation at the plantar fascia insertion and medial aspect of the calcaneus. Pain increases with passive dorsiflexion of the great toe. An x-ray showed the beginning of a heel spur. The athlete was found to have a cavus foot.

Management Plan The athlete was diagnosed as having plantar fasciitis (heel spur syndrome), and a conservative plan was decided on.

Phase I **Acute Injury** GOALS: Minimize inflammation and pain.
ESTIMATED LENGTH OF TIME (ELT): 1 week.

■ **Therapy** RICE plus NSAID as needed to reduce pain and inflammation. Injection therapy for trigger points of a steroid and anesthetic.

■ **Exercise rehabilitation** Toe touch crutch walking. Begin heel cord stretching and rolling pin exercise to increase fascia flexibility.

Phase II **Repair** GOALS: Gain full weight bearing and walking pattern.
ESTIMATED LENGTH OF TIME (ELT): 1 to 3 weeks.

■ **Therapy** Ultrasound to increase blood flow. Cross friction massage over injury site. Apply shock absorption shoe insert with cutout (3 to 5 cm) in the tender area—apply arch taping.

■ **Exercise rehabilitation** Continue heel cord stretching and rolling pin exercise to stretch the plantar fascia. Begin a program of gradual pain-free weight bearing. Begin a program of foot flexor strengthening.

Phase III **Remodeling** GOALS: Focus on full pain-free weight bearing while engaged in running.
ESTIMATED LENGTH OF TIME (ELT): 2 weeks.

■ **Therapy** Ultrasound as warranted. Continue cross friction massage. Use a heel cup when supporting weight along with an arch taping.

■ **Exercise rehabilitation** Heel cord and plantar fascia stretching continues. Shoes must be worn that have a reinforced heel counter for heel control. Foot flexor strengthening against tubular resistance is initiated. General exercise is performed to the lower leg. The athlete begins a running program that is pain free.

Criteria for Returning to Competitive Cross-Country Running

1. Proximal arch and heel are pain free.
2. Heel cord and plantar fascia are stretched.
3. Lower leg has maximum strength.
4. Able to run competitively without pain.
5. Psychologically ready for competition.

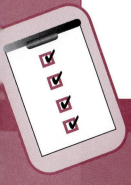

an orthotic device. The physician reduces the subluxation by dorsiflexing the ankle while plantar flexing the forefoot.

Stress Fractures of the Foot

More than 18% of all stress fractures in the body occur in the foot.

Metatarsal Stress Fracture

The most common stress fracture in the foot involves one or more metatarsal shafts. A fracture occurs most commonly to the second or third metatarsal bone (Figure 17-34).

Etiology   It occurs in the runner who has suddenly changed patterns of training such as increasing mileage, running hills, or running on a harder surface. An athlete who has an atypical condition such as a structural forefoot varus, hallux valgus, flatfoot, or a short first metatarsal bone is more easily disposed toward incurring a stress fracture than is the individual whose foot is free of pathological or mechanical defects. A short first metatarsal bone is mechanically unable to make use of its strength and position to distribute the weight properly to the front part of the foot. Therefore excessive pressure and additional weight are transferred to the second metatarsal bone, resulting in traumatic changes and, on occasion, fracture. An x-ray examination may not detect this condition, requiring a bone scan to be performed.

Management   Management of the painful metatarsal stress fracture usually consists of 3 or 4 days of crutch walking or wearing a short-leg walking cast for 1 to 2 weeks. Once the symptoms have significantly subsided, the athlete may resume weight bearing while walking. Shoes with firm soles should be worn. Tape support and therapy for swelling and tenderness should be given. Running should not be resumed for 3 to 4 weeks, with intensity and mileage increased slowly. A more intense day should alternate with an easy day. The athlete must avoid toe running until bone tenderness is gone. Running should be done only on a soft, flat surface.

Calcaneal Stress Fracture

One of the bones of the foot known to develop stress fractures is the calcaneus.

Etiology   A calcaneal stress fracture is most prevalent among distance runners and is characterized by a sudden onset of constant pain in the plantar-calcaneal area.

17-10

Critical Thinking Exercise

A cross-country runner changes her running patterns by increasing distance and performing more hill work. She complains to the athletic trainer of a gradually worsening pain in her forefoot. Inspection reveals point tenderness in the region of the fourth metatarsal bone. X-ray reveals a stress fracture.

? How should this condition be managed?

Figure 17-34

Stress fracture of the third metatarsal bone.

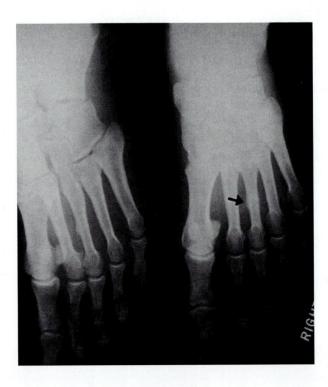

Symptoms and signs   Pressure on the plantar-calcaneal tuberosity causes severe pain. The fracture fails to appear during x-ray examination for 4 to 6 weeks.

Management   Management is usually conservative for the first 2 or 3 weeks and includes rest, elastic wrap compression, elevation, and active range-of-motion exercises of the foot and ankle. After 3 weeks and when pain subsides, activity within pain limits can be resumed gradually, with the athlete wearing a cushioned shoe.

FOOT REHABILITATION

Exercise rehabilitation of the foot must be specific to the injury. The athletic trainer should consider that an injury to the foot can directly or indirectly adversely affect the balance of the entire body. The athletic trainer designs a personalized rehabilitation program that addresses four components: facilitation of healing and repair, identification and correction of tissues that may have predisposed to injury or that could hamper recovery, restoration of optimal function, and successful return of the athlete to competition.[1]

General Body Conditioning

An athlete prevented from physical activity because of a foot condition must enter into a program of deconditioning. Without aggravating the injury the athlete engages in a program that maintains the body's cardiovascular endurance, strength, flexibility, and coordination.

Depending on the sport and individual psychological makeup of the athlete, a variety of options are open. For example, swimming and one-legged stationary bicycle activities can help maintain a degree of cardiovascular endurance, and weight training and stretching exercises will maintain strength and flexibility. Use of a balance board (BAP board) will help in maintaining general balance. An upper-extremity ergometer can be employed for non–weight-bearing cardiovascular endurance training.[4,6]

Weight Bearing

If the athlete is unable walk without a limp, non–weight-bearing or limited weight-bearing crutch walking might be employed. Walking improperly could lead to faulty biomechanics to other body areas and lead to subsequent later injuries.[8]

Foot Joint Mobilization

Manual mobilization techniques are appropriate for foot joints to reduce arthrofibrosis that occurs from immobilization. Examples are anterior and posterior glides of the calcaneocuboid, cuboidmetatarsal, carpometacarpal, talonavicular, and metacarpophalangeal joints[11] (Figure 17-35). (See Chapter 15.)

Flexibility

For the foot to be functional its joints or combination of joints must have full range of motion. Of particular importance is restoring full range of motion to the phalanges (toes). There also has to be restoration of normal motions of supination and pronation in the subtalar joint. Supination implies the foot moving into adduction, plantar flexion, and inversion; pronation is involved with foot eversion, abduction, and dorsiflexion.[6] When motion is restricted manual stretching or proprioceptive neuromuscular facilitation (PNF) stretching techniques can be applied. (See Chapter 15.)

Muscular Strength

Strength exercises for the foot can be directed toward rehabilitation of specific injuries or the amelioration of functional foot dysfunctions such as pronation.

Specific injury muscle rehabilitation can employ a variety of means. Rubber tubing has value in specific rehabilitation (Figure 17-36).

Another approach is a graduated exercise program. In most painful conditions of the foot, weight bearing is prohibited until pain has subsided significantly. During

Figure 17-35

Joint mobilization for the metacarpophylangal joint.

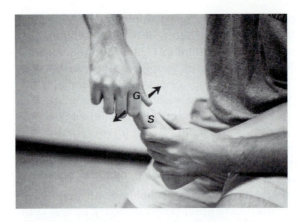

Figure 17-36

Rubber tubing resistance exercise.

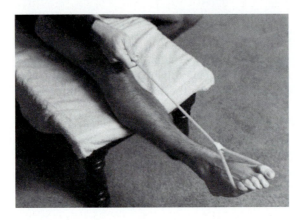

this period and until the athlete is ready to return to full activity, a graduated program of exercise should be instituted.

Beginning and Intermediate Phases

Each exercise should be performed three times a day with non–weight bearing active exercise.

Beginning Phase

In stage 1 primary exercises are used in the non–weight-bearing or early phase of the condition. They include "writing the alphabet," picking up objects, ankle circumduction, and gripping and spreading.

1. *Writing the alphabet*—with the toes pointed, the athlete writes the complete alphabet in the air three times.
2. *Picking up objects*—the athlete picks up 10 small objects such as marbles with the toes and places them in a container.
3. *Ankle circumduction*—the ankle is circumducted in as extreme a range of motion as possible (10 circles in one direction and 10 circles in the other).
4. *Gripping and spreading*—of particular value to toes, gripping and spreading is conducted for up to 10 repetitions (Figure 17-37).

Intermediate Phase

Stage 2 exercises are added to stage 1 when the athlete is just beginning to bear weight. They include the "towel gather" and "scoop" exercises.

1. *Towel gathering*—a towel is extended in front of the feet. The heels are firmly planted on the floor with the forefoot on the end of the towel. The athlete then attempts to pull the towel with the feet without lifting the heels from the floor.

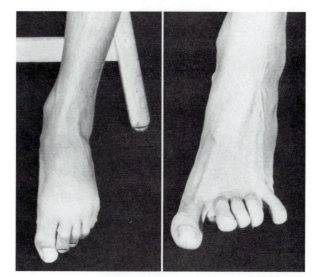

Figure 17-37

Gripping and spreading of the toes can be an excellent rehabilitation exercise for the injured foot.

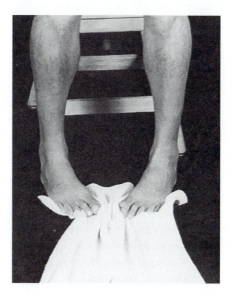

Figure 17-38

The towel gather exercise.

As execution becomes easier, a weight can be placed at the other end of the towel for added resistance. Each exercise should be performed 10 times (Figure 17-38). This exercise can also be used for exercising the foot in abduction and adduction.

2. *Towel scoop*—a towel is folded in half and placed sideways on the floor. The athlete places the heel firmly on the floor and the forefoot on the end of the towel. To ensure the greatest stability of the exercising foot, it is backed up with the other foot. Without lifting the heel from the floor, the athlete scoops the towel forward with the forefoot. As with the towel gather exercise, a weight resistance can be added to the end of the towel. The exercise should be repeated up to 10 times (Figure 17-39).

Rubber tub resistance exercises provide an excellent means for gaining foot strength (see Figure 17-36).[8]

Neuromuscular Control

Neuromuscular control of the foot implies coordination, balance, and position sense (proprioception). Specifically, techniques of PNF, the use of the biomechanical ankle

Figure 17-39

The towel scoop exercise.

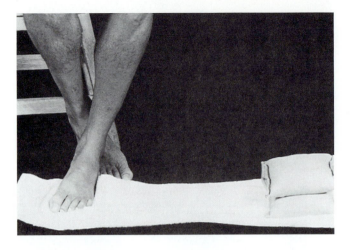

platform (BAP board), and the kinesthetic awareness trainer (KAT) can be used to increase neuromuscular control. (See Figure 15-4.)

Protective Devices

Three approaches are used to enhance the rehabilitation of foot conditions: taping, orthotics, and proper shoe selection.

Foot taping is discussed in detail in Chapter 13. Properly applied tape can protect and support a part. Orthotics is presented in Chapter 5. Orthotics serves to control abnormal compensatory movements of the foot by "bringing the floor to the foot."[6] Shoe selection and fitting (discussed in Chapter 5) is of major importance to the protection and support of the injured foot.

Functional Progressions

A major area in rehabilitation is the reestablishment of normal movement patterns.[8] The purpose of functional progression is to return the athlete to a safe and effective level of activity. In the case of foot injuries the athlete should initiate a succession of activities that simulate actual motor and sport skills. For example, a soccer player who sustained a plantar fasciitis might, when full weight-bearing is allowed, perform the following activities:

- Walking straight ahead (heel-toe).
- Walking backward (toe-heel).
- Toe walking.
- Heel walking.

Return to Activity

The primary criterion for return to full activity is whether full pain-free weight bearing can be initiated. No limp or favoring of the part should be present. The athlete has complete confidence to perform all ambulation activities required in his or her sport.

SUMMARY

- The human foot is a highly complicated anatomical structure, requiring a great deal of strength, flexibility, and coordinated movement. Complaints about foot injuries by athletes call for careful physical examination.
- Common acute injuries are heel and instep bruises, arch strains, and sprains of the midfoot, forefoot, and great toe. Fractures can occur to all areas of the foot.
- Along with the use of other therapy modalities, the use of rehabilitative exercise is important for managing foot conditions.

- To more fully understand chronic and overuse stress injuries in the foot, ankle, and lower leg, biomechanics must be understood in terms of the lower leg linkage system. There must also be an understanding of the foot, ankle, and lower leg as part of the linkage system.
- Chronic and overuse foot conditions can lead to stress problems in the lower extremities. Common chronic problems occur to the arches of the foot, toes, and forefoot. Bunions, a common chronic condition, occur when the great toe becomes deflected laterally. Metatarsalgia also is a chronic condition of the forefoot. Other problems include deformities such as hammer or clawed toes, bony outgrowths, heel bursitis, heel spurs, tendinitis, and stress fractures.

Solutions to Critical Thinking EXERCISES

17-1 The soles of the shoes have opposite wear patterns. The right sole may show a medial wear pattern and the left a more lateral wear pattern.

17-2 This condition is characteristic of a plantar fascial strain. It should be managed symptomatically. A doughnut placed over the epicondyle region along with a heel lift plus wearing of a shoe having a stiff shank may relieve some pain. There should be stretching of the plantar muscles and gastrocnemius along with arch exercises. Application of LowDye taping for pronation can also relieve pain.

17-3 A sprain of the first metatarsal-phalangeal joint (turf toe) stems from hyperextension while playing on artificial turf. This injury is a tear of the joint capsule from the metatarsal head.

17-4 Kicking the locker with the great toe could cause a fracture of the proximal or distal phalanx. In this injury there maybe swelling, discoloration, and point tenderness.

17-5 A lateral sprain can produce an avulsion fracture of the proximal head of the fifth metatarsal bone.

17-6 This condition is a bunion or hallux valgus. It is associated with wearing shoes that are too pointed, narrow, or short. It may begin with an inflamed bursa over the metatarsophalangeal joint. It can be associated with a depressed transverse arch or a pronated foot.

17-7 Metatarsalgia can be caused by a restricted gastrocnemius-soleus complex that produces a pes cavus. It can also be caused by a fallen metatarsal arch abnormally depressing the second or third metatarsal heads, causing a heavy callus to be developed.

17-8 The defensive lineman has an interdigital neuroma. Conservatively it is treated by wearing a broad-toed shoe, a transverse arch support, and a metatarsal bar and injection of lidocaine and steroids.

17-9 Sever's disease is a traction injury to the epiphysis of the calcaneal tubercle where the Achilles tendon attaches. The circulation becomes disrupted, resulting in a degeneration of the epiphyseal region.

17-10 Management of this stress fracture could consist of 3 to 4 days of crutch walking or the wearing of a walking cast for 1 to 2 weeks. With symptoms reduced walking should be performed in firm-soled shoes. Therapy is given to reduce swelling. A return to running occurs in 3 to 4 weeks.

REVIEW QUESTIONS AND CLASS ACTIVITIES

1. Describe the anatomy of the foot.
2. How does the foot function during the gait cycle?
3. The foot, ankle, and lower leg act as a system. How can this fact explain an overuse injury?
4. Demonstrate assessment of the foot.
5. Why is the calcaneus prone to contusion, and how can contusion be prevented? How can it be managed?
6. Identify the types of acute strains that occur in the region of the foot. How can they be prevented? How can they be managed?
7. Where do sprains, dislocations, and fractures commonly occur in the foot? Discuss their symptoms and signs and how they can be cared for.
8. What are the most common foot deformities? How do they occur?
9. Describe where and why exostoses occur in the foot region.
10. Compare postcalcaneal bursitis with apophysitis of the calcaneus in terms of symptoms and signs.
11. What are the possible causes of plantar fasciitis (heel spur syndrome)?
12. Discuss where and why stress fractures occur in the foot.
13. Describe the steps that must be taken during exercise rehabilitation of the foot.
14. Invite a podiatrist to speak to the class about congenital foot abnormalities, major sports injuries and their treatment, and the role of orthotic devices in the control of biomechanical foot problems.
15. Demonstrate rehabilitative exercises that strengthen, stretch, and reeducate the foot after injury.

REFERENCES

1. Benda C: Stepping in the right sock, *Phys Sports Med* 19(12):125, 1991.
2. Cailliet R: *Foot and ankle pain,* Philadelphia, 1986, Davis.
3. Coughlin MJ: Forefoot disorders. In Baxter DE, editor: *The foot and ankle in sports,* St Louis, 1995, Mosby.
4. Davis P et al: Rehabilitation strategies and protocols for the athlete. In Sammarco GJ, editor: *Rehabilitation of the foot and ankle,* St Louis, 1995, Mosby.
5. Hamill J et al: Biomechanics of the foot and ankle. In Sammarco GJ, editor: *Rehabilitation of the foot and ankle,* St Louis, 1995, Mosby.
6. Hunter S: Rehabilitation of foot injuries. In Prentice WE, editor: *Rehabilitation techniques in sports medicine,* ed 2, St Louis, 1994, Mosby.

7. Mann RA: Great toe disorders. In Baxter DE, editor: *The foot and ankle in sports,* St Louis, 1995, Mosby.

8. McGee M: Functional progression in rehabilitation. In Prentice WE, editor: *Rehabilitation techniques in sports medicine,* ed 2, St Louis, 1994, Mosby.

9. Petrizzi MJ: Foot injuries. In Birrer RB, editor: *Sports medicine for the primary care physician,* ed 2, Boca Raton, Fla, 1994, CRC Press.

10. Pfeffer GB: Plantar heel pain. In Baxter DE, editor: *The foot and ankle in sport,* St Louis, 1995, Mosby.

11. Prentice WE, editor: *Rehabilitation techniques in sports medicine,* ed 2, St Louis, 1994, Mosby.

12. Reynolds JC: Functional examination of the foot and ankle. In Sammarco GJ, editor: *Rehabilitation of the foot and ankle,* St Louis, 1995, Mosby.

13. Sammarco GJ: Soft tissue injuries. In Torg JS, Shephard RJ, editors: *Current therapy in sports medicine,* ed 3, St Louis, 1995, Mosby.

14. Tiberio D: Pathomechanics of structural foot deformities, *Phys Ther* 68:1840, 1988.

15. Torg JS: Plantar fasciitis. In Torg JS, Shephard RJ, editors: *Current therapy in sports medicine,* ed 3, St Louis, 1995, Mosby.

16. Welsh RP: Metatarsalgia problems. In Torg JS, Shepard RJ, editors: *Current therapy in sports medicine,* ed 3, St Louis, 1995, Mosby.

ANNOTATED BIBLIOGRAPHY

Baxter DE: *The foot and ankle in sport,* St Louis, 1995, Mosby.

A complete medical text on all aspects of the foot and ankle. It covers common sports syndromes, anatomical disorders in sports, unique problems, athletic shoes, orthoses, and rehabilitation.

Donatelli R: *The biomechanics of the foot and ankle,* Philadelphia, 1990, Davis.

A practical book for the therapist working directly with the patient.

The Ankle and Lower Leg

When you finish this chapter, you should be able to

- Identify the major anatomical components of the ankle and lower leg that are commonly injured in sports.
- Assess ankle and lower leg injuries.
- Discuss the etiology, symptoms and signs, and management of sports injuries occurring to the ankle and lower leg.

Chapter 18 focuses on acute and chronic sports injuries in the ankle and lower leg. As with the foot, the ankle and lower leg are common sites of injury in sports.

THE ANKLE

Ankle injuries, especially to the ligamentous tissue, are the most frequent injuries in sports. For the coach and the athletic trainer, understanding the complex nature of ankle injuries should be a major goal (Figure 18-1).

Bones

The bones that form the ankle joint are the distal ends of the tibia and fibula and the talus. The talus forms a link between the lower leg and the tarsus. This bony arrangement forms the ankle mortise. The ankle works in conjunction with the rear foot or talus and calcaneus.

The talus, the second largest tarsal and the main weight-bearing bone of the articulation, rests on the calcaneus and receives the articulating surfaces of the lateral and medial malleoli. Its almost square shape allows the ankle only two movements: dorsiflexion and plantar flexion. Because the talus is wider anteriorly than posteriorly, the most stable position of the ankle is with the foot in dorsiflexion. In this position the wider anterior aspect of the talus comes in contact with the narrower portion lying between the malleoli, gripping it tightly. By contrast, as the ankle moves into plantar flexion, the wider portion of the tibia is brought in contact with the narrower posterior aspect of the talus, a much less stable position than dorsiflexion.

Articulations

Ankle Joint

The ankle joint, or talocrural joint, is a hinge joint (ginglymus) that is formed by the articular facet on the distal extremity of the tibia, which articulates with the superior articular surface (trochlea) of the talus; the medial malleolus, which articulates with the medial surface of the trochlea of the talus; and the lateral malleolus, which articulates with the lateral surface of the trochlea (Figure 18-2).

The degree of motion for the ankle joint ranges from 20 degrees of dorsiflexion to 50 degrees of plantar flexion depending on the athlete. A normal foot requires 20 degrees of plantar flexion and 10 degrees of dorsiflexion with the knee extended for a normal gait.

Ankle function depends on the joints of the hindfoot, the most important of which is the subtalar joint. The subtalar joint allows for foot pronation and supination. Its range of motion is estimated to be from 20 to 62 degrees. The degree of supination must be twice that of pronation. For normal gait 4 to 6 degrees of pronation and 8 to 12 degrees of supination must be present. The ankle subtalar and transtarsal joints also must work in concert for a normal gait to occur.

Because the talus is wider anteriorly than posteriorly, the most stable position of the ankle is with the foot in dorsiflexion.

Figure 18-1

Figure 18-1

The ankle has the highest incidence of injury in basketball.

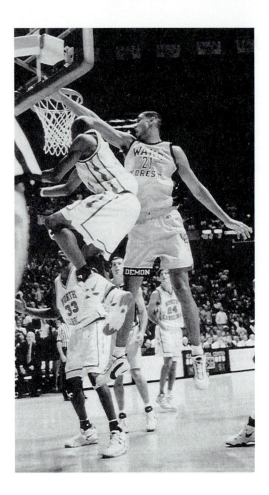

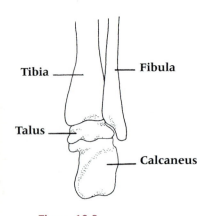

Figure 18-2

The ankle is a hinge joint formed by the tibia, fibula, and talus.

Capsular and Ligamentous Support

The ligamentous support of the ankle additionally fortifies its great bony strength (Figure 18-3). This support consists of the articular capsule, three lateral ligaments, two ligaments that connect the tibia and fibula, and the medial or deltoid ligament. The three lateral ligaments include the anteriotalofibular, the posterior talofibular, and the calcaneofibular (Table 18-1). The anterior and posterior tibiofibular ligaments hold the tibia and fibula together and form the distal portion of the interroseus membrane. A thin articular capsule encases the ankle joint and attaches to the borders of the bone involved. It is somewhat different from most other capsules in that it is thick on the medial aspects of the joint but becomes a thin gauzelike membrane at the back.

The deltoid ligament is triangular, attaching superiorly to the borders of the medial malleolus. It attaches inferiorly to the medial surface of the talus, to the sustentaculum tali of the calcaneus, and to the posterior margin of the navicular bone. The deltoid ligament is the primary resistance to foot eversion. It, along with the plantar calcaneonavicular (spring) ligament, also helps maintain the inner longitudinal arch. Although it should be considered as one ligament, the deltoid ligament includes superficial and deep fibers (Figure 18-4). Anteriorly are the anterior tibiotalar part and the tibionavicular part. Medially is the tibiocalcaneal part, and posteriorly is the posterior tibiotalar part.

Musculature

The movements of the ankle joint are dorsiflexion (flexion) and plantar flexion (extension). It can be generalized that muscles passing posterior to the lateral malleolus

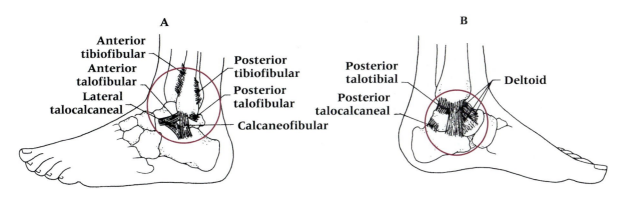

Figure 18-3

Major ligaments of the ankle.
A, Lateral aspect. **B,** Medial
aspect.

will produce ankle plantar flexion along with toe extension. It can also be general-ized that anterior muscles serve to dorsiflex the foot and to produce toe flexion. The anterior muscles include the extensor hallucis longus, the extensor digitorum lon-gus, the peroneus tertius, and the tibialis anterior. The posterior muscle group falls into three layers: at the superficial layer is the gastrocnemius; the middle layer in-cludes the soleus and the plantaris; and the deep layer contains the tibialis posterior, the flexor digitorum longus, and the flexor hallucis longus.

Nerve and Blood Supply

Refer to Chapter 17 for a discussion of nerve and blood supply for the ankle and lower leg.

Functional Anatomy

The motions occurring at the ankle and rear foot are complex. Anatomically the ankle is a very stable hinge joint in which the dome of the talus articulates with the distal end of the tibia. Medial or lateral displacement of the talus is prevented by the mal-leole. Ankle ligaments permit flexion and extension at the ankle joint while limiting inversion and eversion. True inversion and eversion take place in the joints of the midfoot and subtalar joint.[14] (See Chapter 17.)

Ankle Injury Prevention

Many ankle conditions, especially sprains, can be reduced by stretching the Achilles tendon, strengthening key muscles, proprioceptive training, wearing proper footwear, and in some cases proper taping.

Achilles Tendon Stretching

An ankle that can easily dorsiflex at least 15 degrees or more is essential for injury prevention. The athlete, especially one with tight Achilles tendons, should routinely stretch before and after practice (Figure 18-5). To adequately stretch the gastrosoleus Achilles tendon complex, stretching should be performed with the knee extended and then flexed 15 to 30 degrees.

Preventing ankle sprains is
achieved by:
    Stretching the Achilles ten-
    don
    Strengthening key muscles
    Proprioceptive training
    Wearing proper footwear
    Taping when appropriate

TABLE 18-1   **Function of Key Ankle Ligaments**

Ligament	Primary Function
Anterior talofibular	Restrains anterior displacement of talus
Calcaneofibular	Restrains inversion of calcaneus
Posterior talofibular	Restrains posterior displacement of talus
Deltoid	Prevents abduction and eversion of ankle and subtalar joint
	Prevents eversion, pronation, and anterior displacement of talus

Figure 18-4

Medial ankle ligaments.

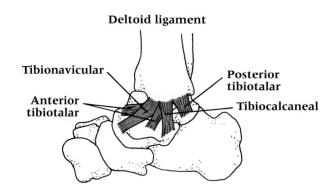

Strength Training

Of major importance in ankle injury prevention is achieving both static and dynamic joint stability (Figure 18-6). A normal range of motion must be maintained, along with strength of the peroneal, plantar flexor, dorsal flexor, and extensor muscles. The peroneals, mainly the peroneus longus muscle, must be exercised to afford eversion strength and to prevent the foot from being forced into inversion.

Proprioceptive Training

Athletes who have ankle injuries or who spend most of their time on even surfaces may develop a proprioceptive deficiency. Ankle ligamentous stability proprioception is also lost. The ankle and foot proprioceptive sense can be enhanced by locomotion over uneven surfaces or by spending time each day on a balance board (wobble board) (Figure 18-7), a BAPS board (Figure 15-4, *A*), or a KAT system (Figure 15-4, *B*).

Footwear

As discussed in Chapter 4, proper footwear can be an important factor in reducing injuries to both the foot and the ankle. Shoes should not be used in activities for which they were not intended—for example, running shoes designed for straight-ahead activity should not be used to play tennis, a sport that demands a great deal of lateral movement. Cleats on a shoe should not be centered in the middle of the sole but should be placed far enough on the border to avoid ankle sprains. High-top shoes, when worn by athletes with a history of ankle sprain, can offer greater support than low-top shoes.

Figure 18-5

Stretching techniques for the heelcord complex: *left*, stretching position for gastrocnemius; *right*, stretching soleus with knee bent.

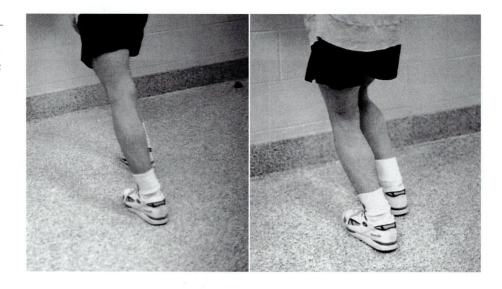

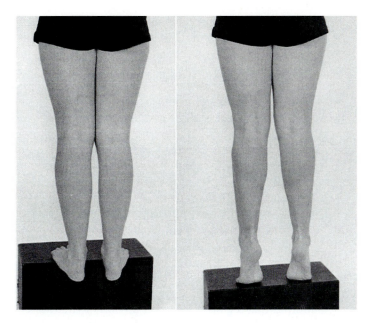

Figure 18-6

Strength training is essential for ankle injury prevention.

Preventive Ankle Taping and Orthoses

As discussed in Chapter 13, there is some doubt as to whether it is beneficial to routinely tape ankles that have no history of sprain. There is some indication that tape, properly applied, can provide some prophylactic protection. Poorly applied tape may do more harm than good. Tape that constricts soft tissue or disrupts normal biomechanical function can create serious injuries. An example of this is that ankle taping can adversely affect the metatarsophalangeal joints by stressing the phalangeal ligaments. Although taping is preferred, a much cheaper cloth muslin wrap may provide some protection. (See Chapter 5.) Lace-up supports and semirigid ankle braces are increasingly being used in place of tape. The sport-stirrup orthosis has been found superior to taping in preventing recurrent ankle sprains.[20] (See Figure 5-24.)

Poorly applied ankle taping can do more harm than good to the athlete.

Ankle Assessment

The injured or painful ankle should be carefully evaluated to determine the possibility of fracture and whether medical referral is necessary.

History

The athlete's history may vary, depending on whether the problem is the result of sudden trauma or is chronic. The athlete with an acute sudden trauma to the ankle should be asked the following questions:
- What trauma or mechanism occurred?
- What was heard when the injury occurred—a crack, snap, or pop?
- What were the duration and intensity of pain?
- How disabling was the occurrence? Could the athlete walk right away, or was he or she unable to bear weight for a period of time?
- Has a similar injury occurred before?
- Was there immediate swelling, or did the swelling occur later (or at all)? Where did the swelling occur?

The athlete with a long-standing painful condition might be asked the following:
- How much does it hurt?
- Where does it hurt?
- Under what circumstances does pain occur—when bearing weight, after activity, or when arising after a night's sleep?

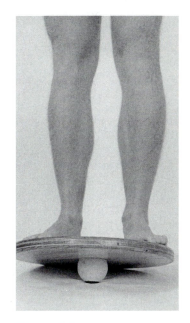

Figure 18-7

The wobble board provides ankle balance training.

- What past ankle injuries have occurred?
- What first aid and therapy, if any, were given for this occurrence?

Observation

In looking initially at the ankle the athletic trainer determines the following[15]:
- Is there an obvious deformity?
- Are the bony contours of the ankle normal and symmetrical, or is there a deviation such as a bony deformity?
- Are the color and texture of the skin normal?
- Is there crepitus or abnormal sound in the ankle joint?
- Is heat, swelling, or redness present?
- Is the athlete in obvious pain?
- Does the athlete have a normal ankle range of motion?
- If the athlete is able to walk, is there a normal walking pattern?

Palpation

Palpation in the ankle region should start with key bony sites and ligaments and progress to the musculature, especially the major tendons in the area. The purpose of palpation in this region is to detect obvious structural defects, swellings, and localized tenderness (Figure 18-8). The following anatomical areas should be palpated:

Bony Palpation

- Medial malleolus
- Lateral malleolus
- Navicular
- Talus
- Calcaneous
- Proximal base of the fifth metatarsal

Soft-tissue Palpation

- Deltoid ligament
- Anterior talofibular ligament
- Calcaneofibular ligament
- Posterior talofibular ligament
- Anterior tibiofibular ligament
- Achilles tendon
- Peroneal tendons
- Posterior tibialis tendon
- Anterior tibialis tendon
- Achilles tendon

If the injury might have impeded blood flow to the ankle area, the pulse should be measured at the dorsal pedal artery and at the posterior tibial artery.

Special Tests—Joint Stability

When there may be ankle joint instability as a result of repeated sprains, tests should be given. The most common sprain is the inversion type, which first involves the talofibular ligament. Because this ligament prevents the talus from sliding forward, the most appropriate test is the one that elicits the anterior drawer sign (Figure 18-9). The athlete sits on the edge of a treatment table with legs and feet relaxed. The athletic trainer or physician grasps the lower tibia in one hand and the calcaneus in the palm of the other hand. The tibia is then pushed backward as the calcaneus is pulled forward. A positive anterior drawer sign occurs when the foot slides forward, sometimes making a clunking sound as it reaches its end point, and generally indicating a tear in the anterior talofibular ligament.

Two other tests that may be used are those that test for torn anterior talofibular and calcaneofibular ligaments on the lateral side. With the foot positioned at 90 degrees to the lower leg and stabilized, the heel is inverted. If the talus rocks in the

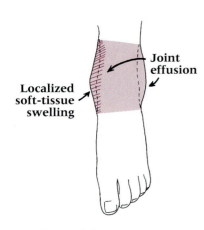

Figure 18-8

Local and diffused ankle swelling.

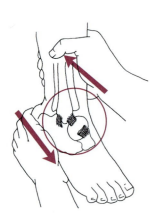

Figure 18-9

Anterior drawer test for ankle ligament instability.

A positive drawer sign of ankle stability is when the foot slides forward, sometimes making a clunking sound as it reaches its end point.

mortise, there is injury to both the anterior talofibular and calcaneofibular ligaments, and there is subsequent lateral ankle instability (Figure 18-10). The deltoid ligament can be tested in the same way, except that the heel is everted. As the heel is moved into eversion, a gap is felt between the medial malleolus and the calcaneus.

Functional Examination

Muscle function is important in evaluating the ankle injury (Figure 18-11). *If the following movements aggravate a recent injury, they should be avoided.* While bearing weight on both feet, the athlete does the following:
- Walks on toes (tests plantar flexion)
- Walks on heels (tests dorsiflexion)
- Walks on lateral border of feet (tests inversion)
- Walks on medial border of feet (tests eversion)

Passive, active, and resistive movements should be manually applied to determine joint integrity and muscle function (Figure 18-12).

The Sprained Ankle

Because of their frequency and the disability that results, ankle sprains present a major problem for the coach, athletic trainer, and team physician. It has been said that in many cases a sprained ankle can be worse than a fracture.

Etiology   Ankle sprains are generally caused by sudden lateral or medial twists (Table 18-2). The inversion sprain, in which the foot turns inward, is the most common type of ankle sprain because there is more bony stability on the lateral side, which tends to force the foot into inversion rather than eversion. If the force is great enough, inversion of the foot continues until the medial malleolus loses its stability and creates a fulcrum to further invert the ankle. The peroneal or everting muscles resist the inverting force, and when they are no longer strong enough, the lateral ligaments become stretched or torn (see Figure 18-12). Generally, most vertically loaded ankle sprains, such as those that occur when an athlete comes down on another athlete's foot, are more significant than horizontally loaded sprains because the vertically loaded sprain involves a greater amount of body weight applied directly to the ankle joint.[23]

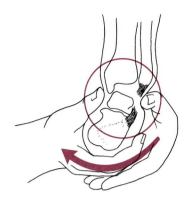

Figure 18-10

Talar tilt testing for lateral ankle instability.

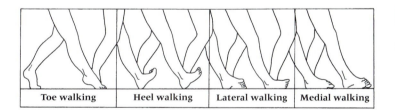

| Toe walking | Heel walking | Lateral walking | Medial walking |

Figure 18-11

Evaluating ankle function during walking.

TABLE 18-2   Mechanisms of Ankle Sprain and Ligament Injury

Mechanisms	Area Injured
Plantar flexion or inversion	Anterior talofibular ligament
	Calcaneofibular ligament
	Posterior talofibular ligament
	Tibiofibular ligament (severe injury)
Inversion (uncommon)	Calcaneofibular ligament (along with anterior or posterior talofibular ligament)
Dorsiflexion	Tibiofibular ligament
Eversion	Deltoid ligament
	Tibiofibular ligament (severe injury)
	Interosseous membrane (as external rotation increases)
	Possible fibular fracture (proximal or distal)

Figure 18-12

Mechanism of an inversion ankle sprain.

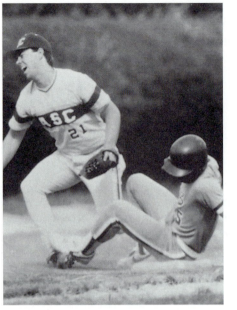
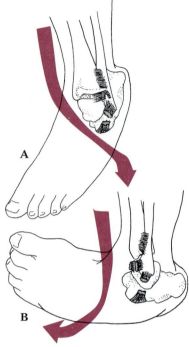

Usually a lateral ankle sprain involves either one or two injured ligaments. If it is a single ligament tear, it usually involves the anterior talofibular ligament, but if it is a double ligament tear with further inversion, the calcaneofibular ligament also tears. The tight heel cord forces the foot into inversion, making it more susceptible to a lateral sprain. In contrast, a foot that is pronated, hypermobile, or has a depressed medial longitudinal arch is more susceptible to medial arch and eversion ankle injuries (Figure 18-13).

The eversion sprain occurs less frequently than the inversion sprain. The usual mechanism is the athlete's having suddenly stepped in a hole on the playing field, causing the foot to evert and abduct and the planted leg to rotate externally.[19] With this mechanism the anterior tibiofibular ligament, interosseous ligament, and deltoid ligament may tear. With a tear of these ligaments, the talus is allowed to move laterally within the mortise, leading to ultimate degeneration within the joint. Also, there is abnormal space between the medial malleolus and the talus (Figure 18-14).

A sudden inversion force could be of such intensity as to produce a fracture of the lower leg. Unexpected wrenching of the lateral ligaments could cause a portion of

Figure 18-13

A pronated foot can lead to an eversion ankle sprain.

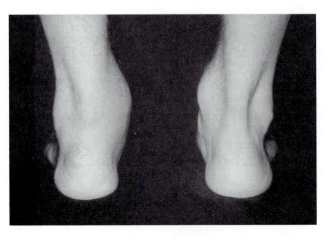
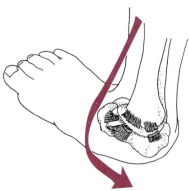

bone to be avulsed from the malleolus[15] (Figure 18-15). One extreme situation is when the lateral malleolus is avulsed by the calcaneofibular bone and the talus rocks up against the medial malleolus to produce a second fracture. This sequence of events is known as the *bimalleolar fracture.*[15]

Lateral Ankle Sprain

Lateral ankle sprains are usually graded by the ligament or ligaments involved. A grade 1 sprain usually involves the anterior talofibular ligament; a grade 2 the anterior talofibular and calcaneofibular ligaments; and a grade 3 the anterior talofibular, calcaneofibular, posterior talofibular, and frequently the anterior tibiofibular ligaments. In each instance of injury, the foot is forcibly turned inward on the leg, such as when a basketball player jumps and comes down on the foot of another player. Inversion sprains can also occur when an individual is walking or running on an uneven surface or suddenly steps into a hole.

Grade 1 inversion ankle sprains   The grade 1 ankle sprain is the most common type of sprain. Lateral sprains are probably the most frequent injury in sports in which running and jumping occur.[2]

Etiology   The inversion sprain occurs with the foot in inversion plantar flexion and adduction with a mild stretching of the anterior talofibular ligament.

Symptoms and signs   Mild pain and disability occur. Weight bearing is not impaired. Signs are slight point tenderness and swelling over the ligament with no joint laxity.[13]

Management   Rest, ice, compression, and elevation (RICE) are used for 20 minutes every few hours for 1 to 2 days. The application of a horseshoe pad may also help control hemorrhage (Figure 18-16). It may be advisable for the athlete to limit weight-bearing activities for a few days. An elastic wrap might provide comfortable pressure when weight bearing begins. When the athlete's ankle is pain free and not swollen, a routine of circumduction is begun. The athlete is instructed to circle the foot first 10 times in one direction then 10 times in the other several times per day. When the athlete returns to weight bearing, application of tape may provide an extra measure of protection. A graduated exercise rehabilitation program is a major requirement in managing the grade 1 inversion sprain.

Grade 2 inversion ankle sprains   Because it has a high incidence among sports participants and causes a great deal of disability with many days of lost time, the grade 2 ankle sprain is a major problem for the coach, athletic trainer, and physician.[18]

Etiology   Moderate force on the ankle while in a position of inversion, plantar flexion, and adduction can cause a grade 2 sprain.

Symptoms and signs   The athlete usually complains that a tearing sensation was felt along with a pop or snap as the tissue gave way on the lateral side of the ankle. There is moderate pain and disability, and weight bearing is difficult. There is tenderness and edema with blood in the joint. Ecchymosis may occur, as well as a positive talar tilt. There is also a positive drawer sign between 4 and 14 mm[2]. NOTE: The grade 2 ankle sprain may be a complete tear of the anterior talofibular ligament and a stretch and tear of the calcaneofibular ligament. The anterior drawer test will elicit slight to moderate abnormal motion. This injury degree can produce a persistently unstable ankle that recurrently becomes sprained and later develops traumatic arthritis.[18]

Management   RICE therapy should be used intermittently for 24 to 72 hours. X-ray examination should be routine for this grade of injury. The athlete should use crutches for 5 to 10 days to avoid bearing weight. The athlete will walk with a dorsiflexion cast or a stirrup for 2 to 4 weeks, followed by taping at 90 degrees for 2 to 4 weeks.[2] Plantar and dorsiflexion exercises, if the athlete is pain free, may begin 48 hours after the injury occurs. Early exercise of this type helps maintain range of motion and normal proprioception. Application of an ice pack for 5 to 10 minutes

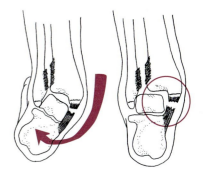

Figure 18-14

An eversion ankle sprain that creates a space between the medial malleolus and the talus.

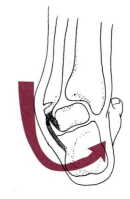

Figure 18-15

The same mechanism that produces an ankle sprain can also cause an avulsion fracture of the malleolus.

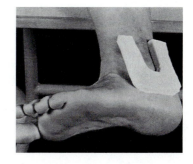

Figure 18-16

A horseshoe-shaped pad provides an excellent compress when held in place by an elastic wrap.

Grade 2 Inversion Ankle Sprain

Injury Situation A male college senior-year lacrosse player stepped into a rut on the field, causing a major twist of the left ankle. At the time of injury the athlete felt a severe pain on the lateral aspect of the ankle before he fell to the ground.

Symptoms and Signs After the injury the athlete complained of moderate pain on the outside of his left ankle. Initially it was painful to move the ankle. Walking on the left foot was very difficult. There was moderate tenderness over the lateral aspect of the ankle. Swelling rapidly occurred around the lateral malleoli. The ankle displayed a slight positive talor tilt and a positive anterior drawer test of 4 mm.

Phase 1   **Acute Injury**   **GOALS:** To control hemorrhage, swelling, pain, and spasm.
                      ESTIMATED LENGTH OF TIME (ELT): 2-3 days.

■ **Therapy** Ice packs are applied (20 minutes) intermittently 6 to 8 times daily. X-ray examination rules out fracture. Athlete wears elastic wrap during waking hours and elevates leg. The leg is elevated during sleep. Nonsteroidal antiinflammatory drugs and analgesics are given. An airsplint is used during this period for support and compression. No weight bearing is allowed. Crutches are used to avoid weight bearing for at least 3 or 4 days or until athlete can walk without a limp with lateral support.

■ **Exercise rehabilitation** The athlete begins exercise by toe gripping and spreading if there is no pain 10 to 15 times every waking hour starting on the second day of injury. General body maintenance exercises are conducted three times a week as long as they do not aggravate the injury.

Phase 2   **Repair**   **GOALS:** To decrease swelling, permit secondary healing to occur, restore full muscle contraction without pain. Restore 50% pain-free movement.
                     ELT: 3 weeks.

■ **Therapy** All treatment is immediately followed by exercise. Use ice pack (5 to 15 minutes), ice massage (7 minutes), cold whirlpool (60° F, 10 minutes), or massage above and below injury site (5 minutes). When hemorrhage is completely controlled, use whirlpool (90° to 100° F, 10 to 15 minutes).

■ **Exercise rehabilitation** Crutch walking with a toe touch if athlete is unable to walk without a limp while wearing an air cast, tape, or both for 3 weeks. First 2 weeks toe griping and spreading (10 to 15 times) every waking hour. Active proprioceptive neuromuscular facilitation ankle patterns three or four times daily for a pain-free range of motion. Avoid any exercise that produces pain or swelling. Ankle circumduction (10 to 15 times each direction) two or three times daily. Achilles tendon stretch from the floor (30 seconds) in each foot position (toe in, toe out, straight ahead) three or four times daily. Toe raises (10 times, one to three sets) three or four times daily. Eversion exercise using a towel or rubber tube or tire resistance three or four times daily. Shifting body weight between injured and noninjured ankle (up to 20 times two or three times daily). Wobble board exercise (1 to 3 minutes) two or three times daily. Progress to straight-ahead short-step walking if it can be done without a limp. General body maintenance exercises are conducted three times a week as long as they do not aggravate injury.

Phase 3   **Remodeling**   **GOALS:** To restore symptom-free full range of motion, power, endurance, speed, and agility.
                     ELT: 3-5 weeks.

■ **Therapy** Therapeutic mobilities such as whirlpool (100° to 105° F) (20 minutes) or ultrasound (0.5 W/cm²) (5 minutes) are used symptomatically.

Continued

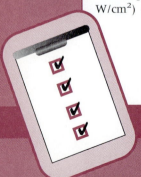

Grade 2 Inversion Ankle Sprain—*cont'd*

■ **Exercise rehabilitation** Achilles tendon stretch using slant board (30 seconds each foot position) two or three times daily. Toe raises using slant board and resistance (10 repetitions, one to three sets) two or three times daily. Resistance ankle device to strengthen anterior, lateral, and medial muscles (starting with 2 lb and progressing to 10 lb) (one to three sets) two or three times daily. Wobble board for ankle proprioception (begin at 1 minute in each direction, progress to 5 minutes) three times daily. Walk-jog routine as long as symptom free, can begin to alternately walk-jog-run-walk 25 yards straight ahead, jog 25 yards straight ahead; progress to walk 25 yards in lazy S or five figure-8s, progress to figure-8 running as fast as possible; when athlete is able to run 10 figure-8s or Z cuts as fast as possible and able to spring up in the air on the injured leg 10 times without pain.

Criteria for Returning to Competitive Lacrosse

1. The ankle is pain free during motion and no swelling is present.
2. Full ankle range of motion and strength have been regained.
3. The athlete is able to run, jump, and make cutting movements as well as before injury.

followed by 5 minutes of proprioceptive neuromuscular facilitation (PNF) exercise improves strength, range of motion, and proprioception. Exercise should include isometrics while immobilized followed by range-of-motion exercises, progressive relaxation exercise (PRE), and balance activities lasting up to 4 weeks.[6]

Taping in a closed basket weave technique may protect the ankle during the early stages of walking (see Figure 13-27). The athlete must be instructed to avoid walking or running on uneven or sloped surfaces for 2 to 3 weeks after weight bearing has begun.

NOTE: The grade 2 sprain, with its torn and stretched ligaments, tends to have a number of serious complications. Because of laxity there is a tendency to twist and sprain the ankle repeatedly. This recurrence over a period of time can lead to joint degeneration and traumatic arthritis. Once a grade 2 sprain has occurred, there must be a major effort to protect the ankle against future trauma.[24]

Grade 3 inversion ankle sprains The grade 3 inversion ankle sprain is relatively uncommon in sports. When it does happen, it is extremely disabling. Often the force causes the ankle to subluxate and then spontaneously become reduced.

Etiology The grade 3 sprain is caused by a severe force to the ankle in inversion, plantar flexion, and adduction. This is a grade 3 injury that involves varying grades of injury to the anterior talofibular, calcaneofibular, and posterior talofibular ligaments, as well as the joint capsule.

Symptoms and signs The athlete complains of severe pain in the region of the lateral malleolus. Swelling is diffused along with discoloration. There is no possible weight bearing and major loss of function. There is a great deal of swelling, with or without pain. Hemorthrosis, discoloration, a positive talar tilt, and a positive anterior drawer test are present.[22]

Management Normally RICE is used intermittently for 2 or 3 days. It is not uncommon for the physician to apply a dorsiflexion cast or weight-bearing brace for 3 to 6 weeks, followed by taping for 3 to 6 weeks.[11,20] Crutches are usually given to the athlete when the cast is removed. Isometric exercise is carried out while the cast

---

18-1

Critical Thinking E x e r c i s e

A basketball player has a history of numerous lateral ankle sprains.

? How may this basketball player reduce the incidence of these ankle sprains?

A tennis player sustains a grade 2 lateral sprain of the left ankle while making a sudden stop.

? Assuming good immediate care was carried out, how should this condition be managed 10 days after injury?

A grade 2 or 3 eversion sprain can adversely affect the medial longitudinal arch.

is on, followed by range-of-motion, PRE, and balance exercises. In some cases surgery is warranted to stabilize the athlete's ankle for future sports participation. NOTE: The grade 3 ankle sprain creates significant joint laxity and instability. Because of this laxity, the ankle joint is prone to severe degenerative forces.

Eversion Ankle Sprains

Eversion ankle sprains represent 5% to 10% of all ankle sprains. It is a more serious injury than the lateral ankle sprain.

Etiology   The mechanism of the eversion ankle sprain is one of eversion, dorsiflexion, and abduction. Athletes with pronated or hypermobile feet are more prone to this injury. Avulsion fracture of the medial malleolus occurs in 15% of the cases.[2]

Symptoms and signs   Depending on the degree of injury, the athlete complains of pain, sometimes severe, that occurs over the foot and lower leg. Usually the athlete is unable to bear weight on the foot. Both abduction and adduction cause pain, but pressing directly upward against the bottom of the foot will not produce pain.

Management   X-ray is necessary to rule out fracture. Initially, RICE and no weight bearing are recommended, and a posterior splint tape is applied. Nonsteroidal antiinflammatory drugs (NSAIDs) and analgesics are given as needed. A grade 1 sprain may be given a weight-bearing cast for up to 3 weeks, followed by taping. A weight-bearing cast is applied to grade 1 and 2 sprains for 3 weeks, followed by taping. The athlete engages in a PRE program for the posteromedial ankle muscles, engages in balance activities, and is fitted with an inner heel wedge shoe insert. NOTE: An eversion sprain of grade 2 or more severity can produce significant joint instability. Because the deltoid ligament is involved with supporting the medial longitudinal arch, a sprain can cause weakness in this area, leading to pronation or a fallen arch. Repeated sprains could lead to pes planus (flatfoot).

Syndesmotic Ankle Sprain

Syndesmotic ankle sprain is a relatively common injury in football. It occurs during games and practice.[3]

Etiology   Two mechanisms can cause a forceful external rotation of the ankle. While the player is lying on the field with his ankle externally rotated, another player falls on the back of the leg and heel of the foot, forcing external rotation.[7] A second cause comes from a lateral blow to the knee or leg with the foot planted, forcing external rotation. The external force can rupture the anterior tibiofibular ligament, the interosseous membrane, and the posterior tibiofibular ligament, or a fracture can occur to the posterior tibial tubercle.[7]

Symptoms and signs   The athlete complains of severe pain and loss of function in the ankle region. When the ankle is passively externally rotated there is a major pain in the lower leg indicating a syndesmotic sprain or a lateral malleolar fracture. Pain normally occurs along the anterolateral leg.

Management   The athlete is out of competition; RICE, NSAIDs, and analgesics are given as required. X-ray examination can reveal fracture or a widening of the ankle mortise. As healing occurs the interosseus membrane tends to ossify. Treatment follows that of a grade 3 lateral sprain. This condition often leads to a chronically unstable ankle. Treatment consists of cryotherapy with active movement and ROM exercises. While protected with bracing and/or tape, the athlete engages in pain-free ambulation. Follow-up treatment may include contrast baths, iontophoresis, and dexamethasone. Goals for full recovery are similar to those for other ankle sprains.[13] Recovery time is approximately 8 weeks.

Injury to the anterior or posterior tibiofibular ligaments   The possibility in both the grade 2 and 3 inversion and eversion sprain of tearing either the anterior or posterior tibiofibular ligament is always present. The anterior tibiofibular ligament can be torn in an inversion sprain; either ligament or both ligaments can be torn in an eversion sprain. In both mechanisms, the tearing of one or both of these ligaments can widen the ankle mortise, leaving it unstable. With the widened mortise, an eversion or inversion motion will allow the talus to move laterally and medially more than 5 degrees. This condition is known as the talar tilt. One method for determining a posterior tibiofibular sprain is having the athlete bend the knee to relax the gastrocnemius muscle and then passively dorsiflex the ankle. A positive reaction to this test is when there is pain in the ankle sulcus.

Ankle Fractures

There are a number of ways in which an ankle can be fractured or dislocated. A foot that is forcibly abducted on the leg can produce a transverse fracture of the distal tibia and fibula. In contrast, a foot that is planted, in combination with a leg that is forcibly rotated internally, can produce a fracture to the distal and posterior tibia (Figure 18-17).

Avulsion fractures, in which a chip of bone is pulled off by resistance of a liga-

18-3

Critical Thinking Exercise

A football player, while lying on the field, has his ankle forced into external rotation by another player.

? What type of injury is sustained by this mechanism? What is a characteristic sign of this injury?

A talar tilt occurs when the ankle mortise is widened.

Figure 18-17

Ankle fractures or dislocations can be major sports injuries.

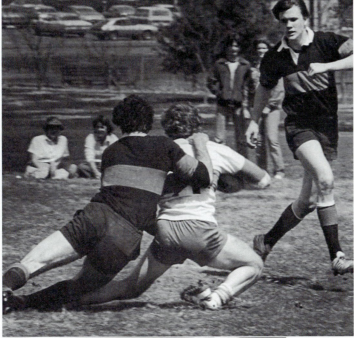

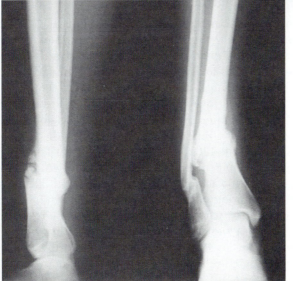

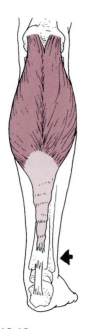

Figure 18-18

Achilles tendon rupture.

A ruptured Achilles tendon usually occurs when inflammation has been chronic.

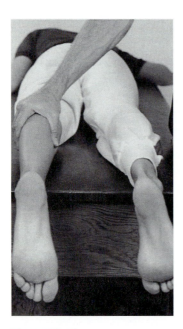

Figure 18-19

The Thompson test to determine an Achilles tendon rupture by squeezing the calf muscle. A positive result to the test is one in which the heel does not move.

ment, are common in grade 2 and 3 degree eversion or inversion sprains. In most cases of fracture, swelling and pain are extreme. There may be some or no deformity; however, if a fracture is suspected, splinting is essential. Rest, ice, compression, and elevation are used as soon as possible to control hemorrhage and swelling. Once swelling is reduced, casting can take place, allowing the athlete to bear weight. Immobilization will usually last for at least 6 to 8 weeks.[15]

Acute Achilles Tendon Injuries

Achilles Tendon Strain

Etiology   Achilles tendon strains are not uncommon in sports and occur most often as a results of a lack of coordination between the agonists and the antagonists after ankle sprains or sudden excessive dorsiflexion of the ankle.

Symptoms and signs   The resulting injury may be mild to severe. A severe injury is a partial or complete avulsion or rupturing of the Achilles tendon. While sustaining this injury, the athlete feels acute pain and extreme weakness on plantar flexion.

Management   Initially, as with other acute conditions, pressure is first applied with an elastic wrap together with the application of cold. Unless the injury is minor, hemorrhage may be extensive, requiring RICE over an extended period of time. After hemorrhaging has subsided, an elastic wrap can be lightly applied for continued pressure.

The tendency for Achilles tendon trauma to develop readily into a chronic condition requires a conservative approach to therapy. Management should be initiated in the following manner:

- More definitive therapy can usually begin on the third day using hydromassage and analgesic packs until soreness has subsided.
- Both heels, affected and unaffected, should be elevated by placing a sponge rubber pad in the heel of each street shoe. Elevation decreases the extension of the tendon and thereby relieves some of the irritation.
- In a few days the athlete will be able to return to activity. The Achilles tendon should be restricted by a tape support and a sponge rubber heel lift placed in each athletic shoe. Heel lifts should be placed in both shoes or taped directly to the bottoms of both heels to avoid leg length asymmetry and subsequent adverse muscle and skeletal stresses.

It should be noted that correcting a rear foot valgus or varus may assist Achilles tendon problems.

Achilles Tendon Rupture

A rupture of the Achilles tendon (Figure 18-18) is a possibility in sports that require stop-and-go action. Although most common in athletes who are 30 years of age or older, rupture of the Achilles tendon can occur in athletes of any age. It usually occurs in an athlete with a history of chronic inflammation and gradual degeneration caused by microtears.[1]

Etiology   The initial insult normally is the result of sudden pushing-off action of the forefoot with the knee being forced into complete extension.

Symptoms and signs   When the rupture occurs, the athlete complains of a sudden snap or that something hit him or her in the lower leg. Pain is felt immediately but rapidly subsides. Point tenderness, swelling, and discoloration are usually associated with the trauma. Toe raising is impossible in an Achilles tendon rupture. The major problem in Achilles tendon rupture is accurate diagnosis, especially in a partial rupture. Any acute injury to the Achilles tendon should be suspected as being a rupture. Signs indicative of a rupture are obvious indentation at the tendon site and a positive Thompson test. The Thompson test (Figure 18-19) is performed by squeezing the calf muscle while the leg is extended and the foot is hanging over the edge of the table. A positive Thompson sign is one in which squeezing the calf muscle does not cause the heel to move or pull upward or in which it moves less when compared with the uninjured leg. An Achilles tendon rupture usually occurs 2 to 6 cm proximal to its insertion onto the calcaneus.

Management   Usual management of a complete Achilles tendon rupture is surgical repair. Nonoperative treatment consists of RICE, NSAIDs, and analgesics with a non–weight-bearing cast for 6 weeks followed by a short-leg walking cast for 2 weeks. With this approach there is 75% to 80% return of normal function.[2] Surgery is usually the choice for serious injuries, providing 75% to 90% return of function. Exercise rehabilitation lasts for about 6 months and consists of range-of-motion exercises, PRE, and the wearing of a 2 cm heel lift in both shoes.[2]

Chronic Ankle Tendon Conditions

Achilles Tendinitis

Covering the Achilles tendon is a paratendon consisting of fatty and areolar tissue that surrounds the tendon and fills the spaces around it.

Etiology   A jerk movement in the gastrocnemius-soleus system in which eccentric contraction is inefficient leads to microtears. Over time repeated injury leads to chronic-inflammation tissue degeneration. In chronic cases of Achilles tendinitis, mucoid nodules occur as a result of tissue degeneration (Figure 18-20). They must be surgically removed for healing to occur.

Other etiological factors are training errors such as hill running, increased mileage, intensive training sessions, and running on uneven surfaces. Wearing a shoe that fails to stabilize the heel adequately, malalignment of the tibia vara, tight hamstrings, and cavus feet, as well as tightness of the gastrocnemius-soleus unit, can predispose an athlete to Achilles tendinitis. Athletes with either a pronated or cavus foot have an increased incidence of Achilles tendinitis (Figure 18-21).

Symptoms and signs   The athlete complains of pain on walking that has increased over time. Examination reveals tenderness, erythema, crepitus, swelling, and weakness on dorsiflexion.

Management   Initially the athlete is treated with RICE, NSAIDs, and analgesics as needed. The athlete engages in range-of-motion exercises and PRE for 1 to 3 weeks. Runners must decrease mileage and avoid hills and uneven surfaces. Foot alignment may be corrected by an orthotic device. A flexible shoe with a molded Achilles pad can be used to prevent irritation, and a 10 to 15 mm heel lift can be used to decrease

18-4

Critical ***Thinking*** Exercise

A 35-year-old racquetball player, while moving backward, experiences a sudden snap and pain in her left Achilles tendon.

? What type of injury does this mechanism describe, and how should it be examined?

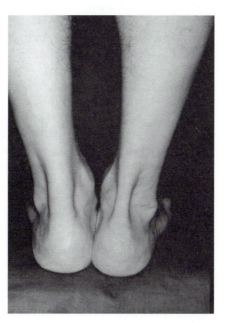

Figure 18-20

A thickened Achilles tendon caused by tendinitis.

Figure 18-21

Common tendinitis of the foot and ankle region.

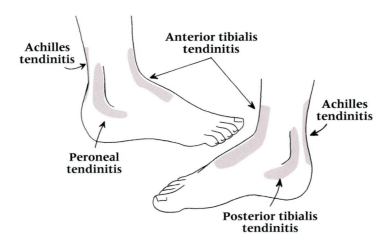

Achilles tendinitis

Anterior tibialis tendinitis

Achilles tendinitis

Peroneal tendinitis

Posterior tibialis tendinitis

tendon excursion. In cases in which there is chronic degeneration, nodules may have to be surgically excised and defects repaired. Surgery is followed by placement in a short-leg cast for 3 to 6 weeks, after which there is a gradual resumption of normal activities. It has been estimated that 15% of individuals suffering from chronic Achilles tendinitis do not respond to conservative treatment.

Peroneal Tendon Subluxation/Dislocation

The peroneus longus and brevis tendons pass through a common groove located behind the lateral malleolus. The tendons are held in place by the peroneal retinaculum.

Etiology   This injury most often occurs in sports that apply major forces (e.g., turning and sharply cutting) to the foot and ankle. Wrestling, football, ice skating, skiing, basketball, and soccer have the highest incidence. Another mechanism is a direct blow to the posterior lateral malleolus. A moderate to severe inversion sprain or forceful dorsiflexion of the ankle can tear the peroneal retinaculum, allowing the peroneal tendon to tear out of its groove. As discussed previously, one of the major functions of the peroneus longus muscle is to pull the first metatarsal bone into plantar flexion. When there is major foot pronation of hypermobility, the peroneus longus tendon becomes overly stressed in its efforts to stabilize the first metatarsal bone.

Symptoms and signs   The athlete complains that in running or jumping the tendons snap out of the groove and then back in when stress is released. Eversion against manual resistance will often replicate the subluxation. The athlete experiences recurrent pain, snapping, and ankle instability. The lateral aspect of the ankle appears with ecchymoses, edema, tenderness, and crepitus over the peroneal tendon.

Management   A conservative approach should be used first, including compression with a felt pad cut in a horseshoe-shaped pattern that surrounds the lateral malleolus. This compression can be reinforced with a rigid plastic or plaster splint until acute signs have subsided, and RICE, NSAIDs, and analgesics are given as needed. The time period for this conservative care is 5 to 6 weeks, followed by a gradual exercise rehabilitation program that includes range-of-motion exercises, PRE, and balance training. If a conservative approach fails, surgery is required.

Anterior Tibialis Tendinitis

Etiology   Anterior tibialis tendinitis is a common condition of athletes and joggers who run downhill for an extended period of time.

Symptoms and signs   There is point tenderness over the anterior tibialis tendon.

Management   The athlete should be advised to rest (or at least decrease running time and distance) and to avoid hills. In more serious cases ice packs, coupled with stretching before and after running, should help reduce the symptoms. A daily strengthening program also should be conducted. Oral antiinflammatory medications may be required.

Posterior Tibial Tendinitis

Etiology   Posterior tibialis tendinitis is a common overuse condition among runners with hypermobility or pronated feet. It is a repetitive microtrauma occurring at the pronation in movements of jumping, running, or cutting.

Symptoms and signs   The athlete complains of pain and swelling in the area of the medial malleolus. Inspection reveals edema and point tenderness directly behind the medial malleolus. Pain becomes more intense when resisting inversion and plantar flexion for the more serious cases.

Management   Initially, RICE, NSAIDs, and analgesics are given as needed. A non–weight-bearing short-leg cast with the foot in inversion may be used. Management consists of correcting the problem of pronation with a LowDye-type taping or an orthotic device.

Peroneal Tendinitis

Etiology   Although not particularly common, peroneal tendinitis can be a problem in athletes with pes cavus because in pes cavus the foot tends to be placed in constant supination, which is resisted by the peroneal tendon. Athletes who constantly bear weight on the outside of the foot also place chronic stress on the peroneal tendon.

Symptoms and signs   The athlete complains of pain over the talar calcaneus when rising on the ball of the foot while jogging, running, cutting, or turning. Tenderness is noted over the tendon located at the lateral aspect of the calcaneus distally to beneath the cuboid bone.[17]

Management   Initially, RICE and NSAIDs as required, taping with elastic tape, and appropriate warm-up and flexibility exercises. LowDye taping (see Figure 13-19) or orthosis to help support the foot and prevent excessive pronation may help.

As with all types of tendinitis in the lower extremities, the mechanics of walking and running should be observed. When faulty mechanics such as running on the outside of the foot occur, realignment with an orthotic device or taping should be used. In some cases a lateral heel wedge may help reduce pain and discomfort. As with the other ankle tendons that are overused, the athlete with peroneal tendinitis should reduce activity, use ice routinely, and stretch and strengthen the tendon through eversion exercise.

THE LOWER LEG

Anatomy

The portion of the lower extremity that lies between the knee and the ankle is defined as the lower leg and consists of the tibia, the fibula, and the soft tissues that surround them.

Bones

Tibia   The tibia, except for the femur, is the longest bone in the body and serves as the principal weight-bearing bone of the leg. It is located on the medial or great toe side of the leg and is constructed with wide upper and lower ends to receive the condyles of the femur and the talus, respectively. The tibia is triangularly shaped in its upper two thirds but is rounded and more constricted in the lower third of its length. The most pronounced change occurs in the lower third of the shaft and produces an anatomical weakness that establishes this area as the site of most of the fractures occurring to the leg. The shaft of the tibia has three surfaces: posterior, medial, and lateral. The posterior and lateral surfaces are covered by muscle; the medial surface is subcutaneous and as a result vulnerable to outside trauma.

18-5

Critical Thinking Exercise

A volleyball player with a history of repeated ankle sprains complains of a snapping sensation in his right ankle.

? What procedures should be followed when managing a subluxated peroneal tendon?

18-6

Critical Thinking Exercise

A jogger, after running downhill for an extended period of time, experiences pain in the anterior medial aspect of her left foot. The condition is diagnosed as anterior tibialis tendinitis.

? How should this condition be managed?

Fibula   The fibula is long and slender and is located along the lateral aspect of the tibia, joining it in an arthrodial articulation at the upper end, just below the knee joint, and as a syndesmotic joint at the lower end. Both the upper and the lower tibiofibular joints are held in position by strong anterior and posterior ligaments. The main function of the fibula is to provide for the attachment of muscles. It serves to complete the groove for the enclosure of the talus in forming the ankle joint.

Articulations   The tibia and fibula articulate with one another superiorly and inferiorly (tibiofibular joints). Joining the tibia and fibula is a strong interosseous membrane. The fibers display an oblique downward-and-outward pattern. The oblique arrangement aids in diffusing the forces placed on the leg. It completely fills the tibiofibular space except for a small area at the superior aspect that is provided for the passage of the anterior tibial vessels. The tibiofibular ligaments form the distal aspect of the interosseous membrane.

The superior tibiofibular joint is diarthrotic, allowing some gliding movements. It articulates with the tibia's lateral condyle and the head of the fibula. It is surrounded by a fibrous capsule reinforced with anterior and posterior ligaments. The superior tibiofibular joint is stronger in front than in back.

The inferior tibiofibular joint is a fibrous articulation. It articulates between the lateral malleolus and the distal end of the tibia. The joint is reinforced by the ankle ligaments.

Compartments

The soft tissue of the leg is contained within four compartments, which are bounded by heavy fascia (Figure 18-22). The *anterior compartment* holds the major structures for ankle dorsiflexion and foot and toe extension, which are the tibialis anterior, extensor hallucis longus, and extensor digitorum longus muscles, the anterior tibial nerve, and the tibial artery. A *lateral compartment* houses the peroneus longus, brevis, and tertius muscles, which evert the ankle, and the superficial branch of the peroneal nerve. The *superficial posterior compartment* is composed of the gastrocnemius muscle and the soleus muscle. These muscles plantar flex the ankle and control foot inversion and toe flexion. The *deep posterior compartment* houses the tibialis posterior, flexor digitorum longus, and flexor hallucis longus muscles and the posterior tibial artery. A major problem resulting from sports traumas can adversely affect these compartments, especially the anterior compartment. Such trauma can lead to swelling and neurological motor and sensory deficits (see further discussion later in this chapter).

Muscles

The lower leg is divided into posterior, anterior, and lateral muscular regions (Figure 18-23). The posterior region is divided into superficial and deep muscles. The superficial muscles include the gastrocnemius, plantaris, and soleus. The deep posterior group includes the tibialis posterior, flexor digitorum longus, and flexor hallucis longus. The anterior muscles consist of the anterior tibialis, extensor digitorum longus, peroneus tertius, and extensor hallucis longus. The lateral muscles are the peroneus brevis and longus.

Nerve Supply and Blood

The major nerves of the lower leg are the tibial and common peroneal, stemming from the large sciatic nerve. The major arteries often accompany the nerves and are the posterior and anterior tibial arteries (Figure 18-24). The primary veins consist of the popliteal peroneal and the anterior and posterior tibial veins.

Functional Anatomy

The lower leg is that part of the anatomy from the knee to the ankle. The tibia and fibula provide attachment points for the thigh and leg muscles. The leg transmits body weight to the ankle and foot.

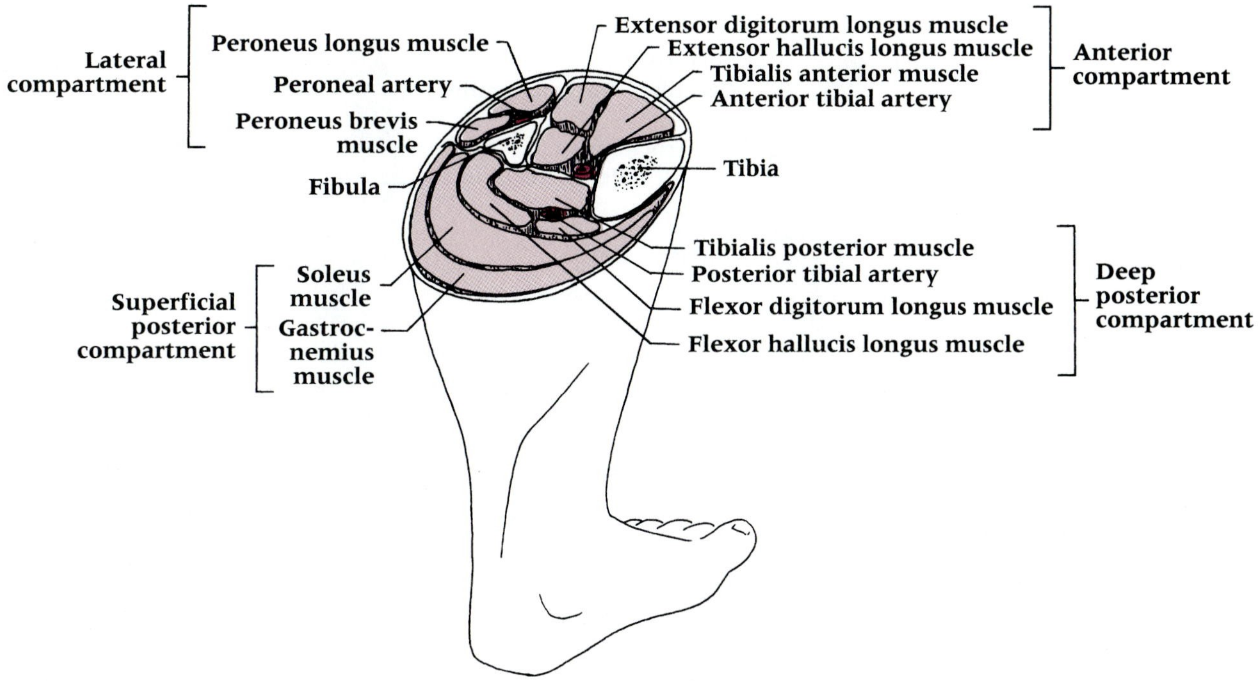

Figure 18-22

The four compartments of the lower leg.

Lower Leg Assessment

An athlete who complains of discomfort in the lower leg region should be asked the following questions:

- How long has it been hurting?
- Where is the pain or discomfort?
- Has the feeling changed or is there numbness?
- Is there a feeling of warmth or coldness?
- Is there any sense of muscle weakness or difficulty in walking?
- How did the problem occur?

Observation

The athlete is generally observed for the following:

- Any postural deviations, such as toeing in, may indicate tibial torsion or genu valgum or varum; foot pronation should also be noted.
- Any walking difficulty should be noted, along with leg deformities or swellings.

Palpation

Palpate the posterior, lateral, anterior, and medial aspects of the leg. Compare both legs as to pain, swelling, and symmetry.

Begin palpation on the posterior aspect of the leg. While the patient is in the prone position with the foot free over the end of the table, the deep posterior compartment, containing the gastrocnemius soleus muscles and the achilles tendon, is palpated.[4]

The lateral aspect of the leg consists of the fibula and lateral compartment with its peroneal muscles. The fibula is gently palpated for fracture. The peroneal muscles are palpated for tenderness followed by a resisted foot eversion for pain sites.

The anterior compartment holds the tibialis anterior, extensor hallucis longus, and extensor digitorum muscles. The muscles are resisted and palpated.[4] The medial aspect of the leg is the shin region. Palpation should be performed over the shin surface and the tibia's anteromedial or anterolateral borders.

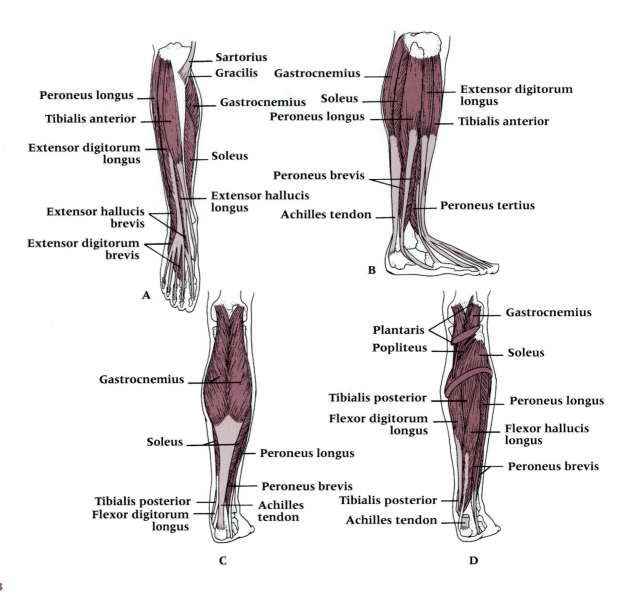

Figure 18-23

Muscles of the lower leg. **A,** Anterior view. **B,** Lateral view. **C,** Posterior view (superficial structures). **D,** Posterior view (deep structures).

Special Tests

Muscle tests   Passive, active, and resistive movement is given to the muscles of the lower leg. Active ankle tests should be repeated for lower leg assessment.

Alignment tests   Determining malalignment of the lower leg can reveal the causes of abnormal stresses applied to the foot, ankle, and lower leg, as well as the knees and hip. A common malalignment of the lower leg is internal or external tibial torsion.

In normal alignment of the lower extremity anteriorly a straight line can be drawn from the anterior superior iliac spine, the patella, and the web between the first and second toes. Laterally normal alignment is when a straight line can be drawn from the greater trochanter of the femur, the center of the patella, and just behind the lateral malleolus. From the rear a straight line can be drawn from the center of the lower leg, through the midline of the Achilles tendon and calcaneus.[4]

Fracture tests   When fracture is suspected, a gentle percussive blow can be given to the tibia or fibula below or above the suspected site. Percussion can also be applied upward on the bottom of the heel. Such blows set up a vibratory force that resonates at the fracture, causing pain.

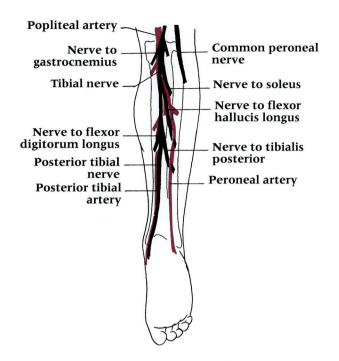

Popliteal artery

Nerve to gastrocnemius

Tibial nerve

Nerve to flexor digitorum longus

Posterior tibial nerve

Posterior tibial artery

Common peroneal nerve

Nerve to soleus

Nerve to flexor hallucis longus

Nerve to tibialis posterior

Peroneal artery

Figure 18-24

Blood and nerve supply of the lower leg.

Acute Leg Injuries

The leg is prone to a number of acute conditions, of which contusions and strains are the most common. Although less common, fractures can occur in relation to direct trauma, such as being struck by a blow, or through torsional forces with the foot fixed to the ground.

Leg Contusions

Shin bruise The shin, lying just under the skin, is exceedingly vulnerable and sensitive to blows or bumps. Because of the absence of muscular or adipose padding here, blows are not dissipated as they are elsewhere, and the periosteum receives the full force of any impact delivered to the shin. The periosteum surrounds bone surfaces, with the exception of the cartilaginous areas, and is composed of two fibrous layers that adhere closely to the bone, acting as a bed for blood vessels and bone-forming osteoblasts.

Etiology A direct force to the shin region is the primary cause of the skin bruise.

Symptoms and signs The athlete complains of pain, swelling, and increased pain when the leg is moved. A hematoma is present with a jellylike consistency.[9] There is decreased range of motion.

Management Give RICE, NSAIDs, and analgesics as needed. The hematoma may be aspirated. The athlete, within pain limitations, engages in range-of-motion and PRE exercises. The athlete is fitted with a doughnut padding under an orthoplast shell.[9]

NOTE: The shin is an extremely difficult area to heal, particularly the lower third, which has a considerably smaller blood supply than the upper portion. An inadequately cared for injury to the periosteum may develop into osteomyelitis, a serious condition that results in the destruction and deterioration of bony tissue (Figure 18-25).

In sports such as football and soccer in which the shin is particularly vulnerable, adequate padding should be provided. All injuries in this area are potentially serious; therefore minor shin lacerations or bruises should never be permitted to go untended.

18-7

Critical Thinking Exercise

A football running back receives a hard low tackle. He hears a loud pop and feels a sharp pain in his right lower leg. Weight bearing is impossible.

? In this situation, what type of injury is suspected?

Severe blows to an unprotected shin can lead to a chronic inflammation.

Figure 18-25

A poorly cared for shin bruise can lead to osteomyelitis.

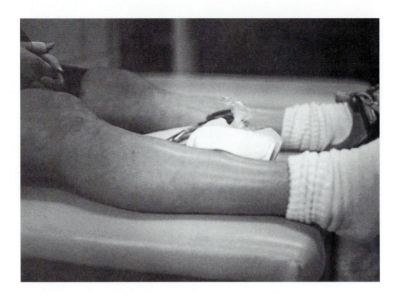

Muscle contusions

Etiology　　Contusions of the leg, particularly in the area of the gastrocnemius muscle, are common in sports.

Symptoms and signs　　A bruise in this area can produce an extremely handicapping injury for the athlete. A bruising blow to the leg will cause pain, weakness, and partial loss of the use of the limb. Palpation may reveal a hard, rigid, and somewhat inflexible area because of internal hemorrhage and muscle spasm.

Management　　When this condition occurs, it is advisable to stretch the muscles in the region immediately to prevent spasm and then, for approximately 1 hour, to apply a compress bandage and cold packs to control internal hemorrhaging.

If cold therapy or other superficial therapy such as massage and whirlpool do not return the athlete to normal activity within 2 to 3 days, the use of ultrasound may be warranted. An elastic wrap or tape support will stabilize the part and permit the athlete to participate without aggravation of the injury.

Leg Spasms and Muscle Strains

Muscle spasms　　Spasms are sudden, violent, involuntary contractions of one or several muscles and may be either clonic or tonic. A *clonic* spasm is identified by intermittent contraction and relaxation. A *tonic* spasm is identified by constant muscle contraction without an intervening period of relaxation. The clonic spasm has a neurological basis and is seen less often in sports.

Etiology　　How and why tonic muscle spasms happen to athletes is often difficult to ascertain. Fatigue, excess loss of fluid through perspiration, and inadequate reciprocal muscle coordination are some of the factors that may predispose an individual to a contracture. The leg, particularly the gastrocnemius muscle, is prone to this condition. It is usually difficult to predict the occurrence of spasm because only the aforementioned criteria can be used as a guide.

Symptoms and signs　　The athlete has considerable muscle tension and pain with the tonic contraction of the calf muscle.

Management　　Management in such cases includes putting the athlete at ease and relaxing the contracted site. Firmly grasping the contracted muscle, together with mild, gradual stretching, relieves most acute spasms. An ice pack or gentle ice massage may also be helpful in reducing spasm. In cases of recurrent spasm, the athletic trainer should make certain that fatigue or abnormal water or electrolyte loss is not a factor.

Calf strain　　The medial head of the gastrocnemius becomes strained and tears near its musculotendinous attachment.

Etiology Sports such as tennis that require quick starts and stops can cause this gastrocnemius strain. Usually the athlete makes a quick stop with the foot planted flat and suddenly extends the knee, placing stress on the medial head of the gastrocnemius (Figure 18-26).

Symptoms and signs A calf strain follows the description given in Chapter 7. Depending on the grade of injury there is a variable amount of pain, swelling, and muscle disability. The athlete may complain of a sensation of having been shot in the calf. Examination reveals edema, point tenderness, and a functional strength loss.[9]

Management Initially, RICE, NSAIDs, and analgesics are given as needed. A grade 1 calf strain should be given a gentle, gradual stretch after muscle cooling. Weight bearing can take place as tolerated. A heel wedge may help reduce stretching of the calf muscle during walking. Appropriate elastic wrap may serve to support the muscle while active. A gradual program of range of motion and PRE should be instituted.

Acute Leg Fractures

Fractures received during sports participation occur most often to the fingers, hands, face, and legs. Of leg fractures, the fibular fracture has the highest incidence and occurs principally to the middle third of the leg. Fractures of the tibia occur predominantly to the lower third.

Etiology Fractures of the shaft of the tibia and fibula result from either direct or indirect trauma during active participation in sports (Figure 18-27). There is often a severe bony displacement with deformity as a result of a strong pull of antagonistic muscles, causing an overriding of the bone ends, particularly if the athlete attempts to move or to stand on the limb after the injury. Crepitus and a temporary loss of limb function are usually present.

Symptoms and signs This injury causes severe soft-tissue insult and extensive internal hemorrhaging. The athlete complains of severe pain and disability. The leg appears hard and swollen, which may indicate the beginning of Volkmann's contracture. Volkmann's contracture is the result of great internal tension caused by hemorrhage and swelling within closed fascial compartments, inhibiting the blood supply and resulting in necrosis of muscles and contractures.

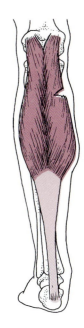

Figure 18-26

Calf strain.

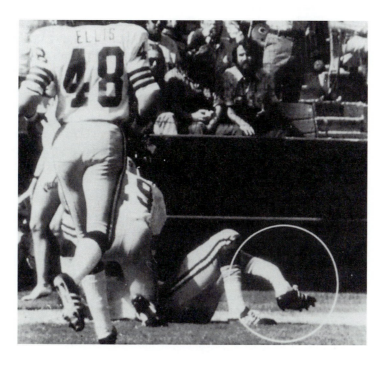

Figure 18-27

Fracture of the tibia.

Management   In most cases, fracture reduction and cast immobilization are applied for 3 to 6 months, depending on the extent of the injury and any complications.

Repetitive and Overuse Leg Problems

A number of problems of the leg can be attributed to repetitive motions and overuse. Three of these conditions are the medial tibial syndrome (shinsplints), exercise-induced compartment compression syndromes, and stress fractures.

Medial Tibial Stress Syndrome

Medial tibial stress syndrome (MTSS) accounts for approximately 10% to 15% of all running injuries and up to 60% of all conditions that cause pain in athletes' legs.

Etiology   Medial tibial stress syndrome is caused by a repetitive microtrauma. It is seen commonly in basketball, running, and gymnastics. A variety of factors can contribute to MTSS, such as weakness of leg muscles, shoes that provide little support or cushioning, and training errors such as running on hard surfaces or overtraining. Malignment problems such as varus foot, a tight heel cord, a hypermobile pronated foot, or a forefoot supination can also lead to MTSS.[12]

The pathological process of this condition is regarded as a myositis or periostitis that occurs either acutely, as in preseason preparation, or chronically, developing slowly throughout the entire competitive season. One should approach this situation through deductive thinking. First, all information about why a certain athlete may have acquired shinsplints must be gathered—examples include changing from a hard gymnasium floor activity to a soft field sport or exhibiting general fatigue after a strenuous season. Second, the athlete should be examined for possible structural body weaknesses. From this information an empirical analysis can be made as to the probable cause of shinsplints. However, persistent shin irritation and incapacitation must be referred to the physician for thorough examination. Conditions such as stress fractures, muscle herniations, and chronic anterior tibial compartment syndromes (a severe swelling within the anterior fascia chamber) may resemble the symptoms of shinsplints. A number of authorities believe that shinsplints involve one of two syndromes: a tibial stress fracture or an overuse syndrome that can progress to an irreversible, exertional compartment syndrome.

Symptoms and signs   Four grades of pain can be attributed to medial tibial syndrome: grade 1 pain occurring after athletic activity; grade 2 pain occurring before and after activity but not affecting performance; grade 3 pain occurring before, during, and after athletic activity and affecting performance; and grade 4 pain, so severe that performance is impossible.

Management   Initially, RICE, NSAIDs, and analgesics are given as needed. Rest is of major importance. Management of medial tibial syndrome is as varied as its etiology. Constant heat in the form of whirlpools and ultrasound therapy gives positive results and, together with supportive taping and gradual stretching, affords a good general approach to the problem. Phonophoresis and iontophoresis also have been effective.

Ice massage to the shin region and aspirin usage have been beneficial before a workout. Ice massage is applied for 10 minutes or until erythema occurs. Ice application should be followed by a gradual stretch to both the anterior and posterior aspects of the leg directly after the massage. Progressive relaxation exercise (PRE) the anterior and posterior leg muscle group. Gradual stretching should be a routine procedure before and after physical activity for all athletes who have a history of MTSS. Exercise must also accompany any therapy program, with special considerations of the calf muscle and the plantar and dorsiflexion movements of the foot. A counterforce circumferential taping of the calf 2 to 4 inches proximal to the malleoli has also been found beneficial.

Exertional Compartment Syndrome

As discussed, the leg is composed of four compartments. Each compartment is bound by fascial sheaths or by fascial sheaths and bone (see Figure 18-22). The anterior compartment contains the anterior tibial muscle, the deep peroneal nerve, the long extensor muscles of the toes, and both the anterior tibial artery and vein. The lateral compartment is composed of the superficial peroneal nerve and the long and short peroneal muscles. Posteriorly, the leg has a deep and superficial compartment. The deep posterior compartment comprises the tibial muscle and flexor muscles of the toes, as well as the peroneal artery and vein, posterior tibial artery and vein, and tibial nerve. The superficial posterior compartment is composed of the soleus muscle and gastrocnemius and plantar tendons.

Etiology   The exercise-induced compartment compression syndrome occurs most frequently among runners and athletes in sports that involve extensive running, such as soccer. The compartments most often affected are the anterior and deep posterior, with the anterior having by far the highest incidence. On occasion, the lateral compartment may be involved. The incidence of bilaterality in chronic exertional compartment syndrome is 50% to 60%.[5]

The chronic exertional compartment syndrome occurs when the tissue fluid pressure has increased because the confines of fascia or bone together with muscle hypertrophy adversely compress muscles, blood vessels, and nerves. With the increase in fluid pressure, muscle ischemia that could lead to permanent disability occurs.

The exercise-induced compartment compression syndrome is classified as either acute or chronic. The rare acute syndrome occurs after being struck a direct blow or after excessive exercise in an untrained individual and is a medical emergency, requiring immediate decompression to prevent permanent damage. The acute exercise-induced compartment compression syndrome resembles a fracture or a severe contusion.

The second type is chronic or recurrent. Internal pressures rise slowly during exercise and subside after discontinuance of exercise. If exercise is not stopped in time, an acute emergency may occur. In chronic exercise-induced compartment compression syndrome, there is a constriction of blood vessels, producing ischemia and pain, but neurological involvement is rare.

The chronic exertional compartment syndrome is often confused with shinsplints by the coach or athletic trainer. It may also be confused with a stress fracture.

Symptoms and signs   The more common chronic exertional compartment syndrome symptoms are usually bilateral. The athlete complains of pain during exercise in the anterolateral region of the leg. Gradually, over time the pain will predictably occur after running a specific distance. The athlete commonly complains of an ache or sharp pain and pressure in the region of the anterior compartment when performing a particular activity. The symptoms subside or go away completely when resting. When major symptoms are present, weakness in foot and toe extension and numbness in the dorsal region may occur.

Management   Often initial symptoms are aided by the application of RICE, NSAIDs, and analgesia as needed. However, recurrent conditions may require surgical release of the associated fascia. Once surgery is performed, the athlete is allowed to return home and begin a light program of exercise in 10 days.

Stress Fracture of the Tibia or Fibula

Stress fractures to the tibia or fibula are a common overuse stress condition, especially among distance runners.

Etiology   Like many other overuse syndromes, athletes who have biomechanical foot problems are more prone to stress fractures of the lower leg (Figure 18-28). Athletes who have hypermobile pronated feet are more susceptible to fibular stress fracture, whereas those with rigid pes cavus are more prone to tibial stress fractures. It

18-8

Critical Thinking Exercise

A gymnast complains of pain in the medial aspect of her right tibia. There is pain before, during, and after activity. Assessment rules out a stress fracture and determines the injury to be a grade III medial tibial stress syndrome.

? What could be the causes of this condition?

Exercise-induced compartment compression syndromes occur most commonly in runners and soccer players.

Figure 18-28

Tibial stress fracture.

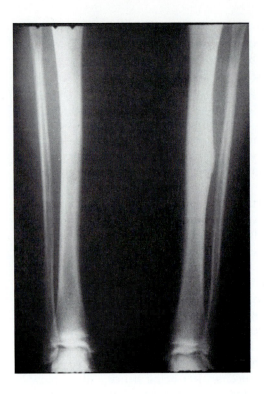

18-9

Critical Thinking Exercise

A soccer player complains of recurrent pain in the anterolateral region of the leg during practice and competition. The pain is described as an ache and a feeling of pressure.

? This condition is determined to be an exertional compartment syndrome. How should it be managed?

The athlete with hypermobile pronated feet is more susceptible to fibular stress fracture. The athlete with rigid pes cavus is more susceptible to tibial stress fractures.

has also been found that the wider the tibia, the lower the incidence of stress fractures. Runners frequently develop a stress fracture in the lower third of the leg; ballet dancers more commonly acquire one in the middle third. Stress fractures often occur to nonexperienced and nonconditioned individuals.[21] Training errors are often the cause.[21] Other reasons include amenorrhea and nutritional deficiencies.

Symptoms and signs   The athlete complains of pain in the leg that is more intense after than during the activity. There is usually point tenderness, but it may be difficult to discern the difference between bone pain and soft-tissue pain. One technique for distinguishing bone pain from soft-tissue pain is bone percussion. The fibula or tibia is tapped firmly above the level of tenderness. Vibration travels along the bone to the fracture, which may respond with pain. Another percussive technique is to hit the heel upward from below causing pain to occur at the fracture site.

Diagnosis of a stress fracture may be extremely difficult. X-ray examination may or may not detect the problem. A bone scan 1 to 3 hours after injection of radioactive material may reflect the stress fracture but does not clearly distinguish between a fracture and periostitis.

Management   The following regimen may be used for a stress fracture of the leg:

- Discontinue running and other stressful locomotor activities for at least 14 days.
- When pain is severe, use crutch for walking or wear a cast.
- Weight bearing may be resumed as pain subsides.
- Bicycling may be done before returning to running.
- After a pain-free period of at least 2 weeks, running can gradually begin again.[8]
- Biomechanical foot corrections should be made.

RELATED REPETITIVE OVERUSE PROBLEMS

Although lower-extremity stress injuries are usually concentrated in the foot, ankle, or lower leg, other body areas also can become involved. This is especially true for long-distance runners. Repetitive use and overuse of the lower extremity, particularly when there are biomechanical and subsequent weight-transmission discrepancies, can lead to problems in other regions of the body. Some of the more commonly affected areas are the knee and hip.

The Knee

A common site for distance runners to have a stress problem is in the region of the knee. In some cases there may be chronic pain and swelling in the knee joint itself, possibly indicating a meniscal tear or degenerative articular cartilage changes. More commonly, the cause is patellar tendinitis, chondromalacia, iliotibial band tendinitis, or pes anserinus tendinitis. (See Chapter 19.)

The Thigh and Hip

As with the knee, the thigh and hip can develop pain that can be attributed to overuse. Two conditions are increasing in incidence because of the popularity of running: trochanteric bursitis and hamstring strain.

Running can place a strain on the middle gluteal muscles and the iliotibial band. When the athlete is in the stand phase, the middle gluteal muscle contracts to stabilize the pelvis. A leg-length discrepancy places additional stress on the hip that may cause the middle gluteal muscle to irritate the trochanteric bursa. The iliotibial band crossing the trochanter of the femur also can cause bursal irritation. (See Chapter 20.)

The hamstring muscles can be irritated by running. After contraction of the quadriceps muscles at heel strike, the hamstring muscle contracts. If there is a significant difference in the strength between the quadriceps muscle and the hamstring muscle or if the athlete overstrides, forcing the hamstring to repeatedly contract from an extreme length, injury may occur. (See Chapter 20.)

Other injuries arising from the repetitive running motion are adductor groin strains and inflammation of the pubis symphysis (osteitis pubis). A foot strike that is too wide from the centerline or a pelvis that abducts excessively can lead to chronic adductor strain or osteitis pubis. (See Chapter 20.)

Running despite constant pain is foolish. Major problems such as stress or avulsion fractures may be present. Any continuous pain over a period of time should be referred for x-ray or bone scan examination.

Ankle and Lower Leg Rehabilitation Techniques

After the acute injury phase when the athlete moves into the phase of repair specific exercise rehabilitation begins. Because of the anatomical and biomechanical nature of the ankle and lower leg, there are many exercises that affect them equally. Many sports physicians and athletic trainers maintain that the best exercise method is the moderately active approach.

General Body Conditioning

The well-conditioned athlete, when unable to effectively bear weight because of injury, will rapidly discondition. This is particularly true of the cardiovascular system.

Stationary bicycles provide an excellent approach to maintaining cardiovascular fitness. Workouts can include slow long-distance training, sprinting, or *interval training*.[16] An athlete unable to use a stationary bicycle may opt for the upper body ergometer (UBE).

Pool exercise is another excellent means to maintain the cardiovascular system. It can be employed using swimming strokes or running in the pool. By using a flotation device the athlete can be kept above the waterline and simulate running patterns.[16]

Athletes with ankle or lower leg injuries must also work to maintain their strength and flexibility. A daily 50% of maximum resistance program will maintain a good percentage of the athlete's strength. A daily stretching program must also take place.

Mobilization

Techniques of mobilization are used to increase the accessory motions of the ankle (Figures 18-29 through 18-31).

18-10

Critical Thinking Exercise

A beginning, poorly conditioned recreational runner with a pes cavus, after 3 weeks of running, experiences pain and discomfort in the lower third of his left lower leg. The pain and discomfort become more intense immediately after running.

? An x-ray shows the beginning of a stress fracture. How should it be managed?

A running foot-strike that is too wide can lead to chronic adductor strain or osteitis pubis.

Medial Tibial Stress Syndrome (Shinsplints)

Injury Situation A female college field hockey player at the end of the competitive season began to feel severe discomfort in the medial aspect of the right shin.

Symptoms and Signs The athlete complained that her shin seemed to ache all the time but became more intense after practice or a game. During palpation there was severe point tenderness approximately 2 inches (5 cm) in length, beginning 4½ inches (11.25 cm) from the tip of the medial malleolus. The pain was most severe along the medial posterior edge of the tibia. Further evaluation showed that the athlete had pronated feet. X-ray examination showed no indication of stress fracture.

Management Plan The injury was considered to be a medial stress syndrome (shinsplints) involving the long flexor muscle, the great toe, and the posterior tibial muscle.

Phase 1 Acute Injury   **GOALS:** To reduce inflammation, pain, and point tenderness.
    ESTIMATED LENGTH OF TIME (ELT): 1-2 weeks.

■ **Therapy** Initially RICE, NSAIDs, and analgesics are given as needed. The athlete is instructed to rest and avoid weight bearing as much as possible. Ice massage (7 minutes) is performed followed by gentle static stretching to the anterior and posterior muscles 2 to 3 times daily. A LowDye taping or orthotic device is applied to the arch to correct pronation during weight bearing.

■ **Exercise rehabilitation** Static stretch of Achilles tendon and anterior part of low leg; hold stretch 30 seconds (two or three times); repeat set three or four times daily (see Figure 17-9). General body maintenance exercises are conducted if they do not aggravate injury, three times weekly.

Phase 2 Repair   **GOALS:** To heal injury, become symptom free, returning to walking, jogging, and finally running.
    ELT: 2-3 weeks.

■ **Therapy** Cold application (5 to 15 minutes) to shin area before and after walking one time daily. Activity is stopped if there is shin pain. Ultrasound (0.5 to 0.075 W/cm^2) (5 to 10 minutes) one to two times daily. Transverse friction massage is given to prevent adhesions. The athlete wears LowDye taping or orthoses when weight bearing. A counterforce bracing with tape is also worn 2 to 4 inches proximal to the malleoli.

■ **Exercise rehabilitation** Ankle range-of-motion exercises plus PRE with rubber tubing to the anterior and posterior leg muscles. Static stretch of lower leg followed by arch and plantar flexion exercises. Towel gather (10 repetitions, one to three sets); progress from no resistance to 10 lb of resistance, three times daily. Towel scoop (10 repetitions, one to three sets); progress to 10 lb, three times daily. Marble pickup, three times daily. General body maintenance exercises are conducted if they do not aggravate injury, three times weekly. Engage in a program of progressive weight bearing and locomotion within pain-free limits starting with slow heel-toe walking, fast walking, jogging, and finally running. As pain decreases activity can increase.

Phase 3 Remodeling   **GOALS:** Return to full-field hockey activity.
    ELT: 3-6 weeks.

■ **Therapy** The athlete carries out cryokinetics before and after practice. The athlete continues to wear counterforce brace and LowDye taping or orthoses for foot pronation.

Continued

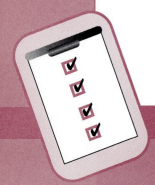

Medial Tibial Stress Syndrome (Shinsplints)—*cont'd*

■ **Exercise rehabilitation** The athlete continues a daily program of lower leg static stretch after ice application before and after activity. The athlete carries out a program of ankle range-of-motion exercises and lower leg PRE 3 days a week.

Criteria for Returning to Competitive Field Hockey

1. Leg is symptom free after prolonged activity.
2. The lower leg and ankle have full strength and range of motion.
3. Hyperpronation is controlled to prevent reoccurrence.

Flexibility

As pain allows, gentle and passive stretching is begun followed by a program of active stretching (Figures 18-32 and 18-33).

Strength

Strength training should include the complete kinetic chain—foot, ankle, and lower leg. Initially, when the injury should be immobilized, isometrics resistance should be performed against plantar flexion, dorsiflexion, inversion, and eversion. Strengthening exercises are performed two to three times daily, progressing from one to three sets of 10 repetitions. Exercise gradually progresses from submaximal resistance to maximum resistance several times per week. Early rehabilitation is performed pain free.

- Gripping and spreading toes—10 repetitions.
- Ankle circumduction—10 circles in one direction and 10 circles in the other.
- Flatfooted Achilles tendon stretching—with the foot flat on the floor, the Achilles tendon is stretched, first with the foot straight ahead, then adducted, and finally abducted. Each stretch is maintained for 20 to 30 seconds and repeated two or three times.

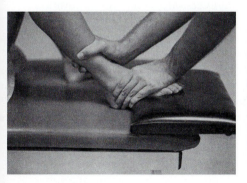

Figure 18-29

Posterior tibial glide for increasing plantar flexion.

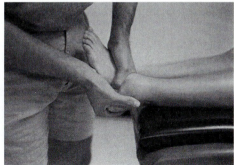

Figure 18-30

Posterior talar glide for increasing dorsiflexion.

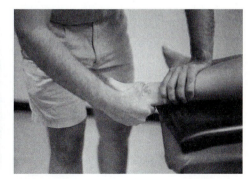

Figure 18-31

Subtalar joint medial/lateral glide (for increasing inversion and eversion).

Figure 18-32

Incline boards can effectively stretch a constricted Achilles tendon.

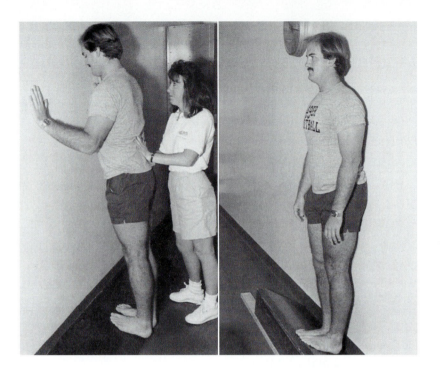

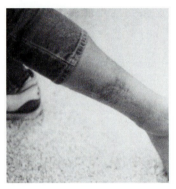

Figure 18-33

Toe stretch for dorsiflexion.

- Toe raises—standing flat on the floor, the athlete rises onto the toes as far as possible, with the toes pointed straight ahead, pointed in, and finally pointed out, for two or three sets of 10 repetitions each.
- Walking on toes and heels—the athlete walks 10 paces forward on toes and 10 paces backward on heels. Repeated two or three times.

Isotonic Resistance Strengthening

Manual resistance   Manual resistance can be applied by the athletic trainer. The exercise is performed in a complete range of motion and in all four ankle movements. Proprioceptive neuromuscular function patterns may be used in place of straight patterns. Exercise is performed until fatigue or pain is felt. (See Figure 19-57.)

Resistance with theraband   Exercise anterior, lateral, and medial leg muscles against a resistance such as surgical tubing or an inner tube strip. The tubing is attached around a stationary table or chair leg. The athlete places the tubing around the foot and pulls the forefoot into dorsiflexion and eversion, then reverses position and exercises the foot in plantar flexion inversion; 10 repetitions, three or four times (Figure 18-34).

Ankle weights and other devices   Ankle weights are excellent devices for ankle rehabilitation (Figure 18-35). An example of heavier resistance is the use of the Elgin machine (Figure 18-36).

Neuromuscular control   Any injury to the ankle or lower leg can disrupt normal proprioception. A variety of both balance and strengthening can be gained by use of the BAP board. (See Figure 15-4, *A*).

Protective Bracing and Orthoses

The athlete may wear protective bracing or an orthotic device throughout the rehabilitation process. An ankle brace may be considered superior to taping. A common ankle brace is the air cast ankle stirrup. (See Figure 5-24.) Orthotics are usually worn to control hyperpronation.

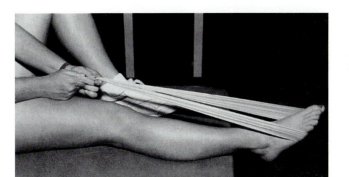

Figure 18-34

Thera band resistance material affords an excellent means to begin an ankle and lower-leg resistance program.

Functional Progressions

A major part of the rehabilitation process is to return to specific requirements of a given sport. The skills required in a sport are broken down into individual subskills. An example might be as follows:

- Heel-toe walking, jogging, and then on-toe running. Distances are gradually increased.
- Backward walking or pedaling.
- Zigzag running.
- Pain-free hopping on affected leg.
- Rope jumping 5 to 10 minutes daily.

Return to Activity

Before returning to a sport the athlete must be pain free. Complete range of motion must exist. The athlete must have at least 80% to 90% of his or her preinjury strength and display the agility required for the sport.[10]

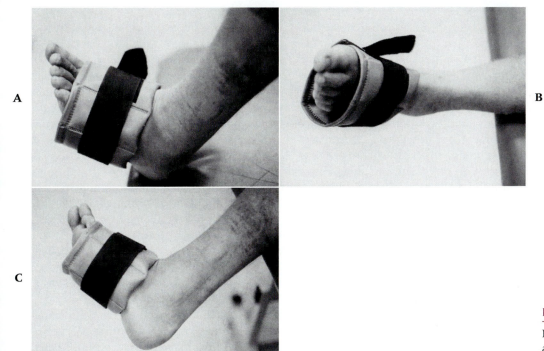

A

B

C

Figure 18-35

Isotonic strengthening using ankle weights. **A,** Dorsiflexion. **B,** Inversion. **C,** Eversion.

Figure 18-36

For heavier ankle and lower-leg resistance training, the Elgin machine is beneficial.

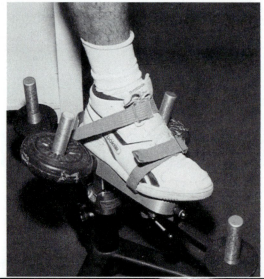

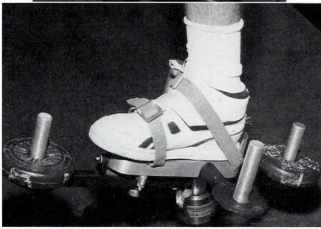

SUMMARY

- The ankle has a high incidence of injury in sports activities. Although it has a relatively strong bony arrangement in terms of its supportive soft tissue, it is very weak laterally. Despite its susceptibility to injuries, preventive procedures can be taken. Many injuries can be prevented through stretching of the Achilles tendon, strength training, wearing proper footwear, and the application of appropriate taping or wrapping.

- First-, second-, and third-degree sprains must be managed by RICE during immediate care. Compression is achieved through application of a doughnut and an elastic wrap. In the early stages, weight bearing should be eliminated or reduced through the use of crutches. A variety of therapeutic modalities, as well as exercise, are used in follow-up management.

- The same mechanisms that strain an Achilles tendon can also cause rupture. The Thompson test is standard for determining a suspected Achilles tendon rupture. Repeated minor Achilles tendon tears can cause tissue degeneration and a subsequent rupture.

- The lower leg is subject to contusion, muscle strains, and fractures. An acute compartment syndrome could lead to serious muscle weakness and paresthesia.

- Chronic ankle conditions include Achilles tendinitis and Achilles tendon bursitis. Peroneal tendon subluxation and tendinitis of the anterior tibial, posterior tibial, and peroneal tendons are relatively common among athletes.

■ Overuse leg problems are common among athletes who engage in repetitive activities over a long period of time. Examples of these conditions are medial tibial syndrome (shinsplints), exercise-induced compartment compression syndromes, and various stress fractures of the lower leg. When there are discrepancies in body weight transmission, overuse problems can also occur in other regions of the body, such as the knee, thigh, and hip. Exercise is an important approach for the rehabilitation of the ankle and the lower leg.

....

Solutions to Critical Thinking EXERCISES

18-1 The athletic trainer takes a multifaceted approach to reducing ankle sprains. The Achilles tendon is stretched to allow at least 15 degrees of dorsiflexion. Strength training is carried out to the peroneals, plantar flexors, and dorsal flexors. Proprioceptive training is carried out using a balance board. The athlete wears high-top shoes. Ankle taping with an orthosis can also be employed.

18-2 The athlete continues to wear a stirrup brace for 1 to 3 weeks longer. Taping at 90 degrees will be conducted for 2 to 4 weeks. The athlete engages in pain-free plantar flexion and dorsiflexion exercises. The athlete also engages in proprioceptive exercises on a balance board.

18-3 The mechanism describes a syndesmotic ankle sprain. The athlete experiences severe pain in the anterolateral leg region when the ankle is externally rotated.

18-4 This is a possible partial or complete rupture of the Achilles tendon. There was pain that then subsided. There is an inability to perform a toe raise. Point tenderness, swelling, and discoloration become apparent. There is an obvious indentation at the tendon site along with a positive Thompson test.

18-5 Compression with a horseshoe-shaped felt pad is used surrounding the lateral malleolus. This pad is reinforced by a rigid splint. RICE, NSAIDs, and analgesics are given as needed. An exercise program is employed to strengthen, stretch, and enhance balance training.

18-6 The athlete is instructed to rest or reduce the stress of running. Application of ice packs followed by stretching is carried out before and after activity. A strengthening program is carried out along with treatment by oral antiinflammatory medications as needed.

18-7 The athlete has sustained a lower leg fracture. The most common site is in the middle third of the fibula.

18-8 In gymnastics athletes often run on hard surfaces wearing shoes with little cushioning. This, combined with overtraining and fatigue, could lead to MTSS. Other reasons are a varus or pronated hypermobile foot.

18-9 The conservative approach is the application of RICE and NSAIDs and rest. With weakness in toe extension and numbness in the dorsal region surgery may be warranted.

18-10 The runner should avoid stressful locomotor activities for at least 14 days. Bicycling and swimming can be engaged in if pain free. Running can be resumed when there is a pain-free period of 2 weeks.

REVIEW QUESTIONS AND CLASS ACTIVITIES

1. Identify and describe the anatomy of the ankle and lower leg.
2. Demonstrate the steps that should be taken when assessing ankle injuries.
3. How can ankle injuries be prevented?
4. Describe how ankle sprains occur. Describe first-, second-, and third-degree ankle sprains.
5. Contrast the management of first-, second-, and third-degree ankle sprains.
6. How can the anterior or posterior tibiofibular ligament be torn?
7. What major overuse tendon problems are associated with the ankle?
8. Describe acute sports injuries to the Achilles tendon. Indicate their etiology and symptoms and signs.
9. Describe the anatomy of the lower leg.
10. How should the lower leg be assessed for possible injuries? What steps should be taken when assessing the lower leg for injuries?
11. Acute injuries to the lower leg are usually contusions or muscle strains. Discuss their etiology, symptoms and signs, and management.
12. Contrast an acute anterior compartment syndrome with the chronic type.
13. How can leg fractures occur?
14. Describe chronic exertional problems that can occur to the lower leg.
15. How may chronic problems of the foot, ankle, or lower leg can be transmitted to the knee, thigh, and hip?
16. Describe the steps that must be taken during exercise rehabilitation of the ankle and the lower leg.

REFERENCES

1. Anderson DL: Surgical management of chronic Achilles tendinitis, *Clin J Sports Med* 2(1):38, 1992.
2. Birrer RB: Ankle injuries. In Birrer RB, editor: *Sports medicine for the primary care physician*, ed 2, St Louis, 1995, Mosby.
3. Booher JM, Thibodeau GA: *Athletic injury assessment*, ed 3, St Louis, 1994, Mosby.
4. Brosky T et al: The ankle ligaments: considerations of syndesmotic injury and implications for rehabilitation, *J Orthop Sports Phys Ther* 21(1):197, 1995.
5. Brown DE: Exertional leg pain. In Brown DE, Neuman RD, editors: *Orthopedic secrets*, Philadelphia, 1995, Hanley & Belfus.
6. Case WS: Recovering from ankle sprains, *Phys Sportsmed* 21(11):43, 1993.

7. Fischer DA: Syndesmotic ankle sprain. In Torg JS, Shephard RJ, editors: *Current therapy in sports medicine,* ed 3, St Louis, 1995, Mosby.

8. Giladi M et al: Stress fractures, *Am J Sports Med* 19(6):647, 1991.

9. Hacut JE: General types of injuries. In Birrer RB, editor: *Sports medicine for the primary care physician,* Boca Raton, Fla, 1994, CRC Press.

10. Hunter S: Rehabilitation of ankle injuries. In Prentice WE, editor: *Rehabilitation techniques in sports medicine,* ed 2, St Louis, 1994, Mosby.

11. Jepson KK: The use of orthoses for athletes. In Birrer RB, editor: *Sports medicine for the primary care physician,* ed 2, Boca Raton, Fla, 1994, CRC Press.

12. Levandowski R, Di Frori JP: Leg injuries. In Birrer RB, editor: *Sports medicine for the primary care physician,* ed 2, Boca Raton, Fla, 1994, CRC Press.

13. McMullen ST: Foot and ankle trauma. In Brown DE, Neumann RD, editors: *Orthopedic secrets,* Philadelphia, 1995, Hanley & Belfus.

14. McPoil Jr TG, Brocoto RS: The foot and ankle: biomechanical evaluation and treatment. In Gould III JA, editor: *Orthopaedic and sports physical therapy,* ed 2, St Louis, 1990, Mosby.

15. Mehlman CT: Ankle fractures: common mechanisms, classifications, complications, *Ath Train* 23(2):110, 1988.

16. Riehl R: Rehabilitation of lower leg injuries. In Prentice WE, editor: *Rehabilitation techniques in sports medicine,* St Louis, 1994, Mosby.

17. Sammarco GJ: Injuries to the tibialis anterior, peroneal tendons, and long flexors and extensions of the toes. In Baxter DE, editor: *The foot and ankle in sport,* St Louis, 1995, Mosby.

18. Scotece SG, Guthrie MR: Comparison of three treatment approaches for grade I and II ankle sprains in active-duty soldiers, *J Orthop Sports Phys Ther* 15(1):819, 1992.

19. Stanish WD: Lower leg, foot, and ankle injuries in young athletes. In Micheli LJ, editor: *The young athlete. Clinics in sports medicine,* vol 14, no 3, Philadelphia, 1995, Saunders.

20. Surve I et al: A fivefold reduction in the incidence of recurrent ankle sprains in soccer players using the sport-stirrup orthosis, *Am J Sports Med* 22(5):601, 1994.

21. Taube RR, Wadsworth LT: Managing tibial stress fractures, *Phys Sports Med* 21(4):123, 1993.

22. Vegso JJ: Ankle sprain: nonoperative management injuries to lower extremity. In Torg JS, Shephard RJ, editors: *Current therapy in sports medicine,* ed 3, St Louis, 1995, Mosby.

23. Wilkerson GB: Treatment of the inversion ankle sprain through synchronous application of focal compression and cold, *Ath Train* 26(3):220, 1991.

24. Zecher SB, Leach RE: Lower leg and foot injuries in tennis and other racquet sports. In Lehman RC, editor: *Racquet sports. Clinic in sports medicine,* vol 14, no 1, Philadelphia, 1995, Saunders.

ANNOTATED BIBLIOGRAPHY

Brown DE, Neumann RD, editors: *Orthopedic secrets,* Philadelphia, 1995, Hanley & Belfus.

Presents an overview of orthopedics in a question-and-answer format. The ankle and lower leg are well presented.

Kwong PK, editor: *Foot and ankle injuries. Clinics in sports medicine,* vol 13, no 4, Philadelphia, 1994, Saunders.

An up-to-date monograph for the practioner on assessing and managing foot and ankle injuries.

The Knee and Related Structures

When you finish this chapter, you should be able to

- Describe the normal structural and functional knee anatomy and relate it to major sports injuries.
- Assess the knee and related structures after injury.
- Establish a knee injury prevention program.
- Discuss etiological factors, symptoms and signs, and management procedures for the major knee joint conditions and related structures.
- Discuss considerations for rehabilitation of the injured knee.

Muscles and ligaments provide the main source of stability in the knee.

The knee is one of the most complex joints in the human body. Because so many sports place extreme stress on the knee, it is also one of the most traumatized joints. The knee is commonly considered a hinge joint because its two principal movements are flexion and extension. However, because rotation of the tibia is an essential component of knee movement, the knee is not a true hinge joint. The stability of the knee joint depends primarily on the ligaments, the joint capsule, and muscles that surround the joint (Figure 19-1). The knee is designed primarily to provide stability in weight bearing and mobility in locomotion; however, it is especially unstable laterally and medially (Figure 19-2).

Figure 19-1

The bony and ligamentous arrangement of the knee.

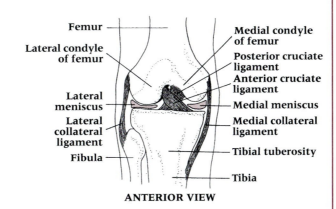

Femur
Lateral condyle of femur
Lateral meniscus
Lateral collateral ligament
Fibula

Medial condyle of femur
Posterior cruciate ligament
Anterior cruciate ligament
Medial meniscus
Medial collateral ligament
Tibial tuberosity
Tibia

ANTERIOR VIEW

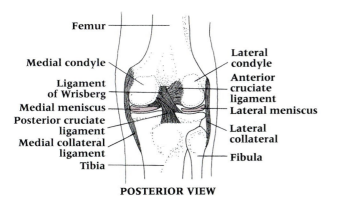

Femur
Medial condyle
Ligament of Wrisberg
Medial meniscus
Posterior cruciate ligament
Medial collateral ligament
Tibia

Lateral condyle
Anterior cruciate ligament
Lateral meniscus
Lateral collateral
Fibula

POSTERIOR VIEW

Figure 19-2

The knee is a highly complicated joint that is often traumatized during competitive sports.

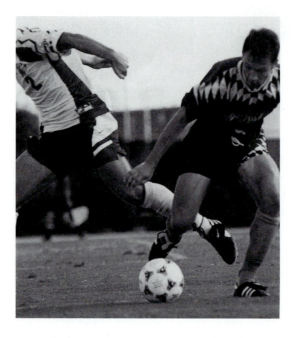

ANATOMY
Bones

The knee joint complex consists of the femur, the tibia, the fibula, and the patella. The distal end of the femur expands and forms the convex lateral and medial condyles, which are designed to articulate with the tibia and the patella. The articular surface of the medial condyle is longer from front to back than is the surface of the lateral condyle. Anteriorly, the two condyles form a hollowed groove to receive the patella. The proximal end of the tibia, the tibial plateau, articulates with the condyles of the femur. On this flat tibial plateau are two shallow concavities that articulate with their respective femoral condyles and are divided by the popliteal notch. Separating these concavities, or articular facets, is a roughened area where the cruciate ligaments attach and from which a process commonly known as the tibial spine arises.

Patella

The patella is the largest sesamoid bone in the human body. It is located in the tendon of the quadriceps femoris muscle and is divided into three medial facets and a lateral facet that articulate with the femur (Figure 19-3). The lateral aspect of the patella is wider than the medial aspect. The patella articulates between the concavity provided by the femoral condyles. Tracking within this groove depends on the pull of the quadriceps muscle, patellar tendon, depth of the femoral condyles, and shape of the patella.

Articulations

The knee joint complex consists of several articulations between the femur and the tibia, the femur and the patella, the femur and the fibula, and the tibia and fibula.

Menisci

The menisci (Figure 19-4) are two oval (semilunar) fibrocartilages that deepen the articular facets of the tibia and cushion any stresses placed on the knee joint. The consistency of the menisci is much like that of the intervertebral disks. They are located medially and laterally on the tibial tuberosity. The menisci transmit one half of the contact force in the medial compartment and an even higher percentage of the

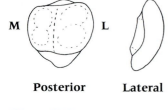

M [L

Posterior   Lateral

Figure 19-3

Patella.

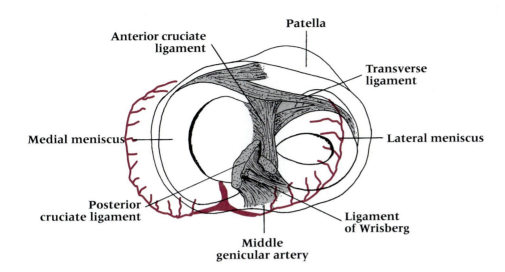

Figure 19-4

Menisci of the knee.

contact load in the lateral compartment. The menisci help stabilize the knee, especially the medial meniscus, when the knee is flexed at 90 degrees.

Medial meniscus   The medial meniscus is a C-shaped fibrocartilage, the circumference of which is attached firmly to the medial articular facet of the tibia and to the joint capsule by the coronary ligaments. Posteriorly, it is also attached to fibers of the semimembranous muscle.

Lateral meniscus   The lateral meniscus is more O-shaped and is attached to the lateral articular facet on the superior aspect of the tibia. The lateral meniscus also attaches loosely to the lateral articular capsule and to the popliteal tendon. The ligament of Wrisberg is the part of the lateral meniscus that projects upward, close to the attachment of the posterior or cruciate ligament. The transverse ligament joins the anterior portions of the lateral and medial menisci.

Meniscal blood supply   Blood is supplied to each meniscus by the medial genicular artery. Each meniscus can be divided into three circumferential zones: the red-red zone is the outer or peripheral one third and has a good vascular supply; the red-white zone is the middle one third and has minimal blood supply; and the white-white zone on the inner one third is **avascular** (Figure 19-5).

Generally the meniscus has a poor blood supply.

avascular
Devoid of blood circulation.

Stabilizing Ligaments

The major stabilizing ligaments of the knee include the cruciate ligaments, the collateral ligaments, and the capsular ligaments (see Figure 19-1).

The Cruciate Ligaments

The cruciate ligaments account for a considerable amount of knee stability. They are two ligamentous bands that cross one another within the joint cavity of the knee. The anterior cruciate ligament (ACL) attaches below and in front of the tibia; then, passing backward, it attaches laterally to the inner surface of the lateral condyle. The

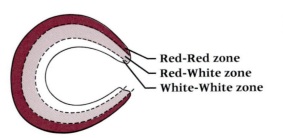

Red-Red zone
Red-White zone
White-White zone

Figure 19-5

The meniscus has three vascular zones.

posterior cruciate ligament (PCL), the stronger of the two and the primary stabilizer of the knee, crosses from the back of the tibia in an upward, forward, and medial direction and attaches to the anterior portion of the lateral surface of the medial condyle of the femur.

The anterior cruciate ligament   The anterior cruciate ligament comprises three twisted bands: the anteromedial, intermediate, and posterolateral bands. In general, the anterior cruciate ligament prevents the femur from moving posteriorly during weight bearing. It also stabilizes the tibia against excessive internal rotation and serves as a secondary restraint for valgus or varus stress with collateral ligament damage.

When the knee is fully extended, the posterolateral section of the cruciate ligament is tight. In flexion the posterolateral fibers loosen and the anteromedial fibers tighten.[42] The anterior cruciate ligament works in conjunction with the thigh muscles, especially the hamstring muscle group, to stabilize the knee joint.

The posterior cruciate ligament   Some portion of the posterior cruciate ligament is taut throughout the full range of motion. It acts as a drag during the gliding phase of motion and resists internal rotation of the tibia. In general, the posterior cruciate ligament prevents hyperextension of the knee and femur, sliding forward during weight bearing.

Capsular and Collateral Ligaments

Additional stabilization of the knee is provided by the capsular and collateral ligaments. Besides stability, they also direct movement in a correct path. Although they move in synchrony, they are divided into the medial and lateral complexes.

Medial collateral ligament   The superficial position of the medial (tibial) collateral ligament (MCL) is separate from the deeper capsular ligament at the joint line. It attaches above the joint line on the medial epicondyle of the femur and below on the tibia, just beneath the attachment of the pes anserinus. The posterior aspect of the ligament blends into the deep posterior capsular ligament and semimembranous muscle. Fibers of the semimembranous muscle go through the capsule and attach to the posterior aspect of the medial meniscus, pulling it backward during knee flexion. Some of its fibers are taut through flexion and extension. Its major purpose is to prevent the knee from valgus and external rotating forces. The medial collateral ligament was thought to be the principal stabilizer of the knee in a valgus position when combined with rotation. It is now known that other structures, such as the anterior cruciate ligament, play an equal or greater part in this function.[21]

Deep medial capsular ligaments   The deep medial capsular ligament is divided into three parts: the anterior, medial, and posterior capsular ligaments. The anterior capsular ligament connects with the extensor mechanism and the medial meniscus through the coronary ligaments. It relaxes during knee extension and tightens during knee flexion. The primary purposes of the medial capsular ligaments are to attach the medial meniscus to the femur and to allow the tibia to move on the meniscus inferiorly. The posterior capsular ligament is sometimes called the posterior oblique ligament and attaches to the posterior medial aspect of the meniscus and intersperses with the semimembranous muscle.[4]

Lateral collateral ligament and related structures   The lateral (fibular) collateral ligament (LCL) is a round, fibrous cord shaped like a pencil. It is attached to the lateral epicondyle of the femur and to the head of the fibula. The lateral collateral ligament is taut during knee extension but relaxed during flexion.

Another stabilizing ligament of importance is the arcuate ligament. It is formed by a thickening of the posterior articular capsule. Its posterior aspect attaches to the fascia of the popliteal muscle and the posterior horn of the lateral meniscus.

Other structures that stabilize the knee laterally are the iliotibial band, popliteus muscle, and biceps femoris of the quadriceps. The iliotibial band, a tendon of the tensor fascia latae and gluteus medius, attaches to the lateral epicondyle of the femur and lateral tibial tubercle (Gerdy's tubercle). It becomes tense during both extension and flexion. The popliteus muscle stabilizes the knee during flexion and, when contracting, protects the lateral meniscus by pulling it posteriorly.

The biceps femoris muscle also stabilizes the knee laterally by inserting into the fibular head, iliotibial band, and capsule.

Joint Capsule

The articular surfaces of the knee joint are completely enveloped by the largest joint capsule in the body. Anteriorly, the joint capsule extends upward underneath the patella to form the suprapatellar pouch. The inferior portion contains the infrapatellar fat pad and the infrapatellar bursa. Medially, a thickened section of the capsule forms the deep portion of the medial collateral ligament. Posteriorly, the capsule forms two pouches that cover the femoral condyles and the tibial plateau. The capsule thickens medially to form the posterior oblique ligament and laterally to form the arcuate ligament.

The joint capsule is divided into four regions: the posterolateral, posteromedial, anterolateral, and anteromedial. Each of these four "corners" of the capsule is reinforced by other anatomical structures. The posterolateral corner is reinforced by the iliotibial band, the popliteus, the biceps femoris, the LCL, and the arcuate ligament. The MCL, the pes anserinus tendons, the semimembranosus, and the posterior oblique ligament reinforce the posteromedial corner. The anterolateral corner is reinforced by the iliotibial band, the patellar tendon, and the lateral patellar retinaculum. The superficial MCL and the medial patellar retinaculum reinforce the anteromedial corner.

Synovial membrane lines the inner surface of the joint capsule, except posteriorly where it passes in front of the cruciates making them extrasynovial (Figure 19-6).

Knee Musculature

For the knee to function properly, a number of muscles must work together in a highly complex fashion. The following is a list of knee actions and the muscles that initiate them (Figure 19-7):

- Knee flexion is executed by the biceps femoris, semitendinous, semimembranous, gracilis, sartorius, gastrocnemius and popliteus, and plantaris muscles.
- Knee extension is executed by the quadriceps muscle of the thigh, consisting of three vasti—the vastus medialis, vastus lateralis, and vastus intermedius—and by the rectus femoris.
- External rotation of the tibia is controlled by the biceps femoris. The bony anatomy also produces external tibial rotation as the knee moves into extension.
- Internal rotation is accomplished by the popliteal, semitendinous, semimembranous, sartorius, and gracilis muscles. Rotation of the tibia is limited and can occur only when the knee is in a flexed position.
- The iliotibial band on the lateral side primarily functions as a dynamic lateral stabilizer.

Bursa

A bursa is a flattened sac or enclosed cleft composed of synovial tissue that is separated by a thin film of fluid. The function of a bursa is to reduce the friction between anatomical structures. Bursae are found between muscle and bone, tendon and bone, tendon and ligament, and so forth. As many as two dozen bursa have been identified around the knee joint. The suprapatellar, prepatellar, infrapatellar, pretibial, and gastrocnemius bursae are perhaps the most commonly injured about the knee joint (Figure 19-8).

Fat Pads

There are several fat pads around the knee. The infrapatellar fat pad is the largest. It serves as a cushion to the front of the knee and separates the patellar tendon from

19-1

Critical Thinking Exercise

A tennis player injures her knee during a match. She is hitting a forehand stroke with her knee in full extension and feels pain in her knee as she rotates on the follow-through. She feels some diffuse pain around her knee joint and is concerned that she has sprained a ligament.

? In a position of full extension, which of the supporting ligaments are taut? Which ligaments are most likely to be injured in this position?

Major actions of the knee:
  Flexion
  Extension
  Gliding
  Rotation

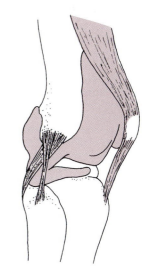

Figure 19-6

Synovial membrane of the knee.

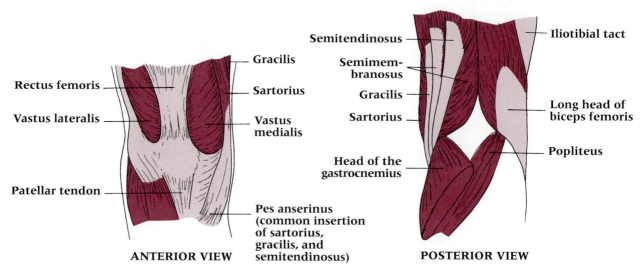

Rectus femoris

Vastus lateralis

Patellar tendon

Gracilis

Sartorius

Vastus medialis

Pes anserinus (common insertion of sartorius, gracilis, and semitendinosus)

ANTERIOR VIEW

Semitendinosus

Semimem-branosus

Gracilis

Sartorius

Head of the gastrocnemius

Iliotibial tact

Long head of biceps femoris

Popliteus

POSTERIOR VIEW

Figure 19-7

Musculature of the knee.

the joint capsule. Other major fat pads in the knee include the anterior and posterior suprapatellar and the popliteal. Some fat pads occupy space within the synovial capsule.

Nerve Supply

The tibial nerve supplies most of the hamstrings and the gastrocnemius. The common peroneal nerve innervates the short head of the biceps femoris and then courses through the popliteal fossa and wraps around the proximal head of the fibula. The femoral nerve innervates the quadriceps and the sartorius muscles (Figure 19-9).

Blood Supply

The main blood supply of the knee consists of the popliteal artery, which stems from the femoral artery. From the popliteal artery, five branches supply the knee: the medial and lateral superior genicular, middle genicular, and medial and lateral inferior genicular arteries (see Figure 19-9).

FUNCTIONAL ANATOMY

Movement between the tibia and the femur involves the physiological motions of flexion, extension, and rotation, as well as arthrokinematic motions, including roll-

Figure 19-8

Common bursae of the knee.

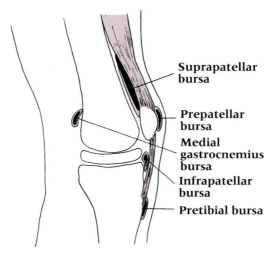

Suprapatellar bursa

Prepatellar bursa

Medial gastrocnemius bursa

Infrapatellar bursa

Pretibial bursa

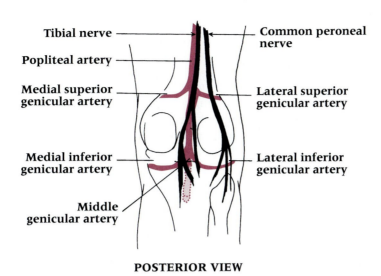

Figure 19-9

Blood and nerve supply to the knee.

Tibial nerve

Popliteal artery

Medial superior
genicular artery

Medial inferior
genicular artery

Middle
genicular artery

Common peroneal
nerve

Lateral superior
genicular artery

Lateral inferior
genicular artery

POSTERIOR VIEW

ing and gliding. As the tibia extends on the femur the tibia glides and rolls anteriorly. If the femur is extending on the tibia, gliding occurs in an anterior direction, whereas rolling occurs posteriorly.

Axial rotation of the tibia relative to the femur is an important component of knee motion. In the "screw home" mechanism of the knee, as the knee extends the tibia externally rotates. Rotation occurs because the medial femoral condyle is larger than the lateral condyle. Thus, when weight bearing, the tibia must rotate externally to achieve full extension. The rotational component gives a great deal of stability to the knee in full extension. When weight bearing, the popliteus muscle must contract and externally rotate the femur to "unlock" the knee so that flexion can occur.

The capsular ligaments are taut during full extension and to some extent relaxed during flexion. This is particularly true of the lateral collateral ligament; however, portions of the medial collateral ligament relax as flexion occurs. Relaxation of the more superficial collateral ligaments allows rotation to occur. In contrast, the deeper capsular ligament tightens to prevent excessive rotation of the tibia.

During extension there is external rotation of the tibia, during the last 15 degrees of which the anterior cruciate ligament unwinds.[34] In full extension the anterior cruciate ligament is taut, and it loosens during flexion. As the femur glides on the tibia, the posterior cruciate ligament becomes taut and prevents further gliding. In general, the anterior cruciate ligament stops excessive internal rotation, stabilizes the knee in full extension, and prevents hyperextension. The posterior cruciate ligament prevents excessive internal rotation, guides the knee in flexion, and acts as a drag during the initial glide phase of flexion.

In complete flexion, approximately 140 degrees, the range of the knee movement is limited by the extremely shortened position of the hamstring muscles, the extensibility of the quadriceps muscles, and the bulk of the hamstring muscles. In this position the femoral condyles rest on their corresponding menisci at a point that permits a small degree of inward rotation.

The patella aids the knee during extension by lengthening the lever arm of the quadriceps muscle. It distributes the compressive stresses on the femur by increasing the contact area between the patellar tendon and the femur.[42] It also protects the patellar tendon against friction. During full extension the patella lies slightly lateral and proximal to the trochlea. At 20 degrees of knee flexion there is tibial rotation, and the patella moves into the trochlea. At 30 degrees the patella is most prominent. At 30 degrees and more the patella moves deeper into the trochlea. At 90 degrees the patella again becomes positioned laterally. When knee flexion is 135 degrees, the patella has moved laterally beyond the trochlea.[42]

Kinetic Chain

As discussed in Chapter 15, the knee is part of the kinetic chain. It is directly affected by motions and forces occurring and being transmitted from the foot, ankle, and lower leg. In turn, the knee must transmit forces to the thigh, hip, pelvis, and spine. Abnormal forces that cannot be distributed must be absorbed by the tissues. When the foot is in contact with the ground, a closed kinetic chain exists. In a closed kinetic chain, forces must either be transmitted to proximal segments or be absorbed in a more distal joint. The inability of this closed system to dissipate these forces typically leads to a breakdown in some part of the system. As part of the kinetic chain, the knee joint is susceptible to injury resulting from absortion of these forces.

ASSESSING THE KNEE JOINT

It is the responsibility of the team physician to diagnose the severity and exact nature of a knee injury. Although the physician is charged with the final evaluation, the coach or athletic trainer is usually the first person to observe the injury; therefore he or she is charged with initial evaluation and immediate care. The most important aspect of understanding what pathological process has taken place is to become familiar with the traumatic sequence and mechanisms of injury, either through having seen the injury occur or through learning its history (Figure 19-10). Often the team physician is not present when the injury occurs, and the athletic trainer must relate the pertinent information.[22]

History

To determine the history and major complaints involved in a knee injury, the following questions should be asked.

Current Injury

- What were you doing when the knee was hurt?
- What position was your body in?
- Did the knee collapse?
- Did you hear a noise or feel any sensation at the time of injury, such as a pop or crunch? (A pop could indicate an anterior cruciate tear, a crunch could be a sign of a torn meniscus, and a tearing sensation might indicate a capsular tear.)
- Could you move the knee immediately after the injury? If not, was it locked in a bent or extended position? (Locking could mean a meniscal tear.) After being locked, how did it become unlocked?

Figure 19-10

It is extremely important to understand the sequence and mechanism of the knee injury before the pathological process can be understood.

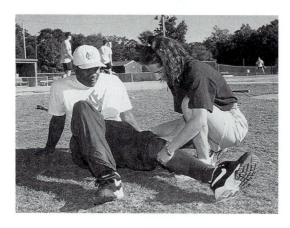

- Did swelling occur? If yes, was it immediate, or did it occur later? (Immediate swelling could indicate a cruciate or tibial fracture, whereas later swelling could indicate a capsular, synovial, or meniscal tear.)
- Where was the pain? Was it local, all over, or did it move from one side of the knee to the other?
- Have you hurt the knee before?

When first studying the injury, the athletic trainer or coach should observe whether the athlete is able to support body weight flatfootedly on the injured leg or whether it is necessary to stand and walk on the toes. Toe walking is an indication that the athlete is holding the knee in a splinted position to avoid pain or that the knee is being held in a flexed position by a wedge of dislocated meniscus. In first-time acute knee sprains, fluid and blood effusion is not usually apparent until after a 24-hour period. However, in an anterior cruciate ligament sprain a hemarthrosis may occur during the first hour after injury. Swelling and ecchymosis will occur unless the effusion is arrested through the use of compression, elevation, and cold packs.

Recurrent or Chronic Injury

- What is your major complaint?
- When did you first notice the condition?
- Is there recurrent swelling?
- Does the knee ever lock or catch? (If yes, it may be a torn meniscus or a loose body in the knee joint.)
- Is there severe pain? Is it constant, or does it come and go?
- Do you feel any grinding or grating sensations? (If yes, it could indicate chondromalacia or traumatic arthritis.)
- Does your knee ever feel like it is going to give way, or has it actually done so? (If yes and often, it may be a capsular, cruciate, or meniscal tear, a loose body, or a subluxating patella.)
- What does it feel like to go up and down stairs? (Pain may indicate a patellar irritation or meniscal tear.)
- What past treatment, if any, have you received for this condition?

Observation

A visual examination should be performed after the major complaints have been determined. The athlete should be observed in a number of situations: walking, half-squatting, and going up and down stairs. The leg also should be observed for alignment and symmetry or asymmetry.

If possible, the athlete with an injured knee should be observed in the following actions:
Walking
Half-squatting
Going up and down stairs

Walking

- Does the athlete walk with a limp, or is the walk free and easy? Is the athlete able to fully extend the knee during heel-strike?
- Can the athlete fully bear weight on the affected leg?
- Is the athlete able to perform a half-squat to extension?
- Can the athlete go up and down stairs with ease? (If stairs are unavailable, stepping up on a box or stool will suffice.)

Leg Alignment

The athlete should be observed for leg alignment. Anteriorly, the athlete is evaluated for genu valgus, genu varum, and the position of the patella. Next, the athlete is observed from the side to ascertain conditions such as the hyperflexed or hyperextended knee.

Deviations in normal leg alignment may or may not be a factor in knee injury but should always be considered as a possible cause. As with any other body segment, leg alignment differs from person to person; however, obvious discrepancies could predispose the athlete to an acute or chronic injury.

Anteriorly, with the knees extended as much as possible, the following points should be noted:

- Are the patellas level with each other?
- Are the patellas facing forward?
- Can the athlete touch the medial femoral condyles and medial malleoli?

Looking at the athlete's knees from the side:

- Are the knees fully extended with only slight hyperextension?
- Are both knees equally extended?

Leg alignment deviations that may predispose to injury   Four major leg deviations could adversely affect the knee and patellofemoral joints: patellar malalignment, genu valgum (knock-knees), genu varum (bowlegs), and genu recurvatum (hyperextended knees).

Patellar malalignment   Kneecaps that are rotated inward or outward from the center may be caused by a complex set of circumstances. For example, a combination of genu recurvatum, genu varum, and internal rotation, or anteversion, of the hip and internal rotation of the tibia could cause the patella to face inward. Internal rotation of the hip also may be associated with knock-knees, along with external rotation of the tibia, or tibial torsion. Athletes who toe-out when they walk may have an externally rotated hip, or retroversion. The normal angulation of the femoral neck after 8 years of age is 15 degrees; an increase of this angle is considered anteversion, and a decrease is considered retroversion. If an abnormal angulation seems to be a factor with the patella, malalignment or tibial torsion angles should be measured.

MEASURING FOR TIBIAL TORSION, FEMORAL ANTEVERSION, AND FEMORAL RETROVERSION   Tibial torsion is determined by having the athlete kneel on a stool with the foot relaxed. An imaginary line is drawn along the center of the thigh and lower leg, bisecting the middle of the heel and the bottom of the foot. Another line starts at the center of the middle toe and crosses the center of the heel. The angle formed by the two lines is measured (Figure 19-11); an angle measuring more or less than 15 degrees is a sign of tibial torsion.

Femoral anteversion or retroversion can be determined by the number of degrees the thigh rotates in each direction. As a rule, external rotation and internal rotation added together equal close to 100 degrees. If internal rotation exceeds 70 degrees, there may be anteversion of the hip.[53]

Hyperextension of the knee may result in internal rotation of the femur and external rotation of the tibia. Internal rotation at the hip is caused by weak external rotator muscles or foot pronation.

Genu valgum   The causes of genu valgum, or knock-knees, can be multiple. Normally, toddlers and very young children display knock-knees. When the legs have strengthened and the feet have become positioned more in line with the pelvis, the condition is usually corrected. Commonly associated with knock-knees are pronated feet. Genu valgum places chronic tension on the ligamentous structures of the medial part of the knee, abnormal compression of the lateral aspect of the knee surface, and abnormal tightness of the iliotibial band. One or both legs may be affected, along with a weakening of the hip's external rotator muscles.

Genu varum   The two types of genu varum, or bowlegs, are structural and functional. The structural type, which is seldom seen in athletes, reflects a deviation of the femur and tibia. The more common functional, or postural, type usually is associated with knees that are hyperextended and femurs that are internally rotated. Often when genu recurvatum is corrected, so is genu varum.

Genu recurvatum   Genu recurvatum, or hyperextended knees, commonly occurs as a compensation for lordosis, or swayback. There is notable weakness and stretching of the hamstring muscles. Chronic hyperextension can produce undue anterior pressure on the knee joint and posterior ligaments and tendons.

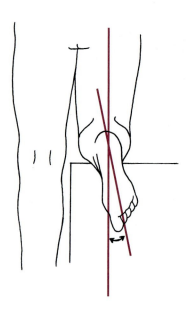

Figure 19-11

Measuring for tibial torsion.

Knee Symmetry or Asymmetry

The athletic trainer must establish whether both of the athlete's knees look the same:

- Do the knees appear symmetrical?
- Is one knee obviously swollen?
- Is muscle atrophy apparent?

Leg-Length Discrepancy

Discrepancies in leg length can occur as a result of many causes. Basically, the causes can be either anatomical or functional. True anatomical leg length can be measured from the anterior superior iliac spine (ASIS) to the lateral malleolus. Functional leg length can be measured from the umbilicus to the medial malleolus.

Anatomical differences in leg length can potentially cause problems in all weight-bearing joints. Functional differences can be caused by rotations of the pelvis or mal-alignments of the spine.

Palpation

Bony Palpation

The bony structures of the knee are palpated for pain and deformities that might indicate a fracture or dislocation. The athlete sits on the edge of the training table or a bench. With the athlete's knee flexed to 90 degrees, the athletic trainer palpates the following bony structures.

Medial Aspect

- Medial tibial plateau
- Medial femoral condyle
- Adductor tubercle

Lateral Aspect

- Lateral tibial plateau
- Lateral femoral condyle
- Lateral epicondyle
- Head of the fibula

Patella

- Superior aspect
- Around periphery with the knee relaxed
- Around periphery with the knee in full extension

Capsular and Ligamentous Tissue Palpation

After palpation of the bony structures, the supportive structures should be palpated for pain and defects (Figure 19-12). The palpation sequence is the anterior capsule, lateral collateral ligament, and medial collateral ligament and capsular structures. Capsular tissue should be palpated at the joint line where most tears occur.

Soft-Tissue Palpation

Soft tissue around the knee should be palpated for symmetry of definition, defects of continuity indicating rupture or tears, and specific pain sites. The quadriceps muscle; patellar tendon; sartorius, gracilis, semitendinosus, and semimembranosus muscles; biceps tendon of the thigh; iliotibial band; popliteal fossa; popliteal muscle; and head of the gastrocnemius muscle should systematically be felt for pain and defects.

Palpation of Swelling Patterns

Of major importance to knee inspection and evaluation is palpating for joint effusion (Figure 19-13). Swelling caused by synovial fluid or by blood in the joint, or **hemar-**

hemarthrosis
Blood in a joint cavity.

Figure 19-12

Typical pain sites around the knee.

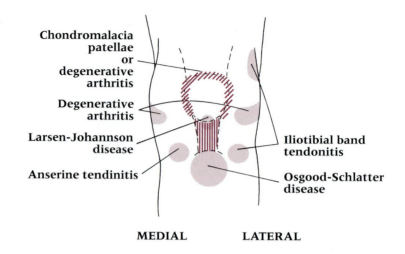

Chondromalacia patellae or degenerative arthritis

Degenerative arthritis

Larsen-Johannson disease

Anserine tendinitis

Iliotibial band tendonitis

Osgood-Schlatter disease

MEDIAL   LATERAL

throsis, must be determined. A hemarthrosis can only be identified by having the team physician aspirate the joint with a needle.

Functional Assessment of Knee Joint Instability

Both acute and chronic injury to the knee can produce ligamentous instability.[57] It is advisable that the injured knee's stability be evaluated as soon after injury as possible. However, tests of this type should be performed only by well-trained professionals. The injured knee and uninjured knee are tested and contrasted to determine any differences in their stability.

Determination of the degree of instability is made by the "endpoint" felt during stability testing. As stress is applied to a joint, there will be some motion, which is limited by an intact ligament. In a normal joint, the endpoint will be abrupt with little or no give and no reported pain. With a grade 1 sprain, the endpoint will still be firm with little or no instability and some pain will be indicated. With a grade 2 sprain, the endpoint will be soft with some instability present and a moderate amount of pain. In a grade 3 complete rupture, the endpoint will be very soft with marked instability, and pain will be severe initially, then mild.[30]

The use of magnetic resonance imaging (MRI) as a diagnostic tool has aided tremendously in the classification of ligamentous sprains. Despite its expense, MRI is being widely used by physicians to detect ligament injuries.

Figure 19-13

Typical swelling sites around the knee.

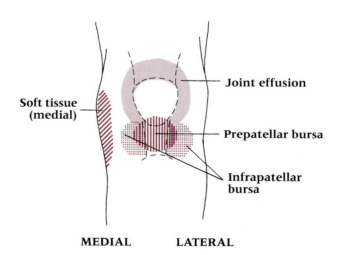

Soft tissue (medial)

Joint effusion

Prepatellar bursa

Infrapatellar bursa

MEDIAL   LATERAL

TABLE 19-1 Knee Stability Tests

Test	If Positive
Valgus stress test at 0°	Torn MCL and possibly ACL, PCL, PMC
Valgus stress test at 20°/30°	Torn MCL (if grade III check ACL, PCL, PMC)
Varus stress test at 0°	Torn LCL and possibly ACL, PCL, PLC
Varus stress test at 20°/30°	Torn LCL (if grade III check ACL, PCL, PLC)
Anterior drawer test (neutral)	Torn ACL
Anterior drawer test (15° ER)	Torn PMC, ACL, and possibly MCL
Anterior drawer test (30° IR)	Torn PLC, ACL
Lachman drawer test (20°/30° flexion)	Torn ACL, PCL (positive more often than anterior drawer because hamstrings are relaxed and medial meniscus/collateral ligaments do not block anterior displacement at 20°)
Pivot-shift tests (Galaway and McIntosh)	Torn ACL, ALC
Extension/IR/valgus (tibia subluxated)→flexion (tibia reduces at 20°)	
Slocum's test	Torn ACL, ALC
Sidelying extension/IR/valgus (tibia subluxated)→flexion (tibia reduces at 20°)	
Jerk test (Hughston)	Torn ACL, ALC
Flexion/IR/valgus (tibia reduced)→extension (tibia subluxates at 20°)	
Losee test	Torn ACL, ALC
45° flexion/ER/valgus (tibia subluxated anteriorly)→extension (tibia reduces at 20°)	
Flexion-rotation drawer test	Torn ACL
15° flex (tibia subluxated anteriorly/femur ER)→flexion (tibia reduces posteriorly/femur IR)	
Posterior drawer test 90°	Torn PCL
External rotation recurvatum test (tibia ER)	Torn PCL, PLC
Posterior sag test 90°	Torn PCL
Reverse pivot-shift test (Jakob)	Torn PCL
Extension (tibia reduced)→flexion (tibia subluxated posteriorly with ER)	
McMurray's test	Torn LM
(IR)	Torn MM
(ER)	
Apley's grinding test	Torn MM

ACL, Anterior cruciate ligament; *ER*, external rotation; *IR*, internal rotation; *LCL*, lateral collateral ligament; *LM*, lateral meniscus; *MCL*, medial collateral ligament; *MM*, medial meniscus; *PCL*, posterior cruciate ligament; *PLC*, posterior lateral corner; *PMC*, posterior medial corner.

Table 19-1 provides a summary of the various tests and what a positive test indicates in terms of the injured structures.

Classification of Knee Joint Instabilities

A good deal of controversy exists over the most appropriate terminology for classifying instabilities in the knee joint.[37] For years the American Orthopedic Society for Sports Medicine has classified knee laxity as either a straight or a rotatory instability. A straight instability implies laxity in a single direction, either medial, lateral, anterior, or posterior. Rotatory instabilities refer to excessive rotation of the tibial plateau relative to the femoral condyles and are identified as anterolateral, anteromedial, posterolateral, or rarely posteromedial. It is not unusual to see combined instabilities depending on the structures that have been injured. This classification system is still the most widely used and accepted by the athletic trainer (Table 19-2).

Recently, the concept of tibial translation has been proposed.[39] **Translation** refers to the amount of gliding of the medial tibial plateau as compared with the lateral tibial plateau relative to the femoral condyles. For example, in anterolateral rotatory

translation
Refers to anterior gliding of tibial plateau.

TABLE 19-2 Classification of Instabilities

Straight Instabilities	Rotary Instabilities
Medial	Anterolateral
Lateral	Anteromedial
Anterior	Posterolateral
Posterior	Posteromedial

instability the anterior translation of the lateral tibial plateau would be much greater than the more stable medial tibial plateau. The amount of anterior translation is determined by the integrity of the anatomical restraints that normally restrict excessive translation. More ligamentous, tendinous, and capsular structures will be damaged as the severity of the injury increases. Classification of knee injury relative to tibial translation is likely to gain popularity among sports medicine professionals.

Valgus and Varus Stress Tests

Valgus and varus stress tests are intended to reveal laxity of the medial and lateral stabilizing complexes, especially the collateral ligaments. The athlete lies supine with the leg extended. To test the medial side, the examiner holds the ankle firmly with one hand while placing the other over the head of the fibula. The examiner then places a force inward in an attempt to open the side of the knee. This valgus stress is applied with the knee fully extended or at 0 degrees and at 30 degrees of flexion (Figure 19-14, *A*). The examination in full extension tests the MCL, posteromedial capsule, and the cruciates. At 30 degrees flexion the MCL is isolated. The examiner reverses hand positions and tests the lateral side with a varus force on the fully extended knee and then with 30 degrees of flexion (Figure 19-14, *B*). With the knee extended the LCL and posterolateral capsule are examined. At 30 degrees of flexion the LCL is isolated.[22] NOTE: The lower limb should be in neutral with no internal or external rotation.

Anterior Cruciate Ligament Tests

A number of tests are currently being used to establish the integrity of the cruciate ligaments.[23] They are the drawer test at 90 degrees of flexion, the Lachman drawer test, the pivot-shift test, the jerk test, and the flexion-rotation drawer test.

Drawer test at 90 degrees of flexion   The athlete lies on the training table with the injured leg flexed. The examiner stands facing the anterior aspect of the athlete's leg, with both hands encircling the upper portion of the leg, immediately below the knee joint. The fingers of the examiner are positioned in the popliteal space of the affected leg, with the thumbs on the medial and lateral joint lines (Figure 19-15, *A*).

Figure 19-14

Valgus and varus knee stress tests. **A,** Valgus. **B,** Varus.

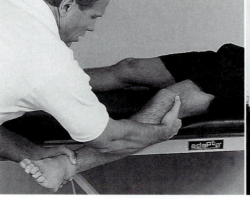
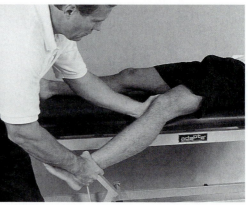

A   B

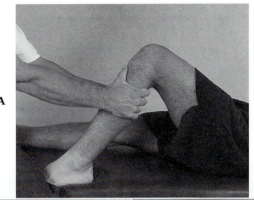

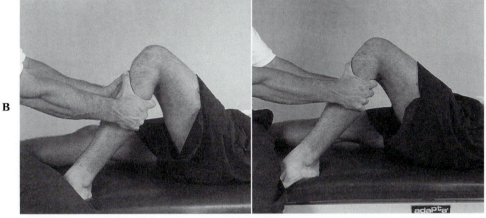

Drawer test for cruciate laxity. **A,** Knee at 90 degrees, with the foot pointing straight. **B,** Knee at 90 degrees, with the leg internally rotated. **C,** Knee at 90 degrees, with the leg externally rotated.

The index fingers of the examiner are placed on the hamstring tendon to ensure that it is relaxed before the test is administered. The tibia's sliding forward from under the femur is considered a positive anterior drawer sign.[34] If a positive anterior drawer sign occurs, the test should be repeated with the athlete's leg rotated internally 30 degrees and externally 15 degrees (Figure 19-15, *B* and *C*). Sliding forward of the tibia when the leg is externally rotated is an indication that the posteromedial aspect of the joint capsule, the anterior cruciate ligament, or possibly the medial collateral ligament could be torn. Movement when the leg is internally rotated indicates that the anterior cruciate ligament and posterolateral capsule may be torn. A normal anterior shear is 5 mm. Cailliet[8] indicates that shears of ½ inch, ½ to ¾ inch, and ¾ inch or more (1.3 cm, 1.3 to 1.9 cm, and 1.9 cm or more) correspond to grades 1, 2, and 3, respectively.

Lachman drawer test   In recent years the Lachman drawer test has become preferred by many over the drawer test at 90 degrees of flexion (Figure 19-16).[54] This is especially true for examinations immediately after injury. One reason for using it immediately after an injury is that it does not force the knee into the painful 90-degree position but tests it at a more comfortable 15 degrees. Another reason for its increased popularity is that it reduces the contraction of the hamstring muscles.[13] The contraction causes a secondary knee stabilizing force that tends to mask the real extent of injury. The Lachman drawer test is administered by positioning the knee in approximately 30 degrees of flexion. One hand of the examiner stabilizes the leg by grasping the distal end of the thigh, and the other hand grasps the proximal aspect of the tibia, attempting to move it anteriorly. A positive Lachman's test indicates damage to the anterior cruciate.

Pivot-shift test   The pivot-shift test is designed to determine anterolateral rotary instability (Figure 19-17). It is most often used in chronic conditions and is a sensitive test when the anterior cruciate ligament has been torn. The athlete lies supine;

Figure 19-16

Lachman drawer test for cruciate laxity.

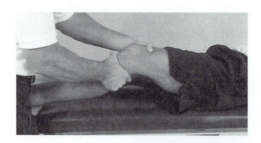

Figure 19-17

Pivot-shift test for anterolateral rotary instability. **A,** The tibia is subluxated in extension. **B,** It reduces at 20 degrees of flexion.

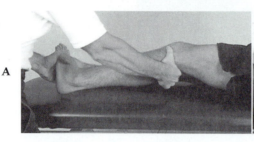 **A**   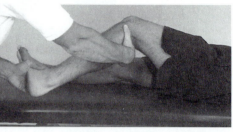 **B**

one hand of the examiner is pressed against the head of the fibula, and the other hand grasps the athlete's ankle. To start, the lower leg is internally rotated and the knee is fully extended. The thigh is then flexed 30 degrees at the hip while the knee is also flexed, and a simultaneous valgus force and axial load are applied by the examiner's upper hand. If the anterior cruciate ligament is damaged, the lateral tibial plateau will be subluxated in the fully extended position. As the knee is flexed to between 20 and 40 degrees, the lateral tibial plateau will reduce itself, producing a palpable shift or "clunk".[4]

Jerk test   The jerk test reverses the direction of the pivot shift.[23] The position of the knee is identical to that for the pivot-shift test except that the knee is moved from a position of flexion into extension with the lateral tibial plateau in a reduced position. If there is anterior cruciate insufficiency, as the knee moves into extension the tibia will subluxate at about 20 degrees of flexion, once again producing a palpable shift or clunk (Figure 19-18).

Flexion-rotation drawer test   With this test the lower leg is cradled with the knee flexed between 15 and 30 degrees. At 15 degrees, the tibia is subluxated anteriorly with the femur externally rotated. As the knee is flexed to 30 degrees the tibia reduces posteriorly and the femur rotates internally[23] (Figure 19-19).

Posterior Cruciate Ligament Tests

Tests for posterior cruciate ligament instability include the posterior drawer test, the external rotation recurvatum test, and the posterior sag test.

Posterior drawer test   The posterior drawer test is performed with the knee flexed at 90 degrees and the foot in neutral. Force is exerted in a posterior direction at the proximal tibial plateau. A positive posterior drawer test indicates damage to the posterior cruciate ligament (Figure 19-20).

19-3

Critical Thinking Exercise

A lacrosse player carrying the ball attempts to avoid a defender by planting his right foot firmly on the ground and cutting hard to his left. His knee immediately "gives way" and he hears a loud pop. He has intense pain immediately, but after a few minutes he feels as if he can get up and walk.

? What ligament has most likely been injured? What stability tests should be done by the athletic trainer to determine the extent of the injury to this ligament?

Figure 19-18

Jerk test for anterolateral rotary instability. **A,** The tibia is reduced in flexion. **B,** It subluxates at 20 degrees of extension.

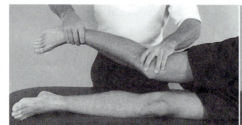 **A**   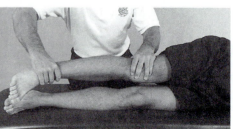 **B**

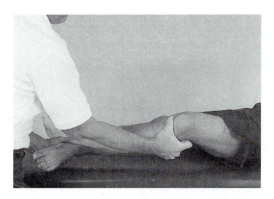

Figure 19-19

Flexion-rotation drawer test.

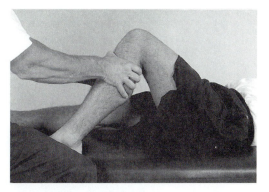

Figure 19-20

Posterior drawer test.

   External rotation recurvatum test   The athletic trainer grasps the great toe and lifts the leg off the table. A posterior sag and external rotation of the tibia indicate damage to the posterior cruciate ligament and posterolateral instability[52] (Figure 19-21).

   Posterior sag test   With the athlete supine, both knees are flexed to 90 degrees. Observing laterally on the injured side, the tibia will appear to sag posteriorly when compared with the opposite extremity if the posterior cruciate ligament is damaged[52] (Figure 19-22).

Instrument Assessment of Cruciate Laxity

Several ligament-testing devices are currently available that objectively quantify the anterior or posterior displacement of the knee joint, thus reducing much of the subjectivity associated with the previously described tests.[19] The KT-2000 arthrometer, the Stryker knee laxity tester, and the Genucom are three such testing devices (Figure 19-23).

   Measurements taken postoperatively and at periodic intervals throughout the rehabilitation process provide an objective indication to the athletic trainer about the effectiveness of the treatment program in maintaining or reducing anterior or posterior translation.[54]

Meniscal Tests

Determining a torn meniscus often can be difficult. The three most commonly used tests are McMurray's test, the Apley compression test, and the Apley distraction test.

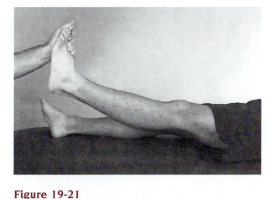

Figure 19-21

External rotation recurvatum test.

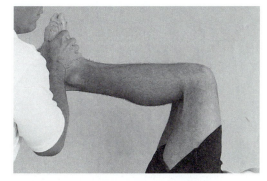

Figure 19-22

Posterior sag test.

Figure 19-23

The KT-2000 knee arthrometer.

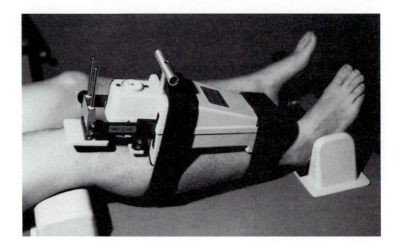

The McMurray meniscal test McMurray's test (Figure 19-24) is used to determine the presence of a displacable meniscal tear within the knee. The athlete is positioned face up on the table, with the injured leg fully flexed. The examiner places one hand on the foot and one hand over the top of the knee, fingers touching the medial joint line. The ankle hand scribes a small circle and pulls the leg into extension. As this occurs, the hand on the knee feels for a "clicking" response. Medial meniscal tears can be detected when the lower leg is externally rotated, and internal rotation allows detection of lateral tears.

The Apley compression test The Apley compression test (Figure 19-25) is performed with the athlete lying face down and the affected leg flexed to 90 degrees. While stabilizing the thigh, a hard downward pressure is applied to the leg. The leg is then rotated back and forth. If pain results, a meniscal injury has occurred. A medial meniscal tear is noted by external rotation, and a lateral meniscal tear is noted by internal rotation of the lower leg.

Figure 19-24

The McMurray meniscal test. **A** and **B,** Internal rotation of the lower leg into knee extension. **C** and **D,** External rotation of the lower leg into knee extension.

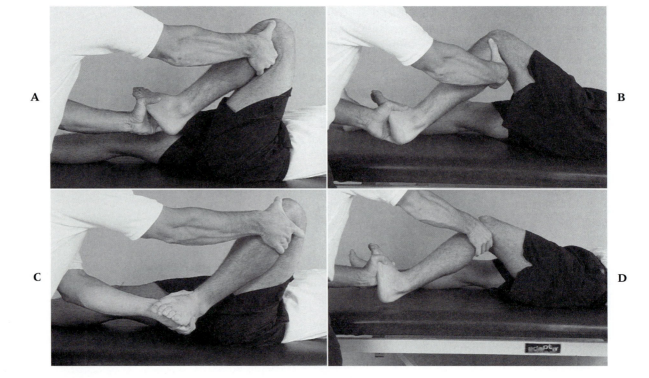

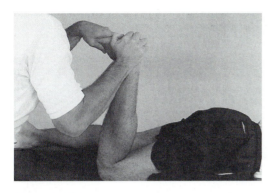

Figure 19-25

The Apley compression test.

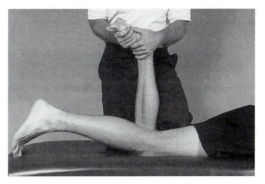

Figure 19-26

The Apley distraction test.

The Apley distraction test   With the athlete in the same position as for the Apley compression test, the examiner applies traction to the leg while moving it back and forth (Figure 19-26). This maneuver distinguishes collateral ligamentous tears from capsular and meniscal tears. If the capsule or ligaments are affected, pain will occur; if the meniscus is torn, no pain will occur from the traction and rotation.[21]

Girth Measurement

A knee injury is almost always accompanied by an eventual decrease in the girth of the thigh musculature. The muscles most affected by disuse are the quadriceps group, which are "antigravity" muscles and assist humans in maintaining an erect, straight-leg position. They are in constant use in effecting movement. Atrophy results when a lower limb is favored and is not used to its potential. Measurement of the circumference of both thighs can often detect former leg injuries or determine the extent of exercise rehabilitation. Five sites have been suggested for girth measurement. These sites are the joint line, 8 to 10 cm above the tibial plateau, the level of the tibial tubercle, the belly of the gastrocnemius muscle measured in centimeters from the tibial tubercle, and 2 cm above the superior border of the patella recorded in centimeters above the tibial tubercle (Figure 19-27).

Because the musculature of the knee atrophies so readily after an injury, girth measurements must be routinely taken.

Functional Examination

It is important that the athlete's knee also be tested for function. The athlete should be observed walking and, if possible, running, turning, performing figure-8s, backing up, and stopping. If the athlete can do a deep knee bend or duck walk without discomfort, it is doubtful that there is a meniscal tear. The resistive strength of the hamstring and quadriceps muscles should be compared with the strength of the knee known to be uninjured (Figure 19-28).

Patellar Examinations

Any knee evaluation should include inspection of the patella. Numerous evaluation procedures are associated with the patella and its surroundings. The following evaluation procedures can provide valuable information about possible reasons for knee discomfort and problems in functioning.[52]

Observation of the Patellar Position, Shape, and Alignment

The first aspect of examining the patella is one of observation. In terms of position, the patella may ride higher than usual (patella alta) or lower than normal (patella infera), causing a tendency toward abnormal articulation when the athlete sits with the legs hanging over the end of a table and with the knees flexed at a 45-degree angle. Observation can also tell the shape and size of the patella. Some patellas are

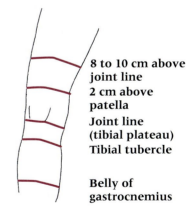

8 to 10 cm above joint line
2 cm above patella
Joint line (tibial plateau)
Tibial tubercle

Belly of gastrocnemius

Figure 19-27

The five sites for girth measurement.

Figure 19-28

A, Testing quadriceps strength.
B, Hamstring strength.

A

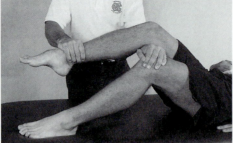
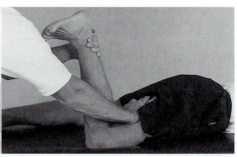

B

A Q angle greater than 20 degrees could predispose the athlete to patellar femoral pathology.

smaller or larger than usual, and some display an abnormal shape, especially at the inferior pole. The symptomatic patella also should be observed for alignment with the nonsymptomatic patella. As discussed earlier, leg alignment problems such as hip anteversion, genu valgum, tibial torsion, and foot pronation can cause the patella to rotate inward, causing a tracking problem within the femoral groove.

The Q Angle

The Q angle is created when lines are drawn from the middle of the patella to the anterosuperior spine of the ilium and from the tubercle of the tibia through the center of the patella (Figure 19-29). It should be measured with the knee fully extended and with it flexed at 30 degrees. The normal angle is 10 degrees for males and 15 degrees for females. Q angles that exceed 20 degrees are considered excessive and could lead to a pathological condition associated with improper patellar tracking in the femoral groove.

The A Angle

The A angle measures the patellar orientation to the tibial tubercle. It is created by the intersection of lines drawn bisecting the patella longitudinally and from the tibial tubercle to the apex of the inferior pole of the patella[2] (Figure 19-30). An A angle of 35 degrees or greater has been correlated with patellofemoral pathomechanics that seems to result in constant patellofemoral pain. The A angle serves as a quantitative measure of patellar realignment after rehabilitative intervention.

Palpation of the Patella

With the quadriceps muscle fully relaxed, the patella is palpated around its periphery and under its sides for pain sites (Figure 19-31).

Patellar Compression, Patellar Grinding, and Apprehension Tests

With the knee held to create approximately 20 degrees of flexion, the patella is compressed downward into the femoral groove; it is then moved forward and backward (Figure 19-32). If the athlete feels pain or if a grinding sound is heard during the patellar grind test, a pathological condition is probably present. With the knee still flexed, the patella is forced forward and is held in this position as the athlete extends the knee (Figure 19-33). A positive Clark's sign is present when pain and grinding are experienced by the athlete. Another test that indicates whether the patella can easily be subluxated or dislocated is known as the patellar apprehension test (Figure 19-34). With the knee and patella in a relaxed position, the examiner pushes the patella laterally. The athlete will express sudden apprehension at the point at which the patella begins to dislocate.[24]

PREVENTION OF KNEE INJURIES

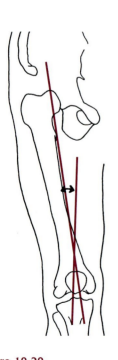

Figure 19-29

Measuring the Q angle of the knee.

Preventing knee injuries in sports is a complex problem. Of major importance are effective physical conditioning, rehabilitation and skill development, and shoe type. A questionable practice may be the routine use of protective bracing.

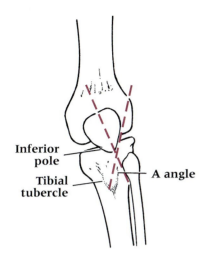

Figure 19-30

Determining the A angle.

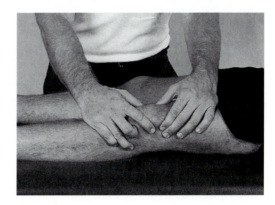

Figure 19-31

Palpating the periphery of the patella while the quadriceps muscle is fully relaxed.

Physical Conditioning and Rehabilitation

To avoid knee injuries the athlete must be as highly conditioned as possible, meaning total body conditioning that includes strength, flexibility, cardiovascular and muscle endurance, agility, speed, and balance.[11] Specifically, the muscles surrounding the knee joint must be as strong as possible and flexible. The joints and soft tissue that make up the kinetic chain of which the knee is a part must also be considered sources of knee injury and therefore must be specifically conditioned for strength and flexibility. Depending on the requirements of a sport, a strength ratio should be acquired between the quadriceps and hamstring muscle groups. For example, in football players the hamstring muscles should have 60% to 70% of the strength of the quadriceps muscles.[47] The gastrocnemius muscle should also be strengthened to help stabilize the knee. Although maximizing muscle strength may prevent some injuries, it fails to prevent rotary-type injuries.

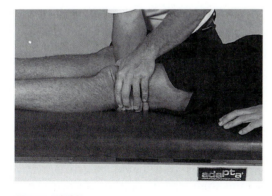

Figure 19-32

Patellar compression test. The patella is pressed downward in the femoral groove and moved forward and backward to elicit pain or crepitus.

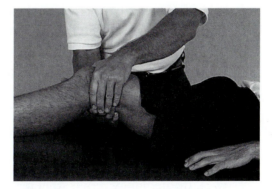

Figure 19-33

Patellar grind test. While the knee is flexed, the patella is forced forward; the athlete then actively contracts the quadriceps. The test reveals a positive Clark's sign if the athlete feels pain or grinding.

Figure 19-34

Patellar apprehension test for the easily subluxated or dislocated patella.

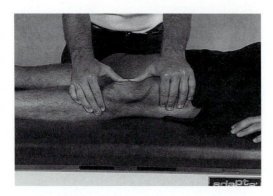

Avoiding abnormal contraction of the muscles through flexibility exercises is a necessary protection for the knee. Gradual stretching of the knee musculature helps the muscle fibers become more extensible and elastic.[11] Of special concern in preventing knee injuries is extensibility of the hamstrings, erector spinae, groin, quadriceps, and gastrocnemius muscles.

Knees that have been injured must be properly rehabilitated. Repeated minor injuries to a knee make it susceptible to a major injury. (See the section on knee joint rehabilitation later in this chapter.)

Shoe Type

During recent years, collision-type sports such as football have been using soccer-style shoes. The change from a few long conical cleats to a large number of cleats that are short (no longer than ½ inch [1.3 cm]) and broad has significantly reduced knee injuries in football. A shoe with more and shorter cleats is better because the foot does not become fixed to the surface and the shoe still allows controlled running and cutting.

Functional and Prophylactic Knee Braces

Functional and prophylactic knee braces are discussed in Chapter 5. These braces have been designed to prevent or reduce the severity of knee injuries.[35] Prophylactic knee braces are worn on the lateral surface of the knee to protect the medial collateral ligament.[17] Functional knee braces are used to protect grade 1 or 2 sprains of the ACL or most commonly a surgically reconstructed ACL. These braces are custom molded and are designed to control rotational stress or tibial translation. The effectiveness of protective knee braces is at best controversial[44,46] (Figure 19-35).

RECOGNITION AND MANAGEMENT OF SPECIFIC INJURIES
Ligamentous Injuries

The major ligaments of the knee can be torn in isolation or in combination. Depending on the application of forces, injury can occur from a direct straight-line or single-plane force, from a rotary force, or from a combination of the two.[2]

Medial Collateral Ligament Sprain

Etiology Most knee sprains affect the medial collateral ligament as a result either of a direct blow from the lateral side, in a medial direction, or of a severe outward twist. Greater injury results from medial sprains than from lateral sprains because of their more direct relation to the articular capsule and the medial meniscus (Figure 19-36). Medial and lateral sprains occur in varying degrees, depending on knee position, previous injuries, the strength of muscles crossing the joint, the force and angle of the trauma, fixation of the foot, and conditions of the playing surface.

The position of the knee is important in establishing its vulnerability to traumatic sprains. Any position of the knee, from full extension to full flexion, can result in

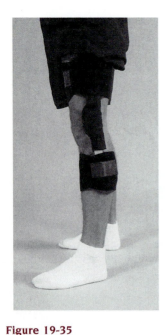

Figure 19-35

Prophylactic knee braces.

injury if there is sufficient force. Full extension tightens both lateral and medial ligaments. However, flexion affords a loss of stability to the lateral ligament but maintains stability in various portions of the broad medial ligament.[20] Medial collateral ligamentous sprains result most often from a violently adducted and internally rotated knee. The most prevalent mechanism of a lateral collateral ligamentous or capsular sprain is one in which the foot is everted and the knee is forced laterally into a varus position.

Speculation among medical authorities is that torn menisci seldom happen as the result of an initial trauma; most occur after the collateral ligaments have been stretched by repeated injury. Many mild to moderate sprains leave the knee unstable and thus vulnerable to additional internal derangements. The strength of the muscles crossing the knee joint is important in assisting the ligaments to support the articulation. These muscles should be conditioned to the highest possible degree for sports in which knee injuries are common. With the added support and protection of muscular strength, a state of readiness may be developed through proper athletic training.

The force and angle of the trauma usually determine the extent of injury that takes place. Even after witnessing the occurrence of a knee injury, it is difficult to predict the amount of tissue damage. The most revealing time for testing joint stability is immediately after injury before effusion masks the extent of derangement.

Grade 1 medial collateral ligamentous sprain   A grade 1 medial collateral ligamentous injury of the knee has the following characteristics (Figure 19-37):

- A few ligamentous fibers are torn and stretched.
- The joint is stable during valgus stress tests.
- There is little or no joint effusion.
- There may be some joint stiffness and point tenderness just below the medial joint line.
- Even with minor stiffness, there is almost full passive and active range of motion.

Management   Immediate care consists of rest, ice, compression, and elevation (RICE) for at least 24 hours. After immediate care, the following procedures should be undertaken:

- Crutches are prescribed if the athlete is unable to walk without a limp.
- Follow-up care may involve cryokinetics, including 5 minutes of ice pack treatment before exercise or a combination of cold and compression or pulsed ultrasound.
- Proper exercise is essential, starting with phase 1 of the knee joint rehabilitation procedures on pp. 506.

Isometrics and straight-leg exercises are important until the knee can be moved without pain. The athlete then graduates to stationary bicycle riding or a high-speed isokinetic program. Exercises for regaining neuromuscular function should also be incorporated.

The athlete is allowed to return to full participation when the knee has regained normal strength, power, flexibility, endurance, and coordination. Usually a period of 1 to 3 weeks is necessary for recovery. When returning to activity, the athlete may require tape support for a short period.

Grade 2 medial collateral ligamentous sprain   Grade 2 medial collateral ligamentous knee sprain indicates both microscopic and gross disruption of ligamentous fibers (Figure 19-38). The only structures involved are the medial collateral ligament and the medial capsular ligament. It is characterized by the following:

- A complete tear of the deep capsular ligament and partial tear of the superficial layer of the medial collateral ligament or a partial tear of both areas.
- No gross instability, but minimum or slight laxity during full extension. However, at 30 degrees of flexion and when the valgus stress test is performed, laxity may be as much as 5 to 15 degrees.

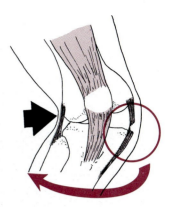

Figure 19-36

A valgus force with the tibia in external rotation injures the medial collateral and capsular ligaments, the medial meniscus, and sometimes the anterior cruciate ligaments.

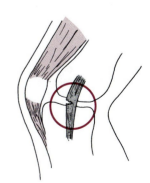

Figure 19-37

Grade 1 medial collateral ligamentous sprain.

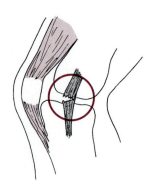

Figure 19-38

Grade 2 medial collateral ligamentous sprain.

- Slight or absent swelling unless the meniscus or anterior cruciate ligament has been torn. An acutely torn or pinched synovial membrane, subluxated or dislocated patella, or an osteochondral fracture can produce extensive swelling and hemarthrosis.
- Moderate to severe joint tightness with an inability to fully, actively extend the knee. The athlete is unable to place the heel flat on the ground.
- Definite loss of passive range of motion.
- Pain in the medial aspect, with general weakness and instability.

Management   Management consists of the following:
- RICE for 48 to 72 hours.
- Crutches are used with a three-point gait until the acute phase of injury is over and the athlete can walk without a limp.
- Depending on the severity and possible complications, a full-leg cast or postoperative knee-immobilizing splint may be applied by the physician (Figure 19-39) for 2 to 5 days, after which range-of-motion exercises are begun.
- Modalities should be used two to three times daily to modulate pain and to control inflammation.
- Isometric exercise emphasizing quadriceps strengthening (quad sets, straight leg lifts) should progress to active resisted full-range exercise as soon as possible.
- Closed kinetic chain exercises such as stationary bike, stair climbing, and resisted flexion and extension should be used as early as possible.
- Functional progression activities should be incorporated early in the rehabilitation program.
- Use of tape or perhaps a hinged brace when attempting to return to running activities is encouraged.

Conservative care of the grade 2 medial collateral ligamentous sprain has been successful. Studies show that there can be spontaneous ligamentous and capsular healing because other structures such as the anterior cruciate ligament also protect the knee against valgus and rotary movement.[20]

Grade 3 medial collateral ligamentous sprain   Grade 3 medial collateral ligamentous sprain means a complete tear of the supporting ligaments. The following are major symptoms and signs (Figure 19-40):
- Complete loss of medial stability.
- Minimum to moderate swelling.
- Immediate severe pain followed by a dull ache.
- Loss of motion because of effusion and hamstring guarding.
- A valgus stress test that reveals some joint opening in full extension and significant opening at 30 degrees of flexion.

Isolated grade 3 sprains of the MCL occur most often when the mechanism of injury involves a direct valgus force with the foot fixed and loaded. Medial collateral ligament tears resulting from rotation combined with valgus stress with the foot fixed but not loaded virtually always result in ACL and occasionally PCL tears. Thus testing must include evaluation of ACL and PCL integrity.[45]

Management   Immediate and follow-up care (RICE for 20 minutes every 2 hours during the waking day) should be performed for at least 72 hours. Conservative nonoperative treatment is now recommended for isolated grade 3 MCL sprains. The question of repair or nonoperative management of MCL tears with associated ACL or PCL tears remains controversial. Recovery times and long-term results regarding knee function and stability appear to be better than with surgical repair. It is necessary to rule out ACL damage before beginning conservative treatment. Conservative treatment usually involves limited immobilization with range of motion and progressive weight bearing for 2 weeks followed by protection with a functional hinged brace for another 2 to 3 weeks. The rehabilitation program would be similar to that for grade 1 and 2 sprains, although recovery time would be greater.

Lateral Collateral Ligament Sprain

Sprain of the lateral collateral ligament of the knee is much less prevalent than sprain of the medial collateral ligament.

Etiology   The force required to tear this ligament is varus, often with the tibia internally rotated (Figure 19-41). Because of the usually inaccessible medial aspect, a direct blow is rare. In skiing, the lateral collateral ligament can be injured when the skier fails to hold a snowplow and the tips cross, throwing the body weight to the outside edge of the ski. If the force or blow is severe enough, both cruciate ligaments, the attachments of the iliotibial band, and the biceps muscle may be torn. This same mechanism could also disrupt the lateral and even the medial meniscus. If the force is great enough, bony fragments can be avulsed from the femur or tibia. An avulsion can also occur through the combined pull of the lateral collateral ligament and biceps muscle on the head of the fibula.

Symptoms and signs   The major symptoms and signs include the following:

1. Pain and tenderness over the LCL. With the knee flexed and internally rotated the defect may be palpated.
2. Swelling and effusion over the LCL.
3. There is some joint laxity with a varus stress test at 30 degrees. If laxity exists in full extension, ACL and possibly PCL injury should be evaluated.
4. Pain will be greatest with grade 1 and grade 2 sprains. In grade 3 sprains pain will be intense initially, and then there will be a dull ache.

An injury can also occur to the peroneal nerve, causing temporary or permanent palsy. The common peroneal nerve originates from the sciatic nerve. It lies behind the head of the fibula and winds laterally around the neck of the fibula, where it branches into deep and superficial peroneal nerves (see Figure 19-9). Tears or entrapment of this nerve can produce varying weaknesses and paralysis of the lateral aspect of the lower leg. Injury of the peroneal nerve requires immediate medical attention.

Management   Management of the lateral collateral ligamentous injury should follow procedures similar to those for the medial collateral ligamentous injuries.

Cruciate Ligamentous Sprains

Anterior cruciate ligamentous sprain   The anterior cruciate ligament is commonly the most serious ligament injury in the knee.[31]

Etiology   The anterior cruciate ligament is most vulnerable to injury when the tibia is externally rotated and the knee is in a valgus position. The anterior cruciate ligament can sustain injury from a direct blow to the knee or from a single-plane force. The single-plane injury occurs when the lower leg is rotated while the foot is fixed (Figure 19-42). In this situation, the anterior cruciate ligament becomes taut and vulnerable to sprain. An example occurs when an athlete who is running fast suddenly decelerates and makes a sharp "cutting" motion, causing an isolated tear of the anterior cruciate ligament. The same mechanism could be true of the skier when his or her ski catches in the snow and the body twists medially or laterally.

Tears of the anterior cruciate ligament combined with injury to other supporting structures in the knee can produce rotatory instabilities. Anterolateral rotatory instability may involve injury to the anterolateral joint capsule, the LCL, and possibly the PCL and structures in the posterolateral corner. Anteromedial rotatory instability usually involves injury to the anteromedial capsule, the MCL, and possibly the PCL and posteromedial corner.

Hyperextension from a force to the front of the knee with the foot planted can tear the anterior cruciate ligament (Figure 19-43) and, if severe enough, can also sprain the medial collateral ligament.

Symptoms and signs   The athlete with a torn ACL will experience a "pop" followed by immediate disability and will complain that the knee feels like it is "coming apart." Anterior cruciate ligament tears produce rapid swelling at the joint line. The athlete

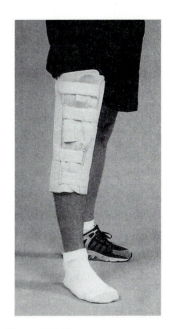

Figure 19-39

Knee immobilizer used after a ligamentous injury.

A lateral knee sprain can be caused by a varus force when the tibia is internally rotated.

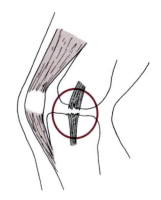

Figure 19-40

Grade 3 medial collateral ligamentous sprain.

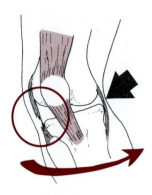

Figure 19-41

A varus force with the tibia internally rotated injures the lateral collateral ligament; in some cases both the cruciate ligaments and the attachments of the iliotibial band and biceps muscle of the thigh may be torn.

Simple surgical repair of the torn anterior cruciate ligament may not establish proper stability.

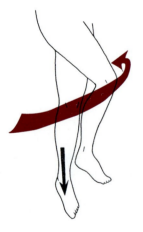

Figure 19-42

A major mechanism causing an anterior cruciate tear occurs when a running athlete suddenly decelerates and makes a sharp "cutting" motion.

with an isolated ACL tear will exhibit a positive anterior drawer sign and a positive Lachman's sign. The pivot-shift test, jerk test, and flexion-rotation drawer test may be positive even with an isolated ACL tear.

Management   Even with application of proper first aid and immediate RICE, swelling begins within 1 to 2 hours and becomes a notable hemarthrosis within 4 to 6 hours.[7] The athlete typically cannot walk without help. If a clinical evaluation is inconclusive, an arthroscopic examination may be warranted to make a proper diagnosis.

Anterior cruciate ligamentous injury could lead to serious knee instability; an intact anterior cruciate ligament is necessary for a knee to function in high-performance situations. Controversy exists among physicians about how best to treat an acute anterior cruciate ligamentous rupture and when surgery is warranted.[38] It is well accepted that an unsatisfactorily treated anterior cruciate ligamentous rupture will eventually lead to major joint degeneration. Therefore a decision for or against surgery must be based on the athlete's age, the type of stress applied to the knee, and the amount of instability present, as well as the techniques available to the surgeon.[6] A simple surgical repair of the ligament may not establish the desired joint stability.

Surgery may involve joint reconstruction, with transplantation of some external structure such as the pes anserinus, semitendinous muscle, tensor fascia lata, or most commonly the patellar tendon to replace the lost anterior cruciate support. This type of surgery involves a brief hospital stay, 3 to 5 weeks in braces, and 4 to 6 months of rehabilitation.[51] A detailed rehabilitation program for an ACL reconstruction is provided in the accompanying management plan.

Little scientific evidence exists to support the use of functional knee braces, yet many physicians feel that they can provide some protection during activity.[9,10]

Posterior cruciate ligamentous sprain   The posterior cruciate ligament has been called the most important ligament in the knee, providing a central axis for rotation.[50] The posterior cruciate ligament provides about 95% of the total restraining force to straight posterior displacement of the tibia.

Etiology   The posterior cruciate ligament is most at risk when the knee is flexed to 90 degrees. Falling with full weight on the anterior aspect of the bent knee with the foot in plantar flexion or receiving a hard blow to the front of the bent knee can tear the posterior cruciate ligament (Figure 19-44). In addition, it can be injured by a rotational force, which also affects the medial or lateral side of the knee.[50]

Symptoms and signs   Major signs and symptoms include the following:
- The athlete will report feeling a "pop" in the back of the knee.
- Tenderness and relatively little swelling will be evident in the popliteal fossa.
- Laxity will be demonstrated in a posterior sag test. The posterior drawer test is fairly reliable; however, an abduction stress test that is positive at both 30 degrees and in full extension is considered to be a definitive test for a torn PCL.

Management   RICE should be initiated immediately. If clinical evaluation is inconclusive, arthroscopic evaluation may be warranted.

Nonoperative rehabilitation of grade 1 and 2 injuries should focus on quadriceps strengthening. As with isolated tears of the ACL, controversy exists as to whether a PCL tear should be treated nonoperatively or with surgical intervention. Satisfactory outcomes achieved by nonoperative means have been reported. Although techniques for repairing the torn PCL are technically difficult, surgery is occasionally recommended. Rehabilitation after surgery generally involves 6 weeks of immobilization in extension with full weight bearing on crutches. Range-of-motion exercises are begun at 6 weeks, progressing to the use of progressive resistive exercise at 4 months.

Meniscal Lesions

The medial meniscus has a much higher incidence of injury than the lateral meniscus. The higher number of medial meniscal lesions is basically a result of the coronary ligament attaching the meniscus peripherally to the tibia and also to the capsular ligament. The lateral meniscus does not attach to the capsular ligament and is more mobile during knee movement. Because of the attachment to the medial structures, the medial meniscus is prone to disruption from valgus and torsional forces.

Etiology   A valgus force can adduct the knee, often tearing and stretching the medial collateral ligament; meanwhile, its fibers twist the medial meniscus outward. Repeated mild sprains reduce the strength of the knee to a state favorable for a cartilaginous tear through lessening its normal ligamentous stability. The most common mechanism is weight bearing combined with a rotary force while extending or flexing the knee. A cutting motion while running can distort the medial meniscus. Stretching of the anterior and posterior horns of the meniscus can produce a vertical-longitudinal, or "bucket-handle," tear (Figure 19-45). Another way a longitudinal tear occurs is by forcefully extending the knee from a flexed position while the femur is internally rotated. During extension the medial meniscus is suddenly pulled back, causing the tear (see Figure 19-45). In contrast, the lateral meniscus can sustain an oblique tear by a forceful knee extension with the femur externally rotated.[7] A large number of medial meniscus lesions are the outcome of a sudden, strong internal rotation of the femur with a partially flexed knee while the foot is firmly planted. As a result of the force of this action, the meniscus is pulled out of its normal bed and pinched between the femoral condyles.

Meniscal lesions can be longitudinal, oblique, or transverse. Because of its blood supply, tears in the outer one third of a meniscus may heal over time if stress in the area is kept to a minimum.[4] Tears that occur within the midsubstance of the meniscus often fail to heal because of lack of adequate blood supply.

Symptoms and signs   An absolute diagnosis of meniscal injury is difficult. For determining the possibility of such an injury, a complete history should be obtained, which consists of information about past knee injury and an understanding of how the present injury occurred. Diagnosis of meniscal injuries should be made immediately after the injury has occurred and before muscle spasm and swelling obscure the normal shape of the knee.

A meniscal tear may or may not result in the following:
- Effusion developing gradually over 48 to 72 hours.
- Joint-line pain and loss of motion.
- Intermittent locking and "giving way."
- Pain when squatting.

Once a meniscal tear occurs, the ruptured edges harden and may eventually atrophy. On occasion, portions of the meniscus may become detached and wedge themselves between the articulating surfaces of the tibia and femur, thus imposing a locking, catching, or giving way of the joint. Chronic meniscal lesions may also display recurrent swelling and obvious muscle atrophy around the knee. The athlete may complain of an inability to perform a full squat or to change direction quickly when running without pain, a sense of the knee collapsing, or a popping sensation. Such

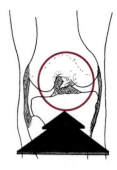

Figure 19-43

An anterior force with the foot planted can tear the anterior cruciate ligament.

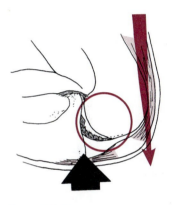

Figure 19-44

A fall or being hit on the anterior aspect of the bent knee can tear the posterior cruciate ligament.

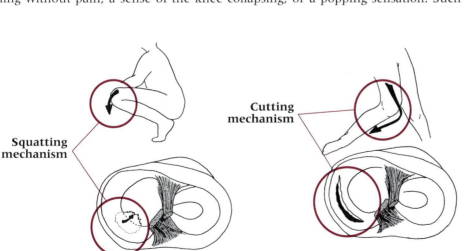

Squatting mechanism

Cutting mechanism

Figure 19-45

Common mechanisms of injury to the meniscus. Forced flexion produces a peripheral tear. Cutting with the foot fixed is likely to produce a "bucket-handle" tear.

Surgical Repair of Anterior Cruciate Ligament

Injury Situation A female college soccer player injured her right knee while cutting to her left with her right foot planted. There was no contact.

Signs and Symptoms She stated that she felt a "pop" and severe pain immediately. A few minutes later she felt that she could walk on it; however, it gave way as she put weight on it. Swelling was apparent at the joint line and over the medial aspect of the knee. Stability tests demonstrated positive anterior drawer, positive Lachman's, positive pivot-shift, positive flexion-rotation drawer, and positive valgus stress test at 0 and 30 degrees.

Management Plan She was diagnosed as having torn the ACL, MCL, and possibly the medial meniscus. Surgical repair was performed using an intraarticular ACL repair with a bone-patellar tendon-bone graft.

Preoperative Phase (3 to 6 weeks after injury) The goal during this phase is resolution of postinjury swelling and pain and restoration of full range of motion. Strengthening exercises through a full pain-free range of motion should begin as soon as can be tolerated. The athlete should be psychologically prepared for surgery during this phase.

Phase **1** Acute Injury **GOALS**: Minimize swelling, pain, and hemorrhage after surgery; establish and maintain full knee extension; achieve good quadriceps control; begin working on regaining knee flexion; regain neuromuscular control. **ESTIMATED LENGTH OF TIME (ELT)**: 1 week.

■ **Therapy** RICE during the entire first week 3 to 4 times per day to control swelling. Electrical muscle stimulation to control pain and elicit muscle contraction. Constant passive motion machine.

■ **Exercise rehabilitation** Achieve full extension by end of first week. Weight shifting on crutches. Early quadriceps activity is important. Perform straight leg raises and multiangle submaximal isometrics at 90, 60, and 40 degrees. Perform knee extensions in 90 to 30–degrees arc. Hip exercises, especially adduction, for VMO function. Active isotonic hamstring contractions to achieve 90 degrees of flexion by end of second week. Mobilize patella. Weight bearing as tolerated with brace locked in full extension.

Phase **2** Repair **GOALS**: Achieve a normal gait pattern; maintain full extension; strengthen quadriceps and hamstrings; increase knee flexion; maintain cardiorespiratory endurance; improve neuromuscular control. Begin light functional activities. **ELT**: 1 to 6 weeks.

■ **Therapy** Electrical muscle stimulation; RICE to control swelling initially and after each treatment session. The amount of swelling will determine the ability to contract the quadriceps. Electrical muscle stimulation to facilitate muscle contraction and for reeducation. Ultrasound to increase blood flow.

■ **Exercise rehabilitation** Ambulate with brace locked in full extension initially. Progressive increase range of motion in brace as tolerated by the patient. Remove brace by week 3 or 4. Full weight bearing without a limp at the end of 4 weeks. Full range of motion should be attained before engaging in intense strength training. Concentrate on hamstring strengthening. Use closed kinetic chain activities and cocontractions as much as possible. Strengthening exercises using minisquats, step-ups, hamstring and hip leg press, knee flexion, and extension standing using surgical tubing. Multidirection patellar mobilization; mobilize tibia. Stationary bike as soon as range of motion permits. Proprioceptive activities on BAPS board and Kinesthetic Awareness Trainer (KAT). KT-2000 test every 2 weeks for up to 12 weeks. Continue bicycling and use step climbing.

Continued

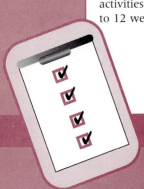

Surgical Repair of Anterior Cruciate Ligament—*cont'd*

Phase 3 Remodeling **GOALS**: Concentrate on functional progressions and return to high-demand activity.
ELT: Week 7 to 4 months.

■ **Therapy** Electrical muscle stimulation to facilitate contraction. Ultrasound to facilitate blood flow. Massage to decrease scar. Mobilization techniques as needed.

■ **Exercise rehabilitation** Isokinetic testing. High-speed training using rubber tubing. Begin hop training. Work on balance. Incorporate sport-specific activities. Begin return to running program at about 4 months. Return to sport activity, injury maintenance.

Criteria for Returning to Competitive Soccer

1. Knee is symptom free.
2. Appropriate isokinetic evaluation.
3. Appropriate arthrometer measurement.
4. Appropriate performance in functional tests.
5. Psychologically prepared for return.

---

symptoms and signs usually warrant surgical intervention. NOTE: Symptomatic meniscal tears can eventually lead to serious articular degeneration with major impairment and disability.

Management If the knee is not locked but shows indications of a tear, the physician might initially obtain an MRI. A diagnostic arthroscopic examination may also be performed.

The knee that is locked by a displaced meniscus may require unlocking with the athlete under anesthesia so that a detailed examination can be conducted. If discomfort, disability, and locking of the knee continue, arthroscopic surgery may be required to remove a portion of the meniscus.

Surgical management of meniscal tears should make every effort to minimize loss of any portion of the meniscus.[26] The menisci are critical in preventing degenerative joint disease. Healing of the torn meniscus is dependent on where the tear has occurred. Tears in the red-red or red-white zones may heal well after surgical repair because they have a good vascular supply. Tears in the inner white-white zone will have to be resected because they are unlikely to heal, even with surgical repair, due to avascularity (see Figure 19-5). Resection or a partial meniscectomy involves removing as little as possible of the meniscus through an arthroscope. Partial meniscectomy of a torn meniscus is much more common than meniscal repair.

Postsurgical management for a partial meniscectomy does not require bracing and allows partial to full weight bearing on crutches as quickly as can be tolerated for about 2 weeks. It is not uncommon for an athlete to return to full activity in as little as 6 to 14 days.

A repaired meniscus requires immobilization in a rehabilitative brace for 5 to 6 weeks. The athlete should be on crutches, progressing from partial to full weight bearing at 6 weeks. During immobilization active range-of-motion (ROM) exercises between 0 and 90 degrees should be done. At 6 weeks full ROM resistive exercises can begin. Rehabilitation should concentrate on endurance.[29]

19-5

Critical Thinking Exercise

A football running back is hit on the lateral surface of his knee by an opponent making a tackle. He has significant pain and some immediate swelling on the medial surface of his knee. The athletic trainer suspects the athlete has sustained a sprain of the MCL.

? What are the most appropriate tests that the athletic trainer should do to determine the exact nature and extent of the injury?

Critical Thinking E x e r c i s e

A wrestler is diagnosed by the team physician as having a torn medial meniscus. On evaluation McMurray's test was positive and a subsequent MRI revealed a longitudinal bucket-handle tear in the posterior horn of the medial meniscus.

? What are the most typical mechanisms of injury that can result in a tear of a meniscus?

Knee plicae that have become thick and hard are often mistaken for meniscal injuries.

Knee Plica

The fetus has three synovial knee cavities whose internal walls, at 4 months, are gradually absorbed to form one chamber; however, in 20% of all individuals, the knee fails to fully absorb these cavities. In adult life these septa form synovial folds known as plicae.

Etiology   The most common synovial fold is the infrapatellar plica, which originates from the infrapatellar fat pad and extends superiorly in a fanlike manner. The second most common synovial fold is the suprapatellar plica, located in the suprapatellar pouch. The least common, but most subject to injury, is the mediopatellar plica, which is bandlike and begins on the medial wall of the knee joint and extends downward to insert into the synovial tissue that covers the infrapatellar fat pad.[5] Because most synovial plicae are pliable, most are asymptomatic; however, the mediopatellar plica may be thick, nonyielding, and fibrotic, causing a number of symptoms. The mediopatellar plica is associated with chondromalacia of the medial femoral condyle and patella[5] (Figure 19-46).

Symptoms and signs   The athlete may or may not have a history of knee injury. If symptoms are preceded by trauma, it is usually one of blunt force such as falling on the knee or of twisting with the foot planted. A major complaint is recurrent episodes of painful pseudolocking of the knee when sitting for a period of time. As the knee passes 15 to 20 degrees of flexion, a snap may be felt or heard. Such characteristics of locking and snapping could be misinterpreted as a torn meniscus. The athlete complains of pain while ascending or descending stairs or when squatting. Unlike meniscal injuries, there is little or no swelling and no ligamentous laxity.

Management   A knee plica that becomes inflamed as a result of trauma is usually treated conservatively with rest, antiinflammatory agents, and local heat. If the condition recurs, causing a chondromalacia of the femoral condyle or patella, the plica will require surgical excision.

Osteochondral Knee Fractures

Etiology   Occasionally the same mechanisms that produce collateral ligamentous, cruciate ligamentous, or meniscal tears can shear off either a piece of bone attached to the anterior cartilage or cartilage alone. Twisting, sudden cutting, or being struck directly in the knee are typical causes of this condition.

Symptoms and signs   The athlete commonly hears a snap and feels the knee give way. Swelling is immediate and extensive because of hemarthrosis, and there is considerable pain.

Figure 19-46

Knee plica.

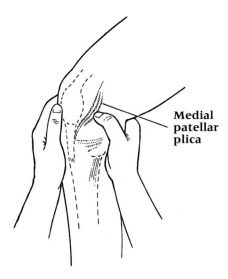

Medial patellar plica

Management   The diagnosis is usually confirmed by arthroscopic examination. Surgery is performed to replace the fragment as soon as possible to avoid joint degeneration and arthritis. The femoral condyles and the patella are affected.

Osteochondritis Dissecans

Osteochondritis dissecans is a painful condition involving partial or complete separation of a piece of articular cartilage and subchondral bone. Both teenagers and adults can have this condition. The vast majority of fragments, over 85%, occur in the lateral portion of the medial femoral condyle.[12] Clinically, osteochondral detachments are seen wherever there is osteochondritis dissecans. Typically the lesion results in normal articular cartilage with dead subchondral bone underneath separated by a layer of fibrous tissue.

Etiology   The exact cause of osteochondritis dissecans is unknown. It usually has a very slow onset. Possible etiological factors include the following:

- Direct or indirect trauma.
- Association with certain familial skeletal or endocrine abnormalities.
- A prominent tibial spine impinging on the medial femoral condyle.
- A facet of the patella impinging on the medial femoral condyle.

Symptoms and signs   The athlete with osteochondritis dissecans complains of a knee that aches, has recurrent swelling, and on occasion may catch or lock. There may be atrophy of the quadriceps muscle and point tenderness.

Management   For children, usually rest and immobilization using a cylinder cast are prescribed. This management affords proper resolution of the injured cartilage and normal ossification of the underlying bone. As with many other osteochondroses, resolution may take as long as 1 year. For the teenager and adult, surgery, such as multiple drilling in the area to stimulate healing, pinning loose fragments, or bone grafting, may be warranted.

Loose Bodies within the Knee

Etiology   Because of repeated trauma to the knee during sports activities, osteochondral fragments or loose bodies ("joint mice") can develop within the joint cavity. Loose bodies can stem from osteochondritis dissecans, fragments from the menisci, pieces of torn synovial tissue, or a torn cruciate ligament.

Symptoms and signs   The loose body may move in the joint space and become lodged, causing locking and popping. The athlete will complain of pain and a feeling of instability with giving way.

Management   When the loose body becomes wedged between articulating surfaces, irritation can occur. If not surgically removed, the loose body can create conditions that lead to joint degeneration.

Injury to the Infrapatellar Fat Pad

The two most important fat pads of the knee are the infrapatellar fat pad and the suprapatellar fat pad. The infrapatellar fat pad lies between the synovial membrane on the anterior aspect of the joint and the patellar tendon, and the suprapatellar fat pad lies between the anterior surface of the femur and the suprapatellar bursa. Of the two pads, the infrapatellar is more often injured in sports, principally as a result of its large size and particular vulnerability during activity.

Etiology   The infrapatellar fat pad may become wedged between the tibia and the patella, irritated by chronic kneeling pressures, or traumatized by direct blows.

Symptoms and signs   Repeated injury to the fat pad produces capillary hemorrhaging and swelling of the fatty tissue; if the irritation continues, scarring and calcification may develop. The athlete may complain of pain below the patellar ligament, especially during knee extension, and the knee may display weakness, mild swelling, and stiffness during movement.

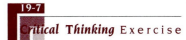

19-7

Critical Thinking Exercise

A gymnast comes to the athletic trainer complaining of knee pain with no history of knee injury. The athlete complains of pain while ascending or descending stairs and when squatting. A major complaint is recurring episodes of painful pseudolocking of the knee when sitting for a period of time. There is little or no swelling and no ligamentous laxity. A palpable tenderness begins on the medial wall of the knee joint and extends downward into the infrapatellar fat pad. As the knee passes 15 to 20 degrees of flexion, a snap may be felt or heard.

? Based on the findings of the evaluation, what might be causing these symptoms and signs?

A knee that locks and unlocks during activity may indicate a fractured meniscus.

Management   Care of acute fat pad injuries involves rest from irritating activities until inflammation has subsided, heel elevation of ½ to 1 inch (1.3 to 1.5 cm), and the therapeutic use of cold. Heel elevation prevents added irritation during full extension; applying hyperextension taping may also be necessary to prevent occurrence of full extension.

Joint Contusions

Etiology   A blow struck against the muscles crossing the knee joint can result in a handicapping condition. One of the muscles frequently involved is the vastus medialis of the quadriceps group, which is primarily involved in locking the knee in a position of full extension.

Symptoms and signs   Bruises of the vastus medialis produce all the appearances of a knee sprain, including severe pain, loss of movement, and signs of acute inflammation. Such bruising is often manifested by swelling and discoloration caused by the tearing of muscle tissue and blood vessels. If adequate first aid is given immediately, the knee will usually return to functional use 24 to 48 hours after the trauma.

Bruising of the capsular tissue that surrounds the knee joint is often associated with muscle contusions and deep bone bruises. A traumatic force delivered to capsular tissue may cause capillary bleeding, irritate the synovial membrane, and result in profuse fluid effusion into the joint cavity and surrounding spaces, thereby producing intraarticular swelling. Effusion often takes place slowly and almost imperceptibly. It is advisable to prevent the athlete from engaging in further activity for at least 24 hours after he or she receives a capsular bruise. Activity causes an increase in circulation and may cause extensive swelling and hematoma at the knee joint. Scar tissue develops wherever internal bleeding with clot organization is present. If this condition is repeated time after time, chronic synovitis or an arthritic sequela may develop.

> Because the knee joint and patella are poorly padded, they are prone to bruising.

Management   Care of a bruised knee depends on many factors. However, management principally depends on the location and severity of the contusion. The following procedures are suggested:
- Apply compression bandages and cold until resolution has occurred.
- Prescribe inactivity and rest for 24 hours.
- If swelling occurs, continue cold application for 72 hours. If swelling and pain are intense, refer the athlete to the physician.
- Once the acute stage has ended and the swelling has diminished to little or none, cold application with active range-of-motion exercises should be conducted within a pain-free range. If a gradual use of heat is elected, great caution should be taken to prevent swelling.
- Allow the athlete to return to normal activity, with protective padding, when pain and the initial irritation have subsided.
- If swelling is not resolved within a week, a chronic condition of either synovitis or bursitis may exist, indicating the need for rest and medical attention.

Bursitis

Bursitis in the knee can be acute, chronic, or recurrent. Although any one of the numerous knee bursae can become inflamed, anteriorly the prepatellar, deep infrapatellar, and suprapatellar bursae have the highest incidence of irritation in sports (see Figure 19-8).

> The knee has many bursae; the prepatellar, deep infrapatellar, and pretibial bursae are most often irritated.

Etiology   The prepatellar bursa often becomes inflamed from continued kneeling, and the deep infrapatellar becomes irritated from overuse of the patellar tendon.

Symptoms and signs   Prepatellar bursitis results in localized swelling above the knee that is ballotable. Swelling is not intraarticular and there may be some redness and increased temperature. Swelling in the popliteal fossa does not necessarily indicate bursitis but could instead be a sign of Baker's cyst (Figure 19-47). A Baker's cyst is connected to the joint, which swells because of a problem in the joint and not because of bursitis. A Baker's cyst is commonly painless, causing no discomfort or disability. Some inflamed bursae may be painful and disabling because of the swelling and should be treated accordingly.

Management   Management usually follows a pattern of eliminating the cause, prescribing rest, and reducing inflammation. Perhaps the two most important techniques for controlling bursitis are the use of elastic compression wraps and antiinflammatory medication. When the bursitis is chronic or recurrent and the synovium has thickened, use of aspiration and a steroid injection may be warranted.

PATELLAR AND EXTENSOR MECHANISM CONDITIONS

The position and function of the patella and the extensor mechanism expose it to a variety of traumas and diseases related to sports activities.

Patellar Injuries

Patellar Fracture

Etiology   Fractures of the patella can be caused by either direct or indirect trauma (Figure 19-48). Most patellar fractures are the result of indirect trauma in which a severe pull of the patellar tendon occurs against the femur when the knee is semiflexed. This position subjects the patella to maximum stress from the quadriceps tendon and the patellar ligament. Forcible muscle contraction may then fracture the patella at its lower half. Direct injury most often produces fragmentation with little displacement. Falls, jumping, or running may result in a fracture of the patella. NOTE: Approximately 3% of the population has a bipartite patella, meaning there are two portions of the patella. This condition can be misdiagnosed as a patellar fracture.

Symptoms and signs   The fracture causes hemorrhage and joint effusion, resulting in generalized swelling. Indirect fracture causes capsular tearing, separation of bone fragments, and possible tearing of the quadriceps tendon. Direct fracture involves little bone separation.

Management   Diagnosis is accomplished through use of the history, palpation of separated fragments, and an x-ray confirmation. As soon as the examiner suspects a patellar fracture, a cold wrap should be applied, followed by an elastic compression wrap and splinting. The athletic trainer should then refer the athlete to the team physician. The athlete will normally be immobilized for 2 to 3 months.

Acute Patellar Subluxation or Dislocation

Etiology   When an athlete plants his or her foot, decelerates, and simultaneously cuts in an opposite direction from the weight-bearing foot, the thigh rotates internally while the lower leg rotates externally, causing a forced knee valgus. The quadriceps muscle attempts to pull in a straight line and as a result pulls the patella laterally—a force that may dislocate the patella. As a rule, displacement takes place outwardly, with the patella resting on the lateral condyle (Figure 19-48).

With this mechanism the patella is forced to slide laterally into a partial or full dislocation. Some athletes are more predisposed to this condition than others because of the following anatomical structures:

- A wide pelvis with anteverted hips.
- Genu valgum, increasing the Q angle.
- Shallow femoral grooves.
- Flat lateral femoral condyles.
- High-riding and flat patellas.
- Vastus medialis and ligamentous laxity with genu recurvatum and externally rotated tibias.
- Pronated feet.
- Externally pointing patellas.

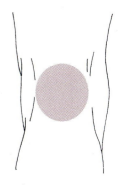

Figure 19-47

Baker's cyst in the popliteal fossa.

Knees that "give way" or "catch" have a number of possible pathological conditions:
   Subluxating patella
   Meniscal tear
   Anterior cruciate ligamentous tear
   Hemarthrosis

Figure 19-48

Fracture and dislocation of the patella.

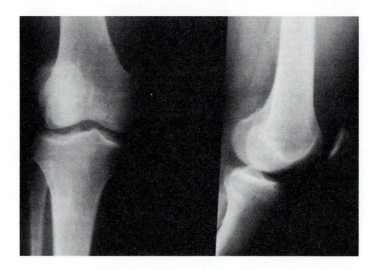

A patella that subluxates repetitively places abnormal stress on the patellofemoral joint and the medial restraints. The knee may be swollen and painful. Pain is a result of swelling but also results because the medial capsular tissue has been stretched and torn. Because of the associated swelling the knee is restricted in flexion and extension. There may also be a palpable tenderness over the adductor tubercle where the medial retinaculum (patellar femoral ligament) attaches.

An acute patellar dislocation is often associated with sudden twisting of the body while the foot or feet are planted and is associated with a painful giving way episode.

Symptoms and signs   The athlete experiences a complete loss of knee function, pain, and swelling, with the patella resting in an abnormal position. The physician immediately reduces the dislocation by applying mild pressure on the patella with the knee extended as much as possible. If a period of time has elapsed before reduction, a general anesthetic may have to be used. After aspiration of the joint hematoma, ice is applied, and the joint is splinted. A first-time patellar dislocation is sometimes associated with a chondral or osteochondral fracture. X-ray evaluation is performed before and after reduction.

Management   To reduce a dislocation, the hip is flexed, and the patella is gently moved medially as the knee is slowly extended. After reduction the knee is immobilized in extension for 4 weeks or longer, and the athlete is instructed to use crutches when walking. During immobilization, isometric exercises are performed at the knee joint. After immobilization the athlete should wear a horseshoe-shaped felt pad that is held in place around the patella by an elastic wrap or that is sewn into an elastic sleeve that is worn while running or performing in sports (Figure 19-49). Commercial braces are also available.

Muscle rehabilitation should be concerned with all the musculature of the knee, thigh, and hip. Knee exercise should be confined to straight-leg raises.

If surgery is performed, it is usually to release constrictive ligaments or to reconstruct the patellofemoral joint. It is important to strengthen and balance the strength of all musculature associated with the knee joint. Postural malalignments must be corrected as much as possible. Shoe orthotic devices may be used to reduce foot pronation, tibial internal rotation, and subsequently to reduce stress to the patellofemoral joint.

Patellofemoral Arthralgia

The patella, in relation to the femoral groove, can be subject to direct trauma or disease, leading to chronic pain and disability.[49] Of major importance among athletes are those conditions that stem from abnormal patellar tracking within the femoral groove, of which the three most common are chrondomalacia patella, degenerative arthritis, and patellofemoral stress syndrome.[21] Patellofemoral arthralgia is a catch-all term that is used to refer to any type of pain that occurs in or around the patellofemoral joint.

Chondromalacia Patella

Etiology   Chondromalacia patella is a softening and deterioration of the articular cartilage on the back of the patella (Figure 19-50). Cailliet[8] describes chondromalacia as undergoing three stages:

- Stage 1—swelling and softening of the articular cartilage.
- Stage 2—fissuring of the softened articular cartilage.
- Stage 3—deformation of the surface of the articular cartilage caused by fragmentation.

The exact cause of chondromalacia is unknown. As indicated previously, abnormal patellar tracking could be a major etiological factor[57]; however, individuals with normal tracking have acquired chondromalacia, and some individuals with abnormal tracking are free of it.[8] Abnormal patellofemoral tracking can be produced by genu valgum, external tibial torsion, foot pronation, femoral anteversion, a quadriceps Q angle greater than 15 to 20 degrees, patella alta, a shallow femoral groove, a shallow articular angle of the patella, an abnormal articular contour of the patella, or laxity of the quadriceps tendon.

Symptoms and signs   The athlete may experience pain in the anterior aspect of the knee while walking, running, ascending and descending stairs, or squatting. There may be recurrent swelling around the kneecap and a grating sensation when flexing and extending the knee.

The patella displays crepitation during the patellar grind test. During palpation there may be pain on the inferior border of the patella or when the patella is compressed within the femoral groove while the knee is passively flexed and extended. The athlete has one or more lower-limb alignment deviations.

Degenerative arthritis occurs on the medial facet of the patella, which makes contact with the femur when the athlete performs a full squat.[8] Degeneration first occurs in the deeper portions of the articular cartilage, followed by blistering and fissuring that stems from the subchondral bone and appears on the surface of the patella.[7,8]

Management   In some cases, patellofemoral arthralgia is initially treated conservatively as follows:

- Avoidance of irritating activities such as stair climbing and squatting.
- Isometric exercises that are pain free to strengthen the quadriceps and hamstring muscles.
- Oral antiinflammatory agents and small doses of aspirin.
- Wearing a neoprene knee sleeve.
- Wearing an orthotic device to correct pronation and reduce tibial torsion.

If conservative measures fail to help, surgery may be the only alternative. Some of the following surgical measures may be indicated[7]:

- Realignment procedures such as lateral release of the retinaculum, moving the insertion of the vastus medialis muscle forward.
- Shaving and smoothing the irregular surfaces of the patella, femoral condyle, or both.
- In cases of degenerative arthritis removing the blister through drilling.
- Elevating the tibial tubercle.
- As a last resort, completely removing the patella.

Patellofemoral Stress Syndrome

Etiology   Patellofemoral stress syndrome results from some lateral deviation of the patella as it tracks in the femoral groove. This tendency toward lateral tracking may be the result of several factors:

- Tightness of the hamstrings and gastrocnemius.
- Tightness of the lateral retinaculum, which compresses the lateral facet of the patella against the lateral femoral condyle.
- Increased Q angle.
- Tightness of the iliotibial band.
- Pronation of the foot.

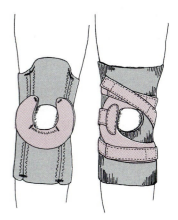

Figure 19-49

Special pads for the dislocated patella.

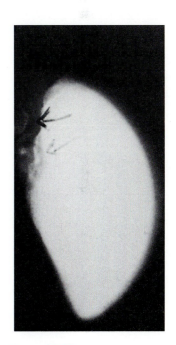

Figure 19-50

Chondromalacia with chipping away of the articular surface of the patella.

A triathlete has been complaining of knee pain for several months. She has never had an acute injury to the knee, but her training regimen is intense, involving 3 hours of training each day. She has been diagnosed by a physician as having chondromalacia patella.

? She has been referred to the athletic trainer for evaluation and rehabilitation. What can the athletic trainer do to help reduce the athlete's symptoms and signs?

Conditions that may be mistaken for one another:
  Osgood-Schlatter disease
  Larsen-Johansson disease
  Jumper's or kicker's knee

- Patella alta (the patellar tendon is longer than the patella).
- Vastus medialis oblique (VMO) insufficiency caused by imbalance with the strength of the vastus lateralis (VL) or inhibition resulting from the presence of 20 to 30 ml of effusion in the knee.[25]
- Weak hip adductors to which the VMO is attached.

Symptoms and signs   There will be tenderness of the lateral facet of the patella and some swelling associated with irritation of the synovium, as well as reports of a dull ache in the center of the knee. Patellar compression will elicit pain and crepitus. The athlete will be apprehensive when the patella is forced laterally.

Management   The athlete must engage in a strengthening program for the adductor muscles and for correcting the imbalance between the VMO and the VL through the use of biofeedback techniques. Stretching exercises for the hamstrings, gastrocnemius, and iliotibial band are also necessary. Orthotics can be used to correct pronation and other malalignments.[1] The McConnell taping technique (see Chapter 13) has been demonstrated to be extremely effective in regaining proper patellar alignment and thus a more symmetrical loading on the lower extremity. Taping is basically designed to correct the orientation of the patella.

If conservative treatment measures fail, lateral retinacular release has been advocated by some physicians.

Extensor Mechanism Problems

Many extensor mechanism problems can occur in the physically active individual. They can occur in the immature adolescent's knee or as a result of jumping and running.

Osgood-Schlatter Disease and Larsen-Johansson Disease

Etiology   Two conditions common to the immature adolescent's knee are Osgood-Schlatter disease and Larsen-Johansson disease. Osgood-Schlatter disease is an apophysitis characterized by pain at the attachment of the patellar tendon at the tibial tubercle seen in adolescents. This condition most often represents an avulsion fracture of the tibial tubercle. This fragment is cartilaginous initially, but with growth a bony callus forms and the tuberosity enlarges. This condition usually resolves when the athlete reaches the age of 18 or 19. The only remnant is an enlarged tibial tubercle.

The most commonly accepted cause of Osgood-Schlatter disease is repeated avulsion of the patellar tendon at the apophysis of the tibial tubercle. Complete avulsion of the patellar tendon is a major complication of Osgood-Schlatter disease.

Larsen-Johansson disease is similar to Osgood-Schlatter disease, but it occurs at the inferior pole of the patella (Figure 19-51). As with Osgood-Schlatter disease, the cause is believed to be excessive repeated strain on the patellar tendon. Swelling, pain, and point tenderness characterize Larsen-Johansson disease. Later, degeneration can be noted during x-ray examination.

Symptoms and signs   Repeated irritation causes swelling, hemorrhage, and gradual degeneration of the apophysis as a result of impaired circulation. The athlete complains of severe pain when kneeling, jumping, and running. There is point tenderness over the anterior proximal tibial tubercle (see Figure 19-51).

Management   Management is usually conservative and includes the following:
- Stressful activities are decreased until the epiphyseal union occurs, within 6 months to 1 year.
- Severe cases may require a cylindrical cast.
- Ice is applied to the knee before and after activities.
- Isometric strengthening of quadriceps and hamstring muscles is performed.

Patellar Tendinitis (Jumper's and Kicker's Knee)

Etiology   Jumping, as well as kicking or running, may place extreme tension on the knee extensor muscle complex. As a result of one or more commonly repetitive

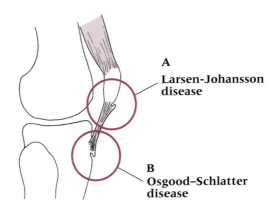

Figure 19-51

Two conditions of the imma-ture extensor mechanism. **A,** Larsen-Johansson disease. **B,** Osgood-Schlatter disease.

A
**Larsen-Johansson
disease**

B
**Osgood–Schlatter
disease**

injuries, tendinitis occurs in the patellar or quadriceps tendon. On rare occasions, a patellar tendon may completely fail and rupture. Sudden or repetitive forceful ex-tension of the knee may begin an inflammatory process that will eventually lead to tendon degeneration.

Symptoms and signs   The athlete will report pain and tenderness at the inferior pole of the patella on the posterior aspect. Patellar tendinitis has been described as having three stages of pain:

- Stage 1—pain after sports activity.
- Stage 2—pain during and after activity (the athlete is able to perform at the ap-propriate level).
- Stage 3—pain during activity and prolonged after activity (athletic performance is hampered); may progress to constant pain and complete rupture.

Management   Any pain in the patellar tendon must preclude sudden explosive movement such as that characterized by heavy plyometric-type exercising. Many ap-proaches to treating athletes with inflammation associated with jumper's knee have been reported, including the use of ice, phonophoresis, iontophoresis, ultrasound, and various forms of superficial heat modalities such as whirlpool together with a program of exercise. A patellar tendon tenodesis brace or strap may also be used (Figure 19-52).

Deep transverse friction massage has been used successfully for treating jumper's knee.[41] Friction is created by firm massage of the patellar tendon at the inferior pa-tellar pole perpendicular to the direction of the fibers. Friction massage is used to increase the process of inflammation so that healing may progress to the fibroblastic phase. Thus when transverse friction massage is used, other techniques for reducing inflammation should not be used.

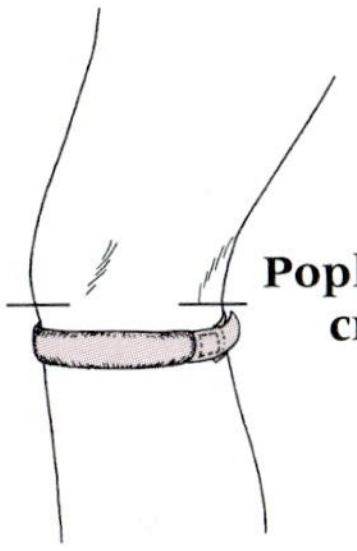

Patellar Tendon Rupture

Etiology   A sudden powerful contraction of the quadriceps muscle with the weight of the body applied to the affected leg can cause a rupture.[56] The rupture may occur to the quadriceps tendon or to the patellar tendon. Usually rupture does not occur unless there has been an inflammatory condition over a period of time in the region of the knee extensor mechanism, causing tissue degeneration. Seldom does a rup-ture occur in the middle of the tendon, but usually it is torn from its attachment. The quadriceps tendon ruptures from the superior pole of the patella, whereas the patellar tendon ruptures from the inferior pole of the patella.

Symptoms and signs   The patella moves upward toward the thigh and the defect can be palpated. The athlete cannot extend the knee. There is considerable swelling with significant pain initially followed by a feeling that the injury may not be all that serious.

Management   A rupture of the patellar tendon usually requires surgical repair. Proper conservative care of jumper's knee can minimize the chances of patellar ten-don rupture. For athletes who use antiinflammatory drugs such as steroids, intense

Lower margin of patella   **Popliteal crease**

Figure 19-52

The chondromalacia brace.

exercise involving the knee must be avoided. Steroids injected directly into these tendons weaken collagen fibers and mask pain.[36]

Runner's Knee (Cyclist's Knee)

Etiology   Runner's knee is a general expression for many repetitive and overuse conditions. Many runner's knee problems can be attributed to malalignment and structural asymmetries of the foot and lower leg, including leg-length discrepancy. Common are patellar tendinitis and patellofemoral problems that may lead to chondromalacia. Two conditions that are prevalent among joggers, distance runners, and cyclists are iliotibial band friction syndrome and pes anserinus tendinitis or bursitis.

ILIOTIBIAL BAND FRICTION SYNDROME   **Iliotibial band friction syndrome** is an overuse condition commonly occurring in runners and cyclists having genu varum and pronated feet.[33] Irritation develops at the band's insertion and, where friction is created, over the lateral femoral condyle.[40] Ober's test (see Chapter 20) will cause pain at the point of irritation. Treatment includes stretching the iliotibial band and performing techniques for reducing inflammation.[28]

PES ANSERINUS TENDINITIS OR BURSITIS   The **pes anserinus** is where the sartorius, gracilis, and semitendinous muscles join to the tibia (see Figure 19-8). Associated with this condition is pes anserinus bursitis. In contrast to iliotibial band friction syndrome, inflammation results from excessive genu valgum and weakness of the vastus medialis muscle. This condition is commonly produced by running on a slope with one leg higher than the other.

Management   Management of runner's or cyclist's knee involves correction of foot and leg alignment problems. Therapy includes cold packs or ice massage before and after activity, proper warm-up and stretching, and avoiding activities such as running on inclines that aggravate the problem. Other management procedures may include administering antiinflammatory medications and using orthotic shoe devices to reduce leg conditions such as genu varum.[49]

The Collapsing Knee

Knee collapse can stem from a variety of reasons. The most common causes of frequent knee collapse include a weak quadriceps muscle; chronic instability of the medial collateral ligament, anterior cruciate ligament, or posterior capsule; a torn meniscus; loose bodies within the knee; a subluxating patella; chondromalacia; and meniscal tears. Frequently the knee will give way in response to pain produced by one of these conditions.

KNEE JOINT REHABILITATION

Rehabilitation of the injured knee joint in an athlete presents a challenge to the athletic trainer who is overseeing the rehabilitation process.[27] The goal of every rehabilitation program is to achieve return to normal activity. For the athlete, "normal" activity involves psychological and physiological stresses that are at a considerably higher level than those on the average person in the population. The athletic trainer must assume the responsibility for rehabilitating the whole athlete and not just the injured knee.

Every athlete who is injured must be treated individually. Attempts to "cookbook" rehabilitation protocols can be frustrating if there is no flexibility to alter a rehabilitation program based on the specific needs of the individual athlete.[32]

It is difficult for anyone supervising rehabilitation programs to stay abreast of the newest techniques and philosophies, which are constantly being updated or altered. This is perhaps more true in the case of injuries involving the knee joint than with any of the other body parts. Rapid advances in technology and surgical techniques, along with an ever-increasing understanding of the physiological, biomechanical, and neural components of knee function, have drastically and repeatedly changed our approach to knee rehabilitation in recent years.

iliotibial band friction syndrome
Runner's knee.

pes anserinus tendinitis
Cyclist's knee.

To best explain the current approach to rehabilitation of the knee, it is necessary to discuss the separate components of a total rehabilitation program.

General Body Conditioning

The athlete must work hard to maintain levels of cardiorespiratory endurance. Full return to activity will be delayed if endurance levels must be improved after the injured knee is rehabilitated. Non–weight-bearing activities such as use of an upper-extremity ergometer, aquatic exercise, and, if range of motion permits, a stationary bicycle can all be performed. It is essential for the athlete to concentrate on maintaining existing levels of strength, flexibility, and proprioception in all other areas of the body throughout the rehabilitation process.

Weight Bearing

Generally, it is best for the athlete to go non–weight bearing on crutches for at least 1 to 2 days after acute injury to the knee. This will allow the healing process to progress well into the inflammatory stage before anything that may interfere with healing is done. Frequently the athlete will be allowed to progress gradually to weight bearing while continuing to wear a rehabilitative brace. The athlete should then progress through touch-down weight bearing, to three-point gait, to four-point gait, and finally to full weight bearing as soon as the healing constraints of the particular injury allow. Injured structures in the knee joint will not heal fully until they are subjected to normal tensile forces and strains.

Knee Joint Mobilization

Mobilization techniques should be incorporated as early as possible to reduce the arthrofibrosis that normally occurs with immobilization.[11] After surgery patellar mobility is generally considered to be the key to regaining normal knee motion. Patellar mobilizations including medial, lateral, superior, and inferior glides should be used along with anterior and posterior tibial glides to ensure the return of normal joint arthrokinematics (Figure 19-53). Constant passive motion (CPM) machines are commonly used to maintain motion in a pain-free arc immediately after surgery (Figure 19-54).

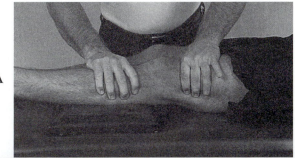

A

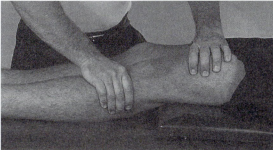

B

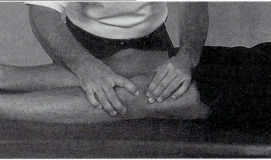

C

Figure 19-53

Knee mobilization techniques. **A,** Posterior femoral glides. **B,** Posterior tibial glides. **C,** Patellar glides.

Figure 19-54

Constant passive motion for the knee.

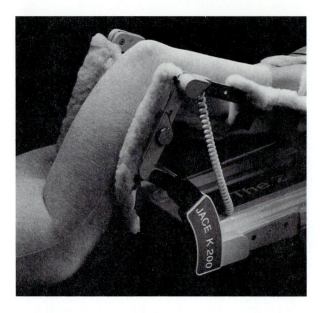

Flexibility

Regaining full range of motion after knee injury is one of the most critical aspects of a knee rehabilitation program. Regardless of whether an injury is treated conservatively or surgically, efforts toward achieving full range of movement are begun on the first day. The athletic trainer should emphasize active range-of-motion exercises throughout the rehabilitation program. Once normal movement of the knee joint has been achieved, efforts should be directed toward maintaining or improving flexibility of each of the muscle groups surrounding the knee joint through stretching. Proprioceptive neuromuscular facilitation (PNF) stretching techniques are most effective.[14,15]

Muscular Strength

Strengthening generally follows a progression from isometric exercise (i.e., straight-leg raises, quad setting) (Figure 19-55), to isotonic exercise stressing both concentric and eccentric components, to isokinetic exercise, to plyometric exercise. In the knee it is essential to concentrate on strengthening all the muscle groups that have some function at that joint, including the quadriceps, hamstrings, abductors, adductors, and gastrocnemius.[48]

Eccentric muscle contraction should be routinely incorporated into strengthening programs with both isotonic and isokinetic exercise. Eccentric contraction of the quadriceps is necessary for deceleration of the lower leg during running. Conversely, the hamstrings must decelerate the lower leg in a kicking motion.[16] Plyometric exercises used during the later phases of rehabilitation use a quick eccentric muscle contraction to facilitate a concentric contraction.

Traditionally, we have tended to make use of the open kinetic chain types of strengthening exercises that use ankle band weights, free weights, machines, and so on. It is important to emphasize closed kinetic chain exercises in which the foot is in contact with the ground. Closed-chain activities are more functional and eliminate many of the stress and shearing forces associated with an open-lever system. Thus they are generally considered to be safer than open-chain exercises. Exercises such as minisquats, step-ups onto a box, leg presses on a machine, use of stationary bicycles, stairmasters, and exercise tubing are examples of closed-chain activities[55] (Figure 19-56). These exercises also emphasize and facilitate cocontraction of antagonistic muscle groups (e.g., quadriceps and hamstrings). This aids in providing appropriate neuromuscular control of opposing muscle groups and thus promotes stability about the joint.[18]

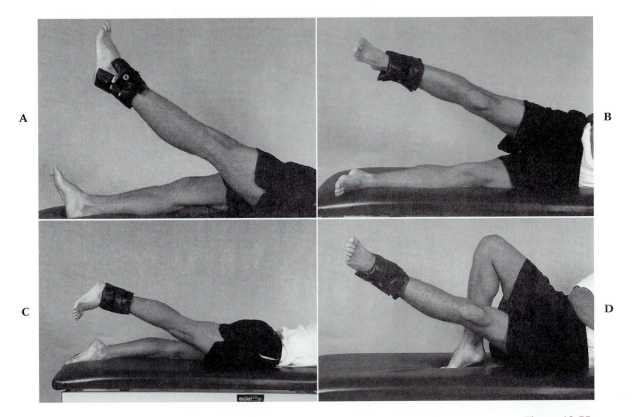

Figure 19-55

Straight-leg raising. **A,** Hip flexion. **B,** Hip abduction. **C,** Hip extension. **D,** Hip adduction.

Proprioceptive neuromuscular facilitation strengthening techniques using D1 and D2 lower-extremity patterns allow the athletic trainer to work on coordinated movement patterns and in particular emphasize the tibial rotation component of knee motion[43] (Figure 19-57).

Neuromuscular Control

Regaining neuromuscular control of joint motion after injury is also important. The athlete quickly "forgets" how to contract a muscle after injury. Loss of neuromuscular control usually occurs because of pain inhibition or swelling. Efforts directed toward proprioceptive control are begun immediately after injury to the knee with weight-shifting exercises on crutches, straight-leg lifts, and quad sets. Strengthening and flexibility exercises mentioned previously will help facilitate return of proprioception. The BAPS board and the KAT system (see Figures 15-4, A and B), a mini tramp, and a slide board can all be used to improve proprioception and balance, as well as the NeuroCom and the Chattex (Figure 19-58).

Bracing

Rehabilitative knee braces have been designed to allow protected motion of either operative or nonoperative knees.[24] Braces enclose the thigh and calf with Velcro straps, are lightweight, and are hinged such that motion can be limited within a specific degree range (see Figure 19-59, A). Depending on the specific injury or the surgical technique used, the knee must be protected in limited ranges for some period of time. The braces are removed during rehabilitation sessions to allow the athlete to work in the greatest range of motion possible. Rehabilitative braces are typically worn for 3 to 6 weeks after surgery.

Functional knee braces are worn to provide some degree of support to the unstable knee on return to activity.[24] All functional braces are custom fitted to some degree and use hinges and posts for support. Some braces use custom-molded thigh and calf enclosures to hold the brace in place whereas others rely on straps for sus-

19-10
Critical Thinking Exercise

A field hockey player is 3 days postop after reconstruction of her knee using a patellar tendon graft. It is essential that she begin active range-of-motion and strengthening exercises as soon as possible.

? What type of strengthening exercises should the athletic trainer recommend?

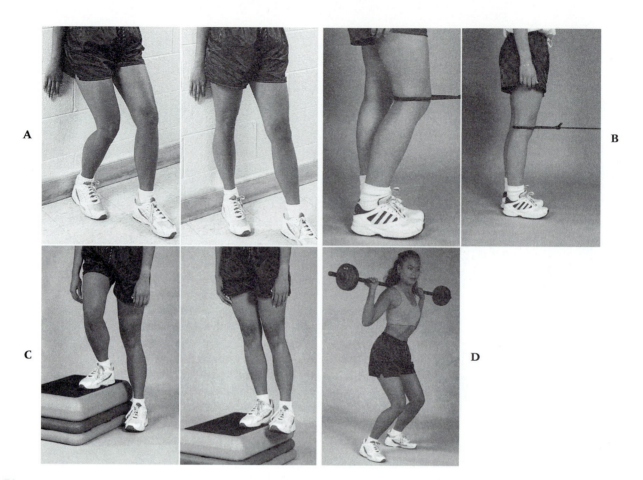

Figure 19-56

Terminal knee extension—closed kinetic chain. **A,** Wall standing—starting position; stopping position. **B,** Using rubber tubing—starting position; stopping position. **C,** Lateral step-ups—starting position; stopping position. **D,** Minisquats.

pension (Figure 19-59, *B, C*). Among the functional braces currently available are the Lennox Hill, CTI, Can-AM, Don Joy RKS, Feaney, Omni TS7, OTI Performer, and the Townsend brace. Braces are designed to improve stability of the ACL-deficient knee by preventing full extension. Some braces attempt to control rotation or varus force. Functional knee braces alone do not seem to be able to control pathological laxity associated with ACL deficiency. However, if combined with an appropriate rehabilitation program, these braces have been shown to restrict anterior-posterior translation of the tibia at low loads.

Functional Progression

Sport-specific skills should be broken down into component parts, and the athlete should be gradually reintroduced to them and progressed through their individual components. For the injured knee a gradual return to running is essential. The athlete should begin with walking (forward, backward, straight line, curve), progressing to jogging (straight, curve, uphill, downhill), running (forward, backward), and then sprinting (straight, curve, large figure-8, small figure-8, zigzag, carioca).

Return to Activity

The decision to permit the athlete to return to full activity should be based on a number of criteria. It is perhaps most important to make sure that the healing process has been given a sufficient chance to repair the injured structure. Objective criteria for return include isokinetic evaluation (torque values at least 90% of the uninjured extremity), arthrometer measurement, and functional performance tests (figure-8s at speed, carioca, hop test, etc.).

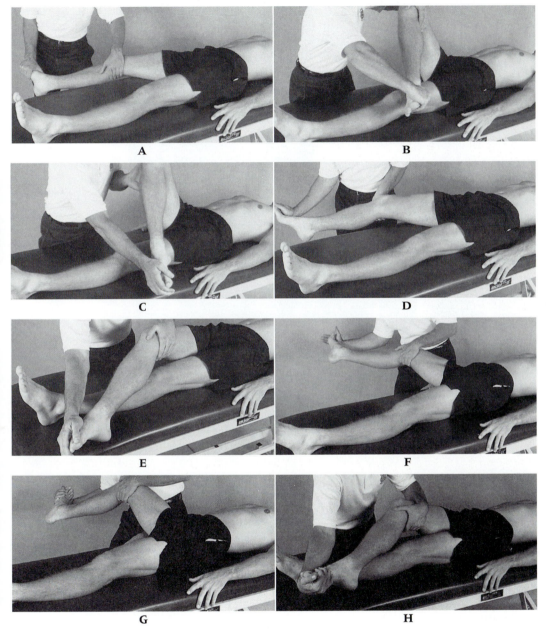

A   B

C   D

E   F

G   H

Figure 19-57

A, D1 lower-extremity pattern moving into flexion-starting position. **B,** D1 lower-extremity pattern moving into flexion-terminal position. **C,** D1 lower-extremity pattern moving into extension-starting position. **D,** D1 lower-extremity pattern moving into extension-terminal position. **E,** D2 lower-extremity pattern moving into flexion-starting position. **F,** D2 lower-extremity pattern moving into flexion-terminal position. **G,** D2 lower-extremity pattern moving into extension-starting position. **H,** D2 lower-extremity pattern moving into extension-terminal position.

Figure 19-58

Balance devices. **A,** Neuro-Com. **B,** Chattex.

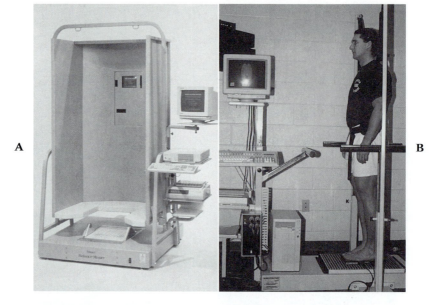

A   B

Figure 19-59

A, Rehabilitative knee brace.
B, C, Functional knee braces.

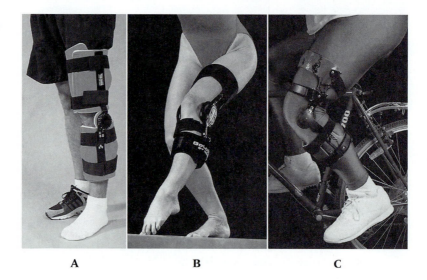

A   B   C

Rehabilitation of Specific Injuries

Throughout this chapter, recommendations and suggestions for management and rehabilitation of specific knee joint injuries have been presented. More detailed rehabilitation protocols are available in other texts that concentrate specifically on rehabilitation of sport-related injuries.

SUMMARY

- The knee is one of the most complex joints in the human body. As a hinge joint that also glides and has some rotation, it is also one of the most traumatized joints in sports. Three structures are most often injured: the medial and lateral collateral capsules and ligaments, the menisci, and the cruciate ligaments.
- Prevention of knee injuries involves maximizing muscle strength and wearing appropriate shoes. Use of protective knee bracing is questionable.
- Acute knee conditions include superficial conditions such as contusions and bursitis. Ligamentous and capsular sprains occur frequently to the medial aspect of the knee and less often to the lateral aspect. The most common ligamentous injury occurs to the anterior cruciate ligament.

- The immediate care of a knee sprain requires rest, ice, compression, and elevation (RICE) for 20 minutes every 1½ hours during waking periods. RICE may be extended for several days, depending on the extent of the injury.
- A meniscus can be injured in a variety of ways, including a rotary force to the knee with the foot planted, a sudden valgus or varus force, or sudden flexion or extension of the knee. There may be severe pain and loss of motion, locking of the knee, and pain in the area of the tear.
- Chronic knee joint problems can occur when the articular cartilage is disrupted. Sometimes pieces of cartilage or bone become loose bodies in the knee joint. These floating pieces can cause chronic knee inflammation, locking, catching, or giving way of the joint.
- The patella and its surrounding area can develop a variety of injuries from sports activities. Some of these injuries are fracture, dislocation, and chronic articular degeneration such as chondromalacia. Other conditions in the region include Osgood-Schlatter disease and jumper's knee.
- The goal of the knee rehabilitation program is to restore the athlete's muscular strength, power, endurance, flexibility, proprioception, and agility. The program varies according to the sport and condition.

Solutions to Critical Thinking EXERCISES

19-1 In full extension when weight bearing, the femur is internally rotated relative to the tibia and is "locked" in this position. The collateral, the cruciates, and the capsular ligaments are tightest in full extension and tend to become more relaxed when moving into flexion. It is possible to injure any of the ligaments in full extension. The posterior cruciate has the least chance of being injured when the knee is fully extended.

19-2 During the evaluation the athletic trainer should look for tightness of the hamstrings or gastrocnemius, tightness of the lateral retinaculum, increased Q angle, tightness of the iliotibial band, pronation of the foot, patella alta, VMO insufficiency, inhibition resulting from the presence of effusion in the knee, or weak hip adductors to which the VMO is attached.

19-3 This is a typical mechanism for a sprain of the anterior cruciate ligament, although other ligamentous, capsular, and meniscal structures may be injured as well. Appropriate stability tests for the ACL include the anterior drawer test done in neutral, internal, and external rotation; Lachman's test; pivot-shift test; jerk test; and the flexion-rotation drawer test.

19-4 It is important to understand that once a ligament has been sprained the inherent stability provided to the joint by that ligament has been lost and will never be totally regained. Thus the athlete must rely on the other structures that surround the joint, the muscles and their tendons, to help provide stability. It is essential for the athlete to work hard on strengthening exercises for all of the muscle groups that play a role in the function of the knee joint.

19-5 A valgus stress test should be used to test the MCL. The examination in full extension tests the MCL, posteromedial capsule, and the cruciates. At 30 degrees of flexion the MCL is isolated. If there is some instability present with the knee in full extension, the athletic trainer should closely evaluate the integrity of the cruciate ligaments.

19-6 The most common mechanism is weight bearing combined with a rotary force while extending or flexing the knee. A large number of medial meniscus lesions are the outcome of a sudden, strong internal rotation of the femur with a partially flexed knee while the foot is firmly planted. Another way a longitudinal tear occurs is by forcefully extending the knee from a flexed position while the femur is internally rotated. During extension the medial meniscus is suddenly pulled back, causing the tear.

19-7 It is likely that the athlete has an inflamed or irritated mediopatellar plica. The mediopatellar plica may be thick, nonyielding, and fibrotic, causing a number of symptoms. The presence of an inflamed mediopatellar plica is sometimes associated with chondromalacia of the medial femoral condyle and patella.

19-8 The athletic trainer should recommend a reduction in the length of the training sessions, in particular limiting the running phase of training. Isometric exercises that are pain free to strengthen the quadriceps and hamstring muscles can be used initially, progressing to closed kinetic chain strengthening exercises. Oral antiinflammatory agents and small doses of aspirin may also be helpful. Wearing a neoprene knee sleeve may also help modulate pain. Use of an orthotic device to correct pronation and reduce tibial torsion can sometimes help eliminate pain.

19-9 A conservative approach would be to use the normal techniques to reduce inflammation, such as rest, ice, ultrasound, and antiinflammatory medications. An alternative and more aggressive technique would be to use a deep transverse friction massage technique to increase the inflammatory response, which will ultimately facilitate healing. If successful, the more aggressive treatment may allow a quicker return to full activity.

19-10 Closed kinetic chain strengthening exercises such as minisquats, lateral or forward step-ups onto a box, leg presses on a machine, use of stationary bicycles, stairmasters or stepping machines, and terminal knee extensions using exercise tubing are all appropriate exercises that can be used safely and effectively almost immediately after surgery. Limitation in range of motion secondary to pain and swelling may restrict the athlete's ability to perform these strengthening exercises.

REVIEW QUESTIONS AND CLASS ACTIVITIES

1. Describe the major structural and functional anatomical features of the knee.
2. Demonstrate the steps that should be taken when assessing the knee.
3. Explain how a knee injury can best be prevented. What injuries are most difficult to prevent?
4. Describe the symptoms, signs, and management of knee contusions and bursitis.
5. Distinguish collateral ligamentous sprains from cruciate sprains.
6. What is the difference between a meniscal lesion and a knee plica?
7. Explain how different fractures (e.g., patellar and epiphyseal fractures) may occur in this region of the knee.
8. Describe the relationship of loose bodies within the knee to osteochondritis dissecans.
9. How do the patella fracture and the patellar dislocation occur?
10. Compare the causes of patellofemoral arthralgia.
11. What types of injuries can occur to the extensor mechanism in a physically immature athlete?
12. Describe and compare the iliotibial band friction syndrome and pes anserinus tendinitis or bursitis.
13. What causes the knee to collapse?
14. Describe knee rehabilitation after conservative treatment of a second-degree medial collateral sprain and after surgical repair of a torn anterior cruciate ligament.

REFERENCES

1. Antich TJ et al: Physical therapy treatment of knee extensor mechanism disorders: comparison of four treatment modalities, *J Orthop Sports Phys Ther* 8:255, 1986.
2. Arno S: The A angle: a quantitive measurement of patella alignment and realignment, *J Orthop Sports Phys Ther* 12(6):237, 1990.
3. Arnosky P: Physiologic principles of ligament injuries and healing. In Scott N, editor: *Ligament and extensor mechanism injuries of the knee: diagnosis and treatment*, St Louis, 1991, Mosby.
4. Arnoczky SP, Warren RF: Microvasculature of the human meniscus, *Am J Sports Med* 10:90, 1982.
5. Blackburn TA Jr et al: An introduction to the plica, *J Orthop Sports Phys Ther* 3:171, 1982.
6. Bergfeld JA: Injury to the anterior cruciate ligament, *Phys Sportsmed* 10:47, 1982.
7. Boland AL Jr: Soft tissue injuries of the knee. In Nicholas JA, Hershman EB, editors: *The lower extremity and spine in sports medicine*, St Louis, 1995, Mosby.
8. Cailliet R: *Knee pain and disability*, ed 2, Philadelphia, 1983, Davis.
9. Colville MR et al: The Lenox Hill brace: an evaluation of effectiveness in treating knee instability, *Am J Sports Med* 14:257, 1986.
10. Coughlin L et al: Knee bracing and anterolateral rotary instability, *Am J Sports Med* 15:161, 1987.
11. Davis M, Prentice W: Rehabilitation of the knee. In Prentice W, editor: *Rehabilitation techniques in sports medicine*, St Louis, 1994, Mosby.
12. DeStefano V: Skeletal injuries of the knee. In Nicholas J, Hirschman E, editors: *The lower extremity and spine in sports medicine*, St Louis, 1995, Mosby.
13. Draper D, Schultheis S: A test for eliminating false positive anterior cruciate ligament injury diagnosis, *J Ath Train* 28(4):355, 1993.
14. Engle B, Canner C: PNF and modified procedures for ACL instability, *J Orthop Sports Phys Ther* 11(6):230, 1990.

15. Engle B, Canner C: Rehabilitation of symptomatic anterolateral knee instability, *J Orthop Sports Phys Ther* 11(6):237, 1990.
16. Engle R: Hamstring facilitation in anterior instability of the knee, *Ath Train* 23(3):226, 1988.
17. Fujiwara L et al: Effect of three lateral knee braces on speed and agility in experienced and nonexperienced wearers, *Ath Train* 25(2):160, 1990.
18. Gryzlo S, Patek R, Pink M: Electromyographic analysis of knee rehabilitation exercises, *J Orthop Sports Phys Ther* 20(1):36, 1994.
19. Harter R et al: A comparison of instrumented and manual Lachman test results in ACL-reconstructed knees, *Ath Train* 25(4):330, 1990.
20. Indelicato P: Isolated MCL tear: nonoperative management. In Torg J, Shepard R, editors: *Current therapy in sports medicine*, St Louis, 1995, Mosby.
21. Inoue M et al: Treatment of the medial collateral ligament injury. I. The importance of anterior cruciate ligament on the varus-valgus knee laxity, *Am J Sports Med* 15:15, 1987.
22. Jensen JE et al: Systemic evaluation of acute knee injuries. In Larson RL, Singer KM, editors: *Clinics in sports medicine*, vol 4, no 2, Philadelphia, 1985, Saunders.
23. Jensen K: Manual laxity tests for anterior cruciate ligament injuries, *J Orthop Sports Phys Ther* 11(10):474, 1990.
24. Johnson C, Bach B: Use of knee braces in athletic injuries. In Scott N, editor: *Ligament and extensor mechanism injuries of the knee: diagnosis and treatment*, St Louis, 1991, Mosby.
25. Kramer PG: Patella malalignment syndrome: rationale to reduce excessive lateral pressure, *J Orthop Sports Phys Ther* 8:301, 1986.
26. Kuhlman K: Meniscal repair. In Torg J, Shepard R, editors: *Current therapy in sports medicine*, St Louis, 1995, Mosby.
27. Leaver D: Rehabilitation of the knee following arthroscopic meniscal repair, *Ath Train* 24(4):349, 1989.
28. Lebsack D et al: Iliotibial band friction syndrome, *Ath Train* 25(4):356, 1990.
29. Lutz G, Warren R: Meniscal injuries. In Griffin L, editor: *Rehabilitation of the injured knee*, St Louis, 1995, Mosby.
30. Lynch M, Henning C: Physical examination of the knee. In Nicholas J, Hirschman E, editors: *The lower extremity and spine in sports medicine*, St Louis, 1995, Mosby.
31. McCarthy M, Buxton B, Hiller D: Current protocols and procedures for anterior cruciate ligament reconstruction and rehabilitation, *J Sport Rehab* 3(3):204, 1994.
32. Mangine R: The knee. In Sanders B, editor: *Sports physical therapy*, Norwalk, Conn, 1990, Appleton & Lange.
33. Martens M: Iliotibial band friction syndrome. In Torg J, Shepard R, editors: *Current therapy in sports medicine*, St Louis, 1995, Mosby.
34. Martin D, Guskiewicz K, Perrin D: Tibial rotation affects anterior displacement of the knee, *J Sport Rehab* 3(4):275, 1994.
35. Montgomery D: Prophylactic knee braces. In Torg J, Shepard R, editors: *Current therapy in sports medicine*, St Louis, 1995, Mosby.
36. Merchant A: Extensor mechanism injuries: classification and diagnosis. In Scott N, editor: *Ligament and extensor mechanism injuries of the knee: diagnosis and treatment*, St Louis, 1991, Mosby.
37. Mont M, Scott N: Classification of ligament injuries. In Scott N, editor: *Ligament and extensor mechanism injuries of the knee: diagnosis and treatment*, St Louis, 1991, Mosby.
38. Nichols C, Johnson R: Cruciate ligament injuries: nonoperative treatment. In Scott N, editor: *Ligament and extensor mechanism injuries of the knee: diagnosis and treatment*, St Louis, 1991, Mosby.
39. Noyes F, Grood E: Classification of ligament injuries: why an anterolateral or anteromedial laxity is not a diagnostic entity. In Griffin P, editor: *Instructional course lectures*, Parkridge, Ill, 1987, American Academy of Orthopaedic Surgeons.
40. Olson DW: Iliotibial band friction syndrome, *Ath Train* 21(1):32, 1986.

41. Pellecchia G, Hame H, Behnke P: Treatment of infrapatellar tendinitis: a combination of modalities and transverse friction massage, *J Sport Rehab* 3(2):125, 1994.

42. Pitman M, Frankel V: Biomechanics of the knee in athletics. In Nicholas J, Hirschman E, editors: *The lower extremity and spine in sports medicine,* St Louis, 1995, Mosby.

43. Prentice W: A manual resistance technique for strengthening tibial rotation, *Ath Train* 23(3):230, 1988.

44. Prentice W, Toriscelli T: The effects of lateral knee stabilizing braces on running speed and agility, *Ath Train* 21(2):112, 1986.

45. Rettig A: Medial and lateral ligament injuries. In Scott N, editor: *Ligament and extensor mechanism injuries of the knee: diagnosis and treatment,* St Louis, 1991, Mosby.

46. Salvaterra G, Wang M, Morehouse C: An in vitro biomechanical study of the static stabilizing effect of lateral prophylactic knee bracing on medial stability, *J Ath Train* 28(2):133, 1993.

47. Scriber K, Matheny M: Knee injuries in college football: an 18-year report, *Ath Train* 25(3):233, 1990.

48. Seto J et al: Rehabilitation of the knee after anterior cruciate ligament reconstruction, *J Orthop Sports Phys Ther* 11(1):8, 1990.

49. Shea K, Fulkerson J: Patellofemoral joint injuries. In Griffin L, editor: *Rehabilitation of the injured knee,* St Louis, 1995, Mosby.

50. Shelbourne D, Klootwyk T, De Carlo M: Ligamentous injuries. In Griffin L, editor: *Rehabilitation of the injured knee,* St Louis, 1995, Mosby.

51. Shelbourne D, Trumper R: Accelerated rehabilitation after ACL reconstruction. In Torg J, Shepard R, editors: *Current therapy in sports medicine,* St Louis, 1995, Mosby.

52. Tria A, Hosea T: Clinical diagnosis of knee ligament injuries. In Scott N, editor: *Ligament and extensor mechanism injuries of the knee: diagnosis and treatment,* St Louis, 1991, Mosby.

53. Wallace L et al: The knee. In Gould J, Davies G, editors: *Orthopaedic and sports physical therapy,* St Louis, 1990, Mosby.

54. Weiss J et al: A functional assessment of anterior cruciate ligament deficiency in an acute and clinical setting, *J Orthop Sports Phys Ther* 11(8):372, 1990.

55. Wilk K, Andrews J: Current concepts in the treatment of anterior cruciate ligament disruption, *J Orthop Sports Phys Ther* 15(6):279, 1992.

56. Woodall W, Welsh J: A biomechanical basis for rehabilitation programs involving the patellofemoral joint, *J Orthop Sports Phys Ther* 11(11):535, 1990.

57. Zarins B, Boyle J: Knee ligament injuries. In Nicholas J, Hershman E, editors: *The lower extremity and spine in sports medicine,* St Louis, 1995, Mosby.

ANNOTATED BIBLIOGRAPHY

Cailliet R: *Knee pain and disability,* ed 2, Philadelphia, 1983, Davis.

Includes both structural and functional anatomy, as well as an in-depth discussion of acute and chronic knee conditions.

Griffin L: *Rehabilitation of the knee,* St Louis, 1995, Mosby.

Incorporates new advances in rehabilitation techniques and equipment and gives emphasis to sport-specific functional rehabilitation programs.

Larson RL, editor: *Symposium on the knee. Clinics in sports medicine,* vol 4, no 2, Philadelphia, 1985, Saunders.

An in-depth monograph about the knee. Presents 15 chapters covering all aspects of the athlete's knee.

Nicholas J, Hershman E: *The lower extremity and spine in sports medicine,* St Louis, 1995, Mosby.

A two-volume set that looks at the entire lower extremity and spine. An excellent comprehensive reference for all joints.

Prentice W: *Rehabilitation techniques in sports medicine,* St Louis, 1994, Mosby.

A comprehensive, well-illustrated text on rehabilitation techniques used in sports medicine. Chapter 14 deals specifically with rehabilitation of the knee and provides up-to-date recommendations for a rehabilitation program.

Scott N: *Ligament and extensor mechanism injuries of the knee,* St Louis, 1991, Mosby.

A comprehensive text that looks at all aspects of the knee joint, including anatomy, biomechanics, ligamentous stability testing, injuries, surgical procedures, bracing, and rehabilitation. Provides an outstanding review of the existing literature on all topics.

The Thigh, Hip, Groin, and Pelvis

When you finish this chapter, you should be able to

- Describe the major anatomical features of the thigh, hip, and pelvis as they relate to sports injuries.
- Identify and evaluate the major sports injuries to the thigh, hip, and pelvis.
- Establish a management plan for a sports injury to the thigh, hip, or pelvis.

Although the thigh, hip, and pelvis have relatively lower incidences of injury than the knee and lower limb, they do receive considerable trauma from a variety of sports activities. Of major concern are thigh strains and contusions and chronic and overuse stresses affecting the thigh and hip.

THE THIGH REGION

Anatomy

The thigh is generally considered that part of the leg between the hip and the knee. Several important anatomical units must be considered in terms of their relationship to sports injuries: the shaft of the femur, musculature, nerves and blood vessels, and the fascia that envelops the thigh.

The Femur

The femur (Figure 20-1) is the longest and strongest bone in the body and is designed to permit maximum mobility and support during locomotion. The cylindrical shaft is bowed forward and outward to accommodate the stresses placed on it during bending of the hip and knee and during weight bearing.

Musculature

The muscles of the thigh may be categorized according to their location: anterior, posterior, and medial.

Anterior Thigh Muscles

The anterior thigh muscles consist of the sartorius and the quadriceps femoris group.

Sartorius The sartorius muscle (Figure 20-2) consists of a narrow band that is superficial throughout its whole length. It stems from the anterosuperior iliac spine and crosses obliquely downward and medially across the anterior aspect of the thigh where it attaches to the anteromedial aspect of the tibial head. It helps flex the thigh at the hip joint, abducts and outwardly rotates the thigh at the hip joint, and inwardly rotates the flexed knee. When the legs are stabilized, both muscles act to flex the pelvis on the thigh. When the sartorius muscle contracts, the pelvis is rotated.

Quadriceps femoris Normally the strongest of the thigh muscles, the quadriceps femoris muscle group (Figure 20-3) consists of four muscles: rectus femoris, vastus medialis, vastus lateralis, and vastus intermedius. These four muscles form a common tendon that attaches distally at the superior border of the patella and indirectly into the patellar ligament, which attaches to the tibial tuberosity.

Rectus femoris The rectus femoris muscle is attached superiorly to the anterior inferior iliac spine and the ilium above the acetabulum and inferiorly to the patella and patellar ligament.

Vastus muscles The vastus medialis and vastus lateralis muscles originate from the lateral and medial linea aspera of the femur. The vastus intermedius muscle originates mainly from the anterior and lateral portion of the femur. Inferiorly, the three

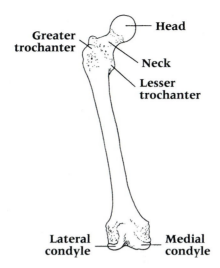

Figure 20-1

Femur (os femoris).

vastus muscles are attached to the rectus femoris muscle and to the lateral and proximal aspects of the patella. Of particular importance is the vastus medialis muscle, which serves as a major stabilizer for patellar tracking.

Functional Anatomy

The function of the quadriceps femoris muscle group is extension of the lower leg or the thigh on the lower leg. The rectus femoris muscle, with its pelvic attachment of the quadriceps muscles, is the only flexor of the thigh at the hip joint. The common peroneal nerve innervates the short head of the rectus femoris muscle, and the tibial portion of the sciatic nerve innervates the long head. This muscle group is innervated by the femoral nerve.

Posterior Thigh Muscles

The posterior thigh muscles include the popliteus and the hamstring muscles.

Hamstring Muscles

Located posteriorly, the hamstring muscle group (Figure 20-4) consists of three muscles: the biceps femoris, semimembranosus, and semitendinosus muscles.

Biceps Femoris

The biceps femoris muscle, as its name implies, has two heads. Its long head originates with the semitendinosus at the medial aspect of the ischial tuberosity. Its short head is attached to the linea aspera below the gluteus maximus attachment on the femur and medial to the attachment of the vastus lateralis. Both muscle heads attach with a common tendon to the head of the fibula.

Semitendinosus

The semitendinosus muscle originates at the medial aspect of the ischial tuberosity along with the biceps femoris muscle. Together with the semimembranosus muscle, the semitendinosus muscle attaches to the medial aspect of the proximal tibia. This attachment is just behind those of the sartorius and gracilis muscles, which all together form the pes anserinus tendon. The tibial branch of the sciatic nerve supplies this muscle.

Semimembranosus

The semimembranosus muscle originates from the lateral aspect of the upper half of the ischeal tuberosity. Moving downward, it attaches into the medial femoral con-

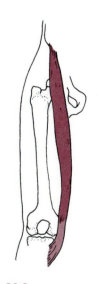

Figure 20-2

Sartorius.

Figure 20-3

Quadriceps femoris.

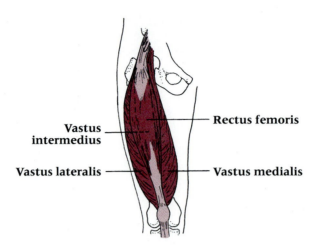

Vastus intermedius

Rectus femoris

Vastus lateralis

Vastus medialis

dyle. It also attaches to the medial side of the tibia, the popliteus muscle fascia, and the posterior capsule of the knee joint. The tibial branch of the sciatic nerve supplies this muscle.

FUNCTIONAL ANATOMY

The hamstring muscles are biarticular, acting as extensors at the hip and flexors at the knee joint. Assisting the hamstrings in knee flexion are the sartorius, gracilis, popliteus, and gastrocnemius muscles. At the hip, hamstrings work in cooperation with the gluteus maximus to extend the hip. Lateral rotation of the leg at the knee is conducted by the biceps femoris muscle. Medial rotation is caused by both the semitendinosus and semimembranosus muscles.

Medial Thigh Muscles

The medial thigh muscles include the gracilis, pectineus, and three adductor muscles.

Gracilis; Pectineus; Adductor Longus, Brevis, and Magnus

Five muscles make up the medial bulk of the thigh: the sartorius; gracilis; and adductor longus, brevis, and magnus muscles. All act as adductors and lateral rotators of the thigh at the hip joint (Figure 20-5).

Gracilis   The gracilis muscle is attached superiorly to the body of the inferior ramus of the pubis and inferiorly to the medial aspect of the proximal tibia. It is a relatively narrow-appearing muscle that adducts the thigh at the hip and flexes and me-

Figure 20-4

Hamstring muscles.

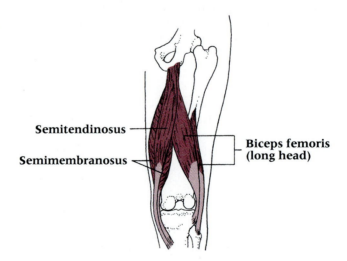

Semitendinosus

Semimembranosus

Biceps femoris (long head)

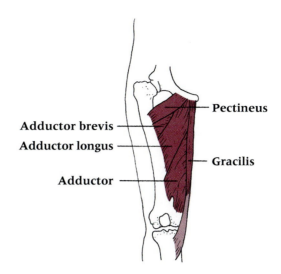

Figure 20-5

Hip adductors.

dially rotates the leg at the knee joint. The anterior branch of the obturator nerve serves this muscle.

Pectineus   The pectineus muscle arises from the pectineal crest of the pubis and attaches distally on the pectineal line of the femur. As one of the adductors, it also flexes and outwardly rotates the thigh.

Adductor longus, brevis, and magnus   The adductor longus, brevis, and magnus muscles originate at the ramus of the pubis and attach inferiorly on the linea aspera of the femur. The muscles adduct the thigh at the hip and outwardly rotate the thigh. All of these muscles assist in the flexion of the thigh.

Nerve Supply

Among nerves that emerge from the sacral plexus are the tibial and common peroneal nerves, which in the thigh form the largest nerve in the body, the greater sciatic nerve. The sciatic nerve supplies the muscles of the thigh and lower leg (see Figure 20-18).

Blood Supply

The main arteries that supply the thigh are the deep medial circumflex femoral, deep femoral, and femoral artery. The two main veins are the superficial great saphenous and the femoral vein (see Figure 20-18).

Fascia

The fascia lata femoris is that part of the deep fascia which invests the thigh musculature. It is relatively thick anteriorly, laterally, and posteriorly but thin on the medial side where it covers the adductors. On its most lateral part, the iliotibial track, an attachment is provided for the tensor fascia lateral and greater aspect of the gluteus maximus.

ASSESSMENT

Thigh injury evaluation is concerned with the femur and the soft tissue that surrounds it.

History

The athletic trainer should ask the following questions:
- Was the onset sudden or slow?
- Has this injury occurred before?
- How was the thigh injured?
- Can the athlete describe the intensity or duration of the pain?

- Is the pain constant? If not, when does it occur?
- Can the athlete specify exactly where the pain is?
- Is the pain related to risk?
- What type of pain is there? Muscle pain is hard to localize, dull, and achy. Vascular pain is sharp, bright, and sometimes burning. Bone pain feels deep, penetrating, and highly localized.

Observation

Compare the thighs:
- Are they symmetrical?
- Are both the same size? Is there swelling?
- Are the skin color and texture normal?
- Is the athlete in obvious pain?
- Is the athlete willing to move the thigh?

Palpation

Both thighs are palpated for comparison with the athlete as relaxed as possible. Feel for the following:
- Tissue tension determing spasm or swelling (hematoma)
- Tissue defects
- Temperature variations
- Point tenderness
- Alteration in skin sensation

Special Tests

NOTE: If a fracture is suspected the following tests are not performed.
- With the knee in extension it is passively flexed. A normal muscle will elicit full range of motion (ROM) that is pain free. One that has swelling or spasm will have restricted passive motion.
- Active movement from flexion to extension that is strong and painful may indicate muscle strain. A movement that is weak and pain free may indicate a third-degree or partial muscle rupture.[12]
- Muscle weakness against an isometric resistance may be indicative of a nerve injury.[12]

PREVENTION OF THIGH INJURIES

As with all muscles in sports the thigh must have maximum strength, endurance, and extensibility to withstand strain. In collision sports such as football thigh guards are mandatory.

Recognition and Management of Specific Thigh Injuries

Injuries to the thigh muscles are among the most common in sports. Contusions and strains occur most often, with the former having the higher incidence.

Quadriceps Contusions

Etiology The quadriceps group is continually exposed to traumatic blunt blows in a variety of vigorous sports. They usually develop as the result of a severe impact to the relaxed thigh, compressing the muscle against the hard surface of the femur. The extent of the force and the degree of thigh relaxation determine the depth of the injury and the amount of structural and functional disruption that take place.

Symptoms and signs Contusions of the quadriceps display all the classic symptoms of most muscle bruises. At the instant of trauma, pain, a transitory loss of function, and immediate capillary effusion usually occur. The athlete usually describes having been hit by a sharp blow to the thigh, which produced intense pain and weakness. Early detection and avoidance of profuse internal hemorrhage are vital, both in effecting a fast recovery by the athlete and in the prevention of widespread scarring. Palpation may reveal a circumscribed swollen area that is painful to the touch.

Grade 1

Grade 1   The grade 1 quadriceps contusion is a superficial intramuscular bruise that produces mild hemorrhage, little pain, no swelling, and mild point tenderness at the site of the trauma. There is no restriction of the range of motion (Figure 20-6, *A*; Table 20-1).

Grade 2   The grade 2 contusion is deeper than grade 1 and produces mild pain, mild swelling, and point tenderness, with the athlete able to flex the knee no more than 90 degrees (Figure 20-6, *B*).

Grade 3   The grade 3, quadriceps contusion is of moderate intensity, causing pain, swelling, and a range of knee flexion that is 90 to 45 degrees with an obvious limp present (Figure 20-6, *C*).

Grade 4   The severe quadriceps, or grade 4, contusion represents a major disability. A blow may have been so intense as to split the fasciae latae, allowing the muscle to protrude (muscle herniation) (Figure 20-6, *D*). A characteristic deep intramuscular hematoma with an intermuscular spread is present. Pain is severe, and swelling may lead to hematoma. Movement of the knee is severely restricted with 45 degrees or less flexion, and the athlete has a decided limp.

Management   The leg should be immediately placed in flexion with an ice pack to avoid muscle shortening (Figure 20-7). Rest, ice, compression, and elevation (RICE), nonsteroidal antiinflammatory drugs (NSAIDs), and analgesics are given as needed. Crutches may be warranted in second- or third-degree contusions. A hematoma that develops may have to be aspirated.[6] One or two units of blood may be lost into the anterior thigh. After exercise or rebumping, RICE must be routinely applied to the thigh. Follow-up care consists of ROM exercises and PRE within a pain-free limitation. Heat, massage, and ultrasound should be avoided to prevent the possibility of myositis ossificans (Figure 20-8).

Generally the rehabilitation of a thigh contusion should be handled conservatively. Cold packs combined with gentle stretching may be the preferred treatment. If heat therapy is used, it should not be initiated until the acute phase of the injury has clearly passed. An elastic bandage should be worn to provide constant pressure and mild support to the quadriceps area. Exercise should be graduated from mild stretching of the quadriceps area in the early stages of the injury to swimming, if possible, and then to jogging and running. Exercise should not be conducted if it produces pain.

Medical care of a thigh contusion may include surgical repair of a herniated muscle or aspiration of a hematoma. Some physicians administer enzymes either orally or through injection for the dissolution of the hematoma.

Once an athlete has sustained a grade 3 or grade 4 thigh contusion, great care must be taken to avoid sustaining another contusion. The athlete should routinely

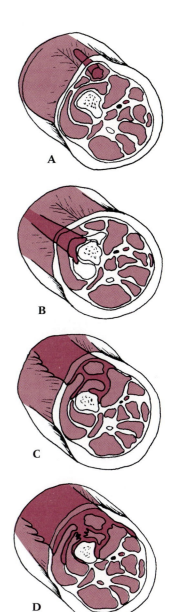

Figure 20-6

Quadriceps contusion. **A,** Grade 1 mild hemorrhage. **B,** Grade 2 mild pain and point tenderness. **C,** Grade 3 moderate pain and swelling. **D,** Grade 4 deep intramuscular hematoma.

TABLE 20-1   Thigh Contusions and Restricted Knee Flexion

Degree of Flexion	Injury Severity
>90°	Grade 1
>45°, <90°	Grade 2
<45°	Grade 3

Figure 20-7

Figure 20-7

Immediate care of the thigh contusion including RICE and a constant stretch of the quadriceps muscle.

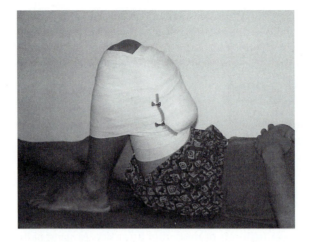

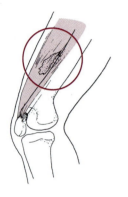

Figure 20-8

Myositis ossificans.

wear a protective pad held in place by an elastic wrap while engaged in sports activity.

Myositis Ossificans Traumatica

Etiology   A severe blow or repeated blows to the thigh, usually to the quadriceps muscle, can lead to ectopic bone production, or **myositis ossificans.** It commonly follows bleeding into the quadriceps muscle and a hematoma. The contusion to the muscle causes disruption of the muscle fibers, capillaries, fibrous connective tissue, and periosteum of the femur. Acute inflammation follows resolution of hemorrhage. The irritated tissue may then produce tissue formations resembling cartilage or bone. Particles of bone may be noted during x-ray examination 2 to 6 weeks after the injury. If the injury is to a muscle belly, complete absorption or a decrease in size of the formation may occur. This is less likely, however, if calcification is at a muscle origin or insertion. In terms of bone attachment, some formations are completely free of the femur, some are stalklike, and some are broadly attached (see Figure 20-8).

Improper care of a thigh contusion can lead to myositis ossificans, the bony deposits or ossification in muscle. The following can initially cause the condition or, once present, aggravate it, causing it to become more pronounced:

- Attempting to "run off" a quadriceps contusion.
- Too-vigorous treatment of a contusion—for example, massage directly over the contusion, ultrasound therapy, or superficial heat to the thigh.

Symptoms and signs   The athlete complains of pain, muscle weakness, soreness, swelling, and decreased muscle function. On examination there is tissue tension and point tenderness along with a decreased ROM.

Management   Once myositis ossificans is apparent, treatment should be extremely conservative. If the condition is painful and restricts motion, the formation may be surgically removed after 1 year with much less likelihood of its return. Too-early removal of the formation may cause it to return. Recurrent myositis ossificans may indicate a blood-clotting problem such as hemophilia, which is a rare condition.

Thigh Muscle Strains

The two major muscle groups in the thigh that are subject to strain are the quadriceps and hamstring groups. (Adductor muscle strain is discussed in the section on hip and pelvic conditions.)

Quadriceps muscle strain   Quadriceps tendon strain is discussed in the section on jumper's problems in Chapter 19.

Etiology   On occasion, the rectus femoris muscle will become strained by a sudden stretch such as falling on a bent knee or a sudden contraction such as occurs during jumping in volleyball or kicking in soccer. Usually it is associated with a muscle that is weakened or one that is overly constricted.

20-1

Critical Thinking Exercise

A basketball player performing a layup shot receives a sharp blow to his right quadriceps muscle.

? How may the grade of this contusion be determined?

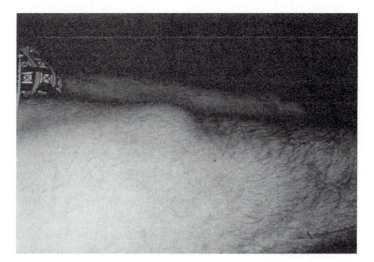

Figure 20-9

Rupture of the rectus femoris.

A tear in the region of the rectus femoris muscle may cause partial or complete disruption of muscle fibers (Figure 20-9). The incomplete tear may be located centrally within the muscle or more peripheral to the muscle.

Symptoms and signs   A peripheral quadriceps femoris muscle tear causes fewer symptoms than the deeper tear. In general, there is less point tenderness and a smaller hematoma. A more centrally located partial muscle tear causes the athlete more pain and discomfort than the peripheral tear. With the deep tear there is a great deal of pain, point tenderness, spasm, and loss of function but with little discoloration from internal bleeding. In contrast, complete muscle tear of the rectus femoris muscle may leave the athlete with little disability and discomfort but with some deformity of the anterior thigh.

Management   Initially, RICE, NSAIDs, and analgesics are given as needed. The extent of the tear should be ascertained as soon as possible before swelling. Swelling can mask the grade of injury. Crutches may be warranted for the first, second, and third days. After the acute inflammatory phase has progressed to resolution and healing has begun, a regimen of isometric muscle contraction, within pain-free limits, can be initiated along with cryotherapy. Other therapy approaches such as cold whirlpool and ultrasound may also be used. Gentle stretching should not be started until the thigh is pain free. A neoprene or elastic sleeve may be worn for support (Figure 20-10).

Hamstring strains   Hamstring strains rank second in incidence of sports injuries to the thigh; of all the muscles of the thigh that are subject to strain, the hamstrings have one of the highest incidences.

Etiology   The exact cause of hamstring strain is not known. It is speculated that a quick change of the hamstring muscle from one of knee stabilization to that of extending the hip when running could be a major cause of strain (Figure 20-11). What leads to this muscle failure and deficiency in the complementary action of opposing muscles is not clearly understood. Possible reasons include muscle fatigue, faulty posture, leg-length discrepancy, tight hamstrings, improper form, or imbalance of strength between hamstring muscle groups. NOTE: Hamstring muscles function as decelerators of leg swing and commonly become injured when an athlete suddenly changes direction or starts to slow. In most athletes the hamstring muscle group should have a strength 60% to 70% of that of the quadriceps group.

It has been theorized that because the short head of the biceps femoris muscle may contract at the same time as the quadriceps muscle as a result of an idiosyncracy of nerve innervation, it is subject to the highest incidence of hamstring strain.

Myositis ossificans can occur from:
  A single severe blow.
  Many blows to a muscle area.
  Improper care of a contusion.

After initial contusion to the anterior thigh, a protective pad should be constructed to disperse the forces occurring with subsequent impacts away from the contused area. This may prevent the development of myositis ossificans altogether.

In order of incidence of sports injury to the thigh, quadriceps contusions rank first and hamstring strains rank second.

Figure 20-10

A neoprene sleeve may be worn for soft-tissue support.

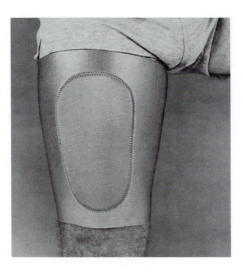

Symptoms and signs Hamstring strain can involve the muscle belly or bony attachment. The extent of injury can vary from the pulling apart of a few muscle fibers to a complete rupture or an avulsion fracture (Figure 20-12).

Capillary hemorrhage, pain, and immediate loss of function vary according to the degree of trauma. Discoloration may occur a day or two after injury.

Grade 1 hamstring strain usually is evidenced by muscle soreness during movement, accompanied by point tenderness. These strains are often difficult to detect when they first occur. Not until the athlete has cooled down after activity do irritation and stiffness become apparent. The soreness of the mild hamstring strain in most instances can be attributed to muscle spasm rather than to the tearing of tissue. Fewer than 20% of fibers are torn in a grade 1 hamstring strain.

A grade 2 hamstring strain represents a partial tearing of muscle fibers, identified by a sudden snap or tear of the muscle accompanied by severe pain and a loss of function during knee flexion. Fewer than 70% of fibers are torn in a grade 2 hamstring tear.

A grade 3 hamstring strain constitutes the rupturing of tendinous or muscular tissue, involving major hemorrhage and disability. With more than 70% of fibers torn, there is severe edema, tenderness, loss of function, ecchymosis, and a palpable mass or palpable gap in the muscle.[11]

Management Initially, RICE, NSAIDs, and analgesics are given as needed. Activity should be reduced until soreness has been completely alleviated.

Figure 20-11

There is a high incidence of hamstring strain in hurdling and sprinting.

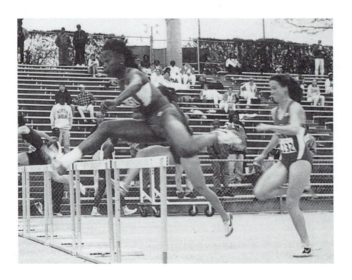

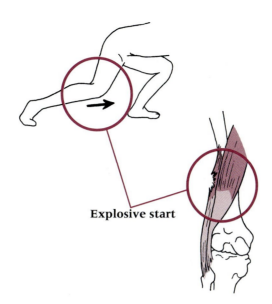

Figure 20-12

Hamstring tear.

Explosive start

In an athlete with a grade 1 hamstring strain, as with the other grades of strain, before he or she is allowed to resume full sports participation, complete function of the injured part must be restored.

Grade 2 and 3 strains should be treated extremely conservatively. For grade 3 strains, RICE should be used for 24 to 48 hours, and for grade 4 strains, for 48 to 72 hours. After the early inflammatory phase of injury has stabilized, a treatment regimen of isometric exercise, cryotherapy, and ultrasound may be of benefit. In later stages of healing, gentle stretching within pain limits, jogging, stationary cycling, and isokinetic exercise at high speeds may be used. After elimination of soreness, the athlete may begin isotonic knee curls. Full recovery may take from 1 month to a full season.

Strains are always a problem to the athlete because they tend to recur as a result of the inelastic, fibrous scar tissue that sometimes forms during the healing process. The higher the incidence of strains at a particular muscle site, the greater the amount of scar tissue and the greater the likelihood of further injury will be. The fear of another pulled muscle becomes, to some individuals, almost a neurotic obsession, which is often more handicapping than the injury itself.

Muscle rehabilitation after injury should emphasize eccentric exercise (Table 20-2).

Femoral Fractures

Acute Fracture

Etiology   In sports, fractures of the femur occur most often in the shaft rather than at the bone ends and are almost always caused by a great force such as falling from a height or being hit directly by another participant. A fracture of the shaft most often takes place in the middle third of the bone because of the anatomical curve at this point, as well as the fact that the majority of direct blows are sustained in this area.

Symptoms and signs   The athlete complains of pain over the fracture site. There is severe pain if weight bearing is attempted. On examination there is swelling and bone movement causing crepitus. Deformity of the thigh may be apparent.

Management   Initially, the athlete is treated for shock. Neurovascular status is verified and a splint applied before being moved. X-ray verifies fracture, followed by reduction and the application of a cast. Analgesics and NSAIDs are given as needed. Shock generally accompanies a fracture of the femur. Bone displacement is usually present as a result of the strength of the quadriceps muscle, which causes overriding of the bone fragments. Direct violence produces extensive soft-tissue injury, with lacerations of the vastus intermedius muscle, hemorrhaging, and major muscle spasms.[14]

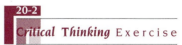

20-2

Critical Thinking Exercise

A sprinter competing in a 100-yard dash experiences a sudden snap, severe pain, and weakness in the left hamstring muscle. Examination reveals a grade 2 strain.

? In terms of exercise, how should this injury be managed?

TABLE 20-2 Management of Muscle-Tendon Injuries of the Hip, Groin and Pelvis

Management	Phase I Acute, 1 to 72 hr	Phase II Healing and Repair	Phase III Maturation and Remodeling
Ice	X		
Compression	X		
Elevation	X		
Rest	X		
Nonsteroidal antiin-flammatory medication	X		
Contrast baths		X	
Whirlpool hydrotherapy		X	
Active range of motion		X	X
Ultrasound		X	X
Muscle stimulation		X	X
Isometric exercise		X	X
Isokinetic/isotonic exercise			X
Stretching			X
Aerobic exercise			X
Proprioceptive activities			X
Agility training			X
Sport-specific activities			X
Jogging			X
Straight-ahead sprint			X
Return to sport			X
Strength and flexibility maintenance			X

Femoral stress fractures are becoming more prevalent because of the increased popularity of repetitive, sustained activities such as distance running.

Femoral stress fracture Femoral overuse fractures represent 10% to 25% of all stress fractures.[11]

Etiology It often stems from excessive downhill or mountain running or in jumping activities. In a compression fracture the fracture occurs more horizontal to the trabeculae. In a distraction type fracture the fracture line occurs perpendicular to the trabeculae of the femoral neck.[10] Stress fractures of the femur are being diagnosed more often than in the past.

Symptoms and signs The athlete complains of a persistent pain in the thigh. X-ray or bone scan reveals the stress fracture. The most common site is in the area of the femoral neck.

Management Analgesics, RICE, and NSAIDs, are given as needed. Range-of-motion exercises and PRE are carried out within pain-free limits. For incomplete fractures rest and limited weight bearing constitute the usual treatment of choice.[7] Complete stress fractures may have to be surgically pinned.

THE HIP, GROIN, AND PELVIC REGION

Normal function of the hip and pelvis is necessary for sports performance. Normal body movement is highly important for sports that predominantly use the lower extremities or the upper extremities. It must be remembered that the hip and pelvis are part of the kinetic chain that transmits a load from the foot to the spine and vice versa in all three planes of movement.

Anatomy

Bones

The pelvis is a bony ring formed by the two innominate bones, the sacrum and the coccyx (Figure 20-13). Each innominate bone is composed of an ilium, ischium, and pubis. The functions of the pelvis are to support the spine and trunk and to transfer their weight to the lower limbs. In addition to providing skeletal support, the pelvis serves as a place of attachment for the trunk and thigh muscles and as protection for the pelvic viscera. The basin formed by the pelvis is separated into a false and a true pelvis. The false pelvis is composed of the wings of the ilium. The true pelvis is composed of the coccyx, the ischium, and the pubis.

The *innominate bones* are three bones that ossify and fuse early in life. They include the ilium, which is positioned superiorly and posteriorly; the pubis, which forms the anterior part; and the ischium, which is located inferiorly. Lodged between the innominate bones is the wedge-shaped *sacrum,* composed of five fused vertebrae.

Articulations

Sacroiliac joint and coccyx   The sacrum is joined to other parts of the pelvis by strong ligaments, forming the sacroiliac joint. A small backward-forward movement is present at the sacroiliac junction. The *coccyx* is composed of four or five small fused vertebral bodies that articulate with the sacrum.

Hip joint   The hip joint is formed by articulation of the femur with the innominate, or hip, bone. The spherical head of the femur fits into a deep socket, the acetabulum, which is padded at its center by a mass of fatty tissue, ligaments, and capsule. The acetabulum, a deep socket in the innominate bone, receives the articulating head of the femur. It forms an incomplete bony ring that is interrupted by a notch on the lower aspect of the socket. The ring is completed by the transverse ligament that crosses the notch. The socket faces forward, downward, and laterally. The femoral head is a sphere fitting into the acetabulum in a medial, upward, and slightly forward direction.

Ligament, joint capsule, and synovial membrane   Surrounding its rim is a fibrocartilage known as the glenoid labrum. A loose sleeve of articular tissue is attached to the circumference of the acetabulum above and to the neck of the femur below. The capsule is lined by an extensive synovial membrane, and the iliofemoral, pubocapsular, and ischiocapsular ligaments give it strong reinforcement. Hyaline cartilage completely covers the head of the femur, with the exception of the fovea capitis, a small area in the center to which the ligamentum teres is attached. The ligamentum

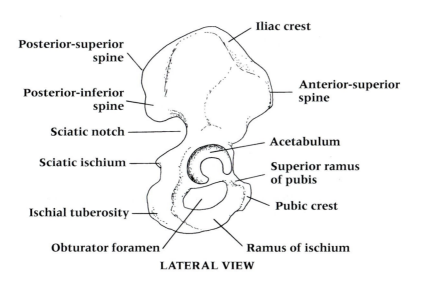

Figure 20-13

Pelvis.

teres gives little support to the hip joint, having as its main function the transport of nutrient vessels to the head of the femur. Because of its bony, ligamentous, and muscular arrangements, this joint is considered by many to be the strongest articulation in the body.

The synovial membrane is a vascular tissue enclosing the hip joint in a tubular sleeve, with the upper portion surrounding the acetabulum. The lower portion is fastened to the circumference of the neck of the femur. Except for the ligamentum teres, which lies outside the synovial cavity, the membrane lines the acetabular socket.

The articular capsule is a fibrous, sleevelike structure covering the synovial membrane, its upper end attaching to the glenoid labrum and its lower end to the neck of the femur. The fibers surrounding the femoral neck consist of circular fibers that serve as a tight collar. This area is called the *zona orbicularis* and acts in holding the femoral head in the acetabulum. Many strong ligaments—the iliofemoral, the pubofemoral, and the ischiofemoral—reinforce the hip joint (Figure 20-14).

The *iliofemoral ligament* (Y ligament of Bigelow) is the strongest ligament of the body. It prevents hyperextension, controls external rotation and adduction of the thigh, and limits the pelvis during any backward rolling of the femoral head during weight bearing. It reinforces the anterior aspect of the capsule and is attached to the anterior iliac spine and the intertrochanteric line on the anterior aspect of the femur.

The *pubofemoral ligament* prevents excessive abduction of the thigh and is positioned anterior and inferior to the pelvis and femur.

The *ischiofemoral ligament* prevents excessive internal rotation and adduction of the thigh and is located posterior and superior to the articular capsule.

Hip Musculature

The muscles of the hip can be divided into anterior and posterior groups. The anterior group includes the iliacus and psoas muscles. The posterior group's muscles include the tensor fasciae latae, gluteus maximus, gluteus medius, gluteus minimus, and the six deep outward rotators—the piriformis, superior gemellus, inferior gemellus, obturator internus, obturator externus, and quadratus femoris.

Anterior hip   The iliacus and psoas muscles are the anterior hip muscles. The triangular-shaped iliacus is contained within the iliac fossa within the abdomen. Its tendon merges with the psoas major muscles, forming a common tendon that is called the iliopsoas. The iliopsoas attaches on the iliac fossa and part of the inner surface of the sacrum proximally, and it attaches distally on the lesser trochanter of the femur. The psoas muscle attaches proximally on the transverse processes and bodies of the lumbar vertebrae. Its distal attachment is on the lesser trochanter. The iliopsoas muscle flexes the thigh at the hip joint and tends to rotate the thigh outwardly and to adduct the thigh when free to move. When fixed, the iliopsoas assists in flexing the trunk and hip.

Posterior hip muscles   The posterior muscles of the hip consist of the tensor fasciae latae, the three gluteal muscles, and the six deep outward rotators.

Figure 20-14

Ligaments of the hip.

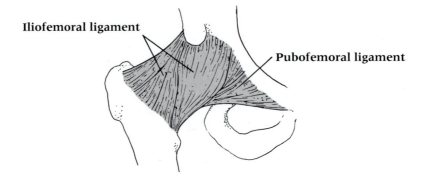

Iliofemoral ligament

Pubofemoral ligament

Tensor fasciae latae   The tensor fasciae latae muscle is located on the upper anterior aspect of the lateral thigh (Figure 20-15). It is attached superiorly to the iliac crest just behind the anterior superior iliac spine and is inserted inferiorly into the iliotibial tract. Its primary action is flexion and medial rotation of the thigh. It is innervated by the superior gluteal nerve.

The gluteal region   The gluteus maximus muscle forms the buttocks in the hip region. Lateral to and underneath the gluteus maximus are the gluteus medius and the gluteus minimus muscles (Figure 20-16). Underneath these larger muscles are much smaller muscles—the piriformis, the obturator internus, and the gemelli (Figure 20-16).

Gluteus maximus   The gluteus maximus muscle is attached above to the posterior aspect of the iliac crest, the sacrum, and the coccyx, as well as to the fascia in the area. Inferiorly, this muscle attaches to the iliotibial tract and into the gluteal tuberosity of the femur between the linea aspera and greater trochanter. It acts as a lateral rotator of the thigh at the hip joint and allows the body to rise from a sitting to a standing position. Through the attachment to the iliotibial tract, it helps extend the flexed knee. The inferior gluteal nerve supplies this muscle.

Gluteus medius   The gluteus medius muscle is located lateral to the hip. It is attached superiorly to the lateral aspect of the ilium and inferiorly to the lateral aspect of the trochanter. The gluteus maximus muscle covers this muscle posteriorly, and it is covered anteriorly by the tensor fasciae latae. It acts primarily as a thigh abductor at the hip, with some flexion and medial rotation occurring from its anterior aspect and some extension and lateral rotation occurring from its posterior aspect. It is innervated by the superior gluteal nerve.

Gluteus minimus   The gluteus minimus muscle originates above the lateral aspect of the ilium and attaches inferiorly to the anterior aspect of the greater trochanter of the femur. Its main action is to cause medial rotation at the hip joint; its secondary action is abduction of the thigh at the hip joint. It is innervated by the superior gluteus nerve.

Deep outward rotators   The six deep outward rotator muscles are positioned behind the hip joint (Figure 20-17). They hold the head of the femur in the acetabulum.

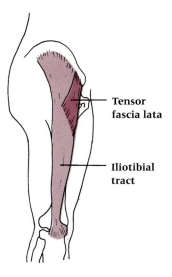

Figure 20-15

Tensor fascia lata.

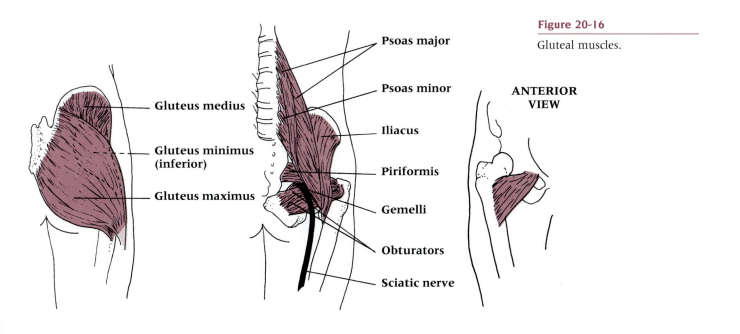

Figure 20-16

Gluteal muscles.

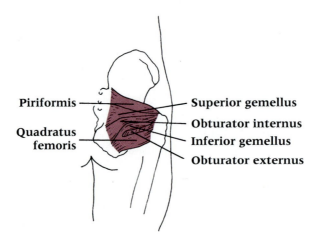

Bursae   The hip joint has many bursae. Clinically, the most important of them are the iliopsoas bursa and the deep trochanteric bursa. The iliopsoas bursa is located between the articular capsule and the iliopsoas muscle on the anterior aspect of the joint. The deep trochanteric bursa lies between the greater trochanter and the deep fibers of the gluteus maximus muscle

Nerve Supply

The lumbar plexus is created by the intertwining of the fibers stemming from the first four lumbar nerves. The femoral nerve, a major nerve emerging from this plexus, later divides into many branches to supply the thigh and lower leg. Nerve fibers from the fourth and fifth lumbar nerves and the first, second, and third sacral nerves form the sacral plexus within the pelvic cavity, anterior to the piriformis muscle. Along with other nerves, the tibial and common peroneal nerves emerge from the sacral plexus and form the large sciatic nerve in the thigh (see Figure 20-18).

Blood Supply

Arteries

Opposite the fourth lumbar vertebra, the aorta divides to become the two common iliac arteries (Figure 20-18). They in turn pass downward to divide, opposite the sacroiliac joint, into the internal and external iliac arteries. Most of the branches of the internal iliac artery supply blood to the pelvic viscera. The external iliac artery is the primary artery to the lower limb.

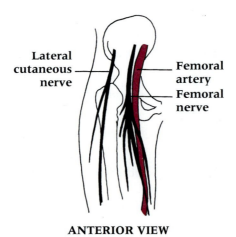

ANTERIOR VIEW

Veins

The major veins in the region of hips, groin, and pelvis include the common iliac vein, which stems from the inferior vena cava on both sides draining the lower body. Next is the internal iliac vein, which ascends behind its iliac artery to the brim of the true pelvis, where it joins the external vein to form the common iliac vein. Its tributaries drain the pelvis and adjoining area. Third is the external iliac vein, which passes upward from the femoral vein behind the inguinal ligament and follows the brim of the true pelvis joining the opposite to the sacroiliac joint and the internal iliac vein.

FUNCTIONAL ANATOMY

The hip joint is a ball-and-socket joint that has maximum stability because of deep insertion into the acetabulum. The acetabulum faces outward, forward, and downward. The capsular pattern of the hip is flexion, abduction, and medial rotation. The forces involved in the hip are as follows: standing—one third of the body weight; standing on one foot—2.4 to 2.6 times the body weight; walking—1.3 to 5.8 times the body weight; and running—4.5 times the body weight.[12]

The sacroiliac joints and symphysis pubis do not have direct control of their movements. They are influenced by the muscles that influence the lumbar spine and hip. Many of these muscles attach to the sacrum and pelvis. Movement occurring in the sacroiliac and symphysis pubis joints is slight when compared with the hip and spinal joints.[11]

ASSESSMENT OF THE HIP AND EXTERNAL PELVIS

The hip and pelvis form the body's major power source for movement. The body's center of gravity is located just in front of the upper part of the sacrum. Injuries to the hip or pelvis cause the athlete major disability in the lower limb, trunk, or both.

Because of the close proximity of the hip and pelvis to the low back region, many evaluative procedures overlap.

History

The following information is determined from the athlete:
- What are your symptoms (e.g., weakness, disability, pain)?
- When did you first notice a problem with the hip or pelvis?
- Describe types of pain (hip pain is felt mainly in the groin and medial or frontal side of thigh; hip pain may also be referred to the knee).
- Describe the sacroiliac pain; does it radiate in the posterior thigh, iliac fossa, or buttock on the affected side?
- When does the pain occur (e.g., during activity, while turning in bed)?
- Age and gender of the athlete (e.g., boys 3 to 12 years old can have Legg-Calvé-Perthes disease; distance-running amenorrheic girls may develop a hip stress fracture).

Observation

The athlete should be observed for postural asymmetry while standing on one leg and during ambulation.

The athlete with an external pelvic pain must be observed for postural asymmetry.

Postural Asymmetry
- From the front view, do the hips look even? A laterally tilted hip could mean a leg-length discrepancy or abnormal muscle contraction on one side of the hip or low back region.
- From the side view, is the pelvis abnormally tilted anteriorly or posteriorly? This tilting may indicate lordosis or flat back, respectively.
- In lower-limb alignment, is there indication of genu valgum, genu varum, foot pronation, or genu recurvatum? The patella should also be noted for relative position and alignment.

■ The posterior superior iliac spines, represented by the skin depressions above the buttocks, should be horizontal to one another. Uneven depressions could indicate that the pelvis is laterally tilted.

Standing on One Leg

Standing on one leg may produce pain in the hip, abnormal movement of the symphysis pubis, or a fall of the pelvis on the opposite side as a result of abductor weakness.

Ambulation

The athlete should be observed during walking and sitting. Pain in the hip and pelvic region will normally be reflected in movement distortions.

Palpation

Bony Palpation

The following bony sites should be palpated for pain and continuity:

Anteriorly	Posteriorly
■ Anterior superior iliac spine	■ Posterior superior
■ Iliac crest	■ Ischial tuberosity
■ Greater trochanter	■ Sacroiliac joint
■ Pubic tubercle	

Soft-Tissue Palpation

The soft-tissue sites of major concern are those lying in the groin region, the femoral triangle, sciatic nerve, and major muscles.

Groin Palpation

Groin pain could result from swollen lymph glands, indicating an infection, or from an adductor muscle strain. The adductors may have point tenderness at any point along their length. Resisted motion may make pain worse.

Muscle Palpation

The following muscles should be palpated for pain, swelling, or fiber disruption:

■ Iliopsoas	■ Adductor longus and brevis
■ Sartorius	■ Adductor magnus
■ Rectus femoris at the hip joint	■ Gluteus medius
■ Gracilis	■ Gluteus maximus
■ Pectineus	■ Hamstring muscles at their origin

Special Tests

Functional Evaluation

The athlete is led through all possible hip movements, both passive and active, to evaluate range of motion and active and resistive strength (Figure 20-19). These movements are as follows: hip abduction, hip adduction, hip flexion, hip extension, and internal and external hip rotation.

Tests for Hip Flexion Tightness

Contractures of the hip flexors are major causes of lordosis and susceptibility to groin pain and discomfort. Two tests can be used: the Kendall test and the Thomas test.

Kendall test   The athlete lies supine on a table with one knee flexed on the chest and the back completely flat (Figure 20-20). The other knee is flexed over the table's

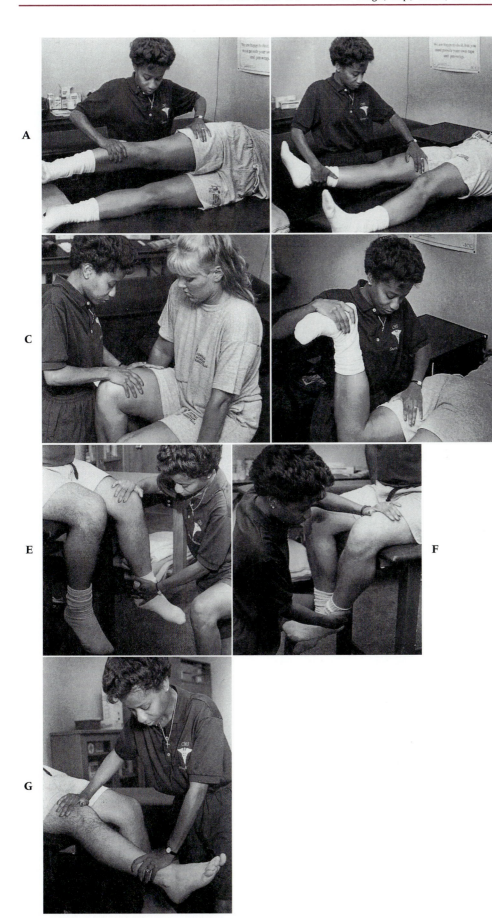

Figure 20-19

Manual muscle tests of the hip. **A,** Abduction. **B,** Adduction. **C,** Flexion (iliopsoas muscle). **D,** Extension. **E,** Internal rotation. **F,** External rotation. **G,** Knee extension to isolate the rectus femoris.

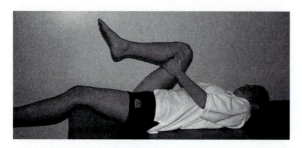

Figure 20-20

Kendall test for hip flexor tightness.

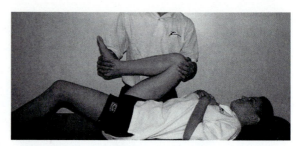

Figure 20-21

Demonstrating tight hip flexors.

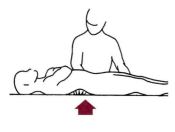

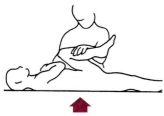

Figure 20-22

Thomas test for hip contractures.

end. Normal extensibility of the hip flexors allows the thigh to touch the table, with the knee flexed approximately 70 degrees. Tight hip flexors are revealed by the inability of the thigh to lie flat on the table. If only the rectus femoris muscle is tight, the thigh will touch the table, but the knee will extend more than 70 degrees (Figure 20-21).

Thomas test   The Thomas test indicates whether hip contractures are present (Figure 20-22). The athlete lies supine on a table, arms across the chest, legs together and fully extended. The athletic trainer places one hand under the athlete's lumbar curve; one thigh is brought to the chest, flattening the spine. In this position the extended thigh should be flat on the table. If not, there is a hip contracture. When the athlete fully extends the leg again, the curve in the low back returns.

Femoral Anteversion and Retroversion

The athlete with a painful hip problem may also have a discrepancy in the relationship between the neck of the femur and the shaft of the femur. The normal angle of the femoral neck is 15 degrees anterior to the long axis of the shaft of the femur and femoral condyles. Athletes who walk in a toe-in manner may be reflecting a hip deformity in which the femoral neck is directed anteriorly (femoral anteversion). In contrast, athletes who walk in a pronounced toe-out manner may be displaying a condition in which the femoral neck is directed posteriorly (femoral retroversion) (Figure 20-23). Internal hip rotation in excess of 35 degrees and (in the case of femoral retroversion) an excess of the normal 45 degrees of external rotation are characteristic of femoral anteversion.

Figure 20-23

A, Anteversion of the femoral neck. When the knee is directed anteriorly, the femoral neck is directed *anteriorly* to some degree. **B,** Retroversion of the femoral neck. When the knee is directed posteriorly, the femoral neck is directed *posteriorly* to some degree.

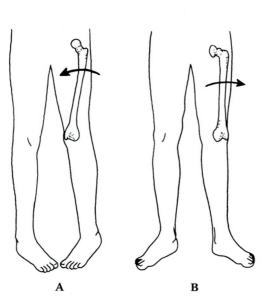

A   B

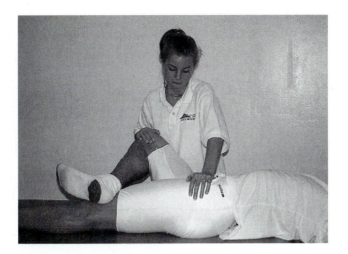

Figure 20-24

Patrick's test for a pathological condition of the hip and sacro-iliac joint.

Test for the Hip and Sacroiliac Joint

Patrick test   The Patrick test detects pathological conditions of the hip and sacro-iliac joint (Figure 20-24). The athlete lies supine on the examining table. The foot on the side of the painful sacroiliac is placed on the opposite extended knee. Pressure is then applied downward on the bent knee. Pain may be felt in the hip or sacroiliac joint.

Testing the tensor fasciae latae and iliotibial band   Three tests that can be used to discern iliotibial band tightness and inflammation of the bursa overlying the lateral femoral epicondyle or direct irritation of the iliotibial band and periosteum are Renne's test, Nobel's test, and Ober's test[2] (Figure 20-25).

Renne's test   While standing, the athlete supports full weight on the affected leg, with the knee bent at 30 to 40 degrees. A positive response of fasciae latae tightness occurs when pain is felt at the lateral femoral condyle.

Nobel's test   The athlete's knee is flexed to 90 degrees, and pressure is applied to the lateral femoral epicondyle while the knee is gradually extended. A positive response occurs when severe pain is felt at the lateral femoral epicondyle with the knee at 30 degrees of flexion.

Ober's test   The athlete lies on the unaffected side. With the knee flexed at 90 degrees, the affected thigh is abducted as far as possible. With the pelvis stabilized,

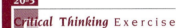

20-3

Critical Thinking Exercise

A gymnast has a history of moderate groin pain. She is susceptible to strains in that region. The athlete also appears to have an exaggerated lumbar lordotic curve.

? What tests should be given to evaluate the tightness of the groin region?

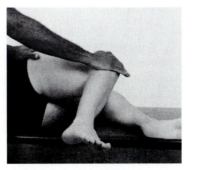

Figure 20-25

Ober's test for iliotibial band tightness.

Figure 20-26

A, Measuring for leg-length discrepancy. **B,** Anatomical discrepancy. **C,** Functional discrepancy.

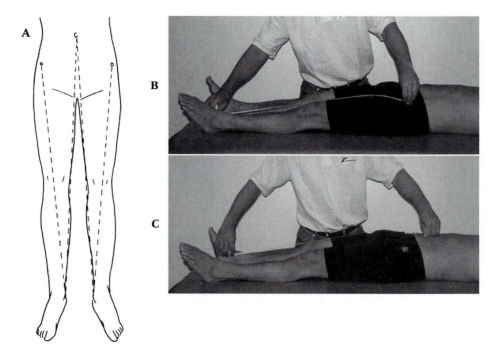

the abducted thigh is then relaxed and allowed to drop into adduction. A contracted tensor fasciae latae or iliotibial band will keep the thigh in an abducted position, not allowing it to fall into adduction.

Measuring Leg-Length Discrepancy

In individuals who are not physically active, leg-length discrepancies of over 1 inch may produce symptoms; however, shortening of as little as 3 mm (⅛ inch) may cause symptoms in highly active athletes. Such discrepancies can cause cumulative stresses to the lower limbs, hip, and pelvis or low back.

There are two types of leg-length discrepancy—true, or anatomical, shortening and apparent, or functional, shortening. X-ray examination is the most valid means of measurement. It is difficult to be completely accurate because of mobility of the soft tissue over bony landmarks (Figure 20-26, *A*).

Anatomical discrepancy   In an anatomical discrepancy, shortening may be equal throughout the lower limb or localized within the femur or lower leg. The athlete lies supine and fully extended on the table. Measurement is taken between the lateral malleoli and the anterior superior iliac spine of each leg (Figure 20-26, *B*).

Functional discrepancy   Functional leg shortening can occur as the result of lateral pelvic tilt (obliquely) or from a flexion or adduction deformity (Figure 20-26, *C*). Measurement is taken from the umbilicus to the medial malleoli of each ankle.

Leg-length discrepancy in an athlete can lead to stress-related physical injuries.

RECOGNITION AND MANAGEMENT OF SPECIFIC HIP, GROIN, AND PELVIC INJURIES
Groin Strain

The groin is the depression that lies between the thigh and the abdominal region. The musculature of this area includes the iliopsoas, the rectus femoris, and the adductor group (the gracilis, pectineus, adductor brevis, adductor longus, and adductor magnus). Any one of these muscles can be torn during sports activity and elicit what is commonly considered a groin strain (Figure 20-27).

Etiology   The adductor longus muscle is most often strained.[5] Running, jumping, or twisting with external rotation can produce such injuries.

Symptoms and signs   The groin strain is one of the most difficult injuries to care for in sports. The strain can be felt as a sudden twinge or feeling of tearing during an

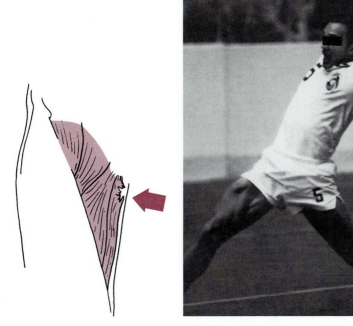

Figure 20-27

Many sports that require severe stretch of the hip region can cause a groin strain.

active movement, or the athlete may not notice it until after termination of activity.[5] As is characteristic of most tears, the groin strain produces pain, weakness, and internal hemorrhage.

Management   If it is detected immediately after it occurs, the strain should be treated by RICE, NSAIDs, and analgesics as needed for 48 to 72 hours.

Passive, active, and resistive muscle tests should be given to ascertain the exact muscle or muscles that are involved. Difficulty is frequently encountered when attempting to care for a groin strain.

In these cases rest has been the best treatment. Daily whirlpool therapy or cryotherapy are palliative; ultrasound offers a more definite approach. Exercise should be delayed until the groin is pain free.[16] Exercise rehabilitation should emphasize gradual stretching and restoration of the normal range of motion. Until normal flexibility and strength are developed, a protective spica bandage or a commercial brace should be applied (Figure 20-28) (see also Figures 13-4 and 13-5). See Table 20-2 for suggestions about managing muscle-tendon injuries of the hip and pelvis.

Trochanteric Bursitis

Trochanteric bursitis is a relatively common condition of the greater trochanter of the femur (Figure 20-29).

Etiology   Although commonly called bursitis, it also could be an inflammation at the site where the gluteus medius muscle inserts or the iliotibial band passes over the trochanter.

Symptoms and signs   The athlete complains of pain in the lateral hip. Pain may radiate down to the knee, causing a limp. Palpation reveals tenderness over the lateral aspect of the greater trochanter. Tests for tensor fascial latae and iliotibial tightness should be carried out.

Management   Therapy initially includes RICE, NSAIDs, and analgesics as needed. Range-of-motion and progressive-resistive exercises directed toward hip abductors and external rotators should follow. Phonophoresis may be added if the athlete does not respond in 3 to 4 days. Returning to running should be cautious; the athlete should avoid running on inclined surfaces. Faulty running form, leg-length discrepancy, and faulty foot biomechanics must be taken into consideration. It is most com-mon among women runners who have an increased Q angle or a leg-length discrepancy.

An increased Q angle or leg-length discrepancy can lead to trochanteric bursitis in women runners.

Figure 20-28

Commercial restraints such as the Sawa groin and thigh braces are increasingly being used by athletic trainers.

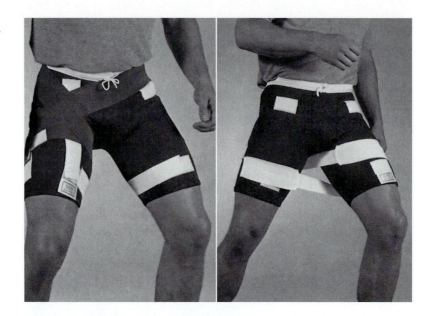

Conditions of the Hip Joint

The hip joint, the strongest and best-protected joint in the human body, is seldom seriously injured during sports activities.

Sprains of the Hip Joint

The hip joint is substantially supported by the ligamentous tissues and muscles that surround it, so any unusual movement that exceeds the normal range of motion may result in tearing of tissue.

Etiology Such an injury may occur as the result of a violent twist, either produced through an impact force delivered by another participant or by forceful contact with another object or sustained in a situation in which the foot is firmly planted and the trunk is forced in an opposing direction.

Symptoms and signs A hip sprain displays all the signs of a major acute injury but is best revealed through the athlete's inability to circumduct the thigh. Symptoms are similar to a stress fracture. There is significant pain in the hip region. Hip rotation increases pain.

Management X-ray or magnetic resonance imaging (MRI) should be done to rule out fracture; RICE, NSAIDs, and analgesics are given as needed. Depending on the grade of sprain, weight bearing is restricted. Crutch walking is used for grade 2 and 3 sprains. Range-of-motion and progressive-resistive exercises are delayed until the hip is pain free.

20-4

Critical Thinking Exercise

A field hockey player has been determined to have a Q angle of 22 degrees. Her left leg is ¾ inch shorter than her right leg. She complains of pain at the point just over the left greater trochanter when she runs.

? Based on the information provided, what could the condition be?

Figure 20-29

Tenderness sites in the region of the hip and pelvis.

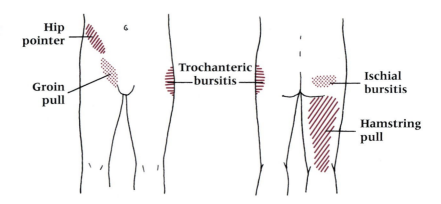

Acute Groin Strain

Injury Situation A woman varsity basketball player had a history of tightness in her groin. During a game she suddenly rotated her trunk while also stretching to the right side. There was a sudden sharp pain and a sense of "giving way" in the left side of the groin that caused the athlete to immediately stop play and limp to the sidelines.

Symptoms and Signs As the athlete described it to the athletic trainer, there was severe pain when rotating her trunk to the right and flexing her left hip. Inspection revealed the following:
1. There was major point tenderness in the groin, especially in the region of the adductor magnus muscle.
2. There was no pain during passive movement of the hip, but severe pain did occur during both active and resistive motion.
3. When the groin and hip were tested for injury, the hip joint, illiopsoas, and rectus femoris muscles were ruled out as having been injured; however, when the athlete adducted the hip from a stretch position, it caused her extreme discomfort.

Management Plan Based on the athletic trainer's inspection, with findings confirmed by the physician, it was determined that the athlete had sustained a grade 2 strain of the groin, particularly to the adductor magnus muscle.

Phase 1 Acute Injury **GOALS:** To stop hemorrhage, reduce pain, and stop muscle spasms.
ESTIMATED LENGTH OF TIME (ELT): 2 to 3 days.

■ **Therapy** Careful physical examination plus MRI to rule out conditions other than a strain. IMMEDIATE CARE: RICE (20 min) intermittently, six to eight times daily. When weight bearing, the athlete wears a 6-inch elastic hip spica

■ **Exercise rehabilitation** No exercise—as complete rest as possible.

Phase 2 Repair **GOALS:** To reduce pain, control spasm, and restore full ability to contract and stretch the adductor longus muscle. Maintain cardiorespiratory fitness.
ELT: 2 to 3 weeks.

■ **Therapy** Ice massage (1 min) three to four times daily followed by hip ROM movements. Muscle electrical stimulation using the surge current at 7 or 8, depending on athlete's tolerance, together with ultrasound, set at 1 W/cm² (7 min) once daily and cold therapy in the form of ice massage (7 min) or ice packs (10-15 min) followed by exercise, two to three times daily.

■ **Exercise** Rehabilitation: Proprioceptive neuromuscular facilitation hip patterns two to three times daily after cold application, progressing to progressive-resistive exercise (PRE) using pulley, isokinetic, or free weights (10 repetitions, three sets) once daily. "Jogging" in chest-level water (10 to 20 min) one or two times daily for first exercise rehabilitation week followed by flutter kick swimming (pain free) once daily during subsequent weeks. General body maintenance exercises are conducted three times a week as long as they do not aggravate the injury.

Phase 3 Remodeling **GOALS:** To restore full power, endurance, and muscle extensibility. The athlete gradually returns to precompetition exercise and finally competition wearing a groin restraint.
ELT: 3 to 6 weeks.

■ **Therapy** If symptom free, precede exercise with ice massage (7 min) or ice pack (5 to 15 min).

Continued

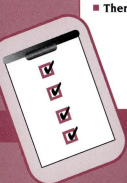

Acute Groin Strain—*cont'd*

■ **Exercise Rehabilitation** Engage in ROM exercise and PRE. Begin a program of jogging on flat course, slowly progressing to a 3-mile run once daily and then progressing to figure-8s, starting with obstacles 10 feet apart and gradually shortening distance to 5 feet, from one-half speed to full speed.

Criteria for Returning to Competitive Basketball

1. As measured by an isokinetic dynamometer, the athlete's injured hip should have strength equal to that of the uninjured hip.
2. Hip has full range of motion.
3. The athlete is able to run figure-8s around obstacles set 5 feet apart at full speed.

20-5

Critical Thinking Exercise

A 15-year-old male football player complains of pain in his hip off and on during the season. There is increasing hip and knee pain during movement. The athlete has a restriction of hip abduction, flexion, and medial rotation. He is beginning to walk with a limp.

? What should the athletic trainer be concerned with in this 15-year-old, and what steps should be taken?

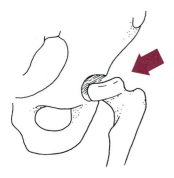

Figure 20-30

Legg-Calvé-Perthes disease (coxa plana). Arrow indicates avascular necrosis of the femoral head.

Subluxation—Dislocated Hip Joint

Dislocation of the hip joint rarely occurs in sports and then usually only as the end result of traumatic force directed along the long axis of the femur.

Etiology Such dislocations are produced when the knee is bent. The most common displacement is one posterior to the acetabulum, with the femoral shaft adducted and flexed.

Symptoms and signs The injury presents a picture of a flexed, adducted, and internally rotated thigh. Palpation will reveal that the head of the femur has moved to a position posterior to the acetabulum. A hip dislocation causes serious pathology by tearing capsular and ligamentous tissue. A fracture is often associated with this injury, accompanied by possible damage to the sciatic nerve.

Management Medical attention must be secured immediately after displacement, or muscle contractures may complicate the reduction. Immobilization usually consists of 2 weeks of bed rest and the use of a crutch for walking for a month or longer.

Complications Complication of the posterior hip dislocation is likely, with the possibilities of a palsy of the sciatic nerve and later the development of osteoarthritis. Hip dislocation also can lead to disruption of the blood supply to the head of the femur, which eventually leads to the degenerative condition known as avascular necrosis.[4]

Immature Hip Joint and Pelvic Problems

The coach or athletic trainer working with a child or adolescent should understand two major problems stemming from the immature hip joint. They are Legg-Calvé-Perthes avascular necrosis (coxa plana) and the slipped capital femoral epiphysis.

Legg-Calvé-Perthes Disease (Coxa Plana)

Legg-Calvé-Perthes disease is avascular necrosis of the femoral head (Figure 20-30). It occurs in children ages 4 to 10 and in boys more often than in girls.

Etiology For the most part this condition is not clearly understood. Trauma accounts for 25% of the cases seen.[1] It is listed under the broad heading of osteochondrosis. Because of a disruption of circulation at the head of the femur, articular cartilage becomes necrotic and flattens.

Symptoms and signs   The young athlete commonly complains of pain in the groin that sometimes is referred to the abdomen or knee. Limping is also typical. The condition can have a rapid onset, but more often it comes on slowly over a number of months. Examination may show limited hip movement and pain.

Management   Care of this condition could mean complete bed rest to alleviate synovitis. A special brace to avoid direct weight bearing on the hip may have to be worn. If treated in time, the head of the femur will revascularize and reossify.

Complications   If the condition is not treated early enough, the head of the femur will become ill shaped, creating problems of osteoarthritis in later life.

Slipped Capital Femoral Epiphysis

The problem of a slipped capital femoral epiphysis (Figure 20-31) is found mostly in boys between the ages of 10 and 17 who are characteristically tall and thin or obese.

Etiology   Although idiopathic, it may be related to the effects of a growth hormone. One quarter of those seen are in both hips. Trauma accounts for 25% of the cases seen.[1] X-ray examination may show femoral head slippage posteriorly and inferiorly.

Symptoms and signs   As with Legg-Calvé-Perthes disease, the athlete has a pain in the groin that comes on suddenly as a result of trauma or over weeks or months as a result of prolonged stress. In the early stages of this condition signs may be minimal; however, in its most advanced stage there is hip and knee pain during passive and active motion; limitations of abduction, flexion, and medial rotation; and a limp.[9]

Management   In minor slippage, rest and non–weight bearing may prevent further slipping. Major displacement usually requires corrective surgery.

Complications   If the slippage goes undetected or if surgery fails to properly restore normal hip mechanics, severe hip problems may occur in later life.

The Snapping Hip Phenomenon

The snapping hip phenomenon is common to young female dancers, gymnasts, and hurdlers, who make similar use of their hips.

Etiology   The problem stems from habitual movements that predispose muscles around the hip to become imbalanced.[13] This condition commonly occurs when the individual laterally rotates and flexes the hip joint as part of the exercise or dance routine. This condition is related to a structurally narrow pelvic width, greater range of motion of hip abduction, and less range of motion in lateral rotation. With hip stability becoming lessened, the hip joint capsule and ligaments and adductor muscles become less stable.

Symptoms and signs   The athlete complains that snapping occurs, especially when balancing on one leg. Such a problem should not go unattended, especially if pain and inflammation are associated with the snapping.

Management   Management should focus on cryotherapy and ultrasound to stretch tight musculature and strengthen weak musculature in the hip region.

Pelvic Conditions

Athletes who perform activities involving jumping, running, and violent collisions can sustain serious acute and overuse injuries to the pelvic region. During running the pelvis rotates along a longitudinal axis proportionate to the amount of arm swing. It also tilts up and down as the leg engages in support and nonsupport. This combination of motion causes shearing at the sacroiliac joint and symphysis pubis. There is also tilting of the pelvis, producing both a decrease and an increase in lumbar lordosis, depending on the slant of the running surface. Running downhill increases lumbar lordosis, and running uphill decreases it.

Contusion (Hip Pointer)

Iliac crest contusion and contusion of the abdominal musculature, commonly known as a hip pointer, occurs most often in contact sports (Figure 20-32).

A young athlete complaining of pain in the groin, abdomen, or knee and walking with a limp may display signs of Legg-Calvé-Perthes disease or a slipped capital femoral epiphysis.

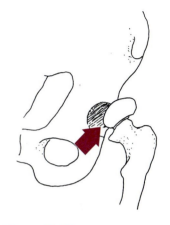

Figure 20-31

Slipped capital femoral epiphysis *(arrow)*.

Figure 20-32

A blow to the pelvic rim can cause a bruise and hematoma known as a hip pointer.

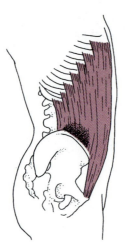
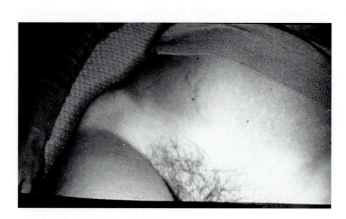

20-6

Critical Thinking E x e r c i s e

A young female gymnast complains to the athletic trainer that her hip snaps when she stands on one leg.

? What is the possible cause of this snapping hip phenomenon?

Etiology   The hip pointer results from a blow to an inadequately protected iliac crest. The hip pointer is considered one of the most handicapping injuries in sports and one that is difficult to manage. A direct force to the unprotected iliac crest causes severe pinching action to the soft tissue of that region.

Symptoms and signs   Such an injury produces immediate pain, spasms, and transitory paralysis of the soft structures. As a result, the athlete is unable to rotate the trunk or to flex the thigh without pain.

Management   RICE should be applied immediately after injury and should be maintained intermittently for at least 48 hours. In severe cases bed rest for 1 to 2 days will speed recovery. It should be noted that the mechanisms of the hip pointer are the same as those for an iliac crest fracture or epiphyseal separation.

Referral to a physician must be made, and an x-ray examination must be performed. A variety of treatment procedures can be used for this injury. Ice massage and ultrasound have been found beneficial. Initially the injury may be injected with a steroid. Later, oral antiinflammatory agents may be used. Recovery time usually ranges from 1 to 3 weeks.

Osteitis Pubis

Because the popularity of distance running has increased, a condition known as osteitis pubis has become more prevalent. It is also caused by the sports of soccer, football, and wrestling.

Etiology   As the result of repetitive stress on the pubic symphysis and adjacent bony structures by the pull of muscles in the area, a chronic inflammatory condition is created (Figure 20-33).

20-7

Critical Thinking E x e r c i s e

A football player who was not wearing hip pads receives a hard compressive hit to his left iliac crest region.

? What injury has this athlete sustained? What are the expected symptoms and signs?

Symptoms and signs   The athlete has pain in the groin region and in the area of the symphysis pubis. There is point tenderness on the pubic tubercle and pain while running, doing sit-ups, and doing squats. Acute osteitis pubis may occur as a result of pressure from a bicycle seat.

Management   Follow-up care usually consists of rest and an oral antiinflammatory agent, with a gradual return to activity.

Stress Fractures

Stress fractures in the pelvic area are seen mostly in distance runners.

Etiology   As with other stress fractures, repetitive cyclical forces created by ground reaction forces can produce stress fractures in the pelvis and the proximal femur. They constitute approximately 16% of all stress fractures and are more common in women than in men. The most common sites are the inferior pubic ramus and the femoral neck and subtrochanteric area of the femur.

Symptoms and signs   Commonly, the athlete complains of groin pain, along with an aching sensation in the thigh that increases with activity and decreases with rest. Standing on one leg may be impossible. Deep palpation will cause severe point tenderness. Pelvic stress fracture has a tendency to occur during intensive interval training or competitive racing. For the ischium and the pubis crutch walking is recommended.[1]

Management   Rest is usually the treatment of choice for 2 to 5 months. X-rays are usually normal for 6 to 10 weeks. Normally a bone scan will pick up osteoclastic activity early.[1] Freestyle swimming can be performed for aerobic exercise. The breast stroke must be avoided.

Avulsion Fractures and Apophysitis

The pelvis has a number of apophyses where major muscles make their attachments. An apophysis, or traction epiphysis, is a bony outgrowth and is contrasted to pressure epiphyses, which are the growth plates for long bones. The three most common sites for avulsion fractures and apophysitis in the pelvic region are the ischial tuberosity and the hamstring attachment, the anterior inferior iliac spine and the rectus femoris muscle attachment, and the anterior superior iliac spine where the sartorius muscle makes its attachment (Figure 20-34).

Etiology   Sports that have sudden acceleration or deceleration such as in football, soccer, and basketball can cause a convulsion, a fracture, or an apophysitis.

Symptoms and signs   The athlete complains of a sudden localized pain with limited movement. On inspection of the injury there is swelling and point tenderness. Muscle testing increases pain.

Management   X-ray examination is routinely given with apophysical pain. Uncomplicated conditions can be treated with RICE and crutches with toe-touch weight bearing for 1 to 2 months.[1] After the control of pain and inflammation (2 to 3 weeks) a gradual stretch program begins. When 80 degrees of range of motion have been returned a progressive-resistive exercise program is instituted.[1] When full range of motion and strength have been regained the athlete can return to competition.

THIGH AND HIP REHABILITATION TECHNIQUES
General Body Conditioning

As with other sports injuries the athlete must retain cardiorespiratory fitness, muscle endurance, and strength of the total body. Pool running and swimming provide a maintenance of total body conditioning. One-legged stationary bicycle and UBE activities can maintain cardiorespiratory fitness.

Flexibility

In the thigh region a major concern of rehabilitation is the restoration of quadriceps and hamstring extensibility. Stretching exercises usually progress from propriocep-

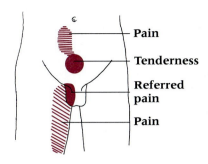

Figure 20-33

Osteitis pubis and other pain sites in the region of the pelvis and groin.

20-8

Critical Thinking Exercise

A cross-country runner complains of pain in her groin and in the area of her symphysis pubis. She says she experienced pain when running and when doing sit-up exercises.

? What conditions might be indicated by this athlete's complaints?

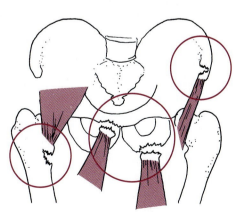

Figure 20-34

Avulsion fractures to the pelvic apophyses.

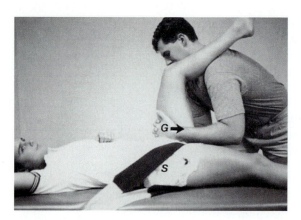

Figure 20-35

Inferior femoral glides. Inferior femoral glides at 90 degrees of hip flexion may also be used to increase abduction and flexion.

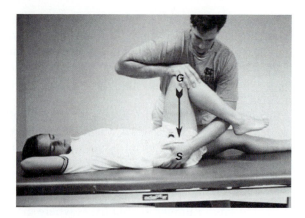

Figure 20-36

Posterior femoral glides. With the athlete supine, a posterior femoral glide can be done by stabilizing underneath the pelvis and using the body weight applied through the femur to glide posteriorly. Posterior glides are used to increase hip flexion.

tive neuromuscular facilitation relaxation stretching to gentle passive stretching to gradual static stretching, all within pain-free limits. When considering the hip and groin region ROM, one must consider its major movements: internal rotation, external rotation, adduction, abduction, extension, flexion, and the combined movement of internal and external circumduction. Stretching of all the ranges of movement must be considered after hip injury. As with the thigh, the hip should undergo a progressive stretching program including proprioceptive neuromuscular facilitation relaxation methods, passive stretching, and active static stretching within pain-free limits.[13]

Mobilization

Mobilizing accessory movements of the hip after injury is essential. Figures 20-35 through 20-38 demonstrate some key hip mobilization techniques.

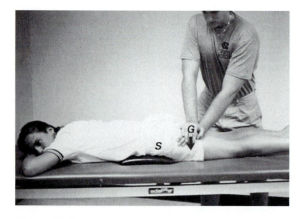

Figure 20-37

Anterior femoral glides. Anterior femoral glides increase extension and are accomplished by using some support to stabilize under the pelvis and applying an anterior glide posteriorly on the femur.

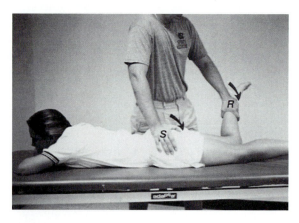

Figure 20-38

Medial femoral rotations. Medial femoral rotations may be used for increasing medial rotation and are done by stabilizing the opposite innominate while internally rotating the hip through the flexed knee.

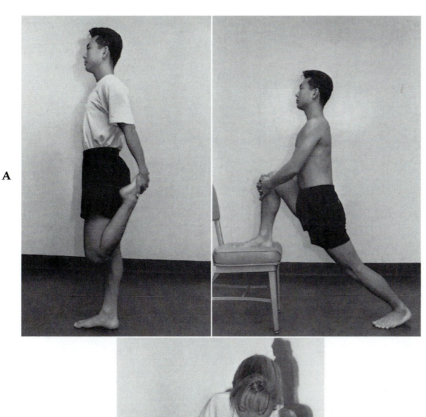

Figure 20-39

Selected basic exercises for hip rehabilitation. **A,** Active hip flexor standing stretch. **B,** Active hip flexor chair stretch. **C,** Manual hip flexor stretch. *(continued)*

Strength

Normally the progression for strength is, first, muscle setting and isometric exercise until the muscle can be fully contracted, followed by active isotonic contraction, and then isotonic progressive-resistive exercise or isokinetic exercise. Proprioceptive neuromuscular facilitation that uses both knee and hip patterns is also an excellent means of thigh rehabilitation. Because of the wide variety of possible movements, it is essential that exercise be conducted as soon as possible after injury, without aggravating the condition. When exercise is begun, it should be practiced within a pain-free range of movement. A program should be organized to start with free movement, leading up to resistive exercises. A general goal is to perform each exercise for up to 10 to 15 repetitions, progressing from one set to three sets two or three times daily

Figure 20-39—cont'd

D, Hip abduction and adduction. **E,** Hip adduction against gravity. **F,** Hip adduction against a resistance.

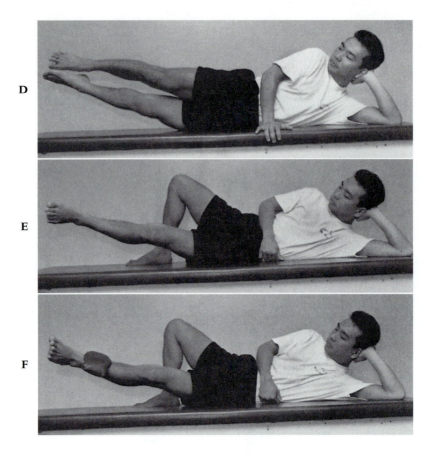

(Figure 20-39). (Because of the relationship of thigh rehabilitation to the knee region, the reader is referred to Chapter 19.)

Neuromuscular Control

In maintaining or restoring neuromuscular control to the thigh or hip region there should be a focus on balance and closed kinetic chain exercises. For balance the athlete can engage in weight bearing on just the affected leg using the balance board. Closed kinetic chain exercise might include minisquats, leg press, and stair climbing or stepping machines.

Functional Progressions

Functional progression might begin in a pool where non–weight-bearing running can be performed. Depending on the sport, weight-bearing progression might consist of walking, jogging, slow running, zigzag running, figure-8 running, and sprinting.

Return to Activity

Before returning to activity and competition the athlete must demonstrate full pain-free function of the thigh and hip region. The athlete must have full range of motion, strength, balance, and agility.

SUMMARY

- The thigh is composed of the femoral bone, musculature, nerves and blood vessels, and fascia that envelops the soft tissue. It is considered that part of the leg between the hip and the knee. The quadriceps contusion and hamstring strain represent the most common sports injuries to the thigh, with the quadriceps contusion having the highest incidence. Of major importance in acute thigh con-

20-9

Critical Thinking Exercise

A soccer player sustains a stress fracture to his right subtrochanter.

? As the stress fracture heals, what should be the neuromuscular control concerns?

20-10

Critical Thinking Exercise

An athlete has successfully completed the rehabilitation process after a hip injury.

? What are the criteria for this athlete's return to activity?

tusion is early detection and the avoidance of internal bleeding. One major complication to repeated contusions is myositis ossificans.

- Jumping or falling on a bent knee can strain the quadriceps muscle. A more common strain is that of the hamstring muscle; however, it is not clearly known why hamstring muscles become strained. Strain occurs most often to the short head of the biceps femoris muscle.
- The femur can sustain both acute fractures and stress fractures. Acute fractures occur most often to the femoral shaft, usually from a direct blow. Femoral stress fractures are most common in the femoral neck.
- The groin is the depression that lies between the thigh and the abdominal region. Groin strain can occur to any one of a number of muscles located in this region. Running, jumping, or twisting can produce a groin strain.
- A common problem among women runners is trochanteric bursitis. An irritation occurs in the region of the greater trochanter of the femur.
- The hip joint, the strongest and best-protected joint in the human body, has a low incidence of acute sports injuries. More common are conditions stemming from an immature hip joint. They include Legg-Calvé-Perthes disease (coxa plana) and the slipped capital femoral epiphysis.
- The snapping hip phenomenon is one in which hip stability is lessened as a result of laxity of the hip joint, ligaments, and adductor muscles.
- A common problem in the pelvic region is the hip pointer. This condition results from a blow to an inadequately protected iliac crest. The contusion causes pain, spasm, and malfunction of the muscles in the area. The pelvis can also sustain overuse conditions such as osteitis pubis, as well as acute fractures and stress fractures.

Solutions to Critical Thinking EXERCISES

20-1 One of the best ways to determine the grade of a contusion to the quadriceps muscle is through the degree of restriction of knee flexion. With grade 1 there is no restriction; with grade 2 more than 90 degrees; with grade 3 between 45 and 90 degrees; and with grade 4 less than 45 degrees.

20-2 Initially, activity is significantly reduced. Isometric exercise is carried out after the early inflammatory phase. In later stages of healing pain-free exercise such as gentle stretching, jogging, stationary cycling, and high-speed isokinetics may be employed.

20-3 The two tests that can be used for hip flexion tightness are the Kendall and Thomas tests. The Kendall test evaluates the athlete's ability to place her thigh flat on the table while the other is flexed on her chest. The Thomas test evaluates whether the athlete can lay on the table with her legs fully extended and at the same time keep her lumbar spine flat.

20-4 This condition could be an inflammation of the gluteus medius muscle or iliotibial band or a trochanteric bursitis caused by the increased Q angle and short leg.

20-5 Because of the age of the athlete, the athletic trainer should consider the possibility of a growth problem. If a growth problem it is most likely a slipped capital femoral epiphysis. The athletic trainer must refer this athlete immediately to a physician for x-ray.

20-6 A likely cause of this problem is a strength imbalance of those muscles that help to stabilize the hip joint while flexing and rotating. There also could be a structurally narrow pelvis, greater than usual ROM of hip abduction, or a restricted ROM during lateral rotation.

20-7 This athlete has sustained a hip pointer or contusion to the skin and musculature in the region of the iliac crest. The athlete most likely will experience severe pain, muscle spasm, and an inability to rotate his trunk or flex his hip without pain.

20-8 This athlete's complaints represent a number of possible conditions. They are osteitis pubis, stress fracture of the inferior pubic ramus, a possible avulsion apophysis fracture, or an apophysitis.

20-9 As the stress fracture heals the athlete must maintain and restore neuromuscular control of the thigh and hip region. The focus should be on balance and closed kinetic chain exercises. Use of a balance board as well as affected leg weight-bearing activities can also be conducted. Minisquats, leg press, and stair climbing and stepping are ot her possible closed kinetic chain exercises.

20-10 The athlete must demonstrate pain-free movement of the thigh and hip. There must be full ROM, strength, balance, and agility along with a preinjury level of cardiorespiratory fitness.

REVIEW QUESTIONS AND CLASS ACTIVITIES

1. Describe the major injuries to the thigh, including how contusions and strains are sustained and cared for.
2. How may hamstring strains be recognized and cared for?
3. How is a groin strain typically recognized and cared for?
4. What are the similarities and differences between coxa plana and a slipped capital femoral epiphysis?

REFERENCES

1. Bielak JM, Henderson JM: Injuries of the pelvis and hip. In Birrer PB, editor: *Sports medicine for the primary care physician,* ed 2, Boca Raton, Fla, 1994, CRC Press.
2. Booher J, Moran B: Evaluation and management of the acute hamstring injury, *Sports Med Guide* 4:2, 1993.
3. Bull RC: Soft tissue injury to the hip and thigh. In Torg JS, Shephard RJ, editors: *Current therapy in sports medicine,* St Louis, 1995, Mosby.
4. Cooper DE: Traumatic subluxation of the hip. In Torg JS, Shephard RJ, editors: *Current therapy in sports medicine,* St Louis, 1995, Mosby.
5. Estwanik JJ et al: Groin strain and other possible causes of groin pain, *Phys Sports Med* 18(2):54, 1990.
6. Hasselman CT et al: When groin pain signals an adductor strain, *Phys Sports Med* 23(7):53, 1995.
7. Hacutt JE: General types of injuries. In Birrer RB, editor: *Sports medicine for the primary care physician,* ed 2, Boca Raton, Fla, 1994, CRC Press.
8. Jackson DL: Stress fracture of the femur, *Phys Sports Med* 19(7):39, 1991.
9. Johnson BC, Klabunde LA: The elusive slipped capital femoral epiphysis, *J Ath Train* 20(2):124, 1995.
10. Kaeding CC: Quadriceps strains and contusions, *Phys Sports Med* 23(1):59, 1995.
11. Levandowski R, Difiori JP: Thigh injuries. In Birrer RB, editor: *Sports medicine for the primary care physician,* ed 2, Boca Raton, Fla, 1994, CRC Press.
12. Magee DJ: *Orthopedic physical assessment,* Philadelphia, 1993, Saunders.
13. Paletta GA et al: Injuries about the hip and pelvis in the young athlete. In Michile LJ, editor: *The young athlete. Clinics in sports medicine,* vol 14, no 3, Philadelphia, 1995, Saunders.
14. Prentice WE: Mobilization and traction techniques in rehabilitation. In Prentice WE, editor: *Rehabilitation techniques in sports medicine* ed 2, St Louis, 1994, Mosby.
15. Strachley DJ: A life-threatening femur fracture, *Phys Sports Med* 19(3):33, 1991.
16. Weicker GG, Munnings F: How to manage hip and pelvis injuries in adolescents, *Phys Sports Med* 21:72, 1993.

ANNOTATED BIBLIOGRAPHY

Jenkins DB: *Hollinshead's functional anatomy of the limbs and back,* ed 6, Philadelphia, 1991, Saunders.

Provides a traditional approach to the study of anatomy.

Garrick JG, Webb DR: *Sports injuries: diagnosis and management,* Philadelphia, 1990, Saunders.

An excellent overview of the recognition, evaluation, and management of sports injuries.

Torg JS, Shephard RJ, editors: *Current therapy in sports medicine,* ed 3, St Louis, 1995, Mosby.

A detailed sports medicine text with extensive coverage of thigh, hip, and pelvic injuries.

The Shoulder Complex

When you finish this chapter, you should be able to

- Identify the major anatomical and functional features of the shoulder complex.
- Discuss how shoulder injuries may be prevented.
- Describe the process for evaluating injuries to the shoulder.
- Explain how shoulder stability is maintained by the joint capsule ligaments and muscles.
- Identify specific injuries that occur around the shoulder joint, and discuss plans for management.
- Discuss rehabilitation techniques for the injured shoulder.

T he shoulder complex, as the name implies, is an extremely complicated region of the body. Because of its anatomical structure, the shoulder complex has a great degree of mobility. To have this mobility there must be some compromise in stability, thus making the shoulder highly susceptible to injury. Many sport activities, in particular those that involve repetitive overhead movements such as throwing, swimming, or serving in tennis or volleyball, place a great deal of stress on the supporting structures (Figure 21-1). Consequently injuries related to overuse in the shoulder are commonplace in the athlete. Some understanding of the anatomy and mechanics of this joint is essential for the coach and the athletic trainer.

ANATOMY
Bones

The bones that make up the shoulder complex and shoulder joint are the clavicle, scapula, and humerus (Figure 21-2).

Clavicle

The clavicle is a slender, S-shaped bone approximately 6 inches (15 cm) long. It supports the anterior portion of the shoulder, keeping it free from the thoracic cage. It extends from the sternum to the tip of the shoulder, where it joins the acromion process of the scapula. The shape of the medial two thirds of the clavicle is primarily circular, and its lateral third assumes a flattened appearance. The medial two thirds bend convexly forward, and the lateral third is concave. The point at which the clavicle changes shape and contour presents a structural weakness, and the largest number of fractures to the bone occur at this point. Lying superficially with no muscle or fat protection makes the clavicle subject to direct blows.

Scapula

The scapula is a flat, triangular shaped bone that serves mainly as an articulating surface for the head of the humerus. It is located on the dorsal aspect of the thorax and has three prominent projections: the spine, the acromion, and the coracoid process. The spine divides the posterior aspect unequally. The superior dorsal aspect is a deep depression called the supraspinous fossa, and the area below, a more shallow depression, is called the infraspinous fossa. The acromion is a process at the lateral tip of the spine. A hooklike projection called the coracoid process arises anteriorly from the scapula. It curves upward, forward, and outward in front of the glenoid fossa, which is the articulating cavity for the reception of the humeral head. The glenoid cavity is situated laterally on the scapula below the acromion.

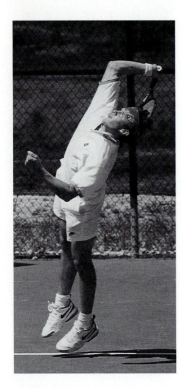

Figure 21-1

Vigorous overhead activities can produce a number of shoulder problems.

Shoulder complex articulations:
    Sternoclavicular
    Acromioclavicular
    Glenohumeral
    Scapulothoracic

Figure 21-2

Skeletal anatomy of the shoulder complex.

Humerus

The head of the humerus is spherical, with a shallow, constricted neck; it faces upward, inward, and backward, articulating with the scapula's shallow glenoid fossa. Circumscribing the humeral head is a slight groove called the anatomical neck, which is the attachment for the articular capsule of the glenohumeral joint. The greater and lesser tuberosities are located adjacent and immediately inferior to the head. The lesser tuberosity is positioned anteriorly and medially, with the greater tuberosity placed somewhat higher and laterally. Lying between the two tuberosities is a deep groove called the bicipital groove, which retains the long tendon of the biceps brachii muscle.

Articulations

There are four major articulations associated with the shoulder complex: the sternoclavicular joint, the acromioclavicular joint, the glenohumeral joint, and the scapulothoracic joint (Figure 21-3).

Sternoclavicular Joint

The clavicle articulates with the manubrium of the sternum to form the sternoclavicular (SC) joint, the only direct connection between the upper extremity and the trunk. The sternal articulating surface is larger than the sternum, causing the clavicle to rise much higher than the sternum. A fibrocartilaginous disk is interposed between the two articulating surfaces. It functions as a shock absorber against the medial forces and also helps prevent any displacement upward. The articular disk is placed so that the clavicle moves on the disk and the disk in turn moves separately on the sternum. The clavicle is permitted to move up and down, forward and backward, in combination, and in rotation.

Acromioclavicular Joint

The acromioclavicular (AC) joint is a gliding articulation of the lateral end of the clavicle with the acromion process. It is a rather weak junction. A fibrocartilaginous disk separates the two articulating surfaces. A thin, fibrous capsule surrounds the joint.

Glenohumeral Joint

The glenohumeral joint (shoulder joint) is an enarthrodial, or ball-and-socket, joint in which the round head of the humerus articulates with the shallow glenoid cavity

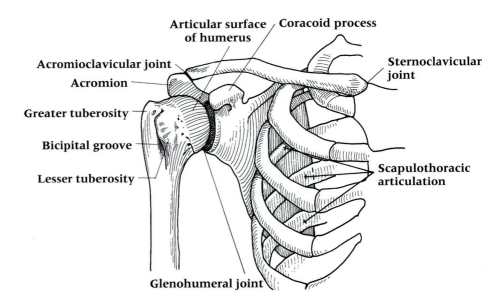

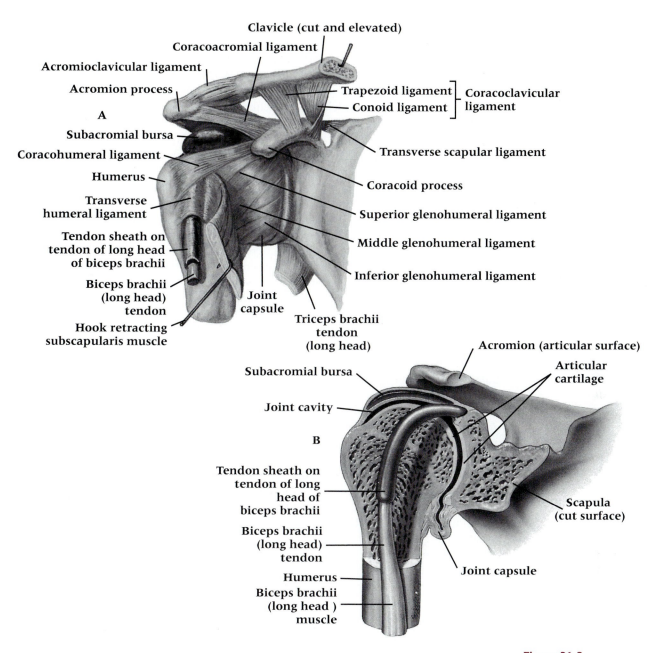

Figure 21-3

Shoulder complex articulations and ligaments. **A,** Anterior view. **B,** Frontal section.

of the scapula. The glenohumeral joint is maintained by both a passive and an active mechanism, the passive mechanism relating to the glenoid labrum and capsular ligaments and the active mechanism relating to the deltoid and rotator cuff muscles. The cavity is deepened slightly by a fibrocartilaginous rim called the glenoid labrum.

Scapulothoracic Joint

The scapulothoracic joint is not a true joint; however, the movement of the scapula on the wall of the thoracic cage is critical to shoulder joint motion. Contraction of the scapular muscles, which attach the scapula to the axial skeleton, is critical in stabilizing the scapula, thus providing a base on which a highly mobile joint can function.

Ligaments

Figure 21-3 shows the ligamentous arrangement of the shoulder complex.

Sternoclavicular Joint Ligaments

The sternoclavicular joint is extremely weak because of its bony arrangement, but it is held securely by strong ligaments that tend to pull the sternal end of the clavicle downward and toward the sternum, in effect anchoring it. The main ligaments are the anterior sternoclavicular, which prevents upward displacement of the clavicle; the posterior sternoclavicular, which also prevents upward displacement of the clavicle; the interclavicular, which prevents lateral displacement of the clavicle; and the costoclavicular, which prevents lateral and upward displacement of the clavicle.[1]

Acromioclavicular Joint Ligaments

The acromioclavicular ligament consists of anterior, posterior, superior, and inferior portions. In addition to the acromioclavicular ligament, the coracoclavicular ligament joins the coracoid process and the clavicle, and helps maintain the position of the clavicle relative to the acromion. The coracoclavicular ligament is further divided into the conoid and trapezoid ligaments. The coracoclavicular ligament, because of the rotation of the clavicle on its long axis, develops some slack, which permits movement of the scapula at the acromioclavicular joint to take place. The coracoacromial ligament connects the coracoid to the acromion. This ligament along with the acromion forms the coracoacromial arch.

Glenohumeral Joint Ligaments

Surrounding the articulation is a loose, articular capsule. This capsule is strongly reinforced by the superior, middle, and inferior glenohumeral ligaments and by the tough coracohumeral ligament, which attaches to the coracoid process and to the greater tuberosity of the humerus.[22] The glenohumeral ligaments appear to produce a major restraint in shoulder flexion, extension, and rotation. The anterior glenohumeral ligament is tense when the shoulder is in extension, abduction, or external rotation. The posterior glenohumeral ligament's greatest tension is in extension with external rotation. The middle glenohumeral ligament is in greatest tension when in flexion and external rotation. The inferior glenohumeral ligament is most tense when the shoulder is abducted, extended, or externally rotated. The posterior capsule is tense when the shoulder is in flexion, abduction, internal rotation, or in any combination of these. The superior and middle segment of the posterior capsule has the greatest tension while the shoulder is internally rotated. The inferior glenohumeral ligament is primarily a check against both anterior and posterior dislocation of the humeral head. The long tendon of the biceps brachii muscle passes across the head of the humerus and then through the bicipital groove. In the anatomical position the long head of the biceps moves in close relationship with the humerus. The transverse ligament retains the long biceps tendon within the bicipital groove by passing over it from the lesser and the greater tuberosities converting the bicipital groove into a canal.

Musculature

Muscles Acting on the Glenohumeral Joint

The muscles that cross the glenohumeral joint produce dynamic motion and establish stability to compensate for a bony and ligamentous arrangement that allows for a great deal of mobility (Figure 21-4). Movements at the glenohumeral joint include flexion, extension, abduction, adduction, and rotation. The muscles acting on the glenohumeral joint may be separated into two groups. The first group consists of muscles that originate on the axial skeleton and attach to the humerus, including the latissimus dorsi and the pectoralis major. The second group originates on the scapula and attaches to the humerus, including the deltoid, the teres major, the coracobrachialis. Additionally, the subscapularis, the supraspinatus, the infraspinatus, and the teres minor muscles constitute the short rotator muscles, commonly called the rotator cuff,

Glenohumeral joint movements:
  Flexion
  Extension
  Abduction
  Adduction
  External rotation
  Internal rotation

Rotator cuff muscles:
  Subscapularis
  Supraspinatus
  Infraspinatus
  Teres minor

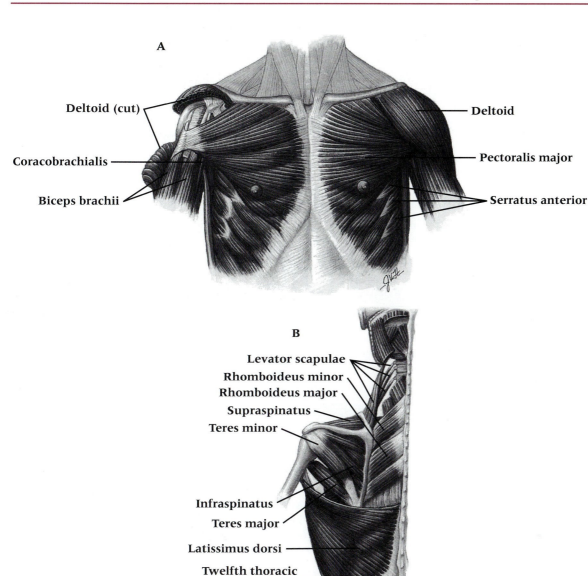

A

Deltoid (cut)

Coracobrachialis

Biceps brachii

Deltoid

Pectoralis major

Serratus anterior

B

Levator scapulae
Rhomboideus minor
Rhomboideus major
Supraspinatus
Teres minor

Infraspinatus
Teres major

Latissimus dorsi

Twelfth thoracic
vertebra

External abdominal
oblique

Figure 21-4

Shoulder musculature. **A,** Anterior. **B,** Posterior.

whose tendons adhere to the articular capsule and serve as reinforcing structures (Figure 21-5). The biceps and triceps muscles attach on the glenoid and effect elbow motion.

Scapular Muscles

A third group of muscles attaches the axial skeleton to the scapula and includes the levator scapula, the trapezius, the rhomboids, and the serratus anterior and posterior. The scapular muscles are important in providing dynamic stability to the shoulder complex.

Figure 21-5

Rotator cuff muscles.

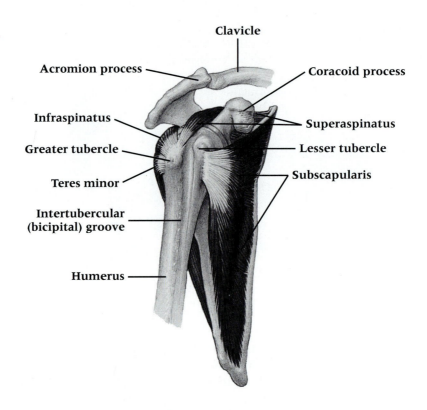

Clavicle

Acromion process

Coracoid process

Infraspinatus

Superaspinatus

Greater tubercle

Lesser tubercle

Teres minor

Subscapularis

Intertubercular
(bicipital) groove

Humerus

21-1

Critical Thinking Exercise

A football quarterback has a multidirectional instability of the glenohumeral joint resulting from a series of two anterior dislocations. He is just beginning preseason practice and wants to know what he can do to strengthen his shoulder so that it does not dislocate again.

? What muscles are important in providing dynamic stability specifically to the glenohumeral joint, and will strengthening these muscle prevent subsequent dislocation?

Bursae

Several bursae are located around the shoulder joint, the most important of which is the subacromial (subdeltoid) bursa (Figure 21-6), located between the coracoacromial arch and the glenohumeral capsule and reinforced by the supraspinous tendon. It is easily subjected to trauma when the humerus is in the overhead position compressing the bursa under the coracoacromial arch.

Nerve Supply

The spinal nerve roots from the fifth cervical vertebra through the first thoracic vertebra create the complex nerve network called the brachial plexus, discussed in Chapter 23 (Figure 21-7). Stemming from this plexus are the peripheral nerves that innervate muscles of the upper extremity, including the axillary nerve (C5-6), the musculocutaneous (C5-7), the subscapular (C5-6), the suprascapular (C5-6), the dorsal scapular (C5), the pectoral (C5-T1), and the radial (C5-T1) nerves.

Blood Supply

The subclavian artery, which lies distal to the sternoclavicular joint, arches upward and outward, passes the anterior scalene muscle, and then moves downward laterally behind the clavicle and in front of the first ribs. The subclavian artery continues on to become the axillary artery at the outer border of the first rib and in the region of the teres major muscle in the upper arm becomes the brachial artery (Figure 21-7).

FUNCTIONAL ANATOMY

The anatomy of the shoulder complex allows for a great degree of mobility.[24] To achieve this mobility, stability of the complex is sometimes compromised. Instability of the shoulder frequently leads to injury, particularly in those sports that involve overhead activity. In the glenohumeral joint, the rounded humeral head articulates with a relatively flat glenoid on the scapula. Thus in movement of the shoulder joint, it is critical to maintain the positioning of the humeral head relative to the glenoid.

The muscles of the rotator cuff, the subscapularis, infraspinatus, supraspinatus, and teres minor, along with the long head of the biceps, function to provide dynamic stability to control the position and prevent excessive displacement of the humeral head relative to the position of the glenoid. The supraspinatus compresses the humeral head into the glenoid while cocontraction of the infraspinatus, teres minor, and subscapularis depresses the humeral head during overhead movements.[21]

The glenohumeral joint capsule also helps control humeral head movement. The tendons of the rotator cuff blend into the glenohumeral joint capsule. As the muscles contract they dynamically tighten the joint capsule, which helps center the humeral head relative to the glenoid.

Dynamic movement, as well as stabilization of the shoulder complex, requires integrated function of not only the glenohumeral joint, but also of the scapulothoracic, acromioclavicular, and sternoclavicular joints.[23] The muscles that produce movement of the scapula on the thorax help maintain the position of the glenoid relative to the moving humerus and include the levator scapula and upper trapezius, which elevate the scapula; the middle trapezius and rhomboids, which adduct the scapula; the lower trapezius, which adducts and depresses the scapula; and the serratus anterior, which abducts and upwardly rotates the scapula.

Scapulohumeral Rhythm

Scapulohumeral rhythm describes the movement of the scapula relative to the movement of the humerus throughout a full range of abduction (Figure 21-8). As the humerus elevates to 30 degrees there is no movement of the scapula. This is referred to as the setting phase, during which a stable base is being established on the thoracic wall. From 30 to 90 degrees, the scapula abducts and upwardly rotates 1 degree for every 2 degrees of humeral elevation. From 90 degrees to full abduction, the scapula abducts and upwardly rotates 1 degree for each 1 degree of humeral elevation.

It should also be noted that for the scapula to abduct and upwardly rotate throughout 180 degrees of humeral abduction, clavicular movement must occur at both the sternoclavicular and acromioclavicular joints. The clavicle must elevate approximately 40 degrees and must rotate in a posterosuperior direction at least 10 degrees.[1]

PREVENTING SHOULDER INJURIES

Proper physical conditioning is of major importance in preventing many shoulder injuries. As with all preventive conditioning, the program should be directed toward general body development and development of specific body areas for a given sport. If a sport places extreme, sustained demands on the arms and shoulders or if the shoulder is at risk for sudden traumatic injury, extensive conditioning must be used. Strengthening through a full range of motion of all the muscles involved in movement of the shoulder complex is essential.

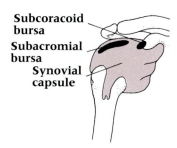

Figure 21-6

Synovial capsule and bursae of the shoulder.

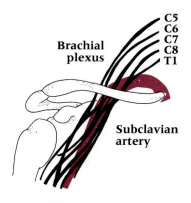

Figure 21-7

Brachial plexus and subclavian artery.

Figure 21-8

Scapulohumeral rhythm.

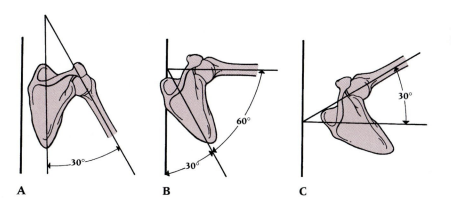

Proper warm-up must be performed gradually before explosive arm movements are attempted. This warm-up includes gaining a general increase in body temperature, followed by sport-specific stretching of selected muscles.

All athletes in collision and contact sports should be instructed and drilled on how to fall properly. They must be taught not to try to catch themselves with an outstretched arm. Performing a shoulder roll is a safer way to absorb the shock of the fall. Specialized protective equipment such as shoulder pads must be properly fitted to help prevent shoulder injuries in tackle football.

To avoid overuse shoulder injuries, it is essential that athletes be correctly taught the appropriate techniques of throwing, spiking, overhead smashing, overhand serving, proper crawl and butterfly swimming strokes, and tackling and blocking.

ASSESSMENT OF THE SHOULDER COMPLEX

The shoulder complex is one of the most difficult regions of the body to evaluate. One reason for this difficulty is that the biomechanical demands placed on these structures during overhand accelerations and decelerations are not yet clearly understood.

History

It is essential that the evaluator understand the athlete's major complaints and the possible mechanism of the injury. It is also necessary to know whether the condition was produced by a sudden trauma or was of slow onset. If the injury was of sudden onset, it must be determined whether the precipitating cause was from external and direct trauma or from some resistive force. The following questions in regard to the athlete's complaints can help the evaluator determine the nature of the injury:

- What happened to cause this pain?
- Have you ever had this problem before?
- What are the duration and intensity of the pain?
- Where is the pain located?
- Is there crepitus during movement, numbness, or distortion in temperature such as a cold or warm feeling?
- Is there a feeling of weakness or a sense of fatigue?
- What shoulder movements or positions seem to aggravate or relieve the pain?
- If therapy has been given before, what, if anything, offered pain relief (e.g., cold, heat, massage, or analgesic medication)?

Observation

The athlete should be generally observed while walking and standing. Observation during walking can reveal asymmetry of arm swing or leaning toward the painful shoulder. The athlete is next observed from the front, side, and back while in a standing position. The evaluator looks for any postural asymmetries, bony or joint deformities, or muscle spasm or guarding patterns.

Anterior Observation

- Are both shoulder tips even with one another, or is one depressed?
- Is one shoulder held higher because of muscle spasm or guarding?
- Is the lateral end of the clavicle prominent (indicating acromioclavicular sprain or dislocation)?
- Is one lateral acromion process more prominent than the other (indicating a possible glenohumeral dislocation)?
- Does the clavicular shaft appear deformed (indicating possible fracture)? Is there loss of the normal lateral deltoid muscle contour (indicating glenohumeral dislocation)?
- Is there an indentation in the upper biceps region (indicating rupture of biceps tendon)?

Lateral Observation

- Is there thoracic kyphosis, or shoulders slumped forward (indicating weakness of the erector muscles of the spine and tightness in the pectoral region)?
- Is there forward or backward arm hang (indicating possible scoliosis)?

Posterior Observation

- Is there asymmetry such as a low shoulder, uneven scapulae, or winging of one scapular wing and not the other (indicating scoliosis)?
- Is the scapula protracted because of constricted pectoral muscles?
- Is there a distracted or winged scapula on one or both sides? (A winged scapula on both sides could indicate a general weakness of the serratus anterior muscles; if only one side is winged, the long thoracic nerve may be injured.)
- Is there normal scapulohumeral rhythm?

Palpation

Bony Palpation

Palpation of the bony structures should be done with the athletic trainer standing in front of and then behind the athlete. Both shoulders are palpated at the same time for pain sites and deformities.

Anterior Structures	Posterior Structures
Sternoclavicular joint	Scapular spine
Clavicular shaft	Scapular vertebral border
Acromioclavicular joint	Scapular lateral border
Coracoid process	Scapular superior border
Acromion process	
Humeral head	
Greater tuberosity of the humerus	
Bicipital groove	

Soft-Tissue Palpation

Palpation of the soft tissue of the shoulder detects pain sites, abnormal swelling or lumps, muscle spasm or guarding, and trigger points. Trigger points are commonly found in the following muscles: levator scapulae, lesser rhomboid, supraspinous, infraspinous, scalene, deltoid, subscapular, teres major, trapezius, serratus anterior, and pectoralis major and minor muscles. As with bony palpation, the shoulder is palpated anteriorly and posteriorly.

Anterior Palpation	Posterior Palpation
Anterior and middle deltoid muscle	Posterior deltoid
Rotator cuff tendons	Rhomboids
Subacromial bursa	Latissimus dorsi
Pectoralis major muscle	Serratus anterior
Sternocleidomastoid muscle	Levator scapulae
Biceps muscle and tendon	Trapezius
Coracoacromial ligament	Supraspinatus
Glenohumeral joint capsule	Infraspinatus
	Teres major and minor
	Latissimus dorsi

Special Tests

A number of special tests can help determine the nature of an injury to the shoulder complex.

Active and Passive Range of Motion

The shoulder's active and passive range of motion should be noted and compared with the opposite side. The following are normal ranges for shoulder motion:

- Flexion = 180 degrees.
- Extension = 50 degrees.
- Abduction = 180 degrees.
- Adduction = 40 degrees.
- Internal rotation = 90 degrees.
- External rotation = 90 degrees.

Muscle Testing

Strength of the shoulder musculature should be assessed by manual muscle testing. Both the muscles that act on the glenohumeral joint and the muscles that act on the scapula should be tested.

Test for Sternoclavicular Joint Instability

With the athlete lying prone, pressure is applied anteriorly, then superiorly, and then inferiorly to the proximal clavicle to determine any instability or increased pain associated with a sprain (Figure 21-9, *A*). Pressure applied to the tip of the shoulder in a medial direction may also increase pain.

Test of Acromioclavicular Joint Instability

The acromioclavicular joint is first palpated to determine if there is any displacement of the acromion process and the distal head of the clavicle. Next, pressure is applied to the distal clavical in all four directions to determine stability and any associated increase in pain (Figure 21-9, *B*). Pressure is applied to the tip of the shoulder, which compresses the acromioclavicular joint and may also increase pain.[21]

Tests for Glenohumeral Instability

Glenohumeral translation (load and shift test) This test may be done with the athlete either sitting or supine. First, one hand is placed over the shoulder to stabilize the scapula (Figure 21-10, *A* and *B*). The other hand grasps the humeral head between the thumb and index finger. A stress load is applied and translation of the humerus is assessed in both an anterior and a posterior direction. Next, the elbow is grasped and traction is applied in an inferior direction. With excessive inferior translation, a depression occurs just below the acromion. This indicates a positive sulcus sign.[16]

Apprehension test (crank test) With the arm abducted 90 degrees, the shoulder is slowly and gently externally rotated as far as the athlete will allow. The athlete

Tests for glenohumeral instability:
    Load and shift
    Apprehension

Figure 21-9

A, Assessing sternoclavicular joint stability. **B,** Assessing acromioclavicular joint stability.

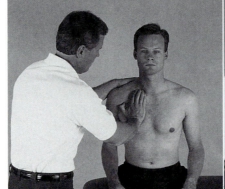
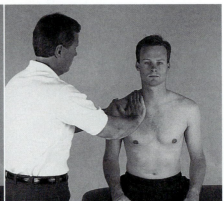

A

B

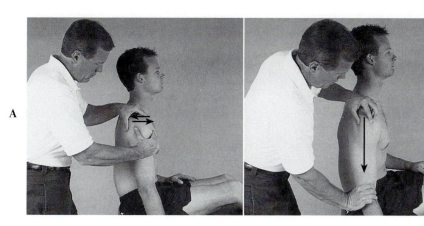

Figure 21-10

A, Test for anterior-posterior translation. **B,** Test for sulcus sign.

with a history of anterior glenohumeral instability will show great apprehension that is reflected by a facial grimace before an end point can be reached. At no time should the evaluator force this movement (Figure 21-11).

Posterior instability also can be determined through an apprehension maneuver. A posterior force is applied to the glenohumeral joint while the arm is internally rotated and moved into various degrees of flexion.

Tests for Shoulder Impingement

Forced flexion of the humerus in the overhead position may cause impingement of soft-tissue structures between the humeral head and the coracoacromial arch. A second test involves horizontal adduction with forced internal rotation of the humerus, which also produces impingement (Figure 21-12). A positive sign is indicated if the athlete feels pain and reacts with a grimace.[17]

Tests for Supraspinatus Muscle Weakness

Drop arm test   The drop arm test is designed to determine tears of the rotator cuff, primarily of the supraspinatus muscle. The athlete abducts the arm as far as possible and then slowly lowers it to 90 degrees. From this position the athlete with a torn supraspinatus muscle will be unable to lower the arm further with control (Figure 23-13, *A*). If the athlete can hold the arm in a 90-degree position, pressure on the wrist will cause the arm to fall.

Empty can test   The empty can test for supraspinatus muscle strength has the athlete bring both arms into 90 degrees of forward flexion and 30 degrees of horizontal abduction (Figure 21-13, *B*). In this position the arms are internally rotated as far as

21-2

Critical Thinking Exercise

A swimmer is complaining of shoulder pain particularly when her arm is in the overhead position during her swimming stroke. She has been diagnosed as having an impingement syndrome and the team physician has referred her to the athletic trainer for rehabilitation.

? What general considerations must the athletic trainer take into account when treating shoulder impingement syndrome?

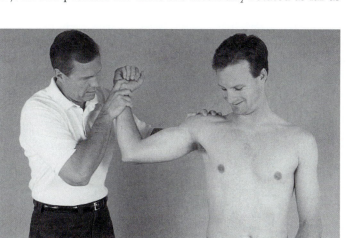

Figure 21-11

Shoulder apprehension test.

Figure 21-12

Shoulder impingement test. **A,** Full elevation. **B,** Horizontal adduction with internal rotation.

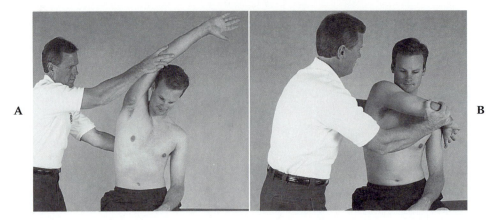

Tests for supraspinatus weakness:
    Drop arm test
    Empty can test

possible, thumbs pointing downward. A downward pressure is then applied by the evaluator. Weakness and pain can be detected, as well as comparative strength between the two arms.

Test for Serratus Anterior Muscle Weakness

The athlete performs a push-up movement against a wall. Winging of the scapula indicates weakness of the serratus anterior muscle. Winging of only one scapula could indicate an injury to the long thoracic nerve.

Tests for Biceps Tendon Irritation

Yergason's test involves keeping the elbow at 90 degrees with the forearm pronated while the athlete attempts to actively supinate against the resistance of the evaluator as the humerus is also being pulled downward (Figure 21-14, *A*). Speed's test is performed with the elbow extended, the forearm supinated, and resistance applied as the humerus elevates to 60 degrees. Both tests are positive if pain is felt in the region of the bicipital groove. If there is instability, the tendon may subluxate out of its groove (Figure 21-14, *B*).

Tests for biceps tendon irritation:
    Yergason's test
    Speed's test

Circulatory Assessment

It is essential that athletes with shoulder complaints be evaluated for impaired circulation. In cases of shoulder complaints pulse rates are routinely obtained over the axillary, brachial, and radial arteries. The axillary artery is found in the axilla against the shaft of the humerus. The brachial artery is a continuation of the axillary artery and follows the medial border of the biceps brachii muscle toward the elbow. The radial pulse is found at the anterior lateral aspect of the wrist over the radius. Taking

Figure 21-13

Supraspinatus tests. **A,** Drop arm test. **B,** Empty can test.

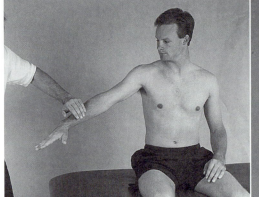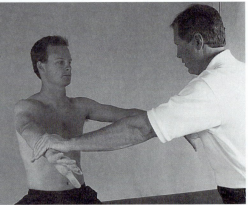

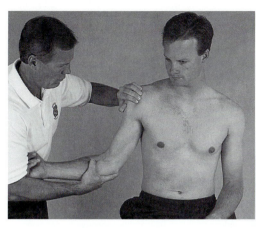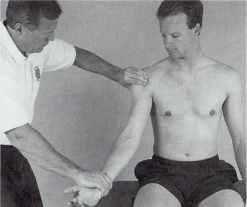

A   B

Figure 21-14

The bicipital tendinitis and subluxation test. **A,** Yergason's test. **B,** Speed's test.

the radial pulse provides an indication of the total circulation of the shoulder and arm.

Skin temperature is subjectively assessed by comparing the back of the athlete's hands. A cold temperature can be an indication of blood vessel constriction.[29]

Tests for Thoracic Outlet Compression Syndrome

Anterior scalene syndrome test (Adson's test)   The purpose of this test is to indicate whether the subclavian artery is being compressed as it enters into the outlet canal that lies between the heads of the anterior and middle scalene muscles. Compression can also occur between the cervical rib and the anterior scalene muscle. This maneuver is performed with the athlete seated on a stool with one hand resting on the thigh. The athlete's radial pulse is taken, first with the arm relaxed and then extended, while at the same time the athlete elevates the chin, turns the face toward the extended hand, and holds the breath (Figure 21-15, *A*). A positive test is one in which the pulse is depressed or stopped completely in the testing position.[13]

Costoclavicular syndrome test   This test indicates whether the subclavian artery is being compressed between the first rib and the clavicle. The radial pulse is taken while the athlete stands in a stiff, military posture. The shoulders are in posterior abduction, the arms are extended, and the neck is hyperextended. A positive test is one in which the pulse is obliterated partially or totally[13] (Figure 21-15, *B*).

Hyperabduction syndrome test   In an athlete with hyperabduction syndrome, the subclavian and axillary vessels and the brachial plexus are compressed as they move behind the pectoral muscle and beneath the coracoid process. To test for this syndrome, the athlete's radial pulse is taken while the arm is fully extended overhead (Figure 21-15, *C*).

Sensation Testing

When there is injury to the shoulder complex, a routine test of cutaneous sensation should be performed. Dermatome levels are tested for pain and light pressure (see Figure 10-9).

RECOGNITION AND MANAGEMENT OF SPECIFIC INJURIES
Fractures

Clavicular Fractures

Etiology   Clavicular fractures (Figure 21-16) are one of the most frequent fractures in sports. Fractures of the clavicle result from a fall on the outstretched arm, a fall on the tip of the shoulder, or a direct impact. The majority of clavicle fractures occur in the middle third from a direct impact. In young athletes these fractures are usually of the greenstick type.

21-3

Critical Thinking Exercise

A wrestler comes into the training room complaining of paresthesia and pain extending down the arm, a sensation of cold, impaired circulation in the fingers, and muscle weakness. During the evaluation it also becomes apparent that he has some muscle atrophy in the affected extremity. The athletic trainer suspects that the wrestler may have thoracic outlet syndrome.

? What specific tests should the athletic trainer do to determine whether thoracic outlet syndrome is present, and what do those tests indicate?

Tests for thoracic outlet compression syndrome:
   Adson's test
   Costoclavicular test
   Hyperabduction test

Figure 21-15

Thoracic outlet syndrome tests. **A,** Adson's test. **B,** Costoclavicular syndrome test. **C,** Hyperabduction syndrome.

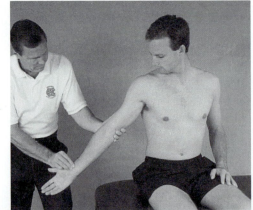

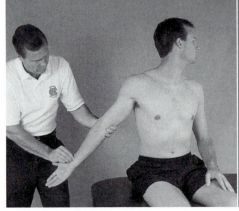
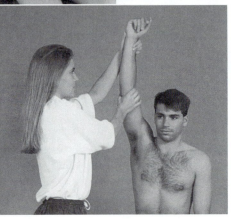

A

B

C

Symptoms and signs   The athlete with a fractured clavicle usually supports the arm on the injured side and tilts his or her head toward that side, with the chin turned to the opposite side. During inspection the injured clavicle appears slightly lower than the unaffected side. Palpation may also reveal swelling, point tenderness, and mild deformity.

Management   The clavicular fracture is cared for immediately by applying a sling and swathe bandage and by treating the athlete for shock, if necessary. If x-ray examination reveals a fracture, a closed reduction should be attempted by the physician followed by immobilization with a figure-8 wrap. Immobilization should be maintained for 6 to 8 weeks. After this period of immobilization, gentle isometric and mobilization exercises should begin with the athlete placed in a sling for an additional 3 to 4 weeks to provide protection. Occasionally, clavicle fractures may require operative management.[8]

Scapular Fractures

Etiology   Fracture of the scapula is an infrequent injury in sports (Figure 21-17). Although the scapula appears extremely vulnerable to trauma, it is well protected by a heavy outer bony border and a cushion of muscle above and below. Those fractures that do occur happen as a result of a direct impact or when the force is transmitted through the humerus to the scapula. Fractures may occur to the body, the glenoid, the acromion, and the coracoid.[6]

Symptoms and signs   Such a fracture may cause the athlete to have pain during shoulder movement, swelling, and point tenderness.

Management   When this injury is suspected, the athlete should be given a supporting sling and sent directly to the physician for x-ray. The arm should be supported in a sling for 3 weeks with overhead strengthening exercises beginning at week 1.

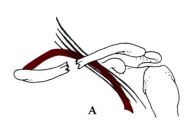

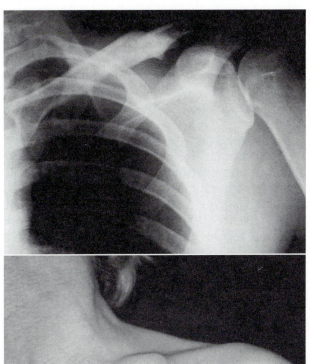

Figure 21-16

Clavicular fracture. **A,** Associated brachial blood vessels and nerves. **B,** X-ray film of a comminuted clavicular fracture. **C,** Typical appearance of clavicular fracture with obvious bone deformity.

B

C

Fractures of the Humerus

Fractures can occur to the humeral shaft, proximal humerus, and head of the humerus (epiphyseal fracture).

Etiology   The etiology of a fracture of the humerus varies with the type of fracture.

HUMERAL SHAFT   Fractures of the humeral shaft (Figure 21-18, *A*) happen occasionally in sports, usually as the result of a direct blow or a fall on the arm. The type of fracture is usually comminuted or transverse, and a deformity is often produced because the bone fragments override each other as a result of strong muscular pull. The pathological process is characteristic of most uncomplicated fractures, except that there may be a tendency for the radial nerve, which encircles the humeral shaft, to be severed by jagged bone edges, resulting in radial nerve paralysis and causing wrist drop and inability to perform forearm supination.

PROXIMAL HUMERUS   Fractures of the proximal humerus (Figure 21-18, *B*) pose considerable danger to nerves and vessels of that area. Fractures of the humerus can result from a direct blow, a dislocation, or the impact received by falling onto the outstretched arm. Various parts of the end of the humerus may be involved, such as the anatomical neck, tuberosities, or surgical neck. This fracture may be mistaken for a shoulder dislocation. The greatest number of fractures take place at the surgical neck.

EPIPHYSEAL FRACTURE   Epiphyseal fracture of the head of the humerus (Figure 21-18, *C*) is much more common in the young athlete than is a bone fracture. An epiphyseal injury in the shoulder region occurs most frequently in individuals 10 years of age and younger. It is caused by a direct blow or by an indirect force traveling along the length of the axis of the humerus. This condition causes shortening of the arm,

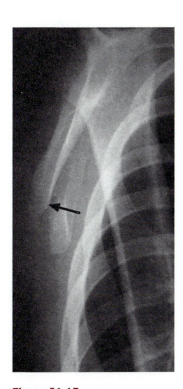

Figure 21-17

Fractures of the scapula are infrequent in sports.

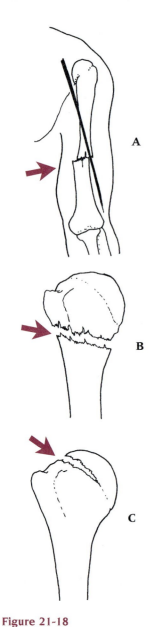

Figure 21-18

Humeral fractures. **A,** Shaft fracture. **B,** Upper humerus. **C,** Epiphyseal fracture.

disability, swelling, point tenderness, and pain. There also may be a false joint. This type of injury should be suspected when the aforementioned signs appear in young athletes.

Symptoms and signs   It may be difficult to recognize a fracture of the humerus by visual inspection alone; therefore x-ray examination gives the only positive proof. Some of the more prevalent signs that may be present are pain, inability to move the arm, swelling, point tenderness, and discoloration of the superficial tissue. Because of the proximity of the axillary blood vessels and the brachial plexus, a fracture to the upper end of the humerus may result in severe hemorrhaging or paralysis.

Management   Recognition of humeral shaft fractures requires immediate application of a splint, treatment for shock, and referral to a physician. The athlete with a fracture to the humeral shaft will be out of competition for approximately 3 to 4 months.

A suspected fracture of the proximal humerus warrants immediate support with a sling and swathe bandage and referral to a physician. Incapacitation may last for 2 to 6 months.

Initial treatment for epiphyseal fractures should include splinting and immediate referral to a physician. Healing is initiated rapidly; immobilization is necessary for only approximately 3 weeks. The main danger of this injury lies in the possibility of damage to the epiphyseal growth centers of the humerus.

Sprains

Sternoclavicular Sprain

Etiology   A sternoclavicular sprain (Figure 21-19) is a relatively uncommon occurrence in sports, but occasionally one may result from one of the various traumas affecting the shoulder complex. The mechanism of the injury can be initiated by an indirect force transmitted through the humerus of the shoulder joint by direct violence such as a blow that strikes the poorly padded clavicle or by twisting or torsion of a posteriorly extended arm. Depending on the direction of force, the medial end of the clavicle can be displaced upward and forward, slightly anteriorly.

Symptoms and signs   Trauma resulting in a sprain to the sternoclavicular joint can be described in three degrees. A grade 1 sprain is characterized by little pain and disability, with some point tenderness but no joint deformity. A grade 2 sprain displays subluxation of the sternoclavicular joint with visible deformity, pain, swelling, point tenderness, and an inability to abduct the shoulder in full range or to bring the arm across the chest, indicating disruption of stabilizing ligaments.

The grade 3 sprain, which is the most severe, presents a picture of complete dislocation with gross displacement of the clavicle at its sternal junction, swelling, and disability, indicating complete rupture of the sternoclavicular and costoclavicular ligaments. If the clavicle is displaced posteriorly, pressure may be placed on the blood vessels, esophagus, or trachea, causing a life-or-death situation.

Management   Rest, ice, compression, and elevation (RICE) should be used immediately after injury. Care of this condition is based on reducing a displaced clavicle to its original position, which is done by a physician, and immobilizing it at that point so that healing may take place. A deformity, primarily caused by formation of scar tissue at that point, is usually apparent after healing is completed. There is no loss of function. Immobilization is usually maintained for 3 to 5 weeks, followed by graded reconditioning exercises. There is a high incidence of recurrence of sternoclavicular sprains.

Acromioclavicular Sprain

Etiology   The acromioclavicular joint is extremely vulnerable to sprains among active sports participants, especially in collision sports[26] (Figure 21-20). The mechanism of an acromioclavicular sprain is most often induced by a direct impact to the tip of the shoulder, pushing the acromion process downward, or by an upward force exerted against the long axis of the humerus (Figure 21-21). The position of the arm

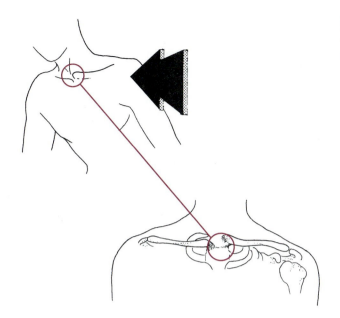

Figure 21-19

Sternoclavicular sprain and dislocation.

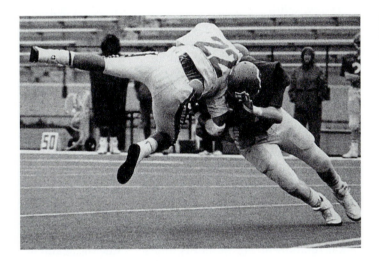

Figure 21-20

Direct impact is a primary mechanism for an acromioclavicular sprain.

during indirect injury is one of adduction and partial flexion. Depending on the extent of ligamentous involvement, the acromioclavicular sprain may be classified as grade 1, 2, or 3. The primary mechanisms of grades 1 and 2 sprains are falling on an outstretched arm or a direct impact to the tip of the shoulder. The mechanism of a grade 3 sprain is most often a direct impact that forces the acromion process downward, backward, and inward while the clavicle is pushed down against the rib cage.

A program of prevention should entail proper fitting of protective equipment, conditioning to provide a balance of strength and flexibility to the entire shoulder complex, and teaching proper techniques of falling and the use of the arm in sports.

CONTUSION TO THE DISTAL END OF THE CLAVICLE   Contusions of this type are often called shoulder pointers and cause a bone bruise and subsequent irritation to the periosteum. During initial inspection this injury may be mistaken for a grade 1 acromioclavicular sprain. In most cases these conditions are self-limiting. When the athlete is able to move the shoulder freely, he or she can return to sports activities.

Symptoms and signs   The grade 1 acromioclavicular sprain reflects point tenderness and discomfort during movement at the junction between the acromion process and the outer end of the clavicle. There is no deformity, indicating only mild stretching of the acromioclavicular ligaments.

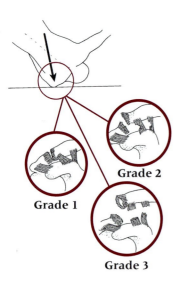

Figure 21-21

Mechanism of an acromioclavicular sprain.

A grade 2 sprain indicates tearing or rupture of acromioclavicular ligaments with associated stretching or tearing of the coracoclavicular ligament. There is definite displacement and prominence of the lateral end of the clavicle when compared with the unaffected side, especially when the acromioclavicular stress test is initiated (Figure 21-22). In this moderate sprain there is point tenderness during palpation of the injury site, and the athlete is unable to fully abduct through a full range of motion or to bring the arm completely across the chest. NOTE: A grade 2 sprain may require surgery to restore stability.

Although occurring less frequently, the grade 3 sprain involves rupture of the acromioclavicular and coracoclavicular ligaments with dislocation of the clavicle. In such an injury there is gross deformity and prominence of the distal clavicle, severe pain, loss of movement, and instability of the shoulder complex.

Management Immediate care of the acromioclavicular sprain involves three basic procedures: (1) application of cold and pressure to control local hemorrhage, (2) stabilization of the joint by a sling and swathe bandage, and (3) referral to a physician for definitive diagnosis and treatment. A grade 1 sprain requires use of a sling for 3 or 4 days. A grade 2 sprain requires 10 to 14 days of protection in a sling. The current recommended management for a grade 3 sprain is nonoperative with approximately 2 weeks of protection in a sling. If there is posterior displacement of the clavicle, surgical reduction and fixation will be necessary. With all grades, an aggressive rehabilitation program involving joint mobilization, flexibility exercises, and strengthening exercises should begin immediately after the recommended period of protection. Progression should be as rapid as the athlete can tolerate without increased pain or swelling. The joint should also be protected with appropriate padding until a pain-free, full range of motion returns.[3]

Glenohumeral Joint Sprain

Etiology The mechanism of this injury is similar to that which produces dislocations and strains. Anterior capsular sprains occur when the arm is forced into abduction (e.g., when making an arm tackle in football). Sprains can also occur from external rotation of the arm. A direct blow to the shoulder could also result in a sprain. The pathological process of a sprain to the glenohumeral joint often involves the rotator cuff muscles.

The infraspinatus–teres minor muscle group is the most effective in controlling external rotation of the humerus and in reducing ligamentous injury.[7] The posterior capsule can be sprained by a forceful movement of the humerus posteriorly when the arm is flexed.

Figure 21-22

Comparison of **A,** a normal shoulder with **B,** a grade 2 acromioclavicular sprain.

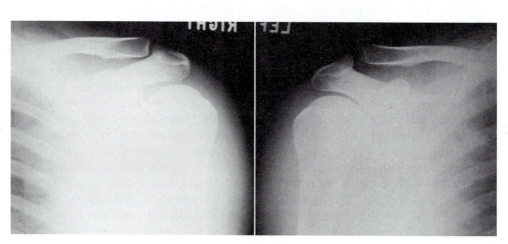

Symptoms and signs   The athlete complains of pain during arm movement, especially when the sprain mechanism is reproduced. There may be decreased range of motion and pain during palpation.

Management   Care after acute trauma to the shoulder joint requires the use of a cold pack for 24 to 48 hours, elastic or adhesive compression, rest, and immobilization by a sling. After hemorrhage has subsided, a program of cryotherapy or ultrasound and massage may be added, and mild passive and active exercise is advocated for regaining full range of motion. Once the athlete can execute full shoulder range of movement without signs of pain, a resistance exercise program should be initiated. Any traumatic injury to the shoulder joint can lead to a subacute and chronic condition of either synovitis or bursitis, which in the absence of shoulder movement will allow muscle contractures, adhesions, and atrophy to develop, resulting in an ankylosed shoulder joint.

Acute Subluxations and Dislocations

Shoulder dislocations account for up to 50% of all dislocations. The extreme range of mobility in the normal shoulder creates an inherent instability in the joint, which is thus susceptible to dislocation. The most common kind of displacement is that occurring anteriorly. Posterior dislocations account for 1% to 4.3% of all shoulder dislocations. Inferior dislocations are extremely rare. Of dislocations caused by direct trauma, 85% to 90% recur.[29]

Etiology

SUBLUXATIONS   With glenohumeral subluxations there is excessive translation of the humeral head without complete separation of the joint surfaces. Subluxation is a brief, transient occurrence in which the humeral head quickly returns to its normal position relative to the glenoid. Subluxation can occur anteriorly, posteriorly, or inferiorly.

ANTERIOR GLENOHUMERAL DISLOCATION   An anterior glenohumeral dislocation may result from direct impact to the posterior or posterolateral aspect of the shoulder. The most common mechanism is forced abduction, external rotation, and extension that forces the humeral head out of the glenoid cavity[9] (Figure 21-23). An arm tackle in football or rugby or abnormal forces created in executing a throw can produce a sequence of events resulting in dislocation.

In an anterior glenohumeral dislocation, the head of the humerus is forced out of its articular capsule in an anterior direction past the glenoid labrum and then downward to rest under the coracoid process. The scope of the pathological process is extensive, with torn capsular and ligamentous tissue, possibly tendinous avulsion of the rotator cuff muscles, and profuse hemorrhage. A tear or detachment of the glenoid labrum may occur. Healing is usually slow, and the detached labrum and capsule can produce a permanent anterior defect on the labrum called a Bankart lesion. Another defect that can occur after dislocation is found on the posterior lateral aspect of the humeral head and is referred to as a Hill-Sachs lesion. It is caused by the compression of the cancellous bone of the head of the humerus against the anterior glenoid rim that creates a divot in the humeral head. Additional complications may arise if the head of the humerus comes into contact with and injures the brachial nerves and vessels. Rotator cuff tears may also occur with anterior dislocations. The bicipital tendon also may be subluxated from its canal as the result of a rupture of its transverse ligament.[29]

POSTERIOR GLENOHUMERAL DISLOCATION   The mechanism of injury is usually forced adduction and internal rotation of the shoulder or a fall on an extended and internally rotated arm. As with anterior dislocations there will be significant soft-tissue damage. Tears of the posterior glenoid labrum are common in posterior dislocation. A fracture of the lesser tuberosity may occur as the subscapularis tendon avulses its attachment.

Symptoms and signs   The athlete with an anterior dislocation displays a flattened deltoid contour. Palpation of the axilla will reveal prominence of the humeral head.

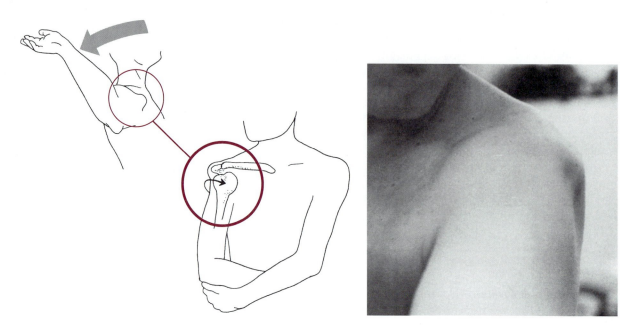

Figure 21-23

Anterior shoulder subluxation and dislocation.

The athlete carries the affected arm in slight abduction and external rotation and is unable to touch the opposite shoulder with the hand of the affected arm. There is often moderate pain and disability.

Posterior glenohumeral dislocation produces severe pain and disability. The arm is often held in adduction and internal rotation. The anterior deltoid muscle is flattened, the acromion and coracoid processes are prominent, and the head of the humerus also may be seen posteriorly. There is limited external rotation and elevation.

Management Initial management of the shoulder dislocation requires immediate immobilization in a position of comfort using a sling with a folded towel or small pillow placed under the arm; immediate reduction by a physician; and control of the hemorrhage by cold packs. The question often arises as to whether a first-time dislocation should be reduced or should receive medical attention. Physicians generally agree that a first-time dislocation may be associated with a fracture, and therefore its treatment is beyond the scope of a coach's or athletic trainer's duties. Ideally, x-rays should be taken before the physician attempts to reduce the dislocated shoulder.[25]

Often a physician will attempt an immediate reduction of anterior dislocations on the field using a method of elevation and internal "derotation" of the arm placed in minimal traction. If unsuccessful, the physician may suggest other methods that use a muscle relaxant. Recurrent dislocations do not present the same complications or attendant dangers as the acute type. However, risk is always involved. Reducing the anterior dislocation usually can be accomplished by applying traction to the abducted and flexed arm.

Reduction of posterior dislocation may have to be performed with the athlete under anesthesia. The procedure usually involves traction on the arm with the elbow bent, followed by adduction of the arm, with posterior pressure being applied to the humeral head anteriorly. While in traction the arm is slowly externally rotated and then internally rotated.

After the dislocation has been reduced and immobilized, muscle reconditioning should be initiated as soon as possible.[27] Protective sling immobilization should continue for approximately 1 week after reduction. In anterior dislocations the arm should be maintained in a relaxed position of adduction and internal rotation. In posterior dislocations the shoulder is immobilized in a position of external rotation and slight abduction. While immobilized, the athlete is instructed to perform isometric exercises for strengthening the internal and external rotator muscles. The strength-

Anterior Glenohumeral Dislocation

Injury Situation A male rugby player was attempting to tackle a ball carrier. At the last second, the ball carrier cut to the right to avoid the tackle. The tackler did not make contact with his left shoulder, but instead with his left arm only. The shoulder was in a position of abduction and external rotation and was forced backward into extension as the ball carrier ran by.

Symptoms and Signs The athlete felt his shoulder give way and felt a pop and a tearing sensation with intense pain. There was a flattened deltoid contour. Palpation of the axilla revealed prominence of the humeral head. The dislocated arm was in slight abduction and external rotation, and the athlete was unable to touch the opposite shoulder with the hand of the affected arm.

Management Plan The athletic trainer should immediately immobilize the dislocated shoulder without attempting reduction. The rugby player should then be referred to a physician for a reduction after x-ray to rule out fracture. After the dislocation has been reduced and immobilized, muscle reconditioning should be initiated as soon as possible.

Phase 1 **Acute Injury**   **GOALS:** Control pain and swelling and begin to regain range of motion. **ESTIMATED LENGTH OF TIME (ELT):** 1 to 5 days.

■ **Therapy** RICE should be applied immediately and should continue to be used for the next several days. Initial management of an anterior shoulder dislocation requires immediate immobilization in a position of comfort using a sling with a folded towel or small pillow placed under the arm. Protective sling immobilization should continue for approximately 1 week after reduction. In anterior dislocations the arm should be maintained in a relaxed position of adduction and internal rotation.

■ **Exercise rehabilitation** While immobilized, the athlete is instructed to perform isometric exercises for strengthening the internal and external rotator muscles. Codman's pendulum exercises and sawing exercises can help with regaining range of motion as pain allows.

Phase 2 **Repair**   **GOALS:** Achieve full range of motion and increase strength. **ELT:** 5 to 12 days.

■ **Therapy** Ice and electrical stimulation should be used to modulate pain. Low-intensity ultrasound may also be used to facilitate healing. The athlete may continue to wear the sling but should be progressively weaned from it as pain allows.

■ **Exercise rehabilitation** Range-of-motion exercises using a T-bar can be instituted as early as tolerated. Wall climbing and rope-and-pulley exercises can also be used to regain motion. Progress the strengthening program from isometrics to resistive rubber tubing and then to dumbbells and other resistance devices as quickly as can be tolerated. Exercises should concentrate on strengthening the rotator cuff. Weight shifting with the hands on the ground can help to begin strengthening the scapular stabilizers and reestablishing neuromuscular control.

Phase 3 **Remodeling**   **GOALS:** Regain normal strength and return to full activity. **ELT:** 12 days to 3 weeks.

■ **Therapy** Electrical stimulation can be used for muscle reeducation. Ultrasound can be used for deep heating to increase blood flow to "clean up" the injured area. Ice should be used after exercise.

■ **Exercise rehabilitation** Strengthening exercise should progress from resisted isotonics to isokinetics at greater speeds. Functional D1 and D2 proprioceptive neuromuscular facilitation strengthening patterns should be used, adjusting resistance to the athlete's capabilities. Plyometric activities using

Continued

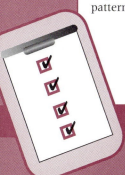

weighted balls can be used to work on more dynamic control. Closed kinetic chain exercises using weight shifting on a ball or balance device improves neuromuscular control. Functional progressions use various activities requiring overhead motion and throwing.

Criteria for Returning to Competitive Rugby

1. The shoulder should have full range of motion and be pain free.
2. Shoulder strength should be near normal.
3. Throwing and catching activities do not produce pain.
4. Protective shoulder braces may be worn to help limit shoulder motion.

21-5

Critical Thinking Exercise

A tennis player has a history of chronic shoulder pain. During an injury evaluation, the athletic trainer notes that as the arm elevates above 90 degrees the athlete seems to be leaning his body toward the side opposite the injured shoulder in an effort to achieve full overhead range of motion. On closer inspection it seems that the scapula is not moving freely above 90 degrees.

? The athletic trainer suspects that for some reason the athlete is not exhibiting a normal scapulohumeral rhythm as the arm moves from adduction to a full overhead position. What is a normal scapulohumeral rhythm?

Recurrent instabilities may be either anterior, posterior, inferior, or multidirectional.

Shoulder instabilities may be attributed to traumatic (macrotraumatic), atraumatic, microtraumatic (repetitive use), congenital, and neuromuscular causes.

ening program should progress from isometrics to resistive rubber tubing and then to dumbbells and other resistance devices as quickly as pain will allow. A major criterion for the athlete's return to sports competition is that there must be internal and external rotation strength equal to 20% of the athlete's body weight. Protective shoulder braces may help limit shoulder motion (see Figure 21-27).

Chronic Recurrent Instabilities of the Shoulder

Chronic or recurrent shoulder instabilities can occur after acute subluxation or dislocation. Recurrent instabilities may be either anterior, posterior, inferior, or multidirectional. Anterior instability accounts for 95% of all recurrent instabilities and usually results after an acute anterior dislocation. With anterior instability, repeated episodes of anterior dislocation have a high probability of occurrence. Posterior instability usually reoccurs as a subluxation rather than a dislocation. Shoulders that have either anterior or posterior instabilities may also subluxate or dislocate inferiorly.[22] If this occurs, a multidirectional instability exists in which there is instability in more than one plane of motion. Multidirectional instabilities most often involve a combination of anteroinferior or posteroinferior laxity but can involve all three directions. It is also possible for a shoulder to dislocate in one direction and subluxate in another.[29]

Etiology The causes of shoulder instabilities may be traumatic (macrotraumatic), atraumatic, microtraumatic (repetitive use), congenital, and neuromuscular. As discussed earlier, traumatic episodes occur from one or more traumatic situations that cause a complete or partial joint displacement. Atraumatic episodes occur in an athlete who either voluntarily or involuntarily displaces the shoulder joint because of inherent ligamentous laxity.[29]

Microtraumatic episodes are created by repetitive use of the shoulder usually involving some faulty biomechanics that leads to soft-tissue laxity. Sports activities such as baseball pitching, tennis serving, and freestyle swimming may produce anterior shoulder instabilities; swimming the back stroke or a backhand stroke in tennis can produce posterior instability. As the supporting tissue becomes increasingly lax, more mobility of the glenohumeral head is allowed, eventually damaging the glenoid labrum. With increased laxity of the supportive capsular and tendinous structures, instability increases, thus increasing the likelihood of recurrent subluxations and dislocations.

Symptoms and signs With recurrent anterior instability the throwing athlete may complain of pain or clicking or experience what is described as a dead arm syndrome in the cocking phase of the overhead throwing motion. Pain is often posterior and may last for several minutes, followed by extreme weakness of the entire arm. Anterior instability may permit excessive translation of the humeral head on the glenoid.[14] This can produce repetitive compression of the rotation cuff, consequently causing impingement of soft tissues under the coracoacromial arch. Tests for apprehension may be positive. Range of motion should be assessed because of the possible decrease in external rotation.[32]

With a recurrent posterior instability, pain may occur posteriorly, anteriorly, or both as a result of subluxation. As with an anterior instability, joint laxity can produce impingement, which is often more of a problem than the subluxation. Crepitation may also be noted on certain movements. There may be a loss of internal rotation when the arm is positioned at 90 degrees of abduction. Stress applied with the arm at 90 degrees of abduction and at 90 degrees of forward flexion, abduction, and internal rotation will allow the degree of posterior humeral head translation to be graded.

In multidirectional instability there will be some inferior laxity, which will exhibit a positive sulcus sign. There is usually some pain and clicking when the arm is held by the side. Any of the symptoms and signs associated with anterior and posterior recurrent instability may be present with multidirectional instability.

Management   Recurrent instabilities may be managed either conservatively or surgically. The initial choice is usually always conservative. Strengthening of all the muscles surrounding the glenohumeral joint, as well as the muscles acting on the scapula, is critical to the success of the rehabilitative program. In particular, strengthening exercises should concentrate on the rotator cuff muscles, which provide dynamic stability in the glenohumeral joint, as well as the scapular stabilizing muscles. With anterior instability strengthening should focus on the internal rotators; the external rotators should be strengthened with posterior instability. Joint mobilization and flexibility exercises should be avoided regardless of the type of recurrent instability. Various types of shoulder harnesses and restraints may be used to limit shoulder motion.[31]

Surgical stabilization may be necessary if the strengthening program fails to improve shoulder function and comfort. Strengthening exercises should be continued for a reasonable period of time before surgery is considered. A physician may choose a variety of surgical techniques or procedures to enhance shoulder stability.

Shoulder Impingement Syndrome

Etiology   Shoulder impingement involves a mechanical compression of the supraspinatus tendon, the subacromial bursa, and the long head of the biceps tendon, all of which are located under the coracoacromial arch (Figure 21-24). This mechanical compression is due to a decrease in space under the coracoacromial arch. Repetitive compression eventually leads to irritation and inflammation of these structures. Impingement most often occurs in repetitive overhead activities such as throwing, swimming, serving a tennis ball, or spiking a volleyball.[20]

Shoulder impingement is closely related to shoulder instability. Athletes involved with overhead activities often exhibit hypermobility and significant capsular laxity. Failure by the rotator cuff muscles to maintain the position of the humeral head relative to the glenoid in overhead activities allows for excessive translation of the humeral head. Eventually this repetitive stress leads to inflammation of those structures under the coracoacromial arch. Prolonged inflammation causes decreased muscular efficiency, and a progressively worsening cycle is created, which can ultimately result in rupture of the supraspinatus or biceps tendons.[17]

Postural malalignments such as a forward head, round shoulders, and an increased kyphotic curve that cause the scapular glenoid to be positioned such that the space under the coracoacromial arch is decreased can also contribute to impingement. Individuals who have a hook-shaped acromion are more likely to have problems with impingement.[10]

Shoulder impingement involves a mechanical compression of the supraspinatus tendon, the subacromial bursa, and the long head of the biceps tendon under the coracoacromial arch.

Figure 21-24

Shoulder impingement compresses soft tissue structures under the coracoacromial arch during humeral elevation.

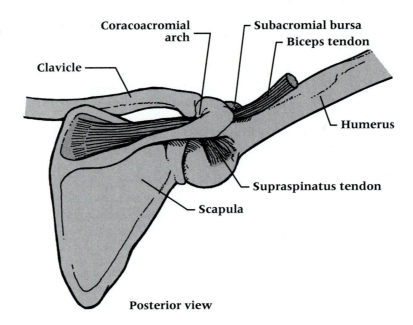

ROTATOR CUFF TEARS   Tears of the rotator cuff muscles are almost always near their insertion on the greater tuberosity. They can be either partial-thickness or complete-thickness tears, with partial-thickness tears occurring twice as often.[17] Most full-thickness tears appear in individuals with a long history of shoulder injury and are relatively uncommon under the age of 40 years. The primary mechanism of injury usually involves either acute trauma or impingement. A rotator cuff tear nearly always involves the supraspinatus muscle.[33] A tear or complete rupture of the other rotator cuff tendons, the subscapularis, infraspinatus, or teres minor, is extremely rare.

Symptoms and signs   The athlete complains of diffuse pain around the acromion. Palpation of the subacromial space increases the pain. Overhead activities also increase the pain.[28] The external rotators are generally weaker than the internal rotators. There may be some tightness in the posterior and inferior joint capsule. There will usually be a positive impingement sign, and both the empty can test and the drop arm test may increase pain.

Neer has described a series of progressive stages of shoulder impingement.[17] Stage I occurs in athletes less than 25 years of age. An initial injury to the supraspinatus or long head of the biceps tendon will produce aching after activity; point tenderness over the supraspinatus or biceps tendons; pain during abduction that becomes worse at 90 degrees; pain during straight-arm full flexion or resisted supination-external rotation; no palpable muscle defect; inflammation with edema; temporary thickening of the rotator cuff and the subacromial bursa; and possible atrophy and constriction of muscles in the region of the shoulder joint.

Stage II involves a permanent thickening and fibrosis of the supraspinatus and biceps tendons and at times the subacromial bursa. Symptoms include aching during activity that becomes worse at night, some restriction of arm movement, and no obvious muscle defect.

Stage III occurs in athletes between the ages of 25 and 40 years. In this stage the athlete has a long history of shoulder problems; shoulder pain during activity with increased pain at night; a tendon defect of 1 cm or less; a possible partial muscle tear; and permanent thickening of the rotator cuff and the acromial bursa with scar tissue.

Stage IV occurs in athletes over the age of 40 years. In this stage there is obvious infraspinatus and supraspinatus wasting; a great deal of pain when abducting the arm

Shoulder Impingement

Injury Situation An 18-year-old female middle distance swimmer is in the third week of her preseason training program. She has significantly increased the distance she has been swimming during the last 3 weeks. Her workouts have increased to twice a day and she has been swimming all freestyle. She is complaining of an aching pain in her left shoulder.

Symptoms and Signs The swimmer complains of diffuse pain around the acromion with point tenderness over the supraspinatus or biceps tendons. Palpation of the subacromial space increases the pain. Overhead activities also increase the pain. There is an achy feeling when she finishes her workout. The external rotators are generally weaker than the internal rotators. There is tightness in the posterior and inferior joint capsule. There is a positive impingement sign, and both the empty can test and the drop arm test increase pain.

Management Plan Management involves restoring normal biomechanics to the shoulder joint in an effort to maintain space under the coracoacromial arch during her swimming workout.

Phase 1 **Acute Injury** GOALS: Control pain and inflammation.
ESTIMATED LENGTH OF TIME (ELT): Day 1 to day 6.

■ **Therapy** RICE and electrical stimulating currents can be used to modulate pain initially. Ultrasound and antiinflammatory medications should be used to reduce inflammation.

■ **Exercise rehabilitation** Her aggressive swimming workout, which caused the problem in the first place, should be modified so that there is some initial control over the frequency and the duration of the workout with a gradual and progressive increase in distance. It may be necessary to keep her out of the pool during phase 1 to allow the inflammation a chance to subside. To maintain her level of fitness, she should substitute running or exercising on a stationary bike for her swimming workout. She may continue her strengthening program, but she must discontinue any strengthening exercise using her sore shoulder.

Phase 2 **Repair** GOALS: Alter joint biomechanics to reduce the likelihood of impingement.
ELT: 1 to 2 weeks.

■ **Therapy** Continue using electrical stimulation and ice to modulate pain. Ultrasound is also helpful in reducing inflammation. Continue antiinflammatory medication.

■ **Exercise rehabilitation** She may now get back into the pool beginning with a short workout initially and then gradually progressing the duration and intensity and using increased pain or stiffness as a guide for progression. Exercises should concentrate on strengthening the rotator cuff. Strengthening of the muscles that abduct, elevate, and upwardly rotate the scapula should also be used. The external rotators should also be strengthened. It may be necessary to limit strengthening exercises in flexion or abduction. Any exercise that places the shoulder in impingement should be avoided. Posterior and inferior glenohumeral joint mobilizations should be done to reduce tightness in the posterior and inferior joint capsule.

Phase 3 **Remodeling** GOALS: Full return to unrestricted activity.
ELT: 2 weeks to full return.

■ **Therapy** Use ultrasound before the workout and ice after completing the workout. Continue antiinflammatory medication.

■ **Exercise rehabilitation** Strengthening exercises should progress to full-range overhead activities.

Continued

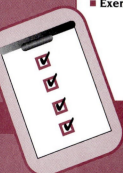

to 90 degrees; a tendon defect greater than 1 cm; limited active and full passive range of motion; weakness during abduction and external rotation; and possible degeneration of the clavicle.

Management Management of stage I and II impingement involves restoring normal biomechanics to the shoulder joint in an effort to maintain space under the coracoacromial arch during overhead activities. Exercises should concentrate on strengthening the rotator cuff muscles, which act to both compress and depress the humeral head relative to the glenoid. Strengthening of the muscles that abduct, elevate, and upwardly rotate the scapula should also be used. The external rotators should also be strengthened. Strengthening of the lower extremity and trunk muscles to reduce the strain placed on the shoulder and arm is also important for the throwing athlete. Posterior and inferior glenohumeral joint mobilizations should be done to reduce tightness in the posterior and inferior joint capsule. Initially, RICE and electrical stimulating currents can be used to modulate pain. Ultrasound and antiinflammatory medications should be used to reduce inflammation. The activity that caused the problem in the first place should be modified so that there is some initial control over the frequency and the level of the activity with a gradual and progressive increase in intensity.

Stages III and IV may require immobilization and complete rest. An athlete who wants to continue activity may require surgical intervention.[12]

Shoulder Bursitis

Etiology The shoulder joint is subject to chronic inflammatory conditions resulting from trauma or from overuse. Inflammation may develop from a direct impact, a fall on the tip of the shoulder, or shoulder impingement. The bursa that is most often inflamed is the subacromial bursa. The pathological process in this condition involves fibrous buildup and fluid accumulation developing from a constant inflammatory state.

Symptoms and signs The athlete has pain when trying to move the shoulder, especially in abduction or with flexion, adduction, and internal rotation. There will also be tenderness to palpation in the subacromial space. Impingement tests will be positive.

21-6

Critical Thinking Exercise

A javelin thrower has been forced to cease his training activity because of pain in his shoulder. He also feels that his shoulder is very loose and unstable. He has been diagnosed by the team physician as having both shoulder impingement syndrome and a multidirectional instability.

? Often, impingement and instability are thought of as being completely separate and unrelated when in fact it is common to find overhead athletes who exhibit signs and symptoms of both problems. How are impingement and instability related to one another?

Management The use of cold, ultrasound, and antiinflammatory medications to reduce inflammation is necessary. If impingement is the primary mechanism precipitating bursitis, measures should be taken to correct this, as previously described. The athlete must maintain a consistent program of exercise, with the emphasis placed on maintaining a full range of motion, so that muscle contractures and adhesions do not immobilize the joint.

Bicipital Tenosynovitis

Etiology Tenosynovitis of the long head of the biceps muscle is common among athletes engaged in overhead activities. Bicipital tenosynovitis is more prevalent among pitchers, tennis players, volleyball players, and javelin throwers. The repeated stretching of the biceps in these highly ballistic activities may eventually cause an irritation of both the tendon and its synovial sheath as it passes under the transverse humeral ligament in the bicipital groove. Complete rupture of the transverse ligament, which holds the biceps in its groove, may take place, or a constant inflammation may result in degenerative scarring or a subluxated tendon.

Symptoms and signs There will be tenderness in the anterior upper arm over the bicipital groove. There may also be some swelling, increased warmth, and crepitus because of the inflammation. The athlete may complain of pain when performing dynamic overhead throwing-type activities.

Management Bicipital tenosynovitis is best cared for by complete rest for several days, with daily applications of cryotherapy or ultrasound to reduce inflammation. Antiinflammatory medications are also beneficial in reducing inflammation. After the inflammation is controlled, a gradual program of strengthening and stretching for the biceps should be initiated.

Contusions of the Upper Arm

Etiology Contusions of the upper arm are frequent in contact sports. Although any muscle of the upper arm is subject to bruising, the area most often affected is the lateral aspect, primarily the brachial muscle and portions of the triceps and biceps muscles. Repeated contusions to the lateral aspect of the upper arm can lead to myositis ossificans, more commonly known as linebacker's arm or blocker's exostosis. Myositis ossificans is a condition in which calcifications or bone fragments occur in a muscle or in soft tissues adjacent to bone.

Symptoms and signs Bruises to the upper arm area can be particularly handicapping, especially if the radial nerve is contused through forceful contact with the humerus, producing transitory paralysis and consequent inability to use the extensor muscles of the forearm.

Management RICE should be applied for a minimum of 24 hours after injury. In most cases this condition responds rapidly to treatment, usually within a few days. The key to treatment is to provide protection to the contused area to prevent repeated episodes that increase the likelihood of myositis ossificans. It is also important to maintain a full range of motion through stretching of the contused muscle.

Biceps Brachii Ruptures

Etiology Ruptures of the biceps brachii (Figure 21-25) can occur in any athlete who is performing a powerful concentric or eccentric contraction of the muscle. The rupture commonly occurs near the origin of the muscle in the bicipital groove.

Symptoms and signs The athlete usually hears a resounding snap and feels a sudden, intense pain at the point of injury. A protruding bulge may appear near the middle of the biceps. When asked to flex the elbow joint of the injured arm and supinate the forearm, the athlete displays a definite weakness.

Management Treatment should include immediately applying a cold pack to control hemorrhage, placing the arm in a sling, and referring the athlete to the physi-

21-7

Critical Thinking Exercise

A volleyball player consistently experiences pain when serving the ball overhead. She also indicates that most of the time when she spikes a ball at the net she experiences pain. During an evaluation the athletic trainer observes that when the humerus is flexed and internally rotated, the pain is worse.

? What is most likely causing the pain when the athlete's shoulder is placed in the overhead position?

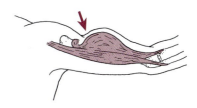

Figure 21-25

Biceps brachii rupture.

cian. In most instances, the athlete with a ruptured bicep will require surgery to repair it. Older individuals may not require surgical repair because the brachialis muscle is the primary flexor of the elbow joint and many nonathletes will be able to function without their biceps.

Frozen Shoulder (Adhesive Capsulitis)

Etiology   Adhesive capsulitis, or frozen shoulder, is a condition more characteristic of an older person, but occasionally it occurs in the younger athlete. The exact cause of adhesive capsulitis is unclear. However, it involves a contracted and thickened joint capsule that is tight around the humeral head with little synovial fluid. There is also chronic inflammation with some fibrosis. The rotator cuff muscles are also contracted and inelastic. Constant, generalized inflammation causes pain on both active and passive motion. Thus the individual will progressively resist moving the joint because of pain. The result is a stiff or frozen shoulder.

Symptoms and signs   Pain is reported in all directions of movement about the shoulder with restriction or limitation of both active and passive movement.

Management   The objectives are to relieve discomfort and restore motion. Treatment usually involves aggressive joint mobilizations and stretching of tight muscles. Electrical stimulating currents may be used to reduce pain. Ultrasound is useful in providing penetrating heat to the area.

Peripheral Nerve Injuries

Etiology   Sports injuries about the shoulder can produce and cause serious nerve injuries. Injuries to shoulder nerves commonly stem from blunt trauma or a stretch type of injury. Nerve injury must be considered when there is constant pain, muscle weakness, paralysis, or muscle atrophy.[18]

Symptoms and signs   Peripheral nerve injuries can result in muscle weakness as follows:

- Suprascapular—supraspinatus and infraspinatus
- Subscapular—subscapularis and teres minor
- Thoracodorsal—latissimus dorsi
- Pectoral—pectoralis major and minor
- Axillary—deltoid and teres minor
- Dorsal scapular—rhomboids and levator scapula
- Long thoracic—serratus anterior
- Musculocutaneous—biceps and coracobrachialis
- Spinal accessory—trapezius

Management   If the injury results from blunt trauma there may also be associated contusion. Thus RICE should be applied immediately. In many instances muscle weakness will be transient with a relatively quick return to normal function. If muscle weakness persists or if there is any muscle wasting or atrophy, referral to a physician is essential.

Thoracic Outlet Compression Syndrome

Etiology   Thoracic outlet compression syndromes involve compression of the brachial plexus, subclavian artery, and subclavian vein (neurovascular bundle) in the neck and shoulder.[15] Neurovascular compression can occur as a result of the following causes:

- Compression of the neurovascular bundle in the narrowed space between the first rib and clavicle (costoclavicular syndrome).
- Compression between the anterior and middle scalene muscles.
- Compression by the pectoralis minor muscle as the neurovascular bundle passes beneath the coracoid process or between the clavicle and first rib.
- The presence of a cervical rib (an abnormal rib originating from a cervical vertebra and the thoracic rib).

Symptoms and signs   Abnormal pressure on the subclavian artery, subclavian vein, and brachial plexus produces a variety of symptoms, including paresthesia and pain, a sensation of cold, impaired circulation in the fingers, muscle weakness, muscle atrophy, and radial nerve palsy. Three tests described earlier can be used to determine thoracic outlet compression syndrome: the anterior scalene test, the costoclavicular test, and the hyperabduction test.

Management   A conservative approach should be taken with early and mild cases of thoracic outlet syndromes. Conservative treatment is favorable in 50% to 80% of cases.[15] It involves correcting the anatomical condition that is responsible for this condition with a series of stretching and strengthening exercises. Exercises should be done to strengthen the trapezius, rhomboids, serratus anterior, and erector muscles of the spine. Stretching exercises for the pectoralis minor and the scalene muscles should also be used.

THROWING DYNAMICS

Throwing activities account for a considerable number of acute and chronic injuries to the shoulder joint. Throwing is a unilateral action that subjects the arm to repetitive stresses of great intensity, particularly in repetitive overhead motions in activities such as throwing a baseball or football, throwing a javelin, serving or spiking a volleyball, and serving or hitting an overhead smash in tennis. If the thrower uses faulty technique, the joints are affected by atypical stresses that result in trauma to the joint and its surrounding tissues.

Throwing is a sequential pattern of movements in which each part of the body must perform a number of carefully timed and executed acts. For example, throwing a ball or javelin uses one particular pattern of movements; hurling the discus or hammer makes use of a similar complex, but with centrifugal force substituted for linear force and the type of terminal movements used in release being different. Putting the shot—a pushing rather than a throwing movement—has in its overall pattern a number of movements similar to those used in throwing.

In the act of throwing, momentum is transferred from the thrower's body to the object that is thrown. Basic physics dictates that the greater and heavier the mass, the greater the momentum needed to move it. Hence, as the size and weight of the object increase, more parts of the body are used to effect the summation of forces needed to accomplish the throw. The same is true in respect to the speed of the object: the greater the speed, the more body parts that must come into play to increase the body's momentum. Timing and sequence of action are of the utmost importance. They improve with correct practice.

In throwing, the arm acts as a sling or catapult, transferring and imparting momentum from the body to the ball. There are various types of throwing, with the overhand, sidearm, and underarm styles being the most common. The act of throwing is fairly complex and requires considerable coordination and timing if success is to be achieved.

In throwing, the most powerful muscle groups are brought into play initially, progressing ultimately to the least powerful but the most coordinated (i.e., the legs, trunk, shoulder girdle, arm, forearm, and finally the hand). The body's center of gravity is transported in the direction of the throw as the leg opposite the throwing arm is first elevated and then moved forward and planted on the ground, thus stopping the forward movement of the leg and permitting the body weight to be transferred from the supporting leg to the moving leg. Initially, the trunk rotates backward as the throwing arm and wrist are cocked, then rotates forward, continuing its rotation beyond the planted foot as the throwing arm moves forcibly from a position of extreme external rotation, abduction, and extension through flexion to forcible and complete extension in the terminal phase of the delivery, bringing into play the powerful internal rotators and adductors. These muscles exert a tremendous force on the distal and proximal humeral epiphysis and over a period of time create cumulative microtraumas that can result in shoulder problems.

Throwing consists of three phases:
Cocking
Acceleration
Follow-through

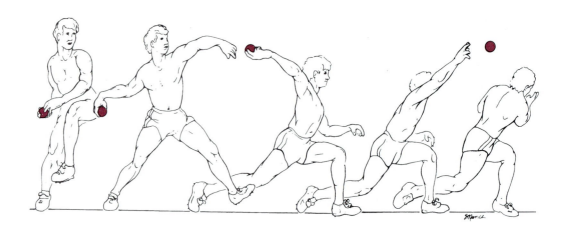

Figure 21-26

Phases of throwing from left to right: windup, early cocking, late cocking, acceleration, follow-through.

Relative to the shoulder complex, throwing or pitching involves three distinct phases: a preparatory, or cocking, phase; the delivery, or acceleration, phase; and the follow-through, or terminal, phase (Figure 21-26).

Cocking Phase

The cocking phase consists of shoulder abduction and extension and external rotation. This phase can cause anterior shoulder pain as a result of strain of the pectoralis major muscle insertion and the origin of the anterior deltoid, long head of the biceps, or internal rotator muscles.

Acceleration Phase

In the acceleration phase the humerus abducts and internally rotates along with a forward flexion, causing some tension on the posterior capsule. The anterior capsule relaxes, and the posterior and inferior capsule tightens.

Follow-through Phase

In the follow-through the humerus moves into adduction and internal rotation, placing the middle and inferior posterior capsule and the anterior superior glenohumeral ligament under tension. In this phase an eccentric load from throwing causes stress to the external rotators and capsule.

REHABILITATION OF THE SHOULDER COMPLEX

Rehabilitation of the shoulder joint after injury requires that the athletic trainer have a sound understanding of the complex anatomical and biomechanical functions of the shoulder girdle. As emphasized earlier, the shoulder is capable of a wide range of movement and consequently sacrifices some degree of stability for the sake of mobility. Achieving the necessary balance between the two is essential in the high-performance athlete.

In recent years the shoulder joint, like the knee joint, has received considerable attention within the sports medicine community. The philosophy of and approach to treatment, management, and rehabilitation continue to change rapidly. Attempts to "cookbook" rehabilitation protocols sometimes fail to allow for essential alteration of protocols in response to the specific needs of the individual athlete. To explain the current approach to rehabilitation of the shoulder most effectively it is necessary to discuss the separate components of a rehabilitation program.

Immobilization after Injury

Rehabilitation programs should be tailored to the individual athlete's needs. An aggressive approach should be used for throwers and swimmers. The length of the immobilization period will vary depending on the structures injured, the severity of the

21-8

Critical Thinking Exercise

A baseball pitcher is throwing a fastball. To effectively execute this motion, the pitcher must develop significant velocity in glenohumeral internal rotation during the acceleration phase. During the follow-through phase this high-velocity internal rotation must quickly decelerate.

? What muscles function to actively internally rotate the glenohumeral joint during the acceleration phase, and what muscles decelerate internal rotation during follow-through?

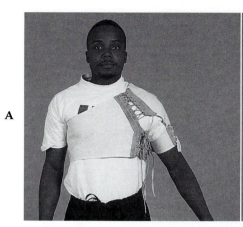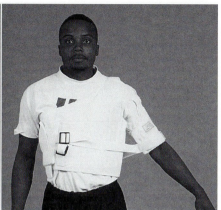

Figure 21-27

Protective braces for the shoulder.

injury, and whether the injury is treated conservatively or surgically by the physician. Regardless of the injury, the injured athlete usually begins to exercise isometrically while wearing an immobilization device (Figure 21-27). For certain injuries it may be unnecessary to wear a sling or brace at all. Other injuries may require that a sling be worn 24 hours a day and removed only for rehabilitative exercises. Certain injuries may require a sling to be worn only at night in the early stages of healing, a motion-limiting brace to be worn during competition only, or in some cases that no sling or brace be worn after the first couple of weeks, but that motion above an angle of 90 degrees be limited for a certain number of weeks. Progression in range of motion and strengthening techniques should be dictated by an understanding of the physiological process of healing and is generally determined by a lack of pain and swelling associated with increased activity.[19]

General Body Conditioning

It is essential for the athlete to maintain a high level of cardiorespiratory endurance throughout the rehabilitation process. In the case of the shoulder joint, activities such as running, speed walking, or riding an exercise bike may be used to maintain cardiorespiratory endurance. Because many athletic activities involve some running, recommending such training would be more useful than recommending swimming for the rehabilitation of an ankle sprain. In sports that require upper-extremity endurance, such as swimming and throwing, the athlete should be progressed to these activities as soon as they can be tolerated. Training and conditioning activities may be modified such that the athlete can continue to maintain strength, flexibility, and neuromuscular control throughout the rest of the body during the period of shoulder rehabilitation.

Shoulder Joint Mobilization

Normal joint arthrokinematics must be maintained to regain normal full-range physiological movement. Mobilization techniques, including inferior, anterior, and dorsal humeral glides; anterior-posterior and inferior-superior glides of the clavicle at both the acromioclavicular and sternoclavicular joints; and generalized scapulothoracic mobilizations, can be incorporated into the early stages of rehabilitation as needed (Figure 21-28).

Flexibility

Regaining a full, nonrestricted, pain-free range of motion is one of the most important aspects of shoulder rehabilitation. Because the shoulder consists of four separate joints that must all function together, the athletic trainer must make certain that normal movement occurs at each joint individually, working toward eventually regaining normal scapulohumeral rhythm. Gentle range-of-motion exercises should begin

Figure 21-28

Shoulder complex joint mobilizations. **A,** Sternoclavicular joint. **B,** Acromioclavicular joint. **C,** Scapular mobilizations. **D,** Anterior humeral glides. **E,** Posterior humeral glides. **F,** Inferior humeral glides.

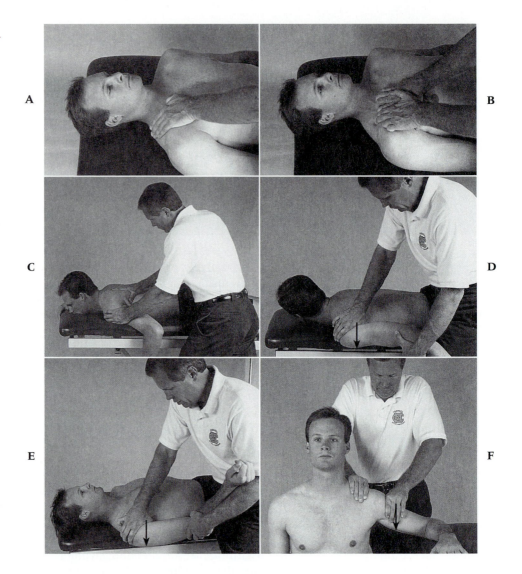

immediately using Codman's pendulum exercises (Figure 21-29) and a "sawing" motion (Figure 21-30). Exercises can be progressed to a series of active-assistive range of motion exercises using a T-bar, done in a pain-free arc for all the cardinal plane movements (Figure 21-31). Cardinal plane movements at the shoulder include flexion, extension, abduction, adduction, internal and external rotation, and horizontal adduction and abduction. Rope-and-pulley exercises (Figure 21-32) or wall-climbing exercises (Figure 21-33) are particularly effective in regaining flexion and abduction.

Muscular Strength

Strengthening exercises in the shoulder generally follow a progression from positional isometrics, to full-range isotonics concentrating on both eccentric and concentric contractions, to isokinetics, to plyometrics. Gentle isometrics should begin immediately after injury or after surgery while the arm is still immobilized at the side.

Isotonic exercise may be incorporated using different types of resistance, including dumbells and barbells (Figure 21-34), surgical tubing or Theraband (Figure 21-35), or manual resistance techniques including PNF strengthening techniques (Figure 21-36).[11] Resistance exercises should include all cardinal plane movements. Particular attention should be given to strengthening the scapular stabilizers by incorporating exercises to resist scapular abduction, adduction, elevation, depression, upward

21-9

Critical Thinking Exercise

After a grade 1 sprain of the acromioclavicular joint, a lacrosse player is having a difficult time regaining full range of motion in both flexion and abduction. When doing his exercises he can elevate his arm above 90 degrees.

? What types of activities should the athletic trainer incorporate in the rehabilitation program to help the athlete regain a full range of motion?

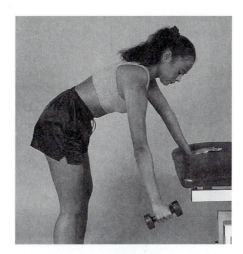

Figure 21-29

Codman's pendulum exercise may begin immediately after injury.

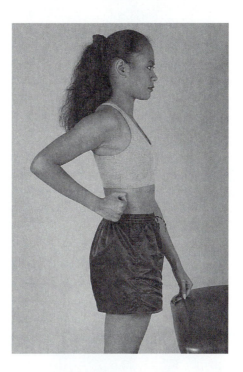

Figure 21-30

"Sawing" exercises are used as a gentle range-of-motion activity for the glenohumeral joint.

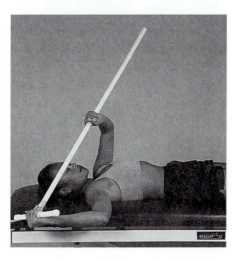

Figure 21-31

T-bar exercises are active-assistive range-of-motion exercises that should be done for each of the cardinal plane movements.

Figure 21-32

Rope-and-pulley exercises for regaining flexion and abduction.

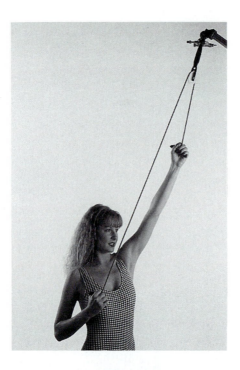

rotation, downward rotation, protraction, and retraction (Figure 21-37). Strengthening the muscles that control the stability of the scapula helps provide a base for the function of the highly mobile glenohumeral joint.

Isokinetic exercises are used to exercise the muscles of the shoulder girdle at varying speeds (Figure 21-38). It must be emphasized that the maximum angular velocities currently available on existing isokinetic devices (approximately 600 degrees per

Figure 21-33

Wall-climbing exercises are useful in regaining abduction and flexion.

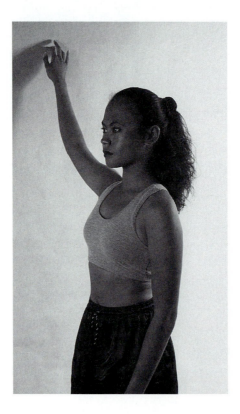

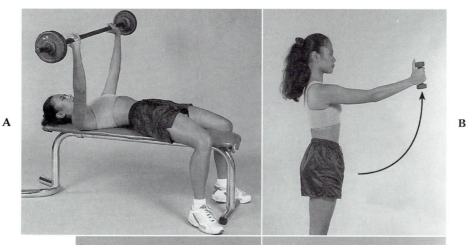

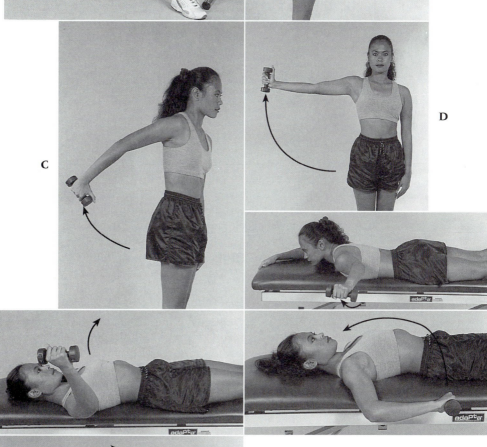

Figure 21-34

Isotonic exercises. **A,** Bench press (pectoralis major, triceps). **B,** Flexion to 90 degrees (anterior deltoid, coracobrachialis, deltoid, pectoralis major, biceps). **C,** Extension (latissimus dorsi, teres major, posterior deltoid). **D,** Abduction to 90 degrees (middle deltoid, supraspinatus, anterior deltoid). **E,** Horizontal abduction (posterior deltoid, infraspinatus, teres minor). **F,** Horizontal adduction (pectoralis major, anterior deltoid). **G,** External rotation (infraspinatus, teres minor, posterior deltoid). **H,** Internal rotation (subscapularis, pectoralis major, latissimus dorsi, teres minor, anterior deltoid).

Figure 21-35

Exercises using surgical tubing are used to emphasize both eccentric and concentric strengthening contractions and can be done in all cardinal planes.

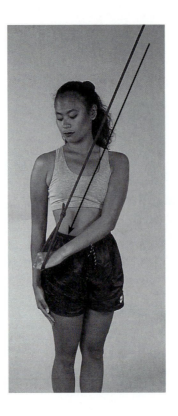

second) do not approach functional speeds of the throwing shoulder; the latter may be as great as 8000 degrees per second of internal rotation.

For both isotonic and isokinetic training, concentric and eccentric components should be emphasized. Eccentric contraction of the external rotators is essential during the deceleration phase of throwing.[4] Plyometric exercises incorporated in the later stages of a rehabilitation program use a quick eccentric stretch of a muscle to facilitate a concentric contraction. Plyometric exercises for the upper extremity can be done using a weighted ball (Figure 21-39).

Regaining Neuromuscular Control

After injury and some period of immobilization, the athlete must "relearn" how to use the injured extremity. Coordinated, highly skilled movement about the shoulder joint is essential for successful return to activity. The athlete must not only regain strength and range of motion but must also develop a firing sequence for the specific muscles that are necessary to perform a highly skilled movement.[5] Biofeedback techniques can help the athlete regain control of specific muscle actions. Efforts toward regaining proprioception should begin immediately in the rehabilitation program.[2]

Closed kinetic chain activities are believed to be important for the lower extremity. However, athletes such as gymnasts, wrestlers, and weight lifters frequently work the upper extremity in a closed kinetic chain. Activities that stress closed kinetic chain function include weight shifting on the hands or on a ball (Figure 21-40) and push-ups. These exercises also emphasize cocontraction of antagonistic muscle groups, thus helping to provide neuromuscular control of opposing muscle groups and promoting stability about the shoulder joint.[30]

Functional Progressions

For the injured shoulder joint, functional progressions usually incorporate some sport-specific skill involving overhead motions such as those required in throwing, swimming, and serving in tennis or volleyball. Strengthening activities should make

(text continues on p. 587)

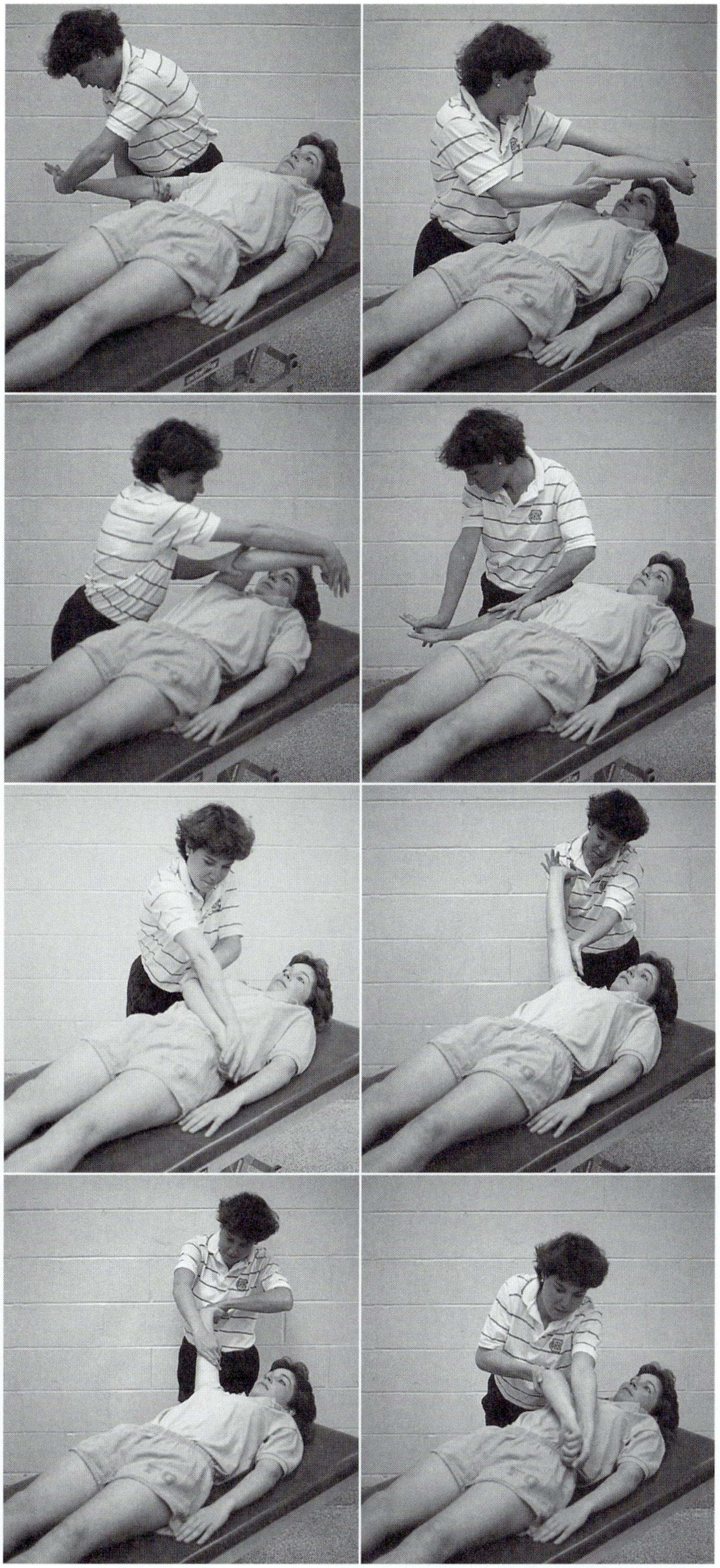

Figure 21-36

Upper-extremity PNF patterns. **A,** D1 upper-extremity pattern moving into flexion-starting position. **B,** D1 upper-extremity pattern moving into flexion-terminal position. **C,** D1 upper-extremity pattern moving into extension-starting position. **D,** D1 upper-extremity pattern moving into extension-terminal position. **E,** D2 upper-extremity pattern moving into flexion-starting position. **F,** D2 upper-extremity pattern moving into flexion-terminal position. **G,** D2 upper-extremity pattern moving into extension-starting position. **H,** D2 upper-extremity pattern moving into extension-terminal position.

Figure 21-37

Strengthening exercises for the scapular stabilizers. **A,** Scapular abduction and upward rotation (serratus anterior). **B,** Scapular elevation (upper trapezius, levator scapulae). **C,** Scapular adduction (middle trapezius). **D,** Scapular depression and adduction (inferior trapezius). **E,** Scapular adduction and downward rotation (rhomboids, inferior trapezius).

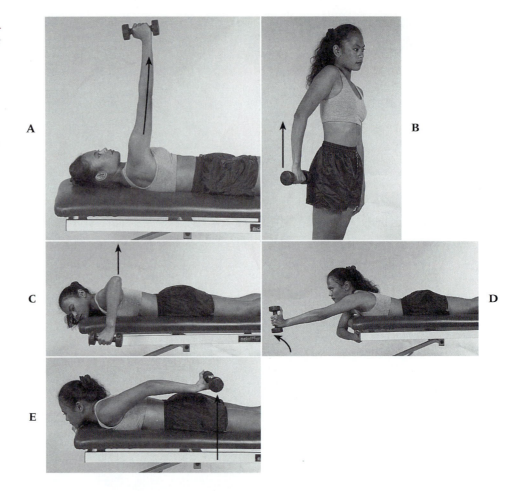

Figure 21-38

Isokinetic exercises may be incorporated in the later stages of a rehabilitation program.

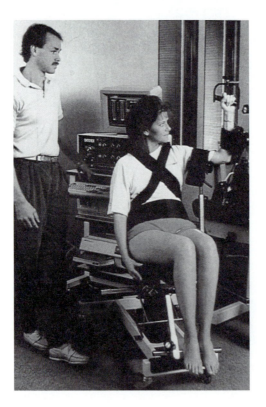

use of the D2 upper-extremity PNF pattern, which closely resembles overhead throwing and serving motions. (See Chapter 15.) Attaching surgical tubing to a baseball or tennis racket and having the athlete move through the throwing or serving motion will help increase the athlete's strength both concentrically and eccentrically (Figure 21-41). Throwing and serving motions require high-speed angular velocities. Thus functional progressions should concentrate on a gradual and progressive increase in these angular velocities. Throwing programs, for example, should increase the throwing distance and the throwing velocity through a series of progressive stages. Progression to a more advanced stage is dictated by lack of pain and swelling at the previous stage.[1]

Return to Activity

Decisions to return an athlete to full activity should be based on preestablished criteria that can be clearly demonstrated by functional performance. Isokinetic testing can provide at least some objective measure of strength. The athletic trainer must have a clear understanding of the healing process and the general time frames re-

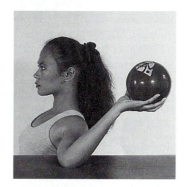

Figure 21-39

Plyometric exercise for shoulder strengthening using a weighted ball.

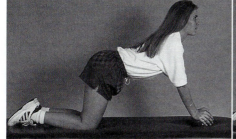

A   B

Figure 21-40

Closed kinetic chain activities such as weight shifting may be functionally important for certain athletes. **A,** Weight shifting on a plyoball. **B,** WS in four-point-position.

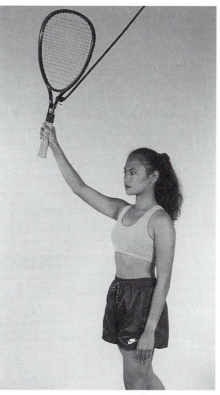

Figure 21-41

Surgical tubing attached to a tennis racket may be used as a functional progression for strengthening overhead motions.

21-10

Critical Thinking E x e r c i s e

A gymnast has a recurrent anterior dislocation of the glenohumeral joint. He has excellent muscular strength in both the glenohumeral muscles and the scapular muscles. He has had no problem regaining full range of motion. He is extremely worried that his shoulder will dislocate again.

? Because strength and range of motion are not a concern in this athlete, what type of activities should the athletic trainer concentrate on during rehabilitation to help reduce the likelihood of a subsequent dislocation?

quired for rehabilitation. Return to full activity should be based on mutual agreement among the athlete, team physician, athletic trainer, and coach.

SUMMARY

- Although the shoulder complex has a great degree of mobility, to have this mobility there must be some compromise in stability, thus making the shoulder highly susceptible to injury. Many sport activities that involve repetitive overhead movements place a great deal of stress on the shoulder joint.

- There are four major articulations associated with the shoulder complex: the sternoclavicular joint, the acromioclavicular joint, the glenohumeral joint, and the scapulothoracic joint. The muscles acting on the shoulder joint consist of those that originate on the axial skeleton and attach to the humerus, muscles that originate on the scapula and attach to the humerus, and a third group of muscles attaching the axial skeleton to the scapula.

- Dynamic movement and stabilization of the shoulder complex require integrated functions of the rotator cuff muscles, the joint capsule, and the muscles that stabilize and position the scapula. In movement of the shoulder joint, it is critical to maintain the positioning of the humeral head relative to the glenoid.

- When evaluating injuries to the shoulder complex, it is necessary to take into consideration all four joints. A number of special tests can provide insight relative to the nature of a particular injury.

- Fractures may occur to the clavicle, scapula, or humerus. Sprains may occur at the sternoclavicular, acromioclavicular, or glenohumeral joints.

- Shoulder dislocations and subluxations are relatively common, with an anterior dislocation and posterior subluxation being the most likely to occur. After a dislocation has been reduced and immobilized, muscle reconditioning should be initiated as soon as possible.

- Chronic or recurrent shoulder instability can occur after acute subluxation or dislocation. Recurrent instabilities may be either anterior, posterior, inferior, or multidirectional. The causes of shoulder instabilities may be traumatic (macrotraumatic), atraumatic, microtraumatic (repetitive use), congenital, or neuromuscular.

- Shoulder impingement is closely related to shoulder instability. Athletes involved with overhead activities often exhibit hypermobility and significant capsular laxity. Shoulder impingement involves a mechanical compression of the supraspinatus tendon, the subacromial bursa, and the long head of the biceps tendon under the coracoacromial arch.

- A number of injuries, including subacromial bursitis, contusions, bicipital tenosynovitis, adhesive capsulitis, peripheral nerve injuries, and thoracic outlet syndromes, are common injuries of the shoulder complex in athletes.

- Rehabilitation after injury to the shoulder joint may require a brief period of immobilization. Joint mobilization, flexibility, and strengthening exercises should be initiated as soon as possible after injury. Progression in range of motion and strengthening techniques should be dictated by a lack of pain and swelling associated with increased activity. Activities that stress closed kinetic chain function emphasize cocontraction of antagonistic muscle groups, thus helping to provide neuromuscular control of opposing muscle groups and promoting stability about the shoulder joint. For the injured shoulder joint, functional progressions usually incorporate some sport-specific skill involving overhead motions.

Solutions to Critical Thinking QUESTIONS

21-1 The athletic trainer should point out that regardless of the strengthening exercises there is still a high probability that a recurrent dislocation will occur. The dynamic stabilizers of the glenohumeral joint include the subscapularis, infraspinatus, teres minor, and supraspinatus. Remember, it is perhaps just as important to strengthen the scapular muscles.

21-2 Restoring normal biomechanics to the shoulder joint in an effort to maintain space under the coracoacromial arch during overhead activities is critical. The athletic trainer should use techniques that strengthen the rotator cuff muscles, which act to both compress and depress the humeral head relative to the glenoid, and strengthen the scapular muscles, which abduct, elevate, and upwardly rotate the scapula. Incorporate posterior and inferior glenohumeral joint mobilizations to reduce tightness in the posterior and inferior joint capsule.

21-3 Thoracic outlet compression syndromes involve compression of the brachial plexus, subclavian artery, and subclavian vein. The anterior scalene syndrome test, or Adson's test, tests for compression by the heads of the anterior and middle scalene muscles or between the cervical rib and the anterior scalene muscle. The costoclavicular syndrome test tests for compression between the first rib and the clavicle. The hyperabduction syndrome test tests for compression behind the pectoral muscle and beneath the coracoid process.

21-4 Falling on the tip of the shoulder is a typical mechanism of injury for a sprain of both the acromioclavicular and sternoclavicular joints. It is also possible that a clavicular fracture has occurred.

21-5 In normal scapulohumeral rhythm, as the humerus elevates to 30 degrees there is no movement of the scapula. From 30 degrees to 90 degrees, the scapula should abduct and upwardly rotate 1 degree for every 2 degrees of humeral elevation. From 90 degrees to full abduction, the scapula should abduct and rotate upward 1 degree for each 1 degree of humeral elevation.

21-6 If the dynamic stabilizers (rotator cuff) and the static stabilizers (joint capsule) of the glenohumeral joint cannot maintain the position of the humeral head relative to the glenoid there will be excessive translation of the humeral head. Excessive translation of the humerus in the overhead position can result in mechanical impingement of those structures under the coracoacromial arch. If the scapular muscles do not function to maintain the position of the glenoid relative to the humerus, impingement can result.

21-7 Her pain is probably due to mechanical impingement or compression of the supraspinatus tendon, the subacromial bursa, or the long head of the biceps under the coracoacromial arch as the arm moves into a fully abducted or flexed position. The space under the arch becomes even more compressed as the humerus is internally rotated, as would occur during the follow-through.

21-8 The subscapularis, pectoralis major, latissimus dorsi, teres major, and anterior deltoid must all contract concentrically to produce internal rotation during the acceleration phase. The infraspinatus, teres minor, and posterior deltoid must contract eccentrically during the follow-through to decelerate internal rotation.

21-9 Because the athlete is having difficulty in regaining active range of motion the athletic trainer might try using diagonal 1 and 2 upper-extremity PNF patterns with rhythmic initiation. This technique involves a progression from passive to active-assistive to active contraction throughout a functional range. The trainer should also utilize joint mobilization techniques for not only the acromioclavicular joint, but also for the sternoclavicular, glenohumeral, and scapulothoracic joints if needed.

21-10 Efforts toward regaining neuromuscular control should begin immediately in the rehabilitation program. Closed kinetic chain exercises emphasize cocontraction of antagonistic muscle groups, thus helping to provide neuromuscular control of opposing muscle groups and promoting stability about the shoulder joint. Activities that stress closed kinetic chain function include weight shifting on the hands or on a ball and push-ups. Biofeedback techniques can help the athlete regain control of specific muscle actions.

REVIEW QUESTIONS AND CLASS ACTIVITIES

1. Explain why a full range of motion of the shoulder joint requires motion at all four joints in the shoulder complex.
2. Explain how the positioning of the humeral head is maintained relative to the glenoid in overhead throwing motions.
3. What is the relationship between shoulder instability and shoulder impingement?
4. What are the mechanisms of an anterior dislocation and a posterior dislocation?
5. How do recurrent instabilities develop?
6. What can be done to minimize the chances of a baseball pitcher developing shoulder impingement?
7. What is myositis ossificans, and how can its development be prevented?
8. How may an athlete acquire bicipital tenosynovitis? How does this condition lead to a ruptured biceps tendon?
9. Describe the various tests for thoracic outlet syndrome.
10. Discuss the mechanics involved in throwing a baseball.
11. Explain why closed kinetic chain exercises are useful in rehabilitation of shoulder injuries.
12. Develop an exercise rehabilitation program for a rotator cuff injury, a glenohumeral dislocation, and an acromioclavicular sprain.

REFERENCES

1. Andrews J, Wilk K: *The athlete's shoulder,* New York, 1994, Churchill Livingstone.
2. Allegrucci M, Whitney S, Lephart S: Shoulder kinesthesia in healthy unilateral athletes participating in upper extremity sports, *J Orthop Sports Phys Ther* 21(4):220, 1995.
3. Bach B, VanFleet T, Novak P: Acromioclavicular joint injuries: controversies in treatment, *Phys Sportsmed* 20(12):87, 1992.
4. Blackburn T, McLeod W: EMG analysis of posterior rotator cuff exercises, *Ath Train* 25(1):40, 1990.
5. Brosa P, Lephart S, Kocher M: Functional assessment and rehabilitation of shoulder proprioception for glenohumeral instability, *J Sport Rehab* 3(1):84, 1994.
6. Butters K: The scapula. In Rockwood C, Masten F, editors: *The shoulder,* Philadelphia, 1990, Saunders.
7. Cain TA et al: Anterior stability of the glenohumeral joint, *Am J Sports Med* 15:144, 1987.
8. Craig E: Fractures of the clavicle. In Rockwood C, Masten F, editors: *The shoulder,* Philadelphia, 1990, Saunders.
9. Grana WA et al: How I manage acute anterior shoulder dislocations, *Phys Sportsmed* 15(4):88, 1987.
10. Greenfield B, Catlin P, Coats P: Posture in patients with shoulder overuse injuries and healthy individuals, *J Orthop Sports Phys Ther* 21(5):287, 1995.

11. Hillman S: Principles and techniques of open kinetic chain rehabilitation: the upper extremity, *J Sport Rehab* 3(4):319, 1994.

12. Irrgang J, Whitney S, Harner C: Nonoperative treatment of rotator cuff injuries in throwing athletes, *J Sport Rehab* 1(3):197, 1992.

13. Karas S: Thoracic outlet syndrome. In Herschman E, editor: *Clinics in sports medicine*, Philadelphia, 1990, Saunders.

14. Li et al: Shoulder function in patients with unoperated anterior shoulder instability, *Am J Sports Med* 19(5):469, 1992.

15. Lutz F, Gieck J: Thoracic outlet compression syndrome, *Ath Train* 21:302, 1986.

16. Masten F, Thomas S, Rockwood C: Glenohumeral instability. In Rockwood C, Masten F, editors: *The shoulder*, Philadelphia, 1990, Saunders.

17. Masten F, Arntz C: Subacromial impingement. In Rockwood C, Masten F, editors: *The shoulder*, Philadelphia, 1990, Saunders.

18. Mendoza F, Main K: Peripheral nerve injuries of the shoulder in the athlete. In Hershman EB, editor: *Neurovascular injuries. Clinics in sports medicine*, vol 9, no 2, Philadelphia, 1990, Saunders.

19. Mendoza F et al: Principles of shoulder rehabilitation in the athlete. In Nicholas JA, Hershman EB, editors: *The upper extremity in sports medicine*, St Louis, 1990, Mosby.

20. Mulligan E: Conservative management of shoulder impingement syndrome, *Ath Train* 23(4):348, 1988.

21. Norris T: History and physical examination of the shoulder. In Nicholas JA, Hershman EB, editors: *The upper extremity in sports medicine*, St Louis, 1990, Mosby.

22. O'Brien S et al: The anatomy and histology of the inferior glenohumeral ligament complex of the shoulder, *Am J Sports Med* 18(5):449, 1990.

23. Perry J et al: The painful shoulder during backstroke: an EMG and cinematographic analysis of 12 muscles, *Clin J Sports Med* 2(1):13, 1992.

24. Pink M et al: The normal shoulder during freestyle swimming, *Am J Sports Med* 19(6):569, 1991.

25. Rofii M et al: Computed tomography (CT) arthrography of shoulder instabilities in athletes, *Am J Sports Med* 16(4):353, 1988.

26. Salter E et al: Anatomical observations on the acromioclavicular joint and supporting ligaments, *Am J Sports Med* 15(3):199, 1987.

27. Sawa T: An alternate conservative management of shoulder dislocations and subluxations, *J Ath Train* 27(4):366, 1992.

28. Scovaggo ML et al: The painful shoulder during freestyle swimming, *Am J Sports Med* 19(6):577, 1991.

29. Skyhar M, Warren R, Altcheck D: Instability of the shoulder. In Nicholas JA, Hershman EB, editors: *The upper extremity in sports medicine*, St Louis, 1990, Mosby.

30. Stone J, Lueken J, Partin N: Closed kinetic chain rehabilitation for the glenohumeral joint, *J Ath Train* 28(1):34, 1993.

31. Terry G et al: The function of passive shoulder restraints, *Am J Sports Med* 19(1):26, 1991.

32. Warner J et al: Patterns of flexibility, laxity, and strength in normal shoulders and shoulders with instability and impingement, *Am J Sports Med* 18(4):366, 1990.

33. Watson K: Impingement and rotator cuff lesions. In Nicholas JA, Hershman EB, editors: *The upper extremity in sports medicine*, St Louis, 1990, Mosby.

ANNOTATED BIBLIOGRAPHY

American Academy of Orthopaedic Surgeons: *Symposium on upper-extremity injuries in athletes*, St Louis, 1986, Mosby.

Covers basic anatomy, biomechanics, surgical and nonsurgical treatment, and detailed rehabilitation relating to upper-extremity injuries in sports.

Andrews J, Wilk K: *The athlete's shoulder*, New York, 1994, Churchill Livingstone.

Concentrates on both conservative and surgical treatment of shoulder injuries occurring specifically in the athletic population.

Cailliet R: *Shoulder pain*, ed 3, Philadelphia, 1991, Davis.

Excellent coverage of the fundamental principles for assessing and treating shoulder pain syndromes.

Hartley A: *Practical joint assessment: a sports medicine manual*, St Louis, 1991, Mosby.

A concise manual of joint assessment, including detailed shoulder evaluation.

Hawkins RJ, editor: *Basic science and clinical application in the athlete's shoulder. Clinics in sports medicine*, vol 10, no 4, Philadelphia, 1991, Saunders.

A detailed monograph dedicated to all aspects of the shoulder in sports.

Nicholas JA, Hershman EB, editors: *The upper extremity in sports medicine*, St Louis, 1995, Mosby.

The text has a great deal of information on the recognition, evaluation, and management of shoulder injuries, in addition to the elbow, wrist, and hand.

Rockwood C, Masten F: *The shoulder*, Philadelphia, 1990, Saunders.

A complete two-volume set that covers essentially every subject relative to the shoulder complex.

The Elbow, Forearm, Wrist, and Hand

When you finish this chapter, you should be able to

- Describe the structural and functional anatomy of the upper arm, elbow, forearm, wrist, and hand and relate it to sports injuries.
- Evaluate the major sports injuries to the elbow, forearm, wrist, and hand.
- Demonstrate proper immediate and follow-up management of upper-limb injuries.

THE ELBOW JOINT
Anatomy
Bones

The elbow joint is composed of three bones: the humerus, the radius, and the ulna (Figure 22-1). The distal end of the humerus forms two articulating condyles. The lateral condyle is the capitulum, and the medial condyle is the trochlea.

Articulations

The convex capitulum articulates with the concave head of the radius. The trochlea, which is spool shaped, fits into an articulating groove, the semilunar notch, which is provided by the ulna between the olecranon and coronoid processes. Above each condyle is a projection called the epicondyle. The structural design of the elbow joint permits flexion and extension through the articulation of the trochlea with the semilunar notch of the ulna. Forearm pronation and supination are made possible because the head of the radius rests against the capitulum freely without any bone limitations.

Ligaments and Capsule

The capsule of the elbow, both anteriorly and posteriorly, is relatively thin and is covered by the brachialis muscle in front and the triceps brachii behind. The capsule is reinforced by the ulnar and radial collateral ligaments. The ulnar collateral ligament is composed of a strong anterior band with weaker transverse and middle sheets. The radial collateral ligament does not attach to the radius, which is free to rotate. The radius rotates in the radial notch of the ulna and is stabilized by a strong annular ligament. The annular ligament is attached to the anterior and posterior margins of the radial notch and encircles the head and neck of the radius.

Valgus elbow stability depends mainly on the integrity of the medial collateral ligament. Lateral elbow stability has two factors: stabilization by the annular ligament maintains the relationship of the radial head to the proximal radioulnar joints. This ligament is of major importance in activities that produce forceful flexion-supination movements. Varus elbow joint forces are uncommon. The main stability of the elbow is contingent on the integrity of radiocapitular articulation, the trochlear-ulnar joint with its coronoid process, and intact medial and lateral ligaments. Additional elbow support is provided by the muscle tendons.

Synovium and Bursa

A common synovial membrane invests the elbow and the superior radioulnar articulations, lubricating the deeper structures of the two joints; a sleevelike capsule surrounds the entire elbow joint. The most important bursae in the area of the elbow are the bicipital and olecranon bursae. The bicipital bursa lies in the anterior aspect of the bicipital tuberosity and cushions the tendon when the forearm is pronated. The olecranon bursa lies between the olecranon process and the skin (Figure 22-2).

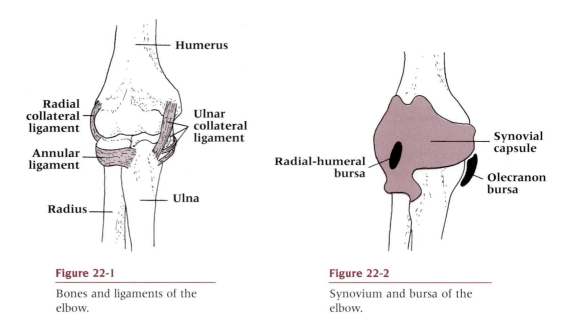

Figure 22-1

Bones and ligaments of the elbow.

Figure 22-2

Synovium and bursa of the elbow.

Musculature

The muscles of the elbow consist of the biceps brachii and the brachialis and brachioradial muscles, all of which in some way act in flexion. Extension is controlled by the triceps brachii muscle (Figure 22-3). The biceps brachii and supinator muscles allow supination of the forearm; the pronator teres and pronator quadratus act as pronators.

Nerve Supply

Nerves stemming from the fifth to eighth cervical vertebrae and the first thoracic vertebra control the elbow muscles. In the cubital fossa these nerves become the musculocutaneous, radial, and median nerves (Table 22-1).

Figure 22-3

Muscles of the elbow joint. **A,** Anterior view. **B,** Posterior view. **C,** Forearm pronators.

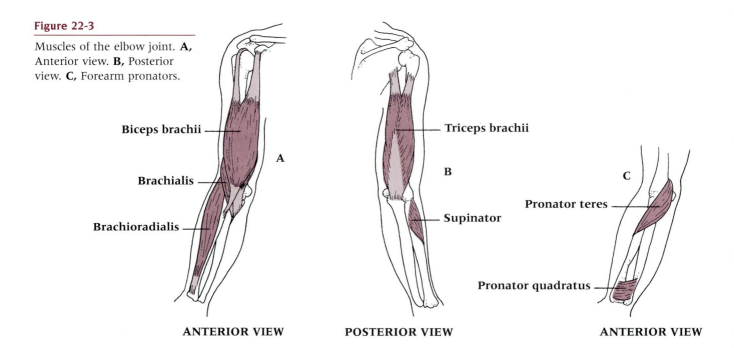

ANTERIOR VIEW   **POSTERIOR VIEW**   **ANTERIOR VIEW**

TABLE 22-1   Resistive Motion to Determine Muscle Weakness Related to Elbow Injury

Resistive Motion	Major Muscles	Involved Nerves
Elbow flexion	Biceps brachii	Musculocutaneous (cervical 5 and 6)
	Brachial	Musculocutaneous (cervical 5 and 6)
	Brachioradial	Radial (cervical 5 and 6)
Elbow extension	Triceps brachii	Radial (cervical 7 and 8)
Forearm supination	Biceps brachii	Musculocutaneous (cervical 5 and 6)
	Supinator	Radial (cervical 6)
Forearm pronation	Pronator teres	Median (cervical 6 and 7)
	Pronator quadratus	Median (cervical 8, thoracic 1)

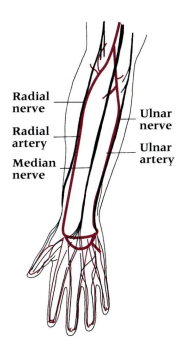

Figure 22-4

Arteries and nerves supplying the elbow joint, wrist, and hand.

Blood Supply

Superficial and close to the skin in front of the elbow lie the veins that return the blood of the forearm to the heart. Deep within the antecubital fossa lie the brachial and medial arteries that supply the area with oxygenated blood (Figure 22-4).

Functional Anatomy

The elbow joint is considered to be a complex rather than a simple joint because the humerus articulates with the radius and ulna. Flexion and extension of the forearm are carried out in the sagittal plane, and supination and pronation occur in the transverse plane.

Assessment of the Elbow

History

As with all sports injuries, the evaluator must first understand the possible mechanism of injury. The following questions are commonly asked in the evaluation of the elbow:
- Is the pain or discomfort caused by a direct trauma such as falling on an outstretched arm or landing on the tip of a bent elbow?
- Can the problem be attributed to sudden overextension of the elbow or to repeated overuse of a throwing-type motion?

The location and duration should be ascertained. As with shoulder pain, elbow pain or discomfort could be from internal organ dysfunction or referred from a nerve root irritation or nerve impingement.
- Are there movements or positions of the arm that increase or decrease the pain?
- Has a previous elbow injury been diagnosed or treated?
- Is there a feeling of locking or crepitation during movement?

Observation

The athlete's elbow should be observed for obvious deformities and swelling. The carrying angle, flexion, and extensibility of the elbow should be observed. If the carrying angle is abnormally increased, a cubitus valgus is present; if it is abnormally decreased, a cubitus varus is present (Figure 22-5). Too great or too little of an angle may be an indication of a bony or epiphyseal fracture. The athlete is next observed for the extent of elbow flexion and extension. Both elbows are compared (Figure 22-6). A decrease in normal flexion, an inability to extend fully, or extending beyond normal extension (cubitus recurvatus) could be precipitating reasons for joint problems (Figure 22-7). Next, the elbow is bent to a 45-degree angle and observed from the rear to determine whether or not the two epicondyles and olecranon process form an isosceles triangle (Figure 22-8).

Bony Palpation

Pain sites and deformities are determined through careful palpation of the epicondyles, olecranon process, distal aspect of the humerus, and proximal aspect of the

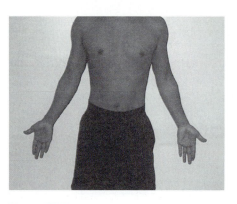

Figure 22-5

Testing for elbow carrying angle and the extent of cubitus valgus and cubitus varus.

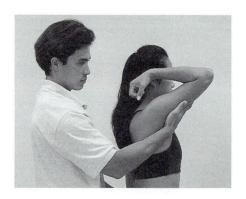

Figure 22-6

Testing for elbow flexion and extension.

ulna (Figure 22-9). The radial head also must be palpated, with the athlete's arm abducted and the elbow bent. The radial head is located approximately 1 inch (2.5 cm) distal to the lateral epicondyle. The athlete supinates and pronates the forearm while pressure is applied to the radial head. Pain during pressure may indicate a sprain of the annular ligament, a fracture, or a chronic articular condition of the radial head.

Soft-Tissue Palpation

Soft tissue includes the following:
- Distal aspect of the wrist flexor muscles
- Pronator teres muscle
- Distal aspect of the wrist extensor muscles
- Medial and lateral collateral ligaments
- Brachioradial muscle
- Biceps tendon
- Antecubital fossa and its contents, including the brachial artery, pulses, and median nerve

22-1

Critical Thinking Exercise

An athlete falls backward, catching himself with the right hand and hyperextending his right elbow.

? What special tests should the athletic trainer perform to determine the nature and extent of this elbow injury?

Figure 22-7

Determining whether the lateral and medial epicondyles, along with the olecranon process, form an isosceles triangle.

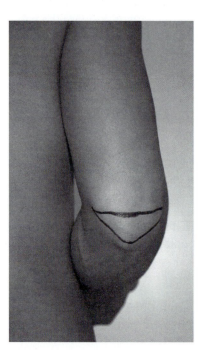

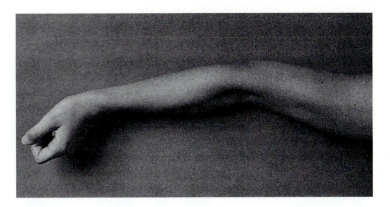

Figure 22-8

Testing for cubitus recurvatus (elbow hyperextension).

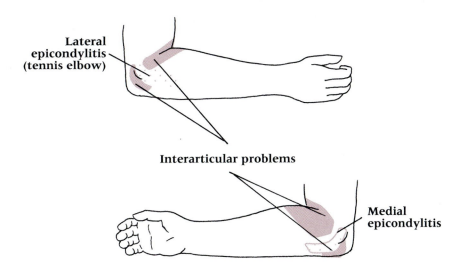

Lateral epicondylitis (tennis elbow)

Interarticular problems

Medial epicondylitis

Figure 22-9

Typical pain sites in the elbow region.

Special Tests

Circulatory and neurological evaluation   With an elbow injury, a pulse routinely should be taken of the brachial artery, which is located in the antecubital fossa, and the radial artery at the wrist.

Alteration of skin sensation also should be noted, which could indicate nerve root compression or irritation in the cervical or shoulder region or in the elbow itself. Additional nerve evaluation is made through testing active and resistive motion (see Table 22-1).

Tests for ligamentous and capsular injury   A test for capsular pain after hyperextension of the elbow is as follows:

- Flex the elbow in a 45-degree position.
- Flex the wrist as far as possible.
- Extend the wrist as far as possible (Figure 22-10).

If joint pain is severe during this test, a moderate to severe sprain or fracture should be suspected.

Lateral and medial collateral ligamentous stability of the elbow is determined as follows:

- The evaluator grasps the athlete's wrist and extends the arm in an anatomical position.
- The other hand of the evaluator is placed over either the lateral or medial epicondyle.
- With the hand over the epicondyle acting as a fulcrum, the hand holding the athlete's wrist attempts to move the forearm.

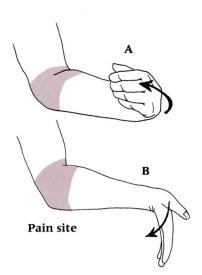

A

B

Pain site

Figure 22-10

Testing for capsular pain after hyperextension of the elbow. **A,** Wrist flexion. **B,** Wrist extension.

Figure 22-11

Collateral ligament test of the elbow.

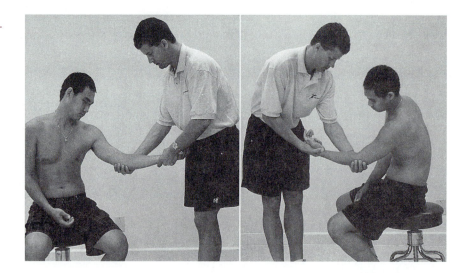

■ In applying the stress, the evaluator notices whether there is an excursion or gapping of the lateral or medial collateral ligament (Figure 22-11).

The athlete complains of severe pain on the medial aspect of the elbow that becomes relieved by flexing the elbow. There is point tenderness on the medial epicondyle, distal aspect of the ulna, or lateral collateral ligament.

Functional Evaluation

The joint and the muscles are evaluated for pain sites and weakness through passive, active, and resistive motions, consisting of elbow flexion and extension (Figure 22-12) and forearm pronation and supination (Figure 22-13). Range of motion is particularly noted in passive and active pronation and supination (Figure 22-14).

Tennis Elbow Test

Resistance is applied to the athlete's extended hand with the elbow flexed 45 degrees. A positive tennis elbow test will be moderate to severe pain at the lateral epicondyle (Figure 22-15).

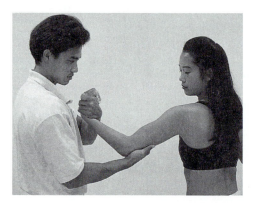

Figure 22-12

Functional evaluation includes performing passive resistance flexion and extension to determine joint restrictions and pain sites.

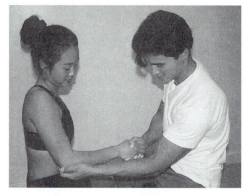

Figure 22-13

Elbow evaluation includes performing passive, active, and resistive forearm pronation and supination.

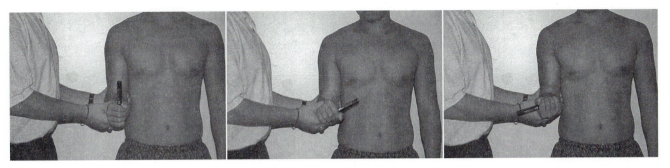

Figure 22-14

The range of motion of fore-arm pronation and supination is routinely observed in athletes with elbow conditions.

The two most common mechanisms of elbow injury:
    Throwing
    Falling on the outstretched hand

Injuries to the Elbow Region

The elbow is subject to injury in sports because of its broad range of motion, weak lateral bone arrangement, and relative exposure to soft-tissue damage.[30] Many sports place excessive stress on the elbow joint. Extreme locking of the elbow in gymnastics or using implements such as racquets, golf clubs, and javelins can cause injuries. The throwing mechanism in baseball pitching can injure the elbow during both the acceleration and follow-through phases.

Soft-Tissue Injuries around the Elbow

Contusions   Because of its lack of padding and its general vulnerability, the elbow often becomes contused during contact sports.

Etiology   Bone bruises arise from a deep penetration or a succession of blows to the sharp projections of the elbow.

Symptoms and signs   A contusion of the elbow may swell rapidly after an irritation of the olecranon bursa or the synovial membrane.

Management   The contused elbow should be treated immediately with cold and pressure for at least 24 hours. If injury is severe, the athlete should be referred to a physician for x-ray examination to determine if a fracture exists.

Olecranon bursitis   The olecranon bursa (Figure 22-16), lying between the end of the olecranon process and the skin, is the most frequently injured bursa in the elbow.

Etiology   Its superficial location makes it prone to acute or chronic injury, particularly as the result of direct blows.

Symptoms and signs   The inflamed bursa produces pain, severe swelling, and point tenderness. Occasionally, swelling will appear almost spontaneously and without the usual pain and heat.

Management   If the condition is acute, a cold compress should be applied for at least 1 hour. Chronic olecranon bursitis requires a program of superficial therapy. In some cases, aspiration will hasten healing. Although seldom serious, olecranon bursitis can be annoying and should be well protected by padding while the athlete is engaged in competition.

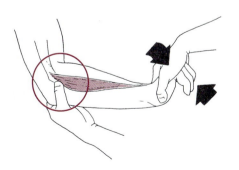

Figure 22-15

Tennis elbow test.

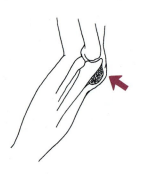

Figure 22-16

Olecranon bursitis.

Strains

Etiology   The acute mechanisms of muscle strain associated with the elbow joint are usually excessive resistive motions such as a fall on the outstretched hand with the elbow in extension, forcing the joint into hyperextension. Repeated microtears that cause chronic injury are discussed in the section on epicondylitis.

The biceps, brachialis, and triceps muscles should be tested through active and resistive movement. The muscles of pronation and supination are also tested.

Symptoms and signs   During active or resistive movement, the athlete complains of pain. There is usually point tenderness in the muscle, tendon, or lower part of the muscle belly.

Management   Immediate care includes rest, ice, compression, and elevation (RICE) and sling support for the most severe cases. Follow-up management may include cryotherapy, ultrasound, and rehabilitative exercises. Conditions that cause moderate to severe loss of elbow function should routinely be referred for x-ray examination. It is important to rule out the possibility of an avulsion or epiphyseal fracture.

Elbow sprains

Etiology   Sprains to the elbow are usually caused by hyperextension or valgus forces.

Symptoms and signs   The athlete complains of pain and an inability to throw or grasp. Inspection displays a point tenderness over the medical collateral ligament. Flexor tendinous injury can also be present. A valgus stress test shows ligamentous disruption.

Management   Immediate care for elbow sprains consists of cold and a pressure bandage for at least 24 hours with sling support fixed at 45 degrees of flexion. After hemorrhage has been controlled, superficial heat treatments in the form of whirlpool may be started and combined with massage above and below the injury. Like fractures and dislocations, strains also may result in abnormal bone proliferation if the area is massaged directly and too vigorously or is exercised too soon. The main concern should be to gently aid the elbow in regaining a full range of motion and then, when the time is right, to commence active exercises until full mobility and strength have returned. Taping can help and should restrain the elbow from further injury, or it may be used while the athlete is participating in sports (see Figure 13-8).[7]

Lateral epicondylitis   Epicondylitis is a chronic condition that may affect athletes who execute repeated forearm flexion and extension movements such as are performed in tennis, pitching, golf, javelin throwing, and fencing. The elbow is particularly predisposed to mechanical trauma in the activities of throwing and striking.[26]

Lateral epicondylitis is one of the most common problems of the elbow occurring in sports. It is most often seen in tennis players and is also seen in baseball, swimming, gymnastics, fencing, golfing, and hammer throwing.[13]

Etiology   The cause of lateral epicondylitis is repetitive microtrauma to the insertion of the extensor muscle of the lateral epicondyle. Hyperpronation is the primary action.[13] *Tennis elbow* is another name for lateral epicondylitis stemming from a backhand stroke involving overextending the wrist.[26]

Symptoms and signs   The athlete complains of an aching pain in the region of the lateral epicondyle during and after activity. The pain gradually becomes worse with weakness in the hand and wrist. Inspection reveals tenderness at the lateral epicondyle and pain on resisted dorsiflexion of the wrist and full extension of the elbow. The elbow has decreased range of motion (ROM).[22]

Management   Treatment includes immediate use of RICE, nonsteroidal antiinflammatory drugs (NSAIDs), and analgesics as needed. Rehabilitation includes range-of-motion exercises, progressive-resistive exercises, deep friction massage, hand grasping while in supination, and avoiding pronation movements. Mobilization and stretching may be used within pain-free limits. The athlete may wear a counterforce or neoprene elbow sleeve for 1 to 3 months. The athlete must be taught proper skill techniques and the proper use of equipment to avoid recurrence of the injury.[13]

Lateral epicondylitis:
   Tennis elbow

Medial epicondylitis Irritation and inflammation of the medial epicondyle may result from a number of different sport activities that require repeated forceful flexions of the wrist and extreme valgus torques of the elbow.[30] *Pitcher's elbow, racquetball elbow, golfer's elbow,* and *javelin-thrower's elbow* are names used to refer to medial epicondylitis.[14]

Etiology Young baseball pitchers learning to throw a curveball or screwball tend to use excessive wrist flexions when imparting a spin on the baseball.[11] A forehand stroke in racquetball requires an explosive wrist flexion at impact to achieve maximum velocity. Golfers may use too much wrist flexion on the trail arm on follow-through. Throwing the javelin requires powerful wrist flexion at release (Figure 22-17).

Symptoms and signs Regardless of the sport or exact location of the injury, the symptoms and signs of epicondylitis are similar. Pain around the epicondyles of the humerus can be produced during forceful wrist flexion or extension. The pain may be centered at the epicondyle, or it may radiate down the arm. There is usually point tenderness and in some cases mild swelling. Passive movement of the wrist into extension or flexion seldom elicits pain, although active movement does.

Management Conservative management of moderate to severe epicondylitis usually includes use of sling rest, cryotherapy, or heat through the application of ultrasound. Analgesics and antiinflammatory agents may be prescribed. A curvilinear brace applied just below the bend of the elbow is highly beneficial in reducing elbow stress. This brace provides a counterforce, disseminating stress over a wide area and relieving the concentration of forces directly on the bony muscle attachments (Figure 22-18). For more severe cases elbow splinting and complete rest for 7 to 10 days may be warranted.

Elbow Osteochondritis Dissecans

Although osteochondritis dissecans is more common in the knee it also occurs in the elbow.

Medial epicondylitis:
  Pitcher's elbow
  Racquetball elbow
  Golfer's elbow
  Javelin-thrower's elbow

Elbow osteochondritis dissecans is similar to that in the knee but is less common.

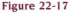

Figure 22-17

Repeated overhand throwing actions can cause epicondylitis.

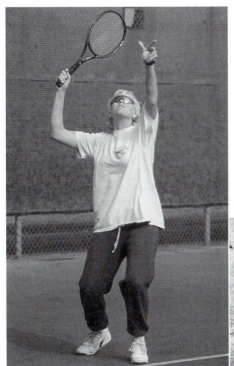

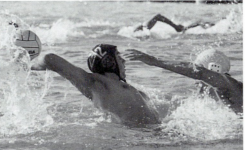

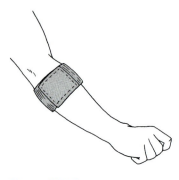

Figure 22-18

Counterforce brace for treatment of elbow epicondylitis.

Etiology   Its cause is unknown; however, impairment of the blood supply to the anterior surfaces leads to fragmentation and separation of a portion of the articular cartilage and bone, creating a loose body within the joint.[4] It is seen in the young athlete 10 to 15 years of age who throws or engages in racquet sports. There is a repetitive microtrauma in the movements of elbow rotation, extension, and valgus stress leading to a compression of the radial head and shearing of the radiocapitular joint.[13]

Symptoms and signs   The child or young adolescent athlete usually complains of sudden pain and locking of the elbow joint. Range of motion returns slowly over a few days. Swelling, pain, and crepitation may also occur. There is a decreased ROM, especially in full extension and tenderness at the radiohumeral joints. There may be a grating sensation on pronation or supination. X-ray examination shows a flattening of the capitellum, a crater in the capitellum, and loose bodies.

Management   In the beginning stage of this condition activity is restricted for 6 to 12 weeks, and NSAIDs are administered. With increased degeneration, activity is restricted and a splint or cast is applied along with physical therapy. If there are loose bodies with repeated locking, fragments are removed surgically.

Little League Elbow

Little League elbow occurs in 10% to 25% of young pitchers.[13] It includes many disorders of growth in the pitching elbow.[28] These disorders may include the following:

- An accelerated apophyseal growth region plus a delay in the medial epicondylar growth plate.
- A traction apophysitis with a possible fragmentation of the medial epicondylar apophysis.
- An avulsion of the medial epicondrosis of the radial head.
- Osteochondrosis of the humeral capitellum.
- A nonunion stress fracture of the olecranon epiphysis.[27,28]

Etiology   Little League elbow is caused by repetitive microtrauma occurring from throwing and not the type of pitch thrown.[13,27]

Symptoms and signs   Injury onset is usually slow. In the beginning the athlete may have a flexion contraction, which includes a tightness of the anterior joint capsule and a weakness of the triceps muscle. The athlete may complain of a locking or catching sensation. There is decreased ROM of forearm pronation and supination.[6]

Management   Initially, RICE, NSAIDs, and analgesics are given as needed.[13] Throwing is stopped until pain is resolved and full ROM is returned. Gentle stretching and triceps strengthening are carried out. Surgical removal of loose bodies may be required.[6] Good throwing mechanics must be taught.

Cubital Tunnel Syndrome

Because of the exposed position of the medial humeral condyle, the ulnar nerve is subject to a variety of problems. The athlete with a pronounced cubitus valgus may develop a friction problem. The ulnar nerve can also become recurrently dislocated because of a structural deformity. The ulnar nerve can become impinged by the arcuate ligament during flexion-type activities. In a problem of the ulnar nerve seen in sports such as baseball, tennis, racquetball, and javelin throwing, fascial bands forming the roof of the cubital tunnel compress the ulnar nerve.[3,23]

Etiology   Normally four factors can lead to this condition: traction injury from a valgus force, irregularities within the tunnel, subluxation of the ulnar nerve because of a lax ligament, or a progressive compression of the ligament on the nerve.

Symptoms and signs   The athlete complains of pain on the medial aspect of the elbow that may be referred proximally or distally. On palpation there is tenderness in the cubital tunnel primarily on hyperflexion. There is intermittent paresthesia reflected by a burning and tingling in the fourth and fifth fingers.[1]

Management   Initially, rest and immobilization for 2 weeks along with NSAIDs. Splinting or surgical decompression or transposition of a subluxating ulnar nerve. The athlete must avoid elbow hyperflexion and valgus stresses.[13]

Dislocation of the Elbow

Etiology   Dislocation of the elbow (Figure 22-19) has a high incidence in sports activity and is caused most often either by a fall on the outstretched hand with the elbow in a position of hyperextension or by a severe twist while it is in a flexed position.[2] The bones of the ulna and radius may be displaced backward, forward, or laterally. By far the most common dislocation is one in which both the ulna and the radius are forced backward. The forward-displaced ulna or radius appears deformed. The olecranon process extends posteriorly, well beyond its normal alignment with the humerus. This dislocation may be distinguished from the supracondylar fracture by observing that the lateral and medial epicondyles are normally aligned with the shaft of the humerus.

Symptoms and signs   Elbow dislocations involve rupturing and tearing of most of the stabilizing ligamentous tissue, accompanied by profuse hemorrhage and swelling. There is severe pain and disability. The complications of such traumas include injury to the median and radial nerves, as well as to the major blood vessels and arteries, and—in almost every instance—myositis ossificans. Elbow dislocation is often associated with a radial head fracture.

Management   The primary responsibility is to apply cold and pressure immediately, then a sling, and to refer the athlete to a physician for reduction. The neurovascular status of the brachial artery and the median and ulnar nerves must be evaluated before and after reduction.[15] Reducing an elbow dislocation should never be attempted by anyone other than a physician. It must be performed as soon as possible to prevent prolonged derangement of soft tissue. In most cases the physician will administer an anesthetic before reduction to relax muscles spasms. After reduction, the physician will often immobilize the elbow in a position of flexion and apply a sling suspension, which should be used for approximately 3 weeks (Figure 22-20). While the arm is maintained in flexion, the athlete should execute hand gripping and shoulder exercises. When initial healing has occurred, heat and gentle, passive exercise may be applied to help regain a full range of motion. Above all, massage and joint movements that are too strenuous should be avoided before complete healing has occurred because of the high probability of encouraging myositis ossificans. Both range of movement and a strength program should be initiated by the athlete, but forced stretching must be avoided.

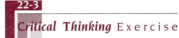

22-3

Critical Thinking Exercise

A female javelin thrower complains of pain on the medial aspect of her elbow that is also referred distally to the forearm. The athlete senses an intermittent paresthesia, a burning sensation, and tingling in the fourth and fifth fingers.

? What condition does this athlete have, and how could it have occurred?

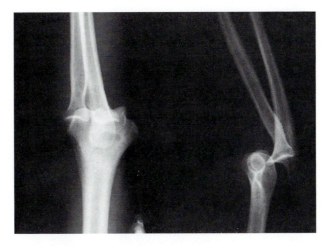

Figure 22-19

Elbow dislocation.

Posterior Elbow Dislocation

Injury Situation A female athlete fell from the uneven bars, landing on her outstretched left hand. The elbow was forced into hyperextension, dislocating the radial head posteriorly.

Symptoms and Signs The athlete complained of extreme pain in the elbow region and numbness in the forearm and hand. From the side view the forearm appeared shortened. An obvious deformity was that the radial head stuck out beyond the posterior aspect of the elbow. The neurovascular status was assessed and found to be normal.

Management Plan The athlete was referred immediately to a physician who performed an x-ray examination of the elbow to rule out fracture. After the x-ray examination, the elbow was reduced by the physician and placed in a cast and sling at 60 degrees for 6 weeks.

Phase 1 **Acute Injury** **GOAL DURING IMMOBILIZATION PHASE:** To maintain wrist and hand strength and shoulder range of motion while elbow is immobilized. **ESTIMATED LENGTH OF TIME (ELT):** 6 weeks.

■ **Exercise rehabilitation** Ball squeeze (10 to 15 repetitions), each waking hour. Shoulder circles in all directions (10 to 15 repetitions), each waking hour. General body maintenance exercises are conducted three times a week as long as they do not aggravate injury.

Phase 2 **Repair** **GOAL AFTER CAST IS REMOVED:** Increase range of motion 50%, strength and coordination 50%. **ELT:** 4 to 6 weeks.

■ **Therapy** Ice (5 to 15 minutes) before and after exercise, electrical stimulation to modulate pain, and low-intensity ultrasound to facilitate healing.

■ **Exercise Rehabilitation** Continue exercises performed during immobilization phase, three to four times daily. Isometric exercise (two to three times), every waking hour. Pain-free active flexion and extension and forearm pronation and supination (10 to 15 repetitions), every waking hour; *avoid forcing movements*. Proprioceptive neuromuscular facilitation (PNF) also can be beneficial. Isokinetic exercise or isotonic exercise against dumbbell resistance, once daily, using daily adjustable progressive resistive exercise (DAPRE). General body maintenance exercises are conducted three times a week as long as they do not aggravate injury.

Phase 3 **Remodeling** **GOALS:** To restore 90% of elbow ROM and strength, including power, endurance, and neuromuscular control, and to reenter competition. **ELT:** 3 to 6 weeks.

■ **Therapy** Electrical stimulation for muscle reeducation. Ultrasound or massage to increase blood flow in the area. Follow exercise with cryotherapy.

■ **Exercise rehabilitation** Continue phase 2 exercises and add isotonic machine resistance or free-weight barbell exercises; bar dips and chin-ups (10 repetitions), three to four times a week, can be added to routine. Return to daily gymnastic practice within pain-free limits. If elbow becomes symptomatic in any way, such as pain, swelling, or decreased range of motion, athlete is to return to phase 2 exercises.

Continued

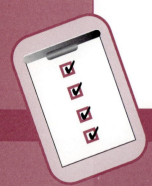

Posterior Elbow Dislocation—*cont'd*

Criteria for Returning to Competitive Gymnastics

The athlete must be able to do the following:
1. Extend and flex the elbow to at least 95% of the uninjured elbow.
2. Pronate and supinate the forearm to at least 95% of the uninjured arm.
3. Perform an elbow curl 10 times, for three sets, against a resistance equal to or greater than that which can be handled by the uninjured elbow (this could be measured by an isokinetic testing device).
4. Perform an elbow extension 10 times, for three sets, against a resistance equal to or greater than that which can be handled by the uninjured elbow (this also can be measured by an isokinetic testing device).
5. Pronate and supinate the forearm against a resistance equal to or greater than that which can be handled by the uninjured forearm.
6. Perform 10 full bar dips.
7. Perform 10 chin-ups.
8. Perform a full routine on the uneven bars without causing discomfort.

Fractures of the Elbow

An elbow fracture can occur in almost any sports event and is usually caused by a fall on the outstretched hand or the flexed elbow or by a direct blow to the elbow (Figure 22-21). Children and young athletes have a much higher rate of this injury than do adults. A fracture can take place in any one or more of the bones that compose the elbow.[7]

Etiology A fall on the outstretched hand often fractures the humerus above the condyles, the condyles proper, or the area between the condyles. The ulna and radius also may be the recipients of trauma, and direct force delivered to the olecranon process of the ulna or a force transmitted to the head of the radius may cause a fracture.

Symptoms and signs An elbow fracture may or may not result in visible deformity. There usually will be hemorrhage, swelling, and muscle spasm in the injured area.

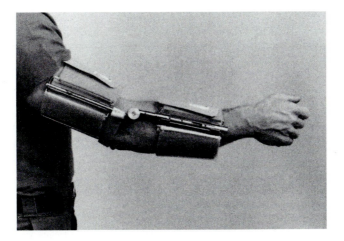

Figure 22-20

Dynasplint for the reduction of elbow flexion contraction.

Figure 22-21

A fall on the outstretched hand can produce an elbow fracture.

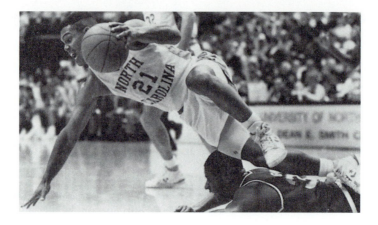

Management   As with a dislocation, an elbow fracture can be associated with certain complications. One major complication is decreased ROM. The neurovascular status of the injury must be continually monitored. Surgery is used to stabilize an adult unstable elbow fracture followed by early ROM. Removable splints are used. Stable fractures do not require surgery. Removable splints are used for 6 to 8 weeks.[21]

Volkmann's Contracture

Volkmann's contracture is a major complication of a serious elbow injury.

It is essential that athletes who sustain a serious elbow injury have their brachial or radial pulse monitored periodically to rule out the possibility of a Volkmann's contracture.

Etiology   It is most often associated with a humeral supracondylar fracture, which causes muscle spasm, swelling, or bone pressure on the brachial artery, inhibiting blood circulation to the forearm, wrist, and hand.

Symptoms and signs   Such a contracture can become permanent. The first indication of this problem is pain in the forearm that becomes greater when the fingers are passively extended. This pain is followed by cessation of the brachial and radial pulses.

Management   Management of the athlete with beginning signs of tissue pressure reflected by pain, coldness, and decreased motion includes the removing of elastic wraps or casts and elevation of the part. Close monitoring must occur.

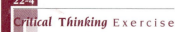

22-4

Critical Thinking Exercise

An athlete sustains a humeral supracondylar fracture that causes severe muscle spasm, swelling, and bone pressure on the brachial artery.

? What should the athletic trainer be concerned with, and what actions should be taken?

Rehabilitation of the Elbow

Rehabilitation of the elbow depends on the type of injury incurred, the specific sport played, and whether conservative or postsurgical care is involved. In general, the entire upper-arm kinetic chain, as well as the trunk and lower extremities, must be considered.

General Body Conditioning

While the elbow is being specifically rehabilitated the athlete is directed to perform general body exercises to main preinjury fitness level.

Elbow Joint Mobilization

An elbow that is immobilized and has restricted motion for a period of time develops an orthrofibrosis and adhesive capsulites, as well as calcific tendinitis. It is therefore important that early ROM and mobilizations be instituted. Hoffman mobilization and traction techniques increase joint mobility and decrease pain by restoring accessory movements (Figures 22-22 and 22-23).

Flexibility

As mentioned, restoring normal ROM is important early in elbow rehabilitation. A variety of approaches can be applied as long as they do not force the joint. Examples

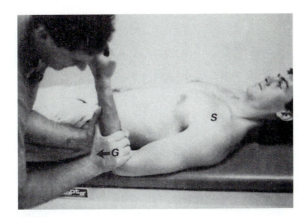

Figure 22-22

Inferior humeroulnar glides. This technique increases elbow flexion and extension. It is performed using the body weight to stabilize proximally with the hand grasping the ulna and gliding inferiorly.

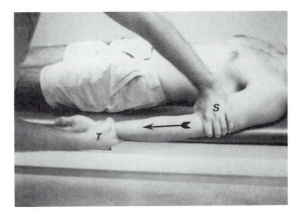

Figure 22-23

Humeroradial inferior glides. This technique increases the joint space and improves flexion and extension.

may be slow passive stretch with a low force and a long duration (Figures 22-24 and 22-25). Active assistive or partner stretching can follow passive stretching. Proprioceptive neuromuscular facilitation (PNF) exercise also aids in restoring a normal ROM.

After a severe injury, such as a dislocation, or after a surgical procedure initial rehabilitation is directed toward regaining or maintaining normal range of motion. After surgery a continuous passive movement could be used.

Strengthening

Beginning strengthening is achieved by low-resistance, high-repetition exercise of the biceps brachialis, triceps, pronators, supinators, wrist flexors, and wrist extensors. Grip and shoulder exercises are also performed to increase strength and range of motion. All activities must be pain free.[10]

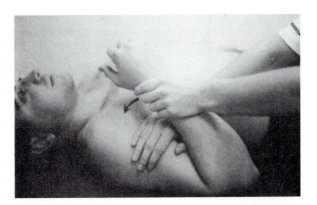

Figure 22-24

Partner stretching of triceps (medial and lateral head) and anconeus. The biceps muscle is stretched when the elbow is moved in the opposite direction.

Figure 22-25

Position for humeroulnar joint traction.

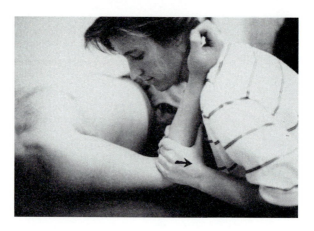

Two procedures may be used to maintain elbow mobility following surgery: namely, the use of the continuous passive machine immediately after surgery, followed by the use of a dynamic splint. In some cases isometric exercise is appropriate while the elbow is immobilized. Maintaining the strength of these articulations will speed the recovery of the elbow. After the elbow has healed and free movement is permitted by the physician, the first consideration should be restoration of the normal range of movement. Proprioceptive neuromuscular facilitation and isokinetic exercises are valuable in the early and intermediate active stage of rehabilitation. Isokinetic exercise is valuable because of its speed control, its use of concentric and eccentric work, and its endurance development. Isokinetic exercise should be begun when the athlete has a full ROM and is a good beginning to functional retraining.

Closed kinetic chain exercises are used for athletes who perform in open kinetic chain sports such as throwing. Closed kinetic chain exercises help provide both static and dynamic stability to the elbow. Proprioceptive conditioning of the elbow must be considered (Figures 22-26 and 22-27).

Figure 22-26

Sitting push-up.

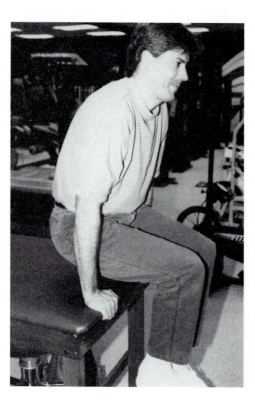

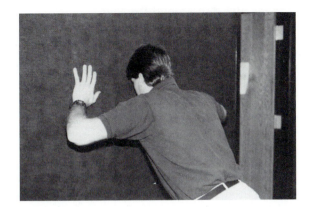

Figure 22-27

Wall push-up.

Functional Progressions

When the athlete has full elbow mobility, no pain or swelling, and 90% of preinjury strength, the following functional progressions can be engaged in:

- Open kinetic chain activities with a controlled range of motion
- Open kinetic chain activities through pain-free ROM
- Closed kinetic chain exercises for stability and neuromuscular control
- Plyometrics
- Mimic functional activity

Return to Activity

The athlete can return to activity after achieving full ROM, joint stability, and functional strength. The athlete must maintain a high level of conditioning. Inadequate rest must be avoided to prevent a recurrence of an overuse injury. When full ROM has been regained (Figure 22-28), a graded, progressive, resistive exercise program should be initiated, including flexion, extension, pronation, and supination (Figure 22-29).

Figure 22-28

Proprioceptive neuromuscular facilitation exercise is an excellent approach to elbow rehabilitation.

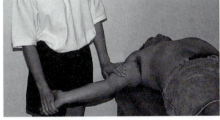 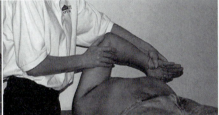 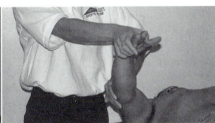

Figure 22-29

A gradual program of progressive resistance is important to elbow rehabilitation.

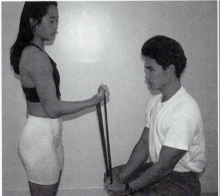 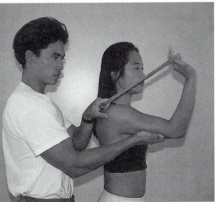

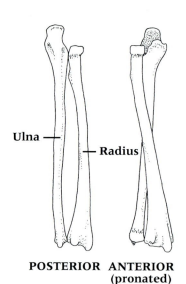

Ulna — — Radius

POSTERIOR ANTERIOR
(pronated)

Figure 22-30

Bones of the forearm.

Protective Taping and Bracing

Protective taping must be continued until full strength and flexibility have been restored. Long-standing chronic conditions of the elbow usually cause gradual debilitation of the surrounding soft tissue. Elbows with conditions of this type should be restored to the maximum state of conditioning without encouraging postinjury aggravation.

THE FOREARM

Anatomy

Bones

The bones of the forearm are the ulna and the radius (Figure 22-30). The ulna, which may be thought of as a direct extension of the humerus, is long, straight, and larger at its upper end than at its lower end. The radius, considered an extension of the hand, is thicker at its lower end than at its upper end.

Articulations

The forearm has three articulations: the superior, middle, and distal radioulnar joints. The superior radioulnar articulation is a pivot joint, moving in a ring that is formed by the ulna and the annular ligament.

Ligaments

The middle radioulnar joint, which is the junction between the shafts of the ulna and the radius, is held together by an oblique ligamentous cord and the interosseous membrane. The oblique cord is a small band of ligamentous fibers that are attached to the lateral side of the ulna and pass downward and laterally to the radius. The interosseous membrane is a thin sheet of fibrous tissue that runs downward from the radius of the ulna and transmits forces directly through the hand from the radius to the ulna. The middle radioulnar joint provides a surface for muscle attachments, and there are openings for blood vessels at the upper and lower ends. The distal radioulnar joint is a pivot joint formed by the articulation of the head of the ulna with a small notch on the radius. It is held securely by the anterior and posterior radioulnar ligaments. The inferior ends of the radius and ulna are bound by an articular, triangular disk that allows radial movement of 180 degrees into supination and pronation.

Musculature

The forearm muscles consist of flexors and pronators that are positioned anteriorly and extensors and supinators that lie posteriorly. The flexors of the wrist and fingers are separated into superficial muscles and deep muscles (Figure 22-31). The deep flexors arise from the ulna, the radius, and the interosseous tissue anteriorly, and the superficial flexors come from the internal humeral condyle. The extensors of the wrist and fingers originate on the posterior aspect and the external condyle of the humerus.

Nerve and Blood Supply

Except for the flexor carpi ulnaris and half of the flexor digitorum profundus, most of the flexor muscles of the forearm are supplied by the median nerve. The majority of the extensor muscles are controlled by the radial nerve. The major blood supply stems from the brachial artery, which divides into the radial and ulnar arteries in the forearm.

Assessment of Forearm Injuries

History

The following questions are asked to determine forearm injuries:
- What caused the injury (e.g., blunt trauma, throwing, or chronic overuse)?
- What were the symptoms at the time of injury? Did symptoms occur later?

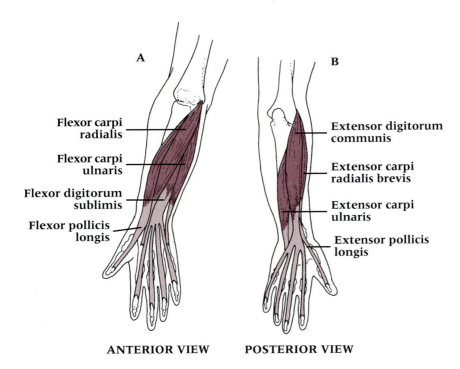

A

Flexor carpi
radialis

Flexor carpi
ulnaris

Flexor digitorum
sublimis

Flexor pollicis
longis

B

Extensor digitorum
communis

Extensor carpi
radialis brevis

Extensor carpi
ulnaris

Extensor pollicis
longis

ANTERIOR VIEW   **POSTERIOR VIEW**

Figure 22-31

Muscles of the forearm. **A,** Anterior view. **B,** Posterior view.

- Were symptoms localized or diffused?
- Was there swelling or discoloration?
- Was there immediate loss of function?
- What treatment was given?
- How does the forearm feel now?

Observation

The entire forearm is first visually inspected, including the wrist and elbow, looking for obvious deformities, swelling, and skin defects. The athlete then is observed pronating and supinating the forearm when a deformity is not present.

Palpation

The injured forearm is palpated at distant sites as well as the point of injury. Palpation can reveal tenderness, edema, fracture deformity, change in skin temperature, a false joint, bone fragments, or a lack of continuity between bones.

Injuries to the Forearm

Lying between the elbow joint and the wrist and hand, the forearm is indirectly influenced by injuries to these areas; however, direct injuries can also occur.

Contusions

Etiology   The forearm is constantly exposed to bruising in contact sports such as football. The ulnar side receives the majority of blows in arm blocks and consequently the greater amount of bruising. Bruises to this area may be classified as acute or chronic. The acute contusion can result in a fracture, but this happens only rarely.

Symptoms and signs   Most often a muscle or bone develops varying degrees of pain, swelling, and hematoma. The chronic contusion develops from repeated blows to the forearm with attendant multiple irritations. Heavy fibrosis may take the place of the hematoma, and a bony callus has been known to arise out of this condition.

Management   Care of the contused forearm requires proper attention in the acute stages through application of RICE for at least 1 hour, followed the next day by cryotherapy. Protection of the forearm is important for athletes who are prone to this condition. The best protection consists of a full-length sponge rubber pad for the forearm early in the season.

Forearm Splints

Etiology   Forearm strain can occur in a variety of sports; most such injuries come from a severe static contraction. Repeated static contraction can lead to forearm splints. Forearm splints, like the medial tibial stress syndrome (shinsplints), are difficult to manage. They occur most often in gymnasts, particularly to those who perform on the side horse, and in wrestlers.[5]

Symptoms and signs   The main symptom is a dull ache between the extensor muscles, which cross the back of the forearm. There also may be weakness and extreme pain during muscle contraction. Palpation reveals an irritation of the interosseous membrane and surrounding tissue. The cause of this condition is uncertain; like shinsplints, forearm splints usually appear either early or late in the season, which indicates poor conditioning or fatigue, respectively. The pathological process is believed to result from the constant static muscle contractions of the forearm (e.g., those required to stabilize the side horse participant). Continued isometric contraction causes minute tears in the area of the interosseous membrane.

Management   Care of forearm splints is symptomatic. If the problem occurs early in the season, the athlete should concentrate on increasing the strength of the forearm through resistance exercises, but if it arises late in the season, emphasis should be placed on rest and cryotherapy or heat and use of a supportive wrap during activity.

Although much less common than in the lower leg, the forearm can also sustain an acute or chronic exertional compartment syndrome. It can occur in sports such as gymnastics and weight lifting and can result from direct injuries such as muscle avulsion, distal radius fracture, or a crush-type injury. The deep forearm compartment containing the flexor digitorum profundus, flexor pollicus longus, and pronator quadratus is most susceptible to changes of muscle and nerve ischemia. Detection and management of this condition are the same as for the lower leg condition.

Forearm Fractures

Etiology   Fractures of the forearm (Figure 22-32) are particularly common among active children and youths and occur as the result of a blow or a fall on the outstretched hand.[12] Fractures to the ulna or the radius alone are much rarer than simultaneous fractures to both. The break usually presents all the features of a long-bone fracture: pain, swelling, deformity, and a false joint. If there is a break in the upper third, the pronator teres muscle has a tendency to pull the forearm into an abduction deformity, whereas fractures of the lower portion of the arm are often in a neutral position. The older the athlete, the greater the danger of extensive damage to soft tissue and the greater the possibility of paralysis from Volkmann's contractures.

Symptoms and signs   The athlete experiences an audible "pop" or crack followed by moderate to severe pain, swelling, and disability. There is localized tenderness, edema, and ecchymosis with possible crepitus.[19]

Management   Initially, RICE is applied followed by splinting until definitive care is available. Definitive care consists of a long-arm plaster or fiberglass cast followed by a program of rehabilitation.

Colles' fracture   Colles' fractures (Figure 22-33) are among the most common types and involve the lower end of the radius or ulna.

Etiology   The mechanism of injury is usually a fall on the outstretched hand, forcing the radius and ulna backward and upward (hyperextension). Much less common is the reverse of Colles' fracture. The mechanism of this fracture is the result of a fall on the back of the hand.

Forearm splints, like shinsplints, commonly occur either early or late in the sports season.

22-5

Critical Thinking Exercise

At the end of the season a gymnast specializing in the side horse experiences a dull ache in the extensor muscles of the forearm. The athlete also complains of weakness and severe pain when these muscles are contracted.

? What is the gymnast's condition, and what is the probable mechanism of injury?

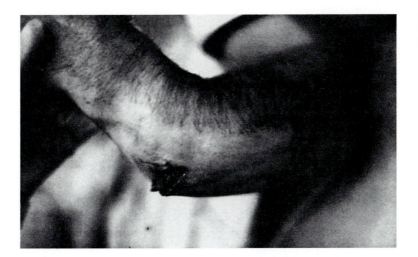

Figure 22-32

An open fracture of the ulna.

Symptoms and signs   In most cases there is forward displacement of the radius that causes a visible deformity to the wrist, which is commonly called a "silver fork" deformity. Sometimes no deformity is present, and the injury may be passed off as a bad sprain—to the detriment of the athlete. Bleeding is profuse in this area with the extravasated fluids causing extensive swelling in the wrist and, if unchecked, in the fingers and forearm. Ligamentous tissue is usually unharmed, but tendons may be torn and avulsed, and there may be median nerve damage.

Management   The main responsibility is to apply a cold compress, splint the wrist, put the limb in a sling, and then refer the athlete to a physician for x-ray examination and immobilization. Severe sprains should always be treated as possible fractures. Lacking complications, the Colles' fracture will keep an athlete out of sports for 1 to 2 months. It should be noted that what appears to be a Colles' fracture in children and youths is often a lower epiphyseal separation.[29]

THE WRIST AND HAND
Anatomy
Bones

The wrist, or carpus, is formed by the union of the distal aspect of the radius and the articular disk (called the triangular fibrocartilage) of the ulna with three of the four proximal (of the eight diversely shaped) carpal bones. Appearing in order from the radial to the ulnar side in the first or proximal row are the navicular, lunate, triquetral, and pisiform bones; the distal row consists of the greater multangular (trapezium), lesser multangular (trapezoid), capitate, and hamate bones (Figure 22-34).

The concave surfaces of the lower ends of the radius and ulna articulate with the convex surfaces of the first row of carpal bones, with the exception of the pisiform, which articulates with the articular disk interposed between the head of the ulna and the triquetral bone. This radiocarpal joint is a condyloid joint and permits flexion, extension, abduction, and circumduction. Its major strength is drawn from the great number of tendons that cross it rather than from its bone structure or ligamentous arrangement. The articular capsule is a continuous cover formed by the merging of the radial and the ulnar collateral, volar radiocarpal, and dorsal radiocarpal ligaments.

Carpal articulations   The carpal bones articulate with one another in arthrodial or gliding joints and combine their movements with those of the radiocarpal joint and the carpometacarpal articulations. They are stabilized by anterior, posterior, and connecting interosseous ligaments.

Metacarpal phalange bones   The metacarpal bones are five bones that join the carpal bones above and the phalanges below, forming metacarpophalangeal (MCP)

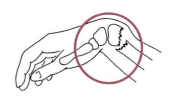

Figure 22-33

Common appearance of the forearm in Colles' fracture.

22-6

Critical Thinking Exercise

A young athlete falls off the parallel bars onto his outstretched left hand, forcing the wrist into hyperextension. There is a visible deformity to the wrist.

? Describe the deformity presented and the actions that should be taken by the athletic trainer.

Figure 22-34

Bones of the wrist and hand.

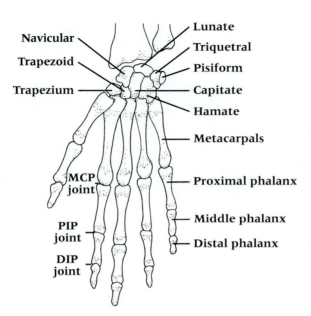

articulations of a condyloid type and permitting flexion, extension, abduction, adduction, and circumduction.

Articulation

As is true for the carpal bones, each joint has an articular capsule that is reinforced by collateral and accessory volar ligaments. The interphalangeal articulations are of the hinge type, permitting only flexion and extension. Their ligamentous and capsular support is basically the same as that of the MCP joints.

The thumb varies slightly at its carpometacarpal joint and is classified as a saddle joint that allows rotation on its long axis in addition to the other metacarpophalangeal movements.

Ligaments

There are numerous wrist and hand ligaments; however, only those concerned with sports injuries are emphasized.

Ligaments of the wrist   The wrist is composed of many ligaments that bind the carpal bones to one another, to the ulna and radius, and to the proximal metacarpal bones. Of major interest in wrist injuries are the collateral ulnar ligament, extending from the tip of the styloid process of the ulna to the pisiform bone, and the triquetral bone and collateral radial ligament that extends from the styloid process to the radius to the navicular bone (scaphoid). Crossing the volar aspect of the carpal bones is the transverse carpal ligament. This ligament serves as the roof of the carpal tunnel, in which the median nerve is often compressed (Figure 22-35).

Ligaments of the phalanges   The proximal interphalangeal (PIP) joints have the same design as the MCP joints. They comprise the collateral ligaments, palmar fibrocartilages, and a loose dorsal capsule or synovial membrane protected by an extensor expansion (Figure 22-36).

Musculature

The wrist and hand are a complex of extrinsic and intrinsic muscles. See Table 22-2 for the major muscles in the hand and wrist (Figure 22-37).

Blood and Nerve Supply

Circulation impairment must be noted as soon as possible in any wrist and hand injury.

The three major nerves of the hand are the ulnar, radial, and median nerves. The ulnar nerve comes to the hand by passing between the pisiform bone and the hook

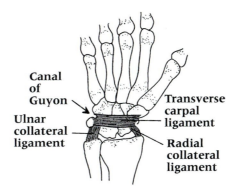

Figure 22-35

Ligaments of the wrist.

of the hamate bone. The radial nerve enters the wrist from the back of the forearm between the superficial and deep extensor muscles where it terminates in the back of the carpus. The median nerve enters the palm of the hand through the carpal tunnel (see Table 22-2). The sensory pattern of peripheral nerves can be seen in Figure 22-38. The radial nerve may or may not follow this pattern.

The arteries that supply the wrist and the hand are the radial and ulnar arteries. They create two arterial arches: the superficial palmar arch, which is the largest and most distal to the hand, and the deep palmar arch.

Assessment of the Wrist and Hand

History

As with other conditions, the evaluator asks about the location and type of pain:

- What increases or decreases the pain?
- Has there been a history of trauma or overuse?
- What therapy or medications, if any, have been given?

Observations

As the athlete is observed, arm and hand asymmetries are noted:

- Are there any postural deviations?
- Does the athlete hold the part in a stiff or protected manner?
- Is the wrist or hand swollen?

Hand usage such as writing or unbuttoning a shirt is noted. The general attitude of the hand is observed (Figure 22-39). When the athlete is asked to open and close the hand, the evaluator notes whether this movement can be performed fully and rhythmically. Another general functional activity is to have the athlete touch the tip of the thumb to each fingertip several times. The last factor to be observed is the color of the fingernails. Nails that are very pale instead of pink may indicate a problem with blood circulation.[20]

Palpation

Bony palpation

Wrist region   The bones of the wrist region are palpated for pain and defects. With the wrist in ulnar flexion, the examiner palpates the radial styloid process, navicular bone (scaphoid) through the anatomical snuffbox, trapezium, and first metacarpal bone. With the wrist straight, the examiner palpates the distal head of the radius, lunate bone, capitate bone, ulnar styloid, triquetral bone, pisiform bone, and hook of the hamate bone.

Hand region   The examiner palpates the first metacarpal bone, MCP joint, and each phalanx, starting with the PIP joint and progressing to the distal interphalangeal (DIP) joint.

Soft-tissue palpation

Wrist region   Each tendon is palpated as it crosses the wrist region. Of major importance is the palpation of the six dorsal wrist tunnels, the carpal tunnel, and the

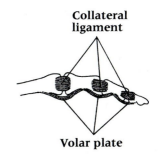

Figure 22-36

Ligaments of the phalanges.

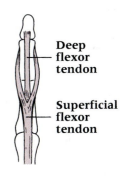

Figure 22-37

Tendons of the phalanges.

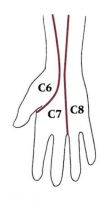

Figure 22-38

Sensory patterns of peripheral nerves in the hand.

TABLE 22-2 **Resistive Motion to Determine Muscle Weakness Related to Wrist and Hand Injury**

Resistive Motion	Major Muscles Involved	Nerves
Wrist flexion	Flexor carpi radialis	Median, cervical 6 and 7
	Flexor carpi ulnaris	Ulnar, cervical 8, thoracic 1
Wrist extension	Extensor carpi radialis longus	Radial, cervical 6 and 7
	Extensor carpi radialis brevis	Radial, cervical 6 and 7
		Radial, cervical 6-8
	Extensor carpi ulnaris	
Flexion of MCP joints of fingers	Lumbricalis manus	Radial, cervical 6-8
	Interossei dorsalis manus	Median, ulnar, cervical 6-8
	Interossei palmares	Ulnar, cervical 8, thoracic 1
		Ulnar, cervical 8, thoracic 1
Flexion of PIP and DIP joints of fingers	Flexor digitorum superficialis	Median, cervical 7 and 8, thoracic 1
Extension of MCP joints of fingers	Extensor digitorum	Radial, cervical 6-8
	Extensor indicis	Radial, cervical 6-8
	Extensor digiti minimi	Radial, cervical 6-8
Finger abduction	Interossei dorsalis	Ulnar
	Abductor digiti	Cervical 8, thoracic 1
Finger adduction	Interossei palmares	Ulnar, cervical 8, thoracic 1
Thumb flexion	Flexor pollicis brevis	Median, cervical 6 and 7
	Lateral portion	Ulnar, cervical 8, thoracic 1
	Medial portion	Cervical 8, thoracic 1
	Flexor pollicis longus	
Thumb extension	Extensor pollicis brevis	Radial, cervical 6 and 7
	Extensor pollicis longus	Radial, cervical 6-8
Thumb abduction	Abductor pollicis longus	Radial, cervical 6 and 7
	Abductor pollicis brevis	Median, cervical 6 and 7
Thumb adduction	Adductor pollicis	Ulnar, cervical 8, thoracic 1
Thumb opposition	Opponens pollicis	Median, cervical 6 and 7
Fifth-finger opposition	Opponens digiti minimi	Ulnar, cervical 6 and 7

tunnel of Guyon on the volar aspect. Pain at the site of the first tunnel may indicate stenosing tenosynovitis, or de Quervain's disease. Point tenderness is an indication for administering the de Quervain's test.

Hand region The examiner palpates the thenar and hypothenar region, palmar aponeurosis, and flexor muscles. On the dorsal aspect, the examiner palpates the extension tendons and phalanges.

Special Tests for the Hand and Wrist

Test for de Quervain's disease The de Quervain's test is also called the Finklestein's test (Figure 22-40). The athlete makes a fist with the thumb tucked inside. The wrist is then deviated into ulnar flexion. Sharp pain is evidence of stenosing tenosynovitis. Pain over the carpal tunnel could mean a carpal tunnel syndrome affecting the median nerve. On occasion the flexor tendons also become trapped, making finger flexion difficult. Any symptoms of carpal tunnel syndrome are an indication for testing, using the tapping sign and wrist press test.

The tapping sign for carpal tunnel syndrome The tapping sign (Tinel's sign) for carpal tunnel syndrome is performed by tapping over the transverse carpal ligament. It is a positive test if pain or paresthesia is elicited (Figure 22-41).

Wrist press Another common test for carpal tunnel syndrome is the wrist press test (Phalen's test). The athlete is instructed to flex both wrists as far as possible and press them together. This position is held for approximately 1 minute. If this test is positive, pain will be produced in the region of the carpal tunnel (Figure 22-42).

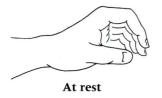

At rest

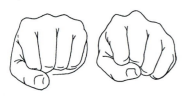

Normal fist   Clenched fist

Figure 22-39

General normal attitudes of the hand.

Circulatory and Neurological Evaluation

The hands should be inspected to determine whether circulation is being impeded. The hands should be felt for their temperature. A cold hand or portion of a hand is a sign of decreased circulation. Pinching the fingernails can also help detect circulatory problems. Pinching will blanch the nail, and on release there should be rapid return of a pink color. Another objective test is the Allen's test.

Testing the radial and ulnar arteries of the hand   The Allen's test is used to determine the function of the radial and ulnar arteries supplying the hand. The athlete is instructed to squeeze the hand tightly into a fist and then open it fully three or four times. While the athlete is holding the last fist, the evaluator places firm pressure over each artery. The athlete is then instructed to open the hand. The palm should now be blanched. One of the arteries is then released, and, if normal, the hand will instantly become red. The same process is repeated with the other artery (Figure 22-43). The hand is next evaluated for sensation alterations, especially in cases of suspected tunnel impingements. Nerve involvements will be further evaluated when active and resistive movements are initiated.

Functional Evaluation

Range of motion is noted in all movements of the wrist and fingers. Active and resistive movements are then compared with those of the uninjured wrist and hand. The following sequence should be conducted:

- Wrist: flexion, extension, radial and ulnar deviation
- MCP joint: flexion, extension
- PIP and DIP joints: flexion, extension
- Finger: abduction, adduction
- MCP, PIP, and DIP joints of the thumb: flexion and extension
- Thumb: abduction, adduction, opposition
- Fifth finger: opposition

Passive, active, and resistive movements are performed in the wrist and hand. Table 22-2 indicates resistive motions to use to determine the extent of strength of the major wrist and hand muscles.

Injuries to the Wrist

The wrist is the region between and including the distal ends of the radius and ulna and the bases of the metacarpals. The wrist area includes the carpal bones and ligaments and the related fibrocartilaginous complex.

The main purposes of the wrist are to position the hand in space and to direct forces from the hand to the forearm and vice versa. To accomplish these purposes there must be both stability and mobility.

The most common wrist injuries in sports are caused by some type of impact. All injuries require immediate on-field evaluation by the athletic trainer or physician. Suspected serious injuries require immediate splinting followed by proper management. Injuries to the wrist usually occur from a fall on the outstretched hand or from repeated flexion, extension, or rotary movements (Figure 22-44).

Sprains

It is often difficult to distinguish between injury to the wrist's muscle tendons and/or to the supporting structure of the carpal region. Emphasis is placed here on the condition of wrist sprain, and tendon injuries will be considered in the discussion of the hand.

A sprain is by far the most common wrist injury and in most cases is the most poorly managed injury in sports. It can arise from any abnormal, forced movement of the wrist.

Etiology   Falling on the hyperextended wrist is the most common cause of wrist sprain, but violent flexion or torsion will also tear supporting tissue. Because the main

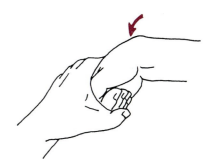

Figure 22-40

De Quervain's test.

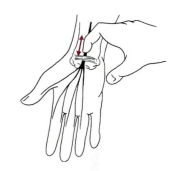

Figure 22-41

Tapping over the transverse carpal ligament to test for carpal tunnel syndrome (Tinel's sign).

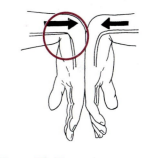

Figure 22-42

Wrist press for carpal tunnel syndrome (Phalen's test).

22-7
Critical Thinking Exercise

An athlete who sustained a major wrist sprain complains of a decrease in her hand circulation.

? How should this injury be evaluated for a circulation problem?

Figure 22-43

Testing the radial and ulnar arteries of the hand (Allen's test).

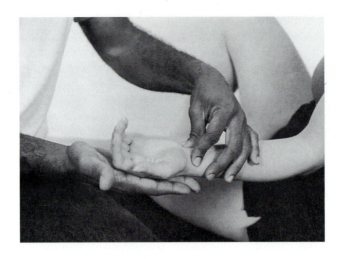

Figure 22-44

Wrist injuries commonly occur from falls on the outstretched hand or from repeated flexion, extension, lateral, or rotary movements.

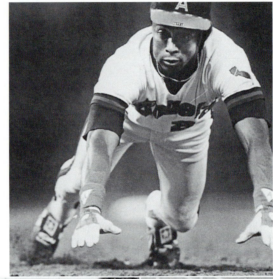

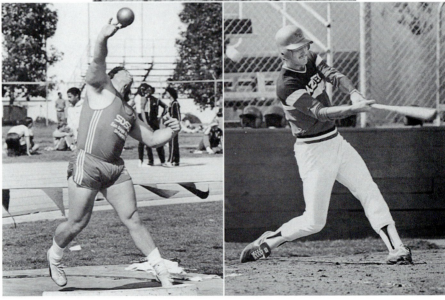

support of the wrist is derived from posterior and anterior ligaments that transport the major nutrient vessels to the carpal bones and stabilize the joint, repeated sprains may disrupt the blood supply and consequently circulation to the carpal bones.

Symptoms and signs   The athlete complains of pain, swelling, and difficulty moving the wrist. On examination there is tenderness, swelling, and limited ROM. All athletes having severe sprains should be referred to a physician for x-ray examination to determine possible fractures.

Management   Mild and moderate sprains should initially be given RICE, splinting, and analgesics. It is desirable to have the athlete start hand-strengthening exercises almost immediately after the injury has occurred. Taping for support can benefit healing and help prevent further injury. (See Chapter 13, Figures 13-40 and 13-41.)

Strains

Tenosynovitis   Wrist tenosynovitis occurs to the extensor carpi radialis longus or brevis in weight lifters and rowers.[18] Other sports that cause wrist tenosynovitis are those that require the athlete to perform repetitive wrist accelerations and decelerations.

Etiology   The cause of tenosynovitis is the repetitive and overuse of the wrist tendons and their sheaths.

Symptoms and signs   The athlete complains of pain with use or pain in passive stretching. There is tenderness and swelling over the tendon.

Management   Acute pain and inflammation are managed by ice massage for 10 minutes four times a day for the first 48 to 72 hours, NSAIDs, and rest. When swelling has subsided range of motion is promoted with contrast baths. Ultrasound or phonophoresis can be used for their antiinflammatory effects. When pain and swelling have subsided, progressive-resistive exercise can be instituted.[18]

Tendinitis   Tendinitis of the flexor carpi radialis is common in racquet sports. Flexor ulnaris pisiform tendinitis is also common. Sports that require repetitive pulling movements and sports that place prolonged pressure on the palms, such as in cycling, can cause flexor digitorum tendinitis.

Etiology   The primary cause of tendinitis is overuse of the wrist.

Symptoms and signs   The athlete complains of pain on active use or passive stretching of the involved tendon. Isometric resistance to the involved tendon produces pain, weakness, or both.

Management   Acute pain and inflammation are managed with ice massage for 10 minutes four times daily for 48 to 72 hours, NSAIDs, and rest. A wrist splint may protect the injured tendon. After swelling has subsided, a program of contrast baths and ROM exercises can be begun. When the athlete is pain free, a high-repetition, low-resistance progressive-resistive exercise program can be instituted.

Nerve Compression

Because of the narrow spaces that some nerves must travel through the wrist to the hand, compression neuropathy or entrapment can occur. The two most common entrapments are of the median nerve, which travels through the carpal tunnel, and the ulnar nerve, which is compressed in the tunnel of Guyon between the pisiform bone and the hook of the hamate bone.

Such compression causes a sharp or burning pain that is associated with an increase or decrease in skin sensitivity or paresthesia. When chronic entrapment may cause irreversible nerve damage, unsuccessful conservative treatment can lead to surgical decompression.

Carpal tunnel syndrome   The carpal tunnel is located on the anterior aspect of the wrist. The floor of the carpal tunnel is formed by the carpal bones and the roof by the transverse carpal ligament (Figure 22-45). A number of anatomical structures course through this limited space, including eight long finger flexor tendons, their synovial sheaths, and the median nerve. Carpal tunnel syndrome results from an in-

Figure 22-45

The transverse carpal ligament lies over the median nerve at the carpal tunnel.

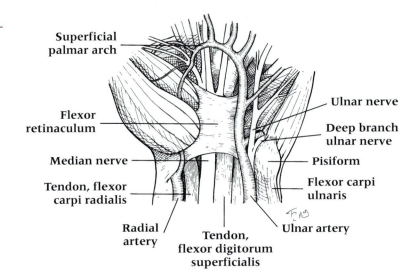

Superficial palmar arch

Flexor retinaculum

Median nerve

Tendon, flexor carpi radialis

Radial artery

Tendon, flexor digitorum superficialis

Ulnar nerve

Deep branch ulnar nerve

Pisiform

Flexor carpi ulnaris

Ulnar artery

flammation of the tendons and synovial sheaths within this space, which ultimately leads to compression of the median nerve.[9]

Etiology   Carpal tunnel syndrome most often occurs in athletes who engage in activities that require repeated wrist flexion, although it can also result from direct trauma to the anterior aspect of the wrist.

Symptoms and signs   Compression of the median nerve will usually result in both sensory and motor deficits. Sensory changes could result in tingling, numbness, and paresthesia in the arc of median nerve innervation over the thumb, index and middle fingers, and palm of the hand. The median nerve innervates the lumbrical muscles of the index and middle fingers and three of the thenar muscles. Thus weakness in thumb movement is associated with this condition.

Management   Initially, conservative treatment involving rest, immobilization, and nonsteroidal antiinflammatory medication is recommended. If the syndrome persists, injection with a corticosteroid and possible surgical decompression of the transverse carpal ligament may be necessary.

de Quervain's disease   de Quervain's disease (also called Hoffman's disease) is a stenosing tenosynovitis in the thumb. The first tunnel of the wrist becomes contracted and narrowed as a result of inflammation of the synovial lining. The tendons that go through the first tunnel are the extensor pollicis brevis and abductor pollicis longus, which move through the same synovial sheath.

Etiology   Because the tendons move through a groove of the radiostyloid process, constant wrist movement can be a source of irritation.

Symptoms and signs   Athletes who use a great deal of wrist motion in their sport are prone to de Quervain's disease. Its primary symptom is an aching pain, which may radiate into the hand or forearm. Movements of the wrist tend to increase the pain, and there is a positive de Quervain's test. There is point tenderness and weakness during thumb extension and abduction, and there may be a painful snapping and catching of the tendons during movement.

Management   Management of de Quervain's disease involves immobilization, rest, cryotherapy, and antiinflammatory medication. Ultrasound and ice massage are also beneficial.

Dislocations

Dislocations of the wrist are relatively infrequent in sports activity. Most occur from a forceful hyperextension of the wrist. Of those dislocations that do happen, the bones

22-8

Critical Thinking Exercise

A shot-putter is beginning to feel tingling, numbness, and paresthesia in the thumb, index, and middle fingers, and palm of the right hand.

? The athlete is demonstrating a carpal tunnel syndrome. What factors could produce this problem?

that could be involved are the distal ends of the radius and ulna (see Figure 22-44) and a carpal bone, the lunate being the most commonly affected.

Dislocation of the lunate bone   Dislocation of the lunate (Figure 22-46) is considered the most common dislocation of a carpal bone.

Etiology   Dislocation occurs as a result of a fall on the outstretched hand, forcing open the space between the distal and proximal carpal bones. When the stretching force is released, the lunate bone is dislocated anteriorly (palmar side).

Symptoms and signs   The primary signs of this condition are pain, swelling, and difficulty in executing wrist and finger flexion. There also may be numbness or even paralysis of the flexor muscles because of lunate pressure on the median nerve.

Management   This condition should be treated as acute, and the athlete should be sent to a physician for reduction of the dislocation. If it is not recognized early enough, bone deterioration may occur, requiring surgical removal. The usual time of disability and subsequent recovery is 1 to 2 months.

Fractures

Fractures of the wrist commonly occur to the distal ends of the radius and ulna and to the carpal bones; the carpal scaphoid bone is most commonly affected, and the hamate bone is affected less often. Serious acute injuries to the wrist are usually caused by impact or by rotational forces. The most common mechanism is a fall on the outstretched hand.

Scaphoid fracture   The scaphoid bone is the most frequently fractured of the carpal bones.

Etiology   The injury is usually caused by a force on the outstretched hand, which compresses the scaphoid bone between the radius and the second row of carpal bones (Figure 22-47). This condition is often mistaken for a severe sprain, and as a result the required complete immobilization is not performed. Without proper splinting, the scaphoid fracture often fails to heal because of an inadequate supply of blood; thus degeneration and necrosis occur. This condition is often called aseptic necrosis of the scaphoid bone. It is necessary to try, in every way possible, to distinguish between a wrist sprain and a fracture of the scaphoid bone because a fracture necessitates immediate referral to a physician.

Symptoms and signs   The signs of a recent scaphoid fracture include swelling in the area of the carpal bones, severe point tenderness of the scaphoid bone in the anatomical snuffbox (Figure 22-48), and scaphoid pain that is elicited by upward pressure exerted on the long axis of the thumb and by radial flexion.

Management   With these signs present, cold should be applied, the area splinted, and the athlete referred to a physician for x-ray study and casting. In most cases, cast immobilization lasts for approximately 6 weeks and is followed by strengthening exercises coupled with protective taping. Immobilization is discontinued for rehabilitation. The wrist needs protection against impact loading for an additional 3 months.[18]

Hamate fracture   A fracture of the hamate bone can occur from a fall but more commonly occurs from contact by an implement such as the handle of a tennis racket, a baseball bat, or a golf club. Wrist pain and weakness are experienced. Pull of the muscular attachments can cause nonunion; therefore casting is usually the treatment of choice.

Wrist Ganglion of the Tendon Sheath

The wrist ganglion (Figure 22-49), which is a synovial cyst, is often seen in sports. It is considered by many to be a herniation of the joint capsule or of the synovial sheath of a tendon; other authorities believe it to be a cystic structure.

Etiology   It usually appears slowly, after a wrist strain, and contains a clear, mucinous fluid. The ganglion most often appears on the back of the wrist but can appear at any tendinous point in the wrist or hand.

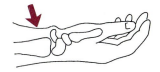

Figure 22-46

Dislocation of the lunate bone.

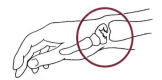
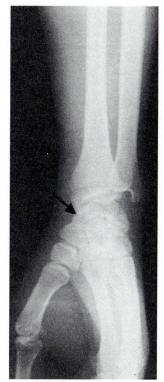

Figure 22-47

Carpal scaphoid fracture.

Figure 22-48

Figure 22-48

Anatomical snuffbox formed by extensor tendons of the thumb.

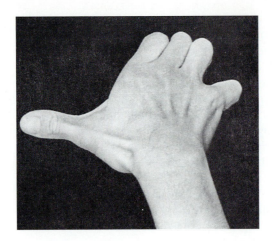

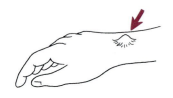

Figure 22-49

Wrist ganglion.

Symptoms and signs The athlete complains of occasional pain with a lump at the site. Pain increases with use. There is a cystic structure that may feel soft, rubbery, or very hard.[18]

Management An old method of treatment was first to break down the swelling through digital pressure and then apply a felt pressure pad for a period of time to encourage healing. A newer approach is the use of a combination of aspiration and chemical cauterization, with subsequent application of a pressure pad. Neither of these methods prevents the ganglion from recurring. Surgical removal is the best of the various methods of treatment.

Injuries to the Hand

The hand is one of the most commonly injured sites in sports, yet it is probably the most poorly managed. Immediate evaluation must be afforded to avoid any delay in proper management. When it comes to improper care the hand is notoriously unforgiving.

Contusions and Pressure Injuries of the Hand and Phalanges

Etiology The hand and phalanges, having an irregular bony structure combined with little protective fat and muscle padding, are prone to bruising in sports.

Symptoms and signs This condition is easily identified from the history of trauma and the pain and swelling of soft tissues.

Management Cold and compression should be applied immediately until hemorrhage has ceased, followed by gradual warming of the part in whirlpool or immersion baths. Although soreness is still present, protection should be given by a sponge rubber pad (see Figure 13-40).

A particularly common contusion of the finger is bruising of the distal phalanx, which results in a *subungual hematoma* (contusion of the fingernail). This is an extremely painful condition because of the accumulation of blood underneath the fingernail. The athlete should place the finger in ice water until the hemorrhage ceases, and the pressure of blood should then be released (Figure 22-50 and the Focus box on the next page.)

Bowler's Thumb

Etiology A perineural fibrosis of the subcutaneous ulnar digital nerve of the thumb can occur from the pressure of a bowling ball thumbhole, with the development of fibrotic tissue around the ulnar nerve.

Symptoms and signs The athlete senses pain, tingling during pressure to the irritated area, and numbness.

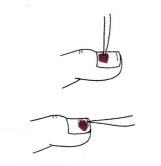

Figure 22-50

Releasing blood from beneath the fingernail, technique no. 1.

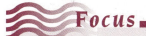

Focus

> **Releasing blood from beneath the fingernail**
>
> The following are two common methods for releasing the pressure of the subungual hematoma.
>
> MATERIALS NEEDED: Scalpel, small-gauge drill or paper clip, and antiseptic.
>
> POSITION OF ATHLETE: The athlete sits with the injured hand palm downward on the table.
>
> TECHNIQUE 1
>
> 1. The injured finger should first be coated with an antiseptic solution.
> 2. A sharp scalpel point, small-gauge drill, or paper clip is used to penetrate the injured nail through a rotary action. If the hematoma extends as far as the end of the nail, it may be best to release the blood by slipping the scalpel tip under the end of the nail.
>
> TECHNIQUE 2
>
> 1. A paper clip is heated to a red-hot temperature.
> 2. The red-hot paper clip or small-gauge drill is laid on the surface of the nail with moderate pressure, resulting in melting a hole through the nail to the site of the bleeding.

Management   Early management includes decreasing the amount of bowling and padding of the thumbhole. If the condition continues, however, surgery may be warranted.

Tendon Conditions

Tendon injuries are common among athletes. As with many other hand injuries occurring in sports, they are characteristically neglected.

Tenosynovitis   The tendons of the wrist and hand can sustain irritation from repeated movement that results in tenosynovitis. An inflammation of the tendon sheath results in swelling, crepitation, and painful movement. Most commonly affected are the extensor tendons of the wrist: the extensor carpi ulnaris, extensor pollicis longus, extensor pollicis brevis, and abductor pollicis longus.

> Two important forms of tenosynovitis:
>   de Quervain's disease
>   Trigger finger or thumb

The trigger finger or thumb is an example of stenosing tenosynovitis. It most commonly occurs in a flexor tendon that runs through a common sheath with other tendons. Thickening of the sheath or tendon can occur, thus constricting the sliding tendon. A nodule in the synovium of the sheath adds to the difficulty of gliding.[16]

Etiology   The cause of trigger finger or thumb is nonspecific overuse.

Symptoms and signs   The athlete complains that when the finger or thumb is flexed, there is resistance to reextension, producing a snapping that is both palpable and audible. During palpation, tenderness is produced, and a lump can be felt at the base of the flexor tendon sheath.

Management   Treatment initially is the same as for de Quervain's disease; however, if it is unsuccessful, steroid injections may produce relief. If steroid injections do not provide relief, splinting the tendon sheath is the last option.

Mallet finger   The mallet finger is common in sports, particularly in baseball and basketball.

Etiology   It is caused by a blow from a thrown ball that strikes the tip of the finger, jamming and avulsing the extensor tendon from its insertion along with a piece of bone.

Symptoms and signs   The athlete complains of pain at the distal interphalangeal joint. X-ray examination may show a bony avulsion from the dorsal proximal distal phalanx. The athlete is unable to extend the finger, carrying it at approximately a

Figure 22-51

Mallet finger.

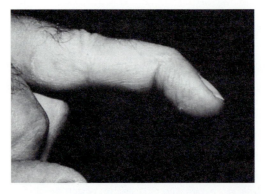
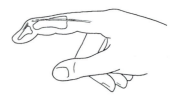

Figure 22-52

Splinting of the mallet finger.

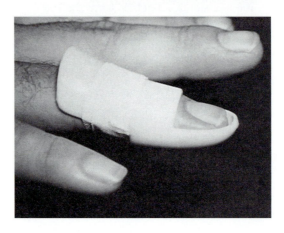
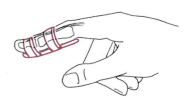

30-degree angle. There is also point tenderness at the site of the injury, and the avulsed bone often can be palpated (Figure 22-51).

Management   RICE is given for the pain and swelling. If there is no fracture the distal phalanx should immediately be splinted in a position of extension for a period 6 to 8 weeks (Figure 22-52).

Boutonnière deformity

Etiology   The boutonnière, or buttonhole, deformity is caused by a rupture of the extensor tendon of the middle phalanx. Trauma occurs to the top of the middle finger, which forces the PIP joint into excessive flexion.

Symptoms and signs   The athlete complains of severe pain and inability to extend the PIP joint. There is swelling, point tenderness, and an obvious deformity (Figure 22-53).

Figure 22-53

Boutonnière deformity.

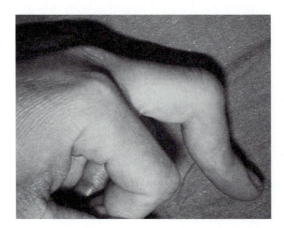
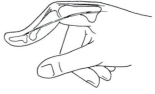

TABLE 22-3 **Conservative Treatment and Splinting of Finger Injuries**

Injury	Constant Splinting	Begin Motion	Additional Splinting during Competition	Joint Position
Mallet finger	6-8 wk	6-8 wk	6-8 wk	Slight DIP hyperextension
Collateral ligament sprains	3 wk	2 wk	4-6 wk	30-degree flexion
PIP and DIP dislocations	3 wk	3 wk	3 wk	30-degree flexion
Phalangeal fractures	4-6 wk	4-6 wk	3 wk	N/A
PIP and DIP fractures	9-11 wk	3 wk	3 wk	30-degree flexion
Pseudoboutonnière volar plate injuries	5 wk	3 wk	3 wk	20- to 30-degree flexion
Boutonnière deformity	6-8 wk	6-8 wk	6-8 wk	PIP in extension; DIP and MCP not included
MCP fractures	3 wk	3 wk	4-6 wk	30-degree flexion
Flexor digitorum profundus repair	5 wk	3 wk	3 wk	Depends on repair

Management   Management of the boutonnière deformity includes cold application followed by splinting of the PIP joint in extension. NOTE: If this condition is inadequately splinted, the classic boutonnière deformity will develop. Splinting is continued for 5 to 8 weeks. While splinted, the athlete is encouraged to flex the distal phalanx (Table 22-3).

Sprains, Dislocations, and Fractures

The phalanges, particularly the thumb (Figure 22-54), are prone to sprains caused by a blow delivered to the tip or by violent twisting. The mechanism of injury is similar to that of fractures and dislocations. The sprain, however, mainly affects the capsular, ligamentous, and tendinous tissues. Recognition is accomplished primarily through the history and the sprain symptoms: pain, severe swelling, and hematoma.

Sprains of the Metacarpophalangeal Joint

Fingers   A sprain of the MCP joint often consists of disruption of the extensor tendon and the athlete's inability to extend the joint fully. There may be obvious slipping of the extensor tendon (see Table 22-3).

22-9

Critical Thinking Exercise

A baseball catcher receives a pitch that jams and avulses his extensor tendon of the distal interphalangeal joint of the second finger.

? How should this condition be managed?

Figure 22-54

Football often places the phalanges at risk of severe injury.

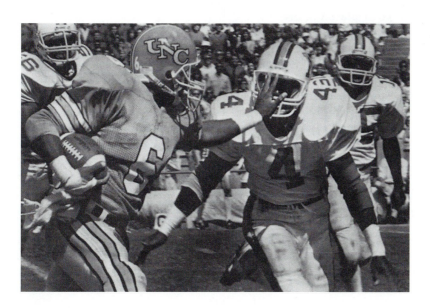

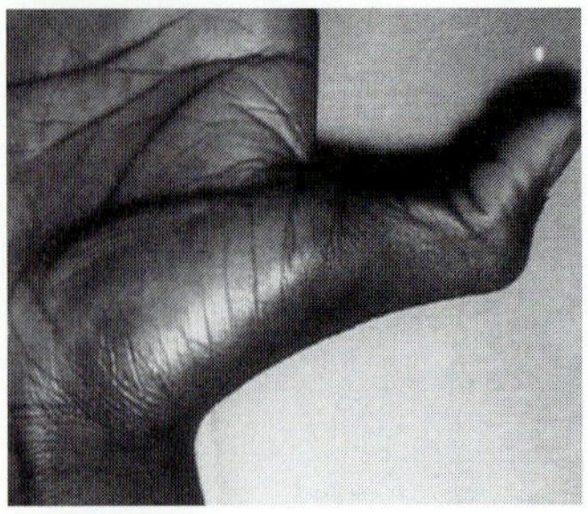

Figure 22-55

Gamekeeper's thumb.

Gamekeeper's thumb   A sprain of the ulnar collateral ligament of the MCP joint of the thumb is common among athletes, especially skiers and tackle football players.

Etiology   The mechanism of injury is usually a forceful abduction of the proximal phalanx, which is occasionally combined with hyperextension[8] (Figure 22-55).

Symptoms and signs   The athlete complains of pain over the ulnar collateral ligament with a weak and painful pinch. Inspection demonstrates tenderness and swelling over the medial aspect of the thumb.[18]

Management   Because the stability of pinching can be severely deterred, proper immediate and follow-up care must be performed. If there is instability in the joints, the athlete should be immediately referred to an orthopedist. If the joint is stable, x-ray examination should routinely be performed to rule out fracture. Splinting of the thumb should be applied for protection over a 3-week period or until it is pain free. The splint, extending from the end of the thumb to above the wrist, is applied with the thumb in a neutral position. After splinting, thumb spica taping should be worn during sports participation (see Figure 13-43).

Sprains of the Interphalangeal Joints of the Fingers

Interphalangeal finger sprains can include the PIP joint or the DIP joint. Injury can range from minor to complete tears of the collateral ligament, a volar plate tear, or a central extensor slip tear (see Table 22-3).

Collateral ligament sprain   A collateral ligament sprain of the interphalangeal joint is common in sports such as basketball, volleyball, and football.

Etiology   A common cause is an axial force producing the jammed finger. This mechanism places valgus or varus stress on the interphalangeal joint.

Symptoms and signs   The athlete complains of pain and swelling at the involved joint. There is severe point tenderness at the joint site, especially in the region of the collateral ligaments. There may be a lateral or medial instability when the joint is in 150 degrees of flexion. Collateral ligamentous injuries may be evaluated by the application of a valgus and varus joint stress test.

Management   Management includes RICE for the acute stage, x-ray examinations, and splinting. Splinting of the PIP joint is usually at 30 to 40 degrees of flexion for 10 days. If the sprain is to the DIP joint, splinting a few days in full extension assists in the healing process. If the sprains are minor, taping the injured finger to a noninjured one will provide protective support. Later, a protective checkrein can be applied for either thumb or finger protection (see Figures 13-42 and 13-43).

Volar plate rupture

Etiology   The volar plate of the PIP joint is most commonly injured in sports from a severe hyperextension force. A distal tear may cause a swan-neck deformity, whereas injury to the proximal part of the plate may cause a pseudoboutonnière deformity.

Symptoms and signs   There is pain and swelling at the PIP. The PIP displays varying degrees of hyperextension. Tenderness is over the volar aspect of the PIP. A major indication of a tear is that the PIP joint can be passively hyperextended in comparison with other PIP joints.

Management   Initially, the athlete is treated with RICE and analgesics as required. Management consists of splinting at 20 to 30 degrees of flexion for 3 weeks and then buddy taping followed by progressive-resistive exercises.

Dislocations of the Phalanges

Dislocations of the phalanges (Figure 22-56) have a high rate of occurrence in sports. A number of joints could be affected such as the PIP dorsal dislocation, PIP palmar dislocation, and the MCP dislocation. Most are seen in collisions or contact sports (Figure 22-57).

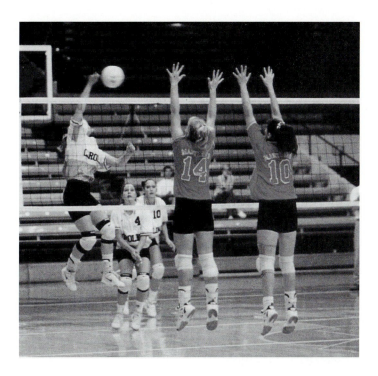

Figure 22-56

Volleyball produces a high percentage of finger injuries.

PIP dorsal dislocation

Etiology   The mechanism is hyperextension that produces a disruption of the volar plate at the middle phalanx.

Symptom and signs   The athlete complains of pain and swelling over the PIP. There is an obvious avulsion deformity and disability.

Management   Initially, the athlete is treated with RICE, splinting, and analgesics, followed by reduction by a physician. After reduction the finger is splinted at 20 to 30 degrees of flexion for 3 weeks. After splint removal buddy taping is used.

PIP palmar dislocation

Etiology   The cause is a twist of a finger while it is semiflexed.

Symptoms and signs   The athlete complains of pain and swelling over the PIP. There is point tenderness over the PIP primarily on the dorsal side. The finger displays an angular or rotational deformity.

Management   The finger is treated with RICE, splinting, and analgesics, followed by reduction. It is then splinted in full extension for 4 to 5 weeks, after which it is protected for 6 to 8 weeks during activity.

MCP dislocation

Etiology   The cause of the MCP dislocation is a twisting or shear force.

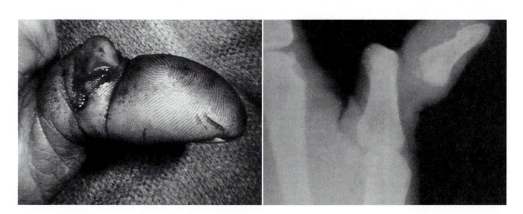

Figure 22-57

Open dislocation of the interphalangeal joint of a thumb.

TABLE 22-4 Avulsion Fractures

Avulsion Fracture	Corresponding Sprain
Corner of base of middle phalanx	Collateral ligament
Volar base of middle phalanx	Volar plate injury
Dorsal base of middle phalanx	Central extensor slip tear
Volar base of distal phalanx	Flexor profundus tear
Dorsal base of distal phalanx	Mallet finger

Symptoms and signs   The athlete complains of pain, swelling, and stiffness at the MCP joint. The proximal phalanx is dorsally angulated at 60 to 90 degrees.[18]

Management   Initially, the injury is treated with RICE, splinting, and analgesics. It is then reduced, buddy taped, and given early ROM.

Metacarpal and Phalange Fractures

As with dislocations, contact and collision sports produce a high number of hand and finger fractures. Presented will be metacarpal fracture, carpometacarpal (CMC) fracture (Bennett's fracture), distal phalangeal fracture, middle phalange fracture, PIP fracture and dislocation, and proximal phalangeal fracture (Table 22-4).

Metacarpal fracture   Fractures of the fifth metacarpal are associated with boxing and the martial arts (Figure 22-58).

Etiology   The cause of metacarpal fractures is commonly a direct axial force or a compressive force, such as being stepped on.

Symptoms and signs   The athlete complains of pain and swelling. The injury may appear to be an angular or rotational deformity.

Management   Initially, RICE and analgesic are given, followed by X-ray examinations. Deformity is reduced, followed by splinting. A splint is worn for 4 weeks, after which early ROM is carried out.

CMC fracture   Another name for a CMC fracture is Bennett's fracture.

Etiology   The athlete experiences an axial and abduction force to the thumb.

Symptoms and signs   The athlete complains of pain and swelling over the base of the thumb. The thumb's CMC appears deformed. X-ray shows fracture.

Management   This condition is structurally unstable and must be referred to an orthopedic surgeon.

Distal phalangeal fracture

Etiology   The primary cause of distal phalangeal fracture is a crushing force.

Symptoms and signs   There is a complaint of pain and swelling of the distal phalanx. A subungual hematoma is often seen in this condition.

Management   Initially, RICE and analgesics are given. A protective splint is applied as a means for relief of pain. The subungual hematoma is drained.

Middle phalange fracture

Etiology   A middle phalange fracture occurs from a direct trauma or twist.

Symptoms and signs   There is pain and swelling with tenderness over the middle phalanx. There may be deformity. X-rays show bone displacement.

Management   RICE and analgesic are given as needed. Depending on the fracture site and whether there is deformity, a buddy tape may be used with a thermoplastic splint for sport activity. If there is deformity, immobilization is applied for 3 to 4 weeks and a protective splint for an additional 9 to 10 weeks.[18]

PIP fracture and dislocation

Etiology   The cause of this combination of fracture and dislocation is an axial load on a partially flexed finger.

Symptoms and signs   This condition causes pain and swelling in the region of the PIP joint. There is localized tenderness over the PIP joint.

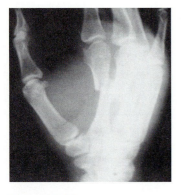

Figure 22-58

Transverse fractures of the second, third, and fourth metacarpals.

Management   RICE and analgesics are given initially, followed by reduction of the fracture. If there is a small fragment buddy taping is used. If there is a large fragment a splint of 30 to 60 degrees of flexion is applied.

Proximal phalangeal fracture

Etiology   There are varying causes of this fracture, including spiral and angular.

Symptoms and signs   The athlete complains of pain, swelling, and deformity. Inspection reveals varying degrees of deformity.

Management   RICE and analgesics are given as needed. Fracture stability is maintained by immobilization of the wrist in slight extension, MCP in 70 degrees of flexion, and buddy taping.

Rehabilitation of the Forearm, Wrist, and Hand

Reconditioning of the hand, wrist, and forearm must commence as early as possible. Immobilization of the forearm or wrist requires that the muscles be exercised almost immediately after an injury occurs if atrophy and contracture are to be prevented.

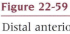
Critical Thinking Exercise

A football player gets into a fistfight on the field and injures his right hand. An injury is produced through an axial force to the fifth metacarpal bone.

? What type of injury should be suspected, and how should it be managed?

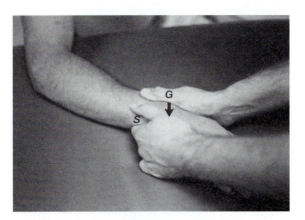

Figure 22-59

Distal anterior-posterior radial glide. Increasing pronation by distal anterior-posterior radial glides, with one hand stabilizing the ulna and the other gliding the radius. Glides are performed in all four directions.

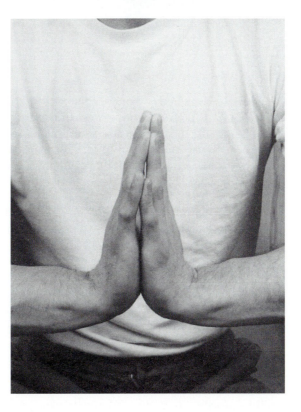

Figure 22-60

Active-assisted wrist extension stretching. Stretching the wrist by using the uninvolved hand to help stretch the involved wrist.

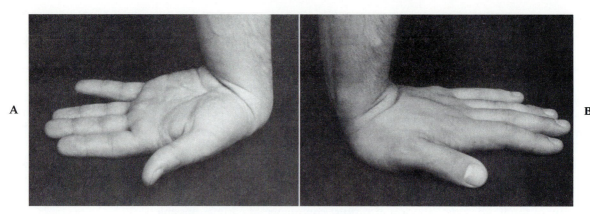

A   B

Figure 22-61

Static wrist stretching.

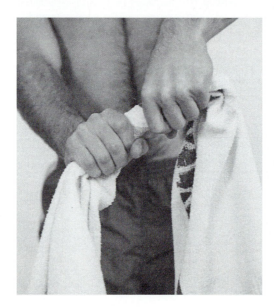

Figure 22-62

Towel twist exercise; the athlete twists the towel in each direction as if wringing out water.

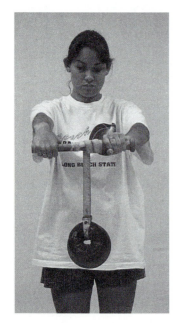

Figure 22-63

Wrist roll; rolling a weight quickly and rolling out slowly.

General Body Conditioning

As with all other body regions, athletes sustaining forearm, wrist, or hand injuries must maintain their preinjury level of conditioning. This includes cardiorespiratory fitness, strength, flexibility, and neuromuscular control.[24] There are many exercise options, such as walking, running, stair climbing, aerobics, cycling, and a variety of resistance and flexibility activities. Modified sports activities can be adapted to the individual injury.[24]

Joint Mobilization

Wrist and hand injuries respond to traction and mobilization techniques. Figure 22-59 represents some of these techniques.[25]

Flexibility

A full pain-free ROM is a major goal of rehabilitation of the lower arm. Working in conjunction with traction and mobilization increases joint function (Figures 22-60 and 22-61). The flexibility program should include active-assisted and active pain-free stretching exercises.[17]

Strength

Strength exercises for the wrist must be cautiously carried out without irritating the healing process. A variety of resistance approaches are available (Figures 22-62

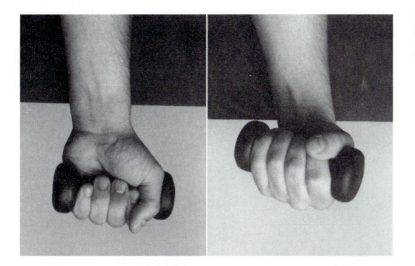

Figure 22-64

Dumbbell wrist flexion exercise.

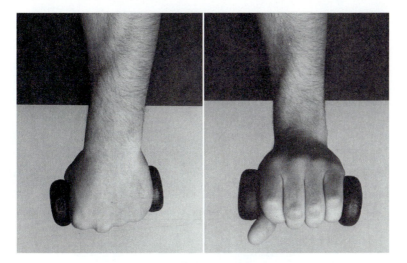

Figure 22-65

Dumbbell wrist extension exercise.

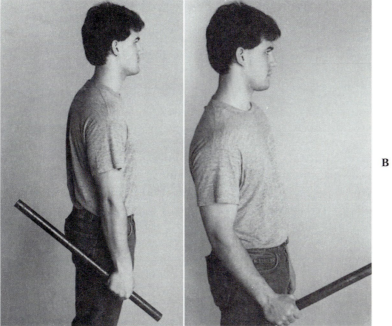

Figure 22-66

Wrist deviation strengthening. **A,** Ulnar deviation. **B,** Radial deviation.

Figure 22-67

Sport-specific wrist- and hand-strengthening exercise.

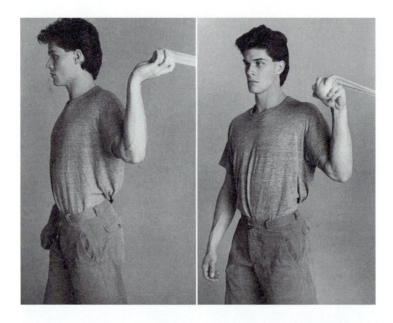

Figure 22-68

A variety of resistance devices are available for restoring hand grip function.

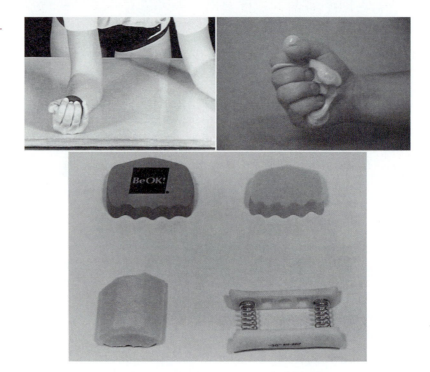

through 22-67). The flexibility program should include active-assisted and active pain-free stretching exercises.[17] The strength principles of hand injuries are consistent with the rehabilitation for most other injuries. Restoring grip strength is essential. It can be regained by gripping a number of different devices (Figure 22-68).

Neuromuscular Control

Hand and finger rehabilitation requires a restoration of dexterity, which includes pinching and other fine motor activities, such as buttoning buttons, tying shoes, and picking up small objects (Figure 22-69). A variety of customized bracing splints and taping techniques are available to protect the injured wrist and hand (see Figure 13-9).

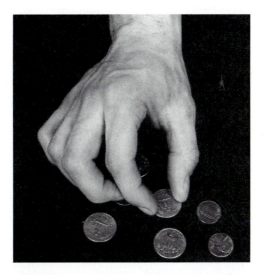

Figure 22-69

Developing finger dexterity.

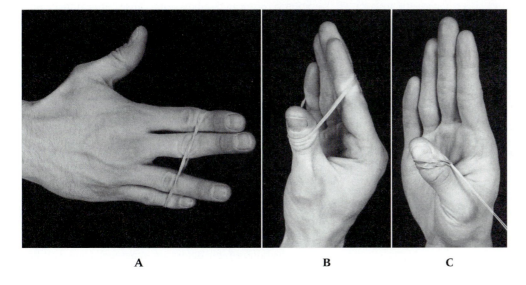

A   B   C

Figure 22-70

Finger strengthening using rubber bands. **A,** Finger abduction exercise. **B,** Thumb abduction exercise. **C,** Thumb opposition exercise.

Return to Activity

Criteria for the return to a sport after wrist or hand injury are grip strength equal to the unaffected limb, full range of motion, and full dexterity. The thumb has unique strength requirements. A manual resistance program can be instituted to strengthen adduction, abduction, flexion, extension, opposition, and circumduction of the thumb. Rubber bands may be used to progressively strengthen the fingers' intrinsic muscles (Figure 22-70). It must be remembered that a primary goal of forearm, wrist, and hand rehabilitation is to return the athlete to preinjury grip strength (Figure 22-71).

SUMMARY

- The upper limb, including the elbow, forearm, wrist, and hand, is second to the lower limb in incidence of sports injuries.
- The elbow is anatomically one of the more complex joints in the human body. The elbow joint allows the movements of flexion and extension, and the radio-ulnar joint allows forearm pronation and supination. The major sports injuries of the elbow are contusions, strains, sprains, and dislocations. Chronic strain, which produces pitcher's, tennis, javelin thrower's, and golfer's elbows, is more formally known as epicondylitis.

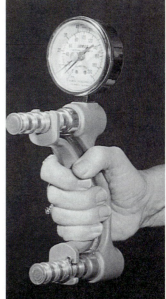

Figure 22-71

The gain of grip strength must be routinely measured.

- The forearm is composed of two bones, the ulna and the radius, as well as associated soft tissue. Sports injuries to the region commonly consist of contusions, chronic forearm splints, acute strains, and fractures.
- Injuries to the wrist usually occur as the result of a fall or repeated movements of flexion, extension, and/or rotation. Common injuries are sprains, lunate carpal dislocation, navicular carpal fracture, and hamate fracture.
- Injuries to the hand occur frequently in sports activities. Common injuries include those caused by contusions and chronic pressure; by tendons receiving sustained irritation, which leads to tenosynovitis; and by tendon avulsions. Sprains, dislocations, and fractures of the fingers are also common.

Solutions to Critical Thinking EXERCISES

22-1 The athletic trainer performs tests for ligamentous and capsular stability. Pulses are taken at the wrist and antecubital fossa. Changes of skin sensation and the athlete's pain reaction to passive, active, and resistive exercise are noted.

22-2 Immediate care consists of RICE and NSAIDs. More definitive management can include ROM, progressive-resistive exercise, friction massage, and hand grasping exercise while in supination. Pronation movements are avoided. Mobilization and stretching can also be employed within pain-free limits.

22-3 This javelin thrower has sustained a cubital tunnel syndrome. Because of a pronounced elbow cubitus valgus, the ulnar recurrently subluxates. Because of ligamentous laxity, there is nerve impingement and compression.

22-4 The concern of the athletic trainer is that this injury can cause a Volkmann's ischemic contracture. The brachial and radial pulses must be monitored for the possibility of a decreasing normal circulation.

22-5 This condition is commonly called forearm splints. Its mechanism is from static contractions of the extensor forearm muscles. As a result, minute tears are produced in the interosseous membrane.

22-6 This is a "silver fork" deformity, which is caused by the fracture displacement of the distal radius. Another name for this injury is Colles' fracture. The athletic trainer applies an ice compress, a splint, and a sling. The athlete is then referred to a physician for an x-ray and definitive treatment.

22-7 The athlete is cold to the touch. Pinching a fingernail makes it blanch, and when released it does not return to a pink color. Allen's test is carried out last, verifying a problem with hand circulation.

22-8 The shot-putter's repeated wrist flexions against a resistance have caused an inflammation of the tendons and synovial sheaths within the carpal tunnel. This inflammation in turn causes a compression of the median nerve and the subsequent symptoms experienced by the athlete.

22-9 RICE is applied immediately. An x-ray is done to rule out a fracture of the distal phalanx. The injury should be splinted in extension.

22-10 The athletic trainer should suspect a fracture of the fifth metacarpal bone. The injury may appear as an angular or rotational deformity. RICE and analgesics are given along with an x-ray examination. The injury is splinted for about 4 weeks along with early ROM exercises.

REVIEW QUESTIONS AND SUGGESTED ACTIVITIES

1. Describe how and why the elbow becomes chronically strained from throwing mechanisms.
2. Describe a dislocated elbow—its cause, appearance, and care.
3. How does the elbow sustain epicondylitis?
4. Compare elbow osteochondritis dissecans and knee osteochondritis dissecans. How does each occur?
5. What causes a Volkmann's contracture? How may it be detected early?
6. Discuss the many aspects of elbow exercise rehabilitation.
7. Compare forearm splints and shinsplints. How does each occur?
8. Describe the Colles' fracture of the forearm—its cause, appearance, and care.
9. What healing problems occur with navicular carpal fractures? Why?
10. How can a subungual hematoma be released?
11. What causes stenosing tenosynovitis in the hand?
12. Describe the circumstances that can produce a mallet finger and the boutonnière deformity in baseball players. What care should each condition receive?
13. A sprained thumb is common in sports activities. How does it occur, and what care should it receive?
14. Should a dislocated finger be reduced by a coach? Explain your answer.

REFERENCES

1. Allman FL, Carlson CA: Rehabilitation of elbow injuries. In Nicholas JA, Hershman EB, editors: *The upper extremity in sports medicine,* St Louis, 1995, Mosby.
2. Andrews JR, Whiteside JA: Common elbow problems in the athlete, *J Orthop Sports Phys Ther* 17(6):289, 1993.
3. Barrett J: Reflex sympathetic ditrophy, *Phys Sportsmed* 23(4):51, 1995.
4. Bennett JB: Acute injuries to the elbow. In Nicholas JA, Hershman EB, editors: *The upper extremity in sports medicine,* St Louis, 1995, Mosby.
5. Black KP et al: Compartment syndrome in athletes. In Hershman EB, editor: *Neurovascular injuries. Clinics in sports medicine,* vol 9, no 2, Philadelphia, 1990, Saunders.
6. Boyd Jr DW: Osteochondritis dissecans of the elbow, *Sports Med Dig* 15(7):2, 1993.
7. Brown DE et al: *Orthopedic secrets,* Philadelphia, 1995, Hanley & Belfus.
8. Campbell JD et al: Ulnar collateral ligament injury of the thumb, *Am J Sports Med* 20(1):29, 1992.

9. Case WS: Carpal tunnel syndrome, *Phys Sportsmed* 33(1):27, 1995.

10. Dickoff-Hoffman S, Foster D: Elbow injuries. In Prentice WE, editor: *Rehabilitation techniques in sports medicine*, ed 2, St Louis, 1994, Mosby.

11. Fleisig GS et al: Kinetics of baseball: pitching with implications about injury mechanisms, *Am J Sports Med* 23(2):233, 1995.

12. Glousman RE: Ulnar nerve problems in the athlete's elbow. In Hershman EB, editor: *Neurovascular injuries. Clinics in sports medicine,* vol 9, no 2, Philadelphia, 1990, Saunders.

13. Halperin BC: Elbow and arm injuries. In Birrer RB, editor: *Sports medicine for the primary care physician,* ed 2, Boca Raton, Fla, 1994, CRC Press.

14. Hocutt JE: General type injuries. In Birrer RB, editor: *Sports medicine for the primary care physician,* ed 2, Boca Raton, Fla, 1994, CRC Press.

15. Hoffman DF: Elbow dislocations, *Phys Sportsmed* 21(11):57, 1993.

16. Kielhaber TR et al: Upper extremity tendinitis and overuse syndrome in the athlete. In Culver JE, editor: *Injuries of the hand and wrist. Clinics in sports medicine,* vol 11, no 1, Philadelphia, 1992, Saunders.

17. Lephart S: Injuries to the hand and wrist. In Prentice WE, editor: *Rehabilitation techniques in sports medicine,* ed 2, St Louis, 1994, Mosby.

18. Lillegrad WA: Hand. In Birrer RB, editor: *Sports medicine for the primary care physician,* ed 2, Boca Raton, Fla, 1994, CRC Press.

19. Lord JL: Forearm injuries. In Birrer RB, editor: *Sports medicine for the primary care physician,* ed 2, Boca Raton, Fla, 1994, CRC Press.

20. Mirabello ST et al: The wrist field evaluation and treatment. In Culver JE, editor: *Injuries of the hand and wrist. Clinics in sports medicine,* vol 11, no 1, Philadelphia, 1992, Saunders.

21. Nuber GW, Bower MK: Olecranon stress fracture in throwing athletes. In Torg JS, Shephard RJ, editors: *Current therapy in sports medicine,* ed 3, St Louis, 1995, Mosby.

22. Parks JC: Overuse injuries of the elbow. In Nicholas JA, Hershman EB, editors: *The upper extremity in sports medicine,* St Louis, 1990, Mosby.

23. Posner MA: Compressive neuropathies of the median and radial nerves at the elbow. In Hershman EB, editor: *Neurovascular injuries. Clinics in sports medicine,* vol 9, no 2, Philadelphia, 1990, Saunders.

24. Prentice WE: Maintenance of cardiorespiratory endurance. In Prentice WE, editor: *Rehabilitation techniques in sports medicine,* ed 2, St Louis, 1994, Mosby.

25. Prentice WE: Mobilization and traction techniques. In Prentice WE, editor: *Rehabilitation techniques in sports medicine,* ed 2, St Louis, 1994, Mosby.

26. Regan WD: Lateral elbow pain in the athlete: a clinical review, *Clin Sports Med* 1(1):53, 1991.

27. Rettig AC et al: Epidemiology of elbow, forearm and wrist. Injuries in the athlete. In Plancher KD, editor: *The athletic elbow and wrist. Part I. Clinics in sports medicine,* vol 14, no 2, Philadelphia, 1995, Saunders.

28. Torg JS: Injuries to the upper extremity—Little League elbow. In Torg JS, Shephard RJ, editors: *Current therapy in sports medicine,* St Louis, 1995, Mosby.

29. Weinstein SM, Herring SA: Nerve problems and compartment syndrome in the hand, wrist and forearm. In Culver JE, editor: *Clinics in sports medicine,* vol 11, no 1, Philadelphia, 1992, Saunders.

30. Werner SL: Biomechanics of the elbow during baseball pitching, *J Orthop Sports Phys Ther* 17(6):274, 1993.

ANNOTATED BIBLIOGRAPHY

Culver JE, editor: *Injuries of the hand and wrist. Clinics in sports medicine,* vol 11, no 1, Philadelphia, 1992, Saunders

A monograph covering all aspects of sports injuries to the hands and wrists.

Plancher KD, editor: *The athletic elbow and wrist. Part I. Clinics in sports medicine,* vol 14, no 2, Philadelphia, 1995, Saunders.

An indepth monograph covering the diagnosis and conservative treatment of athletic elbow and wrist injuries.

Plancher KD, editor: *The athletic elbow and wrist. Part II. Clinics in sports medicine,* vol 15, no 2, Philadelphia, 1996, Saunders.

A detailed discussion of the most common and overuse injuries to the elbow and wrist occurring in sports.

The Spine

When you finish this chapter, you should be able to

- Describe the anatomy of the cervical, thoracic, and lumbar spine.
- Explain how the nerve roots from the spinal cord combine to form specific peripheral nerves.
- Describe a process to assess injuries of the cervical, thoracic, and lumbar spine.
- Explain how to evaluate and identify various postural deformities.
- Describe measures to prevent injury to the spine.
- Identify specific injuries that can occur to the various regions of the spine in terms of their etiology, symptoms and signs, and management.
- Describe the techniques of rehabilitation for the injured neck.
- Describe the rehabilitation goals for managing low back injuries.

T he spine is one of the most complex regions of the body. There are a multitude of bones, joints, ligaments, and muscles, all of which are collectively involved in spinal movement. The proximity to and relationship of the spinal cord, the nerve roots, and the peripheral nerves to the vertebral column adds to the complexity of this region. Injury to the cervical spine has potentially life-threatening implications. Low back pain is one of the most commonly occurring ailments. Thus an in-depth understanding of the anatomy of the spine, the techniques to assess the spine, the various injuries that can occur to different regions of the spine, and the rehabilitative techniques are all essential for the coach or athletic trainer.

ANATOMY

Bones of the Vertebral Column

The spine, or vertebral column, is composed of 33 individual bones called vertebrae. Twenty-four are classified as movable, or true, and nine are classified as immovable, or false. The false vertebrae, which are fixed by fusion, form the sacrum and the coccyx. The design of the spine allows a high degree of flexibility forward and laterally and limited mobility backward. Rotation around a central axis in the areas of the neck and the lower back is also permitted.

The movable vertebrae are separated into three different divisions, according to location and function. The first division comprises the 7 cervical vertebrae; the second, the 12 thoracic vertebrae; and the third, the 5 lumbar vertebrae. As the spinal segments progress downward from the cervical region, they grow increasingly larger to accommodate the upright posture of the body, as well as to contribute in weight bearing. The shape of the vertebrae is irregular, but the vertebrae possess certain characteristics that are common to all. Each vertebra consists of a neural arch through which the spinal cord passes and several projecting processes that serve as attachments for muscles and ligaments. Each neural arch has two laminae and two pedicles. The latter are bony processes that project backward from the body of the vertebrae and connect with the laminae. The laminae are flat bony processes occurring on either side of the neural arch; they project backward and inward from the pedicles. With the exception of the first and second cervical vertebrae, each vertebra has a spinous and transverse process for muscular and ligamentous attachment, and all vertebrae have an articular process.

Regions of the spinal column:
Cervical
Thoracic
Lumbar
Sacrum
Coccyx

The Cervical Spine

The cervical spine consists of seven vertebrae, with the first two differing from the other true vertebrae (Figure 23-1, *A*). These first two are called the atlas and the axis, respectively, and they function together to support the head on the spinal column and to permit cervical rotation. The atlas, named for its function of supporting the head, displays no body or spinous processes and is composed of lateral masses that are connected to the anterior and posterior arches. The upper surfaces articulate with the occipital condyles of the skull and allow flexion and extension along with some lateral movement. The arches of the atlas form a bony ring sufficiently large to accommodate the odontoid process and the medulla of the spinal cord. The axis, or epistropheus, is the second cervical vertebra and is designed to allow the skull and atlas to rotate on it. Its primary difference from a typical vertebra is the presence of a toothlike projection from the vertebral body that fits into the ring of the atlas. This projection is called the odontoid process. The great mobility of the cervical spine is attributed to the flattened, oblique facing of its articular facets and to the horizontal positioning of the spinous processes.

The Thoracic Spine

The thoracic spine consists of 12 vertebrae (Figure 23-1, *B*). Thoracic vertebrae have long transverse processes and prominent but thin spinous processes. Thoracic vertebrae 1 through 10 have articular facets on each transverse process to which the ribs articulate. The head of the rib articulates between two vertebrae, thus sharing half of an articular facet.

Figure 23-1

A, Cervical vertebrae (atlas and axis). **B,** Thoracic vertebrae. **C,** Lumbar vertebrae.

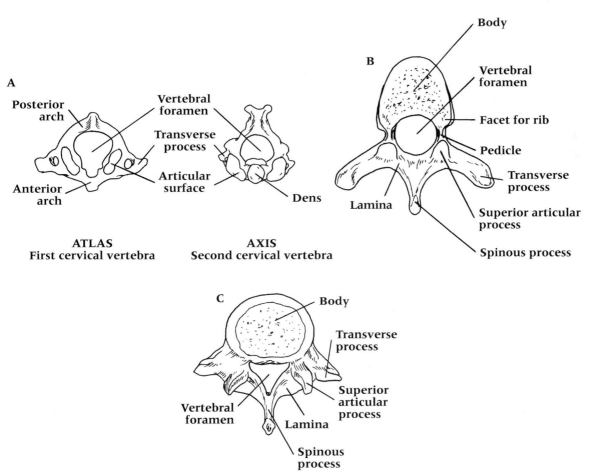

The Lumbar Spine

The lumbar spine is composed of five vertebrae (Figure 23-1, *C*). They are the major support of the low back and are the largest and thickest of the vertebrae, with large spinous and transverse processes. The superior articular processes face medially, and the inferior processes face laterally. The articular processes of the superior vertebrae articulate with the articular processes of the inferior vertebrae. Movement occurs in all of the lumbar vertebrae; however, there is much less flexion than extension.

The Sacrum

The sacrum is formed in the adult by the fusion of five vertebrae and, in addition to the two hip bones, comprises the pelvis (Figure 23-2). The roots of the lumbar and sacral nerves, which form the lower portion of the cauda equina, pass through four foramina lateral to the five fused vertebrae.

The sacrum articulates with the ilium to form the sacroiliac joint, which has a synovium and is lubricated by synovial fluid. During both sitting and standing the body's weight is transmitted through these joints. A complex of numerous ligaments serves to make these joints very stable.

The Coccyx

The coccyx, or tailbone, is the most inferior part of the vertebral column and consists of four or more fused vertebrae. The gluteus maximus muscle attaches to the coccyx posteriorly.

Curves of the Spine

Physiological curves also are present in the spinal column for adjusting to the upright stresses. These curves are, respectively, the cervical, thoracic, lumbar, and sacrococcygeal curves. The cervical and lumbar curves are convex anteriorly, and the thoracic and sacrococcygeal curves are convex posteriorly (Figure 23-3).

Intervetebral Disks

Between each of the cervical, thoracic, and lumbar vertebrae lie fibrocartilaginous intervertebral disks (Figure 23-4). Each disk is composed of the annulus fibrosus and the nucleus pulposus. The annulus fibrosus forms the periphery of the intervertebral disk and is composed of strong, fibrous tissue, with its fibers running in several different directions for strength. In the center is the semifluid nucleus pulposus compressed under pressure. The disks act as important shock absorbers for the spine.

23-1

Critical Thinking E x e r c i s e

In assessing complaints of back pain in a swimmer the athletic trainer notes that on lateral observation the low back appears to be excessively curved and the thoracic spine seems to have a curved, rounded appearance.

? When assessing posture laterally it is normal to have curves in various regions of the spine. What are the normal curves and their shape within the spine?

Figure 23-2

The sacrum.

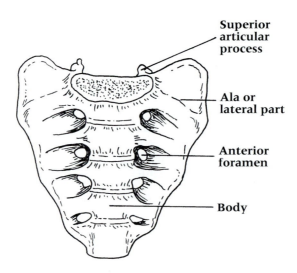

Superior articular process

Ala or lateral part

Anterior foramen

Body

Intervertebral Articulations

Intervertebral articulations are between vertebral bodies and vertebral arches. Articulation between the bodies is of the symphysial type. Besides motion at articulations between the bodies of the vertebrae, movement takes place at four articular processes that derive from the pedicles and laminae. The direction of movement of each vertebra is somewhat dependent on the direction in which the articular facets face.

Ligamentous Structures

The major ligaments that join the various vertebral parts are the anterior longitudinal, the posterior longitudinal, and the supraspinous (Figure 23-5). The anterior longitudinal ligament is a wide, strong band that extends the full length of the anterior surface of the vertebral bodies. The posterior longitudinal ligament is contained within the vertebral canal and extends the full length of the posterior aspect of the bodies of the vertebrae. Ligaments connect one lamina to another. The interspinous, supraspinous, and intertransverse ligaments stabilize the transverse and spinous processes, extending between adjacent vertebrae.

The sacroiliac joint is maintained by the extremely strong dorsal sacral ligaments. The sacrotuberous and the sacrospinous ligaments attach the sacrum to the ischium.

Muscles of the Spine

The muscles that extend the spine and rotate the vertebral column can be classified as either superficial or deep (Figure 23-6). The superficial muscles extend from the vertebrae to the ribs. The erector spinae make up the superficial muscles. The erector spinae muscles are a group of paired muscles made up of three columns or bands, the longissimus group, the iliocostalis group, and the spinalis group. Each of these groups is further divided into regions, the cervicis region in the neck, the thoracis region in the middle back, and the lumborum region in the low back. Generally the erector spinae muscles extend the spine.

The deep muscles extend from one vertebra to another. The deep muscles include the interspinales, multifidus, rotatores, thoracis, and the semispinalis cervicis. These muscles extend and rotate the spine.

Spinal Cord

The spinal cord is that portion of the central nervous system that is contained within the vertebral canal of the spinal column. It extends from the foramen magnum of the cranium to the filum terminale in the vicinity of the first or second lumbar vertebra. The lumbar roots and the sacral nerves form a horselike tail called the cauda equina.

Spinal Nerves and Peripheral Branches

Thirty-one pairs of spinal nerves extend from the sides of the spinal cord: 8 cervical, 12 thoracic, 5 lumbar, 5 sacral, and 1 coccygeal (Figure 23-7). Each of these nerves has an anterior root (motor root) and a posterior root (sensory root). The two roots in each case join together and form a single spinal nerve, which passes downward and outward through the intervertebral foramen. As the spinal nerves are conducted through the intervertebral foramen, they pass near the articular facets of the vertebrae. Any abnormal movement of these facets, such as in a dislocation or a fracture, may expose the spinal nerves to injury. Injuries that occur below the third lumbar vertebra usually result in nerve root damage but do not cause spinal cord damage.

Each pair of spinal nerves with the exception of C1 has a specific area of cutaneous sensory distribution called a dermatome. Figure 10-5 in Chapter 10 shows the dermatomes. Loss of sensation in a specific dermatome can provide information about the location of nerve damage.

The spinal nerve roots combine to form a network of nerves, or a plexus. There are five nerve plexuses, cervical, brachial, lumbar, sacral, and coccygeal. The cervical

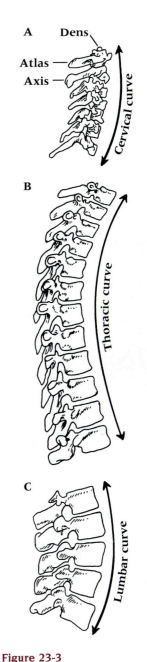

Figure 23-3

A, Cervical curve. **B,** Thoracic curve. **C,** Lumbar curve.

Intervertebral disk.

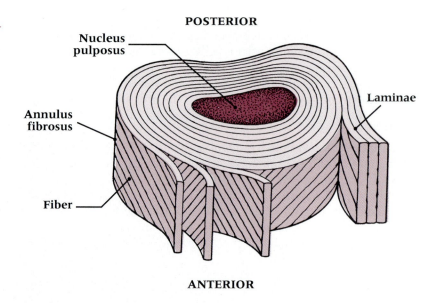

Ligaments of the spine.

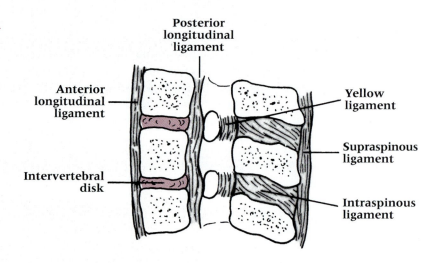

23-2

Critical Thinking E x e r c i s e

A wrestler has normal neck flexion, extension, and lateral flexion but is having difficulty rotating his head toward his left shoulder. The athletic trainer suspects there is a muscle strain of one of the muscles that rotate the head.

? It is important for the athletic trainer to know which muscles rotate the head.

plexus originates from spinal nerves C1-C4. The brachial plexus comes from C5-T1 nerve roots. The lumbar plexus comes form spinal nerves L1-L4. The lumbar plexus comes from L4-S4. The coccygeal plexus comes from S4-S5 and the coccygeal nerve. Tables 23-1 and 23-2 indicate the nerve, nerve roots, muscle innervated and action, and cutaneous innervation for the brachial plexus and the lumbosacral plexus, respectively.

Functional Anatomy

Movements of the Vertebral Column

The movements of the vertebral column are flexion and extension, right and left lateral flexion, and rotation to the left and right. The degree of movement differs in the various regions of the vertebral column. The cervical and lumbar regions allow extension and flexion. Although the thoracic vertebrae have minimal movement, their combined movement between the first and twelfth thoracic vertebrae can account for 20 to 30 degrees of flexion and extension.

Flexion of the cervical region is produced primarily by the sternocleidomastoid muscles and the scalene muscle group on the anterior aspect of the throat. The scalenes flex the head and stabilize the cervical spine as the sternocleidomastoids flex

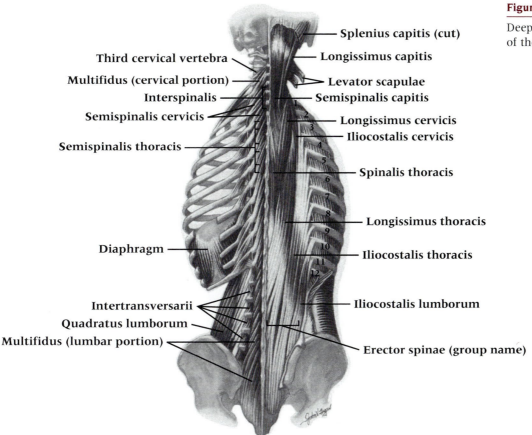

Figure 23-6

Deep and superficial muscles of the spine.

Splenius capitis (cut)
Longissimus capitis
Third cervical vertebra
Multifidus (cervical portion)
Levator scapulae
Interspinalis
Semispinalis capitis
Semispinalis cervicis
Longissimus cervicis
Iliocostalis cervicis
Semispinalis thoracis
Spinalis thoracis
Longissimus thoracis
Diaphragm
Iliocostalis thoracis
Iliocostalis lumborum
Intertransversarii
Quadratus lumborum
Multifidus (lumbar portion)
Erector spinae (group name)

the neck. The upper trapezius, semispinalis capitis, splenius capitus, and splenius cervicis muscles extend the neck. Lateral flexion of the neck is accomplished by all of the muscles on one side of the vertebral column contracting unilaterally. Rotation is produced when the sternocleidomastoid, the scalenes, the semispinalis cervicis, and the upper trapezius on the side opposite to the direction of rotation contract in addition to a contraction of the splenius capitus, splenius cervicis, and longissimus capitus on the same side of the direction of rotation.

Flexion of the trunk primarily involves lengthening of the deep and superficial back muscles and contraction of the abdominal muscles (rectus abdominus, internal oblique, external oblique) and hip flexors (rectus femoris, iliopsoas, tensor fasciae lata, sartorius). Seventy-five percent of flexion occurs at the lumbosacral junction (L5-S1), whereas 15% to 20% occurs between L4 and L5. The rest of the lumbar vertebrae execute 5% to 10% of flexion.[5] Extension involves lengthening of the abdominal muscles and contraction of the erector spinae and the gluteus maximus, which extends the hip. Trunk rotation is produced by the external obliques and the internal obliques. Lateral flexion is produced primarily by the quadratus lumborum muscle, along with the obliques, latissimus dorsi, iliopsoas, and the rectus abdominus on the side of the direction of movement.

PREVENTING INJURIES TO THE SPINE
Cervical Spine

Acute traumatic injuries to the spine can be potentially life threatening, particularly if the cervical region of the spinal cord is involved. Thus the athlete must do everything possible to minimize the possibility of injury. Strengthening of the musculature of the neck is critical. The neck muscles can function to protect the cervical spine by

Movements of the vertebral column:
Flexion
Extension
Lateral flexion
Rotation

Figure 23-7

Spinal cord and spinal nerves.

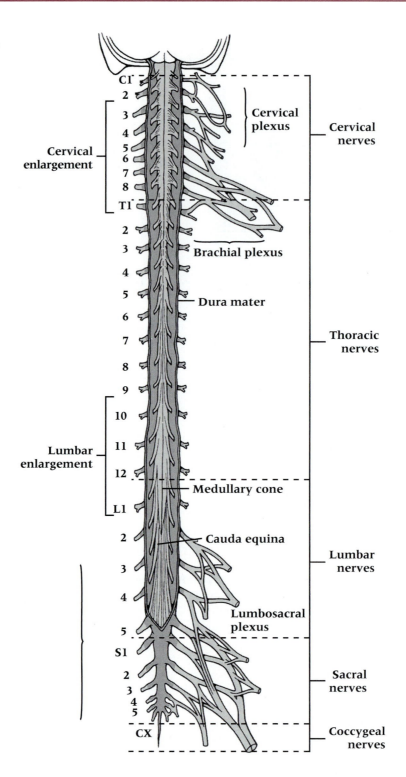

resisting excessive hyperflexion, hyperextension, or rotational forces. During participation the athlete should constantly be in a "state of readiness" and, when making contact with an opponent, should "bull" the neck. This is accomplished by elevating both shoulders and isometrically cocontracting the muscles surrounding the neck. Protective cervical collars can also help limit movement of the cervical spine. Athletes with long, weak necks are especially at risk. Tackle football players and wrestlers must have highly stable necks. Specific strengthening exercises are essential for the development of this stability. A variety of different exercises that incorporate iso-

TABLE 23-1 **Brachial Plexus**

Nerve	Origin	Function, Muscle Innervated	Cutaneous Innervation
Axillary	Posterior cord, C5-C6	Abduct arm 　Deltoid Laterally rotate arm 　Teres minor	Inferior lateral shoulder
Radial	Posterior cord, C5-T1	Extend forearm 　Triceps brachii 　Anconeus Flex forearm 　Brachialis (part) 　Brachioradialis Supinate forearm 　Supinator Extend wrist 　Extensor carpi radialis longus (also abducts wrist) 　Extensor carpi radialis brevis (also abducts wrist) 　Extensor carpi ulnaris (also adducts wrist) Extend fingers 　Extensor digitorum 　Extensor digiti minimi 　Extensor indicis Thumb muscles 　Abductor pollicis longus 　Extensor pollicis longus 　Extensor pollicis brevis	Posterior surface of arm and forearm, lateral two thirds of dorsum of hand
Musculocu-taneous	Lateral cord, C5-C7	Flex arm 　Coracobrachialis Flex forearm 　Biceps brachii (also supinates) 　Brachialis (also small amount of innervation from radial)	Lateral surface of forearm
Ulnar	Medial cord, C8-T1	Flex wrist 　Flexor carpi ulnaris (also adducts wrist) Flex fingers 　Part of flexor digitorum profundus (distal phalanges of little and ring finger) Abduct/adduct fingers 　Interossei Thumb muscle 　Adductor pollicis Hypothenar muscles 　Flexor digiti minimi brevis 　Abductor digiti minimi 　Opponens digiti minimi Midpalmar muscles 　Two medial lumbricals 　Interossei	Medial one third of hand, little finger, and medial one half of ring finger

Continued

tonic, isometric, or isokinetic contractions can be used. One of the best methods is manual resistance by the athlete or by a partner who selectively uses isometric and isotonic resistance exercises. Manual resistance should not be performed just before an individual engages in a collision-type sport such as football or ice hockey to avoid the danger of participating in these activities with fatigued neck muscles.

In addition to strong muscles, the athlete's neck should have a full range of motion. Ideally the athlete should be able to place the chin on the chest and to extend

TABLE 23-1 Brachial Plexus—cont'd

Nerve	Origin	Function, Muscle Innervated	Cutaneous Innervation

Median	Medial and lateral cord, C8-T1	Pronate forearm
		    Pronator teres
		    Pronator quadratus
		Flex wrist
		    Flexor carpi radialis (also abducts wrist)
		    Palmaris longus
		Flex fingers
		    Part of flexor digitorum profundus (distal phalanx of middle and index finger)
		    Flexor digitorum superficialis
		Thumb muscle
		    Flexor pollicis longus
		Thenar muscles
		    Abductor pollicis brevis
		    Opponens pollicis
		    Flexor pollicis brevis
		Midpalmar
		    Two lateral lumbricals
			Lateral two thirds of palm of hand, including lateral half of ring finger and tarsal tips of the same finger

the head back until the face is parallel with the ceiling. There should be at least 40 to 45 degrees of lateral flexion and enough rotation to allow the chin to reach a level even with the tip of the shoulder. Flexibility is increased through stretching exercises and strength exercises that are in full range of motion. Where flexibility is restricted, manual static stretching can be beneficial.

Athletes involved in collision sports, in particular American football and rugby, which involve tackling an opponent, must be taught and required to use techniques that reduce the likelihood of cervical injury. The head, especially one in a helmet, should not be used as a weapon. Football helmets do not protect players against neck injury. In the illegal "spearing" situation, the athlete uses the helmet as a weapon by striking the opponent with its top. Most serious cervical injuries in football result from deliberate axial loading while spearing.[21] In other sports such as diving, wrestling, and bouncing on a trampoline, the athlete's neck can be flexed at the time of contact. Energy of the forward-moving body mass cannot be fully absorbed, and fracture, dislocation, or both can occur. Diving into shallow water causes many catastrophic neck injuries. The diver usually dives into water that is less than 5 feet deep, failing to keep the arms extended in front of the face. The head strikes the bottom, producing a cervical fracture at the C5 or C6 level. Many of the same forces are applied in wrestling. In such trauma, paraplegia, quadriplegia, or death can result. Coaches cannot stress enough to the athlete the importance of using appropriate tackling techniques.

Lumbar Spine

Low back pain is one of the most common and disabling of ailments. However, in the athlete, most cases of low back pain do not involve serious or long-lasting pathology. The athlete, like everyone else in the population, can prevent low back pain by avoiding unnecessary stresses and strains associated with activities of daily living. The back is subjected to these stresses and strains when one is standing, sitting, lying, working, or exercising. Care should be taken to avoid postures and positions that can cause injuries (see the Focus box on page 644).

One should be aware of any postural anomalies that the athletes possess. With this knowledge, one should establish individual corrective programs. Basic conditioning should include an emphasis on trunk flexibility. Every effort should be made to produce maximum range of motion in rotation and both lateral and forward flexion.

TABLE 23-2 Lumbosacral Plexus

Nerve	Origin	Function, Muscle Innervated	Cutaneous Innervation

Obturator	L2-L4	Adduct thigh
		  Adductor magnus
		  Adductor longus
		  Adductor brevis
		  Gracilis (also flexes thigh)
		Rotate thigh laterally
		  Obturator externus
			Superior medial side of thigh

Femoral	L2-L4	Flex thigh
		  Iliacus
		  Psoas major
		  Pectineus
		  Sartorius (also flexes leg)
		Extend leg
		  Rectus femoris (also flexes thigh)
		  Vastus lateralis
		  Vastus medialis
		  Vastus intermedius
			Anterior and lateral branches supply the thigh; the saphenous branch supplies the medial leg and foot

Tibial	L4-S3	Extend thigh, flex leg
		  Biceps femoris (long head)
		  Semitendinosus
		  Semimembranosus
		  Adductor magnus
		Flex leg
		  Popliteus
		Plantar flex foot
		  Gastrocnemius
		  Soleus
		  Plantaris
		  Tibialis posterior
		Flex toes
		  Flexor hallucis longus
		  Flexor digitorum longus
			None

Medial and lateral plantar	Tibial	Plantar muscles of foot	Medial and lateral sole of foot
Sural	Tibial	None	Lateral and posterior one third of leg and lateral side of foot
Common peroneal	L4-S2	Extend thigh, flex leg Bicep femoris (short head)	Lateral surface of knee

Deep peroneal	Common peroneal	Dorsiflex foot
		  Tibialis anterior
		  Peroneus tertius
		Extend toes
		  Extensor hallucis longus
		  Extensor digitorum longus
			Skin over great and second toe

Superficial peroneal	Common peroneal	Plantar flex and evert foot
		  Peroneus longus
		  Peroneus brevis
		Extend toes
		  Extensor digitorum brevis
			Distal anterior third of leg and dorsum of foot

Both strength and flexibility should be developed in the spinal extensors (erector spinae). Abdominal strength is essential to ensure proper postural alignment. In weight lifters, the chance of injury to the lumbar spine can be minimized by using proper lifting techniques. Incorporating appropriate breathing techniques, which involve inhaling and exhaling deeply during lifting, can help stabilize the spine. Weight belts

≈≈≈ *Focus*

Recommended postures to prevent low back pain

Sitting

1. Do not sit for long periods.
2. Avoid sitting forward on a chair with back arched.
3. Sit on a firm, straight-backed chair.
4. The low back should be slightly rounded or positioned firmly against the back of the chair.
5. The feet should be flat on the floor with knees above the level of the hips (if unable to adequately raise the knees, the feet should be placed on a stool).
6. Avoid sitting with legs straight and raised on a stool.

Standing

1. If standing for long periods, shift position from one foot to another or place one foot on a stool.
2. Stand tall, flatten low back, and relax knees.
3. Avoid arching back.

Lifting and carrying

1. To pick up an object, bend at knees and not the waist; do not twist to pick up an object—face it squarely; and tuck in buttocks and tighten abdomen.
2. To carry an object, hold object close to body; hold object at waist level; and do not carry object on one side of the body—if it must be carried unbalanced, change from one side to the other.

Sleeping

1. Do not stay in one position too long.
2. The bed should be flat and firm yet comfortable.
3. Do not sleep on the abdomen.
4. Do not sleep on the back with legs fully extended.
5. If sleeping on the back, a pillow should be placed under the knees.
6. Ideally, sleep on the side with the knees drawn up.
7. Arms should never be extended overhead.
8. The least strain on the back is in the fully recumbent position with the hips and knees at angles of 90 degrees. In the case of a chronic or a subacute low back condition, a firm mattress will afford better rest and relaxation of the lower back. Placing a ¾-inch plywood board underneath the mattress gives a firm, stable surface for the injured back. Sleeping on a water bed will often relieve low back pain. The value of a water bed is that it supports the body curves equally, decreasing abnormal pressures to any one body area.

can also help stabilize the lumbar spine. Spotters can greatly enhance safety by helping lift and lower the weight.

Incorporating dynamic muscular stabilization and dynamic abdominal bracing and finding a neutral position describe a technique used to increase the stability of the trunk. This increased stability will help the athlete maintain the spine and pelvis in the most comfortable and acceptable mechanical position that will control the effects of repetitive microtrauma and protect the structures in the back from further damage. Abdominal muscle control is one key to giving the athlete the ability to stabilize the trunk and control posture.[13]

ASSESSMENT OF THE SPINE

Assessment of injuries to the spine is somewhat more complex than in the joints of the extremities because of the number of articulations involved in spinal movement.

It is also true that injury to the spine, or in particular the spinal cord, may have life-threatening or life-altering implications. Thus the athletic trainer must be systematic and detailed in the evaluation process.

History

The most critical part of the evaluation is to rule out the possibility of spinal cord injury. Questions that address this should first establish the mechanism of injury.

- What do you think happened?
- Did you hit someone with or land directly on the top of your head?
- Were you knocked out or unconscious? Anytime there is an impact sufficient to cause unconsciousness, the potential for injury to the spine exists.
- Do you have any pain in your neck?
- Do you have tingling, numbness, or burning in your shoulders, arms, or hands?
- Do you have equal muscle strength in both hands?
- Are you able to move your ankles and toes? Any sensory or motor changes bilaterally may indicate some spinal cord injury.

A yes response to any of these questions will necessitate extreme caution when moving the athlete. In cases of suspected cervical spine injury, if the athletic trainer is going to make a mistake, the error should be made in being overly cautious. Emergency care of the athlete with suspected cervical spine injury is discussed in detail in Chapter 8.

Once cervical spine injury has been ruled out, other general questions may provide some indication as to the nature of the problem.

- Where is the pain located?
- What kind of pain do you have?
- What were you doing when the pain began?
- Were you standing, sitting, bending, or twisting?
- Did the pain begin immediately?
- How long have you had this pain?
- Do certain movements or positions cause more pain?
- Can you assume a position that gets rid of the pain?
- Is there any tingling or numbness in the arms or legs?
- Is there any pain in the buttocks or the back of the legs?
- Have you ever had any back pain before?
- What position do you usually sleep in? How do you prefer to sit?

It is important to remember that pain in the back may be caused by many different conditions. The source may be musculoskeletal or visceral, or it may be referred.

Observation

Observing the posture and movement capabilities of the athlete during the evaluation can help clarify the nature and extent of the injury.

Posture Evaluation

It is important to observe the athlete's total static posture, with special attention paid to the low back, pelvis, and hips. When observing standing static posture, the athletic trainer must accept the fact that postural alignment varies considerably among individuals; therefore only obvious asymmetries should be considered. The entire body should be observed from all angles—lateral, anterior, and posterior (Figure 23-8). To ensure accuracy of observation, a plumb line or posture screen may be of use (Figure 23-9). A trained observer with a good background in postural observation may not require any special devices. Figure 23-10 shows typical vertical alignment landmarks from a lateral view. Anterior and posterior assessment looks for asymmetries or differences in height between anatomical landmarks on each side (Figure 23-11).

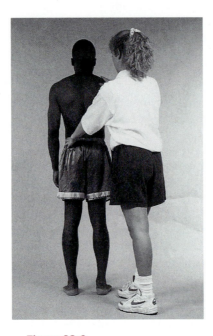

Figure 23-8

Observing spinal alignment.

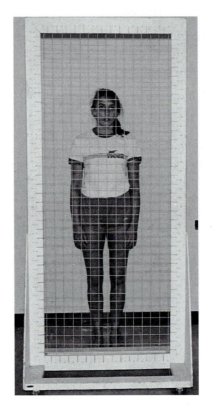

Figure 23-9

Using a grid can produce more accurate results during posture screening.

General observations relative to posture include the following:
- Head is tilted to one side.
- Shoulder is lower on one side.
- One shoulder is carried forward.
- One scapula is lower and more prominent than the other.
- Trunk is habitually bent to one side.
- Space between the body and arm is greater on one side.
- One hip is more prominent than the other.
- Hips are tilted to one side.
- Ribs are more pronounced on one side.
- One arm hangs longer than the other.
- One arm hangs farther forward than the other.
- One patella is lower than the other.

Classic postural deviations include kyphosis, forward head posture, lordosis, flatback posture, swayback posture, and scoliosis.

Kyphosis   Kyphosis is characterized by an increased thoracic curve and scapulae that are protracted, producing a rounded shoulder appearance. Kyphosis is usually associated with a forward head posture (Figure 23-12, *A*).

Scheuerman's disease is a disease of unknown etiology that usually affects adolescent males. This condition is not only painful but also may cause progressive thoracic or lumbar kyphosis.

Forward head posture   If the upper back exhibits a kyphotic posture in standing or sitting, there will be a compensatory change in the position of the head and neck. To keep the eyes level with a slumped or rounded shoulder posture, the cervical spine must extend, which tends to produce short but strong neck extensors and weak long neck flexors. Thus the head will be held in a forward position (Figure 23-12, *B*).

   Flatback posture   Flatback posture is caused by a decreased lumbar curve, with an increase in posterior pelvic tilt and hip flexion (Figure 23-12, *C*).

   Swayback posture   A swayback posture involves an anterior shifting of the entire pelvis, resulting in hip extension. The thoracic segment shifts posteriorly, causing flexion of the thorax on the lumbar spine. Thus there is a decrease in lordosis in the lumbar spine and an increase in kyphosis in the thoracic spine (Figure 23-12, *D*).

   Lordosis   Lordotic posture is characterized by an increased curve in the lumbar spine, with an increase in both anterior tilt of the pelvis and hip flexion. When combined with kyphosis and a forward head posture, this is referred to as a kypholordotic posture (Figure 23-12, *E*).

   Scoliosis   Scoliosis is a lateral curvature of the spine. With scoliosis there is a recognizable abnormal curve in one direction and a compensatory secondary curve in the opposite direction. Scoliosis can be functional or structural. A functional scoliosis can be caused by some nonspinal defect such as unequal leg length, muscle imbalance, or nutritional deficiency. Structural scoliosis is caused by some defect in the bony structure of the spine. In bending forward, the spine may straighten with a functional scoliosis or remain twisted in a structural scoliosis. In this position, one side of the spine may be more prominent than the other (Figure 23-12, *F*).

Cervical Spine Observation

In the case of cervical injury, look at the position of the head and neck. Are the shoulders level and symmetrical? Is the patient willing to move the head and neck freely? Check active range of motion in the neck, including flexion, extension, rotation, and lateral bending.

Thoracic Spine Observation

The athlete is first asked to flex, extend, laterally flex, and rotate the neck (Figure 23-13). Pain accompanying the movement in the upper back region could be referred from a lesion of the cervical disk. Additionally, pain in the scapular area could stem

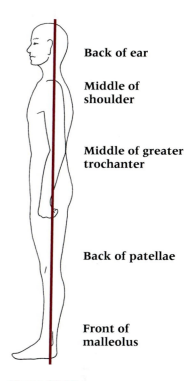

Back of ear

Middle of shoulder

Middle of greater trochanter

Back of patellae

Front of malleolus

Figure 23-10

Typical vertical alignment landmarks.

Figure 23-11

Typical horizontal alignment landmarks. (Colored line indicates vertical landmarks.)

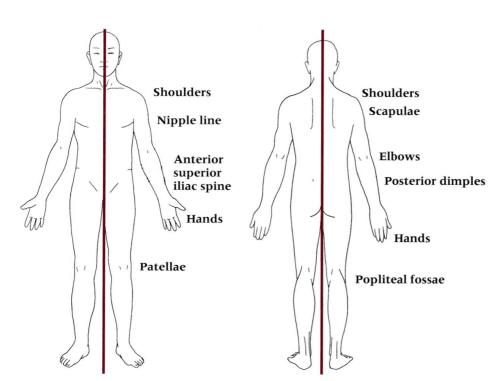

Shoulders
Nipple line
Anterior superior iliac spine
Hands
Patellae

Shoulders
Scapulae
Elbows
Posterior dimples
Hands
Popliteal fossae

Figure 23-12

Postural malalignments. **A,** Kyphosis. **B,** Forward head. **C,** Flatback. **D,** Swayback. **E,** Lordosis. **F,** Scoliosis.

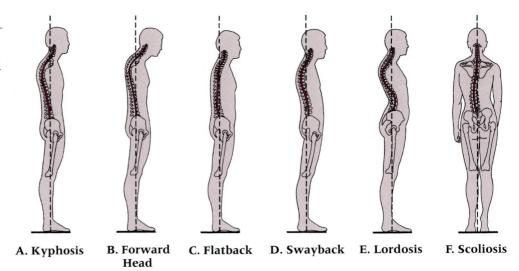

A. Kyphosis   B. Forward Head   C. Flatback   D. Swayback   E. Lordosis   F. Scoliosis

Classic postural deviations include kyphosis, forward head posture, lordosis, flatback posture, swayback posture, and scoliosis.

from an irritation of a myofascial trigger point or from irritation of the long thoracic or suprascapular nerves, requiring evaluation of the shoulder complex. (See Chapter 21.) The athlete should also be asked to flex forward and laterally and to extend and rotate the trunk. Pain felt during movement may indicate nerve root irritation to the lower thoracic region.

The most common cause of thoracic pain is dysfunction of one or more joint articulations usually involving the facet joints. Increased pain in placing the chin on the chest and with deep inspiration is often indicative of a facet joint problem.

Lumbar Spine and Sacroiliac Joint Observation

Normal functional movement in the low back region depends on coordinated motion of the lumbar vertebrae, the sacrum, and the pelvis. The pelvis and shoulders should be level. Both the soft tissue and bony structures on both sides of the midline should be symmetrical. Any unusual curve in the lumbar area observed when the athlete is standing or walking could be due to muscular, capsular, or ligamentous injuries, disk-related problems, or some idiopathic or structural problem. The athlete should be observed in standing, sitting, supine, side-lying, and prone positions. Special tests should be done in each of these positions to determine the nature of the problem.[19]

Palpation

Palpation should be performed with the athlete lying prone and the spine as straight as possible. The head and neck should be slightly flexed. In cases of low back pain a pillow placed under the hips might make the athlete more comfortable. Palpation should progress from proximal to distal, attempting to identify points of tenderness, muscle spasm or guarding, and defects in bone or soft tissue.

The musculature on each side of the spine should be palpated for tenderness or guarding. It should be remembered that referred pain can produce tender areas. At some point in the evaluation of the lumbar spine the abdominal musculature should also be palpated with the athlete performing a partial sit-up to determine symmetry and tone.

The spinous processes are the easiest landmarks to locate. Pressure and release should be applied to the spinous process of each vertebra in an anterior direction to determine if pain is increased either centrally or more laterally. The gaps between the spinous processes should be palpated. Tenderness may indicate some ligamentous or disk-related problem. Each spinous process should be in a direct line with the

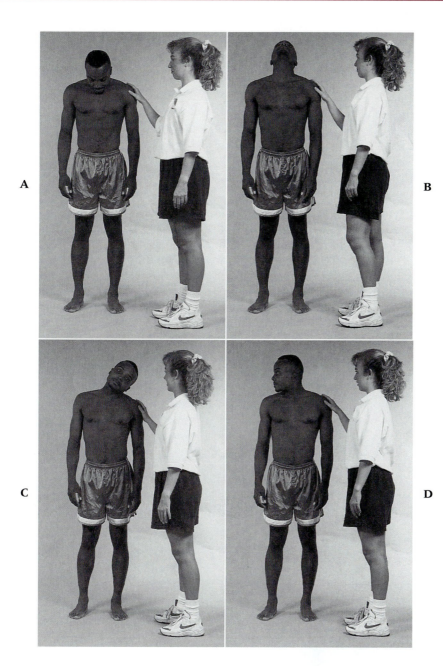

Figure 23-13

Checking neck range of motion. **A,** Flexion. **B,** Extension. **C,** Lateral flexion. **D,** Rotation.

one directly above and directly below (Figure 23-14). Misalignment usually occurs in the cervical or lumbar areas, indicating some rotation of an individual vertebral segment. The transverse processes on both sides of each vertebra can also be palpated. Pressure on one side only produces rotation of that segment, which can increase pain. The facet joints and laminae are difficult to palpate because of the paraspinal muscles.

The sacroiliac joints should be palpated bilaterally for tenderness. Posterior pressure on the sacrum may increase pain if the sacroiliac joint is involved.

Special Tests

Special tests for the lumbar spine should be performed in standing, sitting, supine, side-lying, and prone positions.[13]

Standing position   Observe the gait. Is the patient's trunk bent or are the hips shifted to one side? Is there a limp or any difficulty in walking? Check the alignment

Figure 23-14

Each spinous process should be in a direct line with the one directly above and directly below.

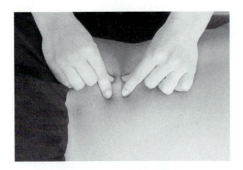

and symmetry of the malleoli, popliteal crease, trochanters, anterior and posterior superior iliac spines (ASIS and PSIS, respectively), and iliac crests.

Forward bending involves stretching of the posterior spinal ligaments (Figure 23-15, A). With forward bending or flexion the PSISs on each side should move together. If one moves further than the other a motion restriction is likely present on the side that moves most. If they move at different times the side that moves first usually has a restriction.

Figure 23-15

Checking lumbar range of motion in standing. **A,** Forward bending. **B,** Backward bending. **C,** Side bending.

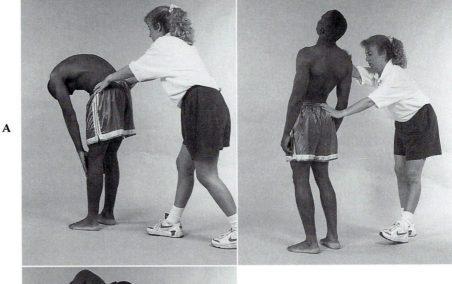

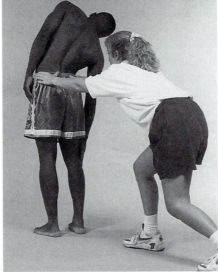

Backward bending places the spine in a hyperextended position, stretching the anterior ligaments of the spine (Figure 23-15, *B*). Restriction or pain present in backward bending is usually associated with a disk problem but may also be related to spondylolysis or spondylolisthesis (discussed later in this chapter).

With a lumbar lesion or with sacroiliac dysfunction, side bending toward the painful side will increase the pain (Figure 23-15, *C*). In the case of a herniated disk, the athlete will usually side bend toward the side of the herniation to relieve the nerve from external compression by the disk.

Sitting position   As in standing, with forward bending or flexion the PSISs should move together. If one moves further than the other a motion restriction is probably present on the side that moves most.

While the athlete is sitting with arms folded across the chest, rotate the athlete's trunk to the left and then to the right, checking the movement of the lumbar spine for symmetry (Figure 23-16, *A*). In this same sitting position, rotate the hip internally and externally (Figure 23-16, *B*). If internal rotation produces pain, this will likely be a piriformis irritation (discussed later in this chapter), and pain is produced as the muscle is stretched.

Supine position   Straight leg raising applies pressure to the sacroiliac joint and may indicate a problem in the sciatic nerve, sacroiliac joint, or lumbar spine (Figure 23-17). Pain at 30 degrees of straight leg raising indicates either a hip problem or an

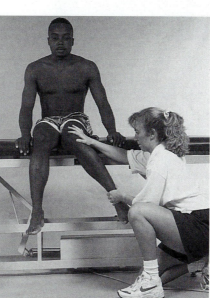
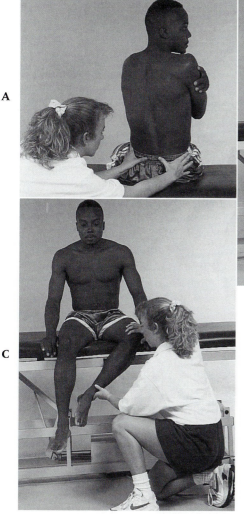

A

B

C

Figure 23-16

Checking lumbar range of motion in sitting. **A,** Rotation. **B,** Internal hip rotation. **C,** External hip rotation.

Figure 23-17

Straight leg raising test.

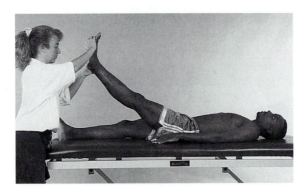

Figure 23-18

Bowstring test for sciatic nerve.

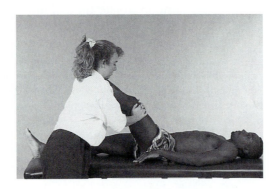

inflamed nerve. Pain from 30 to 60 degrees indicates some sciatic nerve involvement. If dorsiflexing the ankle with maximum straight leg raising increases the pain, it is probably because of some nerve root (L3-4, S1-3) or sciatic nerve irritation (Lasègue's sign). Pain between 70 and 90 degrees is indicative of a sacroiliac joint problem. Straight leg raising of the unaffected side may also produce pain in the low back on the affected side and pain radiating along the sciatic nerve, providing additional proof of nerve root inflammation. Pain on bilateral straight leg raising indicates some problem with the lumbar spine. If pain increases when flexing the neck, there may be either a lumbar disk or some nerve root irritation.[19]

The bowstring test is another way to determine sciatic nerve irritation. The leg on the affected side is lifted until pain is felt. The knee is then flexed until the pain is relieved, at which time pressure is applied to the popliteal fossa. The test result is positive if pain is felt during palpation along the sciatic nerve (Figure 23-18).

To confirm that pain stems from a nerve root involvement and not hamstring tightness, the leg is lowered to a point at which pain ceases. In this position the foot is then dorsiflexed and the neck flexed. If pain returns, it is a verification of a pathological condition of the nerve root.

A Patrick's, or flexion, abduction, external rotation of the hip (FABER) test, indicates a problem with the hip or sacroiliac joint (Figure 23-19, *A*). A flexion, adduction, internal rotation of the hip (FADIR) test indicates a problem in the lumbar area (Figure 23-19, *B*).

Pulling the knees to the chest bilaterally will increase symptoms in the lumbar spine (Figure 23-20, *A*). If pulling a single knee to the chest causes pain in the posterolateral thigh, there may be some irritation to the sacrotuberous ligament (Figure 23-20, *B*). If pain is reported in the area of the PSIS when pulling a single knee to the opposite shoulder, there may be sacroiliac ligament irritation (Figure 23-20, *C*).

Sacroiliac compression and distraction tests are useful in determining if there is a problem in the sacroiliac joint (Figure 23-21).

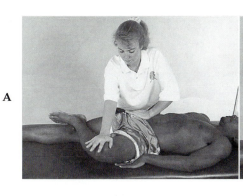
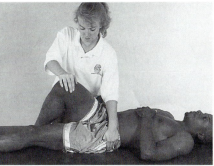

Figure 23-19

A, Patrick's test (FABER). **B,** FADIR test.

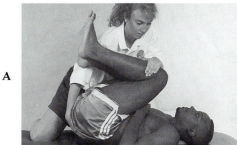
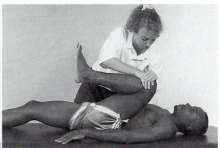
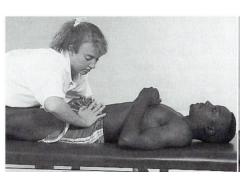

Figure 23-20

A, Bilateral knees to chest. **B,** Single knee to chest. **C,** Knee to opposite shoulder.

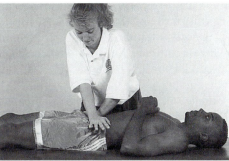

Figure 23-21

A, Sacral compression. **B,** Sacral distraction.

Prone position   Press-ups that extend the spine are done to see if pain radiates into the buttocks or thigh, which may indicate a herniated disk. If pain localizes in this position, conservative care is recommended. If pain is more generalized, surgical care may be required (Figure 23-22).

In a reverse straight leg raise, the athlete lies prone while the examiner lifts the affected leg. If pain occurs in the low back, an L4 nerve root irritation may be present (Figure 23-23).

Side-lying position   Anterior and posterior pelvic tilts that increase the pain on the side being stressed indicate irritation of the sacroiliac joint. Pelvic tilts are more often done lying supine (Figure 23-24).

Figure 23-22

Press-ups.

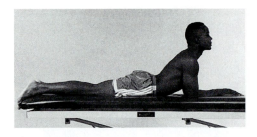

Figure 23-23

Reverse straight leg raise.

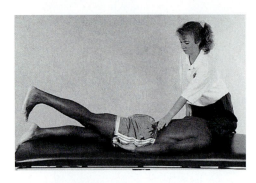

Figure 23-24

A, Anterior pelvic tilt. **B,** Posterior pelvic tilt.

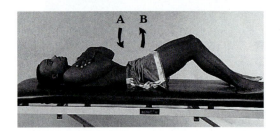

23-3

Critical Thinking Exercise

A cross-country runner was running and stepped in a hole. He immediately felt pain in his left low back below his waist and had to stop running. He comes to the athletic trainer, who suspects that the mechanism of injury has caused a problem with the sacroiliac joint.

❓ What signs should the athletic trainer look for during the evaluation that would likely indicate some injury to the sacroiliac joint?

Neurological examination   The neurological examination is discussed in detail in Chapter 10. In cases of injury to the spine, where the spinal cord and associated nerve roots are potentially injured, sensation testing and reflex testing should be routine aspects of the assessment process.

Sensation testing   When there is a nerve root involvement, sensation can be partially or completely disrupted in dermatomal patterns. Figure 23-25 indicates general disruption or loss of sensation as a result of cervical and lumbosacral nerve root involvement.

Reflex testing   Deep tendon reflexes are discussed in Chapter 10. Three reflexes in the upper extremity are the biceps, brachioradialis, and triceps reflexes. In the biceps reflex the C5 nerve root is being tested. The brachioradialis reflex assesses the C6 nerve root; C7 nerve root dysfunction is indicated by the triceps reflex.

Two reflexes in the lower extremity are the patellar and the Achilles tendon reflexes. A diminished or absent patellar reflex is an indication of an L4, L5, or S1 nerve root problem. The Achilles tendon reflex can determine the presence or absence of an L3, L4, or L5 nerve root problem.

RECOGNITION AND MANAGEMENT OF SPECIFIC INJURIES AND CONDITIONS
Cervical Spine Conditions

Because the neck is so mobile, it is extremely vulnerable to a wide range of sports injuries.[28] Although relatively uncommon, severe sports injury to the neck can produce catastrophic impairment of the spinal cord (Figure 23-26). The neck can be seriously injured by the following traumatic events: an axial load force to the top of

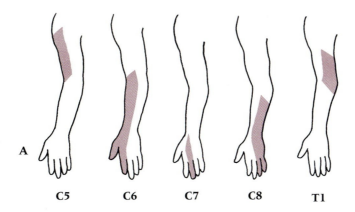
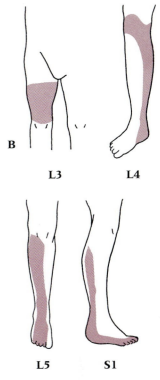

C5   C6   C7   C8   T1

L3   L4

L5   S1

Figure 23-25

A, Upper extremity. **B,** Lower extremity.

the head, a flexion force, a hyperextension force, a flexion-rotation force, a hyperextension-rotation force, or a lateral flexion force[23] (Figure 23-27). The neck is also prone to subtle injuries stemming from stress, tension, and postural malalignments.

Cervical Fractures

Etiology   Fortunately, the incidence of neck fracture is relatively uncommon in athletics. Because the spinal cord is well protected by a bony vertebral canal, a connective tissue sheath, fat, and fluid cushioning, vertebral dislocations and fractures seldom result in paralysis. Nevertheless, the athletic trainer must constantly be prepared to handle such a situation should it arise. The sports having the highest incidence are gymnastics, ice hockey, diving, football, and rugby.[25]

Axial loading of the cervical vertebrae from a force to the top of the head combined with flexion of the neck can result in an anterior compression fracture or possibly a dislocation.[24] Fractures are most common in the fourth, fifth, or sixth cervical vertebrae. If the head is also rotated when making contact, a dislocation may occur

Figure 23-26

The possibility of cervical neck injury is always present in sport.

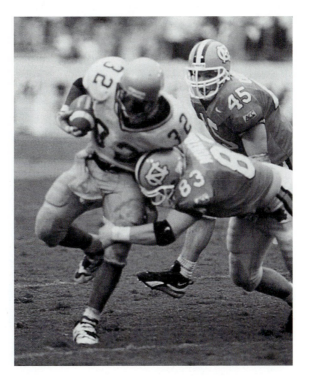

Figure 23-27

Mechanisms of cervical neck injury.

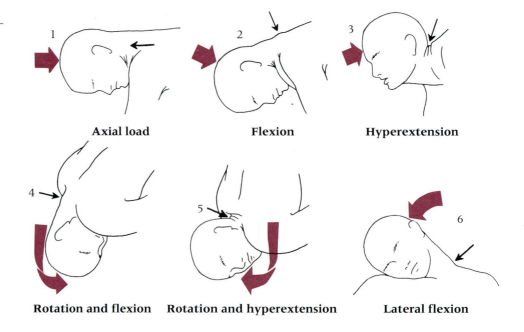

Axial load   **Flexion**   **Hyperextension**

Rotation and flexion   **Rotation and hyperextension**   **Lateral flexion**

along with the fracture. Fractures can also occur during a sudden forced hyperextension of the neck (Figure 23-28).

Symptoms and signs   The athlete may have one or more of the following signs of cervical fracture: neck point tenderness and restricted movement, cervical muscle spasm, cervical pain and pain in the chest and extremities, numbness in trunk or limbs, weakness or paralysis in limbs or trunk, and a loss of bladder or bowel control.

Management   An unconscious athlete should be treated as if a serious neck injury is present until this possibility is ruled out by the physician. Extreme caution must be used in moving the athlete.[1] The athletic trainer must always be aware of the possibility of the athlete's sustaining a catastrophic spinal injury from improper handling and transportation. (See Chapter 8 for emergency care of spinal injuries.)

Cervical Dislocations

Etiology   Cervical dislocations are not common but occur much more frequently in sports than do fractures. They usually result from violent flexion and rotation of

Figure 23-28

Fracture of C3 resulting from a football injury.

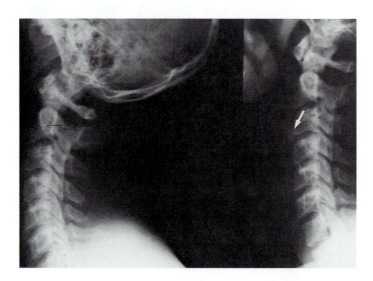

the head. Most injuries of this type happen in pool-diving accidents. The mechanism is analogous to the situation that occurs in football when blocks and tackles are poorly executed. The cervical vertebrae are more easily dislocated than are the vertebrae in other spinal regions, principally because of their horizontally arranged articular facets. The superior articular facet moves beyond its normal range of motion and either completely passes the inferior facet (luxation) or catches on its edge (subluxation). The latter is far more common and, as in the case of the complete luxation, most often affects the fourth, fifth, or sixth vertebra.

Symptoms and signs   For the most part, a cervical dislocation produces many of the same signs as a fracture. Both can result in considerable pain, numbness, and muscle weakness or paralysis. The most easily discernible difference is the position of the neck in a dislocation: a unilateral dislocation causes the neck to be tilted toward the dislocated side with extreme muscle tightness on the elongated side and a relaxed muscle state on the tilted side.

Management   Because a dislocation of a cervical vertebra has a greater likelihood of causing injury to the spinal cord, even greater care must be exercised when moving the patient. The procedures described in Chapter 8 should be applied to cervical dislocations.

Acute Strains of the Neck and Upper Back

Etiology   In a strain of the neck or upper back the athlete has usually turned the head suddenly or has forced flexion, extension, or rotation. Muscles involved are typically the upper trapezius, the sternocleidomastoid, the scalenes, and the splenius capitis and cervicis.

Symptoms and signs   Localized pain, point tenderness, and restricted motion are present. Muscle guarding resulting from pain is common, and there is a reluctance to move the neck in any direction.

Management   Care usually includes use of rest, ice, compression, and elevation (RICE) immediately after the strain occurs and wearing a cervical collar. Follow-up management may include range-of-motion (ROM) exercises followed by isometric progressing to full-range isotonic strengthening exercises, cryotherapy or superficial heat, and analgesic medications as prescribed by the physician.

Cervical Sprain (Whiplash)

Etiology   A cervical sprain can occur from the same mechanism as the strain but usually results from a more violent motion. More commonly the head snaps suddenly, such as when the athlete is tackled or blocked while unprepared (Figure 23-29). Frequently muscle strains occur with ligament sprains. A sprain of the neck produces tears in the major supporting tissue of the anterior or posterior longitudinal ligaments, the interspinous ligament, or the supraspinous ligament.

Symptoms and signs   The sprain displays all the signs of the strained neck, but the symptoms persist longer. There may also be tenderness over the transverse and spinous processes, which serve as sites of attachment for the ligaments.

Pain may not experienced initially but always appears the day after the trauma. Pain stems from the inflammation of injured tissue and a protective muscle spasm that restricts motion.

Management   As soon as possible the athlete should have a physician evaluation to rule out the possibility of fracture, dislocation, or disk injury. Neurological examination is performed by the physician to ascertain spinal cord or nerve root injury. A soft cervical collar may be applied to reduce muscle spasm, and RICE is used for 48 to 72 hours while the injury is in the acute stage of healing. In an athlete with a severe injury the physician may prescribe 2 to 3 days of bed rest, along with analgesics and antiinflammation agents. Therapy might include cryotherapy or heat and massage. Mechanical traction may also be prescribed to relieve pain and muscle spasm.

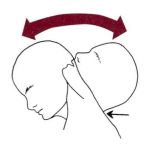

Figure 23-29

Whiplash injury.

Management PLAN

Cervical Sprain (Whiplash)

Injury Situation While at practice, a male ice hockey player was checked hard against the boards. Not being properly set for the force, his head was snapped vigorously backward into extension and forward into flexion. In this process the athlete experienced a sudden sharp pain and a tearing sensation at the base of the posterior neck region.

Symptoms and Signs Initially the athlete complained to the athletic trainer that immediately after the injury there was a dull ache, stiffness, and weakness in the neck region. He also complained of headache, dizziness, and nausea approximately 1 hour after the injury. Palpation revealed severe muscle spasm and point tenderness of the erector spinae muscles and the lateral aspect of the neck and upper shoulder. A neurologic exam did not reveal any changes in motor or sensory abilities. X-ray examination ruled out fracture, dislocation, and spinal cord injury. Gentle passive movement produced some pain. A soft neck collar was applied for immobilization. During further evaluation there was pain during both gentle active and resistive movement. The condition was considered to be a second-degree neck sprain with muscle involvement produced by a whiplash mechanism.

Management Plan The nature of a neck sprain dictates that management should follow a conservative course. A soft cervical collar was to be worn 24 hours a day for comfort or until the athlete was symptom free. Wearing this collar could be followed by wearing the brace just during the waking hours for 1 or 2 additional weeks.

Phase 1 **Acute Injury**   **GOALS:** To control initial hemorrhage, swelling, spasm, and pain.
ESTIMATED LENGTH OF TIME (ELT): 2 to 3 days.

■ **Therapy** Apply ice pack (20 minutes) intermittently six to eight times daily. In some cases, transcutaneous electrical nerve stimulation (TENS) has been used successfully to reduce spasm and pain in the early stages of injury.

■ **Exercise rehabilitation** Wear soft cervical collar. Athlete is taught to hold head in good alignment in relation to shoulder and spine; this should be practiced every waking hour. Begin gentle grade 1 and 2 cervical mobilizations as tolerated.

Phase 2 **Repair**   **GOALS:** To restore 90% neck range of motion and 50% strength
ELT: 7-11 days

■ **Therapy** Ice pack (5 to 15 minutes) or ice massage (7 minutes) three or four times daily; precedes active motion.

■ **Exercise rehabilitation** Active stretching two or three times daily, including neck flexion with depressed shoulders, lateral neck flexion, and right and left head rotation; each position is held for 5 to 10 seconds and repeated five times or within pain-free limits. Gentle passive stretching within pain-free limits (two to three times each direction) once daily; each stretch is held for 20 to 30 seconds. Manual isotonic resistive exercise to the neck is performed once daily by the athlete or athletic trainer (five repetitions). Progress to grade 3 and 4 cervical mobilizations as tolerated.

Phase 3 **Remodeling**   **GOALS:** To restore full range of motion and full strength; to return to ice hockey competition and full neck muscle bulk.
ELT: 4 to 7 days.

■ **Therapy** Ice pack (5 to 15 minutes) or ice massage (7 minutes) once daily preceding exercise.

Continued

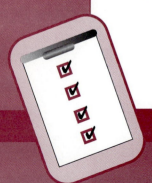

Cervical Sprain (Whiplash)—*cont'd*

■ **Exercise rehabilitation** Continue manual resistive exercise once daily; add resistance devices such as weighted helmet or Nautilus neck strengthener (three sets of 10 repetitions) using DAPRE concept, three times a week. Begin practice daily with a neck roll protective brace during the first few weeks of return. Work on maximum neck resistance three to four times daily.

Criteria for Return to Competition after Whiplash Neck Sprain

The neck of the athlete
1. Is completely symptom free.
2. Has full range of motion.
3. Has full strength and bulk.

Acute Torticollis (Wryneck)

Etiology Acute torticollis is a common condition, more frequently called wryneck or stiffneck. The athlete usually complains of pain on one side of the neck when awakening. This condition usually occurs when a small piece of synovial membrane lining the joint capsule is impinged or trapped within a facet joint in the cervical vertebrae. This problem can also occasionally follow exposure to a cold draft of air or holding the head in an unusual position over a period of time.

Symptoms and signs During inspection, there is palpable point tenderness and muscle spasm. Rotation and side bending are restricted to the side of the irritation with marked muscle guarding. X-ray examination will rule out a more serious injury.

Management Various therapeutic modalities may be used to modulate pain in an attempt to break a pain-spasm-pain cycle. Joint mobilizations involving gentle traction, rotation, and lateral bending first in the pain-free direction and then in the direction of pain can help reduce the guarding. It may be helpful to wear a soft cervical collar to provide for comfort (Figure 23-30). Muscle guarding will generally last for 2 to 3 days as the athlete progressively regains motion.

Cervical Cord and Nerve Root Injuries

Etiology The spinal cord and nerve roots may be injured via four basic mechanisms: laceration by bony fragments, hemorrhage (hematomyelia), contusion, and shock. These mechanisms may be combined into a single trauma or may act as separate conditions.

LACERATION Laceration of the cord is usually produced by the combined dislocation and fracture of a cervical vertebra. The jagged edges of the fragmented vertebral body cut and tear nerve roots or the spinal cord and cause varying degrees of paralysis below the point of injury.

HEMORRHAGE Hemorrhage develops from all vertebral fractures and from most dislocations, as well as from sprains and strains. It seldom causes harmful effects in the musculature, extradurally, or even within the arachnoid space, where it dissipates faster than it can accumulate. However, hemorrhage within the cord itself causes irreparable damage.

CONTUSION Contusion in the cord or nerve roots can arise from any force applied to the neck violently but without causing a cervical dislocation or fracture. Such

The spinal cord and nerve roots may be injured via four basic mechanisms: laceration by bony fragments, hemorrhage, contusion, and shock.

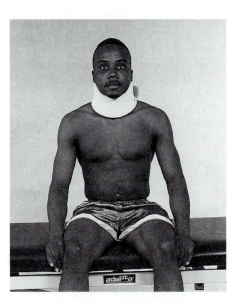

an injury may result from sudden displacement of a vertebra that compresses the cord and then returns to its normal position. This compression causes edematous swelling within the cord, resulting in various degrees of temporary or permanent damage.

SPINAL CORD SHOCK   Occasionally a situation arises in which an athlete, after receiving a severe twist or snap of the neck, has all the signs of a spinal cord injury. The athlete is unable to move or has weakness in certain parts of the body and complains of numbness and a tingling sensation in his or her arms. After a short while all these signs leave. The athlete is then able to move his or her limbs freely and has no other symptoms other than a sore neck. This condition is considered a spinal cord shock and is caused by a mild contusion of the spinal cord or by cervical spine stenosis. In such cases the athlete should be cared for in the same manner used for any severe neck injury.

Symptoms and signs   Each of these situations can result in various types of paralysis affecting the motor or sensory systems. The level of the injury will determine the extent of the functional deficits. Spinal cord lesions may be either complete or incomplete. A complete lesion is one in which the spinal cord has been totally severed and there is a complete loss of all motor function and sensation below the level of the injury. Recovery of significant function below the level of the injury is unlikely, although some nerve root function may eventually recover one to two levels below the injury. Complete cord lesions at or above C3 will impair respiration, resulting in death. Lesions at spinal segment levels below C4 will allow for return of some nerve root function, as follows:

- C4-C5—return of deltoid function.
- C5-C6—return of elbow flexion and wrist extension.
- C6-C7—return of elbow and finger extension and wrist flexion.
- C7-T1—return of grip function.

Incomplete lesions can result in central cord syndrome, Brown-Sequard syndrome, anterior cord syndrome, or posterior cord syndrome.[17] Central cord syndrome is caused by hemorrhage or ischemia in the central portion of the cord and results in complete quadriplegia with nonspecific sensory loss, sexual dysfunction, and bowel-bladder dysfunction. Brown-Sequard syndrome is caused by an injury to one side of the spinal cord, resulting in loss of motor function, touch, vibration, and position sense on one side of the body and loss of pain and temperature sensation on the other side. Anterior cord syndrome is caused by an injury to the anterior two thirds of the cord, resulting in loss of motor function and pain and temperature sensation. However, sexual and bowel-bladder functions are present. Posterior cord syndrome, although rare, is caused by injury to the posterior cord. Motor function is completely intact.

Management   As is the case with suspected cervical fractures and dislocations, suspected injuries to the spinal cord must be handled with extreme caution. With fractures and dislocations care is taken to minimize potential damage to the spinal cord. In cases where evidence of spinal cord damage accompanied by varying degrees of paralysis exists immediately with injury, management efforts must attempt to minimize additional trauma to the cord.[9] Chapter 8 presents a detailed discussion of the recommended procedures for managing athletes with suspected spinal cord injury.

Cervical Spine Stenosis

Etiology   Cervical spine stenosis is a syndrome characterized by a narrowing of the spinal canal in the cervical region that can impinge the spinal cord. This occurs either as a congenital variation or from some change in the vertebrae, including the development of bone spurs, osteophytes, or disk bulges. The presence of cervical stenosis is determined radiographically. From an x-ray, a measurement of the canal diameter is divided by the anteroposterior width of the same vertebral body.[12] A ratio less than 0.80 suggests cervical stenosis.[25]

Symptoms and signs   Transient quadriplegia may occur from axial loading, hyperextension, or hyperflexion. Neck pain may be absent initially. The symptoms may be purely sensory with burning or tingling, or they may have some associated motor weakness in the arms, the legs, or all four extremities. Complete recovery normally occurs within 10 to 15 minutes but may be delayed. After neurological recovery, full neck range of motion is possible.

Management   Cervical spine stenosis may be present without any symptoms and signs. As with any suspected injury to the cervical spine, the presence of transient quadriplegia necessitates extreme caution initially. The athlete must have diagnostic tests, including x-ray or magnetic resonance imaging (MRI), to determine the extent of the problem. Athletes, particularly those in contact sports, who have been identified as having some degree of cervical stenosis should be advised of the potential risks of continued participation in that sport. There is a growing consensus among physicians that continued participation should be discouraged.[5]

Brachial Plexus Neurapraxia (Burner)

Etiology   Transient neurapraxia resulting from stretching or compression of the brachial plexus is the most common of all cervical neurological injuries in the athlete.[17] Neurapraxia involves a disruption in normal function of a peripheral nerve without any degenerative changes occurring. Other terms commonly used to indicate this condition are *stinger, burner,* or *pinched nerve.*[26] The primary mechanism of injury is stretching of the brachial plexus when the neck is forced laterally to the opposite side while the shoulder is depressed, as would occur with a shoulder block in football. A second mechanism compresses the brachial plexus when the neck is extended, compressed, and rotated toward the affected side.

Symptoms and signs   The player complains of a burning sensation, numbness and tingling, and pain extending from the shoulder down to the hand, with some loss of function of the arm and hand that lasts for several minutes. Rarely, symptoms may persist for several days. Neck range of motion is usually normal. Repeated brachial plexus nerve stretch injuries may result in neuritis, muscular atrophy, and permanent damage.[15]

Management   Once the symptoms have completely resolved and there are no associated neurological symptoms, the athlete may return to full activity. Thereafter the athlete should begin strengthening and stretching exercises for the neck musculature. A football player should be fitted with shoulder pads and a cervical neck roll to limit neck range of motion during impact.

Cervical Disk Injuries

Etiology   Herniation of a cervical disk is relatively common and can affect athletes in any sport. A herniation usually develops as an extruded posterolateral disk frag-

23-4

Critical Thinking Exercise

A football linebacker is making a tackle. Initial contact on the ball carrier is with the head, and the neck is forced into hyperflexion. The athlete immediately has transient quadriplegia with burning and tingling and associated motor weakness in the arms and legs. Neck pain is absent initially. Within 15 minutes the athlete recovers completely and has full range of motion.

? What type of injury should the athletic trainer suspect with this athlete, and how should this condition be managed?

ment or from degeneration of the disk. The primary mechanism involves sustained repetitive cervical loading during contact sports.

Symptoms and signs   The symptoms and signs include neck pain with some restriction in neck motion. There is radicular pain (nerve root) in the upper extremity with associated motor weakness or sensory changes.

Management   Initial treatment involves rest and immobilization of the neck to decrease discomfort. Neck mobilizations may help with regaining some range of motion. Cervical traction may also help reduce symptoms. If conservative treatment is not helpful or the neurological deficits increase, surgery may be necessary.

Thoracic Spine Conditions

Injuries to the thoracic region of the spine have a much lower incidence than in the cervical or lumbar regions. This is due to the articulation of the thoracic vertebrae with the ribs, which act to stabilize and limit motion of the vertebrae, thus minimizing the likelihood of injury to this area. Thus thoracic fractures are relatively rare and occur in high-impact sports such as skiing, tobogganing, skydiving, and automobile racing.

Scheuermann's Disease (Dorsolumbar Kyphosis)

Etiology   Scheuermann's disease is characterized by kyphosis resulting from wedge fractures of three or more consecutive vertebral bodies by 5 degrees or greater with associated disk space abnormalities and irregularity of the epiphyseal endplates.[18] This degeneration allows the disk's nucleus pulposus to prolapse into a vertebral body. Characteristically there is an accentuation of the kyphotic curve and backache in the young athlete. Adolescents engaging in sports such as gymnastics and swimming—the butterfly stroke particularly—are prone to this condition. Scheuermann's disease is idiopathic, but the occurrence of multiple minor injuries to the vertebral epiphyses seems to be an etiological factor. These injuries apparently disrupt circulation to the epiphyseal endplate, causing avascular necrosis.

Symptoms and signs   In the initial stages, the young athlete will have kyphosis of the thoracic spine and lumbar lordosis without back pain. In later stages, there is point tenderness over the spinous processes, and the young athlete may complain of backache at the end of a physically active day. Hamstring muscles are characteristically tight.

Management   The major goal of management is to prevent progressive kyphosis. In the early stages of the disease, extension exercises and postural education are beneficial. Bracing, rest, and antiinflammatory medication may also be helpful. The athlete may stay active but should avoid aggravating movements.

Lumbar Spine Conditions

Mechanisms of Low Back Pain

Pain in the low back is second only to foot problems in order of incidence in humans throughout their lifespan. In sports, back problems are relatively common and are most often the result of either congenital or idiopathic (i.e., mechanical or traumatic factors) causes.[3] Congenital back disorders are conditions that are present at birth. Many authorities think that the human back is still undergoing structural changes as a result of its upright position and therefore that humans are prone to slight spinal defects at birth, which later in life may cause pain. The usual cause of back pain among athletes is overuse that produces strains or sprains of paravertebral muscles and ligaments.

Congenital anomalies   Anomalies of bony development are the underlying cause of many back problems in sports. Such conditions would have remained undiscovered had it not been for some abnormal stress or injury in the area of the anomaly. The most common of these anomalies are excessive length of the transverse process of the fifth lumbar vertebra, incomplete closure of the neural arch (spina bifida occulta), nonconformities of the spinous processes, atypical lumbosacral angles or ar-

Low back problems are most often either congenital or idiopathic.

ticular facets, and incomplete closures of the vertebral laminae. All these anomalies may produce mechanical weaknesses that make the back prone to injury when it is subjected to excessive postural strains.

An example of a congenital defect that may develop into a more serious condition when aggravated by a blow or a sudden twist in sports is the condition of spondylolisthesis. Spondylolisthesis is a forward subluxation of the body of a vertebra, usually the fifth lumbar.

Mechanical defects of the spine   Mechanical back defects are caused mainly by faulty posture, obesity, or faulty body mechanics—all of which may affect the athlete's performance in sports. Traumatic forces produced in sports, either directly or indirectly, can result in contusions, sprains, strains, and fractures. Sometimes even minor injuries can develop into chronic and recurrent conditions, which may have serious complications for the athlete. To aid fully in understanding a back complaint, a logical investigation should be made into the history and the site of any injury, the type of pain produced, and the extent of impairment of normal function.

Maintaining proper segmental alignment of the body during standing, sitting, lying, running, jumping, and throwing is of utmost importance for keeping the body in good condition.[16] Habitual violations of the principles of good body mechanics occur in many sports and produce anatomical deficiencies that subject the body to constant abnormal muscular and ligamentous strain.[27] In all cases of postural deformity the athletic trainer should determine the cause and attempt to rectify the condition through proper strength and mobilization exercises.

Back trauma   It is of vital importance that the athletic trainer possess skill in recognizing and evaluating the extent of a sports injury to the back. Every football season there are stories of an athlete who is paralyzed because of the mishandling of a fractured spine. Such episodes could be greatly reduced if field officials, coaches, and athletic trainers would use discretion, exercise good judgment, and be able to identify certain gross indications of serious spine involvement.[9]

Recurrent and chronic low back pain   Repeated strains or sprains in the low back can cause the supporting tissues to lose their ability to stabilize the spine, thus producing tissue laxity. After repeated episodes, the athlete may develop what is referred to as chronic low back pain. Recurrent or chronic low back pain can have many possible causes, including malalignment of the vertebral facets, discogenic disease, and nerve root compression, all of which can result in pain. Gradually this problem could lead to muscular weakness and impairment of sensation and reflex responses. The older the athlete, the more prone he or she is to developing chronic low back pain. The incidence of this condition at the high school level is relatively low but becomes progressively greater with increasing age. An acute back condition is the culmination of a progressive degeneration of long duration that is aggravated or accentuated by sudden flexion, extension, or rotation.

Lumbar Vertebrae Fracture and Dislocation

Etiology   Fractures of the vertebral column, in terms of bone injury, are not serious in themselves, but they pose dangers when related to spinal cord damage. Vertebral fractures of the greatest concern in sports are compression fractures and fractures of the transverse and spinous processes.

The compression fracture may occur as a result of hyperflexion of the trunk (Figure 23-31). Falling from a height and landing on the feet or buttocks may also produce a compression fracture. The vertebrae that are most often compressed are those in the dorsolumbar curves. The vertebrae usually are crushed anteriorly by the traumatic force of the body above the site of injury. The crushed vertebral body may spread out fragments and protrude into the spinal canal, compressing and possibly even cutting the cord.

Fractures of the transverse and spinous processes result most often from kicks or other direct impact to the back. Because these processes are surrounded by large muscles, fracture produces extensive soft-tissue injury. As fractures they present little

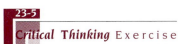

23-5

Critical Thinking Exercise

A volleyball player comes to the athletic trainer complaining of recurring low back pain. She has been seen by a therapist, who has told her that she has a positive straight leg raise test, but the athlete still does not understand what is causing her pain.

? How should the athletic trainer explain what having a positive straight leg raise test means?

Figure 23-31

Lumbar compression fracture.

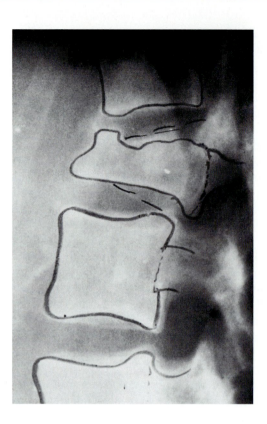

danger and will usually permit the athlete considerable activity within the range of pain tolerance. Most care and treatment will be oriented toward therapy of the soft-tissue pathology.

Dislocations of the lumbar vertebrae in sports are rare, occurring only when there is an associated fracture. This is primarily due to the orientation of the facet joints in the lumbar vertebrae.

Symptoms and signs   Recognition of the compression fracture is difficult without an x-ray examination. A basic evaluation may be made with a knowledge of the history and point tenderness over the affected vertebrae. Fractures of the transverse and spinous processes may be directly palpable. There will be point tenderness with some localized swelling along with muscle guarding to protect the area.

Management   If the symptoms and signs associated with a fracture are present, the injured athlete should be x-rayed. Transporting and moving the athlete should be done on a spine board as described in Chapter 8 in an effort to minimize movement of the fractured segment.

Low Back Muscle Strains

Etiology   There are two mechanisms of the typical lower back strain in sports activities.[4] The first happens from a sudden extension contraction on an overloaded, unprepared, or underdeveloped spine, usually in combination with trunk rotation. The second is the chronic strain commonly associated with faulty posture involving excessive lumbar lordosis. However, other postures such as flat back posture or scoliosis can also predispose one to strain.

Symptoms and signs   Evaluation should be performed immediately after injury to rule out the possibility of fracture. Discomfort in the low back may be diffused or localized in one area. In the case of muscle strain, pain will be present on active extension and with passive flexion. There is no radiating pain farther than the buttocks or thigh and no neurological involvement causing muscle weakness, sensation impairment, or reflex impairments.

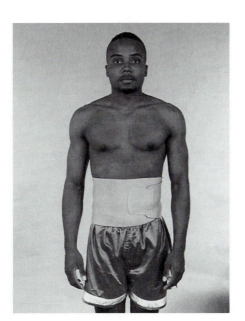

Figure 23-32

An abdominal brace helps support the lumbar area.

Management   In the acute phase of this injury, it is essential that cold packs or ice massage be used intermittently throughout the day to decrease muscle spasm. An elastic wrap or corset-type brace will help compress the area. A graduated program of stretching and strengthening begins slowly during the acute stage. Progressive strengthening exercises should concentrate on extension; stretching should focus on both flexion and extension. Injuries of moderate to severe intensity may require complete bed rest to help break the pain–muscle spasm cycle. The physician may prescribe oral analgesic medication. Cryotherapy, ultrasound, and an abdominal support (Figure 23-32) are often beneficial after the acute phase. Exercise must not cause pain.

Myofascial Pain Syndrome

Etiology   Myofascial pain syndrome is defined as a regional pain with referred pain to a specific area that occurs with pressure or palpation of tender spots or trigger points within a specific muscle.[13] A trigger point is an area of tenderness in a tight band of muscle. Palpation of the trigger point produces pain in a predictable distribution of referred pain. There may also be some restricted range of motion because of pain. Pressure on the trigger point produces a twitch, or "jump," response from the pain. Pain can be increased by passive or active stretching of the involved muscle. In the athlete, painful or active trigger points most often develop because of some mechanical stress to the muscle. This could involve either an acute muscle strain, repetitive motions that fatigue the muscle, or static postural positions that produce constant tension in the muscle. Trigger points occur most typically in the neck, upper back, and lower back. In the lower back there are two muscles in which trigger points commonly occur: the piriformis and the quadratus lumborum.

The piriformis muscle was discussed in Chapter 20. It is an external rotator of the thigh and is located posterior to the hip joint in the sciatic notch. The piriformis muscle is important because of its proximity to the sciatic nerve. The sciatic nerve either pierces the piriformis or courses directly above or below it.

The quadratus lumborum originates on the twelfth rib and the transverse processes of L1-L4. It inserts on the iliac crest. The quadratus functions to elevate the pelvis.

Symptoms and signs   Palpation of or pressure on a trigger point in the piriformis muscle in the sciatic notch refers pain to the posterior sacroiliac region, to the buttocks, and occasionally down the posterior or posterolateral thigh. Pain is a deep ache that increases with exercise or in prolonged sitting with the hip adducted, flexed, and medially rotated. Isometric abduction and passive internal rotation will increase pain. Sciatic pain may also occur with diminished sensation in the leg.

A trigger point in the quadratus lumborum produces a sharp, aching pain in the lateral lower back or flank. Pain may be referred to the upper buttocks and posterior sacroiliac region and sometimes to the abdominal wall. Pain increases when standing for long periods, moving from sitting to standing, or from coughing or sneezing. There will be muscle spasm with pain localized to one side. Pain increases on side bending toward the side of the trigger point.

Management   Rehabilitation exercises should include both stretching and strengthening of the involved muscle. The key in treating myofascial pain is stretching the muscle back to a normal resting length, thus relieving the irritation that created the trigger point. The athlete should be placed in a comfortable position that also stretches the involved muscle. Active stretching should be mild and progressive. The use of electrical stimulation in combination with ultrasound is helpful in relieving the pain associated with a trigger point. A spray and stretch technique has also been used successfully. (See Chapter 14.) Progressive strengthening exercises should also be included.

Lumbar Sprains

Etiology   Sprains may occur in any of the ligaments in the lumbar spine. The most common sprain involves lumbar facet joints. Facet joint sprain typically occurs when bending forward and twisting while lifting or moving some object. It can occur with a single episode or with chronic repetitive stress that causes a gradual onset and becomes progressively worse with activity.

Symptoms and signs   The pain is localized and is located just lateral to the spinous process. Pain becomes sharper with certain movements or postures, and the athlete will limit movement in painful ranges. Passive anteroposterior or rotational movement of the vertebrae will increase pain.

Management   As with sprains to other joints in the body some time will be required for healing. Initial treatment should include RICE to reduce pain. Joint mobilizations using anteroposterior and rotational glides can be used to help decrease pain. Strengthening exercises for abdominals and back extensors, as well as stretching in all directions, should be limited to a pain-free range. The athlete should be instructed in trunk stabilization exercises. A brace or support should be worn to limit movement during early return to activity. It is important to guard against the development of postural changes, which may occur in response to pain.

Back Contusions

Etiology   Back contusions rank second to strains and sprains in incidence. Because of its surface area, the back is vulnerable to bruises in sports. Football produces the greatest number of these injuries. A history indicating a significant impact to the back could indicate an extremely serious condition. Contusion of the back must be distinguished from a vertebral fracture. In some instances this is possible only through an x-ray examination.

Symptoms and signs   The bruise causes local pain, muscle spasm, and point tenderness. A swollen, discolored area may be visible also.

Management   Cold and pressure should be applied immediately for approximately 72 hours or longer along with rest. Ice massage combined with gradual stretching benefits soft-tissue contusion in the region of the lower back. Recovery usually ranges from 2 days to 2 weeks. Ultrasound is effective in treating the deep muscles.

Sciatica

Etiology   Sciatica is an inflammatory condition of the sciatic nerve that can accompany recurrent or chronic low back pain. The term *sciatica* has been incorrectly

23-6

Critical Thinking Exercise

A swimmer complains of an area of tenderness in a tight band of muscle in the middle of her upper back. Palpation of the trigger point refers pain around the chest wall. Pain is increased by both passive and active stretching of the in-volved muscle. Pain is usually increased after a long training workout in the pool.

? What type of muscular problem frequently develops in the middle or low back of athletes who engage in repeti-tive motions, which fatigue a muscle? How is this problem best managed?

Lumbosacral Strain

Injury Situation A high school shot-putter came into the athletic training room complaining of a very sore back. He indicated that he woke up with the problem and was not sure how it occurred. Perhaps he had hurt it by doing dead lifts the day before or by throwing the shot incorrectly.

Symptoms and Signs The athlete complained of a constant dull ache and an inability to flex, extend, or rotate the trunk without increasing the pain. Inspection of the injury indicated the following:

1. The athlete had a pronounced lumbar lordosis.
2. There was an obvious muscle contraction of the right erector spinae.
3. There was severe point tenderness in the right lumbar region.
4. The right pelvis was elevated.
5. Passive movement did not cause pain; however, active and resistive movements produced severe pain.
6. Range of movement in all directions was restricted.
7. All tests for nerve root, hip joint, and sacroiliac joint were negative.
8. Leg length was measured, and the athlete had a functional shortening but no apparent structural shortening.
9. Both the left and right hamstring muscle groups and iliopsoas muscles were abnormally tight.
10. X-ray examination showed no pathological conditions of the lumbar vertebrae.

Based on the examination, it was concluded that the athlete had sustained a first- to second-degree strain of the lumbar muscles, primarily in the right erector spinae region.

Management Plan

Phase 1 **Acute Injury**   **GOALS**: To relieve muscle spasm and pain.
ESTIMATED LENGTH OF TIME (ELT): 2 or 3 days.

■ **Therapy** Ice pack (20 minutes) followed by exercise and then by transcutaneous electrical nerve stimulation (TENS) (15 to 20 minutes) three to four times daily.

■ **Exercise rehabilitation** After cold application, gentle passive stretch of low back region and hamstring and iliopsoas muscles—all within pain tolerance levels—three to four times daily, along with grade 1 and 2 mobilization of affected segments.

Phase 2 **Repair**   **GOALS**: To increase low back, hamstring, and iliopsoas range of motion (ROM) to at least begin postural correction; 50% normal extensibility of the low back hamstring and iliopsoas muscles; appropriate abdominal strength.
ELT: 4 to 12 days.

■ **Therapy** Ice massage followed by exercise two to three times daily. If still painful, TENS therapy should be used. Ultrasound 1 to 1.5 W/cm^2 once daily.

■ **Exercise rehabilitation** Repeat phase 1 exercise and begin proprioceptive neuromuscular facilitation (PNF) to hip and low back regions two to three times daily; or static low back, hamstring, and iliopsoas stretching (two to three repetitions) and lower-abdominal strengthening two to three times daily. Continue grade 1 and 2 mobilizations, progressing to grades 3 and 4 as tolerated. Practice realigning pelvis. General body maintenance exercises are conducted (as long as they do not aggravate the injury) three times a week.

Continued

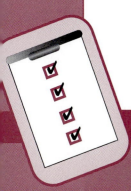

Phase 3   **Remodeling**   GOALS: To restore 90% of ROM, strength, and proper back alignment.

■ **Exercise rehabilitation** Return to weight training and shot-putting program three times a week. Athlete is instructed about proper back alignment when shot-putting. Athlete is to avoid dead lifting and to wear a lifting belt while weight training. Begin spinal stabilization program. Return to normal training three times a week. Gradual reentry into competition. Using an abdominal support belt is advisable during practice and competition.

Criteria for Returning to Competitive Shot-Putting

The athlete's back must be
1. Pain and spasm free.
2. Near normal in hamstring, low back, and iliopsoas extensibility.
3. Making good progress toward correcting lumbar lordosis.
4. Able to perform the shot-put with the spine and pelvis in good alignment.

---

used as a general term to describe all lower back pain, without reference to exact causes. It is commonly associated with peripheral nerve root compression from intervertebral disk protrusion, structural irregularities within the intervertebral foramen, or tightness of the piriformis muscle. This nerve is particularly vulnerable to torsion or direct blows that tend to impose abnormal stretching and pressure on it as it emerges from the spine, thus effecting a traumatic condition.[11]

Symptoms and signs   Sciatica may begin either abruptly or gradually. It produces a sharp shooting pain that follows the nerve pathway along the posterior and medial thigh. There may also be some tingling and numbness along its path. The nerve may be extremely sensitive to palpation. Straight leg raising usually intensifies the pain.

Management   In the acute stage rest is essential. The cause of the inflammation must be identified and treated. If there is a disk protrusion, lumbar traction may be appropriate. Stretching of a tight piriformis muscle may also decrease symptoms. Because recovery from sciatia usually occurs within 2 to 3 weeks, surgery should be delayed to see if symptoms resolve. Oral antiinflammatory medication may help reduce inflammation.

Herniated Lumbar Disk

Etiology   The lumbar disks are subject to constant abnormal stresses stemming from faulty body mechanics, trauma, or both, which over a period of time can cause degeneration, tears, and cracks in the annulus fibrosus.[6] The disk most often injured lies between the L4-L5 vertebrae. The L5-S1 disk is the second most commonly affected.

A herniated lumbar disk can be prolapsed, extruded, or sequestrated.

In sports, the mechanism of a disk injury is the same as for the lumbosacral sprain—forward bending and twisting, which places abnormal strain on the lumbar region. The movement that produces herniation or bulging of the nucleus pulposus may be minimal, and associated pain may be significant. Besides injuring soft tissues, such a stress may herniate an already degenerated disk by causing the nucleus pulposus to protrude into or through the annulus fibrosis (Figure 23-33). As the disk progressively degenerates a prolapsed disk may develop in which the nucleus moves com-

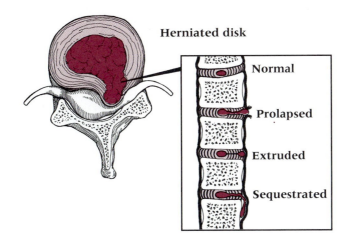

Herniated disk

Normal

Prolapsed

Extruded

Sequestrated

Figure 23-33

A herniated lumbar disk. Further degeneration can lead to a prolapsed disk, an extruded disk, or a sequestrated disk.

pletely through the annulus. If the nucleus moves into the spinal canal and comes in contact with a nerve root, this is referred to as an extruded disk. This protrusion of the nucleus pulposus may place pressure on the cord of spinal nerves, thus causing radiating pains similar to those of sciatica. If the material of the nucleus separates from the disk and begins to migrate, a sequestrated disk exists.

Pressure within the intervertebral disks changes with various positions or posture. When using intervertebral pressure in the standing position as a constant, it was found that pressure was decreased by 75% in the supine position and by 25% in the side-lying position. Pressure was increased by 33% while sitting; by 33% while standing when slightly bent forward; by 45% while sitting when slightly bent forward; by 52% while standing when bent far forward; and by 63% while sitting when bent well forward.

Symptoms and signs   There is usually centrally located pain, which radiates unilaterally in a dermatomal pattern to the buttocks and down the back of the leg, or pain that spreads across the back. Symptoms are worse in the morning when getting out of bed. Onset may be sudden or gradual with pain increasing after sitting and then trying to resume activity. Forward bending and sitting increases pain. Backward bending reduces pain. Posture will exhibit a slight forward bend with side bending away from the side of pain. Side bending toward the side of pain is limited and increases pain. There is tenderness around the painful area. Straight leg raising to 30 degrees increases pain. Tendon reflexes may be diminished. Muscle testing may reveal weakness with bilateral differences.

Management   Initial treatment should involve treatment with pain-reducing modalities such as ice or electrical stimulation. Manual traction combined with passive backward bending or extension makes the athlete more comfortable. The goal is to reduce the protrusion and restore normal posture. Thus the athlete should be taught appropriate posture self-correction exercises. As pain and posture return to normal, back extensor and abdominal strengthening should be used.

If the disk is extruded or sequestrated about the only thing that can be done is to modulate pain with electrical stimulation. Flexion exercises and lying supine in a flexed position may help with comfort. Sometimes the symptoms will resolve with time; however, if there are signs of nerve damage surgery may be necessary.[7]

Spondylolysis and Spondylolisthesis

Etiology   Spondylolysis refers to a degeneration of the vertebrae and, more commonly, a defect in the pars interarticularis of the articular processes of the vertebrae (Figure 23-34). It is often attributed to a congenital weakness with the defect occurring as a stress fracture. It is more common among boys.[14] Spondylolysis may produce no symptoms unless a disk herniation occurs or there is sudden trauma such as hyperextension. Sports movements that characteristically hyperextend the spine,

23-7

Critical Thinking Exercise

A gymnast complains of a centrally located back pain that radiates down her left leg. She describes a sudden onset after a workout that becomes more severe as she tries to rest it. Forward bending and sitting postures increase pain. Backward bending is restricted. Side bending toward the affected side increases pain.

? Based on the athletic trainer's assessment, what would likely be causing this pain?

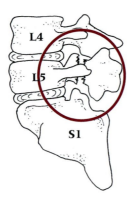

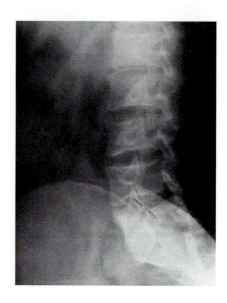

such as the back arch in gymnastics, lifting weights, blocking in football, serving in tennis, spiking in volleyball, and the butterfly stroke in swimming, are most likely to cause this condition.

Commonly, spondylolysis begins unilaterally. However, if it extends bilaterally there may be some slipping of a vertebra on the one below it. This condition is called a spondylolisthesis and is considered to be a complication of spondylolysis often resulting in hypermobility of a vertebral segment.[11] Spondylolisthesis has the highest incidence with L5 slipping on S1 (Figure 23-35). Although pars interarticularis defects are more common among boys, the incidence of slippage is higher in girls. It is possible that a spondylolisthesis may be asymptomatic. The athlete with this condition will usually have a lumbar hyperlordosis postural impairment. A direct blow or sudden twist or chronic low back strain may cause the defective vertebra to displace itself forward on the sacrum. A spondylolisthesis is easily detectable on x-ray.

Symptoms and signs   The athlete complains of persistent aching pain across the low back or stiffness in the lower back, with increased pain after, rather than during,

Spondylolisthesis is considered to be a complication of a spondylolysis.

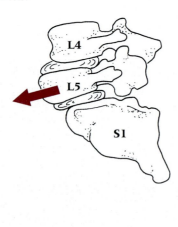

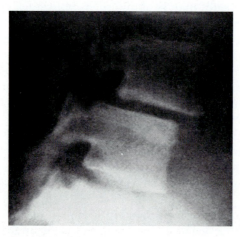

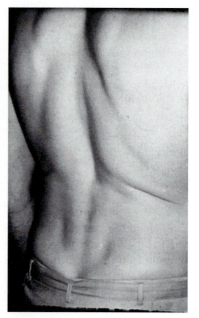

physical activity. The athlete feels a need to change positions frequently or self-manipulate the low back to reduce the pain. Movements of the trunk are full range and painless with some hesitation in forward bending. At extreme ranges held for 30 seconds an aching pain develops. Straightening from forward bending causes a feeling of weakness in the back. There may be tenderness localized to one segment. When applying posteroanterior pressure to the spinous process during palpation some segmental hypermobility may be noted. If displacement is great enough there may be neurological signs.

Management   Initially, bracing and occasionally bed rest for 1 to 3 days will help reduce pain. The major focus in rehabilitation should be directed toward exercises that control or stabilize the hypermobile segment. Progressive trunk-strengthening exercises, especially through the midrange, should be incorporated. Dynamic trunk stabilization exercises that concentrate on the abdominal muscles should also be used. Braces are most helpful during high-level activities. Hypermobility of a lumbar vertebra may make the athlete more susceptible to lumbar muscle strains and ligament sprains. Thus it may be necessary for the athlete to avoid vigorous activity.

Sacroiliac Joint Dysfunction

The sacroiliac is the junction formed by the ilium and the sacrum, and it is fortified by strong ligaments that allow little motion to take place. Because the sacroiliac joint is a synovial joint, disorders can include sprain, inflammation, hypermobility, and hypomobility.

Sacroiliac Sprain

Etiology   A sprain of the sacroiliac joint may result from twisting with both feet on the ground, stumbling forward, falling backward, stepping too far down and landing heavily on one leg, or forward bending with the knees locked during lifting.[20] Any of these mechanisms can produce irritation and stretching of the sacrotuberous or sacrospinous ligaments. They may also cause either an anterior or posterior rotation of one side of the pelvis relative to the other. With rotation of the pelvis there is hypomobility. As healing occurs, the joint on the injured side may become hypermobile, allowing that joint to subluxate in either an anteriorly or a posteriorly rotated position.

Symptoms and signs   With a sprain of the sacroiliac joint there may be palpable pain and tenderness directly over the joint just medial to the PSIS with some associated muscle guarding. On observation, the ASIS or PSIS may be asymmetrical when compared with the opposite side because of either anterior or posterior rotation of one side of the pelvis relative to the other (Figure 23-36). There may also be a measurable leg-length difference. Forward bending reveals a block to normal movement with the PSIS on the injured side moving sooner than on the normal side. Straight leg raising increases pain after 45 degrees. Side bending toward the painful side increases pain.

Management   Modalities can be used to reduce pain. A supportive brace is also helpful in an acute sprain. The sacroiliac joint should be mobilized to correct the existing asymmetry. If one side of the pelvis is posteriorly rotated, it should be mobilized in an anterior direction. Strengthening exercises should be incorporated to improve stability to a hypermobile joint.

Coccyx Injuries

Etiology   Coccygeal injuries in sports are prevalent and occur primarily from direct impact, which may result from forcibly sitting down, falling, or being kicked by an opponent. Injuries to the coccyx include sprains, subluxations, and fractures. With healing the sacrococcygeal joint may become hypermobile, thus restricting passive motion.

Symptoms and signs   Athletes with persistent coccyalgia should be referred to a physician for x-ray and rectal examinations. Pain in the coccygeal region is often pro-

23-8

Critical Thinking Exercise

A gymnast constantly hyperextends her low back. She complains of stiffness and persistent aching pain across the low back with increased pain after, but not usually during, practice. The athlete feels that she needs to change positions frequently or self-manipulate her low back to reduce the pain. She is beginning to develop pain in her buttock and some muscle weakness in her leg.

? What type of injury should the athletic trainer suspect she has? Is there anything that can be done about it?

Figure 23-36

The right PSIS is anteriorly rotated relative to the left.

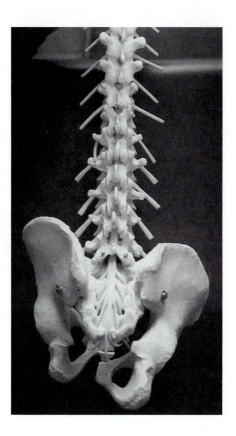

longed and at times chronic. Such conditions are identified by the term *coccygodynia* and occur as a result of an irritation to the coccygeal plexus.

Management   Treatment consists of analgesics and a ring seat to relieve the pressure on the coccyx while sitting. It should be noted that pain from a fractured coccyx may last for many months. Once a coccygeal injury has healed, the athlete should be protected against reinjury by appropriately applied padding.

REHABILITATION TECHNIQUES FOR THE NECK
Joint Mobilizations

Mobilization techniques for the cervical spine are extensively used in rehabilitating the injured neck. Mobilization can decrease pain, restore mobility, and increase range of motion. The most common joint mobilization techniques for the cervical spine include the following (Figure 23-37):
- Cervical flexion mobilizations increase forward bending and flexion.
- Cervical extension mobilizations increase backward bending and extension.
- Cervical rotation mobilizations treat pain or stiffness when there is some resistance in the same direction as the rotation.
- Cervical side-bending mobilizations treat pain and stiffness with resistance when side bending the neck.
- Cervical traction is used to relieve discogenic pain or increase range of motion.

Flexibility Exercises

The first consideration in neck rehabilitation should be restoration of the neck's normal range of motion. If the athlete had a prior restricted range of motion, increasing it to a more normal range is desirable. A second goal is to strengthen the neck as much as possible. All mobility exercises should be performed pain free. Stretching exercises include passive and active movement.[22]

The athlete sits in a straight-backed chair while the athletic trainer applies a gentle passive stretch through a pain-free range. Extension, flexion, lateral flexion, and ro-

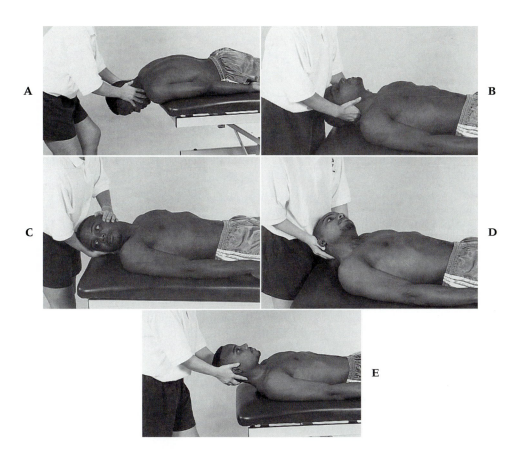

Figure 23-37

Cervical mobilizations. **A,** Cervical flexion. **B,** Cervical extension. **C,** Cervical rotation. **D,** Cervical side bending. **E,** Cervical traction.

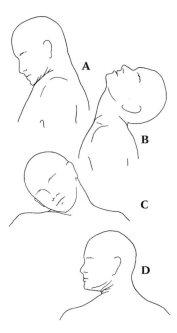

Figure 23-38

Active neck stretching is important in increasing neck mobility after injury. **A,** Forward flexion. **B,** Extension. **C,** Lateral flexion. **D,** Rotation.

tation in each direction is sustained for a count of six and repeated three times. Passive stretching should be conducted daily.

The athlete is also instructed to actively stretch the neck two or three times daily. Each exercise is performed for 8 to 10 repetitions, with each end point held for a count of six. All exercises are performed without force. Figure 23-38 shows forward flexion, extension, lateral flexion, and rotation.

Stretching can progress gradually to a more vigorous procedure such as the Billig procedure. In this exercise the athlete sits on a chair with one hand firmly grasping the seat of the chair and the other hand over the top of the head and placed on the ear on the side of the support hand. Keeping that hand in place, the athlete gently pulls the opposite side of the neck. Stretch should be held for 6 seconds (Figure 23-39). A rotary stretch in each direction can also be applied in the same manner by the athlete.

Strengthening Exercises

When the athlete has gained near-normal range of motion, a strength program should be instituted. All exercises should be conducted pain free. In the beginning each exercise is performed with the head in an upright position facing straight forward. Exercises are performed isometrically, with each resistance held for a count of six, starting with 5 repetitions and progressing to 10 repetitions (Figure 23-40).

1. Flexion—press forehead against palm of hand.
2. Extension—lace fingers behind head and press head back against hands.
3. Lateral flexion—place palm on side of head and press head into palm.
4. Rotation—put one palm on side of forehead and the other at back of the head. Push with each hand, attempting to rotate head. Change hands and reverse direction.

Strengthening progresses to isotonic exercises through a full range of motion using manual resistance, special equipment such as a towel, or weighted devices (Figure 23-41). Each exercise is performed for 10 repetitions and two to three sets. NOTE:

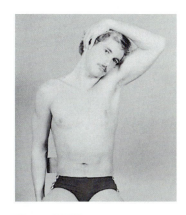

Figure 23-39

Stretching the lateral neck flexors by the Billig procedure.

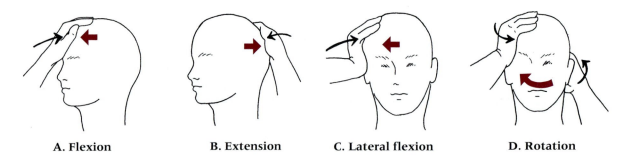

A. Flexion   **B. Extension**   **C. Lateral flexion**   **D. Rotation**

Figure 23-40

Manual neck-strengthening exercises. **A,** Flexion. **B,** Extension. **C,** Lateral flexion. **D,** Rotation.

The athlete must be cautioned against overstressing the neck and must be encouraged to increase resistance gradually.

REHABILITATION TECHNIQUES FOR THE LOW BACK

Over the years many different techniques relative to the treatment and rehabilitation of low back pain have been recommended.[8] Individuals such as Williams, McKenzie, Cyriax, Maitland, Paris, and Saal have proposed effective yet specific philosophical approaches for managing individuals with low back pain. In some instances, a particular approach tended to use the same exercises for all low back pain patients regardless of the existing etiology. Today the techniques for treating low back pain incorporate a more eclectic approach, utilizing a combination of the most applicable and useful aspects of each of the philosophical approaches.[2]

The initial treatment for low back pain should focus on modulating pain. After acute injury ice should be used along with electrical stimulating currents for analgesia. Rest is also helpful in allowing the injured structures to begin the healing process. Avoiding movements or positions that increase pain while positioning the athlete in a posture that minimizes pain and discomfort is essential.

Analgesics and oral antiinflammatory agents are commonly given to inhibit pain and reduce inflammation in the athlete with a low back problem. If muscle spasm or guarding is severe, on occasion muscle relaxants may also be prescribed.

Progressive relaxation techniques can also be useful in treating low back pain. With constant pain comes anxiety and increased muscular tension that compounds the low back problem. By systematically contracting and completely "letting go" of the body's major muscles, the athlete learns to recognize abnormal tension and to relax the muscles consciously. Various relaxation techniques are discussed in Chapter 11.

Figure 23-41

Neck strengthening using resistive devices. **A,** Towel. **B,** Free weight. **C,** Exercise machine.

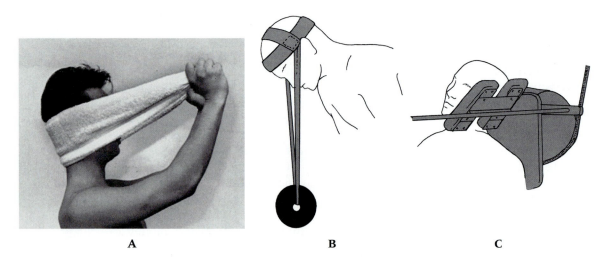

A   **B**   **C**

General Body Conditioning

The low back pain that athletes most often experience is an acute painful experience the rarely lasts longer than 3 weeks. However, in the initial stages of acute injury there can be a great deal of pain and disability. In some of the conditions described previously, any movement at all can produce incapacitating low back pain. Thus with certain conditions, maintaining general body conditioning, particularly during the acute stage of healing, can be difficult. It may be necessary to eliminate any type of conditioning during the first several days. The athlete should resume conditioning activities as soon as the condition has resolved to the point where discomfort can be tolerated. Substituting aquatic exercise as a method for maintaining cardiorespiratory endurance is often helpful in the athlete because pain that may occur with weight bearing may be minimized.

Joint Mobilizations

Joint mobilization of the lumbar spine may be used to improve joint mobility or to decrease joint pain by restoring accessory movements to the joint to achieve a full nonrestricted, pain-free range of motion.[10] Vertebral joints in the lumbar region are capable of both anterior and posterior gliding and rotation, or some combination of the two; mobilization techniques should address all restricted joint motions. Grade 1 and 2 mobilizations may be incorporated early in the rehabilitation program for managing pain. Mobilization may progress to grades 3 and 4 once pain and muscle guarding are decreased. For best results mobilization should be combined with manual traction techniques.

Joint mobilization techniques for the low back are indicated when

- Pain is centralized at a specific joint and increases with activity and decreases with rest.
- Active and passive range of motion are decreased.
- There is muscle tightness.
- Forward and backward bending deviate from the midline.
- Rotation and side bending produce asymmetrical movements.
- Accessory motion at individual spinal segments is decreased.

Specific mobilization techniques for the low back include the following (Figure 23-42):

- Anteroposterior lumbar vertebrae mobilizations to decrease pain and increase mobility of individual vertebrae.
- Lumbar lateral distraction to reduce pain associated with some compression of a spinal nerve.
- Lumbar vertebral rotation mobilizations to decrease pain and increase mobility of individual vertebrae.
- Anterior sacral mobilizations to reduce pain and muscle guarding around the sacroiliac joint.
- Anterior rotation mobilization to correct a unilateral posterior rotation.
- Posterior rotation mobilization to correct a unilateral anterior rotation.

Traction

Traction is the treatment of choice when there is a small protrusion of the nucleus pulposus. Through traction, the lumbar vertebrae are distracted, a subatmospheric pressure is created, tending to pull the protrusion to its original position, and there is tightening of the longitudinal ligament, tending to push the protrusion toward its original position within the disk.[3] Traction may be done manually or using a traction machine. Intermittent traction for at least 30 minutes with a force commensurate with body weight is preferred. An 80 lb (35 kg) force would be the minimum for a small woman, and a 180 lb (80 kg) force would be the minimum for a large man.[3] Traction is usually applied daily (five times per week) for 2 weeks.

Figure 23-42

Low back mobilizations. **A,** Anteroposterior lumbar vertebrae mobilization. **B,** Lumbar lateral distraction. **C,** Lumbar vertebral rotation. **D,** Anterior sacral mobilization. **E,** Anterior rotation mobilization. **F,** Posterior rotation mobilization.

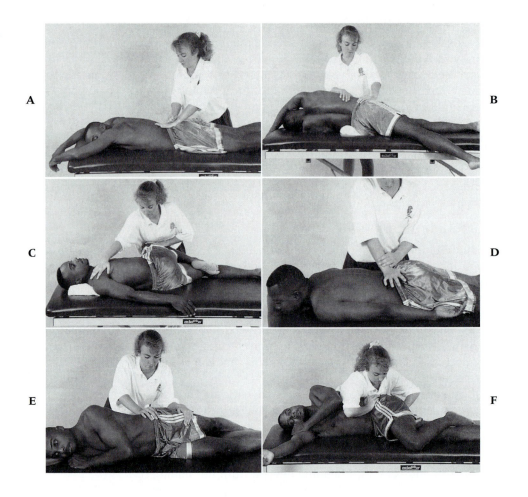

Flexibility Exercises

Back pain may be caused by tightness or a lack of flexibility in a number of different muscle groups related to movement of the low back. Assessing the flexibility of the muscle groups will indicate which ones are tight and need to be stretched. The following muscle groups may need to be stretched (Figure 23-43):

- Low back extensors
- Lumbar rotators
- Lumbar lateral flexors
- Hip adductors
- Hip abductors
- Hip rotators
- Hip flexors
- Hamstrings

Strengthening Exercises

Strengthening exercises should routinely be incorporated into the rehabilitation program to encourage the athlete to remain active and also to regain lumbar motion. It is logical that strengthening exercises that reinforce pain-reducing movements and postures should be used, particularly in cases of low back pain. Any exercise or movement that causes pain to spread over a larger area should be avoided. Thus selecting correct strengthening exercises should centralize or diminish pain.

Generally, strengthening exercises can involve either extension or flexion exercises. Extension exercises are used to strengthen the back extensors, to stretch the

Extension exercises are used to strengthen the back extensors, to stretch the abdominals, and to reduce the pressure on the intervetebral disks.

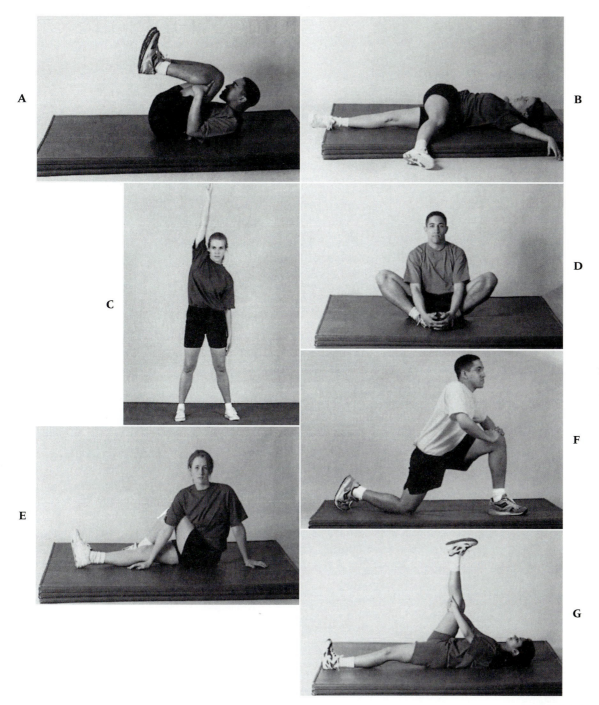

Figure 23-43

Low back stretching exercises. **A,** Low back extensors. **B,** Lumbar rotators and hip abductors. **C,** Lumbar lateral flexors. **D,** Hip adductors. **E,** Hip rotators. **F,** Hip flexors. **G,** Hamstrings.

abdominals, and to reduce the pressure on the intervertebral disks. Extension exercise should be used when (Figure 23-44)

- Back pain is diminished when lying down and increased in sitting.
- Backward bending is limited yet the movement diminishes pain.
- Forward bending is extremely limited and increases pain.
- Straight leg raising is limited and painful.

Flexion exercises are used to strengthen the abdominal muscles, to stretch the back extensors, and to take pressure off of a nerve root by separating the lumbar facet joints and opening the intervertebral foramen. Flexion exercises should be used when (Figure 23-45)

Figure 23-44

Extension strengthening exercises. **A,** Alternating leg extension. **B,** Standing extension. **C,** Supine hip extension. **D,** Prone single hip extension. **E,** Prone double-leg hip extension. **F,** Trunk extension.

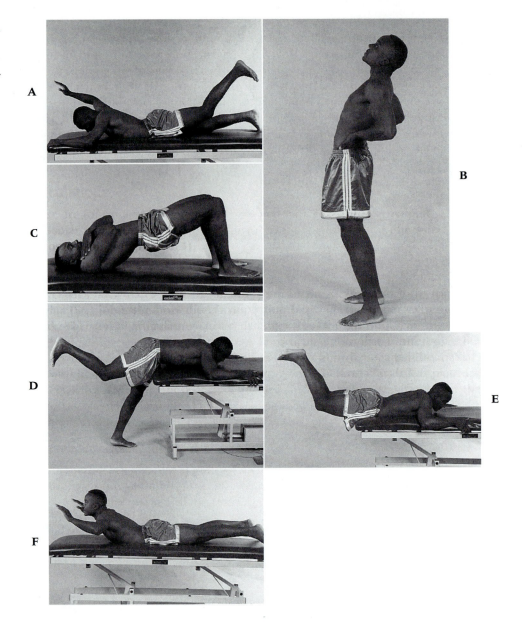

23-9

Critical Thinking Exercise

During a back evaluation on a soccer player, the athletic trainer finds that backward bending is limited yet the movement diminishes pain, straight leg raising is limited and painful, forward bending is extremely limited and increases pain, and back pain is diminished when lying down but increased in sitting.

? What types of rehabilitative exercises should the athletic trainer recommend to the athlete?

- Back pain is diminished when sitting and increased when lying down or standing.
- Forward bending decreases the pain.
- The lordotic curve in the lumbar area does not reverse itself in forward bending.
- Backward bending is painful, especially at the end range.
- There is poor abdominal muscle strength.

Proprioceptive neuromuscular facilitation (PNF) upper trunk chopping and lifting patterns may be used to strengthen the trunk musculature. Besides increasing strength, PNF exercises can help establish neuromuscular control and proprioception. Rhythmic stabilization using isometric exercise can facilitate cocontraction of antagonistic muscle groups. (See Chapter 15.)

Neuromuscular Control

Despite the fact that the athlete may have adequate strength and flexibility, there may be difficulty controlling the spine if the athlete does not learn to contract the

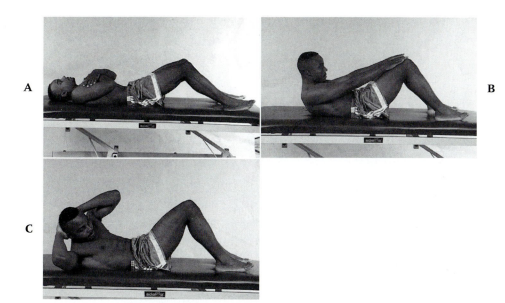

Figure 23-45
Flexion strengthening exercises. **A,** Posterior pelvic tilt. **B,** Partial sit-up. **C,** Partial sit-up with rotation.

appropriate muscles in a desired sequence. Stabilization, especially during complex functional movements, relies heavily on a learned response by the athlete to control the movement. Stabilization exercises for the trunk and spine may help minimize the cumulative effects of repetitive microtrauma to the spine. Spinal stabilization does not mean maintaining a static position. Dynamic stabilization involves maintaining a controlled range of motion that varies with the position and the activity being performed. Dynamic stabilization is achieved by conscious repetitive training, which over time eventually becomes an unconscious natural response. Dynamic stabilization techniques are widely used in rehabilitation programs for the low back.[17]

The first step in dynamic stabilization involves learning to control the position of the pelvis in a neutral position. A posterior tilt of the pelvis causes the lumbar curve to flatten and is caused by a simultaneous cocontraction of the abdominal and gluteal muscles (Figure 23-46). Once the athlete has learned to control pelvic tilt, progressively more advanced movement activities should be incorporated that involve movements of both the spine and extremities while the pelvis is maintained in a neutral position.[17]

Abdominal muscle control is another key to stabilization of the low back. Abdominal bracing exercises focus attention on motor control of the external oblique muscles in different positions. There should also be cocontraction of the abdominal muscles and lumbar extensors to maintain a "corset" control of the lumbar spine.[13]

> Dynamic stabilization involves maintaining a controlled range of motion that varies with the position and the activity being performed.

Functional Progressions

The progression of stabilization exercises should go from supine activities to prone activities, to kneeling activities, and eventually to weight-bearing activities, all performed while actively stabilizing the trunk. The athlete should be taught to perform a stabilization contraction before starting any movement. As the movement begins the athlete will become less aware of the stabilization contraction. The athlete may begin by incorporating stabilization into every movement performed in the strengthening exercises. Stabilization contractions can also be used in aerobic conditioning activities. The exercises should include activities that replicate the demands of the athlete's individual sport. The various components of a sport activity should be broken down into separate activities or skills that allow the athlete to consciously practice the stabilization technique with each drill. Individual athletes will have differences in their degree of control and in the speed at which they can acquire the skills of dynamic trunk stabilization.[13]

Figure 23-46

Dynamic stabilization exercises. **A,** Kneeling. **B,** Standing lunges. **C,** Bridging on a ball. **D,** Wall slides. **E,** Alternating arm and leg extension.

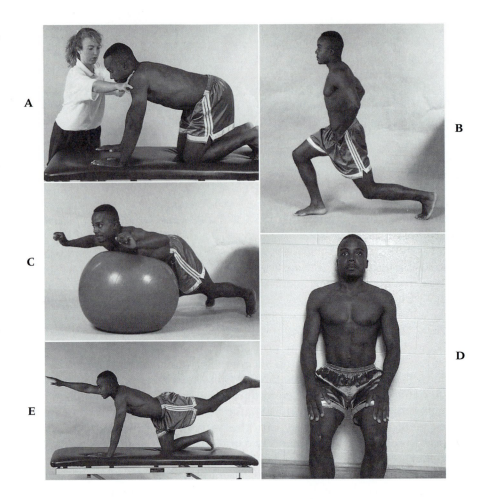

A basketball player has been told by his family physician that he has "an unstable back." The physician referred him to a therapist, who recommended that the athlete perform dynamic stabilization exercises. Unfortunately, the athlete had to leave home and return to college before he had a chance to learn the exercises.

? The athlete asks the athletic trainer to show him the appropriate dynamic stabilization exercises that he should do. What progression should the athletic trainer recommend?

Return to Activity

In most cases of acute injury to the low back involving muscular strain or ligament sprain, the speed at which the athlete can return will be similar to what is expected with similar injuries in the extremities. However, if the injury becomes recurrent or the problem becomes chronic, achieving full return to activity may be frustrating to both the athlete and the athletic trainer. Injuries to the low back can be incapacitating in the athlete as with any other individual in the population. The physical demands of sport activity increase the likelihood of recurrent injury. Thus the athletic trainer must take whatever time is required to fully rehabilitate the athlete with a low back problem and educate the athlete relative to skills and techniques that can help minimize additional injury.

SUMMARY

- The spine, or vertebral column, is composed of 33 individual vertebrae. The design of the spine allows for flexion, extension, lateral flexion, and rotation. The movable vertebrae are separated by intervetebral disks, and position is maintained by a series of muscular and ligamentous supports. The spine can be divided into three different regions, the cervical, thoracic, and lumbar regions. The sacrum and coccyx are fused vertebrae within the vertebral column.
- The spinal cord is that portion of the central nervous system that is contained within the vertebral canal of the spinal column. Thirty-one pairs of spinal nerves extend from the sides of the spinal cord. The spinal nerve roots combine to form the peripheral nerves, which provide motor and sensory innervation. Each pair

of spinal nerves has a specific area of cutaneous sensory distribution called a dermatome.

■ Acute traumatic injuries to the spine can be potentially life threatening, particularly if the cervical region of the spinal cord is involved. Thus the athlete must do everything possible to minimize the possibility of injury. Strengthening of the musculature of the neck is critical. In addition to strong muscles, the athlete's neck should have a full range of motion. Athletes involved in collision sports must be taught and required to use techniques that reduce the likelihood of cervical injury.

■ Low back pain is one of the most common and disabling ailments known. The athlete, like everyone else in the population, can prevent low back pain by avoiding unnecessary stresses and strains associated with standing, sitting, lying, working, and exercising. Care should be taken to avoid postures and positions that can cause injuries.

■ The most critical part of the evaluation is to rule out the possibility of spinal cord injury. Observing the posture and movement capabilities of the athlete during the evaluation can help clarify the nature and extent of the injury. Classic postural deviations include kyphosis, forward head posture, lordosis, flatback posture, swayback posture, and scoliosis. Special tests may be performed in standing, sitting, supine, side-lying, and prone positions.

■ Because the cervical and lumbar regions of the spine are so mobile, they are extremely vulnerable to a wide range of sports injuries, including fractures, dislocations, strains, sprains, contusions, lesions of the intervertebral disks, injuries to spinal nerves, and degenerative conditions. Although relatively uncommon, severe sports injury to the neck can produce catastrophic impairment of the spinal cord.

■ The first consideration in neck rehabilitation should be restoration of the neck's normal range of motion. When the athlete has gained near-normal range of motion, a strength program should be instituted. Mobilization techniques for the cervical spine are extensively used in rehabilitating the injured neck.

■ Rehabilitation of low back pain focuses on learning dynamic stabilization techniques, which involve exercises for the trunk and spine that help minimize the cumulative effects of repetitive microtrauma to the spine. Exercises are designed to strengthen or stretch specific muscles of spinal movement and may be divided into extension and flexion exercises.

. . . .

Solutions to Critical Thinking Exercises

23-1 The normal curves include the cervical, thoracic, lumbar, and sacrococcygeal curves. The cervical and lumbar curves are convex anteriorly, whereas the thoracic and sacrococcygeal curves are convex posteriorly. Lordotic posture is characterized by an increased curve in the lumbar spine with an increase in both anterior tilt of the pelvis and hip flexion. When combined with kyphosis and a forward head posture, this is referred to as a kypholordotic posture.

23-2 Rotation is produced when the sternocleidomastoid, the scalenes, the semispinalis cervicis, and the upper trapezius on the right side contract in addition to a contraction of the left splenius capitus, splenius cervicis, and longissimus capitus.

23-3 The athletic trainer should look for symmetry of the anterior and posterior superior iliac spines (ASIS and PSIS) and iliac crests. Sacroiliac compression and distraction tests and a positive Patrick's, or FABER, test are all useful in determining if there is a problem in the sacroiliac joint. In forward bending or flexion, the PSISs on each side should move together. If one moves further than the other a motion restriction is probably present in the sacroiliac joint on the side that moves most. If they move at different times the side that moves first usually has a restriction.

23-4 The athlete may have cervical spine stenosis, which involves a narrowing of the spinal canal in the cervical region that can impinge the spinal cord. The presence of cervical stenosis is determined by an x-ray, which measures the canal diameter and divides that by the anteroposterior width of the same vertebral body. The athlete should be advised of the potential risks of continued participation in football.

23-5 Straight leg raising applies pressure to the sacroiliac joint and may indicate either a problem in the sciatic nerve, the sacroiliac joint, or lumbar spine. Pain at 30 degrees of straight leg raising indicates either a hip problem or an inflamed nerve. Pain from

30 to 60 degrees indicates some sciatic nerve involvement. Pain between 70 and 90 degrees is indicative of a sacroiliac joint problem. Pain on bilateral straight leg raising indicates some problem with the lumbar spine.

23-6 The athlete has probably developed a myofascial trigger point. The key in treating myofascial pain is stretching the muscle back to a normal resting length, thus relieving the irritation that created the trigger point. Active stretching should be mild and progressive. The use of electrical stimulation in combination with ultrasound is helpful in relieving the pain associated with a trigger point. Progressive strengthening exercises should also be included.

23-7 Pain present in forward bending and restriction in backward bending with radiating pain are usually associated with a disk problem. However, they may also be related to spondylolysis or spondylolisthesis.

23-8 The gymnast probably has a spondylolisthesis that has resulted in hypermobility of a vertebral segment. Initially, rest will help reduce pain. The major focus in rehabilitation should be directed toward exercises that control or stabilize the hypermobile segment. Progressive trunk-strengthening exercises especially to the abdominal muscles through the midrange should be incorporated. A brace can be helpful during practice.

23-9 Given this set of existing conditions the athletic trainer should have the athlete engage in extension exercises to strengthen the back extensors, to stretch the abdominals, and to reduce the pressure on the intervertebral disks.

23-10 The first step in dynamic stabilization involves learning to control the position of the pelvis in a neutral position. Once the athlete has learned to control pelvic tilt, progressively more advanced movement activities should be incorporated that involve movements of both the spine and extremities while the pelvis is maintained in a neutral position. Abdominal muscle control is another key to stabilization of the low back. Stabilization exercises include weight shifting while kneeling, standing lunges, bridging on a ball, wall slides, and alternating arm and leg extensions.

REVIEW QUESTIONS AND CLASS ACTIVITIES

1. Identify the various regions of the spine.
2. Describe the mechanisms of a catastrophic neck injury.
3. What is the relationship between the spinal cord, the nerve roots, and the peripheral nerves?
4. Describe the various postural abnormalities.
5. Describe the special tests used in evaluating the lumbar and sacroiliac portions of the spine.
6. Discuss the various considerations in prevention of cervical injuries.
7. What are the mechanisms of injury to the spinal cord?
8. What can be done to minimize the incidence of low back pain?
9. Describe the various types of herniated disks.
10. How does a spondylolysis become a spondylolisthesis?
11. What is the usual mechanism of injury to the sacroiliac joint?
12. Explain when flexion versus extension exercises should be used in treating conditions of the low back.
13. Explain the rationale for using dynamic stabilization in rehabilitating low back pain.

REFERENCES

1. Anderson C: Neck injuries, backboard, bench, or return to play, *Phys Sports Med* 21(8):23, 1993.
2. Beattie P: The use of an eclectic approach for the treatment of low back pain, a case study, *Phys Ther* 72(12):923, 1992.
3. Binkley J, Finch E, Hall J: Diagnostic classification of patients with low back pain: a survey of physical therapy experts, *Phys Ther* 73(3):138, 1993.
4. Cailliet R: *Low back pain,* ed 3, Philadelphia, 1988, Davis.
5. Cantu R: Functional cervical spinal stenosis: a contraindication to participation in contact sports, *Med Sci Sports Exerc* 25(3):316, 1993.
6. Cibulka M: The treatment of the sacroiliac joint component to low back pain, *Phys Ther* 72(12):917, 1992.
7. Cyriax J: Refresher course for general practitioners: the treatment of lumbar disk lesions, *J Orthop Sports Phys Ther* 12(4):163, 1990.
8. DeRosa C, Poterfield J: A physical therapy model for the treatment of low back pain, *Phys Ther* 72(4):261, 1992.
9. Fourre M: On-site management of cervical spine injuries, *Phys Sports Med* 19:4, 1991.
10. Haldeman S: Spinal manipulative therapy in sports medicine. In Spencer III CW, editor: *Injuries to the spine. Clinics in sports medicine,* vol 5, no 2, Philadelphia, 1986, Saunders.
11. Herring S, Weinstein S: Assessment and neurological management of athletic low back injury. In Nicholas J, Herschman E, editors: *The lower extremity and spine in sports medicine,* St Louis, 1995, Mosby.
12. Holland B, Sacco D: Imaging of the spine. In White A, Schofferman J, editors: *Spine care: diagnosis and conservative treatment,* vol 1, St Louis, 1995, Mosby.
13. Hooker D: Back rehabilitation. In Prentice W, editor: *Rehabilitation techniques in sports medicine,* St Louis, 1994, Mosby.
14. Johnson R: Low back pain in sports: managing spondylolysis in young athletes, *Phys Sports Med* 21(4):53, 1993.
15. Markey K, Benedetto M, Curl W: Upper trunk and brachial plexopathy, *Am J Sports Med* 21(5):650, 1993.
16. Nuber G, Bowen M, Schaffer M: Diagnosis and treatment of lumbar and thoracic spine injuries. In Nicholas J, Herschman E, editors: *The lower extremity and spine in sports medicine,* St Louis, 1995, Mosby.
17. Rapport L, O'Leary P, Cammisa F: Diagnosis and treatment of cervical spine injuries. In Nicholas J, Herschman E, editors: *The lower extremity and spine in sports medicine,* St Louis, 1995, Mosby.
18. Ritz S, Lorren T, Simpson S: Rehabilitation of degenerative disease of the spine. In Hochschuler S, Cotler H, Guyer R, editors: *Rehabilitation of the spine: science and practice,* St Louis, 1993, Mosby.
19. Rodriquez J: Clinical examination and documentation. In Hochschuler S, Cotler H, Guyer R, editors: *Rehabilitation of the spine: science and practice,* St Louis, 1993, Mosby.
20. Saunders D: *Evaluation, treatment and prevention of musculoskeletal disorders,* Bloomington, Minn, 1985, Educational Opportunities.
21. Storey MD: Anterior neck trauma, *Phys Sports Med* 17(9):85, 1993.
22. Teitz CC: Rehabilitation of neck and low back injuries. In Harvey JS, editor: *Symposium on rehabilitation of the injured athlete. Clinics in sports medicine,* vol 4, no 3, Philadelphia, 1985, Saunders.
23. Torg JS et al: The epidemiologic, pathologic, biomechanical, and cinematographic analysis of football-induced cervical spine trauma, *Am J Sports Med* 18(1):50, 1990.
24. Torg JS et al: The axial load teardrop fracture, *Am J Sports Med* 19(4):355, 1991.
25. Torg J, Fay C: Cervical spinal stenosis with cord neurapraxia and transcient quadriplegia. In Torg J, editor: *Athletic injuries to the head, neck, and face,* St Louis, 1991, Mosby.
26. Vereschagin KS et al: Burners, *Phys Sports Med* 1(9):96, 1991.
27. Weber MD, Woodall WR: Spondylogenic disorders in gymnasts, *J Orthop Sports Phys Ther* 14(1):6, 1991.

28. Wilkerson JE, Maroon JC: Cervical spine injuries in athletes, *Phys Sports Med* 18(3):57, 1990.

ANNOTATED BIBLIOGRAPHY

Cailliet R: *Low back pain syndrome*, ed 3, Philadelphia, 1988, Davis.

Presents the subject of low back pain in a clear, concise, and interesting manner.

Hochschuler S, Cotler H, Guyer R, editors: *Rehabilitation of the spine: science and practice*, St Louis, 1993, Mosby.

A comprehensive text that focuses on all aspects of treatment and rehabilitation of the spine. Sport-specific injuries are discussed.

McCulloch J: *Backache*, ed 2, Baltimore, 1990, Williams & Wilkins.

An in-depth text about the evaluation and treatment of back conditions.

Nicholas J, Herschman E, editors: *The lower extremity and spine in sports medicine*, St Louis, 1995, Mosby.

This two-volume text discusses all aspects of injury to the extremities and the spine. The section on evaluation and treatment of spinal conditions is concise but thorough.

Saunders D: *Evaluation, treatment and prevention of musculoskeletal disorders*, Bloomington, Minn, 1985, Educational Opportunities.

This text takes a manual therapy approach to treating and rehabilitating the spine, as well as musculoskeletal injuries in general.

Torg JS, editor: *Head and neck injuries. Clinics in sports medicine*, vol 6, no 1, Philadelphia, 1991, Saunders.

In-depth coverage of head and neck injuries stemming from sports activities.

White A, Schofferman J: *Spine care: diagnosis and conservative treatment*, vol 1, St Louis, 1995, Mosby.

A two-volume set that looks at both conservative and surgical management of back injuries.

The Thorax and Abdomen

When you finish this chapter, you should be able to

- Explain the anatomy of the thorax and abdomen.
- Identify the location and function of the heat and lungs.
- Describe the location and function of the abdominal viscera related to the urinary system, the digestive system, the reproductive system, and the lymphatic system.
- List the techniques for assessing thoracic and abdominal injuries.
- Identify various injuries to the structures of the thorax.
- Identify various injuries and conditions in structures of the abdomen.

This chapter deals with major sports injuries to the thorax and abdomen. In an athletic environment, injuries to the thorax and abdomen have a lower incidence than injuries to the extremities. However, unlike the musculoskeletal injuries to the extremities discussed to this point, injuries to the heart, lungs, and abdominal viscera can be potentially serious and even life threatening if not recognized and managed appropriately. It is imperative for the coach and athletic trainer to be familiar with the anatomy and more common injuries seen in the abdomen and thorax (Figure 24-1).

ANATOMY OF THE THORAX

The thoracic cavity is that portion of the body commonly known as the chest; it lies between the base of the neck and the diaphragm. It consists of the thoracic vertebrae, the 12 pairs of ribs with their associated costal cartilages, and the sternum (Figure 24-2). Its main functions are to protect the vital respiratory and circulatory organs and to assist the lungs in inspiration and expiration during the breathing process. Within the thoracic cage lie the lungs, the heart, and the thymus.

Ribs, Costal Cartilage, and Sternum

The ribs are flat bones that are attached to the thoracic vertebrae in the back and to the sternum in the front. The upper seven ribs are called sternal or true ribs, and each rib is joined to the sternum by a separate costal cartilage. The eighth, ninth, and tenth ribs (false ribs) have a common cartilage that joins the seventh rib before attaching to the sternum. The eleventh and twelfth ribs (floating ribs) remain unat-

The thoracic cage protects the heart and lungs.

Figure 24-1

Collision sports can produce serious trunk injuries.

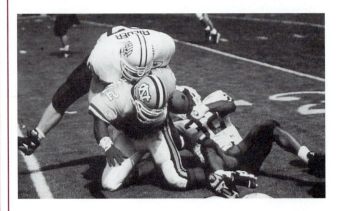

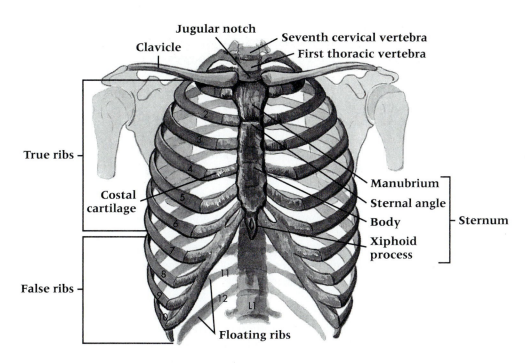

Figure 24-2

The thoracic cage.

tached to the sternum but do have muscle attachments. The individual rib articulation produces a slight gliding action.

The inside of the thoracic cage is lined with the pleura, a thin double-layer membrane filled with pleural fluid that permits the lungs to slide along the thoracic cage.

Thoracic Muscles

There are 11 pairs of both external intercostal muscles and internal intercostal muscles
between the ribs (Figure 24-3). They attach on the inferior border of the rib above
and the superior border of the rib below. The external intercostals function to elevate the diaphragm during inspiration; the internal intercostals depress the rib cage,
assisting with expiration. The intercostal muscles are innervated by the intercostal
nerves.

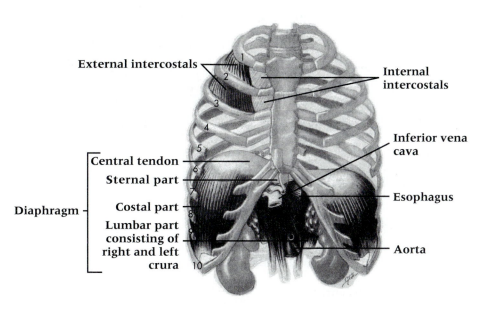

Figure 24-3

Anatomy of the thoracic
muscles.

The pectoralis minor, trapezius, serratus anterior, serratus posterior, levator scapula, and rhomboids are muscles that originate on the thorax. Their primary function is controlling movement of the scapula. (See Chapter 21.)

Lungs

The trachea, or windpipe, branches into right and left primary bronchi, which branch into smaller divisions and ultimately terminate in clusters of air sacs called alveoli within the lungs (Figure 24-4). Alveoli facilitate the exchange of oxygen and carbon dioxide with the capillaries. The lungs are elastic and expand and constrict in response to contraction of the diaphragm muscle.

Respiratory Muscles

The diaphragm is a large dome-shaped muscle that separates the thoracic cavity from the abdominal cavity (Figure 24-3). When the diaphragm contracts, the dome flattens, increasing the volume of the thorax and resulting in inspiration of air. Expiration occurs when the diaphragm relaxes and the elastic components of the lungs and thoracic cage passively decrease thoracic volume.

Blood Supply

Blood flows to the lung through the pulmonary arteries to the alveoli where it is oxygenated and returns to the heart through the pulmonary veins. The bronchi are supplied with oxygenated blood through the bronchial arteries that branch from the aorta. Deoxygenated blood returns to the heart from the bronchi via both the bronchial and pulmonary veins.

Heart

The heart is the main pumping mechanism and functions to circulate oxygenated blood throughout the body to the working tissues. The transport of oxygen involves the coordinated function of the heart, blood vessels, blood, and lungs.

Figure 24-4

Anatomy of the trachea, lungs, and alveoli.

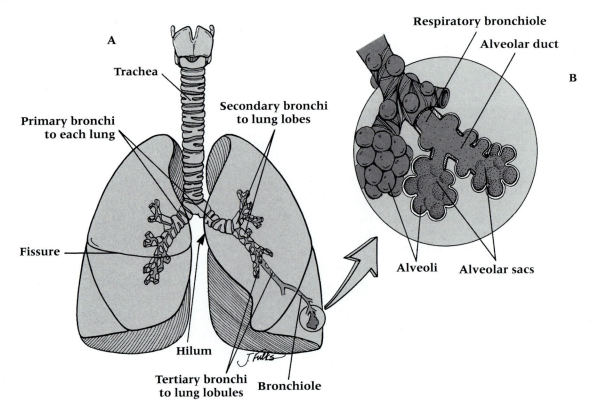

The adult heart lies under the sternum slightly to the left, between the lungs and in front of the vertebral column (Figure 24-5). It is about the size of a clenched fist. It extends from the first rib to the space between the fifth and sixth ribs.

The heart muscle consists of four chambers: the right and left atria and right and left ventricles (Figure 24-6). Deoxygenated blood returns from all parts of the body through the venous system to the right atrium, passing through the tricuspid valve to the right ventricle. The right ventricle pumps the blood through the pulmonary valve to the pulmonary artery and into the lungs, where it is oxygenated. Blood returns from the lungs via the pulmonary vein to the left atrium and passes through the mitral valve into the left ventricle. Blood is ejected past the aortic valve into the aorta, which supplies the entire body through the arterial system.

Figure 24-5

Location of the heart in the thorax.

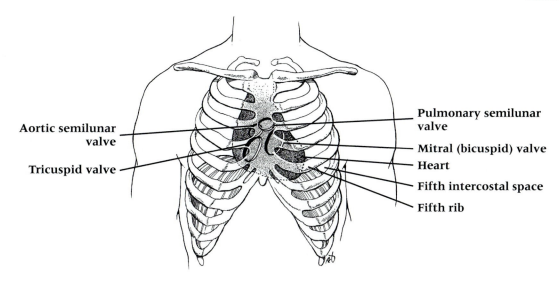

Aortic semilunar valve

Tricuspid valve

Pulmonary semilunar valve

Mitral (bicuspid) valve

Heart

Fifth intercostal space

Fifth rib

Figure 24-6

Anatomy of the heart and blood flow.

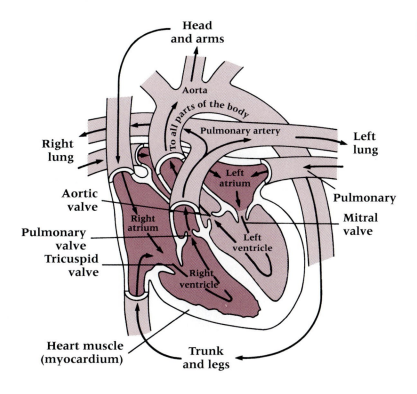

Head and arms

Aorta

To all parts of the body

Pulmonary artery

Right lung

Left lung

Aortic valve

Left atrium

Pulmonary

Right atrium

Mitral valve

Pulmonary valve

Left ventricle

Tricuspid valve

Right ventricle

Heart muscle (myocardium)

Trunk and legs

A single heartbeat consists of a contraction of both atria followed immediately by a contraction of both ventricles. Contraction of the chambers is referred to as systole and relaxation as diastole.

Blood Supply

The heart is supplied by right and left coronary arteries branching from the aorta. Cardiac veins drain into the right atrium.

Thymus

The thymus is located in the thorax just anterior to and above the heart. The function of the thymus is to produce lymphocytes, which migrate to other lymphatic tissues, where they can respond to foreign substances. The thymus is relatively large in the infant and after puberty gradually decreases in size.

ANATOMY OF THE ABDOMEN

The abdominal cavity lies between the diaphragm and the bones of the pelvis and is bounded by the margin of the lower ribs, the abdominal muscles, and the vertebral column. The abdominal cavity is sometimes called the abdominopelvic cavity because there is no physical separation between the abdominal and pelvic cavities.

Abdominal Muscles

The abdominal muscles are the rectus abdominis, the external oblique, the internal oblique, and the transverse abdominis (Figure 24-7). They are invested with both superficial and deep fasciae.

The rectus abdominis muscle, a trunk flexor, is attached to the rib cage above and to the pubis below. It is divided into three segments by transverse tendinous inscriptions; longitudinally it is divided by the linea alba. It functions in trunk flexion, rotation, and lateral flexion and in compression of the abdominal cavity. A heavy fascial sheath encloses the rectus abdominis muscle, holding it in its position but in no way restricting its motion. The inguinal ring, which serves as a passageway for the spermatic cord, is formed by the abdominal fascia.

The external oblique muscle is a broad, thin muscle that arises from slips attached to the borders of the lower eight ribs. It runs obliquely forward and downward and inserts on the anterior two thirds of the crest of the ilium, the pubic crest, and the fascia of the rectus abdominis and the linea alba at their lower front. Its principal functions are trunk flexion, rotation, lateral flexion, and compression.

The internal oblique muscle forms the anterior and lateral aspects of the abdominal wall. Its fibers arise from the iliac crest, the upper half of the inguinal ligament, and the lumbar fascia. They run principally in an obliquely upward direction to the

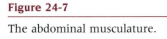

Figure 24-7

The abdominal musculature.

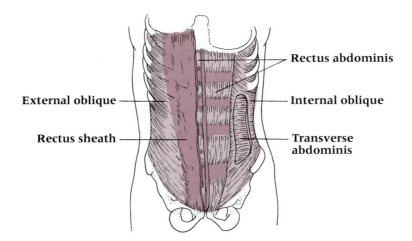

External oblique

Rectus sheath

Rectus abdominis

Internal oblique

Transverse abdominis

cartilages of the tenth, eleventh, and twelfth ribs on each side. The main functions of the internal oblique are trunk flexion, lateral flexion, and rotation.

The transverse abdominis is the deepest of the abdominal muscles. Its fibers run transversely across the abdominal cavity, arising from the outer third of the inguinal ligament, the iliac crest, the lumbar fascia of the back, and the lower six ribs. It inserts into the linea alba and the front half of the iliac crest. The main functions of the transverse abdominis are to hold the abdominal contents in place and to aid in forced expiration. All the abdominal muscles work together in performing defecation, micturition, and forced expiration.

Abdominal Viscera

The abdominal viscera are composed of both hollow and solid organs. The solid organs are the kidneys, spleen, liver, pancreas, and adrenal glands. The hollow organs include vessels, tubes, and receptacles such as the stomach, intestines, gallbladder, and urinary bladder (Figure 24-8). Organs in the abdominal cavity may be classified as being part of the urinary system, the digestive system, the reproductive system, or the lymphatic system.

> Solid internal organs are more at jeopardy from an injury than are hollow organs.
>
> Abdominal viscera are part of the urinary, digestive, reproductive, and lymphatic systems.

Urinary System Organs

The kidneys, the ureters, and the urinary bladder are the urinary system organs.

Kidneys The kidneys are situated on each side of the spine, approximately in the center of the back. They are bean shaped, approximately 4½ inches (11.25 cm) long, 2 inches (5 cm) wide, and 1 inch (2.5 cm) thick. The right kidney is usually slightly lower than the left because of the pressure of the liver. The uppermost surfaces of the kidneys are connected to the diaphragm by strong, ligamentous fibers. As breathing occurs, the kidneys move up and down as much as ½ inch (1.25 cm). The inferior aspect is positioned 1 to 2 inches (2.5 to 5 cm) above the iliac crest. Resting anterior to the left kidney are the stomach, spleen, pancreas, and small and large intestines. Organs that are situated anterior to the right kidney are the liver and the intestines. The kidneys lie posterior to the abdominal cavity. Their primary function is to filter metabolic wastes, ions, or drugs from blood and expel them from the body via urination.[17]

Adrenal glands Although part of the endocrine system rather than the urinary system, the adrenal glands, also called the suprarenal glands, are located on top of each kidney. They secrete the hormones epinephrine, norepinephrine, cortisol, estrogen, aldosterone, and androgen, which have a variety of physiological functions throughout the body.[20]

Ureters and urinary bladder The ureters are small tubes that exend inferiorly from the kidney to the urinary bladder, which functions to store urine. The bladder

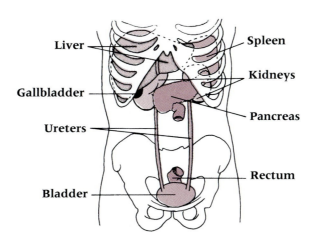

Liver — Spleen
Gallbladder — Kidneys
Ureters — Pancreas
Bladder — Rectum

Figure 24-8

Abdominal viscera.

is a hollow container that lies posterior to the pubic symphysis. In the male it is anterior to the rectum, and in the female it is anterior to the vagina and inferior to the uterus.

Digestive System Organs

The liver, gallbladder, pancreas, stomach, small intestine, and large intestine are digestive system organs.

Liver   The liver is the largest internal organ of the body. It lies in the upper right quadrant of the body against the inferior surface of the diaphragm and weighs about three pounds. It consists of two major right and left lobes. The liver performs both digestive and excretory functions, absorbs and stores excessive glucose, processes nutrients, and detoxifies harmful chemicals. It secretes bile, which is essential in neutralizing and diluting stomach acid and for digesting fat in the small intestine during the digestive process.[20]

Hepatitis is an inflammation of the liver caused by viral infection or alcohol consumption. If it is not corrected, the cells in the liver may die and be replaced by scar tissue, leading to cirrhosis or impaired liver function.[17]

Gallbladder   The gallbladder is a pear-shaped, saclike structure located on the inferior surface of the liver. It serves as a storage reservoir for bile secreted from the liver. Shortly after a meal, the gallbladder secretes the stored bile into the small intestine. Cholesterol, which is secreted by the liver, may cause the gallbladder to produce a gallstone, which can potentially block the release of bile. The gallstone interferes with digestion and must usually be removed surgically.[20]

Pancreas   The pancreas is located between the small intestine and the spleen. It secretes pancreatic juice, which is critical in the digestion of fats, carbohydrates, and proteins. It also produces insulin and glucagon, which are hormones that control the amount of glucose and amino acids in the blood.

Stomach   The stomach is found primarily in the upper left quadrant between the esophagus and the small intestine. It functions mainly as a storage and mixing chamber of food that has been ingested. Some digestion and absorption occur in the stomach. Gastric secretions assist in the partial digestion of protein and the absorption of alcohol and caffeine. Ingested food is mixed with secretions from the stomach glands to form a semifluid material called chyme, which passes from the stomach into the small intestine.[17]

Small intestine   The small intestine connects the stomach to the small intestine via a series of tubelike folds. The small intestine has three portions: the duodenum, the jejunum, and the ileum. In total, it is approximately 6 m in length. In the small intestine, secretions from the liver and pancreas mix with secretions from the small intestine, which are essential to the process of digestion. Mucus is secreted in large amounts to lubricate and protect the wall of the intestine as a mixture of chyme and digestive enzymes is propelled through the small intestine by a series of peristaltic contractions. Chyme moves through the small intestine over a period of 3 to 5 hours. Most of the digestion and absorption of food occurs in the small intestine.[17]

Large intestine   The large intestine is that portion of the digestive tract extending from the small intestine to the anus and is approximately 2 m in length. It has three divisions: the cecum, the colon, and the rectum. The vermiform (wormlike) appendix extends from the cecum. In the colon, chyme is converted to feces through absorption of water, secretion of mucus, and activity of microorganisms. Feces remain in the colon and rectum until the time of defecation.

Lymphatic System Organs

The spleen and thymus (discussed in the section on the thoracic cavity) are organs of the lymphatic system.

Spleen   The spleen is the largest lymphatic organ in the body. It weighs approximately 6 ounces and is approximately 5 inches (12.5 cm) long. It lies under the diaphragm on the left side and behind the ninth, tenth, and eleventh ribs. It is surrounded by a fibrous capsule that is firmly invested by the peritoneum. The spleen's main functions are to serve as a reservoir of red blood cells, to regulate the number of red blood cells in the general circulation, to destroy ineffective red cells, to produce antibodies for immunological function, and to produce lymphocytes.[20]

Reproductive System Organs

Unlike the other organ systems discussed to this point, the male and female reproductive systems differ considerably. The female reproductive organs include the ovaries, the uterus, the uterine tubes (fallopian tubes), and the vagina. The male reproductive organs include the seminal vesicles, the prostate gland, the testes, the vas deferens, the epididymis, the urethra, and the penis.

Female reproductive organs   The reproductive organs in the female are between the urinary bladder and the rectum with the uterus and vagina in the midline and the uterine tubes and ovaries extending to either side (Figure 24-9). Their position is maintained by a group of ligaments, the primary one being the broad ligament. The vagina is a receptacle for sperm, which swim upward into the uterus to fertilize the egg.

The ovaries produce and store the female eggs (ova), which are released one at a time each month into the uterine tubes. The uterine tubes transport the ovum to the uterus, where a fertilized ovum attaches to the uterine wall and becomes a developing embryo. If the ovum is not fertilized the process of menstruation begins.

The reproductive organs in the female are relatively well protected by the pelvis. Thus traumatic injury to these structures is generally rare in the athletic population.

Male reproductive organs   The reproductive organs in the male are found both inside and outside of the abdominal cavity (Figure 24-10). The prostate is dorsal to the pubic symphysis and inferior to the bladder. The urethra and the ejaculatory ducts pass through the prostate, which is made of both glandular and muscular tissue and is similar in size to a walnut. The prostate secretes a milky fluid, which is discharged by 20 to 30 ducts into the prostatic portion of the urethra as a component of semen. The seminal vesicles are also glandular structures found posterior and superior to the prostate gland under the bladder. The seminal vesicles contribute the majority of the fluid to the semen through the ejaculatory ducts.

The remainder of the male reproductive organs are exposed outside of the abdominal cavity and are more susceptible to injury. The testes are the primary male sex organs. They are located within the scrotum and produce spermatozoa and testosterone. The epididymis is a comma-shaped structure connected to the posterior surface of the testis in which the sperm are stored and mature. The vas deferens is a duct running from the epididymis to the ejaculatory duct. The urethra runs from the bladder to the tip of the penis and serves as a pathway through which both urine and semen are ejected through the penis. The penis consists of three layers of erectile tissue, which when engorged with blood cause an erection.

24-1

Critical Thinking Exercise

A soccer player is kicked in the abdomen above the umbilicus. Initially she had the wind knocked out of her. Now she is complaining of pain, and her abdomen is tight on palpation.

? What should the athletic trainer be most concerned about, and what organs may potentially be involved?

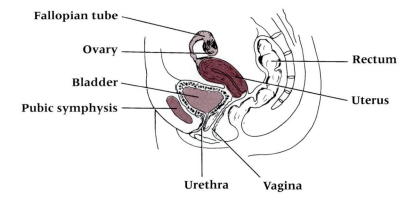

Fallopian tube

Ovary

Bladder

Pubic symphysis

Rectum

Uterus

Urethra   Vagina

Figure 24-9

Female reproductive organs.

Figure 24-10

Male reproductive organs.

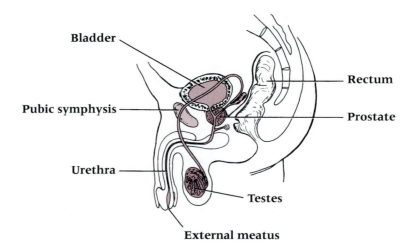

Bladder

Rectum

Pubic symphysis

Prostate

Urethra

Testes

External meatus

PREVENTING INJURIES TO THE THORAX AND ABDOMEN

Injuries to the thorax may be prevented by wearing appropriate protective equipment, particularly in collision sport activities. In football, for example, shoulder pads are usually designed to extend to at least below the level of the sternum. Rib protectors may be worn to cover the entire thoracic cage if necessary.

The muscles of the abdomen should be strengthened to provide protection to the underlying viscera. A consistant regimen of sit-up exercises done in various positions can greatly increase the strength and size of the abdominal musculature.

Making sure that the hollow organs, in particular the stomach and bladder, are emptied before competition can reduce the chance of injury to these structures. Meals should be eaten at least 3 to 4 hours before competition to allow foods to clear the stomach. Urination immediately before stepping onto the field or court will protect the bladder from injury.

ASSESSMENT OF THE THORAX AND ABDOMEN

Injuries to the thorax and abdomen can produce potentially life-threatening situations. An injury that may seem to be relatively insignificant at first may rapidly develop into one that requires immediate and appropriate medical attention. Thus, for the coach or athletic trainer evaluating an injury, the initial primary survey should focus on signs and symptoms that indicate some life-threatening condition. The injured athlete should be continually monitored by the athletic trainer to identify any disruption of normal breathing or circulation or any indication of internal hemorrhage that could precipitate shock.

History

The questions asked to determine a history in the case of thoracic and abdominal injuries are somewhat different than questions that are pertinent to musculoskeletal injuries of the extremities.[15] The primary mechanism of injury should be determined first. What happened to cause this injury? Was there direct contact or a direct blow? What position were you in? What type of pain is there—sharp, dull, localized? Was there immediate or gradual pain? Do you feel any pain other than in the area where the injury occurred? Has there been any difficulty breathing? Are certain positions more comfortable than others? Do you feel faint, light-headed, or nauseous? Do you feel any pain in your chest? Did you hear or feel a pop or crack in your chest? Have you had any muscle spasms? Have you noticed any blood in your urine? Is there any difficulty or pain in urinating? Was the bladder full or empty? How long has it been since you have eaten? Is there a personal or family history of any heart problems, any abdominal problems, or any other diseases involving the thorax and abdomen?

Observation

If the athlete is observed immediately after injury, check for normal breathing and respiratory patterns. Most important, is the athlete breathing at all? Is the athlete having difficulty breathing deeply? Is the athlete catching his or her breath? Does breathing cause pain? Is the athlete holding the chest wall? It there symmetry in movement of the chest during breathing? If the "wind was knocked out" does normal breathing return rapidly or is there prolonged difficulty? This may indicate a more severe injury.

Observe the body position of the athlete. If the athlete has sustained some type of thoracic injury, he or she will often be leaning toward the side that is injured, holding or splinting the area with the opposite hand (Figure 24-11, *A*). In cases of abdominal injury, the athlete will typically lie on the side with the knees pulled up toward the chest (Figure 24-11, *B*). The male who has sustained an injury to the external genitalia will be lying on the side and holding the scrotum (Figure 24-11, *C*).

Check for areas of discoloration, swelling, or deformities that may produce asymmetries. Discoloration or ecchymosis around the umbilicus is indicative of intraabdominal bleeding, and ecchymosis on the flanks may indicate swelling outside of the abdomen. Is there protrusion or swelling of any portion of the abdomen? This may indicate internal bleeding. Does the thorax appear to be symmetrical? Rib fractures can cause one side to appear different. Are the abdominal muscles tight and guarding? Is the athlete holding or splinting a specific part of the abdomen?

There are other observable signs and symptoms that may indicate the nature of a thoracic or abdominal injury. Bright red blood being coughed up indicates some injury to the lungs. Bright red frothy blood being vomited may indicate injury to the esophagus or stomach, although it may also be swallowed from the mouth or nose and then vomited. Cyanosis generally indicates some respiratory difficulty, and pale, cool, clammy skin indicates lowered blood pressure.

It is important to monitor vital signs, including pulse, respirations, and blood pressure. A rapid weak pulse or a significant drop in blood pressure is an indication of some potentially serious internal injury often involving loss of blood.

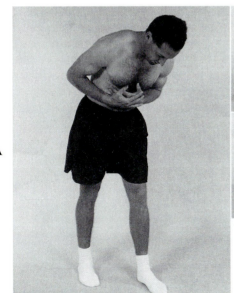

A

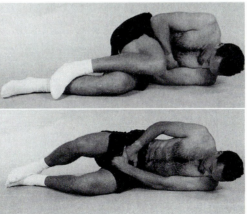

B

C

Figure 24-11

Body positions after injury. **A,** Thoracic injury. **B,** Abdominal injury. **C,** External genitalia injury.

Palpation

Thorax

The hands should first be placed on either side of the chest wall to check for symmetry in chest wall movement during deep inspiration and expiration and to begin to isolate areas of tenderness (Figure 24-12). Once a tender area is identified, the athletic trainer should palpate along the rib, in the intercostal space between the ribs, and at the costochondral junction to locate a specific point of tenderness. Applying anterioposterior compression to the thoracic cage is done to identify potential rib fractures (Figure 24-13, *A*). Transverse compressions applied laterally identify costochondral injuries (Figure 24-13, *B*). If the athlete is having difficulty breathing it may be helpful to use a semireclining position for these tests.

Abdomen

To palpate the abdominal structures, the athlete should be supine with the hips and knees flexed to relax the abdominal muscles with the arms at the side. Begin palpating uninjured areas first using the tips of the fingers to feel for any tightness or rigidity (Figure 24-14). An athlete with an abdominal injury will voluntarily contract the abdominal muscles to guard or protect the tender area. If there is bleeding or irritation inside of the abdominal cavity the abdomen will exhibit boardlike rigidity and cannot be voluntarily relaxed. Rebound tenderness may also accompany intra-abdominal bleeding. This is produced by pressing firmly on the abdomen and then quickly releasing pressure, causing intense pain. If there is only voluntary guarding,

Figure 24-12

Checking asymmetry of the chest wall during breathing.

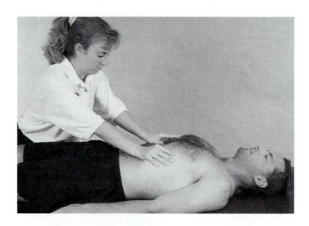

Figure 24-13

A, Checking for rib fractures. **B,** Checking for costochondral injuries.

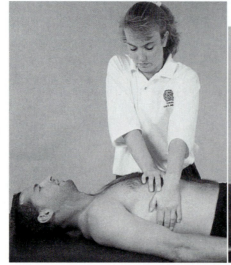

A

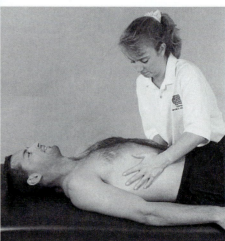

B

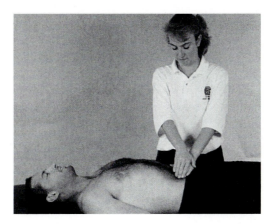

Figure 24-14

Palpating the abdomen for guarding or rigidity.

palpate over the liver, spleen, stomach, small intestine, large intestine, vermiform appendix, and bladder, searching for tenderness, swelling, or enlargement. The kidneys should be palpated with the athlete in a prone position.

Pressure on the abdominal organs may elicit referred pain in predictable patterns away from the source. Figure 24-15 identifies patterns of referred pain.

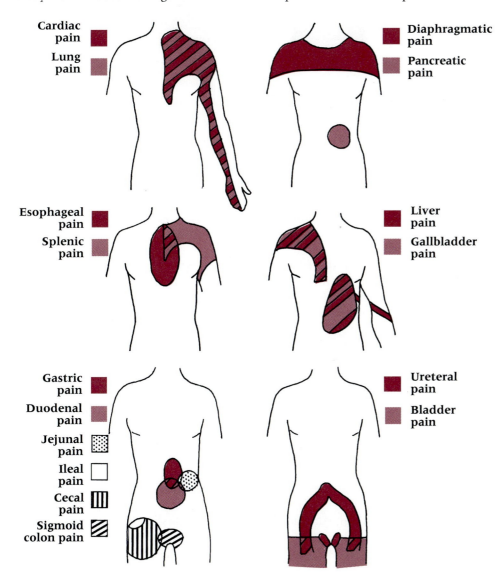

Cardiac pain

Lung pain

Esophageal pain

Splenic pain

Gastric pain

Duodenal pain

Jejunal pain

Ileal pain

Cecal pain

Sigmoid colon pain

Diaphragmatic pain

Pancreatic pain

Liver pain

Gallbladder pain

Ureteral pain

Bladder pain

Figure 24-15

Patterns of referred pain. *(continued)*

Figure 24-15—cont'd

Patterns of referred pain.

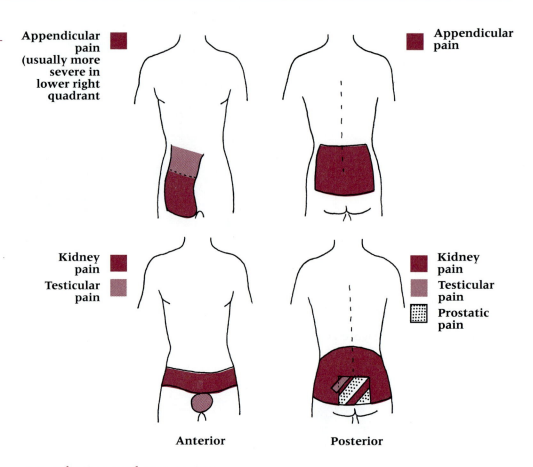

Appendicular pain (usually more severe in lower right quadrant

Appendicular pain

Kidney pain

Testicular pain

Kidney pain

Testicular pain

Prostatic pain

Anterior   Posterior

Auscultation and Percussion

Auscultation involves listening through a stethoscope to heart sounds, breathing sounds, or bowel sounds (Figure 24-16, *A*). Percussion is performed by placing a finger of one hand over an organ and then using one or two fingers from the other hand to strike that finger (Figure 24-16, *B*). The resulting sound may provide some indication as to the status of the organ being percussed. A solid organ such as the liver will produce a dull sound; a hollow organ such as a lung will produce a tympanic or resonant sound.

Some special training is required to know exactly what to listen for. The athletic trainer should know what is "normal" and be able to determine when something is abnormal. The physician is certainly better qualified to make diagnostic decisions based on auscultation and percussion.

RECOGNITION AND MANAGEMENT OF SPECIFIC INJURIES
Thoracic Injuries

The thorax is vulnerable to a variety of injuries to the ribs, costochondral junction, and muscles. Injuries to the lungs and heart are more serious and require special attention.

Rib Contusions

Etiology   A blow to the rib cage can contuse intercostal muscles or, if severe enough, produce a fracture. Because the intercostal muscles are essential for the breathing mechanism, when they are bruised, both expiration and inspiration become painful.

Symptoms and signs   Characteristically the pain is sharp during breathing, there is point tenderness, and pain is elicited when the rib cage is compressed. X-ray examination should be routine in such an injury.

A 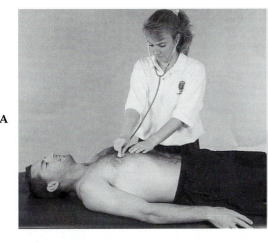 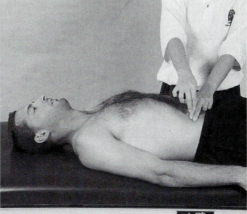 B

Figure 24-16

A, Auscultation. **B,** Percussion.

Management   Rest, ice, compression, and elevation (RICE) and antiinflammatory agents are commonly used. As with most rib injuries, contusions to the thorax are self-limiting, responding best to rest and cessation of sports activities.

Rib Fractures

Etiology   Rib fractures (Figure 24-17) are not uncommon in sports and have their highest incidence in collision sports, particularly wrestling and football. Fractures can be caused by either direct or indirect traumas and can infrequently be the result of violent muscular contractions.[6] A direct injury is the type caused by a kick or a well-placed block, with the fracture developing at the site of force application. An indirect fracture is produced as a result of general compression of the rib cage such as may occur in football or wrestling. Ribs have also been known to fracture from forces caused by coughing and sneezing. Ribs 5 through 9 are the most commonly fractured. Multiple rib fractures can be severe. A flail chest involves a fracture of three or more consecutive ribs on the same side.

The structural and functional disruption sustained in a rib fracture varies according to the type of injury that has been received.[13] The direct fracture causes the most serious damage, because the external force fractures and displaces the ribs inwardly. Such a mechanism may completely displace the bone and cause an overriding of frag-

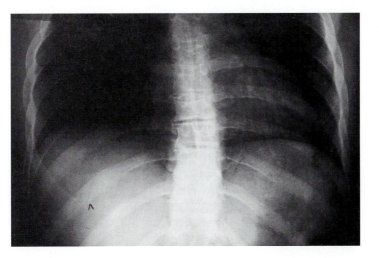

Figure 24-17

A rib fracture.

ments. The jagged edges of the fragments may cut, tear, or perforate the tissue of the pleurae, causing hemothorax, or they may collapse one lung (pneumothorax). Contrary to the pattern with direct violence, the indirect type usually causes the rib to-spring and fracture outward, producing an oblique or transverse fissure. Stress fracture of the first rib is becoming more prevalent. It can result from repeated arm movements such as are used in pitching or in rowing. Stress fractures to other ribs have resulted from repeated coughing or laughing.

Symptoms and signs   The rib fracture is usually easily detected. The history informs the athletic trainer of the type and degree of force to which the rib cage has been subjected. After trauma, the athlete complains of having severe pain during inspiration and has point tenderness. A fracture of the rib will be readily evidenced by a severe sharp pain and possibly crepitus during palpation.

Management   The athlete should be referred to the team physician for x-ray examination if there is any indication of fracture.

An uncomplicated rib fracture is often difficult to identify on x-ray film. Therefore the physician plans the treatment according to the symptoms presented. The rib fracture is usually managed with support and rest. Simple transverse or oblique fractures heal within 3 to 4 weeks. A rib brace can offer the athlete some rib cage stabilization and comfort (Figure 24-18). However, it should also be pointed out that rib supports may predispose the athlete to the development of pneumonia.

Costochondral Separation and Dislocation

Etiology   In sports activities the costochondral separation or dislocation has a higher incidence than fractures. This injury can occur from a direct blow to the anterolateral aspect of the thorax or indirectly from a sudden twist or a fall on a ball, compressing the rib cage. The costochondral injury displays many signs similar to the rib fracture, with the exception that pain is localized in the junction of the rib cartilage and rib (Figure 24-19).

A rib fracture may be indicated by a severe, sharp pain during breathing.

Figure 24-18

A commercial rib brace can provide moderate support to the thorax.

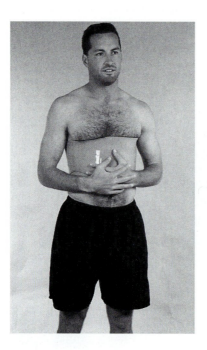

Symptoms and signs   The athlete complains of sharp pain during sudden movement of the trunk, with difficulty in breathing deeply. There is point tenderness with swelling. In some cases there is a rib deformity and a complaint that the rib makes a crepitus noise as it moves in and out of place.

Management   As with a rib fracture, the costochondral separation is managed by rest and immobilization by rib brace. Healing takes anywhere from 1 to 2 months, precluding any sports activities until the athlete is symptom free.

Sternum Fracture

Etiology   Fracture of the sternum results from a high-impact blow to the chest. Sternum fractures are more likely to occur in automobile accidents than in athletics.[5] Injuries to the ribs or the costochondral junction are much more likely in the athlete. An impact severe enough to cause fracture of the sternum may also cause contusion to the underlying cardiac muscle.

Symptoms and signs   There may be point tenderness over the sternum at the site of the fracture that is exacerbated by deep inspiration or forceful expiration. Signs of shock or a weak rapid pulse may indicate more severe internal injury.

Management   The athlete should be sent for x-ray and should be closely monitored for signs of trauma to the heart.

Muscle Injuries

Etiology   The muscles of the thorax are all subject to contusions and strains in sports. The intercostals are especially vulnerable. Traumatic injuries occur most often from direct blows or sudden torsions of the athlete's trunk.[16]

Symptoms and signs   Like other muscle strains, pain occurs on active motion. However, injuries to muscles in this region are particularly painful during inspiration and expiration, laughing, coughing, or sneezing.

Management   Their care requires immediate pressure and application of cold for approximately 1 hour. After hemorrhaging has been controlled, immobilization should be used to make the athlete more comfortable.

Breast Problems

Etiology   It has been suggested that many women athletes can have breast problems in connection with their sports participation. Violent up-and-down and lateral movements of the breasts, such as are encountered in running and jumping, can bruise and strain the breast, especially in large-breasted women. Constant uncontrolled movement of the breast over a period of time can stretch the Cooper's ligament, which supports the breast at the chest wall, leading to premature ptosis of the breasts. (See Figure 5-14.)

Another condition occurring to the breasts is runner's nipples, in which the shirt rubs the nipples, causing an abrasion that can be prevented by placing a Band-Aid over each nipple before participation. Bicyclist's nipples can also occur as the result of a combination of cold and evaporation of sweat, causing the nipples to become painful. Wearing a Windbreaker can prevent this problem.[4]

Management   Wearing a well-designed bra that has minimum elasticity and allows little vertical or horizontal breast movement is most desirable.[8] (See Figure 5-15.) Breast injuries usually occur during physical contact with either an opponent or equipment. In sports such as fencing and field hockey, women athletes should be protected by wearing plastic cup-type brassieres.

Injuries to the Lungs

Fortunately, injuries to the lungs resulting from sports trauma are rare.[23] However, because of the seriousness of this type of injury, the athletic trainer should be able to recognize the basic signs. The most serious of the conditions are pneumothorax, ten-

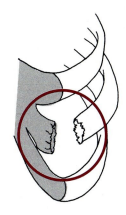

Figure 24-19

Costochondral separation.

24-2

Critical Thinking Exercise

An ice hockey player is checked into the boards by an opponent. He has the wind knocked out of him and on recovery says that there is pain when he tries to take a deep breath. The athletic trainer suspects an injury to the thoracic cage.

? How can the athletic trainer differentiate between a rib fracture and a costochondral injury?

Lung injuries can result in pneumothorax, tension pneumothorax, hemothorax, or traumatic asphyxia.

sion pneumothorax, hemothorax, hemorrhaging into the lungs, and traumatic asphyxia.

Etiology

PNEUMOTHORAX Pneumothorax is a condition in which the pleural cavity becomes filled with air that has entered through an opening in the chest[18] (Figure 24-20, *A*). As the negatively pressured pleural cavity fills with air, the lung on that side collapses. The loss of one lung may produce pain, difficulty in breathing, and anoxia.

TENSION PNEUMOTHORAX A tension pneumothorax occurs when the pleural sac on one side fills with air, displacing the lung and the heart toward the opposite side and compressing the opposite lung (Figure 24-20, *B*). There will be shortness of breath and chest pain on the side of the injury. There may be absence of breath sounds, cyanosis, and distention of neck veins. The trachea may deviate away from the side of injury. Because a total collapse of the opposite lung is possible, medical attention is required immediately.

HEMOTHORAX Hemothorax is the presence of blood within the pleural cavity (Figure 24-20, *C*). It results from the tearing or puncturing of the lung or pleural tissue, involving the blood vessels in the area. As with pneumothorax, pain, difficulty in breathing, and cyanosis develop.

A violent blow or compression of the chest without an accompanying rib fracture may cause a lung hemorrhage. This condition results in severe pain during breathing, dyspnea (difficult breathing), coughing up of frothy blood, and signs of shock. If these signs are observed, the athlete should be treated for shock and immediately referred to a physician.

TRAUMATIC ASPHYXIA Traumatic asphyxia occurs as the result of a violent blow to or a compression of the rib cage, causing a cessation of breathing.[9] Signs include purple discoloration of the upper trunk and head, with the conjunctivae of the eyes displaying a bright red color. A condition of this type demands immediate mouth-to-mouth resuscitation and medical attention.

Management
Each of these conditions is a medical emergency requiring immediate physician attention. Thus the athlete must be transported to the emergency room as quickly as possible.

Heart Contusion

Etiology
A heart contusion may occur when the heart is compressed between the sternum and the spine by a strong outside force, such as being hit by a pitched ball or bouncing a barbell off the chest in a bench press. The right ventricle is most often injured. The most severe consequence of a violent impact to the heart would be a rupture of the aorta, which would be immediately life threatening.[24]

Symptoms and signs
This injury produces severe shock and heart pain. The heart may exhibit certain arrhythmias that cause a decrease in cardiac output, which is followed by death if medical attention is not administered immediately.[11]

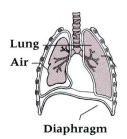

24-3

Critical Thinking Exercise

A lacrosse player is hit in the thorax with an opponent's stick. He has immediate localized pain over his ribs and within minutes begins to develop some respiratory difficulty. The athletic trainer suspects that he has fractured a rib and is extremely concerned that the fracture has damaged the lungs.

? What types of lung injuries are possible, and how should this injury be managed?

Figure 24-20

A, Pneumothorax. **B,** Tension pneumothorax. **C,** Hemothorax.

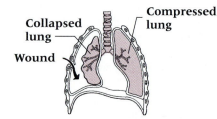
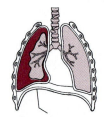

Lung

Air

Diaphragm

A. Pneumothorax

Collapsed lung

Wound

Compressed lung

B. Tension pneumothorax

Pleural space filled with blood

C. Hemothorax

Management   The athlete should be taken immediately to the emergency room. The athletic trainer should be prepared to administer cardiopulmonary resuscitation (CPR) and treat for shock.

Sudden Death Syndrome in Athletes

Etiology   It is catastrophic when a young athlete dies suddenly for no apparent reason. It is estimated that 1 in 280,000 men under age 30 experience sudden death each year.[3] In athletes 35 years old and younger, the most common cause of exercise-induced sudden death is some congenital cardiovascular abnormality.[22] The three most prevalent conditions are hypertrophic cardiomyopathy, anomalous origin of the coronary artery, and Marfan's syndrome.

Hypertrophic cardiomyopathy (HCM) is a condition in which there is thickened cardiac muscle with no evidence of chamber enlargement and extensive myocardial scarring. With this condition there is an increased frequency of ventricular arythmia.[10] In an anomalous origin of the coronary artery, one of the two coronary vessels originates in a different site than normal, thus compromising or obstructing that artery because of its unusual course. In people with Marfan's syndrome, there is an abnormality of the connective tissue resulting in weakening of the structure of the aorta and cardiac valves, which can lead to a rupture of either a valve or the aorta itself.[21]

Other potential cardiac causes of sudden death in athletes include coronary artery disease resulting from atherosclerosis, in which there is a narrowing of the coronary arteries; right ventricular dysplasia, in which there is enlargement of the right ventricle causing a potentially lethal disturbance in heartbeat; cardiac conduction system abnormalities, which can result from abnormalities of the sinus or atrioventricular nodes; aortic stenosis, which is usually associated with a heart murmur that can cause a fall in blood pressure and cardiac collapse during exercise; and myocarditis, an inflammation of the heart associated with a viral condition.[3]

Noncardiac causes of sudden death have also been attributed to the use of certain drugs, including alcohol, cocaine, amphetamines, and erythropoietin (stimulates red blood cell production). A vascular event resulting from bleeding in the brain caused by a cerebral aneurysm or head trauma that causes intracranial bleeding may also result in sudden death. Obstructive respiratory diseases such as asthma can result in sudden death because of drug toxicity or undertreatment.[3]

Symptoms and signs   Common symptoms and signs associated with cardiac causes of sudden death include chest pain or discomfort during exertion, heart palpatations or flutters, syncope, nausea, profuse sweating, heart murmurs, shortness of breath, general malaise, and fever.[19]

Occasionally the symptoms and signs of athletic heart syndrome raise concern when there is no disease present.[2] Athletic heart syndrome is normal for any individual who is exercising. Like skeletal muscle, cardiac muscle will hypertrophy in response to exercise. It is characterized by heart enlargement, systolic heart murmur, slow heart rate, and electrocardiogram changes.

Prevention   It has been suggested that a large number of deaths could be avoided by counseling, screening, and early identification of preventable causes of sudden death.[1] Initial screening should include the following questions:

- Has a physician ever told you that you have a heart murmur?
- Have you had chest pain during exercise?
- Have you fainted during exercise?
- Has anyone in your family under 35 ever died suddenly?
- Has anyone in your family been diagnosed with a thickened heart?
- Does anyone in your family have Marfan's syndrome?

If the answer is yes to any of these questions, a more in-depth medical examination should be performed. Resting and exercise electrocardiograms and echocardiograms may be necessary to determine existing pathology.

The most common causes of sudden death syndrome include hypertrophic cardiomyopathy, anomalous origin of the coronary artery, and Marfan's syndrome.

24-4
Critical Thinking Exercise

A basketball player collapses during a practice session when running sprints. He is conscious and complains of chest pain, heart palpitations or flutters, syncope, nausea, profuse sweating, shortness of breath, and general malaise. The athletic trainer suspects some cardiac-related problem, yet there is no history of such a condition.

? What can cause these symptoms, and what should the athletic trainer do to provide the most appropriate and immediate care for this athlete?

Abdominal Injuries

Although abdominal injuries only make up approximately 10% of sports injuries, they can require long recovery periods and can be life threatening.[7] The abdominal area is particularly vulnerable to injury in all contact sports. A blow can produce superficial or even deep internal injuries, depending on its location and intensity.[7] In internal injuries of the abdomen that occur in sports, the solid organs are most often affected. Strong abdominal muscles give good protection when they are tensed, but when relaxed, they are easily damaged. It is important to protect the trunk region properly against the traumatic forces of collision sports. Good conditioning is essential, as is the use of proper protective equipment and the application of safety rules.

Injuries to Urinary System Organs

Kidney Contusion

Etiology   The kidneys are seemingly well protected within the abdominal cavity. However, on occasion, contusions and even ruptures of these organs occur. The kidney may be susceptible to injury because of its normal distention by blood. An external force, usually one applied to the back of the athlete, will cause abnormal extension of an engorged kidney, resulting in injury. The degree of renal injury depends on the extent of the distention and the angle and force of the blow.[4]

Symptoms and signs   An athlete who has received a contusion of the kidney may display signs of shock, nausea, vomiting, rigidity of the back muscles, and hematuria (blood in the urine). As with other internal organs, kidney injury may cause referred pain to the outside of the body. Pain may be felt high in the costovertebral angle posteriorly and may radiate forward around the trunk into the lower abdominal region. Any athlete who reports having received a severe blow to the abdomen or back region should be instructed to urinate two to three times and to look for the appearance of blood in the urine. If there is any sign of hematuria, immediate referral to a physician must be made.[20]

Management   Medical care of the contused kidney usually consists of a 24-hour hospital observation, with a gradual increase of fluid intake. If the hemorrhage fails to stop, surgery may be indicated. Controllable contusions usually require 2 weeks of bed rest and close surveillance after activity is resumed. In questionable cases complete withdrawal from one active playing season may be required.

Injuries of the Ureters, Bladder, and Urethra

Etiology   On rare occasions a blunt force to the lower abdominal region may avulse a ureter or contuse or rupture the urinary bladder. Injury to the urinary bladder usually occurs only if it is distended by urine. The appearance of red blood cells within the urine is called hematuria. Hematuria is often associated with contusion of the bladder during running and has been referred to as a runner's bladder.[25] Abnormal concentrations of protein in urine is referred to as proteinuria.

Symptoms and signs   After a severe blow to the pelvic region, the athlete may display the following recognizable signs:
- Pain and discomfort in the lower abdomen. With a bladder contusion the athlete will be able to urinate; with a bladder rupture the athlete will be unable to urinate.
- Abdominal rigidity.
- Nausea, vomiting, and signs of shock.
- Blood dripping from the urethra.
- Passing a great quantity of bloody urine, which indicates possible injury to the kidney.

Bladder injury commonly causes referred pain to the lower trunk, including the upper thigh anteriorly and suprapubically.

Prevention   With any impact to the abdominal region, the possibility of internal damage must be considered, and after such trauma the athlete should be instructed

24-5

Critical Thinking Exercise

A basketball player goes for a rebound and is accidentally hit in the abdomen by an opponent's elbow. He is lying on the court on his side with his legs drawn up. The athletic trainer decides to remove him from the court on a stretcher and evaluate him in the training room. On palpation the abdomen feels extremely tight.

? How can the athletic trainer differentiate between muscle guarding, rigidity, and rebound tenderness in the athlete who has sustained an abdominal injury?

Kidney and bladder contusions can cause hematuria.

24-6

Critical Thinking Exercise

A football receiver jumps to catch a high pass thrown over the middle. A defensive back hits the receiver in the low back. The athlete does not seem to have a specific injury. After the game when going to the bathroom he notices blood in his urine and becomes worried.

? Is blood in the urine a cause for concern? What should the athletic trainer do to manage this problem?

to check periodically for blood in the urine. To lessen the possibility of rupture, the athlete must always empty the bladder before practice or game time. The bladder can also be irritated by intraabdominal pressures during long-distance running. In this situation repeated impacts to the bladder's base are produced by the jarring of the abdominal contents, resulting in hemorrhage and blood in the urine.

Injury to the urethra is more common in men because the male's urethra is longer and more exposed than the female's. Injury may produce severe perineal pain and swelling.

Conditions Related to the Digestive System

Like any other individual, the athlete may develop various complaints of the digestive system. The athlete may display various disorders of the gastrointestinal tract as a result of poor eating habits or the stress engendered from competition. The responsibility of the athletic trainer in such cases is to be able to recognize the more severe conditions so that early referrals to a physician can be made.

Gastrointestinal Bleeding

Gastrointestinal bleeding that is reflected in bloody stools occurs in a variety of athletes. Distance runners often have blood in their stools during and after a race. The causes of gastrointestinal bleeding can vary. Possible reasons are gastritis, iron-deficiency anemia, ingestion of aspirin or other antiinflammatory agents, colitis, or even stress and bowel irritation. Athletes displaying gastrointestinal bleeding must be referred immediately to a physician.[15]

Liver Contusion

Etiology   Comparing frequency with other organ injuries from blunt trauma, injuries to the liver rank second.[20] In sports activities, however, liver injury is relatively infrequent. A hard blow to the right side of the rib cage can tear or seriously contuse the liver, especially if it has been enlarged as a result of some disease, such as hepatitis. Hepatitis is an inflammation of the liver caused by either viral infection or alcohol consumption. If not corrected cirrhosis of the liver can occur, in which liver cells die and are replaced by scar tissue thus impairing liver function.

Hepatitis can cause enlargement of the liver.

Symptoms and signs   Liver injury can cause hemorrhage and shock, requiring immediate surgical intervention. Liver injury commonly produces a referred pain that is just below the right scapula, right shoulder, and substernal area and, on occasion, the anterior left side of the chest.

Management   A liver contusion requires immediate referral to a physician for diagnosis and treatment.

Indigestion (Dyspepsia)

Etiology   Some athletes have certain food idiosyncrasies that cause them considerable distress after eating. Others develop reactions when eating before competition. The term given to digestive upset is indigestion (dyspepsia). Indigestion can be caused by any number of conditions. The most common in sports are emotional stress, esophageal and stomach spasms, and inflammation of the mucous lining of the esophagus and stomach.

Indigestion, vomiting, diarrhea, and constipation are common problems in the athlete.

Symptoms and signs   These conditions cause an increased secretion of hydrochloric acid (sour stomach), nausea, and flatulence (gas).

Management   Care of acute dyspepsia involves the elimination of irritating foods from the diet, development of regular eating habits, and avoidance of anxieties that may lead to gastric distress.

Constant irritation of the stomach may lead to chronic and more serious disorders such as gastritis, an inflammation of the stomach wall, or ulcerations of the gastrointestinal mucosa. Athletes who appear nervous and high-strung and suffer from dyspepsia should be examined by the sports physician.

Vomiting

Etiology   Vomiting results from some type of irritation, most often in the stomach. This stimulates the vomiting center in the brain to cause a series of forceful contractions of the diaphragm and abdominal muscles, thus compressing the stomach and forcefully expelling the contents.[17]

Management   Antinausea medications should be administered. (See Chapter 16.) Fluids to prevent dehydration should be administered by mouth if possible. If vomiting persists, fluids and electrolytes must be administered intravenously.

Food Poisoning (Gastroenteritis)

Etiology   Food poisoning, which may range from mild to severe, results from infectious organisms (bacteria of the salmonella group, certain staphylococci, streptococci, or dysentery bacilli) that enter the body in either food or drink. Foods become contaminated, especially during warm weather, when improper food refrigeration permits the organisms to multiply rapidly. Contamination can also occur if the food is handled by an infected food handler.

Symptoms and signs   Infection results in nausea, vomiting, cramps, diarrhea, and anorexia. The symptoms of staphylococcal infections usually subside in 3 to 6 hours. Salmonella infection symptoms may last from 24 to 48 hours or more.

Management   Management requires rapid replacement of lost fluids and electrolytes, which in severe cases may need to be replaced intravenously. Bed rest is desirable in all but mild cases; as long as the nausea and vomiting continue, nothing should be given by mouth. If tolerated, light fluids or foods such as clear, strained broth, bouillon with a small amount of added salt, soft-cooked eggs, or bland cereals may be given.

Peptic Ulcer

Etiology   A peptic ulcer is a condition in which the acids secreted in the stomach destroy the mucous lining either in the stomach or the small intestine. They most often occur in people experiencing severe anxiety for long periods of time.[17]

Symptoms and signs   A "gnawing" pain localized in the epigastric region usually appears between 1 and 3 hours after a meal. Other symptoms include dyspepsia, heartburn, nausea, and vomiting. Pain usually lasts for minutes rather than hours.[20]

Management   Occasionally the symptoms may disappear without the aid of medication. Antacids may be helpful in neutralizing gastric secretions. Altering the diet has not proven to be effective in managing the peptic ulcer. If hemorrhaging or perforation occur surgery may be necessary.

Diarrhea

Etiology   Diarrhea is abnormal stool looseness or passage of a fluid, unformed stool and is categorized as acute or chronic, according to the type present. Diarrhea can be caused by problems in diet, inflammation of the intestinal lining, gastrointestinal infection, ingestion of certain drugs, and psychogenic factors.[17]

Symptoms and signs   Diarrhea is characterized by abdominal cramps, nausea, and possibly vomiting, coupled with frequent elimination of stools, ranging from 3 to 20 a day. The infected person often has a loss of appetite and a light brown or gray, foul-smelling stool. Extreme weakness caused by fluid dehydration is usually present.

Management   The cause of diarrhea is often difficult to establish. It is conceivable that any irritant may cause the loose stool. This can include an infestation of parasitic organisms or an emotional upset. Management of diarrhea requires a knowledge of its cause. Less severe cases can be cared for by omitting foods that cause irritation, drinking boiled milk, eating bland food until symptoms have ceased, and using pectins two or three times daily for the absorption of excess fluid.

Constipation

Etiology   Some athletes are subject to constipation, the failure of the bowels to evacuate feces. There are numerous causes of constipation, the most common of which are lack of abdominal muscle tone; insufficient moisture in the feces, causing it to be hard and dry; lack of a sufficient proportion of roughage and bulk in the diet to stimulate peristalsis; poor bowel habits; nervousness and anxiety; and overuse of laxatives and enemas.[20]

Symptoms and signs   Constipation results in a feeling of fullness with occasional cramping and pain in the lower abdomen. When straining hard to defecate, some vessels may be ruptured in the rectum and bleeding from the anus may occur.

Management   The best means of overcoming constipation is to regulate eating patterns to include foods that will encourage normal defecation. Cereals, fruits, vegetables, and fats stimulate bowel movement, whereas sugars and carbohydrates tend to inhibit it. Some persons become constipated as the result of psychological factors. In such cases it may be helpful to try to determine the causes of stress and, if need be, to refer the athlete to a physician or school psychologist for counseling. Above all, laxatives or enemas should be avoided unless their use has been prescribed by a physician.

Appendicitis

Etiology   Inflammation of the vermiform appendix can be chronic or acute. It is caused by a variety of causes such as a fecal obstruction, lymph swelling, or even a carcinoid tumor. Its highest incidence is in males between the ages of 15 and 25. Appendicitis can be mistaken for a common gastric complaint. In its early stages, the appendix becomes red and swollen; in later stages it may become gangrenous, rupturing into the bowels or peritoneal cavity and causing peritonitis.[20] Bacterial infection is a complication of rupture of the inflamed appendix.

Symptoms and signs   The athlete may complain of a mild to severe pain in the lower abdomen, associated with nausea, vomiting, and a low-grade fever ranging from 99° to 100° F (37° to 38° C). Later, the cramps may localize into a pain in the right side, and palpation may reveal abdominal rigidity and tenderness at a point between the anterior superior spine of the ilium and the umbilicus (McBurney's point), about 2.5 to 5.1 cm above the latter.[20]

A strain of the psoas muscle or an abcess in the sheath of the psoas can sometimes be mistaken for appendicitis.

Management   Surgical removal of the appendix is often necessary. If the bowel is not obstructed there is no need to rush surgery. However, an obstructed bowel with an acute rupture is a life-threatening condition.

Hemorrhoids (Piles)

Etiology   Hemorrhoids are varicosities of the hemorrhoidal venous plexus of the anus. There are both internal and external anal veins. Chronic constipation or straining at the stool may tend to stretch the anal veins, resulting in either a protrusion (prolapse) and bleeding of the internal or external veins or a thrombus in the external veins.

Symptoms and signs   Often hemorrhoids are painful nodular swellings near the sphincter of the anus. There may be slight bleeding and itching. The majority of hemorrhoids are self-limiting and spontaneously heal within 2 to 3 weeks.

Management   The management of hemorrhoids is mostly palliative and serves to eliminate discomfort until healing takes place. The following measures can be suggested:

- Use of proper bowel habits.
- Ingestion of 1 tablespoon of mineral oil daily to assist in lubricating dry stool.

Appendicitis is often mistaken for a common gastric problem.

24-7

Critical Thinking E x e r c i s e

Immediately after finishing a meal, a fencer begins to complain of a mild to severe pain in the lower abdomen. She has nausea, vomiting, and a low-grade fever. The athletic trainer suspects that she may have indigestion. However, in about an hour the cramps begin to localize into a pain in the right side, and palpation reveals abdominal rigidity and tenderness at McBurney's point.

? What should the athletic trainer suspect is wrong with this athlete, and what will probably be necessary in management?

- Application of an astringent suppository (tannic acid).
- Application of a local anesthetic to control pain and itching (dibucaine).

If palliative measures are unsuccessful, surgery may be required.

Injuries to the Reproductive Organs

Injuries to the reproductive organs in sports are much more likely to occur in the male because the genitalia are more exposed.

Scrotal Contusion

Etiology   As the result of its considerable sensitivity and particular vulnerability, the scrotum may sustain a contusion that causes an extremely painful, nauseating, and disabling condition.

Symptoms and signs   As is characteristic of any contusion or bruise, there is hemorrhage, fluid effusion, and muscle spasm, the degree of which depends on the intensity of the impact to the tissue.

Management   Immediately after a scrotal contusion, the athlete must be put at ease, and testicular spasms must be reduced. Increasing or unresolved pain after 15 to 20 minutes requires prompt referral to a physician for evaluation. The following technique is used to relieve testicular spasm: the athlete is placed on his back and instructed to flex his thighs to his chest (Figure 24-21). This position will aid in reducing discomfort and relax the muscle spasm. After the pain has diminished, the athlete is helped from the playing area, and a cold pack is applied to the scrotum.

Spermatic Cord Torsion

Etiology   Torsion of the spermatic cord results from the testicles revolving in the scrotum after a direct blow to the area or as a result of coughing or vomiting.

Symptoms and signs   Cord torsion produces acute testicular pain, nausea, vomiting, and inflammation in the area.

Management   In this case, the athlete must receive immediate medical attention to prevent irreparable complications. Twisting of the spermatic cord may present the appearance of a cluster of swollen veins and may cause a dull pain combined with a heavy, dragging feeling in the scrotum. This condition may eventually lead to atro-

Injuries to the reproductive organs in sports are much more likely to occur in the male because the genitalia are more exposed.

Figure 24-21

Position for reducing testicular spasm.

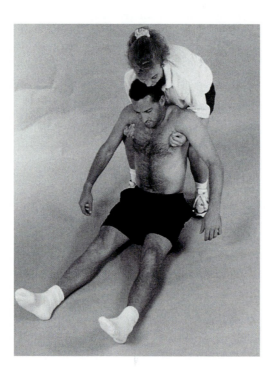

phy of the testicle. A physician should be consulted when this condition is suspected.

Traumatic Hydrocele of the Tunica Vaginalis

Etiology Traumatic hydrocele of the tunica vaginalis is an excess of fluid accumulation caused by a severe blow to the testicular region. The venous plexus on the posterior aspect of the testicle can become engorged, creating a varicocele. A rupture of this plexus results in a rapid accumulation of blood in the scrotum called a hematocele.

Symptoms and signs After trauma the athlete complains of pain. Swelling in the scrotum can significantly increase the size of the sac.

Management Cold packs should be applied to the scrotum, and referral to the physician should be made. Irreversible damage can occur to the testicle if medical treatment is delayed.

Gynecological Injuries

In general the female reproductive organs have a low incidence of injury in sports. By far the most common gynecological injury in the female athlete involves a contusion to the external genitalia or vulva, which includes the labia, clitoris, and the vestibule of the vagina. A hematoma results from the contusion, which most often occurs with a direct impact to this area. A contusion of this area may also injure the pubis symphysis, producing osteitis pubis.

Female water skiers who fall with their legs spread may force water into the vagina and fallopian tubes, potentially tearing the vaginal wall. Vaginal infection in these cases is of some concern.

Injury to Lymphatic Organs

Injury of the Spleen

Etiology Injuries to the spleen are relatively uncommon. If injury does occur it is most often due to a fall or a direct blow to the left upper quadrant of the abdomen when some existing medical condition has caused splenomegaly (enlargement of the spleen). (See Figure 10-3.) Infectious mononucleosis is most likely to cause spleen enlargement. Athletes with mononucleosis should not engage in any activity for 3 weeks because approximately 50% exhibit splenomegaly, or an enlarged spleen, which is difficult to diagnose clinically. (See Chapter 27.)

Infectious mononucleosis can cause spleen enlargement.

Symptoms and signs The gross indications of a ruptured spleen must be recognized so that an immediate medical referral can be made. Indications include a history of a severe blow to the abdomen and possibly signs of shock, abdominal rigidity, nausea, and vomiting. There may be a reflex pain occurring approximately 30 minutes after injury, called Kehr's sign, which radiates to the left shoulder and one third of the way down the left arm.

Athletes who complain of external pain in the shoulders, trunk, or pelvis after a severe blow to the abdomen or back may be describing referred pain from an injury to an internal organ.

Complications The great danger with a ruptured spleen lies in its ability to splint itself and then produce a delayed hemorrhage. Splinting of the spleen is created by a loose hematoma formation and the constitution of the supporting and surrounding structures. Any slight strain may disrupt the splinting effect and allow the spleen to hemorrhage profusely into the abdominal cavity. Potentially the athlete can die of internal bleeding days or weeks after the injury.

Management Conservative nonoperative treatment is recommended initially with a week of hospitalization.[14] At 3 weeks the athlete can engage in light conditioning activities and at 4 weeks full return to activity as long as no symptoms appear. If surgical repair is necessary the athlete will require 3 months to recover. Removal of the spleen will require 6 months before returning to activity.

Injuries to the Abdominal Wall

A number of other abdominal pain sites can be disabling to the athlete. The athletic trainer should be able to discern the pain sites that are potentially more serious and

24-8

Critical Thinking Exercise

A baseball player is hit with a pitch in the left upper quadrant. Initially he appears to be all right, but toward the end of the game becomes nauseous and starts to vomit. He complains of pain in the left upper quadrant and also pain in his left shoulder extending down the arm. The athletic trainer palpates the abdomen and detects rigidity. Within a matter of minutes he begins to develop shocklike symptoms.

? What should the athletic trainer suspect has happened to this athlete, and how should the injury be treated?

Inguinal hernias occur in males; femoral hernias occur in females.

refer the athlete accordingly. Figure 24-22 shows some of the pain sites in the abdomen.

Abdominal Muscle Strains

Sudden twisting of the trunk or reaching overhead can tear an abdominal muscle. These types of injuries can be incapacitating, with severe pain and hematoma formation. The rectus abdominus is the most commonly strained abdominal muscle. Initially, ice and an elastic compression wrap should be used. Treatment should be conservative, with exercise staying within pain-free limits.

Contusions of the Abdominal Wall

Etiology   Compressive forces that injure the abdominal wall are not common in sports. When they do happen, they are more likely to occur in collision sports such as football and ice hockey; however, any sports implements or high-velocity projectiles can injure. Hockey goalies and baseball catchers would be vulnerable to injury without their protective torso pads. Contusion may occur superficially to the abdominal skin or subcutaneous tissue or much deeper to the musculature. The extent and type of injury vary, depending on whether the force is blunt or penetrating.

Symptoms and signs   A contusion of the rectus abdominis muscle can be disabling. A severe blow may cause a hematoma that develops under the fascial tissue surrounding this muscle. The pressure that results from hemorrhage causes pain and tightness in the region of the injury.

Management   A cold pack and a compression elastic wrap should be applied immediately after injury. Signs of possible internal injury must also be looked for in this type of injury.

Hernia

Etiology   The term *hernia* refers to the protrusion of abdominal viscera through a portion of the abdominal wall. Hernias may be congenital or acquired. A congenital hernial sac is developed before birth and an acquired hernia after birth. Structurally a hernia has a mouth, a neck, and a body. The mouth, or hernial ring, is the opening from the abdominal cavity into the hernial protrusion; the neck is the portion of the sac that joins the hernial ring and the body. The body is the sac that protrudes outside the abdominal cavity and contains portions of the abdominal organs.[12]

Hernias resulting from sports most often occur in the groin area. Inguinal hernias (Figure 24-23, *A*), which occur most often in men (over 75%), and femoral hernias (Figure 24-23, *B*), most often occurring in women, are the most prevalent types. Externally the inguinal and femoral hernias appear similar because of the groin protrusion, but a considerable difference is indicated internally. The inguinal hernia results

Figure 24-22

Common sites of abdominal pain.

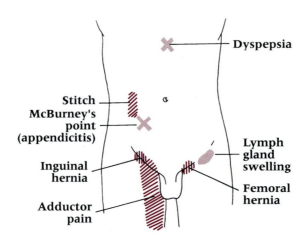

from an abnormal enlargement of the opening of the inguinal canal through which the vessels and nerves of the male reproductive system pass. In contrast to this, the femoral hernia arises in the canal that transports the vessels and nerves that go to the thigh and lower limb.[12]

Under normal circumstances the inguinal and femoral canals are protected against abnormal opening by muscle control. When intraabdominal tension is produced in these areas, muscles produce contraction around these canal openings. If the muscles fail to react or if they prove inadequate in their shutter action, abdominal contents may be pushed through the opening. Repeated protrusions serve to stretch and increase the size of the opening. Most physicians think that any athlete who has a hernia should be prohibited from engaging in hard physical activity until surgical repair has been made.

The danger of a hernia in an athlete is the possibility that it may become irritated by falls or blows. Besides the aggravations caused by trauma, a strangulated hernia may arise, in which the inguinal ring constricts the protruding sac and occludes normal blood circulation. If the strangulated hernia is not surgically repaired immediately, gangrene and death may ensue.

Symptoms and signs   The acquired hernia occurs when a natural weakness is further aggravated by either a strain or a direct blow. Athletes may develop this condition as the result of violent activity. An acquired hernia may be recognized by the following:

- Previous history of a blow or strain to the groin area that has produced pain and prolonged discomfort.
- Superficial protrusion in the groin area that is increased by coughing.
- Reported feeling of weakness and pulling sensation in the groin area.

Management   The treatment preferred by most physicians is surgery. Mechanical devices, which prevent hernial protrusion, are for the most part unsuitable in sports because of the friction and irritation they produce. Exercise has been thought by many to be beneficial to a mild hernia, but such is not the case. Exercise will not affect the stretched inguinal or femoral canals positively.

Blow to the Solar Plexus

Etiology   A blow to the sympathetic celiac plexus (solar plexus) produces a transitory paralysis of the diaphragm ("wind knocked out").

Symptoms and signs   Paralysis of the diaphragm stops respiration and leads to anoxia. When the athlete is unable to inhale, hysteria because of fear may result. These symptoms are usually transitory. It is necessary to allay such fears and instill confidence in the athlete.

Management   In dealing with an athlete who has had his or her wind knocked out, the athletic trainer should adhere to the following procedures:

- Help the athlete overcome apprehension by talking in a confident manner.
- Loosen the athlete's belt and the clothing around the abdomen; have the athlete bend the knees.
- Encourage the athlete to relax by initiating short inspirations and long expirations.

Because of the fear of not being able to breathe, the athlete may hyperventilate. Hyperventilation results in an increased rate of ventilation, resulting in a lowered carbon dioxide level. It causes a variety of physical reactions, such as dizziness, a lump in the throat, pounding heart, and fainting.

There should always be some concern that a blow hard enough to knock out the wind could also cause internal organ injury.

Stitch in the Side

Etiology   A "stitch in the side" is the name given to an idiopathic condition that occurs in some athletes. The cause is obscure, although several hypotheses have been

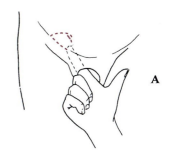
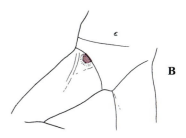

Figure 24-23

A, Inguinal hernia. **B,** Femoral hernia.

24-9

Critical Thinking E x e r c i s e

A wrestler is engaged in a strenuous off-season weight lifting program. Recently he has begun to experience pain in his groin. It seems that whenever he strains hard to lift a weight and especially if he holds his breath the pain appears. He is concerned that he has developed a hernia.

? What symptoms and signs should the athletic trainer look for that would indicate that the athlete does in fact have a hernia?

A blow to the solar plexus can lead to transitory paralysis of the diaphragm and unconsciousness.

advanced. Among the possible causes are constipation, intestinal gas, overeating, diaphragmatic spasm as a result of poor conditioning, lack of visceral support because of weak abdominal muscles, distended spleen, breathing techniques leading to a lack of oxygen in the diaphragm, and ischemia of either the diaphragm or the intercostal muscles.

Signs and symptoms   A stitch in the side is a cramplike pain that develops on either the left or right costal angle during hard physical activity. Sports that involve running apparently produce this condition.

Management   Immediate care of a stitch in the side demands relaxation of the spasm, for which two methods have proved beneficial. First, the athlete is instructed to stretch the arm on the affected side as high as possible. If this is inadequate, flexing the trunk forward on the thighs may be of some benefit.

Athletes with recurrent abdominal spasms may need special study. The identification of poor eating habits, poor elimination habits, or an inadequate athletic training program may explain the athlete's particular problem. It should be noted that a stitch in the side, although not considered serious, may require further evaluation by a physician if abdominal pains persist.

SUMMARY

- Injuries to the heart, lungs, and abdominal viscera can be potentially serious and even life threatening if not recognized and managed appropriately.
- The thorax is that portion of the body commonly known as the chest; it lies between the base of the neck and the diaphragm. Its main functions are to protect the vital respiratory and circulatory organs and to assist the lungs in inspiration and expiration during the breathing process. Within the thoracic cage lie the lungs, the heart, and the thymus.
- The abdominal cavity lies between the diaphragm and the bones of the pelvis and is bounded by the margin of the lower ribs, the abdominal muscles, and the vertebral column. The abdominal viscera are composed of both hollow and solid organs. Organs in the abdominal cavity may be classified as being part of the urinary system, the digestive system, the reproductive system, or the lymphatic system.
- For the coach or athletic trainer evaluating an injury to the abdomen or thorax, the initial primary survey should focus on signs and symptoms that indicate some life-threatening condition. Asking pertinent questions, observing body positioning, and palpation of the injured structures are critical in assessing the nature of the injury.
- Rib fractures and contusions, costochondral junction separations, sternum fractures, muscle strains, and breast injuries are all common injuries to the chest wall.
- Injuries involving the lungs include pneumothorax, tension pneumothorax, hemothorax, and traumatic asphyxia.
- The most common cause of exercise-induced sudden death is some congenital cardiovascular abnormality. The three most prevalent conditions are hypertrophic cardiomyopathy, anomalous origin of the coronary artery, and Marfan's syndrome.
- With any injury to the abdominal region, internal injury to the abdominal viscera must be considered. Injuries to the liver, spleen, and kidneys are among the more common injuries of the abdominal viscera associated with athletics.
- A number of conditions of the digestive system, such as diarrhea, constipation, and gastroenteritis, commonly affect the athletic population.
- Injuries to the reproductive organs in sports are much more likely to occur in the male because the genitalia are more exposed.
- Injuries to the abdominal wall include muscle strains, getting the wind knocked out, and the development of an inguinal or femoral hernia.

24-10

Critical Thinking E x e r c i s e

A cross-country runner complains of a recurring stitch in the side. She has a cramplike pain that develops on the left costal angle during a hard run. She indicates that when she stops running the cramp disappears but seems to come back if she starts to run again.

? What can the athletic trainer recommend that can potentially help this runner alleviate this problem?

Solutions to Critical Thinking Exercises

24-1 The athletic trainer should be concerned about the possibility of injury to an organ that can potentially lead to internal blood loss and eventually result in shock. It is possible that the spleen, liver, stomach, small intestine, pancreas, or gallbladder may all be injured. It is also possible that there may be a contusion to the muscles of the abdominal wall that is causing muscle guarding.

24-2 The athletic trainer should palpate along the rib, in the intercostal space between the ribs, and at the costochondral junction to locate a specific point of tenderness. Applying antero-posterior compression to the thoracic cage is done to identify potential rib fractures. If the athlete complains of increased pain or tenderness on transverse compression applied laterally to the rib cage, a costochondral injury is more likely.

24-3 Injuries severe enough to cause a rib fracture might also result in pneumothorax, tension pneumothorax, hemothorax, or traumatic asphyxia. Any of these conditions should be considered life threatening, and the athletic trainer should access the rescue squad immediately. The trainer should also be prepared to initiate CPR if indicated.

24-4 Potential causes include myocardial infarction, hypertrophic cardiomyopathy, Marfan's syndrome, coronary artery disease resulting from atherosclerosis, right ventricular dysplagia, cardiac conduction system abnormalities, aortic stenosis, and myocarditis. All of these causes have been attributed to sudden death syndrome in athletes. The athletic trainer is dealing with a life-threatening situation and must seek emergency medical care as soon as possible.

24-5 To palpate the abdominal structures, the athlete should be supine with the hips and knees flexed. An athlete with an abdominal injury will voluntarily contract the abdominal muscles to guard or protect the tender area. If there is bleeding or irritation inside of the abdominal cavity the abdomen will exhibit boardlike rigidity and cannot be voluntarily relaxed. Rebound is produced by pressing firmly on the abdomen and then quickly releasing pressure, causing intense pain.

24-6 Anytime blood appears in the urine there is cause for concern. In this case it is likely that the kidneys have been contused, and the blood that appears in the urine will usually disappear over the next couple of days. Nevertheless the athlete should be referred to the team physician for diagnosis.

24-7 It is possible that the athlete has an inflamed vermiform appendix. Most often surgical removal of the appendix is necessary. Occasionally an inflamed appendix results from an obstructed bowel. A rupture of the appendix caused by bowel obstruction becomes a life-threatening emergency.

24-8 The athlete is exhibiting the symptoms and signs of a ruptured spleen. The spleen has the ability to splint itself and stop hemorrhage. However, because of the potential of shock the athletic trainer should treat this injury as life threatening. Usually treatment will be conservative, involving brief hospitalization. Surgical management is necessary when the spleen has ruptured and is hemorrhaging.

24-9 Most often the athlete will have some previous history of a blow or strain to the groin area that has produced pain and prolonged discomfort. There may be a superficial protrusion in the groin area that is increased by coughing or a feeling of weakness and a pulling sensation in the groin area. An inguinal hernia results from an abnormal enlargement of the opening of the inguinal canal through which the abdominal contents may be pushed.

24-10 The athletic trainer should try to modify eating habits that might produce constipation or gas. Cramps can be caused by improper breathing techniques, which may cause a lack of oxygen in the diaphragm, and ischemia of either the diaphragm or the intercostal muscles. They may also be caused by diaphragmatic spasm resulting from poor conditioning or a lack of visceral support because of weak abdominal muscles. Athletes with recurrent abdominal spasms should have further evaluation by a physician if abdominal pains persist.

REVIEW QUESTIONS AND SUGGESTED ACTIVITIES

1. Describe the anatomy of the thorax.
2. Differentiate among rib contusions, rib fractures, and costochondral separations.
3. Compare the signs of pneumothorax, tension pneumothorax, hemothorax, and traumatic asphyxia.
4. Identify the possible causes of sudden death syndrome among athletes.
5. List the abdominal viscera and other structures associated with the urinary system, the digestive system, the lymphatic system, and the reproductive system.
6. What muscles protect the abdominal viscera?
7. What conditions of the abdominal viscera produce pain in the abdominal region?
8. Contrast the signs of a ruptured spleen with signs of a severely contused kidney.
9. What are the most common sports injuries and conditions related to the digestive system?
10. How do you manage an athlete who has had his or her wind knocked out?
11. Distinguish an inguinal hernia or a femoral hernia from a groin strain.
12. Describe the signs of a stitch in the side.

REFERENCES

1. Allison T: Counseling athletes at risk for sudden death, *Phys Sports Med* 20(6):140, 1992.
2. Alpert J, Pape L, Ward A: Athletic heart syndrome, *Phys Sports Med* 17(7):103, 1989.
3. Falsetti H: Sudden death syndrome, *Training and Conditioning* 5(3):24, 1995.
4. Freitas JE: Renal imaging following blunt trauma, *Phys Sports Med* 17(12):59, 1989.
5. Jones H, McBride G, Murphy R: Sternal fractures associated with spinal injury, *J Trauma* 29(3):360, 1989.
6. Hammond S: Chest injuries in the trauma patient, *Nurs Clin North Am* 25(1):35, 1990.
7. Haycock CE: How I manage abdominal injuries, *Phys Sports Med* 14(6):86, 1986.
8. Haycock CE: How I manage breast problems in athletes, *Phys Sports Med* 15(3):89, 1987.
9. Lee M, Wong S, Chu J: Traumatic asphyxia, *Ann Thorac Surg* 51(1):86, 1991.
10. Maron B: Hypertrophic cardiomyopathy in athletes: catching a killer, *Phys Sports Med* 21(9):83, 1993.
11. Maron B et al: Blunt trauma to the chest leading to sudden death from cardiac arrest during sports activities, *N Engl J Med* 333(6):337, 1995.
12. McCarthy P: Hernias in athletes: what you need to know, *Phys Sports Med* 18(5):115, 1990.

13. Miles J, Barrett G: Rib fractures in athletes, *Sports Med* 12(1):66, 1991.
14. Morden R, Berman B, Nagle C: Spleen injury in sports: avoiding splenectomy, *Phys Sports Med* 20(4):126, 1992.
15. Reid D: *Sports injury assessment*, New York, 1992, Churchill Livingstone.
16. Reut R, Bach B, Johnson C: Pectoralis major rupture, *Phys Sports Med* 19(3):89, 1991.
17. Seeley R, Stephens T, Tate P: *Anatomy and physiology*, ed 3, St Louis, 1995, Mosby.
18. Simoneauz S, Murphy B, Tehranzadeh J: Spontaneous pneumothorax in a weight lifter, *Am J Sports Med* 18(6):647, 1990.
19. Steine H: Chest pain and shortness of breath in a collegiate basketball player: case report and literature review, *Med Sci Sports Exerc* 24:504, 1992.
20. *Tabor's Cyclopedic Medical Dictionary*, Philadelphia, 1993, Davis.
21. Van Camp S: Sudden death. In Puffer J, editor: *Clinics in sports medicine*, Philadelphia, 1992, Saunders.
22. Van Camp S, Bloor C, Mueller F: Nontraumatic sports death in high school and college athletes, *Med Sci Sports Exerc* 27(9):641, 1995.
23. Wagner R, Sidhu G, Radcliffe W: Pulmonary contusion in contact sports, *Phys Sports Med* 20(2):126, 1992.
24. Yates M, Aldrete V: Blunt trauma causing aortic rupture, *Phys Sports Med* 19(11):96, 1991.
25. York J: Bladder trauma from jogging, *Phys Sports Med* 18(9):116, 1990.

ANNOTATED BIBLIOGRAPHY

Seeley R, Stephens T, Tate P: *Anatomy and physiology*, ed 3, St Louis, 1995, Mosby.

This anatomy text helps clarify anatomy of the various systems of the abdomen and thorax and also provides clinical correlations for specific injuries and illnesses.

Tabor's Cyclopedic Medical Dictionary, Philadelphia, 1993, Davis.

Despite the dictionary format, this is an excellent guide for the athletic trainer who is searching for clear, concise descriptions of various injuries and illnesses accompanied by brief recommendations for management and treatment.

The Head and Face

When you finish this chapter, you should be able to

- Describe the anatomy of the head and face.
- Recognize major sports injuries to the head and face.
- Manage head and face injuries.

Sports injuries to the head can be life threatening. Facial injuries can lead to disfigurement.

THE HEAD

Head injuries occur from direct and blunt forces to the skull. It is estimated that at least 30 to 40 major head injuries and occasionally a death occur during sport-related activities each year.[20]

Anatomy

Bones

The brain is housed in a skull composed of a series of bones joined together by sutures. The cranial vault is made up of the frontal, ethmoid, sphenoid, parietal, temporal, and occipital bones. The skull's thickness varies in different locations, being thinner over the temporal regions[20] (Figure 25-1).

Scalp

The scalp is the covering of the skull. It has five layers of soft tissue. The skin, connective tissue, and aponeurosis epicranalis are the three outermost tissue layers. They are fused and move as a single layer. The aponeurosis epicranalis is a thick connective tissue sheet that acts as an attachment for the occipitalis and frontalis muscles. Between the first three tissue layers and the periosteum lies a loose connective tissue layer.[20]

The Cerebrum

The *brain,* or encephalon, is the part of the central nervous system that is contained within the bony cavity of the cranium and is divided into four sections: the cerebrum, the cerebellum, the pons, and the medulla oblongata.

Investing the spinal cord and the brain are the *meninges,* which are the three membranes that protect the brain and the spinal cord. Outermost is the dura mater, consisting of a dense, fibrous, and inelastic sheath that encloses the brain and cord. In some places it is attached directly to the vertebral canal, but for the most part, a layer of fat that contains the vital arteries and veins separates this membrane from the bony wall and forms the epidural space. The arachnoid, an extremely delicate sheath, lines the dura mater and is attached directly to the spinal cord by many silklike tissue strands. The space between the arachnoid and the pia mater, the membrane that helps contain the spinal fluid, is called the *subarachnoid space.* The subarachnoid cavity projects upward and, running the full length of the spinal cord, connects with the ventricles of the brain. The pia mater is a thin, delicate, and highly vascularized membrane that adheres closely to the spinal cord and to the brain (Figure 25-2).

Cerebrospinal fluid is contained between the arachnoid and the pia mater membrane and completely surrounds and suspends the brain. Its main function is to act as a cushion, helping to diminish the transmission of shocking forces.

Figure 25-1

Bones of the skull.

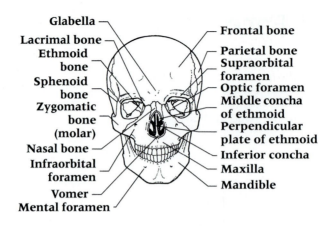

Figure 25-2

Cross section of the head and brain.

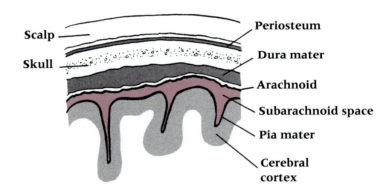

HEAD INJURIES

The head can sustain a variety of injuries in sports. Types of injuries include trauma to the scalp, skull fractures, and cerebral injuries.

Cerebral Injuries

Closed head injuries are common problems in contact and collision sports. They can create neurological, medical, and psychological consequences.[11]

Despite its considerable protection, the brain is subject to traumatic injury, and a great many of the head injuries incurred in sports have serious consequences (Figure 25-3). For this reason it is necessary to give special consideration to this part of the body.

A constant supply of oxygen and blood to the brain is vital and critical to its survival. Although the incidence of serious head injuries from football has decreased in past years when compared with catastrophic neck injuries, the occurrence is still of major concern. Every coach and athletic trainer must be able to recognize the signs of serious head injury in order to act appropriately.

Assessment of Cerebral Injuries

Primary assessment One must be adept at recognizing and interpreting the signs that an unconscious athlete presents. Priority first aid for any head injury must always deal with any life-threatening condition such as impaired airway or hemorrhage. When an athlete is unconscious, a neck injury is also assumed.[5] Without moving the athlete, evaluation includes the following:

1. Look for the possibility of airway obstruction. If breathing is obstructed, do the following:
   a. Remove the face mask by cutting it away from the helmet, but leave the helmet in place.
   b. Stabilize the head and neck.

If neck injuries are suspected in the unconscious athlete, the jaw is brought forward, but the neck is not hyperextended to clear the airway.

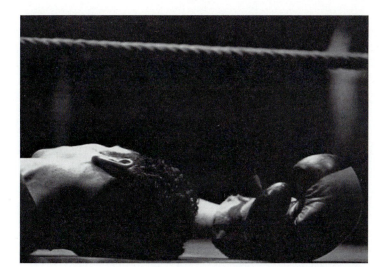

Figure 25-3

Many head injuries incurred in sports have serious consequences.

   c. Bring the jaw forward to clear the air passage (do not hyperextend the neck).
   d. Take the pulse: if absent, cardiopulmonary resuscitation (CPR) is given; if present, oxygen may be given.
   e. NOTE: *Ammonia capsules should not be used for reviving an injured person.* The athlete who is dazed or unconscious, after smelling the pungent ammonia fumes, may jerk the head and exacerbate a spinal fracture.
2. Make a quick observation of the following physical signs of concussion and skull fracture:[23]
   a. Face color may be red or pale.
   b. Skin may be cool or moist.
   c. Pulse, if present, may be strong and slow or rapid and weak.
   d. Breathing, if present, may be deep or shallow.
   e. Pupils may be dilated or unequal.
   f. Head may show swelling or deformity over the area of injury.
3. The athlete is removed carefully from the playing site on a spine board. (See Chapter 8.)

Secondary assessment Athletes with grade 3 or 4 concussions having distinct clinical signs should automatically be sent to the hospital for medical care. In grade 1 and 2 concussions it is often difficult for the athletic trainer to determine exactly how serious the problem is. Also, grade 1 and 2 conditions can slowly—or even quickly—deteriorate to a higher grade. This possibility makes certain evaluative procedures imperative even in apparently minor cases (Table 25-1).

Mental orientation When the athlete regains consciousness, testing for mental orientation and memory should be done. Questions relating to recently acquired information are more sensitive to determining orientation and memory.[13] The following questions are suggested:
- Which team did we play last week?
- Who won the game last week?
- Who scored the last goal?
- What is today's date?

After 5 or 10 minutes, repeat the questions that were previously asked.

Testing eye signs Because of the direct connection between the eye and the brain, pupillary discrepancies provide important information. The athlete should be observed and tested for the following:
1. Dilated or irregular pupils. Checking pupil sizes may be particularly difficult at night and under artificial lights. To ensure accuracy, the athlete's pupil size should be compared with that of an official or another player present. It should

25-1

Critical Thinking Exercise

An athlete falls and hits his head, incurring a possible cerebral injury.

? Initially, what observational signs could be present indicating a cerebral injury?

25-2

Critical Thinking Exercise

A football player sustains a cerebral concussion during a game.

? How should the athletic trainer determine the athlete's level of orientation and memory?

Checking eye signs can yield crucial information about possible brain injury.

TABLE 25-1 Symptoms of Cerebral Concussion

Symptoms	Grade 1	Grade 2	Grade 3	Grade 4
Disorientation	+	+	++	+++
Dizziness		+	++	+++
Retrograde amnesia		+	++	+++
Posttraumatic amnesia			++	+++
Headache			+/++	+++
Loss of consciousness			+/++	+++
Problems in concentrating		+	++	+++
Tinnitus		+	++	+++
Balance problems		+	++	+++
Automatism			+/++	+++
Pupillary discrepancies			+/++	+++

+ Mild.
++ Moderate.
+++ Severe.

be remembered, however, that some individuals normally have pupils that differ in size.

2. Blurred vision determined by difficulty or inability to read a game program or the scoreboard.

3. Inability of the pupils to accommodate rapidly to light variance. Eye accommodation should be tested by covering one eye with a hand. The covered eye normally will dilate, whereas the uncovered pupil will remain the same. When the hand is removed, the previously covered pupil normally will accommodate readily to the light. A slow-accommodating pupil may be an indicator of cerebral injury.

4. Inability of eyes to track smoothly. The athlete is asked to hold the head in a neutral position, eyes looking straight ahead. The athlete is then asked to follow the top of a pen or pencil, first up as far as possible, then down as far as possible. The eyes are observed for smooth movement and any signs of pain. Next, the tip of the pen or pencil is slowly moved from left to right to determine whether the eyes follow the tip smoothly across the midline of the face or whether they make involuntary movements. A constant involuntary back and forth, up and down, or rotary movement of the eyeball is called *nystagmus,* indicating possible cerebral involvement.

Testing balance   If the athlete can stand, the degree of unsteadiness must be noted. A cerebral concussion of grade 2 or more can produce balance difficulties (positive Romberg's sign). To test Romberg's sign the athlete is told to stand tall with the feet together, arms at sides, eyes closed. A positive sign is one in which the athlete begins to sway, cannot keep the eyes closed, or obviously loses balance. Having the athlete attempt to stand on one foot is also a good indicator of balance.

Finger-to-nose test   The athlete stands tall with eyes closed and arms out to the side. The athlete is then asked to touch the index finger of one hand to the nose and then to touch the index finger of the other hand to the nose. Inability to perform this task with one or both fingers is an indication of physical disorientation and precludes reentry to the game.

Babinski's reflex   A major indicator of injury to the brain from trauma is Babinski's reflex. A pointed object is stroked across the plantar aspect of the sole of the foot, from the calcaneus along the lateral aspect of the sole of the forefoot. A positive Babinski's sign is extension of the great toe and, on occasion, spreading of the other toes. A normal reaction is one in which the toes curl downward.

Monitoring the Grade 1 and 2 Head Concussion

An athlete with any degree of concussion should be sent immediately to the sports physician for treatment and observation. Brain injury may not be apparent until hours after the trauma occurs. The athlete may have to be observed closely throughout the night and be awakened approximately every 1 to 2 hours to check the level of consciousness and orientation.

Recognition and Management of Specific Injuries

Skull fracture

Etiology   Skull fractures occur most often from a blunt trauma, such as a baseball to the head, a shot put to the head, or a fall from a height.

Symptoms and signs   The athlete complains of severe headache and nausea. Palpation may reveal a defect such as a skull indentation, blood in the middle ear, blood in the ear canal, bleeding through the nose, or ecchymosis in an eye orbit. Cerebrospinal fluid (straw colored) may seep from the ears and nose.[9]

Management   It must be noted that it is not the skull fracture itself that causes the most serious problem but complications that stem from intracranial bleeding, bone fragments embedded in the brain, and infection.[9] Such an injury requires immediate hospitalization and referral to a neurosurgeon.

Concussion injuries

Etiology   Most traumas of the head result from direct or indirect blows and may be classified as concussion injuries. It has been estimated that more than 250,000 concussions occur annually to football players. Literally, *concussion* means an agitation or a shaking from being hit, and *cerebral concussion* refers to the agitation of the brain by either a direct or an indirect blow (Figure 25-4). Surgeons define concussion as a clinical syndrome characterized by immediate and transient impairment of neural functions, such as alteration of consciousness, disturbance of vision, and equilibrium, caused by mechanical forces. The indirect concussion most often comes from either a violent fall, in which sitting down transmits a jarring effect through the ver-

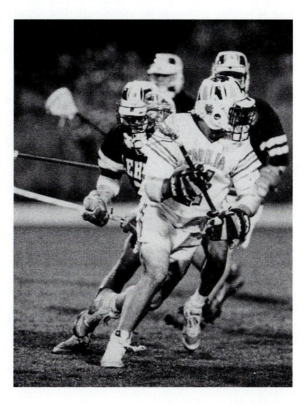

Figure 25-4

Sports using implements can lead to serious head injuries.

tebral column to the brain, or a blow to the chin. In most cases of cerebral concussion there is a short period of unconsciousness, producing a mild to severe outcome.

Symptoms and signs   Most authorities agree that unconsciousness results from brain anoxia that is caused by constriction of the blood vessels. Depending on the force of the blow and the athlete's ability to withstand such a blow, varying degrees of cerebral hemorrhage, edema, and tissue laceration may occur. Because of the fluid suspension of the brain, a blow to the head can effect an injury to the brain either at the point of contact or on the opposite side. After the head is struck, the brain continues to move in the fluid and may be contused against the opposite side. This causes a *contrecoup* type of injury. An athlete who is knocked unconscious by a blow to the head may be presumed to have received some degree of concussion.

Management   In determining the extent of head injury one must be aware of basic gross signs by which concussions may be evaluated. There are many ways to grade cerebral injuries; the following represents one procedure. Concussions are described as mild, moderate, or severe and are graded from 1 through 6 (Table 25-2).

GRADE 1 CONCUSSION   Grade 1 concussions are minimum in intensity and represent the most common type in sports. In general the athlete becomes dazed and disoriented but does not become amnesic or have other signs associated with a more serious condition. There may also be a mild unsteadiness in gait. The athlete is completely lucid in 5 to 15 minutes.

GRADE 2 CONCUSSION   A grade 2 concussion is characterized by minor confusion caused by posttraumatic amnesia. Posttraumatic amnesia is reflected by the inability of the athlete to recall events that have occurred since the time of injury. Unsteadiness, ringing in the ears (tinnitus), and perhaps minor dizziness also occur. A dull headache may follow. The athlete may also develop postconcussion syndrome, which is characterized by difficulty in concentrating, recurring headaches, and irritability. Athletes with postconcussion amnesia should not be permitted to return to play that day. This amnesia may last for several weeks after the trauma, precluding sport participation until symptoms are completely gone.

GRADE 3 CONCUSSION   Grade 3 concussion includes all of the symptoms of grade 2 together with retrograde amnesia. Retrograde amnesia has occurred when the athlete is unable to recall recent events that occurred before the injury. There is also moderate tinnitus, mental confusion, balance disturbance, and headache. With a grade 3 concussion the athlete must not be allowed to return to activity until a thor-

TABLE 25-2   Cerebral Concussion Related to Consciousness and Amnesia

Grade	Symptoms
1	No amnesia and normal consciousness
2	Confusion and amnesia → Normal consciousness with posttraumatic amnesia
3	Confusion and amnesia → Normal consciousness with posttraumatic amnesia and retrograde amnesia
4	**Coma** (paralytic) → Confusion and amnesia
5	**Coma** → Coma vigil
6	→ Death

ough physical examination has been performed. An intracranial lesion that causes a gradual increase in intracranial pressure may be present.

GRADE 4 CONCUSSION   A grade 4 concussion involves that athlete who is "knocked out." This state is considered a paralytic coma, from which the athlete usually recovers in a few seconds or minutes. While recovering, the athlete returns to consciousness through states of stupor and confusion, with or without delirium, to a semilucid state with automatism, and finally to full alertness. Often there is posttraumatic and retrograde amnesia, along with a postconcussion syndrome.

An emergency situation is present whenever there is a loss of consciousness for more than several minutes or when there is a deteriorating neurological state. This situation demands immediate transportation to a hospital, with the athlete carried off the field on a spine board.

GRADE 5 CONCUSSION   A grade 5 concussion has occurred when the athlete is in a paralytic coma that is associated with secondary cardiorespiratory collapse. The Glasgow Coma Scale may be used to determine an athlete's level of consciousness after cervical injury (Table 25-3).[10]

GRADE 6 CONCUSSION—DEATH   The grade 5 concussion and coma may lead to a grade 6 concussion and death.

Cerebral contusion   A cerebral contusion, in comparison with a concussion, constitutes an anatomical brain injury.

Etiology   There is a focal area of cerebral injury with cell damage, edema, and hemorrhage. The cause is variable, such as a contrecoup force or direct blunt trauma to the skull.[9]

Symptoms and signs   Depending on the extent of trauma and injury site, symptoms and signs vary. There may be loss of consciousness, confusion, dizziness, or erratic behavior.

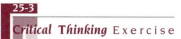

25-3

Critical Thinking Exercise

A football player receives a grade 2 concussion. It is his second concussion this season.

? What guidelines should be followed regarding his return to play?

TABLE 25-3 Glasgow Coma Scale

		Points
Best motor response		
To verbal command	Obeys	6
To painful stimulus*	Localizes pain	5
	Flexion—withdraws	4
	Flexion—abnormal (decerabrate)	3
	Extension (decerabrate)	2
	No response	1
Best verbal response		
With a painful stimulus if necessary	Oriented/converses	5
	Disoriented and converses	4
	Inappropriate	3
	Incomprehensible sounds	2
	No response	1
Eye opening		
	Spontaneously	4
	To verbal command	3
	To pain	2
	No response	1
	TOTAL	3-15**

*Apply knuckles to sternum.
**Score of 7 or less indicates coma.

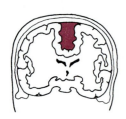

Figure 25-5

Intracranial hemorrhage.

The three major types of intracranial hemorrhage are:
   Epidural
   Subdural
   Intracerebral

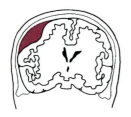

Figure 25-6

Epidural bleeding.

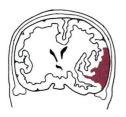

Figure 25-7

Subdural bleeding.

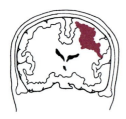

Figure 25-8

Intracerebral bleeding.

Management   Hospitalization with computed tomography (CT) or magnetic resonance imaging (MRI) tests is standard for a cerebral contusion. Treatment varies according to the clinical status of the athlete.[9]

Intracranial hemorrhage   A blow to the head can cause intracranial bleeding. It may arise from rupture of a blood vessel aneurysm or from tearing of a sinus separating the two brain hemispheres (Figure 25-5). Venous bleeding may be slow and insidious; arterial hemorrhage may be evident in a few hours. In the beginning the athlete may be lucid, with few or none of the symptoms of serious head injury, and then gradually display severe head pains, dizziness, nausea, inequality of pupil size, or sleepiness (see the accompanying Focus box). Later stages of cerebral hemorrhage are characterized by deteriorating consciousness, neck rigidity, depression of pulse and respiration, and convulsions. This is a life-threatening situation, necessitating urgent neurosurgical care.

Epidural, subdural, and intracerebral hemorrhage   There are three major types of intracranial hemorrhage: epidural, subdural, and intracerebral.

EPIDURAL BLEEDING   A blow to the head can cause a tear in one of the arteries in the dural membrane that covers the brain (Figure 25-6). It can result from a skull fracture or sudden shift of the brain. Because of arterial blood pressure, blood accumulation and the creation of a hematoma are extremely fast.[15] Often in only 10 to 20 minutes the athlete goes from appearing all right to having major signs of serious head injury. The pressure of the hematoma must be surgically relieved as soon as possible to avoid the possibility of death or permanent disability.

SUBDURAL BLEEDING   In subdural bleeding, veins are torn that bridge the dura mater to the brain.[10] A common mechanism of injury is one of contrecoup, in which the skull decelerates suddenly and the brain keeps moving, tearing blood vessels (Figure 25-7). Because of lower pressure, veins are the primary type of blood vessel injured. Hemorrhage is slow. Signs of brain injury may not appear for many hours after injury. Thus athletes who have sustained a hard blow to the head must be carefully observed for a 24-hour period for signs of pressure buildup within the skull.

INTRACEREBRAL BLEEDING   Intracerebral hemorrhage is bleeding within the brain itself. Most commonly it results from a compressive force to the brain[15] (Figure 25-8). Deterioration of neurological function occurs rapidly, requiring immediate hospitalization.

Returning to Competition after Cerebral Injury

There is always the question of whether an athlete who has been "knocked out" several times should continue in the sport. The team physician must be the final authority on whether an athlete continues to participate in a collision sport after head injury. Each athlete must be evaluated individually.[25] One serious concussion may warrant exclusion from the sport; on the other hand, a number of minor episodes may not. In making this decision, the physician must make sure that the athlete is

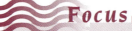

Focus

Conditions indicating the possibility of increasing intracranial pressure

- Headache
- Nausea and vomiting
- Unequal pupils
- Disorientation
- Progressive or sudden impairment in consciousness
- Gradual increase in blood pressure
- Decrease in pulse rate

- Normal neurologically.
- Normal in all vasomotor functions.
- Free of headaches.
- Free of seizure and has a normal electroencephalogram.
- Free of light-headedness when suddenly changing body positions.[15]

Secondary Conditions Associated with Cerebral Injury

In addition to the initial injury to the brain, many secondary conditions can also arise after head trauma. Some of the prevalent ones are cerebral hyperemia (primarily in children), cerebral edema, postinjury epilepsy and seizures, and migraine headaches.

Cerebral hyperemia   A condition common to children with head injuries is cerebral hyperemia, resulting from cerebral blood vessel dilation and a rise in intracranial blood pressure. As a result children develop headache, vomiting, and lethargy. Cerebral hyperemia can occur within a few minutes of injury and can subside in 12 hours.

Cerebral edema   Cerebral edema is a localized swelling at the injury site. Within a 12-hour period the athlete may begin to develop edema, which causes headache and, on occasion, seizures.[15] Cerebral edema may last as long as 2 weeks and is not related to the intensity of trauma.

Seizures   Seizures can occur immediately after head trauma, indicating the possibility of brain injury. They have a higher incidence when the brain has been contused or there is intracranial bleeding. A small number of individuals who have sustained a severe cerebral injury will in time develop epilepsy.[15]

For athletes having a grand mal seizure, the following measures should be taken:

- Maintain airway.
- Make sure the athlete is safe from injury.
- Do *not* put one's fingers into the athlete's mouth in an effort to withdraw the tongue.
- Turn the athlete's head to the side so that saliva and blood can drain out of the mouth once the seizure has ended.

The seizure will normally last only a couple of minutes. The athlete with epilepsy is discussed more fully in Chapter 27.

Migraine headaches   Migraine is a disorder characterized by recurrent attacks of severe headache with sudden onset, with or without visual or gastrointestinal problems.[22] The athlete who has a history of repeated minor blows to the head such as those that may occur in soccer or who has sustained a major cerebral injury may, over a period of time, develop migraine headaches. The exact cause is unknown, but it is believed by many to be a vascular disorder. Flashes of light, blindness in half the field of vision (hemianopia), and paresthesia are thought to be caused by vasoconstriction of intercerebral vessels. Headache is believed to be caused by dilation of scalp arteries. The athlete complains of a severe headache that is diffused throughout the head and often accompanied by nausea and vomiting. There is evidence of a familial predisposition for those athletes who experience migraine headaches after head injury.

Postconcussion syndrome   Postconcussion syndrome is one of the most poorly understood problems resulting from head trauma.

Symptoms and signs   The athlete complains of numerous postconcussion problems, such as impaired memory, lack of concentration, anxiety and irritability, giddiness, fatigue, depression, and visual disturbances.[11]

Management   Any athlete with any of the aforementioned symptoms should not be allowed to return to play. A thorough neurological examination must determine the athlete to be symptom free. Table 25-4 provides guidelines for return to activity after concussion.

Second-impact syndrome

Etiology   The athlete receives a second head injury before symptoms associated with an initial injury have fully cleared.[2] This condition is poorly understood. It is

---

After a cerebral injury, an athlete must be free of symptoms and signs before returning to competition.

Secondary brain injury conditions include:
Cerebral hyperemia
Cerebral edema
Cerebral seizure
Migraine headache

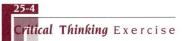
25-4

Critical Thinking Exercise

An athlete with a history of numerous grade I concussions begins to complain of memory difficulty, difficulty in concentrating, and on occasion some irritability, as well as some problems in visual focusing.

? What problem does this athlete have? How should it be managed?

TABLE 25-4 Guidelines for Return to Activity after Concussion

Grade	First Concussion	Second Concussion	Third Concussion
1 (mild)	Return to play if asymptomatic*	Return to play in 2 wk if asymptomatic for 1 wk	Terminate season; may return to play next season if asymptomatic
2 (moderate)	Return to play if asymptomatic for 1 wk	1 mo minimum restriction; may then return to play if asymptomatic for 1 wk; consider terminating season	Terminate season; may return to play next year if asymptomatic
3 (severe)	1 mo minimum restriction; may then return to play if asymptomatic for 1 wk	Terminate season; may return to play next year if asymptomatic	

Adapted from Cantu RC: Guidelines for return to contact sports after a cerebral concussion, *Phys Sportsmed* 14(10):79, 1986.
*No headache or dizziness; no impaired orientation, concentration, or memory during rest or exertion.

thought to be a disruption of the brain's blood autoregulatory system. As a result, there is brain swelling and rapidly increasing intracranial pressure leading to cerebral herniation. The time from second impact to brainstem failure is usually 2 to 5 minutes.[3]

Symptoms and signs   The second impact may be extremely minor. The athlete may appear stunned but does not lose consciousness and may remain on his or her feet such as with a grade 1 concussion. Within 15 seconds to several minutes of the second impact, the athlete collapses with dilated pupils, loss of eye movement, and respiratory failure.[2]

Management   An athlete complaining of headache, light-headedness, visual disturbance, or any other neurological symptoms must not be allowed to return to his or her sport.[2]

Scalp injuries   The scalp can receive lacerations, abrasions, contusions, and hematomas.

Etiology   The cause of scalp injury is usually blunt or penetrating trauma. A scalp laceration could exist in conjunction with a serious skull or cerebral injury.

Symptoms and signs   The athlete complains of being hit in the head. Bleeding is often extensive, making it difficult to pinpoint the exact site. Matted hair and dirt can also disguise the actual point of injury.

Management   The treatment of a scalp laceration poses a special problem because of its general inaccessibility. (See the Focus box on the next page).

THE FACE
Anatomy

The facial skin covers primarily subcutaneous bone with very little protective muscle, fascia, or fat. The supraorbital ridges house the frontal sinuses. In general the facial skeleton is composed of dense bony buttresses combined with thin sheets of bone. The middle third of the face consists of the maxillary bone, which supports the nose and nasal passages. The lower aspect of the face consists of the lower jaw or mandible. Besides supporting teeth, the mandible also supports the larynx, trachea, upper airway, and upper digestive tract (Figure 25-9).

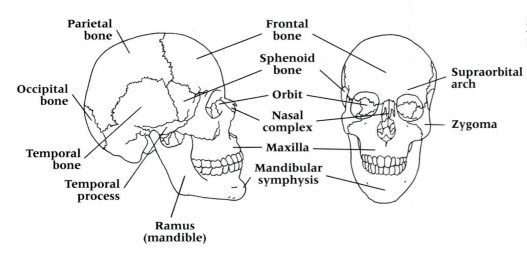

Figure 25-9

Bones of the face.

Facial Injuries

Serious injuries to the face have been reduced significantly by requiring athletes to wear proper protection in high-risk sports. The most prevalent cause of facial injury is a direct blow that injures soft and bony tissue.

Injuries of the Mandible (Jaw)

Jaw fracture   Fractures of the lower jaw or mandible (Figure 25-10) occur most often in collision sports. They are second in incidence of all facial fractures.

Etiology   Because it has relatively little padding and sharp contours, the lower jaw is prone to injury from a direct blow. The most frequently fractured area is near the jaw's frontal angle.

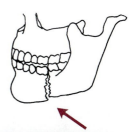

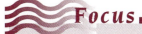

Focus

Care of scalp lacerations

Materials needed

Antiseptic soap, water, antiseptic, 4-inch (10 cm) gauze pads, sterile cotton, and hair clippers.

Position of the athlete

The athlete lies on the table with the wound upward.

Procedure

1. The entire area of bleeding is thoroughly cleansed with antiseptic soap and water. Washing the wound to remove dirt and debris is best done in lengthwise movements.
2. After the injury site is cleansed and dried, it is exposed and, if necessary, the hair is cut away. Enough scalp should be exposed so that a bandage and tape may be applied.
3. Firm pressure or an astringent can be used to reduce bleeding if necessary.
4. Wounds that are more than ½ inch (1.25 cm) in length and ⅛ inch (0.3 cm) in depth should be referred to a physician for treatment. In less severe wounds the bleeding should be controlled and an antiseptic applied, followed by the application of a protective coating such as collodion and a sterile gauze pad. A tape adherent is then painted over the skin area to ensure that the tape sticks to the skin.

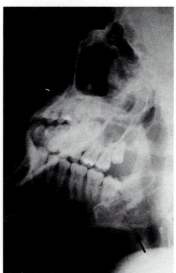

Figure 25-10

Mandibular fracture.

Symptoms and signs   The main indications of a fractured mandible are deformity, loss of normal occlusion of the teeth, pain when biting down, bleeding around teeth, and lower lip anesthesia.[19]

Management   Fracture of the mandible requires temporary immobilization with an elastic bandage followed by reduction and fixation of the jaw by the physician. Mild repetitive activities can be carried out, such as light weight lifting, swimming, or cycling. Fixation is from 4 to 6 weeks. Full activity is resumed in 2 to 3 months with appropriate special headgear and customized mouth guard.[19]

Jaw dislocations   A dislocation of the jaw, or *mandibular luxation,* involves the temporomandibular joint (TMJ), which is formed by the condyle of the mandible and the mandibular fossa of the temporal bone (Figure 25-11). This area has all the features of a hinge-and-gliding articulation. Because of its wide range of movement and the inequity of size between the mandibular condyle and the temporal fossa, the jaw is somewhat prone to dislocation.

Etiology   The mechanism of injury in dislocations is usually initiated by a side blow to the open mouth of the athlete, forcing the mandibular condyle forward out of the temporal fossa. This injury may occur as either a luxation (complete dislocation) or a subluxation (partial dislocation).

Symptoms and signs   The major signs of the dislocated jaw are a locked-open position, with jaw movement being almost impossible, and an overriding malocclusion of the teeth.

Management   Initially, cold is applied along with elastic bandage immobilization and reduction. Follow-up care includes a soft diet, nonsteroidal antiinflammatory drugs (NSAIDs), and analgesic when needed for 1 to 2 weeks. A gradual return to activity can begin 7 to 10 days after the acute period.[19]

Complications   Complications of jaw dislocations are recurrent dislocation, malocclusion, and TMJ dysfunction.

Zygomatic complex (cheekbone) fracture   A fracture of the zygoma represents the third most common facial fracture.[8]

Etiology   The mechanism of injury is a direct blow to the cheekbone.

Symptoms and signs   An obvious deformity occurs in the cheek region, or a bony discrepancy can be felt during palpation. There is usually a nosebleed **(epistaxis),** and the athlete commonly complains of seeing double **(diplopia).** There is also numbness of the cheek.

25-5

Critical Thinking E x e r c i s e

A lacrosse player sustains a severe blow to her cheek by a stick. The blow fractures her maxilla without causing unconsciousness.

? How should the athlete be transported to the hospital and why?

epistaxis
Nosebleed.

diplopia
Seeing double.

Figure 25-11

Dislocation of the jaw (right temporomandibular joint).

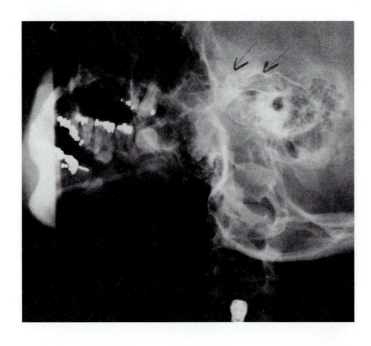

Management   Care by the athletic trainer usually involves cold application for the control of edema and immediate referral to a physician. Healing takes from 6 to 8 weeks. Proper protective gear must be worn when returning to activity.

Maxillary fracture

Etiology   A severe blow to the upper jaw such as would be incurred by being struck by a hockey puck or stick can fracture the maxilla. This ranks fourth in incidence of facial fracture.

Symptoms and signs   After being struck a severe blow to the upper jaw, the athlete complains of pain while chewing, malocclusion, nosebleed, double vision, and numbness in the lip and cheek region.[19]

Management   Because bleeding is usually profuse, airway passages must be maintained. A brain injury may also be associated with this condition, as with all injuries to the face. There must be immediate transportation to a hospital in an upright, forward-leaning position for the conscious athlete. This position allows external drainage of saliva and blood.[18] Fracture reduction, fixation, and immobilization are carried out as specific treatment.[19] The athlete must be referred immediately for medical attention.

Temporomandibular joint dysfunction   The temporomandibular joint is the articulation between the temporal bone and the mandibular condyle.[24] It is a simple hinge joint that also translates anteriorly when the jaw opens. The TMJ is important for both communication and mastication, and it has a high degree of mobility. Because of this extreme mobility, the stability of the joint is compromised. The bony configuration of the joint does not limit its mobility, so the muscles and ligaments provide the primary stability. Within the joint space lies a fibrocartilaginous disk that separates and cushions the bones and provides for a better fit between the articulating surfaces.

Etiology   The most common cause of TMJ dysfunction is a disk-condyle derangement in which the disk is positioned anteriorly with respect to the condyle. This occurs when the jaw is closed. As the jaw opens and the condyle translates forward the disk relocates over the condyle, producing an audible click. A second click may occur when the jaw is closed. This chronic condition eventually leads to deterioration of the posterior stabilizing structures and ultimately anterior dislocation of the disk. This is most typically treated through the use of a custom-designed removable mouthpiece that repositions the condyles anteriorly.[24]

Symptoms and signs   Temporomandibular joint dysfunction has been identified as a cause of various signs and symptoms within the head and neck, including headache, earache, vertigo, signs of inflammation, and neck pain associated with trigger points and muscle guarding. Problems in and about the TMJ are similar to those of other synovial joints in that TMJ dysfunction may result from inflammation of the synovial capsule, internal disk derangement, malocclusion, hypermobility or hypomobility, muscle dysfunction, or limited mandibular joint range of motion.

Management   Traditionally, TMJ dysfunction has been treated by dentists; however, conservative management is certainly within the scope of the athletic trainer.

Facial Lacerations

Facial lacerations are common in contact and collision sports.

Etiology   Lacerations about the face are caused by a direct force to the face with a sharp object or by an indirect compressive force.

Symptoms and signs   The athlete feels pain and skin support. There is bleeding and obvious tearing of the epidermis, dermis, and often the subcutaneous layer of skin (Figure 25-12).

Management   Follow procedures as presented in the section on wound care in Chapter 26. Refer to the physician for definitive care, such as suturing. Athletic trainers should note that with *eyebrow lacerations,* they should not shave the eyebrow because it may not regrow, or if it does it may do so in an irregular pattern.[4] Lip, oral,

Figure 25-12

Facial laceration can be a medical emergency.

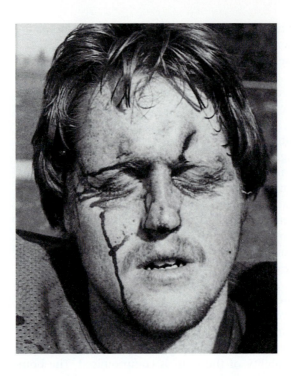

ear, cheek, and nasal lacerations, as with all facial lacerations, are grossly contaminated and must be carefully cleaned before suturing can be successful. Infection must be avoided. Systemic antibiotics and tetanus prophylaxis may be necessary.[4]

Dental Injuries

The tooth is a composite of mineral salts of which calcium and phosphorus are most abundant. The portion protruding from the gum, called the *crown,* is covered by the hardest substance within the body, the enamel. The portion that extends into the alveolar bone of the mouth is called the *root* and is covered by a thin, bony substance known as *cementum.* Underneath the enamel and cementum lies the bulk of the tooth, a hard material known as *dentin.* Within the dentin is a central canal and chamber containing the *pulp,* a substance composed of nerves, lymphatics, and blood vessels

Figure 25-13

Normal tooth anatomy.

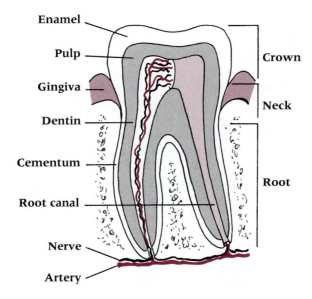

that supply the entire tooth (Figure 25-13). With the use of face guards and properly fitting mouth guards most dental injuries can be prevented. (See Chapter 5.)

Fractured Tooth

Etiology   Any blow to the upper or lower jaw can potentially injure the teeth. Injuries to the tooth below the gum line may repair themselves because of the abundant blood supply. However, fractures of the tooth below the gum line may not heal if there is an injury to the tooth pulp. Even though not obvious, a tooth could sustain a mild blow that disrupts its blood and nerve supply.

Symptoms and signs   Fractured teeth cause pain and bleeding. Teeth may be loose or missing. Missing teeth should be located because they may be replaced if intact. Associated lacerations, brain injury, and jaw fractures should be checked and identified.

Management   Teeth in which the enamel or dentin is chipped fail to rejuvenate because they lack a direct blood supply. They can be capped for the sake of appearance. A tooth that is fractured or loosened may be extremely painful because of the damaged or exposed nerve. In such cases a small amount of calcium hydroxide (Dycol) applied to the exposed nerve area will inhibit the pain until the athlete is seen by a dentist (Figure 25-14).

A fractured tooth is usually extremely sensitive to air and requires the athlete to keep the mouth closed. If there is no bleeding of the gums, the athlete can continue to play and see the dentist after the game.

Partially or Completely Dislocated Tooth

Etiology   A tooth that has been knocked crooked should be manually realigned to a normal position as soon as possible.[12] One that has been totally knocked out should be cleaned with water and replaced in the tooth socket, if possible. If repositioning the dislocated tooth is difficult, the athlete should keep it under the tongue until the dentist can replace it. If this is inconvenient, a dislodged tooth can also be kept in a glass of water. If a completely dislodged tooth is out of the mouth for more than 30 minutes, the chances of saving it are greatly reduced; therefore the athlete should immediately be sent to the dentist for splinting.

> A tooth that has been completely dislocated intact should be rinsed off with water and replaced in the socket.

Nasal Injuries

Nasal Fractures and Chondral Separation

A fracture of the nose is one of the most common fractures of the face.

Etiology   The force of the blow to the nose may come either from the side or from a straight frontal force. A lateral force causes greater deformity than a straight-on blow.

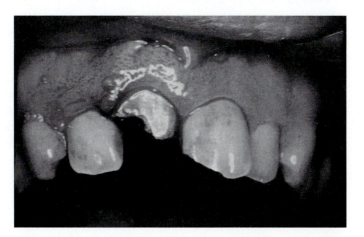

Figure 25-14

Tooth fractures exposing the pulp can predispose the tooth to infection and perhaps death.

Figure 25-15
A nasal fracture may pose a serious medical problem.

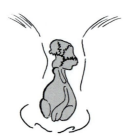

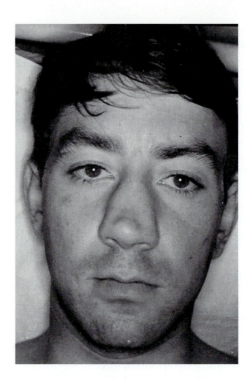

Symptoms and signs   It appears frequently as a separation of the frontal processes of the maxilla, a separation of the lateral cartilages, or a combination of the two (Figure 25-15).

In nasal fractures hemorrhage is profuse because of laceration of the mucous lining. Swelling is immediate. Deformity is usually present if the nose has received a lateral blow. Gentle palpation may reveal abnormal mobility and emit a grating sound (crepitus).

Management   One should control the bleeding and then refer the athlete to a physician for x-ray examination and reduction of the fracture. Simple and uncomplicated fractures of the nose will not hinder or be unsafe for the athlete, and he or she will be able to return to competition within a few days. Fracture deformity reduction must be performed by a trained person.[21] Adequate protection can be provided through splinting (see the Focus box on the next page and Figure 25-16).

Nasal Septal Injuries

A major nasal injury can occur to the septum.

Etiology   As with fracture, the mechanisms are caused by compression or lateral trauma.

Symptoms and signs   A careful evaluation of the nose must be made after the trauma. Injury commonly produces bleeding and in some cases a septal hematoma. The athlete complains of nasal pain.

Management   At the site where a hematoma may occur, compression is applied. When a hematoma is present, it must be drained immediately through a surgical incision through the nasal septal mucosa. After surgical drainage, a small wick is inserted for continued drainage, and the nose is firmly packed to prevent the hematoma from re-forming. If a hematoma is neglected, an abscess will form, causing bone and cartilage loss and ultimately a difficult-to-correct deformity (Figure 25-17).

Nosebleed (Epistaxis)

Nosebleeds in sports are usually the result of direct blows that cause varying degrees of contusion to the septum. Epistaxis is either anterior or posterior. Anterior epistaxis

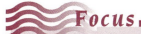

Focus

Nose splinting

The following procedure is used for nose splinting.

Materials needed

Two pieces of gauze, each 2 inches (5 cm) long and rolled to the size of a pencil; three strips of 1½-inch (3.75 cm) tape, cut approximately 4 inches (10 cm) long; and clear tape adherent.

Position of the athlete

The athlete lies supine on the training table.

Procedure

1. The rolled pieces of gauze are placed on either side of the athlete's nose.
2. Gently but firmly, 4-inch (10 cm) lengths of tape are laid over the gauze rolls.

originates from the nasal septum and posterior epistaxis from the lateral wall. Of the two the anterior is more common.

Symptoms and signs Hemorrhages arise most often from the highly vascular anterior aspect of the nasal septum. In most situations the nosebleed presents only a minor problem and stops spontaneously after a short period of time. However, there are persistent types that require medical attention and possibly cauterization.

Management The care of the athlete with an acute nosebleed is as follows:
- The athlete sits upright.
- A cold compress is placed over the nose and the ipsilateral carotid artery.
- The athlete applies finger pressure to the affected nostril for 5 minutes.

If this procedure fails to stop the bleeding within 5 minutes, more extensive measures should be taken. With an applicator, paint the hemorrhage point with an astringent or a styptic such as tannic acid or epinephrine hydrochloride solution. The application of a gauze or cotton pledget will provide corking action and encourage

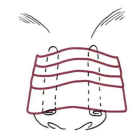

Figure 25-16

Splinting the nose fracture.

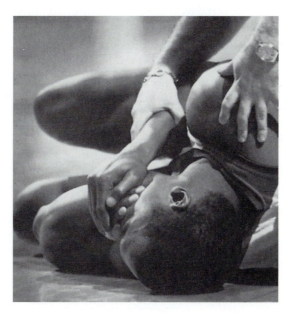

Figure 25-17

Nasal trauma is common in contact and collision sports.

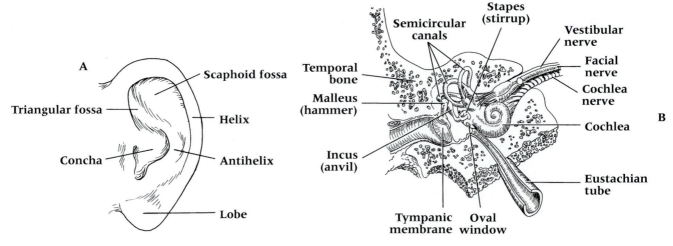

Figure 25-18

Ear anatomy. **A,** External ear. **B,** Inner ear.

blood clotting. If a pledget is used, the ends should protrude from the nostrils at least ½ inch to facilitate removal. After bleeding has ceased, the athlete may resume activity but should be reminded not to blow the nose under any circumstances for at least 2 hours after the initial insult.

Ear Injuries

Anatomy

The ear (Figure 25-18) is responsible for the sense of hearing and equilibrium. It is composed of three parts: the external ear; the middle ear (tympanic membrane) lying just inside the skull; and the internal ear (labyrinth), which is formed in part by the temporal bone of the skull. The middle ear and internal ear are structured to transport auditory impulses to the brain. Aiding the organs of hearing and equalizing pressure between the middle and the internal ear is the eustachian tube, a canal that joins the nose and the middle ear.[17]

Sports injuries to the ear occur most often to the external portion. The external ear is separated into the auricle (pinna) and the external auditory canal (meatus). The auricle, which is shaped like a shell, collects and directs waves of sound into the auditory canal. It is composed of flexible yellow cartilage, muscles, and fat padding and is covered by a closely adhering, thin layer of skin. Most of the blood vessels and nerves of the auricle turn around its borders, with just a few penetrating the cartilage proper.

Hematoma Auris

Hematoma of the ear is common in boxing, rugby, and wrestling. They are most common in athletes who do not wear ear guards (Figure 25-19).

Etiology   This condition usually occurs from a shearing trauma (single or repeated) to the auricle.[7]

Symptoms and signs   Trauma may tear the overlying tissue away from the cartilaginous plate, resulting in hemorrhage and fluid accumulation. A hematoma usually forms before the limited circulation can absorb the fluid. If the hematoma goes unattended, a sequence of coagulation, organization, and fibrosis results in a keloid that appears elevated, rounded, white, nodular, and firm, resembling a cauliflower. Often it forms in the region of the helix fossa or concha; once developed, the keloid can be removed only through surgery.[7] To prevent this disfiguring condition from arising, some friction-reducing agent such as petroleum jelly should be applied to the ears of athletes susceptible to this condition. They should also routinely wear ear guards in practice and in competition.

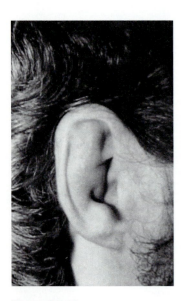

Figure 25-19

Hematoma of the auricle; also called cauliflower ear.

Management   If an ear becomes "hot" because of excessive rubbing or twisting, the immediate application of a cold pack to the affected spot will alleviate hemorrhage. Once swelling is present in the ear, special care should be taken to prevent the fluid from solidifying; a cold pack should be placed immediately over the ear and held tightly by an elastic bandage for at least 20 minutes. If the swelling is still present at the end of this time, aspiration by a physician is required.[22] After drainage, pressure is applied to the area to prevent return of the hematoma. The physician may suture dental rolls into position to ensure uniform pressure.[22] Instead of this procedure a collodion pack may be opted for as follows:

- Cotton is packed into the ear canal.
- The auricle is coated with collodion.
- Small pieces of gauze also coated with collodion are inserted and packed into the auricle of the ear until it is completely filled.
- A ¼-inch-thick felt piece is cut to fit and placed behind the ear.
- A pressure wrap is placed completely around the head, kept in place for 2 days, and then removed.
- The collodion pack is left in place until it can be easily removed.

Rupture of the Tympanic Membrane

Rupture of the tympanic membrane is commonly seen in contact and collision sports, as well as in water polo and diving.[17]

Etiology   A fall or slap to the unprotected ear or sudden underwater variation can rupture the tympanic membrane.

Symptoms and signs   The athlete complains of a loud pop followed by pain in the ear, nausea, vomiting, and dizziness.[17] The athlete demonstrates hearing loss and visible rupture of the tympanic membrane.

Management   Small to moderate perforations of the tympanic membrane usually heal spontaneously in 1 to 2 weeks. Infection can occur and must be continually monitored.

Swimmer's Ear (External Otitis)

A common condition in athletes engaged in water sports is swimmer's ear, or external otitis.

Etiology   *Swimmer's ear* is a general term for infection of the ear canal caused by *Pseudomonas aeruginosa*, a type of gram-negative bacillus. Contrary to current thought among swimming coaches, swimmer's ear is not usually associated with a fungal infection. Water can become trapped in the ear canal as a result of obstructions created by cysts, bone growths, ear wax plugs, or swelling caused by allergies.[14]

Prevention of ear infection can best be attained by drying the ears thoroughly with a soft towel, using ear drops containing a mild acid (3% boric acid) and alcohol solution before and after each swim, and avoiding situations that can cause ear infections such as overexposure to cold wind or sticking foreign objects into the ear.

Symptoms and signs   The athlete may complain of itching, discharge, or even a partial hearing loss. The athlete complains of pain and dizziness.

Management   When the swimmer displays symptoms of external otitis, immediate referral to a physician must be made. Tympanic membrane rupture should be ruled out. Treatment may include acidification through drops into the ear to make an inhospitable environment for the gram-negative bacteria. Antibiotics may be used in athletes with a mild ear infection.[6] In the event of a perforated ear drum custom-made ear plugs must be used.

Eye Injuries

Eye injuries account for approximately 2% of all sports injuries.[16] In the United States, basketball, baseball, boxing, soccer, swimming, and racket sports have a high incidence of eye injuries[18] (Table 25-5).

TABLE 25-5 **Percentage of Sports Eye Injuries in the United States**

Sport	Percent (%)
Baseball	27
Racket sports	20
Basketball	20
Football and soccer	7
Ice hockey	4
Ball hockey	1

Anatomy

The eye has many anatomical protective devices. It is firmly retained within an oval socket formed by the bones of the head. A cushion of soft fatty tissue surrounds it, and a thin skin flap (the eyelid), which functions by reflex action, covers the eye for protection. Foreign particles are prevented from entering the eye by the lashes and eyebrows, which act as a filtering system. A soft mucous lining that covers the inner conjunctiva transports and spreads tears, which are secreted by many accessory lacrimal glands. A larger lubricating organ is located above the eye and secretes heavy quantities of fluid through the lacrimal duct to help wash away foreign particles. The eye proper is well protected by the sclera, a tough white outer layer possessing a transparent center portion called the *cornea* (Figure 25-20).

Eye Protection

The eye can be injured in a number of different ways. Shattered eyeglass or goggle lenses can lacerate; ski pole tips can penetrate; and fingers, racquetballs, and larger projectiles can seriously compress and injure the eye. High-energy sports such as ice hockey, football, and lacrosse require full-face and helmet protection, whereas low-energy sports such as racquetball and tennis require eye guards that rest on the face.[18] Protective devices must provide protection from front and lateral blows.

Sport goggles can be made with highly impact-resistant polycarbonate lenses for refraction. The major problems with sports goggles are distortion of peripheral vision and the tendency to become fogged under certain weather conditions. (See Chapter 5.)

Assessment of the Eye

It is essential that any eye injury be evaluated immediately.

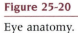

Figure 25-20

Eye anatomy.

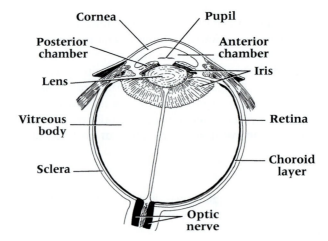

History

- What was the mechanism of injury (sharp and penetrating or blunt)?
- Was loss of vision gradual or immediate?
- What was the visual status before injury?
- Was there loss of consciousness?

Special tests   To make an appropriate eye injury assessment the athletic trainer must have a properly equipped first aid kit.[16] The following is a list of items for use in the immediate care of eye injuries in sports:[16]

- Vision card for testing visual acuity
- Penlight
- Cotton-tipped applicators
- Sterile ocular irrigating solution
- Sterile eye patches
- Plastic eye shields
- Fluorescein strips
- Plunger for removing contact lenses

The first concerns are to understand the mechanism of injury and if there is a related condition to the head, face, or neck. Evaluation steps are as follows:[16]

- Inspect the external ocular structures for swelling and discoloration, penetrating objects, deformities, and movement of the lid.
- Palpate the orbital rim for point tenderness or bony deformity.
- Inspect the globe of the eye for lacerations, foreign bodies, hyphema, or deformities.
- Inspect the conjunctiva and sclera for foreign bodies, hemorrhage, or deformities.
- Determine pupillary response as performed for a possible cerebral injury, including pupil dilation and accommodation by covering the eye and then exposing it to light.
- Determine visual acuity by asking the athlete to report what is seen when looking at some object with the unaffected eye covered. There may be blurring of vision, diplopia, or floating black specks or flashes of light, indicating serious eye involvement.

The Serious Eye Injury

Proper care of eye injuries is essential. The athletic trainer must use extreme caution in handling eye injuries. If there appears to be retinal detachment, perforation of the globe, a foreign object embedded in the cornea, blood in the anterior chamber, decreased vision, loss of the visual field, poor pupillary adaptation, double vision, laceration, or impaired lid function, the athlete should be immediately referred to a hospital or an ophthalmologist.[8] Ideally, the athlete with a serious eye injury should be transported to the hospital by ambulance in a recumbent position (see the Focus box below). Both eyes must be covered during transport. At no time should pressure be applied to the eye. In case of surrounding soft-tissue injury, a cold compress can be applied for 30 to 60 minutes to control hemorrhage (Figure 25-21).

Extreme care must be taken with any eye injury:
    Transport the athlete in a recumbent position.
    Cover both eyes, but put no pressure on the eye.

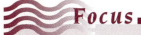

Focus

Symptoms indicating the possibility of serious eye injury

- Blurred vision not clearing with blinking
- Loss of all or part of the visual field
- Pain that is sharp, stabbing, or throbbing
- Double vision after injury

Figure 25-21

A serious eye injury should be treated as a major medical emergency.

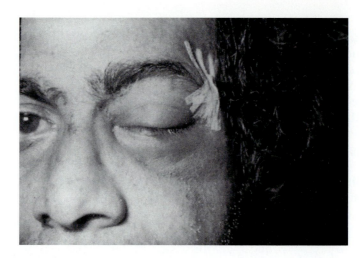

Recognition and Management of Specific Eye Injuries

Orbital hematoma (black eye)

Etiology   Although well protected, the eye may be bruised during sports activity. The severity of eye injuries varies from a mild bruise to an extremely serious condition affecting vision to the fracturing of the orbital cavity. Fortunately, most of the eye injuries sustained in sports are mild. A blow to the eye may initially injure the surrounding tissue and produce capillary bleeding into the tissue spaces. If the hemorrhage goes unchecked, the result may be a classic "black eye."

Symptoms and signs   The signs of a more serious contusion may be displayed as a subconjunctival hemorrhage or as faulty vision.

Management   Care of an eye contusion requires cold application for at least half an hour, plus a 24-hour rest period if the athlete has distorted vision. Under no circumstances should an athlete blow the nose after an acute eye injury. To do so might increase hemorrhaging.

Foreign body in the eye

Etiology   Foreign bodies in the eye are a frequent occurrence in sports and are potentially dangerous.

Symptom and signs   A foreign object produces considerable pain and disability. No attempt should be made to remove the body by rubbing or to remove it with the fingers.

Management   Have the athlete close the eye until the initial pain has subsided, and then attempt to determine if the object is in the vicinity of the upper or lower lid. Foreign bodies in the lower lid are relatively easy to remove by depressing the tissue and then wiping it with a sterile cotton applicator. Foreign bodies in the area of the upper lid are usually much more difficult to localize. Two methods may be used. The first technique is performed as follows: Gently pull the upper eyelid over the lower lid while the subject looks downward. This causes tears to be produced, which may flush the object down onto the lower lid. If this method is unsuccessful, the second technique should be used (see the Focus box on the next page and Figure 25-22). After the foreign particle is removed, the affected eye should be washed with a boric acid solution or with a commercial eyewash. Often after debridement there is a residual soreness, which may be alleviated by the application of petroleum jelly or some other mild ointment. If there is extreme difficulty in removing the foreign body or if it has become embedded in the eye itself, the eye should be closed and "patched" with a gauze pad, which is held in place by strips of tape. The athlete is referred to a physician as soon as possible.

Corneal abrasions

Etiology   An athlete who gets a foreign object in his or her eye will usually try to rub it away. In doing so, the cornea can become abraded.

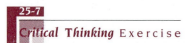

25-7

Critical Thinking Exercise

A wrestler gets a thumb pushed hard into his left eye.

? What symptoms indicate that this may be a serious eye injury?

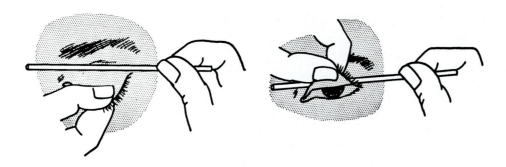

Figure 25-22

Removing a foreign body from the eye.

Symptoms and signs   The athlete will complain of severe pain and watering of the eye, photophobia, and spasm of the orbicular muscle of the eyelid.

Management   The eye should be patched, and the athlete should be sent to a physician. Corneal abrasion is diagnosed through application of a fluorescein strip to the abraded area, staining it a bright green. Once diagnosed the eye is dilated for further assessment. Antibiotic ointment is applied with a semipressure patch placed over the closed eyelid.

Hyphema

Etiology   A blunt blow to the anterior aspect of the eye can produce a hyphema, which is a collection of blood within the anterior chamber. The blood settles inferiorly or may fill the entire chamber. Vision is partially or completely blocked. The athletic trainer must be aware that a hyphema is a major eye injury that can lead to serious problems of the lens, choroid, or retina.

Rupture of the globe

Etiology   A blow to the eye by an object smaller than the eye orbit produces extreme pressure that can rupture the globe. A golf ball or racquetball fits this category; however, larger objects such as a tennis ball or a fist will often fracture the bony orbit before the eye is overly compressed. Even if it does not cause rupture, such a force can cause internal injury that may ultimately lead to blindness.

Symptoms and signs   The athlete complains of severe pain, decreased visual acuity, and diplopia. Inspection reveals irregular pupils, increased intraocular pressure, and orbital leakage.

Management   Treatment requires immediate rest, eye protection with a shield, and antiemetic medication to avoid increasing intraocular pressure. Immediate referral to an ophthalmologist must be made.

25-8

Critical Thinking Exercise

After receiving a blunt blow to her right eye, an athlete has a collection of blood in the anterior chamber.

? What is this type of eye injury and the complications that may follow?

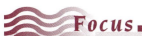

Focus

Removing a foreign body from the eye

Materials needed

One applicator stick, sterile cotton-tipped applicator, eyecup, and eyewash (solution of boric acid).

Position of the athlete

The athlete lies supine on a table.

Procedure

1. Gently pull the eyelid down and place an applicator stick crosswise at its base.
2. Have the athlete look down; then grasp the lashes and turn the lid back over the stick.
3. Holding the lid and the stick in place with one hand, use the sterile cotton swab to lift out the foreign body.

Figure 25-23

A blow to the eye region can detach the retina.

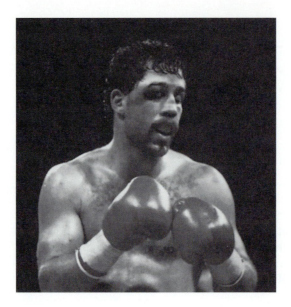

Retinal detachment

Etiology   A blow to the athlete's eye can partially or completely separate the retina from its underlying retinal pigment epithelium. Retinal detachment is more common among athletes who have myopia (nearsightedness).

Symptoms and signs   Detachment is painless; however, early signs include seeing specks floating before the eye, flashes of light, or blurred vision (Figure 25-23). As the detachment progresses, the athlete complains of a "curtain" falling over the field of vision. Any athlete with symptoms of detachment must be immediately referred to an ophthalmologist.

Management   Initially, there is bed rest with patches on both eyes. The athlete should immediately be referred to an ophthalmologist to determine if surgery is required.

Acute conjunctivitis   The conjunctiva is the tissue that lines the back of the eyelid, moves into the space between the eyelid and eye globe, and spreads up over the sclera to the cornea.[1]

Etiology   Acute conjunctivitis is usually caused by various bacteria or allergens. It may begin with conjunctival irritation from wind, dust, smoke, or air pollution. It may also be associated with the common cold or other upper respiratory conditions.

Symptoms and signs   The athlete complains of eyelid swelling, sometimes with a purulent discharge. Itching is associated with allergy. Eyes may burn or itch.

Management   Acute conjunctivitis can be highly infectious. Sodium sulfacetamide 10% is often the treatment of choice.

Hordeolum (sty)   A sty is an infection of the eyelash follicle or the sebaceous gland at the edge of the eyelid.

Etiology   The infection is usually caused by a staphylococcal organism, which has been spread by rubbing or by dust particles.

Symptoms and signs   The condition starts as erythema of the eye. It localizes into a painful pustule within a few days.

Management   Treatment consists of the application of hot, moist compresses and an ointment of 1% yellow oxide or mercury. Recurrent sties require the attention of an ophthalmologist.

Throat Injury

Contusion

Etiology   Blows to the throat do not occur frequently in sports, but occasionally an athlete may receive a kick or blow to the throat. One type of trauma is known as

---

25-9

Critical Thinking Exercise

An athlete develops an eyelash follicle infection.

? What is the cause of this condition, and how should it be treated?

"clotheslining," in which the athlete is struck in the throat region. Such a force could conceivably injure the carotid artery, causing a clot to form that occludes the blood flow to the brain. This same clot could become dislodged and migrate to the brain. In either case, serious brain damage may result.

Symptoms and signs   Immediately after throat trauma the athlete may experience severe pain and spasmodic coughing, speak with a horse voice, and complain of difficulty in swallowing.

Fracture of throat cartilages of the larynx is rare, but it is possible and may be indicated by an inability to breathe and expectoration of frothy blood.[16] Cyanosis may be present. Throat contusions are extremely uncomfortable and are often frightening to the athlete.

Management   If the more severe signs appear, a physician should be called. In most situations cold may be applied intermittently to control superficial hemorrhage and swelling, and after a 24-hour rest period moist hot packs may be applied. For the most severe neck contusions, stabilization with a well-padded collar is beneficial.

SUMMARY

- Injuries to the head are varied. The scalp can sustain soft-tissue injuries; fractures can occur to the skull; and the brain can be contused, concussed, torn, or herniated. Depending on the severity of the concussion, the athlete may display signs of disorientation, dizziness, amnesia, headache, loss of consciousness, problems in concentrating, tinnitus, balance problems, automatism, or pupillary discrepancies.

- Brain concussion is categorized into six grades. In grade 1 the athlete becomes dazed and disoriented. In grade 2 the athlete displays minor confusion caused by a posttraumatic amnesia. There may also be minor dizziness, ringing in the ears, and a dull headache. Grade 3 concussion includes all of the symptoms of grade 2, plus retrograde amnesia. In grade 4 concussion the athlete is "knocked out." Posttraumatic amnesia and retrograde amnesia occur, along with postconcussion syndrome. The grade 5 concussion includes a paralytic coma associated with a secondary cardiorespiratory collapse. A grade 6 concussion is one in which coma leads to death.

- The face is subject to many different types of traumatic sports injuries. The most common are facial wounds, with lacerations ranking at the top. Less common, but usually more serious, are injuries such as jaw fractures and dislocations, dental injuries, and nasal injuries. A potentially disfiguring ear injury is hematoma auris, or cauliflower ear. The eye is also at risk; therefore it is essential that the eye be protected against fast-moving projectiles.

- A throat contusion may occur from a "clotheslining" mechanism or kick. Injury may include carotid artery blood clot and/or a fracture to the throat cartilage.

....

25-10

Critical Thinking Exercise

While carrying the ball, a football back is "clotheslined" and seriously injures his throat.

? What should be the concerns of the athletic trainer in such an injury?

Solutions to *Critical Thinking* EXERCISES

25-1 The athlete's face color is pale and the skin moist, his pulse is rapid with shallow breathing, and his pupils may become dilated.

25-2 The athletic trainer asks the athlete questions that are related to recently acquired information. Examples are the current date, name of last week's opponent, who won that game, and who scored this game's last goal.

25-3 The athlete should be out of play for at least 1 month. After this period he may return to play for 1 week if asymptomatic. The physician may consider terminating the athlete for the rest of the season.

25-4 This athlete is experiencing a postconcussion syndrome. The athlete cannot return completely to his or her sport until cleared by a thorough neurological examination.

25-5 The conscious athlete with a fractured maxilla is transported to the hospital in a forward-leaning position. This position allows external drainage of saliva and blood.

25-6 The athlete sits up with a cold compress placed over the nose and ipsilateral carotid artery. Digital pressure can also be applied to the affected nostril for 5 minutes.

25-7 The symptoms looked for are blurred vision, a loss in the visual field, major pain, and double vision.

25-8 Blood in the anterior eye chamber is known as a hyphema, which could lead to major lens, choroid, or retina problems.

25-9 This sty is caused by a staphylococcal organism that is commonly spread by rubbing or dust particle contamination. It should be managed with hot, moist compresses and a 1% yellow oxide of mercury ointment.

25-10 The compressive force of clotheslining could produce a blood clot in the carotid artery. A large enough force could fracture the larynx, causing a breathing crisis.

REVIEW QUESTIONS AND CLASS ACTIVITIES

1. Pair off with another student, with one acting as the coach or athletic trainer and the other as the injured athlete. The athlete simulates concussions of various grades. The coach or athletic trainer assesses the student, attempting to determine the grade of concussion.
2. List the on-site assessment steps that should be taken when cerebral injuries occur.
3. Demonstrate the following procedures in evaluating a cerebral injury: questioning the athlete, testing eye signs, testing balance, and the finger-to-nose test.
4. List the emergency procedures for treating a serious neck injury.
5. Contrast a grade 2 with a grade 3 concussion.
6. What immediate care procedures should be performed for athletes with facial lacerations?
7. Describe the immediate care procedures that should be performed when a tooth is fractured and when it is dislocated.
8. Describe the procedures that should be performed for an athlete with a nosebleed.
9. How can cauliflower ear be prevented?
10. The eye can sustain an extremely serious injury during some sports activities. What are the major indicators of a possibly serious eye injury?

REFERENCES

1. Berkow R, editor: *The Merck manual,* ed 16, Rahway, NJ, 1992, Merck.
2. Cantu RC: Head and spine injuries in youth sports. In Michelle LJ, editor: *The young athlete. Clinics in sports medicine,* vol 14, no 3, Philadelphia, 1995, Saunders.
3. Cantu RC, Joy R: Second impact syndrome, *Phys Sportsmed* 23(6):27, 1995.
4. Crow RW: Sports-related lacerations, *Phys Sportsmed* 21(2):134, 1993.
5. Curtis SM: Disorders of brain function. In Porth CM, editor: *Pathophysiology,* ed 4, Philadelphia, 1994, Lippincott.
6. Davidson TM, Neuman TR: Managing inflammatory ear conditions, *Phys Sportsmed* 22(8):56, 1994.
7. Davidson TM, Neuman TR: Managing ear trauma, *Phys Sportsmed* 22(7):27, 1994.
8. Eagling EM, Roper-Hall MJ: *Eye injuries: an illustrated guide,* London, 1986, Butterworths.
9. Gennarelli TA, Torg JS: Closed head injuries. In Torg JS, Shephard RJ, editors: *Current therapy in sports medicine,* St Louis, 1995, Mosby.
10. Hargarten KM: Rapid injury assessment, *Phys Sportsmed* 21(2):33, 1993.
11. Henderson JM: Head injuries in sports, *Sports Med Digest* 15(9):1, 1993.
12. Kumamoto DP et al: Oral trauma, *Phys Sportsmed* 23(5):53, 1995.
13. Maddocks DL: The assessment of orientation following concussion in athletes, *Clin J Sports Med* 5(1):32, 1995.
14. Mellion MB et al: Medical problems in athletes. In Birrer RB, editor: *Sports medicine for the primary care physician,* ed 2, Boca Raton, Fla, 1995, CRC Press.
15. McWhorter JM: Concussions and intracranial injuries in athletics, *Ath Train* 25(2):129, 1990.
16. Pashby RC, Pashby TJ: Ocular injuries. In Torg JS, Shephard RJ, editors: *Current therapy in sports medicine,* St Louis, 1995, Mosby.
17. Robinson T, Birrer RB: Ear injuries. In Birrer RB, editor: *Sports medicine for the primary care physician,* ed 2, Boca Raton, Fla, 1995, CRC Press.
18. Robinson T et al: Head injuries. In Birrer RB, editor: *Sports medicine for the primary care physician,* ed 2, Boca Raton, Fla, 1995, CRC Press.
19. Robinson T, Greenberg MD: Nasal injuries. In Birrer RB, editor: *Sports medicine for the primary care physician,* ed 2, Boca Raton, Fla, 1995, CRC Press.
20. Schuller DE, Mountain RE: Auricular injury. In Torg JS, Shephard RJ, editors: *Current therapy in sports medicine,* St Louis, 1995, Mosby.
21. Swenson Jr EJ: Sports medicine emergencies. In Birrer RB, editor: *Sports medicine for the primary care physician,* ed 2, Boca Raton, Fla, 1995, CRC Press.
22. Taylor LP: Neurologic disorders. In Agostini R, editor: *Medical and orthopedic issues of active and athletic women,* Philadelphia, 1994, Hanley & Belfus.
23. Torg JS: Emergency management of head and cervical spine injuries. In Torg JS, Shepard RJ, editors: *Current therapy in sports medicine,* St Louis, 1995, Mosby.
24. Weisberg J, Friedman M: The temporomandibular joint. In Gould J, Davies G, editors: *Orthopaedic and sports physical therapy,* St Louis, 1990, Mosby.
25. Zagelbraum BM: Sports-related eye trauma, *Phys Sportsmed* 21(9):25, 1993.

ANNOTATED BIBLIOGRAPHY

Eagling EM, Roper-Hall MJ: *Eye injuries: an illustrated guide,* London, 1986, Butterworths.

A guide to the recognition and management of eye injuries.

Lehman LB, Ravich SJ: Closed head injuries in athletes. In Hershman EB, editor: *Neurovascular injuries. Clinics in sports medicine,* vol 9, no 2, Philadelphia, 1990, Saunders.

A concise description of cerebral injuries common in sports.

Skin Disorders

When you finish this chapter, you should be able to

- Explain the structure and function of the skin and identify the major lesions that result from skin abnormalities.
- Describe in detail how skin trauma occurs, how it may be prevented, and how it may be managed.
- Identify skin infections that are potentially contagious.
- Describe the correct hygiene practices to use to avoid fungal infections.
- Contrast allergic, thermal, and chemical reactions of the skin.
- Identify infestations and insect bites and contrast them with other skin infections.

It is essential that athletic trainers and coaches understand conditions adversely affecting the skin and mucous membranes, especially highly contagious conditions.

SKIN ANATOMY AND FUNCTION

The skin is the largest organ of the human body. The average adult skin varies in total weight from 6 to 7½ pounds and is from 1/32 to 1/8 inch thick. It is composed of three layers—the epidermis, dermis, and subcutis[19] (Figure 26-1; Table 26-1).

Epidermis

The epidermis has multiple layers. It forms the outer sheath of the body and is composed of the stratum corneum, the pigment melanin, and appendages (hair, nails, and sebaceous and sweat glands). It consists of two types of cells: keratinocytes and melanocytes. As these cells migrate outward toward the surface of the skin, the keratinocytes form the stratum corneum, which offers the greatest skin protection. The epidermis acts as a barrier against invading microorganisms, foreign particles from dirt and debris, chemicals, and ultraviolet rays and also helps contain the body's water and electrolytes. Melanin, produced by melanocytes, protects the body against ultraviolet radiation.

Dermis

The dermis is a skin layer of irregular form, situated underneath the epidermis and composed of connective tissue that contains blood vessels, nerve endings, sweat glands, sebaceous glands, and hair follicles. The dermis forms a series of projections that reach into the epidermis, resulting in an interlocking arrangement and thereby preventing the epidermis from slipping off the dermis.

Hair and Sebaceous Glands

Hair grows from hair follicles contained in the skin. It extends into the dermis, where it is nourished by the blood capillaries. The sebaceous glands, which surround the hair, secrete an oily substance into the hair follicles. Persons who have overactive sebaceous glands may develop blackheads because of plugging of the hair follicle. Small muscles called arrectores pilorum connect to the hair at its root and, when contracted, serve to constrict the hair follicles and cause a "standing-on-end" effect, or goose pimples. Such contractions increase the emission of oil and thereby help protect the body from cold.

Figure 26-1

The skin is the largest organ of the human body, weighing 6 to 7½ pounds in the adult.

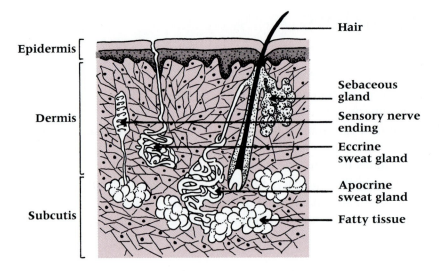

Epidermis

Dermis

Subcutis

Hair

Sebaceous gland

Sensory nerve ending

Eccrine sweat gland

Apocrine sweat gland

Fatty tissue

Sweat Glands

Sweat glands are necessary for cooling the surface of the body and the internal organs. There are two main types of glands: the eccrine glands, which are present at birth and are generally present throughout the skin, and the apocrine glands, which are much larger than the eccrine and mature during adolescence in conjunction with the axillary and pubic hair. Certain individuals with undersecreting sweat glands (dry skin) may be especially susceptible to various diseases. The fluid of the sweat gland contains antibacterial agents that are essential in controlling skin infections.

Nails

The nails are special horny cell structures that come from the phalanges. They are embedded in skin at the base and along their sides and grow approximately ½ inch in 4 months.

Sensory Nerve Endings

Besides its many other functions, the dermis contains sensory nerve endings. These peripheral nerves provide the body with important protective information such as temperature changes and pain.

TABLE 26-1 Outline of the Skin's Structure and Function

Layer	Subregion	Function
Epidermis	Stratum corneum	Prevents intrusion of microorganisms, debris, chemicals, ultraviolet radiation
		Prevents loss of water and electrolytes
		Performs heat regulation for conduction, radiation, convection
	Melanin (pigmentation)	Prevents intrusion of ultraviolet radiation
Dermis		Protects against physical trauma
		Contains sensory nerve endings
		Holds water and electrolytes
	Appendages	Contains eccrine and apocrine sweat glands, hair, nails, sebaceous glands
Subcutis		Stores fat, regulates heat

Subcutis

The subcutis region contains subcutaneous fat. This is the primary area for fat storage, producing internal temperature regulation and mobility of the skin over the internal body core.

SKIN LESIONS DEFINED

Skin that is healthy has a smooth, soft appearance. It is colored by a pigment known as melanin. An increased amount of blood in the skin capillaries may give it a ruddy appearance, and an insufficient amount may give it a pale effect.[1]

The normal appearance of the skin can be altered by external and internal factors. Some changes may be signs of other involvements. The different intensities of paleness or redness of the skin, which is related to the extent of superficial circulation, may be hereditary. Pigment variation may result from an increase of sun exposure or from organic disease; a yellowish discoloration, for example, is indicative of jaundice.

Skin abnormalities may be divided into primary and secondary lesions. Primary lesions include macules, papules, plaques, nodules, tumors, cysts, wheals, vesicles, bullae, and pustules (Figure 26-2; Table 26-2). Secondary lesions usually develop from primary lesions (Figure 26-3; Table 26-3).

MICROORGANISMS AND SKIN INFECTIONS

Skin infections include bacteria, fungi, and viruses.[2]

Bacteria

Bacteria are single-celled microorganisms that can be seen only with a microscope after they are stained with specific dyes. They are of three major shapes: spherical (cocci), which occur in clumps; doublets, or chains, and rods (bacilli); and spirochetes, which are corkscrew shaped.

The three cocci bacteria are staphylococci, which appear in clusters; streptococci, which are divided in chains; and diplococci, which occur in pairs.[12]

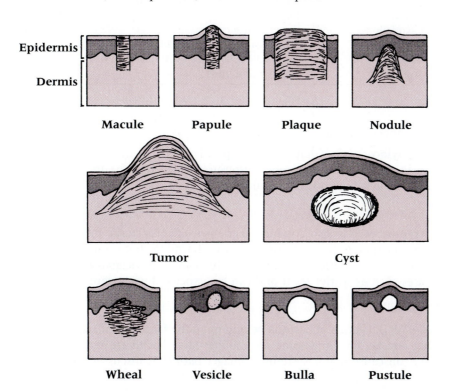

Epidermis
Dermis

Macule   Papule   Plaque   Nodule

Tumor   Cyst

Wheal   Vesicle   Bulla   Pustule

Figure 26-2

Typical primary skin lesions.

TABLE 26-2 **Primary Skin Lesions**

Type	Description	Example
Macule	A small, flat, circular discoloration smaller than 1 cm in diameter	Freckle or flat nevus
Papule	A solid elevation less than 1 cm in diameter	Wart
Plaque or patch	May be a macule or papule larger than 1 cm in diameter	Vitiligo patch (patches of depigmentation)
Nodule	A solid mass less than 1 cm, deeper into the dermis than a papule	Dermatofibroma (fibrosis-tumor–like)
Tumor	Solid mass larger than 1 cm	Cavernous hemangioma (tumor filled with blood vessels)
Cyst	Encapsulated, fluid filled, in dermis or subcutis	Epidermoid cyst
Wheal	A papule or plaque caused by serum collection into the dermis, allergic reactions	Urticaria (hives)
Vesicle	Fluid-filled elevation less than 1 cm, just below epidermis	Smallpox, chickenpox
Bulla	Like a vesicle but larger	Second-degree burn, friction blister
Pustule	Like vesicle or bullae but contains pus	Acne

TABLE 26-3 **Secondary Skin Lesions**

Type	Description	Example
Scales	Flakes of skin	Psoriasis
Crust	Dried fluid or exudates on skin	Impetigo
Fissures	Skin cracks	Chapping
Excoriation	Superficial scrape	Abrasion
Erosion	Loss of superficial epidermis	Scratches (superficial)
Ulcer	Destruction of entire epidermis	Pressure sore
Scar	Healing of dermis	Vaccination, laceration

staphylococcus
Genus of gram-positive bacteria normally present on the skin and in the upper respiratory tract and prevalent in localized infections.

streptococcus
Genus of gram-positive bacteria found in the throat, respiratory tract, and intestinal tract.

Staphylococcus

Staphylococcus is a genus of gram-positive bacteria that commonly appear in clumps on the skin and in the upper respiratory tract. It is the most prevalent cause of infections in which pus is present.

Streptococcus

Streptococcus is also a genus of gram-positive bacteria, but unlike staphylococci, it appears in long chains. Most species are harmless, but some are among the most dangerous bacteria affecting humans. They can be associated with serious systemic diseases such as scarlet fever and can be associated with staphylococci in skin diseases.

Bacillus

Bacillus is a genus of bacteria belonging to the family *Bacillaceae*. They are spore forming and aerobic, and some are mobile. Most bacilli are not pathological; those that are can cause major systemic damage. *Bacillus* is discussed here because of its relationship to the life-threatening disease tetanus, which is introduced through a skin wound. (See the section on punctures later in this chapter.)

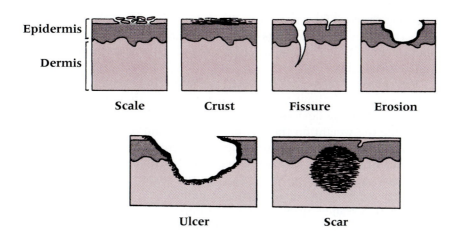

Figure 26-3

Typical secondary skin lesions.

Fungi

Fungi such as mushrooms, yeast, and molds are organisms with a true nucleus that contains chromosomes, but fungi lack chlorophyll and rigid cells walls. In most cases they are not pathogenic; however, some, such as *Trichophyton,* will attack skin, hair, and nails. *Candida,* a yeastlike fungus that is normally part of the flora of the skin, mouth, intestinal tract, and vaginal area, can also lead to a variety of infections.

Viruses

Viruses are minute infectious agents lacking independent metabolism but still having the capacity to reproduce. Reproduction can take place only within a living cell. The individual chemical particle (virion) includes nucleic acid and either deoxyribonucleic acid (DNA) or ribonucleic acid (RNA). The virus can attach to and enter a living cell and may multiply until it kills the cell and bursts out to reinfect other cells. Instead of killing the cell, a budlike growth may occur, with harm to the cell, or the virus may remain within a cell without ever causing an infection.

A number of skin infections are caused by viruses. Two of the most prevalent are herpes virus and the verruca virus.[12] (See Chapters 9 and 27 for discussion of additional viral diseases.)

SKIN TRAUMA

Sports participation can place a great deal of mechanical force on the skin. Mechanical forces that can apply to the skin include friction, compression, shearing, stretching, scraping, tearing, avulsing, and puncturing, all of which can lead to painful and serious injuries.[14]

Friction and Pressure Problems

Excessive rubbing back and forth over the skin, along with abnormal pressure, can cause hypertrophy of the stratum corneum, or horny layer, of the epidermis, especially on the soles of the feet and the palms of the hands. This condition is called *keratoderma.* Another expression for this process is callosity, or **keratosis.** This same mechanism can produce corns and blisters. Usually they occur in association with excessive perspiration (hyperhidrosis).

keratosis
Excessive growth of the horny tissue layer.

Keratosis of the Feet and Hands

Skin, typically the epidermal skin layer, increases in thickness when constant friction and pressure are externally applied. Excessive callus accumulation may occur over bony protuberances.

Etiology Foot calluses may become excessive on an athlete who wears shoes that are too narrow or short. As with the foot, hand calluses can become painful when the subcutaneous fatty layer loses its elasticity, which is an important cushioning effect. The callus moves as a mass when pressure and a shearing force are applied. This movement, coupled with a lack of blood supply, produces rips, tears, cracks, and ultimately infection.

Prevention   Athletes whose shoes are properly fitted but who still develop heavy calluses commonly have foot mechanics problems that may require special orthotics. Special cushioning devices such as wedges, doughnuts, and arch supports may help distribute the weight on the feet more evenly and thus reduce skin stress. Excessive callus accumulation can be prevented by wearing two pairs of socks, a thin cotton or nylon pair next to the skin and a heavy athletic pair over the cotton pair, or a single doubleknit sock; wearing shoes that are the correct size and are in good condition; routinely applying materials such as a lubricant to reduce friction; and shaving the callus with a scalpel, using extreme caution.

Hand calluses can also be controlled by proper toughening procedures and direct protection through the use of a special glove such as is used in batting, or by the application of elastic tape or moleskin. The skin of the hands can be made more resistant to callosity by the routine application of astringents such as tannic acid or by saltwater soaks. In sports such as gymnastics athletic trainers and athletes go to great lengths to protect the athlete's hands against tearing calluses. A protective device is grip, which is a special type of hand covering that may include a wood dowel placed across the grip portion of the hand.

Symptoms and signs   The callus appears as a circumscribed thickening and hypertrophy of the horny layer of the skin. It may be ovular, elongated, brownish, and slightly elevated. Callus may not be painful when pressure is applied.

Management   Athletes who are prone to excess calluses should be encouraged to use an emery callus file after each shower. Massaging small amounts of lanolin into devitalized calluses once or twice a week after practice may help maintain some tissue elasticity. Once excessive formation has occurred, a keratolytic ointment, such as Whitefield's ointment, may be applied. Salicylic acid, 5% to 10%, in a flexible collodion, applied at night and peeled off in the morning, has also been beneficial. Before application of a keratolytic ointment, the athletic trainer might manually decrease the calluses' thickness by carefully pairing with a sharp scalpel, sanding, or pumicing the surface. Great care should be taken not to totally remove the callus and the protection it affords a pressure point. A donut pad may be cut to size and placed on a pressure point to prevent pain.

Blisters

Like calluses, blisters are often a major problem of sports participation, especially early in the season. Shearing forces produce a raised area that contains a fluid collection below or within the epidermis.

Etiology   Blisters are particularly associated with rowing, pole vaulting, basketball, football, and weight events in track and field, such as the shot put and discus. Such activities commonly cause the skin to be subjected to horizontal shearing, which produces a friction blister.

Prevention   Soft feet and hands, coupled with shearing skin stress, can produce severe blisters. A dusting of talcum powder or the application of petroleum jelly can protect the skin against abnormal friction. Wearing tubular socks or two pairs of socks, as for preventing calluses, is also desirable, particularly for athletes who have sensitive feet or feet that perspire excessively. Wearing the correct-size shoe is essential. The shoes must be broken in before they are worn for long periods of time. If, however, a friction area ("hot spot") does arise, the athlete has several options. The athlete can cover the irritated skin with a friction-reducing material such as petroleum jelly, place a "blanked-out" piece of tape tightly over the irritated area, or cover it with a piece of moleskin (Figure 26-4). Another method that has proved effective against blisters is the application of ice over skin areas that have developed abnormal friction.

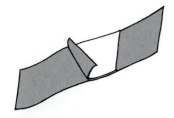

Figure 26-4

A blanked-out tape to prevent a blister.

Symptoms and signs   The athlete normally will feel a hot spot, a sharp, burning sensation as the blister is formed, and the area of sensation should be examined immediately. The blister may be superficial, containing clear liquid. On the other hand, a blood blister may form in which deeper tissue is disrupted, causing blood vessels to rupture. Pain is caused by the pressure of the fluid.

Management   As stated previously, blister prevention is of paramount importance. Once developed, blisters can be a serious problem for the athlete, as well as for the athletic trainer. The following are general rules for managing a blister (OSHA standards must be followed; see Chapter 9):

- The intact blister:
  1. Leave the blister intact for the first 24 hours. Often during that time, many of the symptoms will lessen.
  2. If the blister is large and in a place on the skin that will be continually irritated, clean it thoroughly with antiseptic soap.
  3. With a sterile scalpel, cut a small incision ⅛ to ¼ inch long in the blister along the periphery of the raised tissue. The hole should be large enough that it will not become sealed.
  4. Disperse the fluid by applying a pressure pad, keeping the pad in place to prevent refilling.
  5. Once the fluid has been removed, clean the area again with an antiseptic such as povidone-iodine (Betadine) and cover it with an antibiotic ointment such as Polysporin.
  6. Place a doughnut pad around the dressed blister to avoid further irritation.
  7. Monitor the blistered area daily for the possibility of infection. If infection occurs, refer the athlete to a physician immediately.
  8. Replace the dressing if it becomes wet from fluid seepage. A wet environment encourages growth of staphylococci bacteria and therefore infection.
  9. When the tenderness is completely gone (in approximately 5 to 6 days), denude the area; however, remove no skin if any tenderness persists.
- The open (torn) blister:
  1. Keep the open blister clean to avoid infection. In the beginning of management, carefully and thoroughly wash with soap and water. Once cleaned, apply hydrogen peroxide, benzalkonium chloride, or a combination with a betadine solution. If the blister site is torn along less than one half of its diameter, apply a liquid antiseptic and allow to dry, then apply an antibiotic ointment.
  2. Lay the flap of skin back over the treated tissue; then apply a sterile, nonadhering dressing and a doughnut pad.
  3. As when managing the intact blister, monitor the open blister daily for the possibility of infection.
- The completely denuded blister:
  1. If the blister is torn ½ inch or more, completely remove the flap of skin, using sterile scissors.
  2. Completely clean the exposed tissue with soap and water. Apply an antiseptic liquid such as benzalkonium with occlusive dressing.[7]
  3. If the athlete has completed his or her activity, apply the "second-skin" dressing by Spenco (Spenco Medical Corporation, Waco, Texas) to the raw area. When applied, this gel ensures healing through the night.

Soft Corns and Hard Corns

Soft corns and hard corns are other examples of keratoses caused by abnormal skin pressure and friction.

Etiology   A hard corn (clavus durus) is the most serious type of corn. It is caused by the pressure of improperly fitting shoes, the same mechanism that causes calluses. Hammertoes and hard corns are usually associated with the hard corns that form on the tops of deformed toes (Figure 26-5, *A*). Symptoms are local pain and disability,

26-1

Critical Thinking Exercise

A basketball player wearing new shoes during a game sustains a completely denuded blister on the back of her heel.

? How should this condition be managed during and after the game?

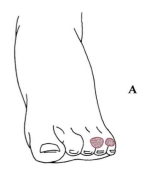

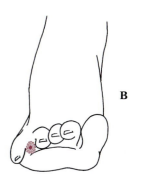

Figure 26-5

A, Hard corn (clavus durus).
B, Soft corn (clavus mollis).

with inflammation and thickening of soft tissue. Because of the chronic nature of this condition, it requires a physician's care.

A soft corn (clavus mollis) is the result of the combination of wearing narrow shoes and having excessive foot perspiration. It is also associated with an exostosis. Because of the pressure of the shoe coupled with the exudation of moisture, the corn usually forms between the fourth and fifth toes (Figure 26-5). A circular area of thickened, white, macerated skin appears between the toes at the base of the proximal head of the phalanges. Both pain and inflammation are likely to be present.[4]

macerated skin
Skin softened by exposure to water.

Prevention   The primary way to prevent a soft or hard corn is to wear properly fitted shoes. Soft corns can be avoided by wearing shoes that are wide enough. Conversely, hard corns can be avoided by wearing shoes that are long enough.

Symptoms and signs   With a soft corn, the athlete complains of pain between the fourth and fifth toes. During inspection, the soft corn appears as a circular piece of thickened, white, **macerated skin** between the fourth and fifth toes at the base of the proximal head of the phalanges. In contrast, a hard corn is on the tops of hammertoes. The bony prominence of the toe is forced up, and it presses on the inner tops of the shoe, causing the corn to form. It appears hard and dry, with a callus that is sharply demarcated.

Management   The corn is difficult to manage. If pain and inflammation are major, referral to a podiatrist for surgical removal may be advisable. The athletic trainer may ameliorate the condition by having the athlete wear properly fitting shoes and socks and may alleviate further irritation of the corn by protecting it with a small felt pad or sponge pad, which can act as a buffer between the shoe and the toe.

In caring for a soft corn the best procedure is to have the athlete wear properly fitting shoes, keep the skin between the toes clean and dry, decrease pressure by keeping the toes separated with cotton or lamb's wool, and apply a keratolytic agent such as 40% salicylic acid in liquid or plasters.

Excessive Perspiration

Excessive perspiration can be a cause of serious skin irritation.

Excessive perspiration (hyperhidrosis) occurs in a small segment of the population. This problem can make the handling of sports objects difficult, causing both performance and safety problems. Emotional excitement often makes the situation worse. The chemical composition of hyperhidrotic perspiration from palms is syruplike in appearance and extremely high in sodium chloride. This problem also increases the possibility of skin irritations and often makes adherence of bandages difficult, especially where adhesive tape is necessary. The condition makes callus development, blisters, and intertrigo (chafing) much more likely to occur. Treatment of excessive perspiration should include using an astringent such as alcohol or an absorbent powder (see the Focus box on the next page).

Chafing of the Skin

Chafing (intertrigo) of the skin is another condition that stems from friction or from rubbing the skin unduly.

Etiology   Chafing occurs particularly in athletes who are obese or heavy limbed. It results from friction and maceration (softening) of the skin in a climate of heat and moisture.

Symptoms and signs   Repeated skin rubbing, as in the groin and axilla, can separate the keratin from the granular layer of the epidermis. This separation causes oozing wounds that develop into crusting and cracking lesions.

Prevention   To prevent intertrigo keep the skin dry, clean, and friction free. For groin conditions the athlete should wear loose, soft, cotton underwear. A male athlete should wear his supporter over a pair of loose cotton boxer shorts.

Management   The chafed area should be cleansed once daily with mild soap and lukewarm water. Treatment of a chafed area includes wet packs, using a medicated

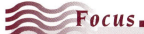

Focus

Foot hygiene for excessive perspiration and odor

Before practice

1. Apply an astringent such as 20% aluminum chloride in anhydrous ethyl alcohol (Drysol) to the skin and allow it to air-dry.
2. Next, liberally apply a powder such as talcum, alum, or boric acid to the skin, socks, and sports footwear.

After practice

1. After thoroughly washing and drying the feet, the same procedure is followed as before practice. An astringent is applied to the skin and an absorbent powder is applied to street socks and shoes.
2. Footwear should be changed frequently.
3. Sports footwear should be liberally powdered after practice to absorb moisture during storage. Ideally, a different pair of shoes should be worn daily.

---

solution such as Burrows for 15 to 20 minutes, three times daily. This is followed by the application of a 1% hydrocortisone cream.

Xerotic (Dry) Skin

Dry skin is a condition that athletes commonly experience during the winter months.[11]

Etiology   Athletes who are exposed to weather and bathe often commonly develop dry or chapped skin. The drying cold of winter tends to dehydrate the stratum corneum. Some athletes naturally may have less skin lipids, which increases the tendency to increase water loss.[11] A decrease in humidity along with cold winds causes the skin to lose water.

Symptoms and signs   The skin appears dry with variable redness and scaling. It occurs first on the shins, forearm, back of the hands, and face. There may be itching. The skin may crack and develop fissures.

Management   The major goals in treatment are to prevent water loss and replace lost water.[11] The following treatment procedures should be followed:

- Bathe in tepid water and shower one time per day.
- Use moisturizing soaps such as Dove or Aveeno. Avoid soaping dry areas. Restrict washing to genitalia, underarms, hands, feet, and face.
- Use emollient lotions, which hydrate the skin. They should be applied after each washing.
- When the condition is more severe the athlete should be referred to a physician for antipruritics, alpha-hydroxy acids, and perhaps topical corticosteroids.[11]

Ingrown Toenails

An ingrown toenail is a common condition among athletes. The large toe is the most often affected. The nail grows into the lateral nailfold and enters the skin.[6]

Etiology   In general, the ingrown nail results from the lateral pressure from poorly fitting shoes, improper toenail trimming, or trauma such as repeated pressure from sliding to the front of the shoe (Color Plate, Figure A).

Prevention   Because of the handicapping nature of this condition, prevention of ingrown toenails is much preferred over management. Properly fitted shoes and socks are essential. The toenails should be trimmed weekly by cutting straight across, avoiding rounding so that the margins do not penetrate the tissue on the side (Figure 26-6).

26-2

Critical Thinking Exercise

A heavy-limbed shot-putter complains of a skin irritation in his groin region. The area appears red and macerated. Some of the tissue is cracked, and there are oozing sores.

? How could this chafing have been prevented?

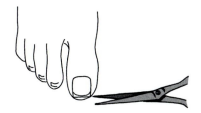

Figure 26-6

Preventing an ingrown toenail requires proper trimming.

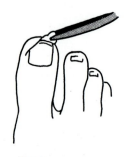

Figure 26-7

Application of a wisp of cotton under the ingrown side.

The nail should be left sufficiently long so that it is clear of the underlying skin, but it should be cut short enough so as not to irritate the skin by pushing against shoes or socks.

Symptoms and signs   The first indications of an ingrown toenail are pain and swelling. If not treated early, the penetrated skin becomes severely inflamed and purulent. The lateral nailfold is swollen and irritated.

Management   There are a number of ways to manage the ingrown toenail. If it is in the first stages of inflammation, more conservative approach can be taken.

- Soak the inflamed toe in hot water (110° to 120°F) for approximately 20 minutes.
- After soaking, the nail will be soft and pliable and may be pried out of the skin. Using sterile forceps or scissors, lift the nail from the soft tissue and insert a piece of cotton to keep the nail out of the skin (Figure 26-7). This also relieves the pain. Perform this procedure daily until the corner of the nail has grown past the irritated tissue.

If the condition becomes chronically irritated, a more aggressive approach is likely to be taken by a physician.

- After applying an antiseptic (e.g., 1% or 2% lidocaine), slip the nail-splitting scissor under the ingrown nail.[9]
- With the scissor inserted to the point of resistance, cut away and remove the wedge-shaped nail. Also remove the granulation tissue in the area. Keep a moist antiseptic compress in place until the inflammation has subsided.
- Athletes with recurrent ingrown nails may require the use of phenol for permanent destruction of the lateral portion of the nail.

Skin Bruises

The consequence of a sudden compressive, blunt force to the skin is a bruise. The skin is not broken, but the soft tissue is traumatized. A first-degree bruise (ecchymosis) causes, in most cases, broken blood vessels and discoloration (black and blue). A great force affects the underlying structures, producing a bone or muscle contusion. Rest, ice, compression, and elevation (RICE) is the treatment of choice to control the hemorrhage that may occur.

Wounds

Traumatic skin lesions, commonly termed *wounds,* are extremely prevalent in sports; abrasions, lacerations, and punctures are daily occurrences (Figure 26-8). To avoid infection, any wound, no matter how slight, must be cared for immediately (Table 26-4). In general all wounds must be cleansed with soap and water to rid them of microorganism contamination. After cleansing, a dressing containing an antiseptic is applied. However, if the wound is to be examined by a physician, no medication should be added to the dressing. Most lacerations and puncture wounds should be treated by a physician. Uninfected abrasions are not usually referred to a physician. They are managed by debridement and thorough cleansing with soap and water, followed by the application of an occlusive dressing.[8] Using an ointment prevents accumulation of a crust and secondary infection. It is advisable that abrasions heal from the inside out to avoid the formation of scabs, which serve only to cover infected areas and are easily torn off by activity. (See Chapter 9.)

Abrasions

Abrasions are common and occur when the skin is scraped against a rough surface. The top layer of skin is worn away, thus exposing numerous blood capillaries. This general exposure, with dirt and foreign materials scraping and penetrating the skin, increases the probability of infection unless the wound is properly debrided and cleansed.

Signs of infection:

   Appear 2 to 7 days after injury

   Red, swollen, hot, and tender wound

   Swollen and painful lymph glands near the area of infection (groin, axilla, or neck)

   Mild fever and headache

26-3

Critical Thinking Exercise

A baseball player slides into second base and sustains a serious slide burn on his left side.

? What are the major concerns with this type of injury, and how should it be managed?

COMMON BACTERIAL INFECTIONS

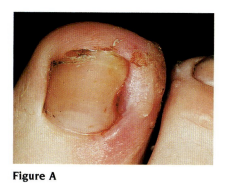

Figure A

Ingrown toenail.

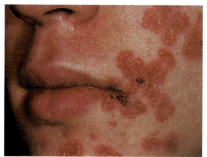

Figure B

Impetigo contagiosa.

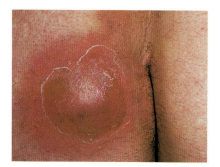

Figure C

Furuncle.

COMMON FUNGAL INFECTIONS

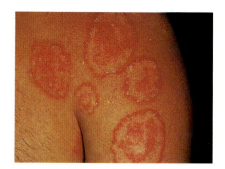

Figure D

Tinea of the body (tinea corporis).

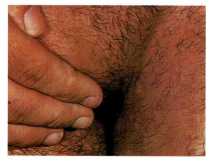

Figure E

Tinea of the groin (tinea cruris).

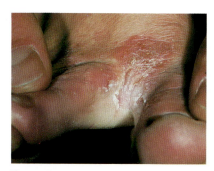

Figure F

Athlete's foot (tinea pedis).

COMMON VIRAL INFECTIONS

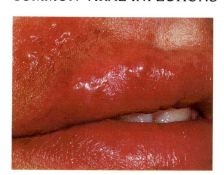

Figure G

Herpes simplex labialis.

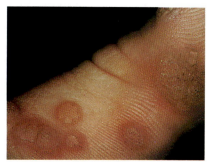

Figure H

Common warts.

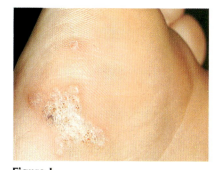

Figure I

Plantar warts on ball of foot.

COMMON SKIN REACTIONS

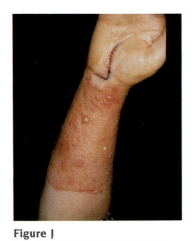

Figure J

Contact dermatitis.

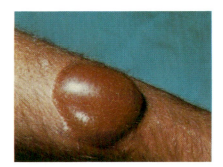

Figure K

Cold reaction.

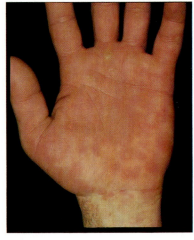

Figure L

Hives.

COMMON SEXUALLY TRANSMITTED INFECTIONS

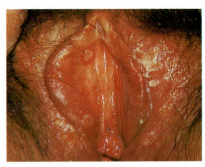

Figure M

Genital herpes simplex.

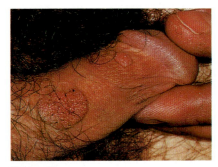

Figure N

Genital warts.

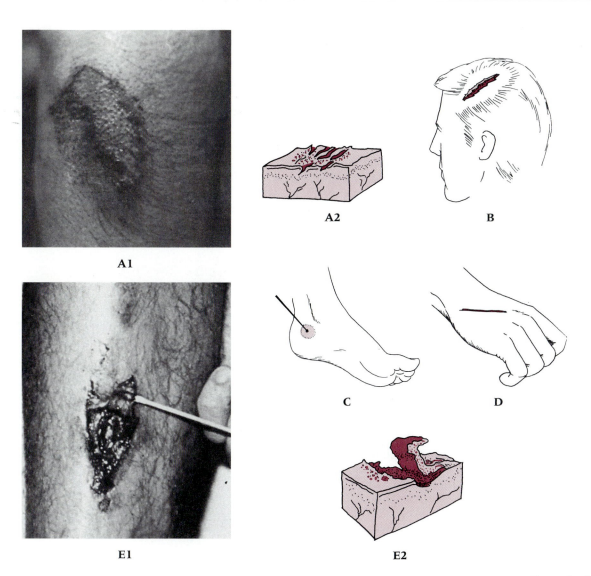

Figure 26-8

Wounds occurring in sports can present a serious problem of infection. **A1** and **A2,** Abrasion. **B,** Laceration. **C,** Puncture. **D,** Incision. **E1** and **E2,** Avulsion.

Punctures

Puncture wounds can easily occur during physical activities and can be fatal. Direct penetration of tissues by a pointed object such as a track shoe spike can introduce the tetanus bacillus into the bloodstream, possibly making the athlete a victim of lock-jaw. All puncture wounds and severe lacerations should be referred immediately to a physician.[15]

Lacerations

Lacerations are also common in sports and occur when a sharp or pointed object tears the tissues, giving the wound the appearance of a jagged-edged cavity. Also, blunt trauma over a sharp bone can cause a wound that is similar in appearance to a laceration. As with abrasions, lacerations present an environment conducive to severe infection. The same mechanism that causes a laceration can also cause a skin avulsion, in which a piece of skin is completely ripped from its source. Specific lacerations are discussed in the body regions they occur.

Skin Avulsions

Avulsion wounds occur when skin is torn from the body; they are frequently associated with major bleeding. The avulsed tissue should be placed on moist gauze that is

TABLE 26-4 **Care of Open Wounds**

Type of Wound	Action of Coach or Athletic Trainer	Initial Care	Follow-Up Care
Abrasion	Provide initial care. Wound seldom requires medical attention unless infected.	Cleanse abraded area with mild Ivory soap and water; debride with brush. Apply solution of hydrogen peroxide over abraded area; continue until foaming has subsided. Follow with Betadine. Apply medicated ointment such as J & J first aid cream to keep abraded surface moist—in sports, it is not desirable for abrasions to acquire a scab. Place a nonadhering sterile pad (Telpha pad) over the ointment.	Change dressing daily; look for signs of infection.
Laceration	Cleanse around wound; avoid wiping more contaminating agents into the area. Apply dry, sterile compress pad; refer to physician.	Complete cleansing and suturing are performed by physician; injections of tetanus toxoid are given if needed.	Change dressing daily; look for signs of infection.
Puncture	Cleanse around wound; avoid wiping more contaminating agents into the area. Apply dry, sterile compress pad; refer to physician.	Complete cleansing and injections of tetanus toxoid, if needed, are performed by physician.	Change dressing daily; look for signs of infection.
Incision	Clean around wound. Apply dry, sterile compress pad to control bleeding; refer to physician.	Cleanse wound. Suturing and injection of tetanus toxoid, if needed, are performed by physician.	Change dressing daily; look for signs of infection.
Avulsion	Clean around wound; save avulsed tissue. Apply dry, sterile compress pad to control bleeding; refer to physician.	Wound is cleansed thoroughly; avulsed skin is replaced and sutured by a physician; tetanus toxoid injection is administered if needed.	Change dressing daily; look for signs of infection.

preferably saturated with saline solution. The tissue and gauze are put into a plastic bag that is then immersed in cold water and taken, along with the athlete, to the hospital for reattachment.

Skin Incisions

Incisions are clearly cut wounds that often occur where a blow has been delivered over a sharp bone or over a bone that is poorly padded. They are not as serious as the other types of exposed wounds.

Infection

tetanus (lockjaw)
An acute, often fatal condition characterized by tonic muscular spasm, hyperreflexia, and lockjaw.

Tetanus   Tetanus (lockjaw) is an acute disease causing fever and convulsions. Tonic spasm of skeletal muscles is always a possibility for any nonimmunized athlete. The tetanus bacillus enters an open wound as a spore and, depending on individual susceptibility, acts on the motor end plate of the central nervous system. After initial childhood immunization by tetanus toxoid, boosters should be given every 10 years. An athlete not immunized should receive an injection of tetanus immune globulin (Hyper-Tet) immediately after injury.

WOUND DRESSINGS

A **bandage,** when properly applied, can contribute decidedly to recovery from sports injuries. Bandages carelessly or improperly applied can cause discomfort, allow wound contamination, or even hamper repair and healing. In all cases bandages must be firmly applied—neither so tight that circulation is impaired nor so loose that the **dressing** is allowed to slip. (See Chapter 13.) Skin lesions are extremely prevalent in sports; abrasions, lacerations, and puncture wounds are almost daily occurrences. It is of the utmost importance to the well-being of the athlete that open wounds be cared for immediately. All wounds, even those that are relatively superficial, must be considered contaminated by microorganisms and therefore must be cleansed, medicated (when called for), and dressed. Wound dressing requires a sterile environment to prevent infections. Individuals who perform wound management in sports often do not follow good principles of cleanliness. To alleviate this problem one must adhere to standard procedures in the prevention of wound contamination.

bandage
A strip of cloth or other material used to cover a wound.

dressing
Covering, protective or supportive, that is applied to an injury or wound.

Training Room Practices in Wound Care

The following are suggested procedures to use in the athletic training room to cut down the possibility of wound infections. See Table 26-4 for more specific suggestions regarding the care of external wounds.

1. Make sure all instruments such as scissors, tweezers, and swabs are sterilized.
2. Clean hands thoroughly.
3. Clean in and around a skin lesion thoroughly.
4. Place a nonmedicated dressing over a lesion if the athlete is to be sent for medical attention.
5. Avoid touching any part of a sterile dressing that may come in contact with a wound.
6. Place medication on a pad rather than directly on a lesion.
7. Secure the dressing with tape or a wrap; always avoid placing pressure directly over a lesion.

In caring for wounds that involve bleeding and other body fluids, the athletic trainer must be concerned with the chance of becoming infected by the human immunodeficiency virus (HIV) or hepatitis B. (See Chapter 9 for OSHA standards on wound care.)

BACTERIAL INFECTIONS

Bacteria are single-celled, plantlike microorganisms that lack chlorophyll and may destroy blood cells. Bacterial infections are common complications of skin insults. Most of them are associated with strains of staphylococci and streptococci, particularly the *Staphylococcus aureus* strain, with the resultant production of purulent matter.

Athletes with bacterial infections associated with pus may pass the infection onto other athletes through direct contact.

Impetigo Contagiosa

Impetigo contagiosa is an extremely common skin disease, primarily observed in young adults, with the greatest number of cases occurring in late summer and early fall.

Etiology   Impetigo contagiosa is caused by group A beta-hemolytic streptococci, *S. aureus*, or a combination of these two bacteria. It is spread rapidly when athletes are in close contact with one another. Wrestling is a sport that is particularly at risk for spreading this disease.[18]

Symptoms and signs   Impetigo contagiosa is first characterized by mild itching and soreness, which are followed by the eruption of small vesicles that form into pustules and later yellow crustations (Color Plate, Figure B). Up to 20% of people carry staphylococcus areus in and about their nostrils. In general impetigo develops in body folds that are subject to friction.[16]

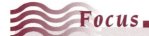

Focus

Management   Impetigo usually responds rapidly to proper treatment. This treatment consists of thorough cleansing of the crusted area, followed by the application of a topical antibacterial agent such as Bactroban (see the Focus box above). Systemic antibiotics also are used.

Furuncles and Carbuncles

Two major skin problems affecting athletes are furuncles and carbuncles. Both, if traumatized, could lead to a serious systemic infection.

Furunculosis

Furuncles (boils) are common among athletes.

Etiology   Furuncles and carbuncles are complications of folliculitis resulting from friction or blunt trauma. The predominant infectious organisms are staphylococci, which produce a pustule.

Symptoms and signs   The areas of the body most affected are the back of the neck, the face, and the buttocks. The pustule becomes enlarged, reddened, and hard from internal pressure. As pressure increases, extreme pain and tenderness develop (Color Plate, Figure C). Most furuncles will mature and rupture spontaneously, emitting the contained pus. NOTE: Furuncles should not be squeezed, because squeezing forces the infection into adjacent tissue or extends it to other skin areas.[10] Furuncles on the face can be dangerous, particularly if they drain into veins that lead to venous sinuses of the brain. Such conditions should immediately be referred to a physician.

Management   Care of the furuncle involves protecting it from additional irritation, referring the athlete to a physician for antibiotic treatment, and keeping the athlete from contact with other team members while the boil is draining. The common practice of hot dressings or special drawing salves is not beneficial to the maturation of the boil.

Carbuncles

Etiology   Carbuncles are similar to furuncles in their early stages, having also developed from staphylococci.

Symptoms and signs   The principal difference between it and a furuncle is that the carbuncle is larger and deeper and usually has several openings in the skin. It may produce fever and elevation of the white cell count. A carbuncle starts as a painful node that is covered by tight, reddish skin that later becomes very thin. The site of greatest occurrence is the back of the neck, where it appears early as a dark red, hard area and then in a few days emerges into a lesion that discharges yellowish-red pus from a number of places.

One must be aware of the dangers inherent in carbuncles—they may result in the athlete's developing an internal infection or may spread to adjacent tissue or to other athletes.

26-4

Critical Thinking Exercise

A wrestler first experiences a mild itching and soreness in his left axillary region. Later, small pustules form that develop into yellow crusts.

? How should the athletic trainer handle this problem?

Management   The most common treatment is surgical drainage combined with the administration of antibiotics. A warm compress is applied to promote circulation to the area.

Folliculitis

Folliculitis is an infection of the hair follicle. It is most prevalent in the hair follicles of the beard and the scalp (Figure 26-9). However, it can occur anywhere that hair exists on the body.

Etiology   Folliculitis can be caused by comedones (blackheads) or, more commonly, by the "ingrown" hair, which grows inward and curls up to form an infected nodule. The infection occurs most often in areas in which hair is shaved or rubs against clothing, such as the neck, face, buttocks, or thigh.[16]

Many hair follicles may become involved through the extension of infection to contiguous sebaceous glands. Such spreading causes a general condition called *sycosis vulgaris,* or "barber's itch." It frequently occurs on the upper lip and forms a red, swollen area, exhibiting tenderness during palpation. Pus collects around the exposed hair, making the hair easy to remove. Sycosis vulgaris should always be referred to a physician for treatment.

Symptoms and signs   The condition starts with inflammation, followed by development of a papule or pustule at the mouth of the hair follicle. This is followed by development of a crust that may later slough off along with the hair. A deeper infection may cause scarring and permanent baldness (alopecia) in that area. The most common microorganism associated with this condition is staphylococcus.

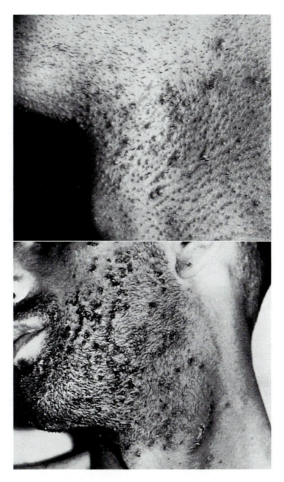

Figure 26-9

Folliculitis.

Management   The management of acute folliculitis is similar to that of impetigo. Moist heat is applied intermittently to increase local circulation. Antibiotic medication may be applied locally, as well as systemically, depending on the scope of the condition.

Hidradenitis Suppurativa

Hidradenitis suppurativa is a chronic inflammatory condition of the apocrine glands or large sweat glands commonly found in the acilla, scrotum, labia majora, and nipples.

Etiology   The exact cause of this condition is unclear. Most authorities believe it is caused by blockage of the apocrine gland ducts as a result of an inflammation. Some authorities believe it is a keratinous plug of a hair follicle. The role of bacteria is not exactly known.

Symptoms and signs   The condition begins as a small papule and grows to the size of a small tumor that is filled with purulent material. Deep dermal inflammation can occur, resulting in large abscesses that result in bands of scar tissue.[6] The contents of this lesion are highly infectious to the athlete and when discharged can infect other members of the team.

Management   Treatment of this problem includes avoiding the use of antiperspirants, deodorants, and shaving creams; using medicated soaps such as those containing chlorhexidine or povidone-iodine (Betadine); and applying a prescribed antibiotic lotion.

Acne Vulgaris

Acne vulgaris is an inflammatory disease that involves the hair follicles and the sebaceous glands. It occurs near puberty and usually is less active after adolescence. Acne is characterized by blackheads, cysts, and pustules.

Etiology   Although most adolescents experience some form of acne, only a few develop an extremely disfiguring case (Figure 26-10). Its cause is not definitely known, but it has been suggested that sex hormone imbalance may be the major causal factor.

Symptoms and signs   Acne begins as an improper functioning of the sebaceous glands with the formation of blackheads and inflammation, which in turn produces pustules on the face, neck, and back in varying depths. The superficial lesions usually dry spontaneously, whereas the deeper ones may become chronic and form disfiguring scars.[6]

The athlete with a serious case of acne vulgaris has a scarring disease and because of it may have serious emotional problems. The individual may become nervous, shy, and even antisocial, with feelings of inferiority in interpersonal relations with peer groups. The athletic trainer's major responsibility in aiding athletes with acne is to help the athlete perform the wishes of the physician and to give constructive guidance and counsel.[6]

Management   The care of acne is usually symptomatic, with the majority of cases following a similar pattern, including hormone therapy given by a physician and a routine of washing three times daily with a mild soap, followed by the application of a drying agent. Other methods may be required such as the nightly application of keratolytic lotions (sulfur zinc or sulfur resorcinol), individual drainage of crusts or blackheads by the physician, and ultraviolet treatment.

Paronychia and Onychia

Fingernails and toenails are continually subject to injury and infection in sports. A common infection is paronychia, which is a purulent infection of the skin surrounding the nail (Figure 26-11).

Etiology   Paronychia and onychia develop from staphylococci, streptococci, and fungal organisms that accompany the contamination of open wounds or hangnails. It is common in football linemen, who regularly stick their fingers in dirt.

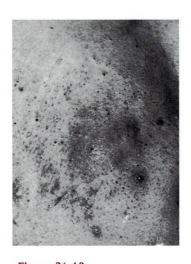

Figure 26-10

Acne vulgaris.

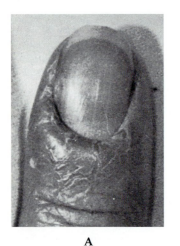

A

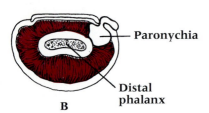

Paronychia

Distal
phalanx

B

Figure 26-11

A, Paronychia is a common infection of the skin surrounding the nail. **B,** Cross section of finger.

Symptoms and signs   Acute paronychia has a rapid onset, with painful, bright red swelling of the proximal and lateral nail. An accumulation of purulent material occurs behind the cuticle.[6] The infection may spread and cause onychia, an inflammation of the nail bed.

Management   One should recognize paronychia early and have the athlete soak the affected finger or toe in a hot solution of Epsom salts or boric acid three times daily. A medicated ointment, preferably penicillin or 5% ammoniated mercury, should be applied between soakings. Every protection must be given the infected nail while the athlete is competing. Uncontrollable paronychia may require medical intervention, consisting of pus removal through a skin incision or the removal of a portion of the infected nail.

FUNGAL INFECTIONS

Fungi cause several of the skin diseases found among athletes because sports produce an environment, at times, that is beneficial to their cultivation. Fungi grow best in unsanitary conditions combined with warmth, moisture, and darkness. Three categories of superficial fungal infections are discussed: dermatophytes, candidiasis (moniliasis), and tinea versicolor. The fungus attacks mainly the keratin of the epidermis but may go as deep as the dermis through hair follicles. These organism are given the common name of ringworm (tinea) and are classified according to the area of the body infected. Infection takes place within superficial keratinized tissue such as hair, skin, and nails. The extremely contagious spores of these fungi may be spread by direct contact, contaminated clothing, or dirty locker rooms and showers.

Dermatophytes (Ringworm Fungi)

Etiology   Dermatophytes, also known as *ringworm fungi,* are the cause of most skin, nail, and hair fungal infections. They belong to three genera: *Microsporum, Trichophyton,* and *Epidermophyton.*

Tinea of the Scalp (Tinea Capitis)

Symptoms and signs   Tinea (ringworm) of the scalp (tinea capitis), beginning as a small papule of the scalp and spreading peripherally, is most common among children. The lesions appear as small grayish scales, resulting in scattered bald patches. The primary sources of tinea capitis infection are contaminated animals, barber clippers, hairbrushes, and combs.

tinea (ringworm)
Common name given to many superficial fungal infections of the skin.

Management   Griseofulvin is usually the treatment of choice. It is given in small doses over a period of time or in one large dose. A topical cream such as 1% clotrimazole (Micatin, Tinactin) may be used to help prevent the spread of the disease.

Tinea of the Body (Tinea Corporis)

Symptoms and signs   Tinea of the body (tinea corporis) mainly involves the upper extremities and the trunk. The lesions are characterized by ring-shaped, reddish, vesicular areas that may be scaly or crusted (Color Plate, Figure D) Excessive perspiration and friction increase susceptibility to the condition.

Management   Treatment usually consists of antifungal medication such as 2% miconaxole cream or 1% clotrimazole cream or lotion.

Tinea of the Nail (Tinea Unguium)

Symptoms and signs   Tinea of the nail (tinea unguium) is a fungus infection of the toenails and fingernails. It is often seen among athletes who are involved in water sports or who have chronic athlete's foot. Trauma predisposes the athlete to infection. It is often difficult for a physician to determine accurately what is the real cause of the disease. Many different organisms can adversely affect the nail plate. When infected, the nail becomes thickened, brittle, and separated from its bed (Figure 26-12).

Management   The treatment of tinea unguium can be difficult. Oral therapy has not been found effective, and topical creams of lotions do not penetrate the nail. Sur-

Figure 26-12

Tinea of the nail (tinea unguium).

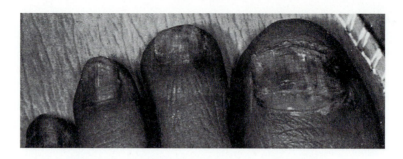

Figure 26-13

When managing a fungal infection it is essential to break the chain of infection.

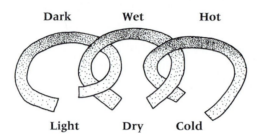

Dark   Wet   Hot

Light   Dry   Cold

gical removal of the nail may have to be performed on the athlete with extremely infected nails.[13]

Tinea of the Groin (Tinea Cruris)

Etiology   Tinea of the groin (tinea cruris), more commonly called jock itch, appears as a bilateral and often symmetrical brownish or reddish lesion resembling the outline of a butterfly in the groin area.

Symptoms and signs   The athlete complains of mild to moderate itching, resulting in scratching and the possibility of a secondary bacterial infection (Color Plate, Figure E).

Management   One must be able to identify lesions of tinea cruris and handle them accordingly. Conditions of this type must be treated until cured (Figure 26-13). Infection not responding to normal management must be referred to the team physician. Most ringworm infections will respond to many of the nonprescription medications that contain such ingredients as undecylenic acid, triacetin, or propionate-caprylate compound, which are available as aerosol sprays, liquids, powders, or ointments. Powder, because of its absorbent qualities, should be the only medication vehicle used in the groin area. Medications that are irritating or tend to mask the symptoms of a groin infection must be avoided.

Atypical or complicated groin infection must receive medical attention. Many prescription medications that may be applied topically or orally and have dramatic effects on skin fungus are presently on the market.

Athlete's Foot (Tinea Pedis)

Etiology   The foot is the most common area of the body that is infected by dematophytes, usually by tinea pedis, or athlete's foot. *Tricophyton mentagrophytes* infect the space between the third and fourth digits and enter the plantar surface of the arch. The same organism attacks toenails. *Trichophyton rubrum* causes scaling and thickening of a sole. Toe webs that become macerated and infected are an infection that is mixed with *Candida* yeast or gram-negative rods in addition to or replacing the original dermatophyte[17] (Figure 26-14). The athlete wearing shoes that are enclosed will sweat, encouraging fungal growth. However, contagion is based mainly on the athlete's individual susceptibility. There are other conditions that may also be thought to be athlete's foot, such as a dermatitis caused by allergy or an eczema-type skin infection (Color Plate, Figure F).

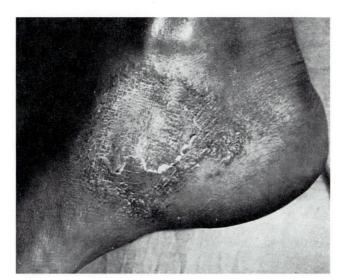

Figure 26-14
Athlete's foot (tinea pedis).

Symptoms and signs   Athlete's foot can reveal itself in many ways but appears most often as an extreme itching on the soles of the feet and between and on top of the toes. It appears as a rash, with small pimples or minute blisters that break and exude a yellowish serum (see Figure 26-14). Scratching because of itchiness can cause the tissue to become inflamed and infected, manifesting a red, white, or gray scaling of the affected area.

Management   Grisefulvin is the most effective management for tinea pedis. Of major importance is good foot hygiene. Topical medications used for tinea corporis can be beneficial (see the Focus box on the next page).[11]

Candidiasis (Moniliasis)

Candidiasis is a yeastlike fungus, which can produce skin, mucous membrane, and internal infections.

Etiology   Candidiasis is caused by the yeastlike fungus *Candida albicans* and some other species. It will attack the skin, as well as other structures, if the environment is right. Weather that is hot and humid, tight clothing that rubs, and poor hygiene provide the ideal environment for fungal growth.

Symptoms and signs   Among athletes, candidiasis can occur anywhere there is intertrigo, especially under the arm and in the groin area. In other words, it can occur anywhere skin touches skin when accompanied by heat and moisture. The coach or athletic trainer may mistake this condition for simple intertrigo. It appears with a bright red, moist, glistening base.[9] The border of this lesion, in contrast to that of intertrigo, is commonly rimmed with small red pustules. In cases in which it occurs where the skin is folded, a white, macerated border may surround the red area. Later, deep painful fissures may develop where the skin creases. Of major importance to the coach or athletic trainer is that *Candida albicans* can cause a systemic disease that may be life threatening. Therefore, when suspected, immediate referral to a physician must be made.

Management   The first concern in treatment is to maintain a dry area. A cool, wet, medicated compress may be applied for 20 to 30 minutes several times per day to promote dryness. Depending on the site of the disease, an antibiotic salve or lotion containing miconaxole may be applied. (NOTE: Genital candidiasis is discussed in Chapter 27 in the section on sexually transmitted diseases.)

Tinea Versicolor

Tinea versicolor is a unique fungal infection and therefore is dealt with separately. It is a common fungal infection among young adults.

26-5

Critical Thinking Exercise

Fungal infections are commonly found among athletes. Fungi grow best in unsanitary conditions, along with an environment of warmth, moisture, and darkness.

? What are the symptoms and signs of the fungal infection tinea pedis?

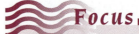

Focus

> **Basic care of athlete's foot**
> - Keep the feet as dry as possible through frequent use of talcum powder.
> - Wear clean white socks to avoid reinfection, changing them daily.
> - Use a standard fungicide for specific medication. Over-the-counter medications such as Desenex and Tinactin are useful in the early stages of the infection. For stubborn cases see the team physician; a dermatologist may need to make a culture from foot scrapings to determine the best combatant to be used.
>
> The best cure for the problem of athlete's foot is *prevention*. To keep the condition from spreading to other athletes, the following steps should be faithfully followed by individuals in the sports program:
> - All athletes should powder their feet daily.
> - One should dry the feet thoroughly, especially between and under the toes, after every shower.
> - One should keep sports shoes and street shoes dry by dusting them with powder daily.
> - All athletes should wear clean sports socks and street socks daily.
> - The shower and dressing rooms should be cleaned and disinfected daily.

Etiology   Tinea versicolor is caused by a yeast called *Pityrosporum orbiculare*. It is a normal part of the skin's flora, appearing commonly in areas in which sebaceous glands actively secrete body oils.

Symptoms and signs   The fungus characteristically produces multiple, small, circular macules that are pink, brown, or white. In black persons, they appear hyperpigmented. They commonly occur on the abdomen, neck, and chest. The lesions do not tan when exposed to the sun and are usually asymptomatic.

Management   Treatment of tinea versicolor usually provides only temporary relief, and recurrences are common. The medication of choice is usually selenium sulfide (Selsun shampoo).

VIRAL INFECTIONS

As discussed previously, viruses are ultramicroscopic organisms that do not have enzyme systems but parasitize living cells. Entering a tissue cell, the virus exists as nucleic acid. Inside, the virus may stimulate the cell chemically to produce more virus until the host cell dies or the virus is ejected to infect additional cells. Of the many viral infections that can directly infect the athlete, these common ones will be discussed: herpesvirus, wart-causing verrucas, and poxvirus (molluscum contagiosum).

Herpes Simplex: Labialis and Gladiatorum

Herpes simplex is a strain of virus that is associated with skin and mucous membrane infection. Types 1 and 2 cause cutaneous lesions and are indistinguishable from one another (Color Plate, Figure G); however, type 1 is found, for the most part, extragenitally and type 2 genitally.[1] Both can, however, be found anywhere on the skin or mucous membrane.

Etiology   Herpes simplex is highly contagious and is usually transmitted directly through a lesion in the skin or mucous membrane. After the initial outbreak, it is thought to move down a sensory nerve's neurilemmal sheath to reside in a resting state in a local ganglion. Recurrent attacks can be triggered by sunlight, emotional disturbances, illness, fatigue, infection, or other situations that may stress the organism.[5] However, sunlight does not adversely affect the reactivation rate if a sunscreen of sun protection factor (SPF) 15 is used.

Common viruses that attack the skin of athletes:
  Herpes virus
  Verruca
  Poxvirus (molluscum contagiosum)

Symptoms and signs Not all individuals infected with the virus develop overt symptoms.[5] An early indication that a herpes infection is about to erupt is a tingling or hypersensitivity in the infected area 24 hours before the appearance of lesions. Local swelling occurs, followed by the appearance of vesicles. The athlete may feel generally ill with a headache and sore throat, lymph gland swelling, and pain in the area of lesions. The vesicles generally rupture in 1 to 3 days, spilling out a serous material that will form into a yellowish crust. The lesions will normally heal in 10 to 14 days. Of the two areas of the body affected, herpes labialis (cold sore) is usually the least symptomatic. Herpes simplex gladiatorum is the more serious, with lesions commonly on the side of the face, neck, or shoulders. Genital herpes is discussed in Chapter 27. Herpes simplex infection is so highly contagious that it may run rampant through an entire team in a short time. Wrestlers having any signs of a herpes infection should be disqualified from body contact for at least 120 hours (5 days).

Management Herpes simplex lesions are self-limiting. Therapy usually is directed toward reducing pain and promoting early healing. Application of ice or liquid nitrogen during the early symptoms, before the appearance of lesions, effectively reduces later symptoms. Oral acyclovir is the treatment of choice for herpes simplex 1.[5]

Complications Herpes simplex, if not carefully managed, can lead to secondary infection. A major problem is keratoconjunctivitis, an inflammation of the cornea and conjunctiva that could lead to loss of vision and that must be considered a medical emergency.

Verruca Virus and Warts

Numerous forms of verruca exist, including the verruca plana (flat wart), verruca plantaris (plantar wart), and the condyloma acuminatum (venereal wart).

The verruca virus uses the skin's epidermal layer for reproduction and growth. The verruca wart enters the skin through a lesion that has been exposed to contaminated fields, floors, or clothing. Contamination can also occur from exposure to other warts.

Common Wart

Etiology Verruca plana is associated with the common wart and is prevalent on the hands of children (Color Plate, Figure H).

Symptoms and signs This wart appears as a small, round, elevated lesion with rough, dry surfaces. It may be painful if pressure is applied. These warts are subject to secondary bacterial infection, particularly if they are located on the hands or feet, where they may be constantly irritated.

Management Vulnerable warts must be protected until they can be treated by a physician. Application of a topical salicylic acid preparation or liquid nitrogen and electrocautering are the most common ways of managing this condition.

Plantar Warts

Etiology Plantar warts are associated with the virus verruca plantaris and are usually found on the sole of the foot, on or adjacent to areas of abnormal weight bearing; however, they can spread to the hands and other body parts. They most commonly result from a fallen metatarsal arch or bruises to the ball of the foot, such as may be sustained during excessive jumping or running on the ball of the foot. Other names for this condition are *papilloma* and *seed warts*.

Symptoms and signs Plantar warts are seen as areas with excessive epidermal thickening and cornification (Color Plate, Figure I). They produce general discomfort and point tenderness in the areas of excessive callus formation. Commonly the athlete complains that the condition feels as though he or she has stepped on broken glass. A major characteristic of the plantar wart is its punctuation of hemorrhages, which look like a cluster of small black seeds.

26-6

Critical Thinking Exercise

An athlete experiences a tingling and sometimes painful sensation in the upper lip region. Twenty-four hours later, swelling occurs followed by the formation of vesicles. The athlete also experiences a mild headache, sore throat, and lymph gland swelling.

? What condition does this scenario describe, and how could the later symptoms have been prevented?

Management There are many different approaches to the treatment of warts. In general, while the athlete is competing, a conservative approach is taken. Concern is to protect the wart against infection and to keep the growth of the warts under control. A common approach to controlling plantar warts is the careful paring away of accumulated callous tissue and application of a keratolytic such as 40% salicylic acid plaster. When the competitive season is over, the physician may decide to remove the wart by freezing it with liquid nitrogen or by electrodesiccation. Until its removal, a wart should be protected by a doughnut pad.

Molluscum Contagiosum

Etiology Molluscum contagiosum is a poxvirus infection. It is more contagious than warts, particularly during direct body contact activities such as wrestling.

Symptoms and signs Molluscum contagiosum appears as a small, pinkish, slightly raised, smooth-domed papule. When this condition is identified, it must be referred immediately to a physician.

Management Treatment often consists of cleansing thoroughly and using a destructive procedure. Destructive procedures include the use of a powerful counterirritant such as cantharidin (Cantharone), surgical removal of the lesion, or cryosurgery, using nitrogen.

ALLERGIC, THERMAL, AND CHEMICAL SKIN REACTIONS

The skin can react adversely to a variety of nonpathogenic influences. Among the most common affecting athletes are allergies, temperature extremes, and chemical irritants.

Allergic Reactions

The skin displays allergic reactions in various ways (Color Plate, Figures K and L). An allergy is caused by an allergen, a protein toward which the body is hypersensitive. Causative factors may be food, drugs, clothing, dusts, pollens, plants, animals, heat, cold, or light, or the cause may be psychosomatic. The skin may reflect an allergy in several ways such as reddening, elevated patches (urticaria or hives), or eczema. Reddening and swelling of the tissue may occur either locally or generally from an increased dilation of blood capillaries. Urticaria occurs as a red or white elevation (wheal) of the skin, characterized by a burning or an itching sensation. Eczema is a skin reaction in which small vesicles are produced, accompanied by itching and a crust formation.

The athletic trainer should be able to recognize gross signs of allergic reactions and should then refer the athlete to the physician. Treatment usually includes avoidance of the sensitizing agents and use of an antipruritic agent (such as calamine location) and antihistamine drugs.

Allergic Contact Dermatitis

There are many substances in the sports environment to which the athlete may be allergic, causing a skin reaction.

Etiology The most common plants that cause allergic contact dermatitis are poison ivy, poison oak, sumac, ragweed, and primrose. Over time the athlete may become allergic to topical medications such as antibiotics, antihistamines, anesthetics, or antiseptics. Chemicals commonly found in soaps, detergents, and deodorants can create a reaction. Some athletes are allergic to materials in the adhesive used in athletic tape. Also, the countless chemicals used in the manufacture of shoes and clothing and other materials have been known to produce allergic contact dermatitis.

Symptoms and signs The period of onset from the time of initial exposure may range from 1 day to 1 week. Skin that is continually warm will develop signs earlier. The skin reacts with redness, swelling, and the formation of vesicles that ooze fluid and form a crust. A constant itch develops that is increased with heat and made worse

---

26-7

Critical Thinking Exercise

A tennis player complains to the athletic trainer that she has a sharp pain in the ball of her right foot. She says that the pain resembles having stepped on a piece of glass. On inspection the athletic trainer observes excessive callus formation on the ball of the foot that is dotted with a cluster of black specks.

? What is this condition, and how should it be managed?

Skin reactions to allergy:
  Reddening
  Elevated patches
  Eczema

by rubbing. Secondary infection is a common result of scratching (Color Plate, Figure J).

Management   The most obvious treatment approach is to determine the irritant and avoid it. This may not always be simple and may require extensive testing. In the acute phase, tap water compresses or soaks soothe and dry the vesicles. In the nonacute stage topical corticosteroids may be beneficial.

Actinic Dermatitis (Sunburn)

Serious skin damage can occur from overexposure to the sun's rays. Actinic dermatitis (sunburn) is a precursor to this damage.

Etiology   Sunburn is a dermatitis caused by the ultraviolet radiation from the sun, and it varies in intensity from a mild erythema (pink color) to a severe, second-degree burn represented by itching, swelling, and blistering. Every protection should be given to athletes who have thin, white skin. Such persons are called *heliopaths;* their skin tends to absorb a greater amount of ultraviolet radiation than more pigmented individuals. Individuals who may be taking photosensitizing drugs such as thiazide diuretics, some tetracyclines, and phenothiazine are also sensitive. The chemical psoralen in oil of limes, parsnips, and celery, as well as other foods, can produce a severe adverse reaction in some individuals who expose themselves to sunlight.

Symptoms and signs   If a large area of the skin is sunburned, the athlete may display all the symptoms of severe inflammation accompanied by shock. A sunburn can cause malfunctioning of the organs within the skin, which in turn may result in infection of structures such as hair follicles and sweat glands.

Sunburn appears 2 to 8 hours after exposure. Symptoms become most extreme in approximately 12 hours and dissipate in 72 to 96 hours. After once receiving a severe sunburn, the skin is more susceptible to burning. The skin remains injured for months after a severe sunburn has been sustained. Prevention of sunburn should be accomplished by a gradual exposure to the rays of the sun, combined with use of a sunburn medication that will filter out most of the ultraviolet light. Individuals prone to burning should routinely wear a sunscreen such as para-aminobenzoic acid (PABA). The amount of protection provided by sunscreens is determined by the sun protection factor. The SPF refers to the length of time a person can stay in the sun without getting sunburned. An SPF of 15 means a person can be expected to be exposed to the sun 15 times longer than when exposed to the sun without sunscreen. Constant overexposure to the sun can lead to chronic skin thickening and damage.[3]

Management   A sunburn is treated according to the degree of inflammation present. Mild burns can be aided by a soothing lotion that contains a mild anesthetic. Boric acid solution has also proved beneficial. Moderate and severe burns can be relieved by a tub bath in which a pound of cornstarch is used; a vinegar solution will also help. Severe sunburn may be treated by the physician with corticosteroids and other antiinflammatory drugs.

It must be noted that ultraviolet radiation is damaging—it can prematurely age the skin and can increase the chances of skin cancers. Basal cell and squamous cell carcinomas are the most common cancers.[17]

Miliaria (Prickly Heat)

Prickly heat is common in sports and occurs most often during the hot season of the year in those athletes who perspire profusely and who wear heavy clothing.

Etiology   Continued exposure to heat and moisture causes retention of perspiration by the sweat glands and subsequent miliaria.

Symptoms and signs   Miliaria results in itching and burning vesicles and pustules.[3] It occurs most often on the arms, trunk, and bending areas of the body.

Management   Care of prickly heat requires avoidance of overheating, frequent bathing with a nonirritating soap, wearing loose-fitting clothing, and the use of antipruritic lotions.

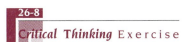

26-8

Critical Thinking Exercise

Actinic dermatitis, or sunburn, occurs from overexposure to the sun's rays.

? What should an athlete who is a heliopath be told about the sun's rays?

Chilblains

Etiology   Chilblains is a common type of dermatitis caused by excessive exposure to cold.

Symptoms and signs   The tissue does not freeze but reacts with edema, reddening, possibly blistering, and a sensation of burning and itching. The parts of the body most often affected are the ears, face, hands, and feet.

Management   Treatment consists of exercise and a gradual warming of the part. Massage and application of heat are contraindicated in cases of chilblains. (See Chapter 12 for more information about reactions to cold.)

INFESTATION AND BITES

Certain parasites cause dermatoses or skin irritations when they suck blood, inject venom, and even lay their eggs under the skin. Athletes who come in contact with these organisms may develop various symptoms such as itching, allergic skin reactions, and secondary infections from insult or scratching. The more common parasitic infestations in sports are caused by mites, crab lice, fleas, ticks, mosquitoes, and stinging insects such as bees, wasps, hornets, and yellow jackets.

Depending on the part of the country in which the athlete resides, parasites such as mites, crab lice, fleas, ticks, mosquitoes, and stinging insects can cause serious discomfort and infection.

Seven-Year Itch (Scabies)

Etiology   Seven-year itch (scabies) is a skin disease caused by the mite *Sarcoptes scabiei,* which produces extreme nocturnal itching. The parasitic itch mite is small, with the female causing the greatest irritation. The mite burrows a tunnel approximately ¼ to ½ inch (1.25 cm) long into the skin to deposit its eggs.

Symptoms and signs   The mite's burrows appear as dark lines between the fingers, toes, body flexures, nipples, and genitalia. Excoriations, pustules, and papules caused by the resulting scratching frequently hide the true nature of the disease. The young mite matures in a few days and returns to the skin surface to repeat the cycle. The skin often develops a hypersensitivity to the mite, which produces extreme itching.

Management   Gamma benzene hexachloride (Lindane) has been identified as the most effective scabicide. It is available as a cream or a shampoo. Because of the athlete's itching and scratching, secondary infections are common and must also be treated (see the Focus box on the next page for treatment).

Lice (Pediculosis)

Etiology   Pediculosis is an infestation by the louse, of which three types are parasitic to humans. The *Pediculus humanus capitis* (head louse) infests the head, where its eggs (nits) attach to the base of the hair shaft. The *Phthirus pubis* (crab louse) lives in the hair of the pubic region and lays its eggs at the hair base. The *Pediculus humanus corporis* (body louse) lives and lays its eggs in the seams of clothing.

Symptoms and signs   The louse is a carrier of many diseases; its bite causes an itching dermatitis, which, through subsequent scratching, provokes pustules and excoriations.

Management   Cure is rapid with the use of any of a number of parasiticides or lotions such as one composed of chlorophenothane 5 g, isopropyl alcohol 50 ml, and propylene glycol 50 ml, rubbed into the infected areas at night before retiring and again the following morning when arising. The area should not be washed for 7 to 10 days; then the lotion is reapplied. The lice cannot survive dryness. Good hygiene is of paramount importance in all infestations. All clothing, bedding, and toilet seats must be kept clean and sterile.

Fleas

Etiology   Fleas are small wingless insects that suck blood. Singly, their bites cause only minor discomfort to the recipient, unless the flea is a carrier of some contagious disease.

Symptom and signs   When there is a large number of biting fleas, a great deal of discomfort can occur. After attaching themselves to some moving object such as a

---

26-9

Critical Thinking Exercise

A cross-country runner complains to the athletic trainer of extreme nocturnal itching. Observation of the athlete's skin reveals dark lines in the area of the finger and toes.

? What insect infestation does this scenario describe? What type of infection should be expected?

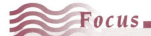

Treatment of scabies
- The entire body should be thoroughly cleansed, with attention to skin lesions.
- Bedding and clothing should be disinfected.
- The coating of gamma benzene hexachloride (Lindane) should be applied on the lesions for 3 nights.
- All individuals who have come in contact with the infected athlete should be examined by the physician.
- Locker and game equipment must be disinfected.

dog or a human, most fleas bite in patterns of three. Fleas seem to concentrate their bites on the ankle and lower leg.

Management   Once the flea bite has been incurred, the main concern is to prevent itching with an antipruritic lotion such as calamine. Scratching the bite should be avoided to prevent a secondary infection. Areas in which fleas abound can be sprayed with selected insecticides containing malathion or some other effective insecticide.

Ticks

Etiology   Ticks are parasitic insects that have an affinity for the blood of many animals, including humans. They are carriers of a variety of microorganisms that can cause Rocky Mountain spotted fever or Lyme disease. Because ticks are commonly found on grass and bushes, they can easily become attached to the athlete who brushes against them.

Symptoms and signs   Rocky Mountain spotted fever and Lyme disease are characterized by headache, fever, malaise, myalgia, and a rash about the wrist and forearms.

Management   To remove a tick, mineral oil or fingernail polish is applied to its body, at which time it will withdraw its head. At no time should one attempt to pull the tick from the body; doing so may result in leaving the head of the tick embedded in the skin.

Mosquitoes

Etiology   Unless it is the carrier of a disease, the mosquito, as a blood sucker, produces a bite that causes only mild discomfort. Generally mosquitoes are attracted to lights, dark clothing, and warm, moist skin.

Symptoms and signs   The mosquito bite produces a small reddish papule. Multiple bites may lead to a great deal of itching.

Management   Itching is most often relieved by the application of a topical medication such as calamine lotion. In climates where mosquitoes are prevalent, repellents should be used directly on the skin.

Stinging Insects

Etiology   Bees, wasps, hornets, and yellow jackets inflict a venomous sting that is temporarily painful for most individuals; however, some hypersensitive individuals may respond with an allergic reaction that may be fatal. Stings to the head, face, and neck are particularly dangerous to the athlete. Athletes having a history of allergic reactions from stings must be carefully scrutinized after a sting to prevent an anaphylactic reaction. To avoid stings, the athlete should not wear scented lotions or shampoos; should not wear brightly colored clothes; should not wear jewelry, suede, or leather; and should not go barefoot.[3]

Symptoms and signs The allergic athlete may respond with an increase in heart rate, fast breathing, chest tightness, dizziness, sweating, and even loss of consciousness.

Management In uncomplicated sting cases, the stinging apparatus must be carefully removed with tweezers, followed by the application of a soothing medication. Detergent soap applied directly on the sting often produces an immediate lessening of symptoms. In severe reactions to a sting the athlete must be treated for severe shock and referred immediately to a physician. For sensitive athletes who perform outdoors, it should be suggested that they avoid using scented cosmetics, scented soap, colognes, or aftershave lotions and colorful, floral, or dark-colored clothing.

SUMMARY

- The skin is the largest organ of the human body. In the average adult, skin varies in weight from 6 to 7½ pounds and is from ⅟₃₂ to ⅛ inch thick. It is composed of three layers: the epidermis, the dermis, and the subcutis. The outermost layer, the epidermis, acts as protection against infections from a variety of sources. The dermis contains sweat glands, sebaceous glands, and hair follicles. The subcutis layer is the major area for fat storage and temperature regulation.

- Primary skin lesions include macule, papule, plaque, nodule, tumor, cyst, wheal, vesicle, bulla, and pustule. Secondary skin lesions include scale, crust, fissure, erosion, ulcer, and scar. Microorganisms, trauma, allergies, temperature variations, chemicals, infestations, and insect bites can cause skin lesions.

- Sports participation can place a great deal of mechanical force on the skin, which can lead to many different problems. Abnormal friction causes keratosis, blisters, and intertrigo. Hyperhidrosis adds to the problems of skin friction and infections. A tearing force can lacerate or avulse skin. Compression can bruise, scraping abrades, and a pointed object can puncture.

- Providing immediate proper care is essential to avoid skin infections. Streptococcal and staphylococcal bacteria are associated with wound contamination, and the tetanus bacillus can cause lockjaw. All athletes should be immunized by the tetanus toxoid before they participate in sports.

- Impetigo contagiosa is a highly infectious disease among athletes and is associated with both the staphylococcal and streptococcal bacteria. Furuncles, carbuncles, and folliculitis are streptococcal-caused afflictions and can be spread by direct contact. Other bacterial skin conditions are hidradenitis suppurativa, acne vulgaris, and paronychia and onychia.

- The sports environment, which is often one of excessive moisture, warmth, and darkness, is conducive to fungal growth. An extremely common fungus, ringworm, is under the general heading of dermatophytes. The three genera of fungus for this condition are *Microsporum*, *Trichophyton*, and *Epidermophyton*. Under the right conditions, these fungi can attack a wide variety of body tissues. Candidiasis is a more serious form of infection caused by a yeastlike fungus, *Candida albicans*.

- Herpes simplex is a virus associated with herpes labialis and herpes gladiatorum. The verruca virus commonly is related to a variety of warts such as the plantar wart or the papilloma. The poxvirus causes molluscum contagiosum, a highly contagious wart spread by direct contact.

- Athletes are also subject to many other causes of skin conditions, including allergies, extremes of heat or cold, and chemical irritations. One major problem that produces an insidious destruction of the skin is prolonged overexposure to sunlight.

- Different parts of the country have problems with insect infestations and bites. Two of these problems are scabies (caused by mites) and pediculosis (from lice), and there are others that may be produced by fleas, ticks, mosquitoes, and stinging insects.

26-10

Critical Thinking Exercise

An athlete who is allergic to bee stings is stung.

? What physical reactions should the athlete be expected to have?

Solutions to Critical Thinking Exercises

26-1 Initially, the skin flap is completely removed. The area is cleaned with soap and water and the antiseptic liquid benzalkonium is applied along with an occlusive dressing. After the game the "second-skin" dressing by Spenco is applied to the raw area.

26-2 To prevent intertrigo the skin is kept dry, clean, and friction free. The athlete who is prone to this problem should wear loose cotton underwear. Males should wear a supporter over underwear.

26-3 A major concern of this abrasion is infection. The abraded area is cleaned with mild Ivory soap and debrided with a brush. Hydrogen peroxide is applied to the injury, followed by Betadine. A medicated salve is then applied to prevent scabbing. Finally, a nonocclusive dressing is applied.

26-4 This skin condition is the highly contagious disease impetigo contagiosa. The athlete must not have physical contact with other athletes until the disease is resolved. It is managed with daily thorough cleansing of crusted material followed by an application of an antibiotic salve.

26-5 With tinea pedis there is severe itching on the top of and between the toes and on the soles of the feet. A rash occurs with blisters that secrete a yellow serum. Scratching can cause an infection. A red, white, or grayish scaling may also be present.

26-6 This condition is a herpes simplex labialis viral infection. Many of the later symptoms could have been prevented by the application of ice or liquid nitrogen.

26-7 The black specks are plantar warts. The accumulated callus is pared down followed by the application of a 40% salicylic acid plaster. A doughnut pad is applied to protect the area.

26-8 The athlete who is a heliopath has thin white skin and tends to absorb a greater amount of the sun's radiation compared with the more pigmented athlete. The athlete must be instructed that a sunburn produces irreversible damage to the skin.

26-9 This scenario describes infestation by the mite *Sarcoptes scabiei.* Another name for this condition is the seven-year itch or scabies. The mite burrows a tunnel under the skin to deposit her eggs. The eggs hatch, and the young mites return to the skin surface to repeat the cycle. A hypersensitivity develops that causes extreme itching at night.

26-10 The athlete may be expected to experience an anaphylactic reaction. There is an increase in heart rate, fast breathing, chest tightness, dizziness, sweating, and possibly a loss of consciousness. This is a medical emergency.

REVIEW QUESTIONS AND CLASS ACTIVITIES

1. Describe the skin's anatomy, functions, and lesions that are indicative of infection.
2. Contrast the microorganisms that are related to skin infections.
3. Relate the mechanical forces of friction, compression, shearing, stretching, scraping, tearing, avulsing, and puncturing to specific skin injuries.
4. List the steps to take in managing major skin traumas.
5. How should wounds be managed to avoid serious infections?
6. Characterize the different viruses that are associated with common skin infections that occur in sports.
7. What bacterial skin infections are commonly seen in athletes?
8. Tinea (ringworm) is a fungus that can be present on different parts of the body. Name the body parts.
9. How may skin infections related to microorganisms be avoided?
10. Why is candidiasis considered one of the most serious fungal infections in sports?
11. What allergic, thermal, and chemical skin reactions could an athlete sustain in the typical sports environment?
12. Different parts of the United States have their own problems with insects that infect the skin of humans. Identify the insects in your area that can cause problems to athletes. How may they be avoided?

REFERENCES

1. Allen AC: Skin. In Kissane JM, editor: *Anderson's pathology,* vol 2, ed 9, St Louis, 1990, Mosby.
2. American Academy of Orthopaedic Surgeons: *Athletic training and sports medicine,* ed 2, Park Ridge, Ill, 1991, American Academy of Orthopaedic Surgeons.
3. Arntizen KR: Dermatologic issues. In Agostini R, editor: Philadelphia, 1994, Hanley & Belfus.
4. Baxter DE: *The foot and ankle in sport,* St Louis, 1995, Mosby.
5. Bergfeld WF, Munnings F: How to manage herpes in active patients, *Sportsmedicine* 22(9):71, 1994.
6. Conklin RJ: Acne vulgaris in the athlete, *Phys Sportsmed* 16(10):65, 1988.
7. Fletcher SB et al: Medicated compress for blister treatment, *J Ath Train* 28(1):81, 1993.
8. Foster DT et al: Management of wounds, *J Ath Train* 30(2):135, 1995.
9. Habif TP: *Clinical dermatology,* St Louis, 1990, Mosby.
10. Hamann BP: *Disease: identification, prevention and control,* St Louis, 1994, Mosby.
11. Mackey S: Relieving winter skin discomfort, *Phys Sportsmed* 23(1):53, 1995.
12. Ramsey ML: Clearing up fungal infections of the nail plate, *Phys Sportsmed* 21(2):70, 1993.
13. Rheinecker SB: Wound management: the occlusive dressing, *J Ath Train* 30(2):143, 1995.
14. Sammarco GJ: Soft tissue injuries. In Torg JS, editor: *Current therapy in sports medicine,* ed 3, St Louis, 1995, Mosby.
15. Scheinberg RS: Exercise-related skin infection, *Phys Sportsmed* 22(6):47, 1994.
16. Scheinberg RS: Stopping skin assailants: fungi, yeasts, and viruses, *Phys Sportsmed* 22(7):33, 1994.
17. Simandl G: Alterations in skin function and integrity. In Porth CM, editor: *Pathophysiology,* Philadelphia, 1994, Lippincott.
18. Thibodeau GA, Patton KT: *Anatomy and physiology,* ed 2, St Louis, 1993, Mosby.
19. Williams JGP: *Color atlas of injuries in sports,* Chicago, 1990, Year Book.

ANNOTATED BIBLIOGRAPHY

Douglas LG: Facial injuries. In Torg JS, Welsh RP, Shepard RJ, editors: *Current therapy in sports medicine,* vol 2, Philadelphia, 1990, Decker.

An excellent overview of the major open skin wounds that occur among athletes.

Habif TP: *Clinical dermatology,* St Louis, 1990, Mosby.

An excellent, in-depth text about skin disease, diagnosis, and therapy. Contains extensive color photos and illustrations.

Williams JGP: *Color atlas of injury in sports,* Chicago, 1990, Year Book.

Presents extensive color illustrations for all aspects of sports injuries, including the area of dermatology.

Additional Health Conditions

When you finish this chapter, you should be able to

- Describe symptoms and signs of respiratory infections.
- Describe common gastrointestinal tract conditions.
- Explain diabetes mellitus and contrast diabetic coma and insulin shock.
- Identify the causes of epilepsy and explain how to perform the appropriate action when a seizure occurs.
- Describe hypertension in athletes.
- Describe anemias common to athletes.
- Describe the symptoms and signs of the most common venereal diseases.
- Describe menstrual irregularities and their effect on the athlete.
- Explain female reproduction and pregnancy as they relate to the athlete.

B esides the skin and musculoskeletal conditions already addressed, the athlete is subject to many other conditions. The athletic trainer, as a health and safety practitioner, should be able to recognize and give advice on a vast array of health problems. This chapter presents many prevalent important additional health problems that may confront the coach and athletic trainer.

RESPIRATORY CONDITIONS

Respiratory tract infections can be highly communicable among sports team members.

Because of the nature of sports the athlete may be prone to conditions of the respiratory tract, which includes the nose, sinuses, throat, larynx, trachea, and bronchi. Specific conditions to be discussed are the common cold, sinusitis, pharyngitis, influenza, rhinitis, infectious mononucleosis, bronchitis, and asthma.[14]

Common Cold

The common cold is the most prevalent of all communicable diseases. It is referred to as an upper respiratory infection.

Etiology There are more than 100 different rhinoviruses that cause colds. Colds are transmitted by either direct or indirect contact. They are spread by droplets expelled by a person with a cold who sneezes, coughs, or speaks. One method of infection is by touching a contaminated article and then rubbing one's eyes.[8]

Symptoms and signs Frequently the cold begins with a scratchy or sore throat, watery discharge or stopped-up nose, and sneezing. Not all colds follow the same pattern. In some instances a secondary bacterial infection occurs producing a thickened yellowish nasal discharge, watering eyes, mild fever, sore throat, headache, **malaise,** myalgia, and dry cough. Additional to the secondary infection can be laryngitis (hoarseness), tracheitis (irritation of trachea), acute bronchitis, sinusitis, and even an inflammation of the middle ear (otitis media).

malaise
Discomfort and uneasiness caused by an illness.

Management Treatment of the common cold is symptomatic. Most colds last for 5 to 10 days regardless of treatment. Nonprescription cold medications may help ease some symptoms. To avoid colds one should stay out of crowds, wash hands frequently, avoid sharing personal items, eat a balanced diet, and drink at least eight 8-ounce glasses of water per day. Emotional stress and extreme fatigue should be avoided as much as possible.

Sinusitis

Sinusitis is an inflammation of the paranasal sinuses.

Etiology   Sinusitis can stem from an upper respiratory infection caused by a variety of bacteria. As a result, nasal mucous membranes swell and block the ostium oft he paranasal sinus. A painful pressure occurs from an accumulation of mucus, producing pain.[4]

Symptoms and signs   The skin area over the sinus may be swollen and painful to the touch. A headache and malaise may be present. A purulent nasal discharge may also occur.

Management   Where there is a purulent infection antibiotics may be warranted. Steam inhalation and other nasal topical vasoconstrictors, such as phenylephrine 0.25% spray, can produce vasoconstriction and drainage.

Pharyngitis (Sore Throat)

Acute inflammation of the throat or pharyngitis can be related to the common cold, influenza, or a more serious condition such as mononucleosis.

Etiology   Pharyngitis can be caused by a virus such as the Epstein-Barr virus of mononucleosis or the streptoccus bacteria in the condition of scarlet fever or tonsillitis.[4] Approximately 95% of all bacterial pharyngitis is caused by a streptococcal infection.[8] Transmission is often by direct contact with an actively infected person or one who is a carrier. Ingestion of contaminated food can lead to a streptococcal sore throat.[8]

Symptoms and signs   Pharyngitis is characterized by pain on swallowing, fever, swollen lymph glands and tonsils, malaise, weakness, and anorexia. The mucous membranes of the throat may be severely inflamed with a covering of purulent matter.[4] A throat culture for determining the presence of a streptococcal bacterial infection may be warranted.

Management   Topical gargles and rest may be warranted. Antibiotic therapy is given for a streptococcal infection to prevent scarlet fever and rheumatic fever.[4]

Influenza

Influenza, commonly known as the flu, is one of the most persistent and debilitating diseases. It usually occurs in various forms as an annual epidemic, causing severe illness among the populace.

Etiology   Influenza is caused by myoviruses classified as types A, B, and C. Type A influenza is the most common, causing serious and widespread epidemics. The virus enters the cell through its genetic material. The virus multiplies and is released from the cell by a budding process, to be spread throughout the body. Not all athletes need influenza vaccines; however, athletes engaging in winter sports, basketball, wrestling, and swimming may require them.[21]

Symptoms and signs   The athlete with the flu will have the following symptoms: fever, cough, headache, malaise, and inflamed respiratory mucous membranes with **coryza.** It should be noted that certain viruses can increase the body's core temperature. Flu generally has an incubation period of 48 hours and comes on suddenly, accompanied by chills and a fever of 102° to 103° F (39° to 39.5° C), which develops over a 24-hour period. The athlete complains of a headache and general aches and pains—mainly in the back and legs. The headache increases in intensity, along with **photophobia** and aching at the back of the skull. There is often sore throat, burning in the chest, and in the beginning a nonproductive cough, which later may develop into bronchitis. The skin is flushed, and the eyes are inflamed and watery. The acute stage of the disease usually lasts up to 5 days. Weakness, sweating, and fatigue may persist for many days. Flu prevention includes staying away from infected persons and maintaining good resistance through healthy living. Vaccines, including prevalent strains, may be given to individuals who are at risk such as pregnant women or people in frail health.

Management   If the flu is uncomplicated, its management consists of bed rest. During the acute stage, the temperature often returns to normal. Symptomatic care such

coryza
Profuse nasal discharge.

photophobia
Unusual intolerance to light.

as aspirin should be avoided because of Reye's syndrome for all individuals under 18 years of age. Amantadine vaccine is given for influenza A for individuals at risk. It also is beneficial for fever and respiratory symptoms.[4] Steam inhalation, cough medicines, and gargles may be given.

Seasonal Atopic (Allergic) Rhinitis

Hay fever, or pollinosis, is an acute seasonal allergic condition that results from airborne pollens.

Etiology   Hay fever can occur during the spring as a reaction to tree pollens such as oak, elm, maple, alder, birch, and cottonwood. During the summer grass and weed pollens can be the culprits. In the fall, ragweed pollen is the prevalent cause. Airborne fungal spores also have been known to cause hay fever. These substances act as allergens and cause an allergic reaction in susceptible people. The body's immune system produces allergic antibodies that release the chemical histamine, which produces the symptoms of hay fever.

Symptoms and signs   In the early stages, the athlete's eyes, throat, mouth, and nose begin to itch, followed by watering of the eyes, sneezing, and a clear, watery, nasal discharge. The athlete may complain of a sinus-type headache, emotional irritability, difficulty in sleeping, red and swollen eyes and nasal mucous membranes, and a wheezing cough.[4] It should be noted that other common adverse allergic conditions are asthma, anaphylaxis, urticaria, angioedema, and rhinitis.[5]

Management   Most athletes obtain relief from hay fever through oral antihistamines. To avoid the problem of sedation stemming from these drugs, the athlete may ingest a decongestant during the day and a long-acting antihistamine before going to bed.

Infectious Mononucleosis

Infectious mononucleosis is an acute viral disease that affects mainly young adults and children.

Etiology   Infectious mononucleosis, commonly called "mono," is caused by the Epstein-Barr virus (EBV), a member of the herpes group. It has major significance to athletes because it can produce severe fatigue and raise the risk of spleen rupture.[21] Incubation is 4 to 6 weeks. The EBV is carried in the throat and transmitted to another person through saliva. It has been called the kissing disease.[8]

Symptoms and signs   The EBV syndrome usually starts with a 3- to 5-day prodrome of headache, fatigue, loss of appetite, and myalgias. From days 5 to 15 there is fever, swollen lymph glands, and a sore throat.[8] By the second week 50% to 70% of those infected with EBV will have an enlarged spleen, 10% to 15% will have jaundice, and 5% to 15% will have a skin rash, a pinkish flush to the cheeks, and puffy eyelids.[21] Complications include ruptured spleen, meningitis, encephalitis, hepatitis, and anemia.[8]

Management   Treatment is supportive and symptomatic. Acetaminophen is often given for headache, fever, and malaise. Mellion[21] indicates that "athletes may resume easy training in 3 weeks after the onset of illness if: (1) the spleen is not markedly enlarged or painful, (2) he or she is afebrile, (3) liver function tests are normal, and (4) pharyngitis and any complication have resolved."

Acute Bronchitis

An inflammation of the mucous membranes of the bronchial tubes is called bronchitis. It occurs in both acute and chronic forms. If occurring in an athlete, bronchitis is more likely to be in the acute form.

Etiology   Acute bronchitis usually occurs as an infectious winter disease that follows a common cold or other viral infection of the nasopharynx, throat, or tracheobronchial tree. Secondary to this inflammation is a bacterial infection that may follow overexposure to air pollution. Fatigue, malnutrition, or becoming chilled could be predisposing factors.

27-1

Critical Thinking Exercise

A swimmer complains of a fever, cough, headache, malaise, aching in the back of the head, and a sore throat, along with light sensitivity.

? What is this scenario describing, and how could it be managed?

Symptoms and signs   The symptoms of an athlete with acute bronchitis usually start with an upper respiratory infection, nasal inflammation and profuse discharge, slight fever, sore throat, and back and muscle pains. A cough signals the beginning of bronchitis. In the beginning, the cough is dry, but in a few hours or days, a clear mucus secretion begins, becoming yellowish, indicating an infection. In most cases, the fever lasts 3 to 5 days, and the cough lasts 2 to 3 weeks or longer. The athlete may wheeze and rale when auscultation of the chest is performed. Pneumonia could complicate bronchitis. To avoid bronchitis, it is advisable that an athlete not sleep in an area that is extremely cold or exercise in extremely cold air without wearing a face mask to warm inhaled air.

Management   Management of acute bronchitis involves rest until fever subsides, drinking 3 to 4 L of water per day, and ingesting an antipyretic analgesic, a cough suppressant, and an antibiotic (when severe lung infection is present) on a daily basis.

Bronchial Asthma

Etiology   As one of the most common respiratory diseases, bronchial asthma can be produced from a number of stressors such as a viral respiratory tract infection, emotional upset, changes in barometric pressure or temperature, exercise, inhalation of a noxious odor, or exposure to a specific allergen.

Symptoms and signs   Bronchial asthma is characterized by a spasm of the bronchial smooth muscles, edema, and inflammation of the mucous membrane. In addition to asthma's narrowing of the airway, copious amounts of mucus are produced. Difficulty in breathing may cause the athlete to hyperventilate, resulting in dizziness. The attack may begin with coughing, wheezing, shortness of breath, and fatigue (see the Focus box on the next page).

Exercise-Induced Bronchial Obstruction (Asthma)

Exercise-induced bronchial obstruction is also known as exercise-induced asthma (EIA). It is a disease that occurs almost exclusively in asthmatic persons.[26]

Etiology   An exercise-induced asthmatic attack can be stimulated by exercise in some individuals and can be provoked in others, only on rare occasions, during moderate exercise. The exact cause of EIA is not clear. Metabolic acidosis, postexertional hypocapnia, stimulation of tracheal irritant receptors, adrenergic abnormalities such as a defective catecholamine metabolism, and psychological factors have been suggested as possible causes. Loss of heat and water causes the greatest loss of airway reactivity. Eating certain foods such as shrimp, celery, and peanuts can cause EIA. Sinusitis can also trigger an attack in an individual with chronic asthma.

Symptoms and signs   The athlete with EIA often displays an airway narrowing caused by bronchial-wall thickening and excess production of mucus. Athletes who have a chronic inflammatory asthmatic condition (bronchiectasis) characteristically have a constant dilation of the bronchi or bronchioles. There is chest tightness, breathlessness, coughing, and wheezing.[19] The athlete with EIA may show signs of swelling of the face (angioedema), swelling of the palms and soles of the feet, nausea, hypertension, diarrhea, fatigue, itching, respiratory stridor (high-pitched noise on respiration), headaches, and redness of the skin. It may occur within 3 to 8 minutes of strenuous activity.[2]

Management   Swimming is the least bronchospasm-producing exercise, which may be a result of the moist, warm air environment. It is generally agreed that a regular exercise program can benefit asthmatics. Conditioning and running longer distances reduce EIA bouts.[13] There should be gradual warm-up and cool-down. The duration of exercise should build slowly to 30 to 40 minutes, four or five times a week. Exercise intensity and loading also should be graduated slowly. An example would be 10 to 30 seconds of work, followed by 30 to 90 seconds of rest. Many athletes with chronic or exercise-induced asthma use the inhaled bronchodilator. Exercise is best performed in warm, humid conditions. Wearing a mask or scarf may be beneficial in avoiding cold, dry air. Slow nasal breathing is suggested with the avoid-

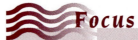
Focus

Management of the acute asthmatic attack

Athletes who have a history of asthma usually know how to care for themselves when attack occurs. However, the athletic trainer must be aware of what to look for and what to do if called on.

Early symptoms and signs
- Anxious appearance
- Sweating and paleness
- Flared nostrils
- Breathing with pursed lips
- Fast breathing
- Vomiting
- Hunched-over body posture
- Physical fatigue unrelated to activity
- Indentation in the notch below the Adam's apple
- Sinking in of rib spaces as the athlete inhales
- Coughing for no apparent reason
- Excess throat clearing
- Irregular, labored breathing or wheezing

Actions to take
- Attempt to relax and reassure the athlete.
- If medication has been cleared by the team physician, have the athlete use it.
- Encourage the athlete to drink water.
- Have the athlete perform controlled breathing along with relaxation exercises.
- If an environmental factor triggering the attack is known, remove it or the athlete from the area.
- If these procedures do not help, immediate medical attention may be necessary.

27-2

Critical Thinking Exercise

A soccer player has a history of exercise-induced asthma (EIA).

? How should the athlete avoid incidences of EIA?

---

ance of exercise in areas with high levels of air pollution or high pollen counts.[13] The most commonly prescribed B_2 agonist for EIA is albuterol, which acts for about 2 hours. Salmeterol provides a prophylaxis for up to 12 hours. Albuterol should be administered 15 minutes before exercise and salmeterol 30 to 60 minutes before exercise. Cromolyn sodium should be inhaled 30 minutes before exercise. Metered-dose inhalers are preferred for administration.[19] It has also been found that prophylactic use of the bronchodilator 15 minutes before exercise delays the symptoms by 2 to 4 hours.[4] Asthmatic athletes who receive medication for their condition should make sure that what they take is legal for competition.

DIABETES MELLITUS

Diabetic athletes engaging in vigorous physical activity should eat before exercising and if the exercise is protracted should have hourly glucose supplementation. As a rule, the insulin dosage is not changed, but food intake is increased. The response of diabetics varies among individuals and depends on many variables. Although there are some hazards, with proper medical evaluation and planning by a professional, diabetics can feel free to engage in most physical activities. The most common types of diabetes are type I, insulin-dependent diabetes mellitus (IDDM), and type II, non–insulin-dependent diabetes mellitus (NIDDM). Insulin-dependent diabetes is found in individuals under 35 years of age and represents between 5% and 10% of all cases. Non–insulin-dependent diabetes is most commonly detected after 30 or 40 years of age, represents 80% of all cases, and is associated with obesity.[27]

Etiology   Diabetes is a syndrome that results from an interaction of physical and environmental factors. Its etiology is not distinct. There is a complete or partial decrease in the secretion of insulin by the pancreas.

Symptoms and signs   Insulin-dependent diabetes is the most commonly seen in childhood. It may occur suddenly, with frequent urinating, constant thirst, weight loss, constant hunger, tiredness and weakness, itchy dry skin, and blurred vision. Non–insulin-dependent diabetes occurs later in life when the patient is 40 years old or older. It is usually associated with being overweight. The pancreas does not produce enough insulin or the body resists the insulin that is produced. As with IDDM, NIDDM can be a threat to the heart, kidneys, blood vessels, and eyes.

Management   It is essential that blood glucose levels be controlled to acceptable levels. This includes a balanced diet and, when needed, daily doses of insulin. It must also be noted that regular vigorous exercise can be effective in increasing peripheral insulin action to enhance glucose tolerance. Exercise, in general, improves the diabetic person's quality of life. It helps increase type I insulin sensitivity and utilization and may reduce long-term complications. In persons with type II diabetes, exercise decreases insulin resistance, improves glycemia control, and reduces or eliminates the need for insulin.[13] The athletic trainer should be aware that the diabetic athlete can adversely respond to extreme temperature variations or an unpredictable level of activity duration or intensity and may require rapid-acting carbohydrates.

Diabetic Coma and Insulin Shock

It is important that coaches and athletic trainers who work with athletes who have diabetes mellitus be aware of the major symptoms of diabetic coma and insulin shock and the proper actions to take when either one occurs.[27]

Diabetic Coma

If not treated adequately through proper diet or intake of insulin, the diabetic athlete can develop acidosis.

Etiology   A loss of sodium, potassium, and ketone bodies through excessive urination produces a problem of ketoacidosis that can lead to coma.

Symptoms and signs   Symptoms and signs include labored breathing or gasping for air, fruity-smelling breath caused by acetone, nausea and vomiting, thirst, dry mucous membrane of the mouth, flushed skin, and mental confusion or unconsciousness followed by coma.

Management   Because of the life-threatening nature of diabetic coma, early detection of ketoacidosis is essential. The injection of insulin into the athlete will normally prevent coma.

Insulin Shock

Etiology   Unlike diabetic coma, insulin shock occurs when too much insulin is taken into the body and hypoglycemia results.

Symptoms and signs   The athlete complains of tingling in the mouth, hands, or other body parts; physical weakness; headaches; and abdominal pain. It may be observed that the athlete has normal or shallow respirations, rapid heartbeat, and tremors, along with irritability and drowsiness.

Management   The diabetic athlete who engages in intense exercise and metabolizes large amounts of glycogen could inadvertently take too much insulin and thus have a severe reaction. To avoid this problem the athlete must adhere to a carefully planned diet that includes a snack before exercise. The snack should contain a combination of a complex carbohydrate and protein such as cheese and crackers. Activities that last for more than 30 to 40 minutes should be accompanied by snacks of simple carbohydrates. Some diabetics carry with them a lump of sugar or have candy or orange juice readily available in the event an insulin reaction seems imminent.[26]

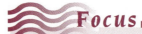

Focus

Management during a seizure

- Be emotionally composed.
- If possible, cushion the athlete's fall.
- Keep the athlete away from injury-producing objects.
- Loosen restrictive clothing.
- Prevent the athlete from biting the mouth by placing a soft cloth between the teeth.
- Allow the athlete to awaken normally after the seizure.
- Do not restrain the athlete during seizure.

SEIZURE DISORDERS (EPILEPSY)

epilepsy
Recurrent paroxysmal disorder characterized by sudden attacks of altered consciousness, motor activity, sensory phenomena, or inappropriate behavior.

Berkow[4] defines seizure disorders as "a recurrent paroxysmal disorder of cerebral function characterized by sudden, brief attacks of altered consciousness, motor activity, sensory phenomena, or inappropriate behavior caused by an abnormal excessive discharge of cerebral neurons." Any recurrent seizure pattern is termed **epilepsy**. Epilepsy is not a disease but is a symptom that can be caused by a large number of underlying disorders.

Etiology   For some types of epilepsy there is a genetic predisposition and a low threshold to having seizures. In others, altered brain metabolism or a history of injury may be the cause. A seizure can range from extremely brief episodes lasting 5 to 15 seconds (petit mal seizures) to major episodes (grand mal seizures) lasting a few minutes, with unconsciousness and uncontrolled tonic-clonic muscle contractions. There are approximately 1 million epileptics in the United States, most of whom can participate in some form of physical activity.[13] Sports-related injuries are not increased, nor is the sudden death syndrome linked to strenuous activity by the epileptic.[13]

Symptoms and signs   Each person with epilepsy must be considered individually as to whether he or she should engage in competitive sports. It is generally agreed that if an individual has daily or even weekly major seizures, collision sports should be prohibited. This prohibition is not because hitting the head will necessarily trigger a seizure, but because unconsciousness during participation could result in a serious injury. If the seizures are properly controlled by medication or occur only during sleep, little if any sports restriction should be imposed except for scuba diving, swimming alone, or participation at a great height.[13]

For individuals who have major daily or weekly seizures, collision-type sports may be prohibited.

Management   The athlete commonly takes an anticonvulsant medication that is specific for the type and degree of seizures that occur. On occasion the athlete may experience some undesirable side effects from drug therapy such as drowsiness, restlessness, nystagmus, nausea, vomiting, problems with balance, skin rash, or other adverse reactions.

When an athlete with epilepsy becomes aware of an impending seizure, measures should be taken to avoid injury such as immediately sitting or lying down. When a seizure occurs without warning, the steps in the Focus box above should be taken by the athletic trainer.

HIGH BLOOD PRESSURE (HYPERTENSION)

Excessive pressure applied against arterial walls while blood circulates is known as hypertension or high blood pressure (HBP). A normal average pressure is 120 systolic and 80 diastolic where the upper limits at rest for the older adolescent and adult HBP is 140/90 mm Hg and over (Table 27-1).

TABLE 27-1 Age and Blood Pressure Limits

Age	Upper Blood Pressure Limits at Rest*
<10	120/75 mm Hg
10-12	125/80 mm Hg
13-15	135/85 mm Hg
16-18	140/90 mm Hg
>18	140/90 mm Hg

*If the upper limits of blood pressure are exceeded during three measurements, the athlete may have hypertension.

Etiology   Hypertension is classified as primary, or essential, and secondary. Primary hypertension accounts for 90% of all cases, with no disease being associated. Secondary hypertension is related to a specific underlying cause, such as kidney disorders, overactive adrenal glands (increase blood volume), hormone-producing tumor, narrowing of the aorta, pregnancy, and medications (oral contraceptives, cold remedies, etc.). The presence of prolonged high blood pressure increases the chances of premature mortality and morbidity, such as coronary artery disease, congestive heart failure, and stroke.[1]

Symptoms and signs   Primary hypertension is usually asymptomatic until complications occur.[4] Uncomplicated high blood pressure may cause dizziness, flushed facies, headache, fatigue, epistaxis, and nervousness.

Management   High blood pressure is not determined until many pressure readings are recorded at various times. A thorough examination must be conducted to ascertain the type of hypertension. Primary hypertension may be controlled with lifestyle changes such as weight loss, salt restriction, and aerobic exercise. Commonly in secondary hypertension, when the underlying condition is cured the blood pressure returns to normal.

Endurance exercise training can lower systolic and diastolic blood pressure by 10 mm Hg in mild hypertensives (140/90 to 180/105 mm Hg). Individuals with blood pressures over 180/105 mm Hg carry out endurance exercises after pharmacological therapy. Resistive strength training, especially isometrics, is not recommended as the only form of exercise.[1]

> Hypertension may be a factor excluding players from sports participation.

ANEMIA IN ATHLETES

Anemia has been identified as the most common medical condition among athletes. It is more common in females than males and most common among female athletes.

Iron-Deficiency Anemia

Iron deficiency is the most common form of true anemia among athletes. Stores of iron are depleted before clinical signs occur. Iron is mainly stored in hemoglobin (64%) and bone marrow (27%).[10] Iron-deficiency anemia is most prevalent among menstruating women and males 11 to 14 years old.[9]

Etiology   Three conditions occur during anemia: erythrocytes (red blood cells) are too small, hemoglobin is decreased, and ferritin concentration is low. Ferritin is an iron-phosphorous-protein complex that normally contains 23% iron. There are many ways that athletes can be iron deficient. Gastrointestinal (GI) losses are common in runners because of bowel ischemia. Aspirin or nonsteroidal antiinflammatory drugs (NSAIDs) may cause GI blood loss. Runners absorb 16% of iron from the GI tract as compared with 30% in nonathletes who are iron deficient. Menstrual losses account for most iron loss in female athletes. Average menstrual iron loss is 0.6 to 1.5 mg per day. Inadequate dietary intake of iron is the primary cause of iron deficiency. The recommended daily allowance (RDA) is 15 mg per day for females and 10 mg per day for males. The average diet contains 5 to 7 mg of iron per 100 kcal. Because female athletes often eat less than they need, they also fail to consume enough iron. If the athlete is a vegetarian, he or she might lack iron.

Symptoms and signs   In the first stages of iron deficiency, the athlete's performance begins to decline. The athlete may complain of burning thighs and nausea from becoming anaerobic. Ice craving is also common. Athletes with mild iron-deficiency anemia may display some mild impairment in their maximum performance. Determining serum ferritin is the most accurate test of iron status. Two factors must be checked by the physician: the athlete's mean corpuscular volume (MCV), which is the average volume of individual cells in a cubic micron, and the relative sizes of the erythrocytes.

Management   The following are some ways to manage iron deficiency: ensure proper diet, including more red meat or dark poultry; avoid coffee and tea, which hamper iron absorption from grains; ingest vitamin C sources, which enhance iron absorption; and take an iron supplement, consisting of ferrous sulfate 325 mg, three times daily.

Footstrike Anemia

hemolysis
Destruction of red blood cells.

Footstrike anemia, or **hemolysis,** is secondary to iron deficiency in athletes.

Etiology   The cause of footstrike anemia, as its name implies, is the impact of the foot as it strikes the floor surface. Impact forces serve to destroy normal erythrocytes within the vascular system.

Symptoms and signs   Hemolysis is characterized by mildly enlarged red cells, an increase in circulatory reticulocytes, and a decrease in the concentration of haptoglobin, which is a glycoprotein bound to hemoglobin and released into the plasma. Even if the athlete wears a well-designed and well-constructed running shoe, this condition can occur. Footstrike anemia varies according to the amount of running performed.

Management   Footstrike anemia can be managed by running on soft surfaces, wearing well-cushioned shoes and insoles, and running "light on the feet."

Sickle Cell Anemia

Sickle cell anemia is a chronic hereditary hemolytic anemia. Approximately 35% of the black population in the United States has this condition; 8% to 13% are not anemic but carry this trait in their genes. If both parents carry the defective gene, the child will have sickle cell anemia; if only one parent carries the gene, the child will have sickle cell trait.[8] The person with sickle cell anemia or trait can have sicklemia. The person with the sickle cell trait may participate in sports and never encounter problems until symptoms are brought on by some unusual circumstance.

Etiology   In individuals with sickle cell anemia the red cells are sickle or crescent shaped. Within the red cells, an abnormal type of hemoglobin exists. It has been speculated that the sickling of the red blood cells results from an adaptation to malaria, which is prevalent in Africa.

The sickle cell has less potential for transporting oxygen and is fragile when compared with normal cells. A sickle cell's life span is 15 to 25 days, compared with the 120 days of a normal red cell; the short life of the sickle cell can produce severe anemia in individuals with acute sickle cell anemia. The cell's distorted shape inhibits its passage through the small blood vessels and can cause clustering of the cells and consequently clogging of the blood vessels, producing **thrombi,** which block circulation. For individuals having this condition, death can occur (in the severest cases of sickle cell anemia) from a stroke, heart disease, or an **embolus** in the lungs. Conversely, persons with sickle cell anemia may never experience any problems. Four factors of exercise can cause sickling: acidosis; hyperthermia; dehydration of red blood cells, increasing hemoglobin concentration; and severe hypoxemia.

thrombi
Plural of "thrombus"; a blood clot that blocks small blood vessels or a cavity of the heart.

embolus
A mass of undissolved matter.

Symptoms and signs   An athlete may never experience any complications from having the sickle cell trait. However, a sickle cell crisis can be brought on by exposure to high altitudes or by overheating of the skin, as is the case with a high fever. Crisis symptoms include fever, severe fatigue, skin pallor, muscle weakness, and severe pain in the limbs and abdomen. Abdominal pain in the right upper quadrant may indicate a splenic syndrome in which there is an infarction.[7] This is especially characteristic of a crisis triggered by a decrease in ambient oxygen while flying at high altitudes. The athlete may also experience headache and convulsions.

Management   Treatment of a sickle cell crisis is usually symptomatic. The physician may elect to give anticoagulants and analgesics for pain.

SEXUALLY TRANSMITTED DISEASES

Sexually transmitted diseases are of major concern in sports because many athletes are at an age during which they are more sexually active than they will be at any other time in their lives. The venereal diseases with the highest incidence among the relatively young are nonspecific sexually transmitted infection (NSI), genital herpes, gonorrhea, genital candidiasis, condyloma acuminata, hepatitis, and the human immunodeficiency virus (HIV) leading to the acquired immunodeficiency syndrome (AIDS).

Nonspecific Sexually Transmitted Infection

Nonspecific sexually transmitted infection, although not required to be reported to health officials, is considered by many the most common venereal disease in the United States. It is more common than gonorrhea.[4]

Etiology   The two organisms associated with NSI are **Chlamydia trachomatis** and *Ureaplasma urealyticum.* Nonspecific sexually transmitted infection is most commonly called chlamydia. In females, chlamydia may result in pelvic inflammatory disease and is an important cause of infertility and ectopic pregnancy.

Symptoms and signs   In the male, inflammation occurs along with a purulent discharge, 7 to 28 days after intercourse.[2] On occasion, painful urination and traces of blood in the urine occur. Most females with this infection are asymptomatic, but some may experience a vaginal discharge, painful urination, pelvic pain, and pain and inflammation in other sites.

Management   A bacteriological examination is given to determine the exact organisms present. Once identified, the infection must be treated promptly to prevent complications. Organism identification and treatment must take place immediately in women who are pregnant. Chlamydial ophthalmia neonatorum can cause conjunctivitis and pneumonia in the newborn from an infected mother.[2] Uncomplicated cases are usually treated with antibiotics. Approximately 20% of the sufferers have one or more relapses.

Genital Herpes

Genital herpes is a venereal infection that is currently widespread.

Etiology   Type 2 herpes simplex virus is associated with genital herpes infection, which is now the most prevalent cause of genital ulcerations. Signs of the disease appear approximately 4 to 7 days after sexual contact. Primary genital herpes crusts in 14 to 17 days, and secondary cases crust in 10 days.

Symptoms and signs   The first signs in the male are itching and soreness, but women may be asymptomatic in the vagina and cervix. It is estimated that 50% to 60% of individuals who have had one attack of herpes genitalis will have no further episodes, or if they do, the lesions are few and insignificant. Like herpes labialis and gladiatorum, lesions develop that eventually become ulcerated with a red areola. Ulcerations crust and heal in approximately 10 days, leaving a scar (Color Plate, Figure M). Of major importance to a pregnant woman with a history of genital herpes is whether there is an active infection when she is nearing delivery. Herpes simplex can be fatal to a newborn child. There is also some relationship (although this is un-

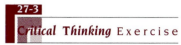

27-3
Critical Thinking Exercise

A female athlete complains of burning thighs and having nausea when she exercises. The athlete also craves ice.

? What should the athletic trainer expect from this scenario, and how should it be handled?

Chlamydia trachomatis
A genus microorganism that can cause a wide variety of diseases in humans, one of which is venereal and causes nonspecific urethritis.

clear) between a higher incidence of cervical cancer and the incidence of herpes genitalis.[4]

Management At this time there is no cure for genital herpes. Recently systemic medication, specifically antiviral medications such as acycloguanosine (Zovirax, Acyclovir) and vidarabine (Vira-A), are being used to lessen the early symptoms of the disease.[4]

Trichomoniasis

Trichomoniasis is an infection that affects 20% of all females during their reproductive years and 5% to 10% of males.

Etiology Trichomoniasis is caused by the flagellate protozoan *Trichomonas vaginalis*.

Symptoms and signs The female with trichomoniasis typically has a vaginal discharge that is greenish yellow and frothy. The disease causes irritation of the vulva, perineum, and thighs. The female may also experience painful urination. Males are usually asymptomatic, although some may experience a frothy, purulent urethral discharge.

Management Metronidazole, 2 g in one dose, is usually the drug of choice in the treatment of trichomoniasis, curing up to 95% of women. Men, in contrast, should be treated with 500 mg bid for 7 days. The sexual partner is treated concurrently. Complete cure is required before the individual can again engage in sexual intercourse.

Genital Candidiasis

As discussed in Chapter 26, *Candida* (a genus of yeastlike fungi) is commonly part of the normal flora of the mouth, skin, intestinal tract, and vagina.

Etiology The *Candida* organism is one of the most common causes of vaginitis in women of reproductive age. The infection is usually transmitted sexually but also can stem from the intestine.

Symptoms and signs As with other related conditions, the female complains of vulval irritation beginning with redness and severe pain and a vaginal discharge (scanty). The male is usually asymptomatic but could develop some irritation and soreness of the glans penis, especially after intercourse. Rarely, a slight urethral discharge may occur.

Management Because of the highly infectious nature of this disease, all sexual contact should cease until completion of treatment. The drug nystatin (a fungicide) is usually inserted high into the vagina for 14 nights at bedtime. This treatment is immediately followed by application of nystatin cream to the labia, perineum, and perianal region.

Condyloma Acuminata (Venereal Warts)

Another sexually transmitted disease that should be recognized and referred to a physician is condyloma acuminata, or venereal warts.

Etiology These warts are transmitted through sexual activity and commonly occur from poor hygiene. They appear on the glans penis, vulva, or anus.

Symptoms and signs This form of wart virus produces nodules that have a cauliflower-like lesion or can be singular. In their early stage they are soft, moist, pink or red swellings that rapidly develop a stem with a flowerlike head. They may be mistaken for secondary syphilis or carcinoma (Color Plate, Figure N).

Management Moist condylomas are often carefully treated by the physician with a solution containing 20% to 25% podophyllin. Dry warts may be treated with a freezing process such as liquid nitrogen.

Gonorrhea

Gonorrhea, commonly called "clap," is an acute venereal disease that can infect the urethra, cervix, and rectum.

Etiology   The organism of infection is the gonococcal bacteria *Neisseria gonorrhoea,* which is usually spread through sexual intercourse.

Symptoms and signs   In men the incubation period is 2 to 10 days. The onset of the disease is marked by a tingling sensation in the urethra, followed in 2 or 3 hours by greenish-yellow discharge of pus and painful urination. Sixty percent of infected women are asymptomatic. For those who have symptoms, onset is between 7 and 21 days. In these cases symptoms are mild, with some vaginal discharge. Gonorrheal infection of the throat and rectum are also possible.

Management   Because of embarrassment, some individuals fail to secure proper medical help for treatment of gonorrhea, and, although the initial symptoms will disappear, such an individual is not cured and can still spread the infection. Untreated gonorrhea becomes latent and will manifest itself in later years, usually causing sterility or arthritis. Treatment consists of large amounts of penicillin or other antibiotics. Recent experimental evidence suggests an increasing resistance of the gonococci to penicillin. Evidence of any of the symptoms should result in immediately remanding the individual to a physician for testing and treatment. *All sexual contact must be avoided* until it has been medically established that the disease is no longer active. Because of the latent residual effects that are the end result of several diseases in this group, including sterility and arthritis, immediate medical treatment is mandatory. Although outward signs may disappear, the disease is still insidiously present in the body. Additionally, such treatment will alleviate the discomfort that accompanies the initial stages of the disease.

Syphilis

A sexually transmitted disease that is on an increase is syphilis. A reason for this increase is high-risk sexual behavior, drug usage, and lack of knowledge about preventing infection.[8]

Etiology   *Treponema pallidum,* a spirochete bacteria, is the organism related to syphilis. It enters the body through mucous membranes or skin lesions.[4]

Symptoms and signs   Untreated syphilis may have a course of four stages within the body: primary, secondary, latent, and late, or tertiary. The incubation period of syphilis is normally 3 to 4 weeks but can range anywhere from 1 to 13 weeks. A painless chancre or ulceration develops and heals within 4 to 8 weeks. This stage is highly contagious. Ulcerations can occur on the penis, urethra, vagina, cervix, mouth, around the eye, or on the hand or foot.

The secondary stage of syphilis occurs within 6 to 12 weeks after the initial infection. It is characterized by a skin rash, lymph swelling, body aches, and mild flulike symptoms. Hair may fall out in patches.

Latent syphilis follows the secondary stage and is characterized by no or few symptoms. If untreated, approximately one third of persons with latent syphilis will develop late, or tertiary, syphilis.

The late stage of syphilis is characterized by a deep penetration of spirochetes damaging skin, bone, and the cardiovascular and nervous systems. Tertiary syphilis can develop within 3 to 10 years of infection. Neurosyphilis can progress into severe muscle weakness, paralysis, and various types of psychoses.

Management   Penicillin is the antibiotic for all stages of syphilis. Those allergic to penicillin may be treated with erythromycin. Because *T. pallidum* can exist only in body fluids, air-drying and cleaning with soap and water will destroy it. Because of the rise of penicillin resistance, ceftriaxone may be the drug of choice.

MENSTRUAL IRREGULARITIES AND THE FEMALE REPRODUCTIVE SYSTEM

There are special menstrual and reproductive concerns related to the female who engages in intense physical activity. This section addresses some of the more prevalent issues.

27-4

Critical Thinking Exercise

A male college basketball player confides in the athletic trainer about a greenish-yellow urethral discharge and painful urination.

? How should this situation be managed by the athletic trainer?

Physiology of the Menstrual Cycle

Menstruation refers to the periodic discharge of bloody fluid from the uterus usually at regular intervals during the life of a woman from the age of puberty to menopause.

Menarche

During the prepubertal period, girls are the equal of, and often superior to, boys of the same age in activities requiring speed, strength, and endurance.

Menarche, the onset of the menses, and puberty normally occur between ages 9 and 17, with the majority of girls usually entering it between ages 13 and 15. Puberty is that period of life in which either sex becomes able to reproduce. There is indication that strenuous sports training and competition will delay the onset of menarche. The greatest delay is related to the higher-caliber competition. In itself, a delay in the first menses does not appear to pose any significant danger to the young female athlete. Delayed menarche, or primary amenorrhea, is defined as menstruation not occurring by age 16 or a failure to develop secondary sexual characteristics by age 14. The late-maturing girl commonly has longer legs, narrower hips, and less adiposity and body weight for her height, all of which are more conducive to sports.

The onset of menarche may be delayed by strenuous training and competition.

Menstruation

The effects of sustained and strenuous training and competition on the menstrual cycle and the effects of menstruation on performance still cannot be fully explained with any degree of certainty.

The classic 28-day cycle consists of the follicular and luteal phases, each of which is approximately 14 days long. The menses vary from 3 to 7 days, with an average of 4 to 7 days. The majority of women tend to show some variation in the length of their cycles, with these differences occurring principally because of differences in duration of the preovulatory phase rather than the premenstrual phase.

With the onset of menarche a cyclic hormone pattern commences, which establishes the menstrual cycle. These hormonal changes result from complex feedback mechanisms and specifically controlled interactions that occur between the hypothalamus, ovaries, and pituitary gland. Two gonadotropins induce the release of the egg from the mature follicle at midcycle (ovulation): follicle-stimulating hormone (FSH), which stimulates the maturation of an ovarian follicle, and luteinizing hormone (LH), which stimulates the development of the corpus luteum and the endocrine structure that secretes progesterone and estrogens. The control and eventual inhibition of the production of FSH when the follicle reaches maturity is brought about by the estrogenic steroids produced by the ovaries. Progesterone, a steroid hormone produced within the corpus luteum—a small body that develops within a ruptured ovarian follicle after ovulation—eventually inhibits production of LH. Estrogen is secreted principally by the luteal cells. Before onset of a new menstrual period, FSH levels are already rising, probably to initiate maturation of new follicles to reinstitute the next cycle.

Menstrual Cycle Irregularities

The highly active female athlete, such as those participating in ballet, gymnastics, and long-distance running, can experience irregularities in the normal menstrual cycle of 25 to 38 days. *Oligomenorrhea* (diminished flow) refers to fewer than 3 to 6 cycles per year.[3] A short luteal phase of 10 days' duration and anovulation can occur with regular menstrual bleeding, both in the absence of ovulation and in cycles with a short luteal phase. **Amenorrhea** is the complete cessation of the cycle with ovulation occurring seldom or not at all because of the low level of circulating estrogen.[3] Approximately 10% to 20% of vigorously exercising women have amenorrhea.

amenorrhea
Absence or suppression of menstruation.

Etiology   The cause of exercise-related amenorrhea, or "athlete's amenorrhea," is often a hypothalamic dysfunction. The gonadotropin-releasing hormone (GnRH) produced by the hypothalamus is often deficient.[20] Many factors must be ruled out by a physical examination before athlete's amenorrhea is determined. Pregnancy and ab-

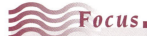

Focus

Suggested factors in exercise-induced amenorrhea
- Competition such as long-distance running, gymnastics, professional ballet dancing, cycling, or swimming
- Low body weight with weight loss after beginning of training
- Total calorie intake inadequate for energy needs
- An eating disorder
- High incidence of menstrual abnormalities before vigorous training
- Higher levels of stress when compared with those experiencing normal menses
- Likely to have begun training at an early age
- A rapid increase in high-intensity exercise

normalities of the reproductive or genital tract must be ruled out, as well as ovarian failure and pituitary tumors.[11,20]

Symptoms and signs   The Focus box above includes some factors of exercise-related amenorrhea.

Management   The ideal treatment of exercise-induced amenorrhea is the reestablishment of normal hormone levels and the return of the normal menstrual cycle.[3] It is important that a medical evaluation be given first before other intervention procedures are given. Cleared of any physical abnormalities, nutritional counseling is given as to balancing calorie output and intake and proper amount of nutrients. Reducing exercise intensity and counseling to reduce emotional stress can be helpful. Estrogen replacement may be considered.[3]

Dysmenorrhea

Dysmenorrhea (painful menstruation) apparently is prevalent among more active women; however, it is inconclusive whether specific sports participation can alleviate or produce dysmenorrhea. For girls with moderate to severe dysmenorrhea, gynecological consultation is warranted to rule out a pathological condition.[3]

Dysmenorrhea is caused by ischemia (a lack of normal blood flow to the pelvic organs) or by a possible hormonal imbalance. This syndrome, which is identified by cramps, nausea, lower abdominal pain, headache, and on occasion emotional lability, is the most common menstrual disorder. Mild to vigorous exercises that help ameliorate dysmenorrhea are usually prescribed by physicians. Physicians generally advise a continuance of the usual sports participation during the menstrual period, provided the performance level of the individual does not drop below her customary level of ability. Among athletes, swimmers have the highest incidence of dysmenorrhea; it, along with menorrhagia, occurs most often, probably as the result of strenuous sports participation during the menses. Generally, oligomenorrhea, amenorrhea, and irregular or scanty flow are more common in sports that require strenuous exertion over a long period of time (e.g., long-distance running, rowing, cross-country skiing, basketball, tennis, field hockey, and soccer). Because great variation exists among female athletes with respect to menstrual pattern, its effect on physical performance, and the effect of physical activity on the menstrual pattern, each individual must learn to make adjustments to her cycle that will permit her to function effectively and efficiently with a minimum of discomfort or restriction. Evidence to date indicates that top performances are possible in all phases of the cycle.

Bone Health

The athlete who has a prolonged decrease of FSH, LH, estrogen, and progesterone shows a profile similar to that of a postmenopausal woman.[12] Osteoporosis is most

Girls who have moderate to severe dysmenorrhea require examination by a physician.

27-5

Critical Thinking Exercise

A female athlete has been diagnosed as having a serious eating disorder and amenorrhea.

? Why may these two medical disorders lead eventually to osteoporosis?

common in women older than 50 years whose bone mass (bone mineral density) has fallen below a critical threshold. Athletic women who have irregular menses because of endocrine changes are strong candidates for bone loss. Low bone mass leads to bone fragility and increased susceptibility to stress fractures in female athletes with premature osteoporosis, especially athletes with late menarche.[15] There is evidence of estrogen receptors on bone cells causing a direct relation on growth and bone function.[12] Calcium nutrition is also needed with a recommended daily allowance for adolescents through age 24 of 1200 mg daily.[18]

An athlete experiencing loss of periods with low bone mass should decrease training intensity and volume, increase total calories, and ingest 1200 to 1500 mg of calcium daily. A program of resistance training designed for both muscle mass and strength may enhance the skeletal profile and protect against muscle injury. Estrogen replacement therapy may be warranted if other means fail.[15]

The Female Athlete Triad

The relationship of three medical disorders has been termed *the female athlete triad*. It includes disorded eating, amenorrhea, and osteoporosis, a bone disease marked by softening and increased porosity.[22,23]

Etiology As stated by Nattiv and co-workers,[22,23] "The young woman athlete, driven to excel in her chosen sport and pressured to fit a specific athletic image in order to reach her goals, is at risk for the development of disordered patterns of eating," which "may lead to menstrual dysfunction and subsequent premature osteoporosis." This triad has the potential for serious illness and risk of death.[23]

Symptoms and signs The components of the triad are disorded eating, amenorrhea, and osteoporosis. Disordered eating follows the same patterns of eating characteristics of anorexia nervosa and bulimia. (See Chapter 4.) Amenorrhea is discussed earlier in this chapter. Osteoporosis in young women athletes refers to premature bone loss and inadequate bone development resulting in low bone mass, microarchitectural destruction, increased skeletal fragility, and increased risk of fracture.[23] Physicians, athletic trainers, and coaches must be aware of the athlete's potential for being at risk. Special concern must be directed toward those sports that focus on an ideal body type and weight, the signs of disorded eating, and disruption in menarche or the menstrual cycle.

Management Management of this triad lies in prevention. Those concerned with the athlete's total health must be educated. A concerted effort must be made to identify and screen athletes who are at risk.

Contraceptives and Reproduction

Female athletes have been known to take extra oral contraceptive pills to delay menstruation during competition. This practice is not recommended. Such practices can cause nausea, vomiting, fluid retention, amenorrhea, hypertension, double vision, and thrombophlebitis. It should be noted that some oral contraceptives make women hypersensitive to the sun. Any use of oral contraceptives related to physical performance should be under the express direction and control of a physician. However, oral contraceptive use is acceptable for females with no medical problems who have coitus at least twice a week. The new low-dose preparations, containing less than 50 mg of estrogen, add negligible risks to the healthy woman.

In general, athletes who wear intrauterine devices are free of such problems. However, intrauterine devices are not recommended for nulliparous (never borne a viable child) adolescents because of the associated risk of pelvic inflammatory disease. On occasion the athlete may complain of a lower-abdominal cramp while being active. In such cases referral to a physician should be made.

Pregnancy

During pregnancy, women athletes exhibit high levels of muscle tonicity. It has been determined that women who suffer from a chronic disability after childbirth usually

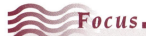

Focus

have a record of little or no physical exercise in the decade immediately preceding pregnancy. Generally, competition may be engaged in well into the third month of pregnancy unless bleeding or cramps are present and can frequently be continued until the seventh month if no handicapping or physiological complications arise.[17] Such activity may make pregnancy, childbirth, and postparturition less stressful. Many women athletes do not continue beyond the third month because there is a drop in their performance. This decline may result from a number of causes, some related to the pregnancy, others perhaps psychological. It is during the first 3 months of pregnancy that the dangers of disturbing the pregnancy are greatest. After that period there is less danger to the mother and fetus because the pregnancy is stabilized. There is no indication that mild to moderate exercise during pregnancy is harmful to fetal growth and development or causes reduced fetal mass, increased perinatal or neonatal mortality, or physical or mental retardation.[6,25] It has been found, however, that extreme exercise may lower birth weight. (See the Focus box above.) Many athletes compete during pregnancy with no ill effects. Most physicians, although advocating moderate activity during this period, believe that especially vigorous performance, particularly in activities in which there may be severe body contact or heavy

In general, childbirth is not adversely affected by a history of hard physical exercise.

jarring or falls, should be avoided.[16] Contraindications to exercise include the following:

- Pregnancy-induced hypertension
- Preterm rupture of membranes
- Preterm labor during the prior or current pregnancy or both
- Incompetent cervix or cerclage
- Persistent second- or third-trimester bleeding
- Intrauterine growth retardation

SUMMARY

- Athletes may be prone to a variety of respiratory conditions, such as the common cold, sinusitis, pharyngitis, flu, and seasonal allergies. Infectious mononucleosis, acute bronchitis, and exercise-induced asthma are some of the more serious conditions of the respiratory tract.
- Athletes are also subject to various gastrointestinal conditions that can adversely affect their performances. These conditions include mouth, gum, and tooth problems and digestive conditions such as dyspepsia, diarrhea, constipation, and hemorrhoids. Gastrointestinal bleeding may or may not be a serious medical problem. Food poisoning can occur from various bacterial infections.
- Diabetes mellitus is a complex hereditary or developmental disease of carbohydrate metabolism. Athletes under 30 years of age usually have insulin-dependent diabetes mellitus, whereas non–insulin-dependent diabetes mellitus usually occurs after 40 years of age. Athletes with this condition must carefully balance their diet, exercise, and insulin ingestion. Diabetics must be extremely cautious about the possibility of going into diabetic coma or insulin shock. Diabetic coma can occur if there is too little insulin in the system; conversely, insulin shock can occur from too much insulin in the body.
- Some athletes have a history of epilepsy that could lead to an alteration of consciousness. Epilepsy is not a disease, and each person with epilepsy must be considered individually.
- The athlete with high blood pressure may have to be carefully monitored by the physician. Hypertension may require the avoidance of heavy resistive activities.
- Anemia in athletes usually is one of three types: iron-deficiency anemia, foot-strike anemia, and sickle cell anemia. Most often, iron-deficiency anemia is a condition found in women. In an athlete with iron-deficiency anemia, hemoglobin is decreased and the ferritin concentration is low. The athlete with foot-strike anemia is usually heavyset and engages in an activity such as running in which the sustained impact forces destroy erythrocytes. The athlete with the sickle cell trait may have an adverse reaction at high altitudes, where the sickle-shaped blood cell is unable to transport oxygen adequately.
- Sexually transmitted disease has its highest incidence among younger, sexually active persons. Because the highest number of athletes are in this highest-risk age group, there should be great concern about the spread of these diseases. To avoid these infections, "safe sex" is suggested, which involves the use of a condom, the elimination of multiple partners, or even complete abstinence from sexual intercourse.
- The highly active female may have menstrual irregularities, including dysmenorrhea, amenorrhea, or oligomenorrhea. Menstrual irregularities could lead to a thinning of bone and subsequent fractures. Contraception and pregnancy are issues the female athlete may have to address.

Solutions to Critical Thinking EXERCISES

27-1 This scenario describes flu symptoms. There should be symptomatic care and the avoidance of aspirin.

27-2 The athlete maintains a high level of conditioning, including the running of longer distances. There should be always a gradual warm-up and a cool-down. All exercise intensity and loading should be graduated slowly. A bronchodilator may be employed. A mask or scarf is used when there is cold, dry air. The athlete should avoid exercising in areas with high levels of air pollution or when there is a high pollen count.

27-3 The athlete appears to have iron-deficiency anemia. After verification by a physician, the athlete should eat a diet rich in iron, avoid coffee and tea, eat foods high in vitamin C, and take a daily iron supplement.

27-4 This situation must be handled with the strictest confidentiality. Because this condition could be gonorrhea, immediate medical referral must be made. All sexual contact must be avoided until this condition has been resolved.

27-5 These medical disorders make up the female athlete triad. Osteoporosis is the softening and increased porosity of bones with subsequent fracturing. Athletes who have anorexia nervosa or bulimia to establish a perceived body image are at risk. Athletes who train so hard that they stop menstruating also stop their estrogen production, which results in a loss of calcium in the bones.

REVIEW QUESTIONS AND CLASS ACTIVITIES

1. Contrast the symptoms and signs of the following respiratory tract conditions: the common cold, influenza, and allergic rhinitis.
2. Discuss mononucleosis in detail, including prevention and etiology.
3. Discuss and contrast bronchial obstructive diseases such as bronchitis and asthma. How do you care for an athlete with an acute asthmatic attack?
4. Describe the most common gastrointestinal complaints. How are the conditions which produce them acquired and managed?
5. What is diabetes mellitus? What value might exercise have for the person with diabetes mellitus? How are diabetic coma and insulin shock managed?
6. In a sports setting, what are some major indications that an athlete has a contagious disease?
7. What is epilepsy? How should a grand mal seizure be managed?
8. Define hypertension. What dangers does it present to the athlete?
9. Describe the anemias that most often affect the athlete. How should each be managed?
10. Discuss the etiology, symptoms and signs, and management of the most common sexually transmitted diseases. How can they be prevented?
11. Discuss menstrual irregularities that occur in highly active athletes. Why do they occur? How should they be managed? How do they relate to reproduction?
12. What are the implications of pregnancy for extensive physical activity?

REFERENCES

1. American College of Sports Medicine: Position stand: physical activity, physical fitness and hypertension, *Med Sci Sports Exerc* 25(10):1, 1993.
2. Bartimole J: Exercise-induced asthma: pre-treating for prevention, *NATA News* 4, 1995.
3. Benson MT, editor: *1994-95 NCAA sports medicine handbook: menstrual-cycle dysfunction,* Overland Park, Kans, 1994, National Collegiate Athletic Association.
4. Berkow R, editor: *The Merck manual,* ed 16, Rahway, NJ, 1992, Merck.
5. Blumenthal MN: Sports-aggravated allergies, *Phys Sportsmed* 18(12):70, 1990.
6. Clapp III JF: A clinical approach to exercise during pregnancy. In Agostini R, editor: *The athletic woman. Clinics in sports medicine,* vol 13, no 2, Philadelphia, 1994, Saunders.
7. Eichner ER: Sickle cell trait, heroic exercise, and fatal collapse, *Phys Sportsmed* 21(7):51, 1993.
8. Hamann B: *Disease: identification, prevention, and control,* St Louis, 1994, Mosby.
9. Harris SS: Exercise-related anemias. In Agostini R, editor: *Medical and orthopedic issues of active and athletic women,* St Louis, 1994, Mosby.
10. Harris SS: Helping active women avoid anemia, *Phys Sportsmed* 23(5):34, 1995.
11. Harter-Snow C: Athletic amenorrhea and bone health. In Agostini R, editor: *Medical and orthopedic issues of active and athletic women,* St Louis, 1994, Mosby.
12. Harter-Snow CM: Bone health and prevention of osteoporosis in active and athletic women. In Agostini R, editor: *The athletic woman. Clinic in sports medicine,* vol 13, no 2, Philadelphia, 1994, Saunders.
13. Howe WB: The athlete with chronic illness. In Birrer RB, editor: *Sports medicine for the primary care physician,* ed 2, Boca Raton, Fla, 1994, CRC Press.
14. Jong EC: Infections. In Agostini R, editor: *Medical and orthopedic issues of active and athletic women,* St Louis, 1994, Mosby.
15. Karpalcka J et al: Recurrent stress fracture in a female athlete with primary amenorrhea, *Clin J Sports Med* 4(2):136, 1994.
16. Kulpa P: Exercise during pregnancy and post partum. In Agostini R, editor: *Medical and orthopedic issues of active and athletic women,* St Louis, 1994, Mosby.
17. LeBrun CM: Effects of the menstrual cycle and birth control pills on athletic performance. In Agostini R, editor: *Medical and orthopedic issues of active athletic women,* St Louis, 1994, Mosby.
18. Lemcke DP: Osteoporosis and menopause. In Agostini R, editor: *Medical and orthopedic issues of active and athletic women,* St Louis, 1994, Mosby.
19. Mahler DA: Exercise-induced asthma, *Med Sci Sports Exerc* 25(5):554, 1993.
20. Marshall LA: Clinical evaluation of amenorrhea. In Agostini R, editor: *Medical and orthopedic issues of active and athletic women,* St Louis, 1994, Mosby.
21. Mellion MB et al: Medical problems in athletes. In Birrer RB, editor: *Sports medicine for the primary care physician,* Boca Raton, Fla, 1994, CRC Press.
22. Nattiv A, Lynch L: The female athlete triad, *Phys Sportsmed* 22(1):60, 1994.
23. Nattiv A et al: The female athletic triad. In Agostini R, editor: *Medical and orthopedic issues of active and athletic women,* St Louis, 1994, Mosby.
24. *PACOG Technical Bulletin 189. Exercise during pregnancy and postpartum period,* Washington, DC, 1994, The American College of Obstetricians and Gynecologists.
25. Partin N: The diabetic athlete, *Ath Train* 24(4):381, 1989.

26. Robbins DC, Carleton S: Managing the diabetic athlete, *Phys Sportsmed* 17(12):45, 1989.

27. Taunton JE, McCargarl EL: Staying active with diabetes, *Phys Sportsmed* 23(3):55, 1995.

ANNOTATED BIBLIOGRAPHY

Agostini R, editor: *Medical and orthopedic issues of active and athletic women,* St Louis, 1994, Mosby.

An excellent overview of health issues facing the physically active female.

Berkow R, editor: *The Merck manual of diagnosis and therapy,* Rahway, NJ, 1992, Merck.

A major reference book on etiology, symptoms and signs, and treatment of disease.

Birrer RB, editor: *Sports medicine for the primary care physician,* ed 2, Boca Raton, Fla, 1994, CRC Press.

A comprehensive review of the important medical, orthopedic, and scientific aspects of caring for athletes.

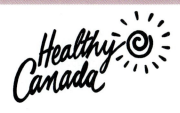

CANADA'S

Food Guide

TO HEALTHY EATING

 Health and Welfare Canada   Santé et Bien-être social Canada

Enjoy a variety of foods from each group every day.

Choose lower-fat foods more often.

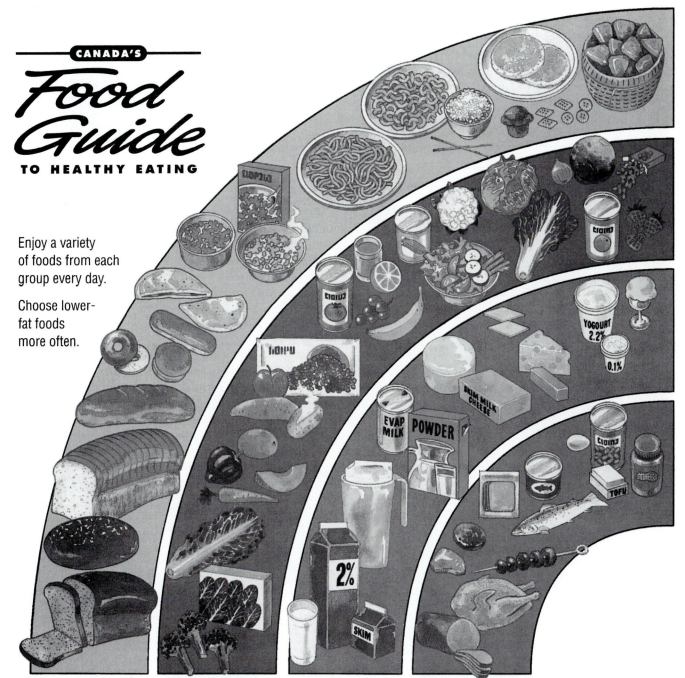

Grain Products
Choose whole grain and enriched products more often.

Vegetables & Fruit
Choose dark green and orange vegetables and orange fruit more often.

Milk Products
Choose lower-fat milk products more often.

Meat & Alternatives
Choose leaner meats, poultry and fish, as well as dried peas, beans and lentils more often.

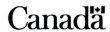 Canada

Continued

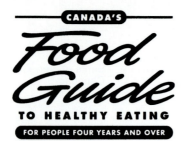

Different People Need Different Amounts of Food

The amount of food you need every day from the 4 food groups and other foods depends on your age, body size, activity level, whether you are male or female and if you are pregnant or breast-feeding. That's why the Food Guide gives a lower and higher number of servings for each food group. For example, young children can choose the lower number of servings, while male teenagers can go to the higher number. Most other people can choose servings somewhere in between.

Grain Products
5-12 SERVINGS PER DAY

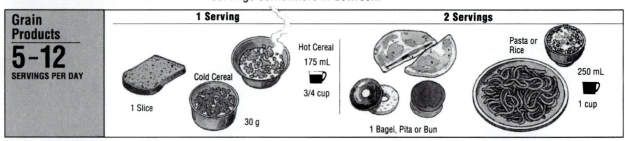

1 Serving — 1 Slice; Cold Cereal 30 g; Hot Cereal 175 mL 3/4 cup

2 Servings — 1 Bagel, Pita or Bun; Pasta or Rice 250 mL 1 cup

Vegetables & Fruit
5-10 SERVINGS PER DAY

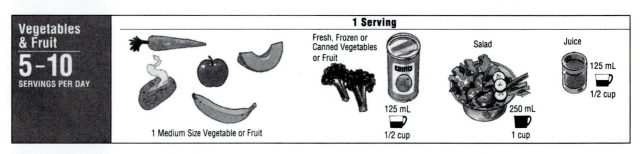

1 Serving — 1 Medium Size Vegetable or Fruit; Fresh, Frozen or Canned Vegetables or Fruit 125 mL 1/2 cup; Salad 250 mL 1 cup; Juice 125 mL 1/2 cup

Milk Products
SERVINGS PER DAY
Children 4–9 years: 2–3
Youth 10–16 years: 3–4
Adults: 2–4
Pregnant & Breast-feeding Women: 3–4

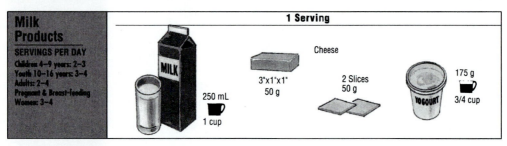

1 Serving — MILK 250 mL 1 cup; Cheese 3"x1"x1" 50 g; 2 Slices 50 g; YOGOURT 175 g 3/4 cup

Meat & Alternatives
2-3 SERVINGS PER DAY

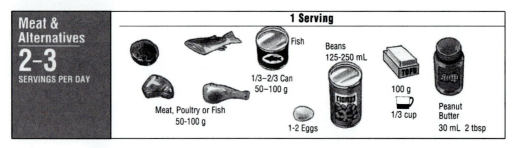

1 Serving — Meat, Poultry or Fish 50-100 g; Fish 1/3–2/3 Can 50–100 g; 1-2 Eggs; Beans 125–250 mL; TOFU 100 g 1/3 cup; Peanut Butter 30 mL 2 tbsp

Other Foods

Taste and enjoyment can also come from other foods and beverages that are not part of the 4 food groups. Some of these foods are higher in fat or Calories, so use these foods in moderation.

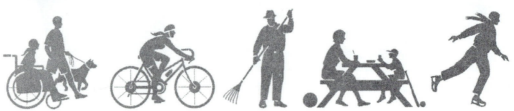

Enjoy eating well, being active and feeling good about yourself. That's VITALITÉ®

© Minister of Supply and Services Canada 1992 Cat. No. H39-252/1992E No changes permitted. Reprint permission not required.
ISBN 0-662-19648-1

Nutrient Recommendations for Canadians

Recommended Nutrient Intake

Age	Sex	Weight (kg)	Protein (g)	Vit. A (RE[a])	Vit. D (μg)	Vit. E (mg)	Vit. C (mg)	Folate (μg)	vit. B$_{12}$ (μg)	Calcium (mg)	Phos-phorus (mg)	Mag-nesium (mg)	Iron (mg)	Iodine (μg)	Zinc (mg)
Months															
0-4	Both	6.0	12[b]	400	10	3	20	25	0.3	250[c]	150	20	0.3[d]	30	2[d]
5-10	Both	9.0	12	400	10	3	20	40	0.4	400	200	32	7	40	3
Years															
1	Both	11	13	400	10	3	20	40	0.5	500	300	40	6	55	4
2-3	Both	14	16	400	5	4	20	50	0.6	550	350	50	6	65	4
4-6	Both	18	19	500	5	5	25	70	0.8	600	400	65	8	85	5
7-9	M	25	26	700	2.5	7	25	90	1.0	700	500	100	8	110	7
	F	25	26	700	2.5	6	25	90	1.0	700	500	100	8	95	7
10-12	M	34	34	800	2.5	8	25	120	1.0	900	700	130	8	125	9
	F	36	36	800	2.5	7	25	130	1.0	1100	800	135	8	110	9
13-15	M	50	49	900	2.5	9	30	175	1.0	1100	900	185	10	160	12
	F	48	46	800	2.5	7	30	170	1.0	1000	850	180	13	160	9
16-18	M	62	58	1000	2.5	10	40[e]	220	1.0	900	1000	230	10	160	12
	F	53	47	800	2.5	7	30[e]	190	1.0	700	850	200	12	160	9
19-24	M	71	61	1000	2.5	10	40[e]	220	1.0	800	1000	240	9	160	12
	F	58	50	800	2.5	7	30[e]	180	1.0	700	850	200	13	160	9
25-49	M	74	64	1000	2.5	9	40[e]	230	1.0	800	1000	250	9	160	12
	F	59	51	800	2.5	6	30[e]	185	1.0	700	850	200	13	160	9
50-74	M	73	63	1000	5	7	40[e]	230	1.0	800	1000	250	9	160	12
	F	63	54	800	5	6	30[e]	195	1.0	800	850	210	8	160	9
75+	M	69	59	1000	5	6	40[e]	215	1.0	800	1000	230	9	160	12
	F	64	55	800	5	5	30[e]	200	1.0	800	850	210	8	160	9
Pregnancy (additional)															
1st Trimester		5	0	2.5	2	0	200	0.2	500	200	15	0	25	6	
2nd Trimester		20	0	2.5	2	10	200	0.2	500	200	45	5	25	6	
3rd Trimester		24	0	2.5	2	10	200	0.2	500	200	45	10	25	6	
Lactation (additional)		20	400	2.5	3	25	100	0.2	500	200	65	0	50	6	

[a]Retinol equivalents
[b]Protein is assumed to be from breast milk and must be adjusted for infant formula.
[c]Infant formula with high phosphorus should contain 375 mg calcium.
[d]Breast milk is assumed to be the source of the mineral.
[e]Smokers should increase vitamin C by 50%.
SOURCE: Scientific Review Committe: *Nutrition Recommendations,* Ottawa, Canada: Health and Welfare, 1990.
Reproduced with permission of the Minister of Supply and Services Canada, 1996.

Continued

Nutrient Recommendations for Canadians—cont'd

Energy Expressed as Daily Rates

Age	Sex	Energy (Cal)	Thiamin (mg)	Riboflavin (mg)	Niacin (NE[b])	n-3 PUFA[a] (g)	n-6 PUFA (g)
Months							
0-4	Both	600	0.3	0.3	4	0.5	3
5-12	Both	900	0.4	0.5	7	0.5	3
Years							
1	Both	1100	0.5	0.6	8	0.6	4
2-3	Both	1300	0.6	0.7	9	0.7	4
4-6	Both	1800	0.7	0.9	13	1.0	6
7-9	M	2200	0.9	1.1	16	1.2	7
	F	1900	0.8	1.0	14	1.0	6
10-12	M	2500	1.0	1.3	18	1.4	8
	F	2200	0.9	1.1	16	1.2	7
13-15	M	2800	1.1	1.4	20	1.5	9
	F	2200	0.9	1.1	16	1.2	7
16-18	M	3200	1.3	1.6	23	1.8	11
	F	2100	0.8	1.1	15	1.2	7
19-24	M	3000	1.2	1.5	22	1.6	10
	F	2100	0.8	1.1	15	1.2	7
25-49	M	2700	1.1	1.4	19	1.5	9
	F	1900	0.8	1.0	14	1.1	7
50-74	M	2300	0.9	1.2	16	1.3	8
	F	1800	0.8[c]	1.0[c]	14[c]	1.1[c]	7[c]
75+	M	2000	0.8	1.0	14	1.1	7
	F[d]	1700	0.8[c]	1.0[c]	14[c]	1.1[c]	7[c]
Pregnancy (additional)							
1st Trimester		100	0.1	0.1	1	0.05	0.3
2nd Trimester		300	0.1	0.3	2	0.16	0.9
3rd Trimester		300	0.1	0.3	2	0.16	0.9
Lactation (additional)		450	0.2	0.4	3	0.25	1.5

[a]PUFA, polyunsaturated fatty acids.
[b]Niacin equivalents.
[c]Level below which intake should not fall.
[d]Assumes moderate physical activity.
SOURCE: Scientific Review Committe: *Nutrition Recommendations,* Ottawa, Canada: Health and Welfare, 1990.
Reproduced with permission of the Minister of Supply and Services Canada, 1996.

A

abduction Movement of a body part away from the midline of the body.

accident Occurring by chance or without intention.

acute injury An injury with sudden onset and short duration.

ad libitum Amount desired.

adduction Movement of a body part toward the midline of the body.

adipose cell Stores triglyceride.

afferent nerves Nerves that transport messages toward the brain.

agonist muscles Muscles directly engaged in contraction as related to muscles that relax at the same time.

ambient Environmental (e.g., temperature or air that invests one's immediate environment).

ambulation Move or walk from place to place.

ameboid action Cellular action like that of an amoeba, using protoplasmic pseudopod.

amenorrhea Absence or suppression of menstruation.

analgesia Pain inhibition.

analgesic Agent that relieves pain without causing a complete loss of sensation.

anaphylaxis Increased susceptibility or sensitivity to a foreign protein or toxin as the result of previous exposure to it.

androgen Any substance that aids the development and controls the appearance of male characteristics.

anemia Lack of iron.

anesthesia Partial or complete loss of sensation.

anomaly Deviation from the normal.

anorexia Lack or loss of appetite; aversion to food.

anorexia nervosa Eating disorder characterized by a distorted body image.

anoxia Lack of oxygen.

antagonist muscles Muscles that counteract the action of the agonist muscles.

anterior Before or in front of.

anteroposterior Refers to the position of front to back.

anteversion Tipping forward of a part as a whole, without bending.

antipyretic Agent that relieves or reduces fever.

anxiety A feeling of uncertainty or apprehension

apophysis Bony outgrowth to which muscles attach.

apophysitis Inflammation of an apophysis.

arrhythmical movement Irregular movement.

arthrogram Radiopaque material injected into a joint to facilitate the taking of an x-ray.

arthrokinematics Physiological and accessory movements of the joint.

arthroscopic examination Viewing the inside of a joint through an arthroscope, which uses a small camera lens.

asymmetry (body) Lack of symmetry of sides of the body.

atrophy Wasting away of tissue or of an organ; diminution of the size of a body part.

attenuation Decrease in intensity as ultrasound enters deeper into tissues.

autogenic inhibition The relaxation of the antagonist muscle during contractions.

aura Preepileptic phenomenon, involving visual sensation of fire or glow, along with other possible sensory hallucinations and dreamlike states.

automatism Automatic behavior before consciousness or full awareness has been achieved after a brain concussion.

avascular Devoid of blood circulation.

avascular necrosis Death of tissue caused by the lack of blood supply.

avulsion Forcible tearing away of a part or a structure.

axilla Armpit.

B

bacteria Morphologically, the simplest group of nongreen vegetable organisms, various species of which are involved in fermentation and putrefaction, the production of disease, and the fixing of atmospheric nitrogen; a schizomycete.

bacteriostatic Halting the growth of bacteria.

ballistic stretching Older stretching technique that uses repetitive bouncing motions.

bandage Strip of cloth or other material used to cover a wound.

beam nonuniformity ratio (BNR) Amount of variability of the ultrasound beam.

beta-endorphin Chemical substance produced in the brain.

biomechanics Branch of study that applies the laws of mechanics to living organisms and biological tissues.

bipedal Having two feet or moving on two feet.

BMR Basal metabolic rate.

body composition Percent body fat plus lean body weight.

bradykinin Peptide chemical that causes pain in an injured area.

buccal Pertaining to the cheek or mouth.

bulimia Binge-purge eating disorder.

bursitis Inflammation of a bursa, especially those bursae located between bony prominences and a muscle or tendon such as those of the shoulder and knee.

C

calcific tendinitis Deposition of calcium in a chronically inflamed tendon, especially the tendons of the shoulder.

calisthenic Exercise involving free movement without the aid of equipment.

calorie (large) Amount of heat required to raise 1 kg of water 1°C; used to express the fuel or energy value of food or the heat output of the organism; the amount of heat required to heat 1 lb of water to 4°F.

cardiorespiratory endurance Ability to perform activities for extended periods of time.

catastrophic injury Relates to a permanent injury of the spinal cord, leaving the athlete quadriplegic or paraplegic.

catecholamine Active amines, epinephrine and norepinephrine, that affect the nervous and cardiovascular systems.

cerebrovascular accident Stroke.

chafing Superficial inflammation that develops when skin is subjected to friction.

chemotaxis Response to influence of chemical stimulation.

chiropractor One who practices a method for restoring normal condition by adjusting the segments of the spinal column.

Chlamydia trachomatis A genus microorganism that can cause a wide variety of diseases in humans, one of which is venereal and causes nonspecific urethritis.

chondromalacia Abnormal softening of cartilage.

chronic injury Injury with long onset and long duration.

cicatrix Scar or mark formed by fibrous connective tissue; left by a wound or sore.

circadian rhythm Biological time clock by which the body functions.

circuit training Exercise stations that consist of various combinations of weight training, flexibility, calisthenics, and aerobic exercises.

circumduct Act of moving a limb such as the arm or hip in a circular manner.

clonic muscle contraction Alternating involuntary muscle contraction and relaxation in quick suspension.

coenzymes Enzyme activators.

collagen Main organic constituent of connective tissue.

collision sport Sport in which athletes use their bodies to deter or punish opponents.

colloid Liquid or gelatinous substance that retains particles of another substance in a state of suspension.

commission (legal liability) Person commits an act that is not legally his or hers to perform.

communicable disease Disease that may be transmitted directly or indirectly from one individual to another.

concentric (positive) contraction The muscle shortens while contracting against resistance.

conduction Heating through direct contact with a hot medium.

conjunctiva Mucous membrane that lines the eyes.

contact sport Sport in which athletes do make physical contact but not with the intent to produce bodily injury.

contrast bath procedure Two minutes of immersion in ice slush, followed by 30 seconds in tepid water.

contrecoup brain injury After head is struck, brain continues to move within the skull, resulting in injury to the side opposite the force.

convection Heating indirectly through another medium such as air or liquid.

conversion Heating by other forms of energy (e.g., electricity).

convulsions Paroxysms of involuntary muscular contractions and relaxations.

core temperature Internal, or deep, body temperature monitored by cells in the hypothalamus, as opposed to shell, or peripheral, temperature, which is registered by that layer of insulation provided by the skin, subcutaneous tissues, and superficial portions of the muscle masses.

corticosteroid Steroid produced by the adrenal cortex.

coryza Profuse nasal discharge.

counterirritant Agent that produces mild inflammation and acts, in turn, as an analgesic when applied locally to the skin (e.g., liniment).

crepitation Crackling sound heard during the movement of ends of a broken bone.

cryokinetics Cold application combined with exercise.

cryotherapy Cold therapy.

cubital fossa Triangular area on the anterior aspect of the forearm directly opposite the elbow joint (the bend of the elbow).

cyanosis Slightly bluish, grayish, slatelike, or dark purple discoloration of the skin caused by a reduced amount of blood hemoglobin.

D

DAPRE Daily adjustable progressive resistive exercise.

debride Removal of dirt and dead tissue from a wound.

deconditioning State in which the athlete's body loses its competitive fitness.

degeneration Deterioration of tissue.

dermatome Segmental skin area innervated by various spinal cord segments.

diagnosis Identification of a specific condition.

diapedesis Passage of blood cells through ameboid action through the intact capillary wall.

diarthrodial joint Ball-and-socket joint.

diastolic blood pressure The residual pressure when the heart is between beats.

DIP Distal interphalangeal joint.

diplopia Seeing double.

distal Farthest from a center, from the midline, or from the trunk.

DNA Deoxyribonucleic acid.

doping The administration of a drug that is designed to improve the competitor's performance.

dorsiflexion Bending toward the dorsum or rear; opposite of plantar flexion.

dorsum The back of a body part.

dressing Covering, protective or supportive, that is applied to an injury or wound.

drug Any substance that, when taken into the living organism, may modify one or more of its functions.

dysrhythmia Irregular heartbeats.

E

eccentric (negative) contraction The muscle lengthens while contracting against resistance.

ecchymosis Black-and-blue skin discoloration caused by hemorrhage.

ectopic calcification Calcification occurring in an abnormal place.

edema Swelling as a result of the collection of fluid in connective tissue.

effective radiating area Portion of the transducer that produces sound energy.

effleurage Stroking.

electrolyte Solution that is a conductor of electricity.

embolus A mass of undisolved matter.

emetic Agent that induces vomiting.

endurance Body's ability to engage in prolonged physical activity.

enthesitis Group of conditions characterized by inflammation, fibrosis, and calcification around tendons, ligaments, and muscle insertions.

enzyme An organic catalyst that can cause chemical changes in other substances without being changed itself.

epidemiological approach Study of sports injuries, involving the relationship of as many factors as possible.

epilepsy Recurrent paroxymal disorder characterized by sudden attacks of altered consciousness, motor activity, sensory phenomena, or inappropriate behavior.

epiphysis Cartilaginous growth region of a bone.

epistaxis Nosebleed.

etiology Science dealing with causes of disease.

ethics Principles of morality.

eversion of the foot To turn the foot outward.

excoriation Removal of a piece or strip of skin.

exostoses Benign bony outgrowths, usually capped by cartilage, that protrude from the surface of a bone.

extraoral mouth guard Protective device that fits outside the mouth.

extravasation Escape of a fluid from its vessels into the surrounding tissues.

exudate Accumulation of fluid in an area.

F

facilitation To assist the progress of.

fascia Fibrous membrane that covers, supports, and separates muscles.

fasciitis Inflammation of fascia.

fibrinogen Blood plasma protein that is converted into a fibrin clot.

fibroblast Any cell component from which fibers are developed.

fibrocartilage Type of cartilage (e.g., intervertebral disks) in which the matrix contains thick bundles of collaginous fibers.

fibrosis Development of excessive fibrous connective tissue; fibroid degeneration.

foot pronation Combined foot movements of eversion and abduction.

foot supination Combined foot movements of inversion and abduction.

force couple Depressor action by the subscapularis, infraspinatus, and teres minor muscles to stabilize the head of the humerus and to counteract the upward force exerted by the deltoid muscle during abduction of the arm.

friction Heat producing.

FSH Follicle-stimulating hormone.

G

GAS theory General adaptation syndrome.

genitourinary Pertaining to the reproductive and urinary organs.

genu recurvatum Hyperextension at the knee joint.

genu valgum Knock-knee.

genu varum Bow leg.

GH Growth hormone.

glycogen loading High-carbohydrate diet.

glycosuria Abnormally high proportion of sugar in the urine.

H

hemarthrosis Blood in a joint.

hematolytic Pertaining to the degeneration and disintegration of the blood.

hematoma Blood tumor.

hematuria Blood in the urine.

hemoglobin Coloring substance of the red blood cells.

hemoglobinuria Hemoglobin in the urine.

hemolysis Destruction of red blood cells.

hemophilia Hereditary blood disease in which coagulation is greatly prolonged.

hemopoietic Forming blood cells.

hemorrhage Discharge of blood.

hemothorax Bloody fluid in the pleural cavity.

hertz (Hz) Number of sound waves per second.

hirsutism Excessive hair growth or the presence of hair in unusual places.

homeostasis Maintenance of a steady state in the body's internal environment.

hunting response Causes a slight temperature increase during cooling.

hyperemia Unusual amount of blood in a body part.

hyperextension Extreme stretching of a body part.

hyperflexibility Flexibility beyond a joint's normal range.

hyperhidrosis Excessive sweating; excessive foot perspiration.

hyperkeratosis Increased callus development.

hypermobility Extreme mobility of a joint.

hyperpnea Hyperventilation; increased minute volume of breathing; exaggerated deep breathing.

hypertension High blood pressure; abnormally high tension.

hyperthermia Elevated body temperature.

hypertonic Having a higher osmotic pressure than a compared solution.

hypertrophy Enlargement of a part caused by an increase in the size of its cells.

hyperventilation Abnormally deep breathing that is prolonged, causing a depletion of carbon dioxide, a fall in blood pressure, and fainting.

hyperallergenic Low allergy producing.

hypoxia Lack of an adequate amount of oxygen.

I

idiopathic Cause of a condition is unknown.

iliotibial band friction syndrome Runner's knee.

injury Act that damages or hurts.

innervation Nerve stimulation of a muscle.

interosseous membrane Connective tissue membrane between bones.

intertrigo Chafing of the skin.

interval training Alternating periods of work with active recovery.

inunctions Oily or medicated substances (e.g., liniments) that are rubbed into the skin to produce a local or systemic effect.

inversion of the foot To turn the foot inward; inner border of the foot lifts.

ions Electrically charged atoms.

ipsilateral Situated on the same side.

ischemia Local anemia.

isokinetic muscle resistance Accommodating and variable resistance.

isometric exercise Contracts the muscle statically without changing its length.

isotonic exercise Shortens and lengthens the muscle through a complete range of motion.

J

joint capsule Saclike structure that encloses the ends of bones in a diarthrodial joint.

joint play Movement that is not voluntary but accessory.

K

keratolytic Loosening of the horny skin layer.

keratosis Excessive growth of the horny tissue layer.

kilocalorie Amount of heat required to raise 1 kg of water 1°C.

kinesthesia; kinesthesis Sensation or feeling of movement; the awareness one has of the spatial relationships of his or her body and its parts.

kyphosis Exaggeration of the normal curve of the thoracic spine.

L

labile Unsteady; not fixed and easily changed.

lactase deficiency Difficulty digesting dairy products.

LASER Light amplification by stimulated emission of radiation.

leukocytes Consist of two types—granulocytes (e.g., basophils and neutrophils) and agranulocytes (e.g., monocytes and lymphocytes).

LH Luteinizing hormone.

liability Legal responsibility to perform an act in a reasonable and prudent manner.

load An outside force or forces acting on tissue.

lordosis Abnormal lumbar vertebral convexity.

luxation Complete joint dislocation.

lysis To break down.

M

macerated skin Skin that has been softened through wetting.

malaise Discomfort and uneasiness caused by an illness.

margination Accumulation of leukocytes on blood vessel walls at the site of injury during early stages of inflammation.

mast cells Connective tissue cells that contain heparin and histamine.

MCP Metacarpophalangeal joint.

mechanical failure Elastic limits of tissue are exceeded, causing tissue to break.

menarche Onset of menstrual function.

metatarsalgia A general term to describe pain in the ball of the foot.

microtrauma Microscopic lesion or injury.

muscle contracture Permanent contraction of a muscle as a result of spasm or paralysis.

muscular endurance The ability to perform repetitive muscular contractions against some resistance.

muscular strength The maximal force that can be applied by a muscle during a single maximal contraction.

myocarditis Inflammation of the heart muscle.

myoglobin Respiratory protein in muscle tissue that is an oxygen carrier.

myositis Inflammation of muscle.

myositis ossificans Myositis marked by ossification of muscles.

N

necrosin Chemical substance that stems from inflamed tissue, causing changes in normal tissue.

negative resistance Slow eccentric muscle contraction against a resistance.

nerve entrapment Nerve compressed between bone or soft tissue.

neuritis Inflammation of a nerve.

neuroma Tumor consisting mostly of nerve cells and nerve fibers.

nociceptor Receptor of pain.

noncontact sport Sport in which athletes are not involved in any physical contact.

nystagmus Constant involuntary back and forth, up and down, or rotary movement of the eyeball.

O

obesity Excessive amount of body fat.

omission (legal) Person fails to perform a legal duty.

orthopedic surgeon One who corrects deformities of the musculoskeletal system.

orthosis Used in sports as an appliance or apparatus to support, align, prevent, or correct deformities or to improve function of a movable body part.

orthotics Field of knowledge relating to orthoses and their use.

osteoarthritis Chronic disease involving joints in which there is destruction of articular cartilage and bony overgrowth.

osteochondral Refers to relationship of bone and cartilage.

osteochondritis Inflammation of bone and cartilage.

osteochondritis dissecans Fragment of cartilage and underlying bone is detached from the articular surface.

osteochondrosis Disease state of a bone and its articular cartilage.

osteoporosis A decrease in bone density.

P

palpation Feeling an injury with the fingers.

paraplegia Paralysis of lower portion of the body and of both legs.

paresis Slight or incomplete paralysis.

paresthesia Abnormal or morbid sensation such as itching or prickling.

pathogenic Disease producing.

pathology Science of the structural and functional manifestations of disease.

pathomechanics Mechanical forces that are applied to a living organism and adversely change the body's structure and function.

pediatrician Specialist in the treatment of children's diseases.

pes anserinus tendinitis Cyclist's knee.

permeable Permitting the passage of a substance through a vessel wall.

pétrissage Kneading.

phagocytosis Destruction of injurious cells or particles by phagocytes (white blood cells).

phalanges Bones of the fingers and toes.

phalanx Any one of the bones of the fingers and toes.

pharmacology Science of drugs, their preparation, uses, and effects.

phonophoresis Introduction of ions of soluble salt into the body through ultrasound.

photophobia Unusual intolerance to light.

piezoelectric Production of an electric current as a result of pressure on certain crystals.

PIP Proximal interphalangeal joint.

plyometric exercise Type of exercise that maximizes the myotatic or stretch reflex.

pneumothorax Collapse of a lung as a result of air in the pleural cavity.

podiatrist Practitioner who specializes in the study and care of the foot.

point tenderness Pain is produced when an injury site is palpated.

polymers Natural or synthetic substances formed by the combination of two or more molecules of the same substance.

posterior Toward the rear or back.

primary assessment Initial first aid evaluation.

prognosis Prediction as to probable result of a disease or injury.

prophylactic Refers to prevention, preservation, or protection.

prophylaxis Guarding against injury or disease.

proprioception The ability to determine the position of a joint in space.

proprioceptive neuromuscular facilitation (PNF) Stretching techniques that involve combinations of alternating contractions and stretches.

proprioceptor One of several receptors, each of which responds to stimuli elicited from within the body itself (e.g., the muscle spindles that invoke the myotatic or stretch reflex).

prostaglandin Acidic lipid widely distributed in the body; in musculoskeletal conditions it is concerned with vasodilation, a histamine-like effect; it is inhibited by aspirin.

prosthesis Replacement of an absent body part with an artificial part; the artificial part.

prothrombin Interacts with calcium to produce thrombin.

proximal Nearest to the point of reference.

psychogenic Of psychic origin; that which originates in the mind.

purulent Consisting of or containing pus.

Q

quadriplegia Paralysis affecting all four limbs.

R

radiation Emission and diffusion of rays of heat.

Raynaud's phenomenon Condition in which cold exposure causes vasospasm of digital arteries.

regeneration Repair, regrowth, or restoration of a part such as tissue.

residual That which remains; often used to describe a permanent condition resulting from injury or disease (e.g., a limp or a paralysis).

resorption Act of removal by absorption.

retroversion Tilting or turning backward of a part.

retrovirus A virus that enters a host cell and changes its RNA to a proviral DNA replica.

revascularize Restoration of blood circulation to an injured area.

RICE Rest, ice, compression, and elevation.

ringworm (tinea) Common name given to many superficial fungal infections of the skin.

RNA Ribonucleic acid.

rotation Turning around an axis in an angular motion.

rubefacients Agents that redden the skin by increasing local circulation through dilation of blood vessels.

S

SAID principle Specific adaptation to imposed demands.

scoliosis Lateral rotary curve of the spine.

secondary assessment Follow-up; a more detailed examination.

seizure Sudden attack.

septic shock Shock caused by bacteria, especially gram-negative bacteria commonly seen in systemic infections.

sequela Pathological condition that occurs as a consequence of another condition or event.

serotonin Hormone and neurotransmitter.

sign Objective evidence of an abnormal situation within the body.

spica A figure-8 bandage, with one of the two loops larger than the other.

Staphylococcus Genus of gram-positive bacteria normally present on the skin and in the upper respiratory tract and prevalent in localized infections.

stasis Blockage or stoppage of circulation.

static stretching Passively stretching an antagonist muscle by placing it in a maximal stretch and holding it there.

Streptococcus Genus of gram-positive bacteria found in the throat, respiratory tract, and intestinal tract.

stress Positive and negative forces that can disrupt the body's equilibrium.

strain Extent of deformation of tissue under loading.

stressor Anything that affects the body's physiological or psychological condition, upsetting the homeostatic balance.

subluxation Partial or incomplete dislocation of an articulation.

symptom Subjective evidence of an abnormal situation within the body.

syndrome Group of typical symptoms or conditions that characterize a deficiency or disease.

synergy To work in cooperation with.

synovitis Inflammation of the synovium.

synthesis To build up.

systolic blood pressure The pressure caused by the heart's pumping.

T

tapotement Percussion.

tendinitis Inflammation of a tendon.

tenosynovitis Inflammation of a tendon synovial sheath.

tetanus (lockjaw) An acute, often fatal condition characterized by tonic muscular spasm, hyperreflexia, and lockjaw.

tetanus toxoid Tetanus toxin modified to produce active immunity against *Clostridium tetani.*

thermotherapy Heat therapy.

thrombi Plural of "thrombus"; a blood clot that blocks small blood vessels or a cavity of the heart.

tinea (ringworm) Superficial fungal infections of the skin.

tonic muscle spasm Rigid muscle contraction that lasts over a period of time.

torsion Act or state of being twisted.

training effect Stroke volume increases while heart rate is reduced at a given exercise load.

transitory paralysis Temporary paralysis.

translation Refers to anterior gliding of tibial plateau.

trauma (plural—traumas or traumata) Wound or injury.

traumatic Pertaining to an injury or wound.

trigger points Small hyperirritable areas within a muscle.

V

valgus Position of a body part that is bent outward.

varus Position of a body part that is bent inward.

vasoconstriction Decrease in the diameter of a blood vessel.

vasodilation Increase in the diameter of a blood vessel.

vasospasm Blood vessel spasm.

vehicle The substance in which a drug is transported.

verruca Wart caused by a virus.

vibration Rapid shaking.

viscoelastic Any substance having both viscous and elastic properties.

viscosity Resistance to flow.

volar Referring to the palm or the sole.

Y

yield point Elastic limits of tissue.

Chapter **1** *Focus boxes, pp. 4, 7, 17, 24, 26 & Table 1-1, p. 9,* Courtesy, The National Athletic Trainers Association.

Chapter **2** *Figures 2-3, 2-4, 2-6, 2-9, pp. 39, 40, 42, 48,* Courtesy, The University of North Carolina at Chapel Hill; *Table 2-1, p. 43,* Adapted from Myers GC, Garrick JG: The preseason examination of school and college athletes. In Strauss RH, ed: *Sports medicine,* Philadelphia, 1984, WB Saunders; *Figure 2-7, p. 46,* Courtesy, D Bailey, California State University at Long Beach.

Chapter **3** *Figures 3-2, 3-11, 3-12, pp. 65, 77, 78,* From Prentice WE: *Get fit stay fit,* St Louis, 1996, Mosby; *Figures 3-6, 3-14, 3-15, 3-16, 3-17, 3-18, 3-19, pp. 70, 82-85,* From Prentice WE: *Fitness for college and life,* ed 5, St Louis, 1997, Mosby; *Figures 3-7, 3-9, 3-10, 3-13, pp. 71, 75, 79,* From Prentice WE: *Rehabilitation techniques in sports medicine,* ed 2, St Louis, 1994, Mosby.

Chapter **4** *Tables 4-1, 4-2, Figures 4-1, 4-4, pp. 95-96, 101, 108,* From Prentice WE: *Get fit stay fit,* St Louis, 1996, Mosby; *Table 4-3, pp. 98,* Modified from *Recommended dietary allowances,* copyright 1989 by the National Academy of Sciences, National Academy Press, Washington, DC; *Figure 4-2, p. 102,* US Dept of Agriculture/US Dept of Health & Human Services, August, 1992; *Figure 4-3, p. 106,* From Prentice WE: *Fitness for college and life,* ed. 5, St Louis, 1997, Mosby.

Chapter **5** *Figure 5-1 (top), p. 116,* Courtesy, Robert Freligh, California State University at Long Beach; *Figures 5-12 and 5-13, pp. 122, 123,* From Nicholas JA, Hershman EB: *The upper extremity in sports medicine,* ed 2, St Louis, 1995, Mosby; *Figure 5-15, p. 124,* Photos courtesy, Denise Fandel, The University of Nebraska at Omaha; *Figures 5-19, 5-26, 5-29, pp. 126, 131, 132,* Courtesy, Mueller Sports Medicine; *Figure 5-20, p. 127,* From Prentice WE: *Fitness for college and life,* ed 5, St Louis, 1997, Mosby; *Figures 5-23, 5-31, 5-32, 5-33, 5-34, 5-35, 5-36, 5-37, pp. 130, 133, 134, 135, 136,* From Nicholas JA, Hershman EB: *The lower extremity and spine in sports medicine,* ed 2, St Louis, 1995, Mosby.

Chapter **6** *Figures 6-2, 6-3, 6-4, pp. 143, 144,* Art by Donald O'Connor.

Chapter **7** *Figure 7-1, p. 167,* Focus on Sports; *Figure 7-2, p. 168,* Steve Powell/ Allsport; *Figure 7-6, p. 179,* From Prentice WE: *Therapeutic modalities in sports medicine,* ed 3, St Louis, 1994, Mosby.

Chapter **8** *Table 8-1, p. 187,* Modified from *International medical guide for ships,* Geneva, World Health Organization; *Figure 8-17, p. 202,* Courtesy, Hartwell Medical Corp, Carlsbad, Calif.

Chapter **9** *Figure 9-2, p. 216,* Art by Don O'Connor; *Focus box, p. 218,* From Hahn DB, Payne WA: *Focus on health,* ed 3, St Louis, 1997, Mosby.

Chapter **10** *Table 10-1, p. 229,* Adapted from Post M: *Physical examination of the musculo-skeletal system,* Chicago, 1987, Year Book Medical Publishers; *Table 10-2, p. 236,* Modified from Veterans Administration Standard Form A, Washington, DC, US Government Printing Office; *Figure 10-7, p. 242,* From Nicholas JA, Hershman, EB: *The lower extremity and spine in sports medicine,* ed 2, St Louis, 1995, Mosby.

Chapter **11** *Figures 11-1, 11-2, 11-3, pp. 247, 249, 253,* Courtesy Ken Bartlett, California State University at Long Beach.

Chapter **12** *Table 12-3, p. 267,* Modified from Berkow R: *The Merck manual of diagnosis and therapy,* ed 14, Rahway, NJ, 1982, Merck & Co; *Focus box, p. 270,* Courtesy,

ER Buskirk, WC Grasley, Human Performance Laboratory, The Athletic Institute, The Pennsylvania State University.

Chapter 13 *Figures 13-2, 13-6, 13-10, 13-18, 13-21, 13-25, 13-28, 13-38, 13-39, pp. 284, 286, 288, 294, 296, 297, 300, 304, 305,* From Arnheim DD: *Essentials of athletic training,* ed 3, St Louis, 1995, Mosby; *Figures 13-22, 13-37, pp. 296, 304,* Art by Donald O'Connor.

Chapter 14 *Figure 14-6, p. 319,* Courtesy, Hygenic Corp, Akron, Ohio; *Figure 14-7, p. 319,* Courtesy, Maxxim Medical, Sugarland, Tex; *Figure 14-9, p. 321,* Courtesy, International Medical Electronics, Kansas City, Mo; *Figures 14-13, 14-14, 14-15, pp. 329, 331,* From Prentice WE: *Therapeutic modalities in sports medicine,* ed 3, St Louis, 1994, Mosby; *Figure 14-24, p. 338,* Chattanooga Corp, Hickson, Tenn; *Figure 14-25, p. 338,* Courtesy, Winchesters Inc, Daytona Beach, Fla; *Figure 14-26, p. 339,* Courtesy, Country Technologies, Inc., Gay Mills, Wis.

Chapter 15 *Figure 15-4B, p. 351,* Courtesy, BREG, Inc, Vista, Calif; *Figure 15-4C, p. 351,* Courtesy, Biodex Medical Systems, Inc, Shirley, NY; *Figures 15-5G, 15-9, pp. 353, 360,* From Prentice WE: *Get fit stay fit,* St Louis, 1996, Mosby; *Figure 15-5H, p. 353,* Courtesy, Contemporary Design, Glacier, Wash; *Figure 15-5I, p. 353,* Courtesy, Fitter International, Calgary, Alberta; *Figures 15-6, 15-14, pp. 354, 362,* From Prentice WE: *Rehabilitation techniques in sports medicine,* ed 2, St Louis, 1994, Mosby; *Figure 15-7, p. 358,* Aqua Jogger courtesy Excel Sport Science, Inc, Eugene, Ore; *Figure 15-12, p. 362,* Adapted from Maitland G: *Extremity manipulation,* London, 1977, Butterworth, and Maitland G: *Vertebral manipulation,* London, 1978, Butterworth.

Chapter 16 *Figure 16-2, p. 370,* Courtesy Mueller Sports Medicine; *Figure 16-3, p. 372,* From Arnheim DD: *Essentials of athletic training,* ed 3, St Louis, 1995, Mosby; *Focus box, p. 374,* Adapted from Lombardo JA: *Drugs in sports.* In Krakurer LJ: *The yearbook of sports medicine,* Chicago, 1986, Year Book Medical Publishers.

Chapter 17 *Figures 17-17, 17-18, pp. 415, 416,* From Arnheim DD: *Essentials of athletic training,* ed 3, St Louis, 1995, Mosby; *Figures 17-20, 17-29, pp. 418, 423,* From Williams JPG: *Color atlas of injury in sport,* ed 2, Chicago, 1990, Year Book Medical Publishers; *Figures 17-35, 17-36, p. 430,* From Prentice WE: *Rehabilitation techniques in sports medicine,* ed 2, St Louis, 1994, Mosby.

Chapter 18 *Figures 18-3, 18-25 (bottom), pp. 437,* From Arnheim DD: *Essentials of athletic training,* ed 3, St Louis, 1995, Mosby; *Table 18-2, p. 441,* Adapted from Singer KM, Jones DC: *Ligament injuries of the ankle and foot.* In Nicholas JA, Hershman EB, eds: *The lower extremity and spine in sports medicine,* vol 1, ed 2, St Louis, 1995, Mosby; *Figures 18-13 (left), 18-20, 18-28, pp. 442, 449, 460,* From Williams JPG: *Color atlas of injury in sport,* ed 2, Chicago, 1990, Year Book Medical Publishers; *Figure 18-17 (top), p. 447,* Courtesy, Cramer Products, Gardner, Kan; *Figure 18-27 (top), p. 457,* From Nicholas JA, Hershman EB: *The lower extremity and spine in sports medicine,* vol 2, ed 2, St Louis, 1995, Mosby; *Figures 18-33, 18-35, pp. 464, 465,* From Prentice WE: *Rehabilitation techniques in sports medicine,* ed 2, St Louis, 1994, Mosby.

Chapter 19 *Figures 19-5, 19-30, 19-46, pp. 471, 489, 498,* Art by Donald O'Connor; *Figure 19-23, p. 486,* Courtesy, Medmetric Corp, San Diego, Calif; *Figure 19-54, p. 508,* Courtesy, Thera-Kinetics and JACE Systems, Mount Laurel, NJ.

Chapter 20 *Figures 20-7, 20-20, 20-21, 20-24, 20-25, 20-26B and C, pp. 522, 534, 535, 536,* Courtesy Ken Bartlett, California State University at Long Beach; *Figures 20-9, 20-32 (right), pp. 523, 542,* From Williams JPG: *Color atlas of injury in sport,* ed 2, Chicago, Year Book Medical Publishers; *Figure 20-10, p. 524,* Courtesy, Mueller Sports Medicine; *Table 20-2, p. 526,* From Boland AL, and Hosea JM: *Hip and back pain in runners, Postgraduate Advances in Sports Medicine I-XII,* Pennington, NJ, Forum Medicus, 1986; *Figure 20-19, p. 533,* Courtesy, Robert Barclay, Renee Reavis Shingles, Central Michigan University; *Figure 20-27 (right), p. 537,* From Nicholas JA, Hersh-

man EB: The lower extremity and spine in sports medicine, vol 2, ed 2, St Louis, 1995, Mosby; *Figure 20-28, p. 538,* Courtesy, BRACE International, Phoenix, Ariz; *Figures 20-35, 20-36, 20-37, 20-38, pp. 544,* From Prentice WE: *Rehabilitation techniques in sports medicine,* ed 2, St Louis, 1994, Mosby.

Chapter **21**   *Figures 21-2, 21-26, pp. 550, 555,* From Nicholas JA, Hershman EB: *The upper extremity in sports medicine,* ed 2, St Louis, 1995, Mosby; *Figures 21-3, 21-4, 21-5, pp. 551, 553, 554,* From Seeley RR, Stephens TD, Tate P: *Anatomy & physiology,* ed 3, St Louis, 1995, Mosby; Art by David Mascaro *(Figure 21-3A),* Scott Bodell *(Figure 21-3B),* John V Hagen *(Figures 21-4, 21-5); Figures 21-8, 21-24, pp. 555, 572,* Art by Donald O'Connor; *Figure 21-31, p. 581,* Courtesy, PrePak Products, Carlsbad, Calif; *Figure 21-38, p. 586,* Courtesy, Healthsouth Rehabilitation Program, Birmingham, Ala.

Chapter **22**   *Figures 22-5, 22-6, 22-7, 22-11, 22-12, 22-13, 22-14, 22-17, 22-28, 22-29, 22-63, 22-68, pp. 594, 596, 597, 599, 607, 628, 630,* Courtesy Ken Bartlett, California State University at Long Beach; *Figures 22-8, 22-20, 22-45, 22-51 (left), 22-52 (left), 22-53, 22-54, 22-55, 22-57, 22-68, 22-71, pp. 595, 603, 618, 622, 623, 624, 625, 630, 631,* From Nicholas JA, Hershman EB: *The upper extremity in sports medicine,* ed 2, St Louis, 1995, Mosby; *Figures 22-22, 22-23, 22-24, 22-25, 22-26, 22-27, 22-59, 22-60, 22-61, 22-64, 22-65, 22-66, 22-67, 22-69, 22-70, pp. 605, 606, 607, 627, 628, 629, 630, 631,* From Prentice WE: *Rehabilitation techniques in sports medicine,* ed 2, St Louis, 1994, Mosby.

Chapter **23**   *Figures 23-4, 23-12, 23-33, pp. 638, 648, 669,* Art by Donald O'Connor; *Figures 23-6, 23-7, pp. 639, 640,* From Seeley RR, Stephens TD, Tate P: *Anatomy & physiology,* ed 3, St Louis, 1995, Mosby; *Tables 23-1, 23-2, pp. 635, 636,* From Seeley RR, Stephens TD, Tate P: *Anatomy & physiology,* St Louis, 1989, Mosby; *Figure 23-31, p. 664,* From Nicholas JA, Hershman EB: *The lower extremity and spine in sports medicine,* vol 2, ed 2, St Louis, 1995, Mosby; *Figure 23-35 (middle & right), p. 670,* From Williams JPG: *Color atlas of injury in sport,* ed 2, Chicago, Year Book Medical Publishers, 1990; Prentice WE: *Get fit stay fit,* St Louis, 1996, Mosby.

Chapter **24**   *Figures 24-2, 24-3, 24-4, 24-5, pp. 685, 686, 687,* From Seeley RR, Stephens TD, Tate P: *Anatomy & physiology,* ed 3, St Louis, 1995, Mosby; Art by David Mascaro *(Figure 24-2),* John V Hagen *(Figure 24-3),* Jody L Fulks *(Figure 24-4),* Rusty Jones *(Figure 24-5); Figure 24-6, p. 687,* From Prentice WE: *Fitness for college and life,* ed 5, St Louis, 1997, Mosby; *Figure 24-15, p. 695,* From Boyd CE: Referred visceral pain in athletics, *Ath Train* 15:20, 1980.

Chapter **25**   *Figure 25-1, p. 714,* Art by Donald O'Connor; *Figure 25-3, p. 715,* Allsport; *Table 25-2, Focus box, pp. 718, 720,* Adapted from Vegso JJ, Lehman RC: *Field evaluation and management of head and neck injuries.* In Torg JS, ed: *Head and neck injuries, Clinics in Sports Medicine,* vol 6, no 1, Philadelphia, 1987, WB Saunders; *Table 25-4, p. 722,* Adapted from Cantu RC: Guidelines for return to contact sports after a cerebral concussion, *Phys Sportsmed* 14(10): 79, 1986; *Figures 25-14, 25-15, 25-19, pp. 727, 728, 730,* From Williams JPG: *Color atlas of injury in sport,* ed 2, Chicago, 1990, Year Book Medical Publishers; *Figure 25-17, p. 729,* Focus on Sports; *Table 25-5, p. 732,* Adapted from Pashby RC, Pashby TJ: *Ocular injuries in sport.* In Welsh PR, Shepard RJ, eds: *Current therapy in sports medicine, 1985-1986,* Philadelphia, 1985, BC Decker; *Focus box, p. 733,* Adapted from Vinger PF: How I manage corneal abrasions and lacerations, *Phys Sportsmed* 14(5): 170, 1986; *Figure 25-23, p. 736,* Allsport.

Chapter **26**   *Figure 26-8 (top left), p. 749,* From Booher JM, Thibodeau GA: *Athletic training assessment,* St Louis, 1994, Mosby; *Figure 26-8 (bottom left), p. 749,* Courtesy, Dr James Garrick; *Figures 26-9, 26-10, 26-12, 26-14, pp. 753, 754, 756, 757,* From Stewart WD, Danto JL, Madden S: *Dermatology: diagnosis and treatment of cutaneous disorders,* ed 4, St Louis, 1978, Mosby; *Color plates,* From Habif TP: *Clinical dermatology,* ed 3, St Louis, 1996, Mosby.

Checklist for Athletic Trainer's Kit*

Item	Amount	Item	Amount
Accident reports		Forceps (tweezers)	1
Adhesive tape		Germicide (solution)	2 ounces
½-inch (1.25 cm)	1 roll	Skin lube	
1 inch (2.5 cm)	2 rolls	Heel cups	2
1½-inch (3.75 cm)	3 rolls	Insurance information	
2-inch (5 cm)	1 roll	Instant cold pack	2
Alcohol (isopropyl)	4 ounces	Mirror (hand)	1
Ammonia ampules	10	Moleskin	6 by 6 sheet
Analgesic balm	½ pound	Nonadhering sterile pad (3 by 3)	12
Ankle wraps	2	Oral thermometer	1
Antacid tablets or liquid	100	Paper and pencil	
Antiglare salve	4 ounces	Peroxide	2 ounces
Band-Aids (assorted sizes)	2 dozen	Plastic cups	
Butterfly bandages (sterile strip)		Sponge rubber	
Medium	6 dozen	⅛-inch (0.3 cm)	6 by 6 sheet
Small	6 dozen	¼-inch (0.6 cm)	6 by 6 sheet
Contact case		½-inch (1.25 cm)	6 by 6 sheet
Cotton-tipped applicators	2 dozen	Sterile gauze pads (3 by 3)	6
Elastic bandages		Sun lotion	2 ounces
3-inch (7.5 cm)	2 rolls	Surgical scissors	1
4-inch (10 cm)	2 rolls	Tape adherent	6-ounce spray can
6 inch (15 cm)	2 rolls	Tape remover	2 ounces
Elastic tape roll (3-inch)	2 rolls	Tape scissors (pointed)	1
Eyewash	2 ounces	Tongue depressors	5
Felt		Triangular bandages	2
¼-inch (0.6 cm)	6 by 6 sheet	Waterproof tape (1-inch)	1 roll
½-inch (1.25 cm)	6 by 6 sheet		

*Extra amounts of items such as tape and protective padding are carried in other bags.